Maxillofacial Surgery

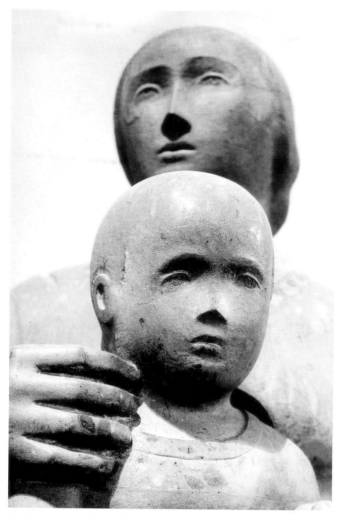

Madonna and child, by Henry Moore, 1943.
Sculpture in Hornton stone, in the Church of St Matthew,
Northampton, UK

Maxillofacial Surgery

Volume 2

EDITED BY

Peter Ward Booth FDS, FRCS

Consultant Surgeon, Department of Maxillofacial Surgery, Queen Victoria Hospital, East Grinstead, UK

Stephen A Schendel MD DDS FACS

Professor and Chairman, Department of Functional Restoration, Stanford University,
School of Medicine, Division of Plastic and Reconstructive Surgery
California, USA

Jarg-Erich Hausamen MD DDS PhD

Professor and Chairman, Klinik f. Mund-, Kiefer- u. Gesichtschirurgie
Medizinische Hochschule Hannover, Hannover, Germany

Illustrations by Ian Ramsden

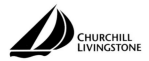
CHURCHILL
LIVINGSTONE

EDINBURGH LONDON NEW YORK PHILADELPHIA SAN FRANCISCO SYDNEY 1999

CHURCHILL LIVINGSTONE
A division of Harcourt Brace & Co Limited

© Harcourt Brace & Co Ltd 1999

ISBN 0 443 05853 9

British Library Cataloguing in Publication Data
A catalogue record for this book is available from the British Library.

Library of Congress Cataloging in Publication Data
A catalog record for this book is available from the Library of Congress.

Medical knowledge is constantly changing. As new information becomes available, changes in treatment, procedures, equipment and the use of drugs become necessary. The editors/authors/contributors and the publishers have, as far as it is possible, taken care to ensure that the information given in the text is accurate and up to date. However, readers are strongly advised to confirm that the information, especially with regard to drug usage, complies with latest legislation and standards of practice.

The
publisher's
policy is to use
**paper manufactured
from sustainable forests**

Printed in Hong Kong

Contents

Volume 2

SECTION 3: CRANIOFACIAL DEFORMITY

Section Editors: Stephen A Schendel, Peter Ward Booth

SECTION 4: ORAL SURGERY

Section Editor: Peter Ward Booth

Contributors

Peter R Ayliffe FRCS (Eng) FDS RCS (Eng) MBBS
BDS
Specialist Registrar in Maxillofacial Surgery
South Thames Training Scheme UK
King's College Hospital, UK
Royal Surrey County Hospital, Guildford
Queen Victoria Hospital, East Grinstead, UK

Karl-Heinz Austermann MD DDS PhD
Professor and Chairman
Klinik f. Mund-, Kiefer- u. Gesichtschirurgie
Phfilipps-Universität Marburg
Marburg, Germany

Nick Baker MBBS FDSRCS FRCS
Consultant in Oral and Maxillofacial Surgery
Maxillofacial Unit
Southampton University Hospitals
Southampton, UK

Shivaram Bharathwaj MB BS Dip NB(Surgery), FRCS
(Edin)
Specialist Registrar in Plastic Surgery
Queen Victoria Hospital
East Grinstead, UK

Remy H Blanchaert Jr MD DDS
Maxillofacial Oncology Fellow
Department of Oral and Maxillofacial Surgery
University of Maryland
Baltimore, USA

Henry G Bone MD
Institute for Craniofacial and Reconstructive Surgery
Southfield
Michigan, USA

John G Boorman MB CHB FRCS(Plast)
Consultant Plastic Surgeon
The Queen Victoria Hospital NHS Trust
East Grinstead, UK

A Mark Boustred MB BCh, FCS (SA), FRCS (Edin),
FCS(SA)(Plast)
Fellow in Plastic and Reconstructive Surgery
Emory University Hospital, Scottish Rite Childrens'
Hospital
The Cleft and Craniofacial Unit of the Red Cross
Children's Hospital
University of Cape Town
South Africa

Nicolas B Bowley MB BS DMRD FRCR
Consultant Radiologist
Head of Department of X-ray
The Queen Victoria Hospital NHS Trust
East Grinstead, UK

J Brian Boyd MB ChB MD FRCS FRCS(C) FACS
Professor of Surgery, Ohio State University
Chairman of Plastic Surgery
Cleveland Clinic Florida
Fort Lauderdale, Florida, USA

Jay O Boyle MD
Fellow, Head and Neck Surgical Oncology
Head and Neck Service,
Department of Surgery,
Memorial Sloan-Kettering Cancer Center
New York, USA

Burt Brent MD
Consultant
Woodside, California, USA

Andrew E Brown FRCS FDSRCS
Consultant Maxillofacial Surgeon
Regional Centre for Maxillofacial Surgery
Queen Victoria Hospital
East Grinstead, UK

James S Brown MD FRCS FDSRCS
Consultant Oral and Maxillofacial Surgeon
University Hospital Aintree
Liverpool, UK

Roberto Brusati MD
Head of Department of Maxillofacial Surgery
Member of the Cleft Palate Center
Department of Maxillofacial Surgery
San Paolo University Hospital
Milan, Italy

Harry J Buncke MD
Director
Department of Microsurgical Replantation and
Transplantation
Davies Medical Center
San Fancisco
California, USA

Roderick Cawson MD FRCPath FDS RCPS FDS RCS
Professor of Oral Pathology
Department of Oral Medicine
Eastman Dental Insitute of Oral Health Care Sciences
University of London, London, UK

Stephen R Cohen MD
Center for Craniofacial Surgery
Scottish Rite Children's Medical Center
Atlanta, Georgia, USA

William A Crawley MD DDS FACS
Consultant
6565 North Charles Street
Suite 401
Baltimore, USA

Colin Cryer PhD, Csat
Statistician
South East Institute of Public Health
King's College, London, UK

Susan J Cunningham BChD FDSRCS Msc MOrthRCS
Lecturer
Department of Orthodontics
Eastman Dental Institute
University of London
London, UK

Joy E Curran MB FRCA
Consultant Anaesthetist
Queen Victoria Hospital
East Grinstead, UK

Jeffrey S Dean DDS MD
Chief Resident
Division of Oral and Maxillofacial Surgery
The University of Texas Southwestern Medical Center
Texas, USA

M Franklin Dolwick DMD PhD
Department of Oral, Maxillofacial Surgery and Diagnostic
Sciences
College of Dentistry
University of Florida, Gainesville
Florida, USA

I P Downie
Specialist Registrar
Department of Maxillofacial Surgery
Southampton University Hospital
Southhampton, UK

M Stephen Dover BDS FDSRCS, MBChB, FRCS
Consultant Maxillofacial Surgeon
Queen Elizabeth Hospital
United Hospitals NHS Trust
Birmingham, UK

André Eckardt MD DDS PhD
Klinik für Mund-, Kiefer- u. Gesichtschirurgie
Medizinsche-Hochschule, Hannover, Germany

Uwe Eckelt MD DDS PhD
Professor and Chairman
Department of Maxillo-Facial Surgery
University of Dresden
Dresden, Germany

Alfons Erle MD DDS PhD
Universitatsklinik für Mund-, Kiefer- und
Gesichtschirurgie
Otto-von-Guericke-Universitat Magdeburg
Magdeburg, Germany

Barry T Evans
Consultant in Oral and Maxillofacial Surgery
Maxillofacial Unit
Southampton University Hospitals
Southampton, UK

Charlotte Feinmann MD Msc FRCPsych FDS (Hon)
Senior Lecturer
Behavioural Sciences and Dentistry
Eastman Dental Institute
University of London
London, UK

R Theodore Fields DDS
Oral and Maxillofacial Surgery
Resident at Baylor College of Dentistry
Texas A&M University System
Texas, USA

Patricia M Finlay BDS FDSRCPS
Associate Specialist in Oral and Maxillofacial Surgery
Department of Oral and Maxillofacial Surgery
Canniesburn Hospital, Glasgow, UK

David E Frost DDS MS
Oral and Maxillofacial Surgeon
401 Providence Road, Chapel Hill
North Carolina, USA

Nils-Claudius Gellrich MD DDS PhD
Assistant Professor
Department of Oral and Maxillofacial Surgery
Albert-Ludwigs-University Freiburg
Freiburg, Germany

Klaus-Louis Gerlach MD DDS PhD
Professor and Chairman
Universitatsklinik für Mund-, Kiefer- und
Gesichtschirurgie
Otto-von-Guericke-Universität Magdeburg
Magdeburg, Germany

Sabine C Girod MD DDS PhD
Klinik und Poliklinik fur Mund-, Kiefer-, Gesichtschirurgie
Friedrich-Alexander-Universität Erlangen-Nürnberg
Erlangen, Germany

Karsten K H Gundlach MD DDS PhD
Professor and Chairman
Klinik f. Mund-, Kiefer- u. Gesichtschirurgie
Universität Rostock
Rostock, Germany

Franz Härle MD DDS PhD
Professor and Chairman
Department of Oral and Maxillofacial Surgery
University Hospital of the Christian-Albrechts Universtitat
Kiel, Kiel, Germany

Jarg-Erich Hausamen MD DDS PhD
Professor and Chairman
Klinik f. Mund-, Kiefer- u. Gesichtschirurgie
Medizinische Hochschule Hannover
Hannover, Germany

A P Heise
Consultant
Lancaster, Pennsylvania, USA

Michael C Hill FDS MScD MSc
Consultant
Department of Oral and Maxillofacial Surgery
University of Wales College of Medicine
Cardiff, UK

Bodo Hoffmeister MD DDS PhD
Professor and Chairman, Department of Maxillofacial
Surgery and Facial Plastic Surgery
University Hospital Benjamin Franklin
Free University of Berlin
Berlin, Germany

Hans-Peter Howaldt MD DDS PhD
Professor and Chairman
Department of Maxillofacial and Plastic Surgery
University Hospital Giessen
Giessen, Germany

Ian T Jackson MD Dsc (Hon) FRCS FACS FRACS (Hon)
Institute for Craniofacial and Reconstructive Surgery
Southfield, Michigan, USA

Hemen Jaju MS Mch DNB
Institute for Craniofacial and Reconstructive Surgery
Southfield, Michigan, USA

Johnathan S Jacobs DMD MD FACS
Associate Professor
Eastern Virginia Medical School
Virginia Beach, Virginia, USA

Alistair Jenkins MB CHB MD FRCS (Edin)
Consultant and Honorary Senior Lecturer in
Neurosurgery
Regional Neurosciences Centre
Newcastle General Hospital
Newcastle Upon Tyne, UK

Vishwanath S Jigjinni MS FRCS
Fellow in Craniofacial Surgery
Department of Plastic Surgery
Eastern Virginia Medical School
Norfolk, Virginia, USA

Ulrich Joos MD DMD PhD DHC
Professor and Chairman
Department of Oral, Craniomaxillofacial, Plastic and
Reconstructive Surgery
University of Münster
Münster, Germany

Gernot Jundt MD
Associate Professor of Pathology
Bone Tumor Reference Center at the Institute of
Pathology
Kantonsspitafsl/University Hospital
Basel, Switzerland

Julian Eamonn Kabala MRCP FRCR
Consultant Radiologist
Directorate of Clinical Radiology
Bristol Royal Infirmary
Bristol, UK

Leonard Kaban DDS MD
Chief of Department
Oral and Maxillofacial Surgery
Massachusetts General Hospital
Boston, USA

Gerry Kearns
Consultant Oral and Maxillofacial Surgeon
Limmerick Ireland

Cyrus Kerawala FRCS (OMFS) FDSRCS
Senior Registrar, Sub-Region Oral and Facial Unit
Sunderland Royal Hospital
Sunderland, UK

Andrew K M Khoo MBBS FRCS(Edin) FRCS(Glasg.)
Consultant
Department of Plastic Surgery
UT MD Anderson Cancer Center
Houston, Texas, USA

David Koppel
Senior Registrar in Oral and Maxillofacial Surgery
Department of Oral and Maxillofacial Surgery
Canniesburn Hospital, Glasgow, UK

Norbert R Kübler MD DMD PhD
Senior Physician of the Department of Cranio-Maxillo-
Facial Surgery
Bavarian Julius-Maximilians-University
Würzberg

D A Lang
Consultant
Wessex Neurological Centre
Southampton University Hospitals
Southampton, UK

Thomas J Laney MD DDS
Director,
Laney Surgical Arts
Seattle, USA

James A A Langtry MRCP
Consultant Dermatologist
Sunderland Royal Hospital
Sunderland, UK

Ken M Lavery
Consultant Maxillofacial Surgeon
The Queen Victoria Hospital NHS Trust
East Grinstead, UK

Juergen Lentrodt MD DDS PhD
Professor and Chairman of the Clinic for Maxillofacial and
Facial Plastic Surgery
University Hospital
Düsseldorf, Germany

Jeffrey S Lewis MD DMD
Specialist Maxillofacial Surgeon
Ithaca
New York, USA

Christian Lindqvist MD DDS PhD
Head of Department of Oral and Maxillofacial Surgery
Helsinki University Central Hospital
Helsinki
Finland

Michael T Longaker MD
John Marquis Converse Professor of Plastic Surgery
Research
Institute of Reconstructive Plastic Surgery
NYU School of Medicine
New York City, USA

H Peter Lorenz MD
Assistant Professor of Plastic Surgery
University of California, Los Angeles School of Medicine
Los Angeles, USA

Hans-Georg Luhr MD, DMD PhD
Professor and Chairman
Department of Maxillofacial Surgery
University Hospital of Göettingen
Göettingen, Germany

Egbert Machtens MD DDS PhD
Professor and Chairman
Department of Oral and Maxillofacial Surgery
and Facial Plastic Surgery
University of Bochum
Bochum, Germany

R Geir Madland BSc FDS RCS
Eastman Dental Institute for Oral Health Care Sciences
University of London
London, UK

Nicola Mannucci MD
Assistant Professor
Department of Maxillofacial Surgery
San Paolo University Hospital
Milan, Italy

Paul Manson MD
Professor
Johns Hopkins University Medical School
Baltimore, USA

Anthony F Markus FDSRCS
Consultant Maxillofacial Surgeon and Director
Dorset Cleft Centre
Poole Hospital Trust
Dorset, UK

Ian C Martin FDSRCS FRCS
Consultant Oral and Facial Surgeon
Oral and Facial Unit
Sunderland Royal Hospital
Sunderland, UK

Robert E Marx DDS
Professor of Maxillofacial Surgery
Chief, Division of Oral/Maxillofacial Surgery
Deering Medical Plaza
Miami
Florida, USA

Mark E Mason MD DDS
Department of Functional Restoration
Stanford Univeristy School of Medicine
Division of Plastic and Reconstructive Surgery
California, USA

Joseph McCarthy MD
Professor
Department of Plastic Surgery
New York University Medical Center
New York, USA

Maurice Y Mommaerts LDS MD DMD FEBOMS
Surgeon – Consultant
Division of Maxillofacial Surgery
General Hospital St John
Bruges, Belgium

Khursheed Moos
Consultant Oral and Maxillofacial Surgeon
Canniesburn Hospital
Glasgow, UK

Joachim Mühling MD DDS PhD
Professor and Chairman
Department of Maxillofacial Surgery
University of Heidelberg
Heidelberg, Germany

Friedrich-Wilhelm Neukam MD DDS PhD
Professor and Chairman
Klinik und Poliklinik für Mund-, Kiefer-, Gesichtschirurgie
Friedrich-Alexander-Universität Erlangen-Nürnberg
Erlangen, Germany

G Neil-Dwyer
Wessex Neurological Center
Southampton University Hospitals
Southampton, UK

Laurence Newman MB FDSRCS FRCS
Consultant Oral and Maxillofacial Surgeon
University College Hospital
London, UK

Robert A Ord MD DDS FRCS FACS MS
Associate Professor
Department of Oral and Maxillofacial Surgery
University of Maryland Cancer Center
University of Maryland
Baltimore, USA

Juha Paatsama MD DDS
Department of Oral and Maxillofacial Surgery
Helsinki University Central Hospital
Helsinki
Finland

Bonnie Padwa DMD MD
Children's Hospital
Boston, Massachusetts, USA

Maxine Partridge PhD FDSRCS
Consultant Oral Surgeon
King's College Hospital
Denmark Hill
London, UK

Manu Patel FRCS FDSRCS
Consultant Oral and Maxillofacial Surgeon
Department of Oral and Maxillofacial Surgery
South Manchester University Hospitals NHS Trust
Withington Hospital
Manchester, UK

Michael Perry FRCS, FDS, Bsc
Senior Registrar in Oral and Maxillofacial Surgery
King's College Healthcare
UK

Stephen Porter MD PhD FDS RCS FDS RCSE
Consultant
Department of Oral Medicine
Eastman Dental Hospital
London, UK

Jeffrey C Posnick DMD MD FRCS(C), FACS
Clinical Professor of Surgery, Pediatrics
Otolaryngology, and Maxillofacial Surgery
Georgetown University
USA

Olda A Pospisil MD FRCSEd FDSRCSEd
Consultant Craniomaxillofacial Surgeon
Regional Unit for Maxillofacial Surgery
Aintree Hospitals NHS Trust
University Hospital Aintree
Liverpool, UK

Joachim Prein MD DDS PhD
Professor of Maxillofacial Surgery
Kantonsspital/University Hospital
Basel, Switzerland

Peter Reichart DDS PhD
Professor and Chairman
Abt f. Oralchirurgie u.Zahnärztl
Röntgenologie
Universitatsklinikum Charité
Berlin, Germany

Torsten E Reichert MD DDS PhD
Department of Oral and Maxillofacial Surgery
Johannes-Gutenberg University of Mainz
Mainz, Germany

Siegmer Reinert MD DDS PhD
Professor and Chairman
Department of Oral and Maxillofacial Surgery
and Plastic Surgery
University of Tübingen
Tübingen, Germany

Jürgen F Reuther MD DMD PhD
Professor and Chairman of Department of Cranio-
Maxillo-Facial Surgery
Bavarian Julius-Maximilians-University
Würzburg, Germany

David Richardson FRCS FDSRCS
Consultant Oral and Maxillofacial Surgeon
Regional Unit for Maxillofacial Surgery
Aintree Hospitals NHS Trust
University Hospital Aintree
Liverpool, UK

Dieter Riediger MD DDS PhD
Professor and Chairman
Department of Maxillofacial and Plastic Facial Surgery
University of Technology Aachen
Aachen, Germany

Ramon L Ruiz DMD, MD
Department of Oral and Maxillofacial Surgery
University of North Carolina
North Carolina, USA

Stephen A Schendel MD DDS FACS
Professor and Chairman
Department of Functional Restoration
Division of Plastic and Reconstructive Surgery
Stanford University School of Medicine
Stanford, California, USA

Henning Schliephake MD DDS PhD
Klinik für Mund-, Kiefer- u. Gesichtschirurgie
Medizinische Hochschule Hannover
Hannover, Germany

Rainer Schmelzeisen MD DDS PhD
Professor and Chairman
Department of Oral and Maxillofacial Surgery
Albert-Ludwigs-University Freiburg
Freiburg, Germany

R Schön MD DDS PhD
Consultant
Department of Oral and Maxillofacial Surgery
Albert-Ludwigs-University of Freiburg
Freiburg, Germany

Mark Schusterman MD
The Ermosa Center for Plastic Surgery
The Hermann Professional Building
Houston, Texas, USA

Jatin P Shah MD FACS FRCS(Hons)
Professor of Surgery
E W Strong Chair in Head and Neck Oncology
Chief, Head and Neck Service
Department of Surgery
Memorial Sloan-Kettering Cancer Center
New York, USA

Kirt E Simmons DDS PhD
Craniofacial Orthodontics Director
Assistant Professor, Department of Surgery
University of Arkansas for Medical Sciences
Arkansas Children's Hospital
Little Rock
Arkansas, USA

Alistair G Smyth BDS MBBS FDSRCS FRCS
Consultant Oral and Maxillofacial Surgeon
Department of Oral and Maxillofacial Surgery
Middlesbrough General Hospital
Cleveland, UK

Wayne Smith MBChB, MMed (plastics)
Professor
Head of Department
The University of the Orange Free State
Department of Plastic and Reconstructive Surgery
Faculty of Medicine
Republic of South Africa

Clark M Stanford DDS PhD
Associate Professor
Dows Institute for Dental Research, and
Department of Prosthodontics
College of Dentistry
University of Iowa
Iowa City, USA

Leo F A Stassen FRCS (Ed) FDSRCS M.A
Consultant Oral and Facial Surgeon
Sunderland Royal Hospital
Sunderland, UK

David Sutton BDS FDSRCS(Ed) MBChB FRCS(Ed)
Specialist Registrar in Maxillofacial Surgery
Department of Maxillofacial Surgery
University Hospital Aintree, Liverpool, UK

Riita Suuronen MD DDS PhD
Department of Oral and Maxillofacial Surgery
Helsinki University Central Hospital
Helsinki, Finland

Jean Claude Talmant MD
Plastic Surgeon
Nantes, France

Clark O Taylor MD DDS
Assistant Professor
Department of Maxillofacial Surgery
University of Nebraska, Omaha, Loma Linda University
California, USA

David W Thomas FDS MScD PhD
Senior Lecturer
Department of Oral and Maxillofacial Surgery
University of Wales College of Medicine
Cardiff, UK

Andrew E Turk MD
Assistant Professor
Division of Plastic and Reconstructive Surgery
Stanford University Medical Center
California, USA

Timothy A Turvey DDS
Professor and Chair
Department of Oral and Maxillofacial Surgery
University of North Carolina School of Dentistry
USA

Joseph E Van Sickels DDS
Professor and Senior Surgeon
Department of Oral and Maxillofacial Surgery
University of Texas Health Science Center at San Antonio
San Antonio, Texas, USA

E David Vaughan
Consultant Maxillofacial Surgeon
Department of Maxillofacial Surgery
University Hospital Aintree/Phase 2 building
Liverpool, UK

Peter J H Venn MB FRCA
Consultant Anaesthetist
The Queen Victoria Hospital
East Grinstead, UK

Wilfried Wagner MD DDS PhD
Professor and Chairman
Department of Oral and Maxillofacial Surgery
Johannes-Gutenberg University of Mainz
Mainz, Germany

Saman Warnakulasuriya PhD FDSRCS
Consultant, Oral Medicine/Oral Pathology
King's College Hospital
London, UK

Peter Ward Booth FDS FRCS
Consultant Surgeon
Department of Maxillofacial Surgery
Queen Victoria Hospital
East Grinstead, UK

Laurence D Watkins
Senior Registrar in Neurosurgery
Regional Neurosciences Centre
Newcastle General Hospital
Newcastle Upon Tyne, UK

Rosemary Watts DipCSLT, MRCSLT
Senior Specialist Speech and Language Therapist
Dorset Healthcare NHS Trust
Dorset Centre for Cleft Lip and Palate
Poole Hospital, Dorset, UK

Thomas G Wendt MD PhD
Professor and Chairman
Department of Radiation Oncology
Friedrich Schiller University Jena
Jena, Germany

Kerwin J Williams MD
Assistant Professor and Attending Surgeon
Division of Craniofacial, Plastic and Reconstructive
Surgery
Children's Hospital and Regional Medical Center
Seattle, USA

Alan W Wilson BDS FDS RCS(Ed) BM(Hons)
FRCS(Lon)
Specialist Registrar
Department of Oral and Maxillofacial Surgery
Dorset Healthcare NHS Trust
Poole
Dorset

Lindsay J Winchester BDS MSc FDSRCS(Eng)
MOrthRCS(Eng)
Consultant
Department of Orthodontics
The Queen Victoria Hospital
East Grinstead, UK

Larry Wolford DDS
Clinical Professor
Department of Oral and Maxillofacial Surgery
Baylor College of Dentistry – Texas A&M University
System, Dallas, Texas

Wai Lup Wong MRCP FRCR
Consultant Radiologist
Mount Vernon Hospital
Northwood, Middlesex, UK

Stephen F Worrall MD FRCS FDSRCS
Consultant and Senior Lecturer
Department of Oral and Maxillofacial Surgery
North Staffordshire Hospital
Stoke-on-Trent, UK

David R Young BDS Sc FRSRCS(Eng) MOrthRCS(Eng)
Department of Orthodontics
Guy's Hospital Trust, London, UK

Michael F Zide DMD
Associate Director
Facial and Oral Surgery
John Peter Smith Hospital
Fort Worth
Texas, USA

Preface

Great opportunities and challenges exist in the complex realm of maxillofacial surgery. Certainly, few anatomic areas are so vital to our patients as the maxillofacial region. Disorders of any one of the many intricate structures within it can be potentially devastating. In addition to the importance of disorders affecting sight, hearing, speech or the masticatory structures, the accompanying esthetic considerations are equally important. Keeping pace with the rapidly growing sphere of knowledge in this field and developing expertise in the most modern surgical techniques, is of utmost importance for both surgeons and their patients.

It is our hope that this book will make an important contribution to the knowledge of maxillofacial surgery. Our goal has been to assemble a group of distinguished international specialists who, regardless of their professional backgrounds, have not only made this field of surgery their main interest, but have also made noteworthy contributions. Indeed, we feel the rich diversity of our contributors' experiences is an exceptional asset, bringing fresh perspectives to this book. In presenting advances in technology and ever increasing biologic knowledge, this book reflects the vibrant nature of our speciality. While it was never our intention to cover every aspect of maxillofacial surgery, it was our aim that the significant information contained in these volumes, will stimulate further progress and inspire closer cooperation among specialists and readers.

Finally, we would like to use this page to express our great gratitude to those many people, particularly secretaries, who have done so much hard work to support the production of this book. In particular, Nora Naughton our Project Manager, who took such a pivotal role managing the book after the takeover of Churchill Livingstone. She has encouraged, coaxed and, when necessary, bullied us all, but always with charm, patience and palpable enthusiasm. Others whose contributions have been so important are Jennifer Hardy, Deborah Russell and Teresa Phillips.

Principles of Craniofacial Deformity

Classification, diagnosis and etiology of craniofacial deformities

51

IAN T. JACKSON/A. WAYNE SMITH

CLASSIFICATION AND DIAGNOSIS

Despite the fact that an accurate clinical diagnosis does not usually influence the management of patients with congenital anomalies, it does contribute to enhanced patient management. It also helps to alleviate some of the parents' concerns and enables the physician to direct them, complete with an accurate diagnosis, for appropriate counseling. Until now, the diagnosis of congenital anomalies has mainly been made on grounds of clinical presentation and physician experiences. This was due to the fact that genetic diagnosis and the use of molecular biology techniques to diagnose these anomalies have not been readily accessible, have been expensive, and up until the present time have not been particularly reliable. However, with new genetic information and laboratory techniques, in addition to molecular biology diagnosis procedures, not only will classification systems change (these have previously been based on laborious clinical presentations), but so also will the ability to accurately diagnose what are often confusing and complex clinical presentations consisting of multiple clinical signs with associated multiorgan involvement. These are frequently associated with variable degrees of phenotypic expressivity which makes the clinical diagnosis of these conditions more difficult. It appears, however, that in the foreseeable future, with the explosion of data relating to abnormal fibroblast growth factors (FGF) and the appropriate fibroblast growth factor receptors that are presently being assessed, diagnosis will be simplified. An accurate diagnosis will be obtained within hours by simply sending off tissue and blood specimens to the molecular biology laboratory. At this time, however, this is not the case; until that time the tried and tested methods, albeit imperfect and cumbersome, still need to be used (Fig. 51.1).

When a patient presents to the craniofacial clinic with a congenital anomaly he enters the flow diagram at point A. If the disorder is isolated and not familial, it is usually multifactorial in origin and the parents are counseled accordingly. Many of the conditions previously considered multifactorial will probably be diagnosed utilizing molecular biology techniques, and this limb of the diagnostic approach may expand considerably. If the disorder is isolated and familial, it may be multifactorial (including environmental factors) or monogenic. A pedigree analysis is then performed on these patients and the parents are appropriately counseled. If the anomaly is not isolated and is part of a recognizable clinical pattern for which a confirmatory test is available, this test is carried out. If the results of this clinical presentation and confirmatory test are complementary and the inheritance pattern is known, the parents are counseled accordingly. If the result of the confirmatory test does not confirm or correlate with a recognizable clinical picture, a karyotype is carried out to assess the chromosomes and status of the patient, and the patient re-enters the diagnostic hierarchy as shown. If the anomaly is not isolated and is not part of a recognizable clinical pattern, a karyotype is performed. If the chromosomes are abnormal, parental karyotyping may be carried out to assess the inheritance pattern and the chance of recurrence. The parents are then counseled based on this information. If, however, the karyotype reveals normal chromosomes, further work-up is considered depending on whether the condition appears familiar or not. If it is familial a pedigree analysis is performed and the parents counseled appropriately.

If an anomaly is not isolated but does form part of a recognizable pattern and there is no confirmatory test but the inheritance pattern is known, a pedigree analysis is completed and the parents are appropriately counseled. If the inheritance pattern is not known and the condition is

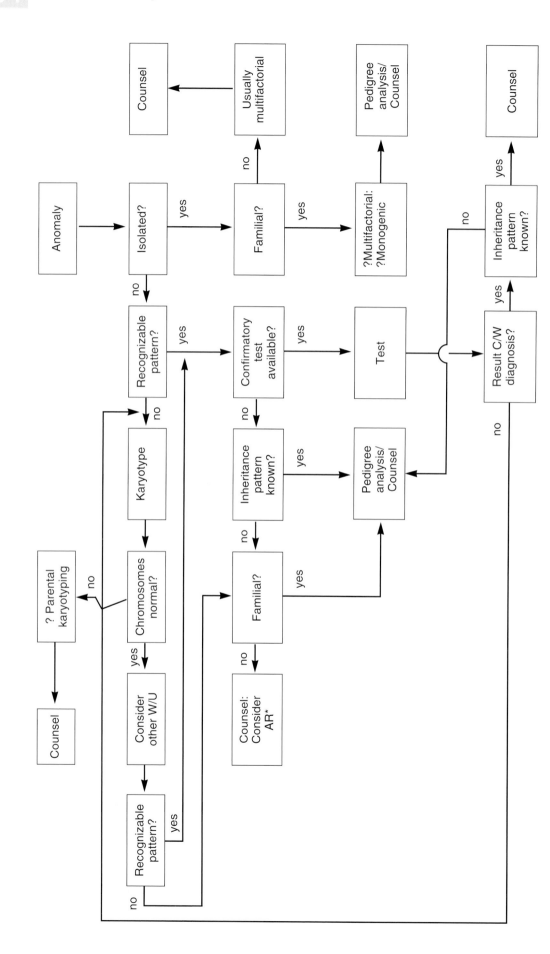

*AR = autosomal recessive

Fig. 51.1 A diagnostic approach to congenital anomalies.

familial, a pedigree analysis is performed with the appropriate parental counseling. If the condition is not familial the parents are counseled and it is assumed that the mode of inheritance is autosomal recessive.

ETIOPATHOGENESIS

The etiology and pathogenesis of the various craniofacial conditions and syndromes has, until very recently, been speculative at best. It has been based on a limited amount of basic research data. Most of the evidence utilized to investigate the causes and development of the multiple and often complex conditions frequently encountered by craniofacial surgeons in clinical practice was provided in the early and mid 1900s by anatomists and embryologists such as Virchow,[1] Veau,[2] and later Moss,[3] Park and Powers,[4] and Ross.[5] Despite all these efforts, it was not until the late 1980s with breakthroughs in techniques of genetic investigation in the new and expanding field of molecular biology that the pathogenesis and etiology of these conditions became more clearly understood.

Of all the craniofacial conditions it is the etiology of the craniofacial clefting syndromes which is probably best understood. The evolution of this understanding can probably be traced back to the work of Dursy (1869) and His (1892), which became known as the classic theory of Dursy and His. These authors were of the opinion that craniofacial clefting conditions resulted from the failure of fusion of various facial processes; at this time all macroanatomists were aware of this. They further proposed that unknown factors caused the advancing ectoderm of these facial processes not to fuse. Wherever this occurred, a cleft resulted. This theory was simple and attractive, but could not adequately describe the very complex facial clefts that were frequently seen. In 1910, Pohlman, later supported by Veau (1938),[1] suggested an alternative mechanism, proposing that it was mesodermal migration to the edge of the advancing facial process followed by mesenchymal penetration and support for the advancing ectodermal ridge that resulted in normal fusion and maintenance of the fusion of the facial processes and established facial form rather than fusion of the two adjacent advancing ectodermal ridges. This mesenchymal migration and penetration theory was further propagated by Stark (1954).[6] Stark claimed that epithelial fusion does actually take place but then breaks down, and a facial cleft is produced if mesenchymal migration and advancement fails to take place. The severity of the cleft is then inversely proportional to the quality of mesodermal penetration. This theory has been further supported as the understanding of the role of the neural crest cells has increased. The neural crest cells arise from the lateral edges of the neural plate as it folds to form the neural tube on the dorsal aspect of the developing embryo. The cells from this region then migrate laterally and anteriorly to lie under the epithelial surfaces of the facial processes. The neural crest cells which migrate to the head and neck region under the influence of the effects of tissue hyaluronidase and fibronectin form the skeletal and connective tissue of the head and neck.[7] The above theory is attractive and elegant, however it does not describe the frequently seen bizarre clefting defects which appear to be due to intrauterine amniotic bands causing a direct restriction over that portion of the head and neck which, as a result, becomes clefted. The cleft appears to be caused by direct constriction of the amniotic band with a subsequent arrest of growth in this region. These amniotic bands are thought to occur as a result of low-grade intrauterine chorioamnionitis with adhesion formation in utero. A recent experimental study of the face where constrictions were formed by suture material placed on the fetus in utero adds some credence to this theory.

The etiopathogenesis of isolated craniosynostosis is still under investigation. Since Virchow[1] first suggested that the site of the pathology lay in the suture which was synostosed and that the deformity in the skull base was secondary to the sutural abnormality many other theories have been proposed. Most authors now agree with Moss[3] that the cranial base is the site of the primary anomaly and that the calvarial deformity is secondary to skull base sutural synostosis. The particular cranial base suture which has been proposed is the sphenozygomatic. Park and Powers[4] suggested that the defect is located in the mesenchymal blastema of both the cranial base and the sutures of the cranial vault. Clinically, irradiation to the sphenoid area, e.g. for orbital rhabdomyosarcoma and retinoblastoma in infants, produces a deformity similar to hemifacial microsomia, often with more of a cranial deformity. In the laboratory, irradiation of the sphenoid area in kittens has produced a similar widespread deformity.[8]

Despite these advances, isolated craniosynostosis appears to occur sporadically and therefore is possibly of multifactorial origin.[9] There is possibly both a genetic and/or environmental cause. Some environmental causes have indeed been associated with isolated craniosynostosis: the most commonly cited is the association of microcephaly with first trimester viral infections (especially rubella) and the initiation of microcephaly by irradiation of experimental animals. Isolated craniosynostosis has also been noted with increasing frequency in Hurler syndrome (inborn error of metabolism).[10] Some cases of craniosynostosis have been shown to be related to the deformational process or molding to which the cranial vault is exposed when passing through the maternal pelvis at the completion of pregnancy and during the process of childbirth. The external deformational forces are applied once the period of embryogenesis is complete (usually by day 56). It is most commonly seen in coronal and/or lambdoid plagiocephaly[11] which, if deformational in origin, is usually self-correcting over time. these two forms of plagiocephaly produce quite different clinical pictures and on most occasions can be easily differentiated clinically.

The investigation of craniofacial syndromes associated with syndromal craniosynostosis has recently produced some exciting developments due to the relatively new field of molecular biology. There has recently been tremendous interest in the role of human fibroblast growth factor (FGF) and human fibroblast growth factor receptors (FGFR) since possible anomalies of these may be the cause of various craniofacial syndromes. Recently, mutations in the fibroblast growth factor receptor (FGFR) have been associated with three skeletal dysplasias and four craniosynostotic syndromes.

The following craniofacial syndromes and skeletal dysplasias have been found to have FGFR anomalies:

1. achondroplasia
2. Apert syndrome
3. Crouzon syndrome
4. Jackson–Weiss syndrome
5. Pfeiffer syndrome
6. thanatophoric dysplasia and hypochondroplasia.

The fibroblast growth factor family consists of structurally related polypeptides that play a key role in numerous aspects of embryogenesis, growth, and homeostasis. Fibroblast growth factors have a potent growth-stimulating (mitogenic) and/or differentiation-inducing effect on cells such as those derived from the early embryonic mesodermal ectoderm. Fibroblast growth factors also stimulate chemotaxis, cell survival, and angiogenesis.[9]

FGF mediates cellular responses on binding to and activation of FGFRs. In mammals, nine FGFs and four FGFRs have been identified that are genetic and distinct, and expressed in specific spatial temporal patterns in the developing embryo. The number of different polypeptides produced from these genes is considerably larger as a result of alternative RNA splicing for FGFRs and translational initiation for FGFs. This large family of proteins allow for diversity in addition to some redundancy in function. FGF receptors are transmembrane receptors of the tyrosine kinase group. FGFR consists of three extracellular immunoglobulin-like domains (designated I, II and III), a transmembrane domain, and intracellular tyrosine kinase domains (S M M). Immunoglobulin-like domains II and III are necessary for ligand binding. Most FGFR2 mutations discovered so far in craniosynostotic syndromes have been located in that portion of the gene that codes for Ig-like domain III and the region binding If II and III (S S M).

The first human disorder characterized by FGFR mutation was the most common form of dwarfism (achondroplasia). Achondroplasia is inherited as an autosomal dominant trait, although most cases are sporadic.[12] The prevalence of ACH is between 1:15 000 and 1:77 000. A gene for ACH was localized to 4p16.3 by linkage analyses.[13] The ACH candidate region included the gene encoding FGFR3 with point mutations in the FGFR3 gene in both ACH heterozygotes and homozygotes. The mutation found was $G \rightarrow A$ transition at nucleotide 1138 of the cDNA. Less often a mutation at the same position but with $G \rightarrow C$ transversion was found.[13]

Both the above mutations resulted in the substitution of an arginine residue for a glycine at position 380 of the mature protein. This is the transmembrane domain of FGFR3. Bellus et al[12] evaluated 154 unrelated individuals with ACH for mutations in the FGFR3 transmembrane domain. All but one of the cases assessed were found to have glycine to arginine substitution at codon 380. Stoilov et al[14] did not find the common G38OR mutation in eight hypochondroplasia chromosomes studied. They suggested that some cases of hypochondroplasia are caused by mutation in a gene other than FGFR3.

Apert syndrome is a well-known autosomol dominant condition which includes craniosynostosis (usually brachycephaly) and associated complex syndactyly of both hands and feet as the main components of this disorder. Other abnormalities seen include mental retardation and cleft palate.[3] The birth prevalence is 1:65 000.[15–20] The presence of both craniosynostosis and associated skeletal deformities does increase the index of suspicion of several causative genetic abnormalities. Wilkie et al[20] studied 40 unrelated patients with Apert syndrome. Only 11 recorded cases exist where patients with Apert syndrome have had children – hence the paucity of appropriate pedigrees and a resultant lack of a classical genetic linkage approach to this disorder. Wilkie et al[20] identified mis-sense mutations in FGFR2 in all 40 patients but in none of 23 normal controls or in patients with Crouzon syndrome. In three families from whom mRNA was available from both unaffected parents, they demonstrated that the mutation (C934G in one case, C937G in two cases) had arisen de novo. They conclude that their observations indicate that specific non-conservative substitutions (Ser 252 Trp or Pro 253 Arg) of adjacent amino acids of FGFR2 cause the great majority of cases of Apert syndrome. They postulated that different mutations may occur in occasional patients. They end by stating, and we quote, 'Apert Syndrome is a disorder caused largely by two (2) alternative mutations. It will be of great interest to determine the molecular bases of this disorder and whether further distinctive phenotypes associated with FGFR2 mutation await discovery'.[20] We concur.

Crouzon syndrome has various classical clinical features which include shallow orbits with varying degrees of proptosis due to maxillary hypoplasia.[21] This autosomal dominant condition has fewer variable craniofacial anomalies and no limb deformities.

Reardon et al[22] identified FGFR2 mutations in patients with Crouzon syndrome. They also identified identical mutations in the FGFR2 gene causing Pfeiffer and Crouzon syndrome phenotypes. Jabs et al[23] found two further mutations in the FGFR2 gene in Crouzon patients where each new mutation introduced an additional cysteine residue in the Ig domain. They propose that the mechanism of the reported FGFR2 mutations may be receptor activation. In 1996 Steinberger et al[21] reported on the as yet unrecognized deletion, duplication and point mutation within the FGFR2 gene in Crouzon patients.

The Jackson–Weiss syndrome is a clinically distinct autosomal dominant condition characterized by foot, hand and other skull abnormalities first described in 1976.[24] In affected families the variability and penetrance are high with some patients having foot anomalies with no craniofacial deformities. This syndrome has been mapped to the same chromosomal region (10q25–q26) as Crouzon syndrome (FGFR2).[24–26] The molecular basis of Crouzon syndrome involves mutations of FGFR2.[21] Jabs[23] described a mutation in the same conserved immunoglobulin IIIc domain where FGFR2 mutations were found for Crouzon syndrome in Jackson–Weiss syndrome patients. Jabs further identified an Arg 344 Gly mutation in the FGFR2 gene. This substitution was detected in all family members who were affected with Jackson–Weiss syndrome. It was not found in any normal patient studied. Thus, two clinically distinct craniosynostotic conditions (Crouzon and Jackson–Weiss syndrome) are due to allelic mutations in the FGFR2 gene, suggesting that FGFR2 mutations might have variable phenotypic effects.[23]

Pfeiffer syndrome is an autosomal dominant form of acrocephalosyndactyly. It classically consists of craniosynostosis (often brachycephaly) with deviation and enlargement of the thumbs and great toes and varying degrees and forms of syndactyly and interphalangeal ankylosis.[25] Utilizing single strand conformation polymorphism and sequence analyses of amplified exons in a sporadic case of Pfeiffer syndrome, Lajeunie et al[25] found an A → G transition in the 3′ acceptor splice site of the intron adjacent to exon B of FGFR2 thereby disrupting the consensus sequence required for the normal processing of the RNA transcript. This mutation may result in an aberrant protein. In the familial form of Pfeiffer syndrome an A → C transition at nucleotide 974 (condon B21) of the coding sequence (exon B), creating an Eael site and changing an aspartic acid into an alanine in the third Ig-like domain of the protein, was found. These base substitutions were not found in 80 normal controls.[25] This information where Pfeiffer syndrome mutations are found in FGFR2 expands by Muenke et al[26] the discovery of Pfeiffer syndrome mutation mapping to the FGFR1 region.

In 1997 Muenke et al[26] presented 61 individuals from 20 unrelated families where coronal synostosis was due to an amino acid substitution (Pro 25 Arg) that results from a single point mutation in the FGFR3 gene on chromosome 4p. They hereby defined a new clinical syndrome based on this molecular finding. Utilizing this information, they suggest that all patients with coronal synostosis should be tested for this mutation.

In summary, FGFRs are essential at many different stages of development. All human mutations identified to date are mis-sense or splice site mutations. These mutations may permit early human developmental abnormalities but they also interfere with later developmental processes affecting primordial bone cells involved in sutural closure, rib and long bone development, and limb formation. The pathogenesis of the mutations can be explored by analysis, either by chemical function in transferred cells or of its phenotype in transgenic animals. Clearly, it would be helpful to develop transgenic animals with a known human mutation as a model for craniosynostosis and the skeletal dysplasias. These animal models could then be further utilized to elucidate the signals and pathways implicated in normal human skeletal development as well as to assess the reasons why anomalies occur.[8]

In spite of the exciting developments at the molecular biology level in etiopathogenesis of the craniodysostosis syndromes, a great deal of work is still necessary before this information can have any major impact on the clinical management of these cases. However, with further development and accumulation of information about the etiology and pathogenesis of these craniofacial syndromes it may one day be possible to eliminate the development of these syndromes using gene therapy and gene manipulation. However, to be absolutely realistic, that day is a very long way off.

REFERENCES

1. Virchow R 1981 Uber don Cretinismus, nomentlich in Franken und uber pathologische Schadoiformen. Verh Phys Med Gesellsoh 2:230
2. Veau V, Politzer J 1936 Embryology du bec de liévre. Annals of Anatomy and Pathology 13:278
3. Moss ML 1959 The pathogenesis of premature cranial synostosis in man. Acta Anatomica 37:351
4. Park E A, Powers G F 1920 Acrocephaly and scaphocephaly with symmetrically distributed malformations of the extremities. American Journal of Diseases of Childhood 20:235
5. Ross R B, Johnson M C 1972 Cleft lip and palate. Williams & Wilkins, Baltimore
6. Stark RB, Kaplan JM 1973 Development of the cleft lip nose. Plastic and Reconstructive Surgery 51:413
7. Noden DM 1983 The role of the neural crest in patterning of avian cranial skeletal, connective and muscle tissue. Developmental Biology 96:144
8. Carls FR, Çelebiler Ö, Narayana V, Robertson P, McLaughlin W, Jackson IT 1998 Craniofacial deformities created by highly selected spheno-irradiation in cats. (in preparation)
9. Vander Kolk CA, Beaty T 1994 Etiopathogenesis of craniofacial anomalies. Clinics in Plastic Surgery 21:4
10. Cohen MM Jr 1986 Craniosynostosis: Diagnosis, evaluation and management. Raven Press, New York
11. Hanson M, Mulliken JB 1994 Frontal plagiocephaly: Diagnosis and treatment. Clinics in Plastic Surgery 21:4
12. Bellus GA, Hefferon TW, Ortiz de Luna RI et al 1996 Achondroplasia is defined by recurrent G380R mutations of FGFR3. American Journal of Human Genetics 56:368–373
13. Shiang R, Thompson LM, Zhu Y et al 1994 Mutations in the transmembrane domain of FGFR3 cause the most common genetic form of dwarfism, achondroplasia. Cell 78:335–342
14. Stoilov I, Kirkpatrick MW, Tsipouras P 1995 A common FGFR3 gene mutation is present in achondroplasia but not in hypochondroplasia. American Journal of Human Genetics 55:127–133
15. Blank OE 1960 Apert's syndrome (a type of acroscaphalosyndactyly) observations on a British series of thirty-nine cases. Annals of Human Genetics 24:151–164
16. Cohen MM Jr, Kreiborg S 1990 The central nervous system in the Apert syndrome. American Journal of Medical Genetics 35:36–45
17. Upton J, Zuker RM (eds) 1991 Apert syndrome. Clinics in Plastic Surgery 18:1–435
18. Cohen MM Jr, Kreiborg S 1993 Visceral anomalies in the Apert syndrome. American Journal of Medical Genetics 45:758–760
19. Cohen MM Jr, Kreiberg S 1993 Skeletal abnormalities in the Apert syndrome. American Journal of Medical Genetics 47:624–632
20. Wilkie AOM, Slaney SF, Odridge M et al 1995 Apert syndrome results from localized mutations of FGFR2 and is allelic with Crouzon syndrome. Nature Genetics 9
21. Steinberger D, Mulliken JB, Muller U 1996 Crouzon syndrome: Previously unrecognized deletion, duplication and point mutation with FGFR2 gene. Human Mutation 8:388–390
22. Reardon W, Winter RM, Rutland P, Pulleyn LJ, Jones SM, Malcolm S 1900 Mutations in the fibroblast growth factor receptor 2 gene cause Crouzon syndrome. Nature Genetics 8:98–103
23. Jabs EW, Scott AF, Meyers G et al 1900 Jackson-Weiss and Crouzon syndromes are allelic with mutations in fibroblast growth factor receptor 2. Nature Genetics 8:275–279
24. Jackson CE, Weiss L, Reynolds WA, Forman TF, Peterson JA 1975 Craniosynostosis, midface hypoplasia and foot abnormalities: An autosomal dominant phenotype in a large Amish kindred. Journal of Pediatrics 88:963–968
25. Lejeunie E, Wei Ma H, Bonaventure J, Munnich A, Le Merrer M 1995 FGFR2 mutations in Pfeiffer syndrome. Nature Genetics 9
26. Muenke M, Griff KW, McDonald-McGinn UM et al 1997 A unique point mutation in the Fibroblast Growth Factor Receptor 3 gene (FGFR3) defines a new craniosynostosis syndrome. American Journal of Human Genetics 60:665–564

Principles of surgical management

TIMOTHY A. TURVEY/RAMON L. RUIZ

INTRODUCTION

Tessier introduced the concept of craniofacial surgery in 1967, and since then the principles and operative techniques of this unique surgical discipline have continued to evolve.[1] Tessier's original work with craniofacial surgical techniques involved children and adults with congenital malformations including craniofacial dysostosis and facial clefts. Experience with the correction of craniofacial anomalies in infants then required modification of the original principles. Subsequent modifications of Tessier's techniques now provide the craniofacial surgeon with improved access for tumor resection, management of post-traumatic deformities, and superior esthetic outcomes in the correction of congenital anomalies.[2,3] Further technical refinements continue to build upon the original principles of craniofacial surgery and expand the applications of these techniques for the correction of facial deformities. The purpose of this chapter is to present principles that may be applied during craniofacial surgical procedures undertaken in the management of a variety of conditions.

PRINCIPLES

DEFINING THE PROBLEM AND DEVELOPING A TREATMENT PLAN

Comprehensive management of patients with craniomaxillofacial malformations is best accomplished by a multidisciplinary team of experienced healthcare providers, including the surgeon. Patients with craniofacial syndromes often have defects involving other organ systems, therefore careful evaluation of the patient's overall medical condition and identification of potential surgical risk factors must be part of the preoperative work-up. In addition, detailed examinations of neurologic and visual function, speech, and airway status are essential early in life and then longitudinally as the child grows and undergoes treatment. Other non-surgical issues including the patient's emotional state, familial support and structure, and other psychosocial stress factors must not be overlooked.

Poor outcomes in craniomaxillofacial surgery occur for many reasons, the most common being inadequate preoperative evaluation and lack of an organized treatment plan. From a surgical perspective, the establishment of an accurate diagnosis is a critical initial step in the management of patients with craniofacial malformations; because there are substantial variations in the expression of these conditions, formulation of the problem list must clearly define specific dysmorphic features and their associated functional and esthetic impairments. A description of a patient as having facial features consistent with a particular diagnostic entity such as Crouzon or Treacher Collins syndrome is of limited therapeutic value.

Preoperative physical examination is composed of both subjective evaluations of facial esthetics and quantitative anthropometric measurements of craniomaxillofacial proportions and symmetry. Measurement analysis of anatomic landmarks using lateral and posteroanterior cephalometric radiographs is invaluable to understand the relationships of the different structures within the craniomaxillofacial complex. More recently, the use of computed tomography scans for preoperative evaluation and quantitative postoperative assessment has become routine. Anatomic dental casts mounted on a semiadjustable articulator document occlusal and jaw relationships, and constitute another important component of the presurgical database. Articulated casts are also employed to confirm proposed surgical movements (model surgery) and to fabricate splints used during the corrective surgical procedures.

Information collected during the presurgical evaluation must then be integrated into a surgical treatment plan. Operations should be designed to improve the specific dysmorphic features of an individual, and not the syndrome. For example, middle face deficiency is not expressed uniformly in the orbits and at the occlusal plane in patients with Crouzon syndrome. Consequently, a 'standard' operation should not be employed for every patient with this condition. If a basic operation is used, variations should be tailored to address specific dysmorphic features, enhance esthetic outcomes, and meet the functional goals. Development of the final surgical treatment plan also requires input from the patient and family.

PLACEMENT OF INCISIONS

Utilization of incisions that minimize visible scars is another principle of craniomaxillofacial surgery. To accomplish this, the coronal incision and intraoral incisions should be used whenever possible. The transconjunctival approach to the orbit is useful, but rarely necessary. Facial incisions, no matter how well camouflaged, should if possible be avoided. Sometimes the resulting facial scar is more obvious than the soft-tissue problem which it was intended to correct. For instance, midline forehead scars secondary to skin excision may appear as unsightly as widened eyebrows.

Coronal incision

The coronal incision is a versatile and cosmetically acceptable approach for access to the cranial vault, cranial base, forehead, nose, upper middle face, and orbits. With the use of this incision, inferior eyelid or transconjunctival access to the orbit in most cases is not necessary.

The incision is placed from one supra-auricular area to the other and the degree of skeletal exposure required for a given procedure dictates the inferior extent of the incision. When access to the zygoma and infraorbital rims is necessary, the incisions must be extended further inferiorly. The hairline of the patient is the primary consideration in the placement of the incision. Although anterior extension at the midportion of the coronal flap may enhance flap retraction and access to the midface, the resulting scar may subsequently become obvious with male pattern baldness. The authors' preference is to place the incision across the top of the head rather than carrying it toward the forehead. The use of a postauricular coronal incision eliminates visible scars in the preauricular area and decreases the risk to the frontal branch of the facial nerve in reoperated patients, but it may also limit exposure anteriorly.[4] Placement of this incision further posterior in the scalp is also beneficial in children, where migration of the coronal scar may occur with growth. When secondary operations are performed, it is preferable to reincise through the original scar. Although it may be tempting to place the incision in a different location, consideration must be given to the effect of the previous scar on flap perfusion and wound healing. Use of a zigzag (stealth) incision avoids a straight-line scar and is particularly useful in patients with short hair.[5] The additional blood loss associated with a greater incision length and longer closure time may offset the benefit.

After a 1 cm strip has been shaved along the proposed incision line, the area of the incision is injected with a diluted solution of 1% lidocaine with epinephrine (1:200 000). This reduces bleeding and helps dissection along the subaponeurotic plane. Sterile saline is injected freely into the subgaleal plane from the incision line to the forehead with the use of a spinal needle. Cross-hatch markings aid in the reapproximation of wound margins during flap closure. The scalp has a rich vascular supply, and so the incision is carried out in segments with application of hemoclips. Bipolar electrocautery is utilized to obtain hemostasis; this has a minimal effect on the adjacent peripheral hair follicles. The use of monopolar electrocautery is contraindicated because of the increased risk of destroying regional hair follicles which results in a visible scar. Adequate hemostasis is especially important in infants and young children because of the potential loss of their blood volume. Once the pericranium is identified, a plane of dissection is established above it. Dissection proceeds rapidly and bloodlessly to the forehead in this supraperiosteal plane. At the hairline, an incision is made through the pericranium and dissection is then continued subperiosteally to expose the facial skeleton. It is critical to remain within the subperiosteal plane during dissection over the facial skeleton in order to avoid injury to the facial nerve. Bleeding from vessels perforating the cranium can be controlled with bone wax. In infants and young children, care must be exercised when dissecting over open sutures, especially midline sutures, to avoid venous sinus hemorrhage and injury to the meninges. Care must also be exercised when establishing a plane of dissection over the temporalis muscle. The natural plane of dissection is subgaleal. Within the region over the temporalis muscle, the plane should be deepened to the level of the muscle fascia (superficial layer of the deep temporal fascia). The temporoparietal fascia, which is superficial to the fascia of the temporalis muscle and is an extension of the superficial musculoaponeurotic system, invests the temporal branch of the facial nerve. Deepening the incision to the level of the temporalis muscle fascia avoids the nerve and leads to subperiosteal dissection of the facial skeleton. The supraorbital nerves sometimes restrict flap mobility and dissection of the periorbita. Removal of the bony floor of the foramina utilizing a small osteotome is often required to release the supraorbital neurovascular bundles and permit further mobility of the flap. Closure of the incision in layers, even after facial advancement exceeding 15 mm, is usually not a problem. The lateral canthus is resuspended to the fascia over the temporalis muscle in an upward and posterior direction. Dissection of the posterior scalp in the subgaleal plane is sometimes necessary to facilitate closure.

Oral incisions

The use of transoral approaches to the facial skeleton provides wide exposure while concealing scars, and this is a useful component of sound craniofacial surgical principles. By combining oral incisions with the coronal incision, the entire craniofacial skeleton may be dissected and visualized.

In general, a horizontal incision from the molar region of the maxilla to the opposite molar region adequately exposes the lateral walls of the maxilla, inferior orbital rim pterygomaxillary juncture, zygomatic buttress, and nasal cavity. When the maxilla is mobilized at the Le Fort I level, a circumvestibular incision under the upper lip is utilized. The bilateral cleft maxilla is an exception, and an anterior mucosal pedicle on the premaxilla must be maintained, even if previous bone grafting has united the segments. When Le Fort III and Le Fort I osteotomies are combined, the preservation of an anterior soft-tissue pedicle provides additional perfusion to the middle face which is already vascularly compromised by the Le Fort III osteotomy.

The entire facial aspect of the mandible may also be accessed through oral mucosal incisions. An incision through the mucosa of the lower lip is normally utilized to approach the anterior mandible, such as when a genioplasty or a mandibular subapical osteotomy is performed. If access to the mandibular body or ramus is necessary, incisions along the external oblique ridge may be extended. The lingual soft tissues provide adequate perfusion to the mandible during dissection and retraction of the buccal tissues. It is, therefore, important to maintain these lingual attachments during mandibular osteotomies. When inferior border osteotomies are undertaken, preservation of the attached genial musculature assures better long-term survival of the mobilized segment. If this procedure is conducted as a free bone graft, resorption of the segment is predictable.

SUBPERIOSTEAL DISSECTION

Of importance to craniofacial skeletal operations is generous subperiosteal dissection of the facial skeleton, sufficient to permit visualization and instrumentation. This is the case when the facial skeleton is exposed through a coronal incision and in any transoral approach to the maxilla, zygomatic complex, and mandible.

When the orbit is involved in the osteotomy, complete subperiosteal dissection is necessary to relax tension on the globe as well as to permit adequate access. Flap relaxation may be achieved by releasing the supraorbital neurovascular bundle and freeing the periorbita around the circumference of the orbit. When additional periosteal stripping and uncovering of the medial orbital wall is required, the anterior and posterior ethmoidal arteries may be cauterized and divided. It is seldom necessary to dissect more than 15 mm toward the apex from the orbital rim. Although further posterior dissection is possible, the risk of optic nerve injury increases proportionately. The attachment of the medial canthal tendon to the frontal process of the maxilla is identified and protected during the dissection, unless repositioning is planned. Preservation of this structure on the anterior lacrimal crest avoids the uncertainties of reattaching it. If the medial canthus is abnormally located, it should be repositioned at the completion of the surgery.

Subperiosteal dissection of the nasal bridge is of importance when onlay bone grafts are placed or when a portion of interorbital bone is to be excised, as with correction of hypertelorism. Similarly, dissection of the lateral walls of the maxilla, zygomatic buttress, and arch is necessary for placement of contour bone grafts. It is also very important for coronal flap relaxation and to permit facial advancement and soft-tissue redraping at the completion of surgery. Confining the dissection of the facial skeleton to the subperiosteal plane minimizes the possibility of facial nerve injury. When facial nerve injury occurs during craniofacial procedures, it is the frontal and temporal branches that are most frequently involved. Identification of the subperiosteal plane posteriorly and anteriorly prior to dissection around the zygomatic arch further assists in the prevention of this injury.

ADEQUATE COOLING WHEN UTILIZING POWER CUTTING INSTRUMENTS

A basic principle of performing surgery on bone is to prevent overheating which damages the cells adjacent to the osteotomy. Overheating is common, however, and is felt by some to be trivial. Osteocyte damage from overheating, especially when autogenous bone grafts are used, probably has more significant histologic effects than clinical ramifications. Relapse associated with some craniofacial procedures may however be related to bone healing problems secondary to heat damage to the bone.

Today there is a greater reliance on screw and plate fixation of osteotomies. Inadequate use of coolants at the time of screw hole placement may result in thermal bone injury, poor hardware retention, and unstable osteotomized segments.

Harvesting of bone grafts with the use of power instruments was the likely reason for the poor initial success rates of cranial bone grafts to the cleft maxilla.[6] When the cranial diploe is harvested with a curette rather than a craniotome, success is similar to that observed with the ilium as the donor site.[7] It is apparent that using power instruments without adequate cooling damages the cells and diminishes the osteogenic potential of the bone graft.

In no other aspect of craniofacial surgery has the importance of using adequate coolant and slow speed rotary instrumentation become more apparent than with the placement of craniofacial endosseous implants. In this setting, it is crucial to maintain the viability of the cells adjacent to the implant to allow for osseointegration. Reduction of heat damage by adequate irrigation and use of slow speed rotary instruments is critical to success.

COMPLETION OF OSTEOTOMIES UNDER DIRECT VISUALIZATION

Adequate mobilization of skeletal segments during total midfacial advancements can only be accomplished when osteotomies are complete. The combination of intracranial and subcranial (anterior) approaches to the craniomaxillofacial region allows retraction and protection of the brain and globes so that the procedure may be carried out safely under direct visualization.

The craniotomy provides access for visualization and protection of the brain throughout the operative procedure. When operations are conducted in the temporal fossa, adequate dissection of the fossa below the sphenoid wing affords protection to the temporal lobe during the osteotomy. This is especially important in Apert syndrome where the temporal lobe tip may extend forward into the lateral orbital rim.

As previously described, wide exposure of the orbits and middle face is accomplished through a coronal incision. Meticulous dissection and retraction of soft-tissue structures is important for visualization and thorough instrumentation at the osteotomy sites.

Once an osteotomy is completed, the bone cuts should be tested with a thin osteotome in order to identify areas of incomplete separation and prevent unintended fractures. Attempts to mobilize facial bones after incomplete osteotomies may result in fracture disruption of the segments, inadequate advancement, and relapse. This most frequently occurs during movements at the Le Fort III or frontofacial (monobloc) levels. Inadequate separation of the posterior maxillary walls and perpendicular portion of the palatine bone, which are impossible to visualize completely, contributes to this problem and may result in disruption of the zygomatic portion of the orbit. The use of osteotomes and specially designed bone spreaders assists in the completion of pterygomaxillary separation and minimizes the risk of associated fractures. When fractures occur, complete mobilization must still be accomplished. Repair of the involved segments by plate fixation is indicated; when this is appropriately performed it seldom results in a problem.

Simultaneous intracranial and subcranial approaches to the craniofacial region are also utilized for direct visualization during midline procedures. With the use of magnification, this exposure allows removal of interorbital bone and preservation of olfactory nerve filaments in the correction of hypertelorism.[8]

OVERCORRECTION

Relapse is a problem familiar to those involved with osteotomies of the craniofacial skeleton. Three types of postoperative skeletal relapse may occur. The first is movement of the bones towards their original position. This occurs mostly because of inadequate mobilization and stabilization. The osteotomized segments must be adequately mobilized and positioned to achieve the desired result. Additionally, associated soft tissues must be adequately relaxed to accommodate the skeletal movements. The use of rigid internal fixation devices provides better stability of the cranial and midfacial regions. This is less true in the mandible where musculoskeletal adaptation is required for stability.[9] The second type of relapse occurs because of disproportionate growth. This growth may involve the operated skeleton and/or adjacent structures. The third mechanism for relapse is related to bone remodeling or pathologic changes such as condylar resorption. In all three conditions, the result is similar (return to the original condition).

Overcorrection of the mobilized skeleton is more important in children since continued growth is expected. The amount of overcorrection is variable and dependent upon the skeletal unit operated, the vector and magnitude of the movement, and expectation of growth. In children, overcorrection of the occlusion should be employed since postsurgical growth is the key to the result. Overcorrection of the mobilized skeletal segments in adults is more controversial. In the adult, occlusion should determine the position of the maxilla and mandible, providing that the patient has undergone appropriate orthodontic preparation.

STABILIZATION AND FIXATION

Appropriate stabilization of skeletal segments and bone grafts is necessary for successful outcomes in craniofacial surgery. Inadequate stabilization contributes to relapse and infection, and the use of rigid fixation may minimize problems.

The use of bone plates and screws has significantly improved the outcome of most craniomaxillofacial surgical procedures. This is more true of surgery in the adult patient than is the case with pediatric patients. Problems with the use of plate and screw fixation in children arise from cranial remodeling (endocranial bone resorption, exocranial bone deposition), damage to developing teeth, and restriction of growth.[10,11] An added concern is the unknown long-term effect of the implanted metals over the lifespan of the patient. When plates and screws are used in pediatric patients, removal should be considered within 9 months following surgery. Even in this short time, the removal may be difficult because of osseointegration of the hardware.

PLACEMENT OF BONE GRAFTS

The use of fresh autogenous bone grafts provides the most predictable results in craniofacial surgery. As a general rule, all bony defects should be grafted in order to assure adequate regeneration and continuity. Ilium and rib were formerly the most frequently utilized donor sites, and the site was chosen according to the desired bone consistency. The cranium has now become the most favored site.[12] The proximity to the surgical site, ease of harvesting, and quantities of bone available make the calvaria an attractive alternative. Additionally, the consistency of the bone in the cranium (dense cortical) and its rich haversian network allow it to revascularize quickly and resorb minimally.[13] Consequently, cranial bone grafts are excellent for use in recontouring the craniomaxillofacial skeleton. Although the ilium remains the favored donor source for grafting of clefts, adequate quantities of cancellous bone may also be harvested from the cranium when necessary with equally good results.[14]

Allogeneic bone, lyophilized cartilage, and alloplastic materials have all been used in craniofacial surgery. Although success has been achieved with the use of these materials in certain instances, none has the same success rate or predictability of fresh autogenous bone.

MANAGEMENT OF DEAD SPACE

The elimination of dead space during closure of the craniomaxillofacial region is critical for sound surgical practice. Dead space resulting from craniofacial procedures is resolved by meticulous closure of tissues, placement of bone grafts, and obliteration with soft-tissue flaps or free fat.

Forward advancements of the craniofacial skeleton and anterior cranial vault result in the creation of extradural retrofrontal dead space and communication with the nasal cavity.[15] Potential complications of residual dead space include delayed healing, cerebrospinal fluid leaks, and infection.[16,17] The management of this space in the anterior cranium following frontofacial or forehead advancement remains controversial. Expansion of the frontal lobes and relatively rapid filling of the residual intracranial space has been well demonstrated in infants and young children.[15,18] This observation supports the conservative management of dead space in younger patients. More gradual, and less complete, filling occurs in the adult and this may be particularly troublesome when the space communicates directly with the nasal cavity. Sealing the nasal cavity from the cranial fossa is accomplished with primary repair of the nasal mucosa. When this is not feasible, an anteriorly based pericranial flap may be inserted for coverage of the anterior cranial base. The use of fibrin glue in the reconstruction of the anterior cranial floor also provides a temporary seal between the cavities and allows for re-epithelialization of the nasal mucosa.[19] When forehead procedures are performed and the frontal sinuses are present, management of the dead space is achieved by cranialization, complete removal of the mucosal lining, and obliteration of the nasofrontal ducts with bone grafts or free fat.

The placement of bone grafts into bony defects is important for closure of dead space and facilitates rapid healing. These bone grafts should be wedged or stabilized with screws to prevent migration. Additionally, defects within the temporal fossa following facial advancements or orbitozygomatic reconstruction in Treacher Collins syndrome should be filled by advancement of temporalis muscle flaps. This eliminates the dead space, and the defect is confined to the hair-bearing area of the scalp.

A layered closure of the coronal incision is required for elimination of dead space and an optimal esthetic result.[20] The lateral canthus is stripped during exposure of the orbital rims, and these structures must be resuspended. Sutures are passed through the canthus and secured to the lateral orbital rim or temporalis muscle fascia. When the temporalis muscle is stripped from the lateral temporal crest or fossa, it should be reattached to the lateral orbital wall and temporal ridge in order to prevent bitemporal defects. Closure of the subcutaneous tissues and galea is accomplished as a separate layer. Sutures or surgical staples are used for cutaneous closure. The use of chromic gut on the skin in children is effective and may obviate the need for postoperative suture removal.

Until the nasopharyngeal mucosa seals, communications with the nasal cavity allow air leaks that may result in subcutaneous emphysema or a pneumocephalus. To prevent this type of airflow, postoperative endotracheal intubation may be extended or bilateral nasopharyngeal airways placed for a 3–5-day period.[21] In addition, sinus precautions and restriction of nose blowing further limit reflux of air and fluid during the postoperative period.

PERIOPERATIVE MANAGEMENT

Preoperative evaluation of the craniofacial surgical patient must include a complete physical examination, appropriate laboratory tests, and compatibility studies for blood transfusion. Recent advances in transfusion medicine have made possible the use of autologous blood donated preoperatively by the patient.

Standard intraoperative monitoring consists of electrocardiographic leads, pulse oximetry, capnography, temperature probe, and a precordial stethoscope. Central venous catheters are useful for perioperative hemodynamic monitoring and provide additional vascular access. The use of an arterial blood pressure line is required during long procedures or when controlled hypotensive anesthetic techniques are employed. Arterial lines provide constant blood pressure measurements and access for obtaining serial blood gas samples. Hourly evaluation of urine output, using a catheter, is a useful and easily quantifiable indicator of renal perfusion and volume status. When extensive dural lacerations or cerebrospinal fluid leaks occur, primary repair or patch grafts should be accomplished. Lumbar drains in the subarachnoid space during the perioperative period are sometimes helpful.

At the completion of surgery, the patient is transported directly to a critical care unit (pediatric or surgical) by the anesthesiologist, surgeon, and intensivist. Joint management by the surgeon and critical care specialist allows close monitoring of the patient's respiratory, hemodynamic, and neurologic status. In the intubated patient, sedation must be carefully administered to allow serial neurologic examinations during the immediate postoperative period. Measurement of serum electrolytes and blood counts must be performed frequently during the initial 24 hours following operation. In patients who have received large blood transfusions, evaluation of platelets, prothrombin time, and partial thromboplastin time is needed because of the potential for dilutional coagulopathies. The decision to extubate the patient is based upon alertness, respiratory parameters (level of ventilator support, tidal volume, negative inspiratory force), and degree of edema.

Administration of short-term, high-dose steroids during the immediate perioperative period is useful in reducing postoperative edema. Recollection of the massive edema seen in patients undergoing orthognathic procedures who were not treated with steroids is sufficient for the authors to recommend their perioperative use for craniofacial surgery. By reducing edema of the craniofacial region, the risk of excessive pressure on the globes is reduced, as is discomfort. The patient's mental status must be monitored closely as periods of euphoria, psychosis, and mild depression are possible during and immediately after steroid administration.

Perioperative antibiotic coverage is indicated for craniomaxillofacial surgery, and the exact regimen is determined by the type of surgical procedure. The duration of the antibiotic administration also varies. When facial osteotomies are performed without bone grafts, 24-hour coverage is sufficient. For major procedures involving bone grafts, or operations that result in the creation of dead space within the craniofacial region, antibiotics are continued for at least 10 days postoperatively.

Penicillin remains the antibiotic prophylaxis of choice for procedures that are done through transoral incisions. For operations utilizing coronal or other cutaneous incisions a first generation cephalosporin is effective against most Staphylococcus, Streptococcus, enteric Gram-negative species, and some anaerobes. First generation cephalosporins, however, have variable activity against *H. influenzae*. Aminoglycosides provide additional coverage of Pseudomonas and Enterobacteriaceae. They do not cover streptococci or Listeria, but act synergistically with penicillins against these organisms.

REFERENCES

1. Tessier P 1967 Osteotomies totales de la face. Syndrome de Crouzon, syndrome d'Apert: Oxycephalies, scaphocephalies, turriciphalies. Annales de Chirurgie Plastique 12(4):273–286
2. Jackson IT, Marsh WR 1983 Anterior cranial fossa tumors. Annals of Plastic Surgery 11:479
3. Posnick JC 1994 Craniomaxillofacial fractures in children. Oral Maxillofacial Surgical Clinics 6;1:169–184
4. Posnick JC, Goldstein JA, Clokie C 1992 Advantages of the postauricular coronal incision. Annals of Plastic Surgery 29:114
5. Munro IR, Fearon JA 1994 The coronal incision revisited. Plastic and Reconstructive Surgery 93:185
6. Sadove AM, Nelson CL, Jones EL et al 1985 Alveolar cleft donor sites: A caution. Presented at the 42nd Annual Meeting of the American Cleft Palate Association. Miami, May 1985
7. Turvey TA 1987 Donor sites for alveolar cleft bone grafts. Letter to the editor. Journal of Oral and Maxillofacial Surgery 45:834 October
8. Sailer HF, Landolt AM 1987 A new method for the correction of hypertelorism with preservation of the olfactory nerve filaments. Journal of Cranio-Maxillofacial Surgery 15(3):122–124
9. Proffit WR, Turvey TA, Phillips C 1996 Orthognathic surgery: A hierarchy of stability. Adult Orthodontic and Orthognathic Surgery 16:191–209
10. Fearson JA, Munro IR, Bruce DA 1995 Observations on the use of

rigid fixation for craniofacial deformities in infants and young children. Plastic and Reconstructive Surgery 95:634–637

11. Manson P 1991 Commentary on the long term effects of rigid fixation on the growing craniomaxillofacial skeleton. Journal of Craniofacial Surgery 2:69

12. Tessier P 1982 Autogenous bone grafts taken from the calvarium for facial and cranial applications. Clinics in Plastic Surgery 9;4:531–538

13. Marx RE 1993 Philosophy and particulars of autogenous bone grafting. Oral and Maxillofacial Surgical Clinics 7:599–612

14. Peleaux RD, Turvey TA 1993 Cranium and ilium for cleft grafting. A comparison of five year results. American Association of Oral and Maxillofacial Surgeons 75th Annual Meeting Educational Summaries and Outline. Journal of Oral and Maxillofacial Surgery 51 (suppl):102

15. Posnick JC, Al-Qattan MM, Armstrong D 1996 Monobloc and facial bipartition osteotomies for reconstruction of craniofacial malformations: A study of extradural dead space and morbidity. Plastic and Reconstructive Surgery 97;6:1118–1128

16. Whitaker LA, Munro IR, Salyer KE et al 1979 Combined report of problems and complications in 793 craniofacial operations. Plastic and Reconstructive Surgery 64:198

17. David DJ, Cooter RD 1987 Craniofacial infection in 10 years of transcranial surgery. Plastic and Reconstructive Surgery 80:213

18. Marsh JL, Galic M, Vannier MW 1991 Surgical correction of craniofacial dysmorphology of Apert syndrome. Clinics in Plastic Surgery 18:251

19. Saltz R, Sierra D, Feldman D et al. 1991 Experimental and clinical applications of fibrin glue. Plastic and Reconstructive Surgery 88:1005

20. Ellis E, Zide MF 1995 Surgical approaches to the facial skeleton. Williams and Wilkins, Baltimore, pp 65–93

21. Tessier P 1993 The monobloc frontofacial advancement: Do the pluses outweigh the minuses? (Discussion.) Plastic and Reconstructive Surgery 91:988

Psychological aspects of facial deformity

CHARLOTTE FEINMANN/SUSAN J. CUNNINGHAM

Facial attractiveness is a complex concept. The measurement of esthetics is difficult as it is a subjective commodity. In addition, the perception of facial attractiveness varies between cultures and different societies are known to show preferences for certain facial or dental characteristics. Esthetic attitudes were recorded 5000 years ago by the Egyptians: kings were portrayed with perfectly proportioned faces and lesser nobles had less perfect faces. Woolnoth[1] was the first person to classify faces as being straight, convex or concave in profile and stated that a straight face was thought to be the most attractive. Shortly after this the famous orthodontist, Edward Angle,[2] studied the skull of the Apollo Belvedere and noted that 'every feature is in balance with every other feature and all the lines are wholly incompatible with mutilation or malocclusion'.

FACIAL ATTRACTIVENESS

Facial attractiveness is extremely important to all of us and facial disfigurements are ranked among the least desirable handicaps by both children and adults.[3] A person's physical appearance is the characteristic which is most obvious to others in social interactions. It is not only the individual's own perception of his or her appearance which contributes to these psychosocial effects but also the reaction of others.[4,5] Self-concept, the way an individual perceives him- or herself, is a major influence on the way an individual behaves.[6] Individuals with unattractive facial esthetics may perceive themselves negatively and may then behave in a negative manner, particularly in social interactions. Physical attractiveness stimulates different expectations according to the degree of attractiveness perceived. Evidence suggests that physically attractive persons are differentiated from their less attractive peers at various stages during their life and in a range of different settings ranging from school to dating and marriage.[7] Clifford and Walster[8] found that attractive schoolchildren were more likely to be highly evaluated by their teachers and Efran[9] found that attractive persons were treated more generously than unattractive individuals when punishment was assigned for a social transgression.

Social responses to an individual's appearance may occur at a subconscious level or may be more obvious and manifest themselves in teasing and nicknames, which in itself can be particularly distressing, especially in childhood. Indeed, the Hopi Indians deliberately drove offenders in their community insane by the simple punishment of laughing at them.[10] Shaw et al[11] found that 60% of children who were teased about their teeth admitted to being upset by it. This was reinforced by the second part of the same study in which schoolchildren were asked to study 12 faces, to describe them and give the person a nickname. The dental condition was commented on in a large number of cases, with dental features increasing in salience where the deviation was most obvious. A study by Shaw[12] upheld the hypothesis that photographs of children with a normal dental appearance would be judged by both peers and by lay adults as being more attractive, more desirable as a friend and less likely to behave in an aggressive manner than children with dental anomalies. Background attractiveness of the face was, however, of greater importance than the dental appearance. There can be little doubt that facial anomalies which are sufficient to affect an individual's appearance may well put the individual at a social disadvantage.

FACIAL DEFORMITY AND PSYCHOLOGICAL IMPLICATIONS

Facial deformity is a term which may be used to cover a whole range of variations from a dental malocclusion to a cleft of the lip and palate through to other disfiguring craniofacial syndromes as well as traumatically induced deformities. Much of the work which has been undertaken in this area has involved individuals with clefts of the lip and/or palate, and improved mental wellbeing is cited as the major benefit for those who undergo corrective surgery.

Those who advocate reconstructive surgery of craniofacial deformities in early childhood believe that it is important that an individual does not develop a sense of deformity and that early treatment prevents such a sense developing.[13] It is also argued that it may improve the child's interactions with the parents and thus increase the chances of healthy psychological development. Barden et al[14] found that although the mothers of facially deformed infants rated their parental satisfaction more positively than mothers of non-facially deformed infants, they consistently behaved in a less nurturing manner and this may alter the infant–mother relationship.

The role of the face in social interactions is crucial to understanding the difficulties of individuals with facial disfigurements. The face is a primary means of non-verbal communication and a face which deviates from the 'norm' becomes a stigma. The reaction of the general public to an individual with a facial disfigurement depends on the combination of a large number of factors including the type of disfigurement, the type of interaction and the expected duration of the interaction. Research suggests that the difference in a person's reaction to a facially disfigured individual as compared with a non-disfigured individual lies in non-verbal communication, e.g. averting one's gaze or pretending the person is not there. The importance of this field of research has been established through a range of experiments investigating responses to facially deformed individuals: more money was collected in a charity box when the researcher appeared without a port-wine birthmark than with one.[15] Helping behavior is also influenced by facial deformities. An investigator appeared on a New York subway train with and without a port-wine birthmark; the investigator pretended to be blind and fell when the train stopped. Help was offered on 61% of occasions when the birthmark was present and 86% of cases when it was not present.[16] A birthmark is not a major craniofacial anomaly and this finding may suggest that those with more severe problems will experience greater alienation in social interactions. Further experimentation in this area may help to ascertain whether this theory is correct.

Many authors have attempted to examine the proposed relationship between external appearance and inner psychological characteristics, and a number have suggested that there is an important interdependence between the two areas. Closely related to this is the theory that the reaction of others to an individual's appearance leads to the development of certain social characteristics within that individual. Those with facial handicaps frequently complain that they are rejected by others and that people behave in a negative manner in social interactions.[17,18] Rumsey et al[18] showed that, although in certain situations people behave in a negative manner, this is frequently influenced by the fact that facially disfigured individuals may exhibit shyness, apprehension and defensiveness. Facially disfigured individuals often feel that their privacy is violated – whereas most people can enter a social situation and 'blend into the crowd', those with facial deformity remain conspicuous.[19]

FACIAL DEFORMITY AND THE CRANIOFACIAL PATIENT

In the United Kingdom, surgeons, orthodontists and speech therapists are frequently represented on the craniofacial team, however it is less common to include a specialist to address the specific psychosocial issues which may affect the patient with a craniofacial deformity. In the United States, mental health professionals are more likely to be included in the team. Such specialists play a vital role in counseling, assessment and support for both the patient and the family, particularly during hospitalization. The mental health professional, usually a psychologist, plays a major role in the management of cleft lip and palate patients as well as those with craniofacial malformations.[20]

Improved mental wellbeing is cited as a major benefit of facial reconstruction in patients with craniofacial malformation; those who support early surgery do so on the grounds that normalization of appearance before the child develops a sense of deformity has major benefits.[13] A further important factor in the development of a facially deformed child is the attitude of the parents and family: those who have a positive family background may be more likely to develop higher self-esteem.[21,22]

There are four domains where individuals are particularly affected by their deformity:[23]

1. Cognitive development – some craniofacial patients may have mental retardation or learning disabilities which create problems. In other cases there may be a negative perception of their abilities, leading to lack of educational stimulation despite normal intelligence levels.
2. Emotional attachment between child and parents – it may be that the attachment formed between mother and child is not as positive as that with a non-disfigured child, thus affecting future psychological development.[14] This is an area which requires further research.

3. Development of peer relationships – peer acceptance is essential for normal development; failure to form such relationships may lead to social withdrawal and negative social behavior.
4. Experience of shame – this certainly does not occur in all cases, however facially disfigured individuals may be at greater risk of such feelings.

THE CLEFT LIP AND/OR PALATE PATIENT

A number of the research projects investigating the psychological implications of facial deformity have centered on cleft lip and/or palate patients. However, differences in psychosocial variables between children with clefts and control populations have often been small and statistically non-significant. Brantley and Clifford[24] proposed that overall an adolescent with a cleft could be classified as a normal subject rather than belonging to a unique 'cleft group'. The same authors proposed that the cleft experience may have a more general effect on the adolescent than the mother, and such children were not judged as having any more adjustment or behavioral problems than the control group of the same age and social class.[25] In their study of 98 cleft patients, Clifford et al[26] concluded that individuals with clefts perceived the cleft had relatively little influence on their lives, particularly with respect to education, dating, teasing and occupation. It may be that the parents and siblings of the child experience problems which the child manages to overcome; this reinforces the need for counseling and support services to be made available to the families of patients.[20,27]

Other studies have shown that adolescents with clefts show greater concern and higher stress levels over interpersonal reactions and that children with clefts have psychological as well as physical sequelae.[28,29] Cleft subjects have been found to show significantly lower global self-concept when compared to non-cleft subjects and also to report significantly less global happiness and satisfaction.[29,30] With society's emphasis on facial attractiveness it would seem likely that cleft patients would experience some limitations, particularly socially and in their attempts to secure employment.

Adolescence is a time when patients with clefts are particularly likely to experience psychological difficulties. They face the typical developmental tasks of this age group: development of a sense of identity, growth of interpersonal peer relationships and achievement of independence, but with the added burden of their condition and the treatment required. They may reject further medical intervention in an attempt to accept themselves as they are and also to take charge of their own future, but at the same time they are aware of their own limitations and still have serious worries about their appearance. Such conflicts may manifest in a variety of ways including anxiety or depression.[31,32] Some individuals may benefit from cognitive therapy or the teaching of social skills, e.g. role playing skills to make them acceptable as part of a group, or communication and assertion skills, alongside the surgical intervention required.[31]

A major goal is the development of reliable and valid measures to identify those children at elevated risk for subsequent psychosocial maladjustment.[33] This would allow targeting of interventions to high-risk children and may reduce the chance of social maladjustment at a later stage. Bennett and Stanton[34] proposed that, in order to develop successful psychotherapy programs, cleft palate centers should work with social scientists outside the cleft area and also with researchers who focus on other stigmatizing conditions, e.g. obesity. The information and insight gained from these groups may be put to use with cleft patients. They also reinforced the need for more longitudinal field studies of cleft children. Mental health intervention will be successful only if it is understood how the social environment of the cleft patient differs from that of the non-cleft individual. Other studies focusing on individual differences and risk factors, such as individual coping styles, may also provide useful information.

CASE REPORT

A 21-year-old Bosnian refugee presented with a history of extensive facial surgery. She had undergone 12 surgical attempts to improve her appearance with very limited success. Following counseling she reported that she had become sufficiently confident to return intrusive stares with a gesture of defiance such as sticking out her tongue. Other patients become hostile and aggressive when confronted with similar unwanted attention. It is important that there is time and support for patients and their families to air their feelings and that counseling should be readily available if required.

The difficulties involved in the management of these patients and the problems which they face are not easily overcome. Only by establishing centralized units with clinicians from all specialties will the expertise be readily available for collaboration in the assessment and treatment of the wide range of presenting problems.

FACIAL DEFORMITY AND ORTHOGNATHIC SURGERY

Orthognathic surgery has evolved over a number of years to correct facial abnormalities and also dental abnormalities arising from skeletal disproportion and as such beyond the scope of routine orthodontic treatment. As orthognathic surgery has become more widely available and more socially acceptable, the demand for treatment has increased enormously. What used to be accepted as a variant of normal appearance is now no longer acceptable in society. This has led to surgery being carried out for less severe defects and to more extensive surgery being undertaken. The aim of surgery is not to create beauty but to correct the problem as the patient perceives it. The importance of careful patient assessment to ascertain what he or she expects from the procedure cannot be overemphasized.

It is easy to imagine that there is a linear relationship between the severity of psychological disturbance and the degree of the deformity. Clinical experience has shown, however, that a mild deformity may be harder to cope with than one that is more severe.[10,35] Reich[36] postulated that severely deformed individuals can confidently predict a negative response, whereas those with milder abnormalities are less confident in their predictions, leading to raised anxieties. Many of the patients who present requesting orthognathic surgery fall into the milder deformities group and may be more severely affected psychologically than is apparent at initial consultation. They therefore need sympathetic understanding of their problems.

PATIENT SELECTION AND PATIENT MANAGEMENT

Orthognathic treatment is usually undertaken for esthetic or functional reasons. It has been suggested that some patients believe that clinicians will be more likely to accept them for treatment if there is a functional element or that a functional complaint is somehow more legitimate than an esthetic one and therefore fail to disclose dissatisfaction with a certain area of their appearance.[37,38] It is important to reassure the patient at the start of treatment that there is no stigma attached to requesting treatment for esthetic reasons and to ascertain the exact objectives of treatment from the patient's perspective if dissatisfaction is to be avoided.

The selection of appropriate patients for orthognathic surgery has been the subject of much debate. A means of detecting those patients who will respond poorly to treatment would be ideal but does not appear to exist as yet. A number of studies have shown that the majority of orthognathic patients are essentially well adjusted and do not exhibit psychological disturbances.[39–43] However, it is still very important to assess carefully those patients presenting for treatment (Table 53.1).

Patients who have a reasonable 'body image' are usually better surgical risks than those with a negative body image.

Table 53.1 Prognostic indicators in orthognathic surgery

Good prognostic indicators	Poor prognostic indicators
Reasonable 'body image'	Minimal, or no, deformity
Realistic expectations of what surgery can achieve	Unrealistic expectations of what surgery will achieve
Patient has felt unhappy for some time about the particular feature he/she wants corrected	Those who have recently become concerned about some aspect of their appearance – especially if it coincides with a major life event
Answers positively to questions such as 'What do you think is wrong?' and 'What do you want from treatment?'	Those who have been persuaded to have surgery by someone else – parent, spouse, etc.
No previous surgical opinions	Multiple opinions sought in the past
No accessories to the history	Presenting with pictures, photographs, etc., showing their 'deformity' or showing how they would like to look

Those who know what they want from the treatment and can answer positively to 'What do you think is wrong?' and 'Why do you want treatment?' usually make better surgical candidates than those who can only answer vaguely.[39] Patients with a long history of unhappiness about a particular feature are usually better surgical candidates than those who have only just decided they have a problem; the latter group may be undergoing some crisis which has precipitated this unhappiness and it may be better to delay treatment until the clinician is convinced that surgery is the best option.[39,44] Care must also be taken with those individuals who want secondary gain from the operation (e.g. a better job, a new relationship) and with those who present with 'subjective deformities' which are minimal and would be tolerated by the majority of individuals.

Edgerton and Knorr[44] described two types of motivation in patients seeking orthognathic surgery:

External

These patients may seek treatment to please others, e.g. a parent or spouse. Alternatively, they may believe that surgery will please others and make their external environment easier. These patients need very careful evaluation before agreeing to treatment, and referral for psychiatric assessment may be appropriate.

Internal

Internal motivation is usually a more valid form of motivation. The patients frequently have longstanding feelings about a defect in their appearance and feel that the deformity blocks their enjoyment of life. In general, these patients make better candidates for surgery. It is important for the clinician to realize that not all patients can be placed into these two discreet categories: some patients will exhibit characteristics of both external and internal motivation.

SATISFACTION AND DISSATISFACTION WITH OUTCOME

Patient satisfaction and dissatisfaction have become favored methods of assessing surgical outcome.[38,45–47] An overall review of the literature suggested that between 92% and 100% of patients are happy with the outcomes of their surgery.[48] The largest longitudinal investigation of pre- and postoperative patients was that undertaken by Kiyak and colleagues at the University of Washington, Seattle, and a number of papers report the data from this study. It was found that patients who underwent bimaxillary procedures were just as likely to report satisfaction as those who underwent single jaw procedures; minor problems such as temporomandibular joint clicking and discomfort did not appear to affect outcome.[49] High levels of satisfaction were found postoperatively and if patients perceived an esthetic improvement their satisfaction was high regardless of functional problems. Profile body image increased significantly beyond presurgery levels at 24 months, therefore patients perceived considerable improvements in their profile.[50] It is frequently believed that females are less likely than males to be satisfied with the outcome of treatment. However, Kiyak et al[40] found levels of satisfaction to be high among males and females and there were no significant sex differences in postsurgical satisfaction. Ostler and Kiyak[51] showed high levels of satisfaction in esthetics and function at all ages. They also noted that, following operation, a number of patients reported that they had motives fulfilled that preoperatively they had failed to mention. This reinforces the necessity to assess prior to surgery exactly what it is that the patient desires and expects from treatment.

Postoperative dissatisfaction does occur despite the reported satisfaction rates being high. It is frequently the result of a failure in communication between patient and clinician rather than a poor technical result and this further reinforces the importance of good preoperative explanations.[39,46,52,53] There is little doubt that dissatisfaction can be minimized by describing accurately all aspects of treatment. Recent changes within the National Health Service have increased emphasis on information regarding treatment and the associated problems. However, a study by Cunningham et al[53] found that almost a quarter of patients felt that the postoperative problems had not been

adequately explained and several patients stated that they were alarmed by the degree of swelling or bleeding experienced. These features are also upsetting to relatives and friends if they are not warned of them in advance.

Involvement of the relatives in preoperative discussions may reduce anxiety and also avoid feelings of alienation. This is illustrated in the following case report:

CASE REPORT

A 26-year-old female presented requesting treatment for her class II division 1 malocclusion. Her main complaint was that she did not like the appearance of her teeth and profile. The patient was married with two young children. A combined surgical–orthodontic approach was advised and the surgery, side-effects and complications were fully explained. The initial orthodontic phase was followed by bimaxillary surgery utilizing rigid fixation. At one of the follow-up visits, the patient showed some concern about her ability to adapt to her new situation and it was assumed that this was due to the trauma of the recent surgery and also that she was missing her children who were being cared for by relatives for several weeks. No further concerns were raised at later visits and it was not until several months later that the patient said that she and her husband had separated and were planning to divorce. Subsequent discussions with the patient raised the following issues: her husband felt unable to cope with the dramatic change in her appearance and also the apparent change in her personality (she now felt more confident in social situations where she had previously felt shy and intimidated). Although the planned surgery had been discussed in detail with the patient and she had been encouraged to discuss it with her husband, he felt isolated from the decisions being made and felt completely unprepared to cope with the postoperative sequelae – from the degree of swelling experienced to the postoperative depression. The patient also felt confused and unprepared for the emotions she experienced, in particular her need to seek affirmation that she looked good and had made the right decision to undergo surgery. When it first became apparent to the patient and her husband that they were having problems, they felt isolated and were unsure where to seek help. Although neither of them blamed the surgery for their break-up, both felt it was a contributing factor.

© 1995 Journal of Clinical Orthodontics.
Psychological problems following orthognathic surgery.
Cunningham et al[54]

PREPARATION FOR SURGERY

When preparing patients for surgery, the importance of explaining psychological aspects should not be overlooked. Parents, partners or spouses should be encouraged to attend certain key appointments and ask questions if they wish. In addition, there must be some way for patients and families to seek help urgently if they feel the situation is out of

Eastman Dental Hospital
Special Health Authority

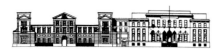

Information on

ORTHOGNATHIC SURGERY

Fig. 53.1 A typical information sheet. See Appendix 1 for details included in the information leaflet.

their control. Holman et al[55] studied the influence of interpersonal support on patient satisfaction and found that availability of support and satisfaction with support from specific members of the patient's support group were significantly associated with satisfaction in the early postoperative period. The support of close friends who backed the patient's decision to proceed with surgery was also found to be associated with satisfaction during the early months after surgery.

Verbal information should always be backed up with a written leaflet (Fig. 53.1). This should be designed to look as attractive as possible in order to encourage patients to read it – a plain sheet of A4 paper covered in printing will frequently deter them before they even start to read it! Patients frequently fail to take in all the information provided at outpatient appointments, particularly if they have been seen in a large joint orthodontic/maxillofacial clinic where there are a number of clinicians present and the patient feels nervous and uneasy. The leaflet should back up the information provided and may also answer worries which the patient has failed to ask about (see Appendix 1). It should provide advice regarding what will happen in the presurgical phase as well as explaining some of the common postoperative problems. There must be some mention of postoperative depression and other psychological difficulties which may occur, along with an emergency telephone number in case of urgent problems.

The orthodontist plays an important part in the counseling of orthognathic patients, as he or she sees them over a protracted time period and comes to know them well. The patient will frequently ask the orthodontist questions which they do not feel able to ask in larger joint clinics.

Imaging tools which provide useful information for treatment planning include CT scans, laser scans,[56] and video imaging.[57] Three-dimensional reconstructions utilizing CT and laser scans[56] are expensive and expose the patient to a significant radiation dose but do have an important role to play, particularly in the reconstructive surgery of complex craniofacial deformities. Recent advances in technology have resulted in the development of computer software which allows manipulation of video images to give some indication of the post-surgical outcome. Although these systems are popular in the United States, in the United Kingdom there has been a certain amount of resistance because of the difficulty in producing an accurate assessment of the surgical outcome, particularly with respect to the soft tissues. Refinement of the software has resulted in more accurate estimations and some clinicians now believe that video imaging may be beneficial as part of the initial patient consultation as it acts as a communication tool and also allows the patient to make an informed decision about whether to proceed with treatment.[57,58] It is important to explain to the patient that this is not a guarantee as to how they will look, but rather an estimation to help them make a decision regarding treatment.

ADAPTATION TO CHANGES IN FACIAL APPEARANCE

Surgery produces sudden and dramatic changes in facial appearance and the individual must suddenly incorporate this new image into his or her own self-concept. This puts great demands on adaptation skills and contrasts with the very gradual changes produced by orthodontic treatment.[41] Patients who are undergoing surgery must be thoroughly prepared for these changes and should the clinician have any doubt about their ability to cope with sudden and dramatic changes, then the patient should be referred for further assessment.

Depression is not uncommon following any surgical procedure and it is hardly surprising that the orthognathic patient may feel depressed with the difficulties involved in speaking, eating and drinking, not to mention those who may have to be placed in intermaxillary fixation. Kiyak et al[41] found that patients mentioned depression even at 9 months after surgery, a time when they are not receiving the support and counseling available to them immediately following surgery. This reinforces the importance of support from friends, family and medical personnel for at least a year following surgery. Any patient who shows signs of depression should be assessed and treated. It is important that this should be available as an emergency measure and that patients who do require help do not have to wait long periods of time to see personnel trained in this form of management. In some cases, a short course of antidepressants may produce dramatic improvements. By forewarning patients that a transient period of depression is likely, the impact on patient and family may be reduced. The response of others also affects how individuals feel about their postoperative appearance and there is a strong correlation with satisfaction and those who report positive comments from friends and relatives[41,46,55]

There has been little research on anxiety in orthognathic patients. It is likely that they experience feelings of anxiety, at least in the immediate pre- and postoperative phases. The postoperative discomfort, as well as difficulties involved in eating and communicating, may well result in an anxious patient. The instruments available for studying depression and anxiety in facial surgery patients are very limited; the majority of questionnaires available were designed for use with populations who are more psychologically disturbed. Cunningham et al[53] used the Hospital Anxiety and Depression Scale[59] to study patients before and after surgery but found no significant difference between the two groups for either anxiety or depression. This may reflect a psychologically well-adjusted group of patients or it may be that the instrument used is inappropriate for that sample, in which case further study of anxiety and depression in orthognathic patients would require the development of a scale for this group of individuals.

'INAPPROPRIATE' SURGICAL PATIENTS

It is difficult, if not impossible in some cases, to detect those patients who may be inappropriate to undergo orthognathic procedures or who may need the support of a psychiatrist or psychologist during treatment. It is because of this that careful assessment of these patients by experienced clinicians is of paramount importance.

USE OF RATING SCALES IN PATIENT ASSESSMENT

Researchers and clinicians are often unaware of the many health measurements available for use in the assessment and management of patients. Psychological measures with a clinical emphasis, e.g. those measuring anxiety or depression or quality of life, are numerous but many have been designed for use with severely disturbed patients and are therefore not appropriate for use with craniofacial or orthognathic patients who may present with some psychological problems but are not usually severely affected.

The most important features of any rating scale or health measure are reliability and validity. Reliability is the extent to which measurements can be replicated and validity assesses whether the scale measures what it is intended to measure. Establishing the validity of any rating measure is difficult and the method of validation is frequently open to debate.[60,61]

The concept of using rating scales in the initial assessment of patients to establish their suitability for treatment is an attractive proposition. A number of scales may have limited use in this respect but nearly all demand that a provisional diagnosis has been made in allowing the correct scale to be selected. For example, the Body Dysmorphic Disorder Examination (BDDE) Scale is a semistructured interview and self-completion questionnaire which was developed to assess those patients with the initial presenting features of BDD.[62] This, however, obviously relies on these features being noted at initial presentation. The Hospital Anxiety and Depression Scale[59] was developed to facilitate the task of detecting emotional disturbances in those patients attending hospital medical and surgical departments but it may be that facially deformed patients present with different psychological disturbances to those detected by this scale.

Questionnaires used in the social sciences frequently rely on self-reporting of feelings and attitudes; this may be in an interview situation or in response to a self-administered questionnaire. Response formats are commonly in the form of category rating scales with labeled tick boxes for responses. Sometimes visual analog scales are also used. The measurement instrument may be in the form of single-item questions, which are easy to administer and analyze but give low levels of precision, or may be multi-item scales, which improve the quality of data collection.[63]

The major difficulties associated with the use of rating scales are that they are frequently time consuming to complete and difficult for the clinician to analyze. These difficulties reinforce the need for close liaison between clinicians and psychologists or psychiatrists who can offer advice in this area.

BODY DYSMORPHIC DISORDER (BDD)

The majority of maxillofacial surgeons and orthodontists will be familiar with the patient who requests treatment for a small or non-existent defect and the patient who is unhappy with the results of technically good treatment. Both scenarios may suggest a diagnosis of dysmorphophobia, which was first defined by Morselli[64] as 'the sudden onset and subsequent persistence of an idea of deformity; the individual fears he has become or may become deformed and feels tremendous anxiety of such an awareness'. The term dysmorphophobia has now been replaced by the diagnosis of 'Body dysmorphic disorder'. The Diagnostic and Statistical Manual of Mental Disorders IV[65] and ICD-10[66] redefined dysmorphophobia into delusional and non-delusional variants and it is the latter non-delusional variant which is known as body dysmorphic disorder. In order for a patient to be defined as suffering from this condition he or she must fulfil the following criteria:

1. There is a preoccupation with an imagined or minor defect in the appearance.
2. The preoccupation causes significant distress in social, occupational and other important areas of functioning.
3. The preoccupation is not better accounted for by another mental disorder (e.g. anorexia nervosa).

Concerns frequently involve non-existent or minor flaws of the face and head. As a result of this, maxillofacial surgeons, plastic surgeons, orthodontists and general dental practitioners are particularly likely to encounter this group of patients. This compounds the pre-existing problems with diagnosis and treatment of such patients as these clinicians are frequently not used to dealing with complicated and fragile patients. It is important that clinicians who may encounter these patients are familiar with the presenting symptoms and the possible treatment options. Further research into the cause, features and treatment response of body dysmorphic disorder is necessary in view of the significant distress this disorder may cause.

Clinical importance and presenting features

The secretive nature of body dysmorphic disorder, its late presentation and the fact that affected patients are seen by a number of different specialties make the collection of demographic data difficult. The onset is usually during adolescence and the condition may persist over a number of years with the symptoms fluctuating in intensity.[67,68] There is nearly always a considerable time delay between the onset of symptoms and the patient seeking treatment.[67] Body dysmorphic disorder affects both sexes and it seems probable that males and females are equally affected. It may be that women present for treatment more frequently than men and this may affect the collected data. The majority of individuals are unmarried and unemployed, which may reflect the time consuming behavior of affected individuals or alternatively it may be a reflection of the personality damage of body dysmorphic disorder.

Patients become obsessed with an imagined or greatly exaggerated defect in their appearance to such an extent that they may spend hours studying the imagined defect in a mirror or they may avoid social contact because they believe that other people are laughing at and ridiculing them. Some may even become housebound or attempt suicide. Patients frequently see surgery as a means of improving their appearance and solving all their problems, and some go from surgeon to surgeon ('doctor shopping') until they find a clinician who is prepared to operate on them. Such treatment rarely improves the situation and, indeed, the problem may become worse with the patient finding a 'new' defect.

Management

Clinicians should be alerted by patients requesting treatment for minor or non-existent deformities and by those patients who have already sought several opinions elsewhere or had previous cosmetic-type surgical procedures. A good history, taken by an experienced clinician, is essential. Many body dysmorphic disorder patients have coexisting psychiatric problems, the most common being depression. When depression exists it must be treated, as this alone may produce major improvements.

Many patients are secretive about their symptoms and embarrassed by what they see as a dreadful defect. Others are intrusive and talk constantly about their problem; they may also bring previous photographs and diagrams in an attempt to show that they do have a problem (Fig. 53.2). These patients frequently demand a second opinion. Clinicians need to be extremely sensitive when interviewing body dysmorphic disorder patients. They must also avoid drawing attention to other areas of the appearance and suggesting that these could be improved. Well meaning but inappropriate remarks may cause considerable distress to the patient.

Treatment of body dysmorphic disorder patients depends partly on the services available in the local area. There are three main treatment modalities:

1. surgery
2. counseling and behavioral therapy
3. pharmacological treatment.

Surgery alone rarely improves the situation and, indeed, may worsen it. There are reports of successful surgical outcome in minimally deformed patients but the clinician must bear in mind that unless a defect is actually corrected the outcome is unlikely to be successful. Patients who are operated on for minimal defects should be prepared initially by a psychiatrist or psychologist with an understanding of body dysmorphic disorder and its associated problems. The vast majority of clinicians believe that surgery should be withheld in those with no evident defect. The general opinion is that surgery is not helpful in the long term and will often result in a new defect or in intensified concern

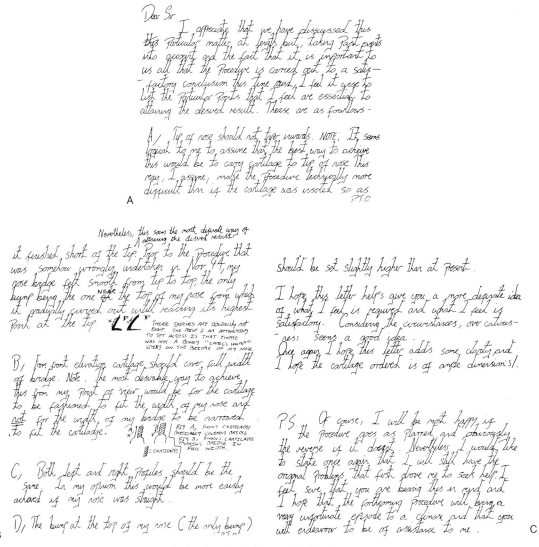

Fig. 53.2 Letter sent by a patient suffering from body dysmorphic disorder.

about the original 'defect'.[69,70] Many of these patients can be very persuasive and it is essential that the clinician is not forced into treatment against his or her better judgement. It is unfortunate that the literature is almost exclusively concerned with severe cases of body dysmorphic disorder as it is possible that some of the milder cases may benefit from surgical treatment with appropriate psychological support.

Counseling and behavioral therapy have shown encouraging results. A number of treatment options exist including psychoanalytical psychotherapy, systematic desensitization or a cognitive behavioral approach. Thompson[71] and Rosen et al[72] have had successful results using cognitive-behavioral body image therapy. This involves methods such as exposure therapy, thought stopping and relaxation to prevent distress at the sight of the feature the individual is concerned about; exposure therapy to overcome avoidance of feared body image situations; response prevention to decrease body checking behavior and recording relevant situations in a body image diary.[72]

Pharmacological treatment in body dysmorphic disorder has been difficult to evaluate because of the lack of controlled clinical trials. A number of recent reports indicate the effectiveness of antidepressants in general and selective serotonin reuptake inhibitors (SSRIs) in particular. Phillips et al[73] found that patients with non-delusional body dysmorphic disorder as well as those with the delusional variant both responded to SSRIs, with a response rate of approximately 60% in each group. As previously discussed, a high proportion of body dysmorphic disorder patients are also suffering from depression and in the majority of cases the SSRIs are successful in treating both the depressive symptoms and the symptoms of body dysmorphic disorder.

The complicated nature of the disorder is illustrated in the following case history:

CASE REPORT

A 25-year-old male presented to the maxillofacial department complaining of 'hollow cheeks and sunken eyes'. As a teenager he had become involved in a fight and subsequently became preoccupied with the size of his nose, feeling that it had become broader after this incident. He requested referral for a rhinoplasty which was subsequently undertaken at another unit after consultation with a psychiatrist. The patient was dissatisfied with the results and repeatedly wrote letters to the surgeon explaining which features he was unhappy about. In the letters he reported 'unkind comments' about his facial appearance, these included 'you look older now' and 'What has happened to your eyes?'. The comments precipitated a request for orthognathic surgery. At his initial consultation he insisted that he had photographic evidence that his face was 'chubbier' prior to the rhinoplasty and produced a diagram to illustrate that his cheekbones were now flattened, leading to 'hollows and rugged lines'. Examination revealed very mildly hypoplastic zygomas, however this could not have resulted from previous surgery. Photographs prior to the rhinoplasty revealed no gross differences in the contour of the eyes or the cheeks as the patient claimed. A diagnosis of BDD was made and his request for surgery was refused. He was referred to the liaison psychiatrist for treatment and remains under her care.

© 1996 British Journal of Maxillofacial Surgery. Dysmorphophobia: recent developments of interest to the maxillofacial surgeon. Cunningham et al[74]

THE FUTURE

A review of the published evidence supports the clinical observation that most patients are happy with the outcome of orthognathic treatment or craniofacial surgery. However, there remains a great deal of research to be undertaken in this field. Methods of patient assessment, detection of those patients who are inappropriate for surgery or who would benefit from associated counseling, and delineating the indications for surgery and psychiatric treatment are all areas which warrant further research.

The most effective methods of providing information to patients considering surgery must also be studied. A small but vociferous group of patients become dissatisfied, unfortunately as a result of poor communication between clinician and patient, even when the results are technically good. It is only by good communication and provision of information that dissatisfaction in this group will be avoided.

There is an urgent need for changes in clinical practice. Facially deformed patients, especially those with clefts and severe-deformities, will only have sufficient expertise available to them if services are centralized and 'craniofacial support teams', including all appropriate specialists, can be established. Establishing one-to-one care would appear to be the ideal situation for the patient and it may be that in such a setting patients could be allocated a 'primary carer' who would follow their care and be available to provide counseling to patients and families as required.

The authors recommend collaborative surgical, orthodontic and psychiatric assessment to consider not only surgery but also antidepressants and cognitive treatment.

APPENDIX 1 EXAMPLE OF INFORMATION TO BE INCLUDED IN AN INFORMATION LEAFLET (© Eastman Dental Institute)

The type of surgery that you are considering is known as Orthognathic surgery. Its purpose is:-

(a) To align your teeth and to improve the way they meet/function
(b) To improve the relationship between your upper and lower jaws
(c) To improve your facial appearance

It is essential to plan these changes so that the result remains stable.

BEFORE SURGERY each patient's case has to be planned individually in order to determine which method of treatment is best for you. A number of investigations need to be carried out, which include a full examination of your face and mouth, special X-rays of your face and jaws, impressions to make casts of your teeth and photographs of your face and mouth.

Using this information, the team of orthodontists and surgeons will decide the treatment options. You will require several appointments before a final decision is made and explained to you.

Prior to surgery, you may require 12–18 months of orthodontic treatment to get your teeth into position for the best surgical result. This usually involves braces which are fixed to your teeth. Orthodontic treatment after the operation is normally required too.

Just before your operation an appointment is necessary to check all these details and to discuss any problems you may have and also to arrange for routine blood tests. The plastic wafer which will be attached to your teeth during and after the operation will also be checked.

You will be admitted to hospital the day before your

operation. Please bring a child's small toothbrush with you to help you clean your teeth after the operation.

AFTER SURGERY several things will happen which may concern you:-

(a) Pain and discomfort is worst during the first 24 hours and will be carefully controlled with medication.

(b) Your face will become swollen but most of this will subside in the first two to three weeks. Please note that it can take up to six months for the face to look its best.

(c) You may experience numbness or tingling of your face, especially your lower lip. This is usually temporary, but may persist for six months or more. Rarely, it may be permanent.

(d) Initially it will be difficult to swallow. This rapidly improves over a few days. During your operation you will have a narrow feeding tube passed down your nostril into your stomach in case you have difficulty drinking afterwards.

(e) Your teeth may be wired together or you may have elastic bands between the upper and lower teeth. This is not particularly uncomfortable and you will adjust very quickly. Speech may be difficult at first but soon becomes much easier. The dietitian will visit you and give advice. If you have your teeth wired together a liquidiser at home would be useful.

(f) The stay in hospital is usually 3–6 days.

(g) In some cases, more than one operation is planned – such as surgery to your nose or chin. These are usually smaller procedures and do not involve wiring of the jaws.

Most patients are able to return to office or light work after two weeks. Sporting activities and foreign travel should be avoided during the first two months following surgery.

You will need to attend regular Outpatient appointments at first frequently and then at yearly intervals. This is to check that all is stable and also so that further X-rays, models and photographs can be taken. These visits also allow you to talk to us about any problems you may have.

PSYCHOLOGICAL PROBLEMS ASSOCIATED WITH ORTHOGNATHIC SURGERY

Your surgery has been explained to you, but it is also very important to know something about the psychological problems which may arise. Orthognathic surgery changes more than facial features. It also has a significant effect on your psychological well-being and on the way your friends and relatives react to you as a person.

Your face is the 'window on the world'; it is your focal point and the site of all your special senses. It is very important to realise that changes in facial appearance vary with the complexity of the surgery. The greater the change in appearance, the greater the amount of adjustment required.

All previous studies suggest that patients may become anxious and depressed a few weeks after surgery. The anxiety is associated with many factors, such as:-

(1) Restriction of eating
(2) 'Pins and needles' sensation
(3) Swollen face
(4) Wiring of the jaws (where this is necessary)
(5) Difficulty with speech
(6) Pain and discomfort

This kind of anxiety and slight degree of depression is very transient and will disappear within a few weeks. Your face will not be improved immediately after surgery although this improvement is one of the main aims of surgery. Your face will improve gradually, most of the swelling will settle within a month but needs at least 6 months to settle fully.

Orthodontic treatment also needs to be continued following surgery to produce the ideal 'bite'. So you need to be realistic in your expectations and please be patient....

Sometimes it takes 2 years following surgery to become really content with the appearance of your face.

If you have any problems please contact:-
09.00–17.00 hrs ....
Out of hours ....

REFERENCES

1. Woolnoth T 1865 The study of the human face. W Tweedie, London
2. Angle EH 1900 The treatment of malocclusion of the teeth and fractures of the maxillae, 6th edn. S S White, Philadelphia
3. Hill-Beuf A, Porter JD 1984 Children coping with impaired appearance: social and psychologic influences. General Hospital Psychiatry 6:294–301
4. Clifford MM 1975 Physical attractiveness and academic performance. Child Study Journal 5:201–209
5. Edwards M, Watson ACH 1980 Psychosocial aspects of cleft lip and palate. In: Edwards M, Watson ACH (eds) Advances in the management of cleft palate. Churchill Livingstone, New York
6. Kinch J 1968 Experiments on factors related to self-concept change. Journal of Social Psychology 74:251–258
7. Adams GR 1977 Physical attractiveness research. Toward a developmental social psychology of beauty. Human Development 20:217–239
8. Clifford MM, Walster E 1973 The effects of physical attractiveness on teacher expectations. Sociology and Education 46:248–258
9. Efran MG 1974 The effect of physical appearance on the judgment of guilt, interpersonal attraction and severity of recommended punishment in a simulated jury task. J Res Pers 8:45–54
10. Macgregor FC 1970 Social and psychological implications of dentofacial disfigurement. Angle Orthodontist 40:231–233

11. Shaw WC, Meek SC, Jones DS 1980 Nicknames, teasing, harassment and the salience of dental features among school children. British Journal of Orthodontics 7:75–80

12. Shaw WC 1981 The influence of children's dentofacial appearance on their social attractiveness as judged by peers and lay adults. American Journal of Orthodontics 79:399–415

13. Lefebvre A, Munro I 1978 The role of psychiatry in a craniofacial team. Plastic and Reconstructive Surgery 61:564–569

14. Barden RC, Ford ME, Jensen AG, Rogers-Salyer M, Salyer KE 1989 Effects of craniofacial deformity in infancy on the quality of mother-infant interactions. Child Development 60:819–824

15. Bull RHC 1990 Society's reactions to facial disfigurements. Dental Update 202–205

16. Piliavin I, Piliavin J, Rodin J 1975 Costs, diffusion and the stigmatized victim. Journal of Personal and Social Psychology 32:429–438

17. Bull R, Stevens J 1981 The effects of facial disfigurement on helping behaviour. Italian Journal of Psychology 8:25–33

18. Rumsey N, Bull R, Gahagan D 1982 The effect of facial disfigurement on the proxemic behaviour of the general public. Journal of Applied and Social Psychology 12:137–150

19. Macgregor FC 1990 Facial disfigurement: problems and management of social interaction and implications for mental health. Aesthetic and Plastic Surgery 14:249–257

20. Clifford E 1982 Psychologist in a Plastic Surgery Service. Annals of Plastic Surgery 8:79–82

21. Clifford E, Crocker E 1971 Maternal responses: The birth of a normal child as compared to the birth of a child with a cleft. Cleft Palate Journal 8:298–306

22. Palkes HS, Marsh JL, Talent BK 1986 Pediatric craniofacial surgery and parental attitudes. Cleft Palate Journal 23:137–143

23. Pruzinsky T 1992 Social and psychological effects of major craniofacial deformity. Cleft Palate-Craniofacial Journal 29:578–584

24. Brantley HT, Clifford E 1979a Cognitive, self-concept and body image measures on normal, cleft palate and obese adolescents. Cleft Palate Journal 16:177–182

25. Brantley HT, Clifford E 1979b Maternal and child locus of control and field-dependence in cleft palate children. Cleft Palate Journal 16:183–187

26. Clifford E, Crocker EC, Pope BA 1972 Psychological findings in the adulthood of 98 cleft lip-palate children. Cleft Lip-Palate Psychology 50:234–237

27. Heller A, Tidmarsh W, Pless IB 1981 The psychosocial functioning of young adults born with cleft lip or palate. Clinical Pediatrics 20:459–465

28. Harper DC, Richman LC 1978 Personality profiles of physically impaired adolescents. Journal of Clinical Psychology 34:636–642

29. Jones JE 1984 Self-concept and parental evaluation of peer relationships in cleft lip and palate children. Pediatric Dentistry 6:132–138

30. Kapp K 1979 Self concept of the cleft lip and or palate child. Cleft Palate Journal 16:171–176

31. Kapp-Simon KA 1995 Psychological interventions for the adolescent with cleft lip and palate. Cleft Palate-Craniofacial Journal 32:104–108

32. Whitehead TD, Tobiasen JM, Hebert JM 1996 Presurgical anxiety treated with cognitive behavioral therapy in a 13-year old female with cleft lip and palate: A psychological Case Report. Cleft Palate-Craniofacial Journal 33:258–261

33. Speltz ML, Greenberg MT, Endriga MC, Galbreath H 1994 Developmental approach to the psychology of craniofacial anomalies. Cleft Palate-Craniofacial Journal 31:61–67

34. Bennett ME, Stanton ML 1993 Psychotherapy for persons with craniofacial deformities: Can we treat without theory? Cleft Palate-Craniofacial Journal 30:406–410

35. Lansdown R, Lloyd J, Hunter J 1991 Facial deformity in childhood: severity and psychological adjustment. Child: Care, Health and Development 17:165–171

36. Reich J 1969 The surgery of appearance: psychological and related aspects. Medical Journal of Australia 2:5–8

37. Wictorin L, Hillerström K, Sörenson S 1969 Biological and psychosocial factors in patients with malformation of the jaws: A study of 95 patients prior to treatment. Scandinavian Journal of Plastic and Reconstructive Surgery 3:138–143

38. Jacobson A 1984 Psychological aspects of dentofacial aesthetics and orthognathic surgery. Angle Orthodontist 54:18–35

39. Peterson LJ, Topazian RG 1976 Psychological considerations in corrective maxillary and midfacial surgery. Journal of Oral Surgery 34:157–164

40. Kiyak HA, Hohl T, Sherrick P, West RA, McNeill RW, Bucher F 1981 Sex differences in motives for and outcomes of orthognathic surgery. Journal of Oral Surgery 39:757–764

41. Kiyak HA, West RA, Hohl T, McNeill RW 1982a The psychological impact of orthognathic surgery: A 9 month follow-up. American Journal of Orthodontics 81:404–412

42. Auerbach SM, Meredith J, Alexander JM, Mercuri LG, Brophy C 1984 Psychological factors in adjustment to orthognathic surgery. Journal of Oral and Maxillofacial Surgery 42:435–440

43. Flanary CM, Barnwell GM, Van Sickels JE, Littlefield JH, Rugh AL 1990 Impact of orthognathic surgery on normal and abnormal personality dimensions: A 2 year follow-up study of 61 patients. American Journal of Orthodontics and Dentofacial Orthopedics 98:313–322

44. Edgerton MT, Knorr NJ 1971 Motivational patterns of patients seeking cosmetic (aesthetic) surgery. Plastic and Reconstructive Surgery 48:551–557

45. Hutton CE 1967 Patients' evaluation of surgical correction of prognathism: survey of 32 patients. Journal of Oral Surgery 25:225–228

46. Reich J 1975 Factors influencing patient satisfaction with the results of aesthetic plastic surgery. Plastic and Reconstructive Surgery 55:5–13

47. Finlay PM, Atkinson JM, Moos KF 1995 Orthognathic surgery: patient expectations; psychological profile and satisfaction with outcome. British Journal of Oral and Maxillofacial Surgery 33:9–14

48. Flanary CM, Barnwell GM, Alexander JM 1985 Patient perceptions of orthognathic surgery. American Journal of Orthodontics 88:137–145

49. Kiyak HA, McNeill RW, West RA, Hohl T, Bucher F, Sherrick P 1982b Predicting psychological responses to orthognathic surgery. Journal of Oral and Maxillofacial Surgery 40:150–155

50. Kiyak HA, Hohl T, West RA, McNeill RW 1984 Psychological changes in orthognathic surgery patients: A 24 month follow-up. Journal of Oral and Maxillofacial Surgery 42:506–512

51. Ostler S, Kiyak HA 1991 Treatment expectations versus outcomes among orthognathic surgery patients. International Journal of Adult Orthodontic and Orthognathic Surgery 6:247–255

52. Rittersma J, Casparie AF, Reerink E 1980 Patient information and patient preparation in orthognathic surgery: A medical audit study. Journal of Maxillofacial Surgery 8:206–209

53. Cunningham SJ, Hunt NP, Feinmann C 1996 Perceptions of outcome following orthognathic surgery. British Journal of Oral and Maxillofacial Surgery 34:210–213

54. Cunningham SJ, Feinmann C, Horrocks EN 1995 Psychological problems following orthognathic surgery. Journal of Clinical Orthodontics 29:755–757

55. Holman AR, Brumer S, Ware WH, Pasta DJ 1995 The impact of interpersonal support on patient satisfaction with Orthognathic surgery. Journal of Oral and Maxillofacial Surgery 53:1289–1297

56. Moss JP, Grindrod SR, Linney AD, Arridge SR, James D 1988 A computer system for the interactive planning and prediction of

maxillofacial surgery. American Journal of Orthodontic and Dentofacial Orthopedics 94:469–475

57. Sarver DM 1993 Videoimaging: The pros and cons. Angle Orthodontist 63:167–170

58. Phillips C, Hill BJ, Cannac C 1995 The influence of video imaging on patients' perceptions and expectations. Angle Orthodontist 65:263–270

59. Zigmond AS, Snaith RP 1983 The Hospital Anxiety and Depression Scale. Acta Psychiatrica Scandinavica 67:361–370

60. McDowell I, Newell C 1987 Measuring Health – A guide to rating scales and questionnaires. Oxford University Press, Oxford

61. Fitzpatrick R 1990 Measurement of patient satisfaction. In: Hopkins A, Costain D (eds) Measuring the outcomes of medical care. Royal College of Physicians, London

62. Rosen JC, Reiter J, Orosan P 1995 Assessment of body image disorders with the BDD examination. Behaviour Research and Therapy 33:77–84

63. Bowling A 1995 Measuring disease. Open University Press, Buckingham

64. Morselli E 1891 Sulla dismorfofobia e sulla tafefobia. Boll Accad Med Geneva 6:110–119

65. American Psychiatric Association 1994 Diagnostic and Statistical Manual of Mental Disorders, 4th edn. American Psychiatric Press, Washington DC, pp 466–469

66. World Health Organization 1992 The ICD-10 Classification of Mental and Behavioural Disorders: Clinical Descriptions and Diagnostic Guidelines. WHO, Geneva

67. Phillips KA 1991 Body dysmorphic disorder: The distress of imagined ugliness. American Journal of Psychiatry 148:1138–1149

68. Phillips KA, McElroy SL, Keck PE, Hudson JI, Pope HG 1994 A comparison of delusional and nondelusional body dysmorphic disorder in 100 cases. Psychopharmacology Bulletin 30:179–186

69. Thomas CS 1984 Dysmorphophobia: A question of definition. British Journal of Psychiatry 144:513–516

70. Phillips KA, McElroy SL, Hudson JI, Pope HG 1995 Body dysmorphic disorder: An obsessive-compulsive spectrum disorder, a form of affective spectrum disorder, or both? Journal of Clinical Psychiatry 56(suppl 4):41–51

71. Thompson JK 1991 Body image disturbance, assessment and treatment. Pergamon Press, New York

72. Rosen JC, Reiter J, Orosan P 1995 Cognitive-behavioral body image therapy for body dysmorphic disorder. Journal of Consulting and Clinical Psychology 63:263–269

73. Phillips KA, McElroy SL, Keck PE, Pope HG, Hudson JI 1993 Body dysmorphic disorder: 30 cases of imagined ugliness. American Journal of Psychiatry 150:302–308

74. Cunningham SJ, Bryant CJ, Manisali M, Hunt NP, Feinmann C 1996 Dysmorphophobia: recent developments of interest to the maxillofacial surgeon. British Journal of Oral and Maxillofacial Surgery 34:368–374

Surgical management of Crouzon, Apert and related syndromes

54

JEFFREY C. POSNICK

INTRODUCTION

Virchow coined the term 'craniosynostosis' and formulated the classic theory known as Virchow's law.[1] This states that premature fusion of a cranial vault suture (synostosis) inhibits normal skull growth perpendicular to the fused suture and that compensatory growth occurs at the open sutures. The general direction of growth after synostosis is parallel to the fused suture.

The term 'craniofacial dysostosis' is used in a generic way to describe familial forms of craniosynostosis involving not only the cranial vault but also various cranial base and midface sutures. Familial types of craniofacial dysostosis were described by Apert in 1906,[2] Crouzon in 1912,[3] Pfeiffer in 1964,[4] Saethre–Chotzen in 1931[5] and Carpenter in 1901.[5] Cloverleaf skull (Kleeblattschadel) anomaly refers to the overall shape of the skull and face when specific cranial vault and cranial base sutures fuse prematurely.[5]

The birth prevalence of craniosynostosis is about 343:1 000 000.[6] Most cases of simple craniosynostosis are sporadic. If both parent and child are affected, however, the risk for a subsequent child approaches 50%. Syndromic craniosynostosis is usually genetic and may be autosomal dominant as in Crouzon or Apert syndrome.

A large group of patients with familial or sporadic craniosynostosis do not have one of the classical craniosynostosis syndromes. Muenke et al recently reported on 61 individuals from 20 unrelated families where coronal synostosis was due to an amino acid substitution (Pro 250 Arg) that results from a single point mutation in the fibroblast growth factor receptor 3 gene on chromosome 4p.[7] In addition to the skull findings (unilateral or bilateral coronal synostosis) some patients in this group also have abnormalities of the hands and feet including thimble-like middle phalanges, coined epiphyses, and carpal or tarsal fusions. Brachydactyly is seen in some patients; none with clinically significant syndactyly or deviation of the great toe. Neurosensory hearing loss is present in some and developmental delay may be seen in a minority. It is likely that many of these patients with bicoronal synostosis and minimal hand and foot deformities have been misdiagnosed as Pfeiffer or Jackson–Weiss syndrome in the past. Many patients labeled as 'Crouzon syndrome presenting with bicoronal synostosis and minimal midface involvement' also fit into this category, which has now been termed 'FR3 associated coronal synostosis syndrome'.[8]

The treatment of these conditions is surgical, but the indications, timing, type and effectiveness of reconstruction have not been well evaluated. This chapter describes a personal philosophy and rationale for treatment intervention.

CROUZON SYNDROME

The incidence of Crouzon syndrome is 1:25 000 in the general population. The inheritance pattern is autosomal dominant and the trait is variably expressed.[9–15] Crouzon described an affected family pedigree in 1912.[3] He listed four major characteristics of the syndrome: exorbitism; retromaxillism; inframaxillism; and paradoxic retrogenia. Premature fusion of sutures may occur at the level of the cranial vault, with bilateral coronal suture fusion being the most common. When this occurs early in childhood the result is a brachycephalic (short and wide skull) head shape. In addition to cranial vault synostosis, there is a poorly defined effect on the anterior cranial base and facial sutures which results in a variable degree of symmetric hypoplasia of the orbits, zygomas and maxilla.[3,9,13,14,16–28] The mandible has normal growth but may become secondarily deformed with an obtuse angle formed by the ramus and the inferior border and with a vertically long chin.[29] In patients with classic findings, the cranial vault is either brachycephalic or oxycephalic (pointed skull), the orbits are shallow with proptotic eyes, and the midface is flat with an Angle class III malocclusion.

APERT SYNDROME

Most cases of Apert syndrome have occurred sporadically[4,6,30] but autosomal dominant family pedigrees have been described.[30] The incidence is thought to be 1:100 000 in the general population.[6]

Postmortem histologic and radiographic studies suggest that skeletal deficiencies in the Apert face result from a cartilage dysplasia at the cranial base, leading to premature fusion of the midline sutures from the occiput to the anterior nasal septum.[25,28,31–34] Apert first described the syndrome as a combination of physical findings including severe mis shapenness of the skull, mitten hand and foot deformities (compound complex syndactylism), mental retardation and blindness.[2] We now know that the craniofacial skeletal abnormality of Apert syndrome is complex and includes fusion of the coronal sutures and abnormal formation/fusion of the anterior cranial base and midface sutures and synchondrosis. Limited formation of the metopic and sagittal sutures is also a component of the cranial vault deformity. In addition, the syndrome is characterized by 4-limb symmetric complex syndactylies of the hands and feet. Fusion and malformation of other joints, including the elbows and shoulders, often occurs. Although the syndrome has some similar features in the general craniofacial skeletal dysmorphology as Crouzon syndrome there are distinct differences:[31] expressivity of the trait in Apert syndrome is generally more severe and there is less variation in expression; shallow hyperteloric orbits and proptotic eyes are more severe. The midface hypoplasia is often more marked, both vertically and horizontally, with a greater upper face transverse width than that seen in Crouzon syndrome. The soft-tissue drape also varies from that seen in Crouzon syndrome, with a greater downward slant to the lateral canthi and a distinctive, S-shaped upper eyelid ptosis. Apert syndrome is frequently associated with a degree of developmental delay and often hyperactivity. Cohen has clarified some of these issues by documenting distinctive central nervous system malformations in the Apert syndrome patient.[35–38]

OTHER SYNDROMES

CARPENTER SYNDROME

Carpenter syndrome is characterized by craniosynostosis, often associated with pre-axial polysyndactyly of the feet, short fingers with clinodactyly and variable soft-tissue syndactyly.[5]

It is recognized to be an autosomal recessive syndrome.

PFEIFFER SYNDROME

In 1964, Pfeiffer described a syndrome consisting of craniosynostosis, broad thumbs, broad great toes and, occasionally, partial soft-tissue syndactyly of the hand.[5] This is an autosomal dominant inherited syndrome with complete penetrance and variable expressivity.

SAETHRE–CHOTZEN SYNDROME

Saethre–Chotzen syndrome has an autosomal dominant inheritance pattern with a high degree of penetrance and expressivity.[5] Its pattern of malformations may include craniosynostosis, low-set frontal hairline, ptosis of the upper eyelids, facial asymmetry, brachydactyly, partial cutaneous syndactyly, and other skeletal anomalies.

CLOVERLEAF SKULL ANOMALY

Kleeblattschadel anomaly (cloverleaf skull) is a trilobular-shaped skull secondary to complex craniosynostosis.[5] The cloverleaf skull anomaly is known to be both etiologically and pathogenetically heterogeneous.

FUNCTIONAL CONSIDERATIONS

BRAIN GROWTH

Brain volume in the normal child almost triples within the first year of life. By 2 years, the cranial capacity is 4 times that at birth. For this rapid brain growth to proceed unhindered, the open cranial vault and base sutures must spread during phases of rapid growth, resulting in marginal ossification. In craniosynostosis, premature suture fusion is combined with continued attempts towards normal brain growth. The shape of the cranial vault, cranial base, and upper orbit is determined by Virchow's law.[1] In theory, depending on the number and location of prematurely fused sutures and the timing of closure, the growth of the brain may be restricted. The objective of surgical intervention is to increase intracranial volume for the otherwise restricted brain and to reshape the skull toward an acceptable configuration.[39]

INTRACRANIAL PRESSURE

Elevated intracranial pressure is the most worrisome functional problem associated with premature suture fusion. Its late and devastating effect is indirectly identified on plain radiographs from the fingerprinting or beaten copper appearance along the inner table of the cranial vault and base. When raised intracranial pressure goes untreated, it affects brain function. The sensitivity of an indirect fundoscopic examination as an indicator of elevated intracranial pressure is unclear, while papilledema and later optic atrophy are significant findings.

Intracranial hypertension can be documented invasively by means of a craniotomy used to place an epidural pressure sensor or by lumbar puncture monitoring.[39,40] Increased intracranial pressure is most likely to affect those with the greatest disparity between brain growth and intracranial capacity. When using standard measurements as an indication of significantly elevated intracranial pressure (> 15 mm of mercury) Renier et al determined that 42% of untreated children with more than one suture and 14% with just one suture prematurely fused fall into this category.[39] A specific head shape in conjunction with radiographic findings of synostosis is not definitively associated with decreased intracranial volume or increased intracranial pressure.[41,42]

OTHER FUNCTIONAL CONCERNS

If increased intracranial pressure is left untreated, papilledema with eventual optic atrophy develops, resulting in partial or complete blindness. When the eyes are proptotic because of hypoplastic orbits, the cornea may be exposed and abrasions or ulcerations may occur. When the orbits are extremely shallow, herniation of the globes themselves may occur and require emergency reduction followed by tarsorrhaphies or urgent orbital decompression. Divergent or convergent non-paralytic strabismus or exotropia occurs frequently and should be looked for in every patient. This may result from congenital anomalies of the extraocular muscles themselves. Hydrocephalus affects as many as 10% of the patients with a craniofacial dysostosis syndrome.[43–45] The etiology is not always clear. Hydrocephalus may be secondary to a generalized cranial base hypoplasia with constriction at

the base of the skull resulting in venous congestion. A percentage of infants born with a craniofacial dysostosis syndrome that includes hypoplasia of the midface may also have diminished nasal and nasopharyngeal spaces with increased nasal airway resistance. An affected infant expends greater energy respiring and that may push the child into a catabolic state unless supportive treatment is undertaken (i.e. tracheostomy and gastrostomy). There is a higher incidence of dental and oral anomalies than is seen in unaffected children. In Apert syndrome in particular the palate is high and constricted in width, and the incidence of isolated cleft palate approaches 40%. Anomalies of the extremities ranging from simple to complex syndactylism, polydactyly, and fusion of more proximal joints may occur in specific syndromes. Hearing deficits are more frequent than in the general population with conductive hearing deficit being common in Crouzon and Apert syndrome.

ESTHETIC ASSESSMENT

Examination of the entire craniofacial region should be meticulous and systematic. The skeleton and soft tissues are assessed in the standard way to identify all normal and abnormal anatomy. Specific findings tend to occur in particular malformations, but each patient is unique. Quantitative analysis of measurements taken from computed tomographic (CT) scans, surface anthropometry, cephalometry and dental models are valuable components of the craniofacial assessment.[19,23,46–56] The achievement of symmetry, proportionality and balance and the reconstruction of specific esthetic units is critical to forming an unobtrusive face in a child born with one of the craniofacial dysostosis syndromes. Specific esthetic units to consider include the fronto-upper orbital region, the posterior cranial vault region, the orbitonasozygomatic region, and the maxillomandibular region.

QUANTITATIVE MORPHOLOGIC ASSESSMENT

The purpose of quantitative assessment by CT scan analysis,[19,23,51–56] anthropometric surface measurements,[46–49] cephalometric analysis[50] or dental model analysis is to help predict growth patterns, confirm or refute clinical impressions, aid in treatment planning and provide a framework for objective assessment of immediate and long-term results. These methods of assessment rely on the measurement of linear distances, angles and proportions based on accurate, reliable and reproducible anatomical landmarks found to be useful for patient evaluation.

SURGICAL APPROACH

HISTORICAL PERSPECTIVE

The first recorded surgical approaches to craniosynostosis were performed by Lannelongue in 1890[57] and Lane in 1892,[58] who completed strip craniectomies of fused sutures. Their aim was to control the problem of brain compression by removing the prematurely fused suture. The classic neurosurgical techniques developed over the ensuing decades were geared toward resecting the synostotic suture(s), the objective being 'release' of fused suture(s) to allow for creation of a new suture line at the site of the previous synostosis. Spontaneous normalization of cranial vault growth and symmetry was then to occur.[15] With the realization that this goal was rarely achieved, attempts were made to fragment the cranial vault surgically, replacing segments of flat bone over the dura–brain as free grafts to encourage an improvement on the preoperative cranial vault shape. These techniques occasionally result in cerebral decompression but they rarely produce an adequate and symmetric shape. Furthermore, uncontrolled postoperative skull moulding during the healing process often resulted in skull distortions. Skull reossification by this technique of skull fragmentation is unpredictable, either with rapid reossification or with significant residual cranial vault defects.

In 1967, Tessier described a new approach to the management of Crouzon and Apert syndrome.[59] His landmark presentation and publications were the beginning of modern craniofacial surgery. Tessier combined an intracranial–extracranial approach, the use of a coronal (skin) incision, 360 degree periorbital dissection, autogenous bone grafting and ingenious osteotomy sites.[60–66] The concept of suture release combined with skull reshaping carried out in infancy was later pioneered by Hoffman,[67] Whittaker[68] and Marchac.[69]

CURRENT SURGICAL APPROACH: STAGING OF RECONSTRUCTION

Primary cranio-orbital decompression–reshaping in infancy

Once a craniofacial dysostosis syndrome is recognized, the child should be assessed by a craniofacial team. Planning of

the timing and type of surgical interventions must consider the functions, future growth and development of the craniofacial skeleton as well as the achievement of a satisfactory body image and self-esteem.

Branchycephaly results from bilateral premature coronal suture fusion which extends into the cranial base. This is the most common basic cranial vault synostosis pattern associated with Apert, Crouzon and Pfeiffer syndromes. In infancy and early childhood it is not always possible to separate isolated bilateral coronal synostosis from Crouzon syndrome unless either midface hypoplasia is evident or a family pedigree with an autosomal dominant inheritance pattern is known. The extent of midface deficiency associated with Crouzon syndrome is variable and genetically programmed. It is not always obvious until later in childhood.

With early bilateral coronal synostosis, the supraorbital ridge is recessed and the overlying eyebrows sit posterior

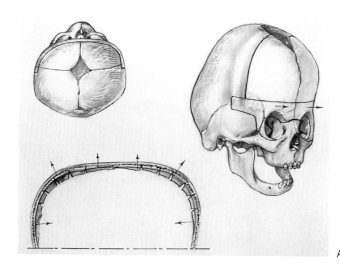

A

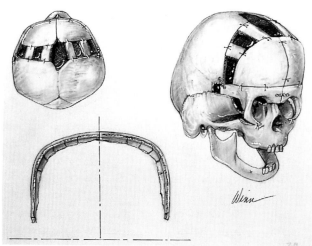

B

Fig. 54.1 The craniofacial skeleton in a child with bilateral coronal synostosis before and after cranio-orbital reshaping as carried out by the author. **(A)** The site of osteotomies indicated. **(B)** After osteotomies, reshaping and fixation of the cranio-orbital regions. (From Posnick)[73]

to the cornea of the eyes. The anterior cranial base is short in the anterior–posterior (AP) dimension and wide transversely. The overlying cranial vault is high in the superior – inferior dimension, with anterior bulging of the upper forehead resulting from compensatory growth through the open metopic and sagittal sutures. The orbits are often shallow and the eyes proptotic and abnormally separated (orbital hypertelorism). The sphenoid wings are elevated bilaterally, producing the harlequin appearance often described on the anteroposterior skull radiographs or CT scans. In

the craniofacial dysostosis syndromes, in addition to premature fusion of multiple cranial vault sutures there is a poorly defined effect on the anterior cranial base and facial sutures that results in a variable degree of symmetrical hypoplasia of the orbits, zygomas and maxilla.

Initial treatment for the craniofacial dysostosis syndromes generally consists of suture release, decompression and simultaneous cranial vault and upper orbital osteotomies with reshaping and advancement carried out in infancy (Figs 54.1–3).[67–73] The author's preference is to carry this

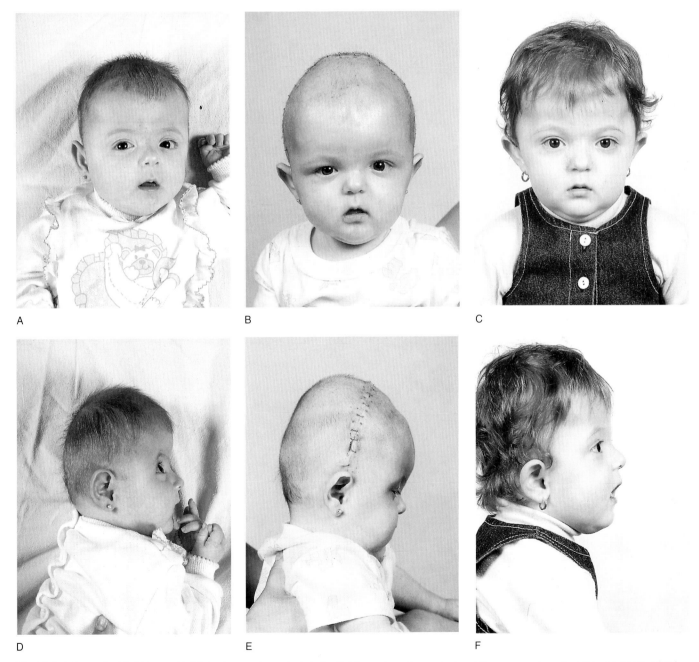

Fig. 54.2 A 6-month-old girl born with bilateral coronal synostosis (a familial form of craniosynostosis not Crouzon syndrome) underwent cranio-orbital reshaping by the technique described. **(A)** Preoperative frontal view. **(B)** Frontal view 10 days postoperatively. **(C)** Frontal view 3 years later. **(D)** Preoperative profile view. **(E)** Profile view 10 days after surgery. **(F)** Profile view 3 years later. (From Posnick et al)[23]

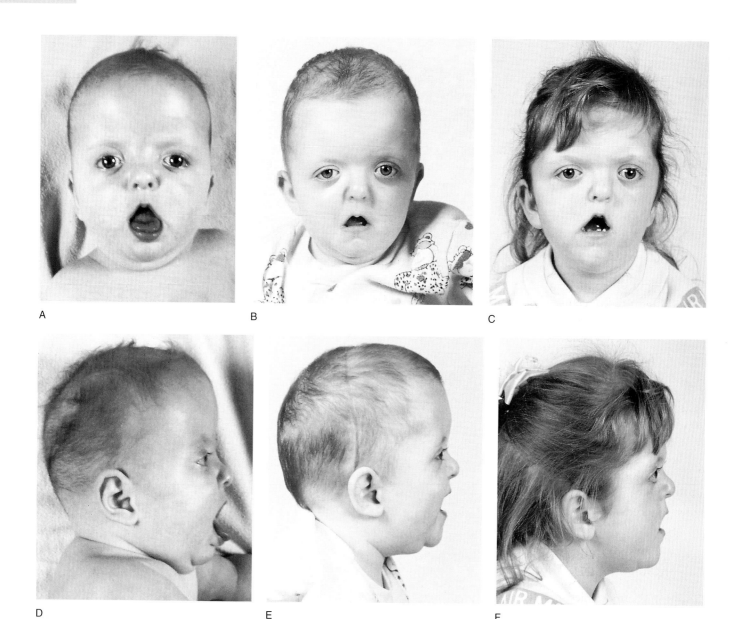

Fig. 54.3 A 6-month-old girl with Apert syndrome underwent cranio-orbital reshaping by the technique described. **(A)** Preoperative frontal view. **(B)** Frontal view 1 year postoperatively. **(C)** Frontal view 2 years postoperatively. **(D)** Preoperative profile view. **(E)** Profile view 1 year postoperatively. **(F)** Profile view 2 years postoperatively. (From Posnick et al)[54]

out between 9 and 11 months of age unless signs of increased intracranial pressure are identified early in life,[73] when decompression and reshaping is carried out as soon as the problem is recognized. The reshaping of the upper three quarters of the orbital rims and supraorbital ridge component is geared to a slight decrease of the bitemporal and anterior cranial base width with simultaneous horizontal advancement to increase the anterioposterior dimension. The depth of the upper orbits is increased, resulting in some improvement of the proptosis. Once the orbits are stabilized, the overlying forehead is reconstructed. The overall improved shape also provides a needed increase in

intracranial volume within the anterior cranial vault. A degree of overcorrection is preferred at the level of the supra-orbital ridge. The general range of advancement is between 1.5 and 2.5 cm.

Repeat craniotomy–decompression–reshaping in young children

After the initial suture release, decompression and reshaping carried out during infancy, the young child is followed clinically at intervals by the pediatric craniofacial/plastic surgeon, pediatric neurosurgeon, pediatric neuro-ophthalmologist, developmental specialist and neuroradiologist; interval CT scanning is performed. Should signs of increased intracranial pressure develop then urgent decompression with further reshaping to expand the intracranial volume is performed.[8,74] When increased intracranial pressure is suspected, the location of cranial vault constriction influences the region of the skull earmarked for decompression and reshaping. Head shape and CT scan findings are helpful in determining the location requiring decompression.

If the problem is judged to be anterior, then further anterior cranial vault and upper orbital osteotomies with reshaping and advancement are carried out. The technique is similar to that described above. Decompression and expansion of the posterior cranial vault may be required. If so, this is completed with the patient in the prone position. The second (redo) craniotomy carried out for further decompression and reshaping is often complicated by brittle cortical bone, bony spicules piercing the dura, previous fixation devices in the operative field (i.e. Silastic sheeting with metal clips, stainless steel wires, microplates and screws) and convoluted dura compressed (herniated) through the inner table of the skull resulting in a higher incidence of dural tears during the calvarectomy than would occur during a primary procedure. A greater amount of blood loss should be anticipated when re-elevating the scalp flaps, completing the craniotomies, and dissecting the dura free of the inner table of the skull and cranial base at the time of the second procedure.

MANAGEMENT OF THE TOTAL MIDFACE DEFORMITY IN CHILDHOOD

The type of osteotomies selected to manage the total midface deficiency and residual cranial vault dysplasia should depend on the presenting deformity rather than a fixed universal approach to the midface malformation.[22,24,59,75–81] In 1971, Tessier described a single-stage intracranial frontofacial advancement in which the orbitofrontal bandeau was advanced as a separate element but in conjunction with the Le Fort III complex below and the frontal bones above.[62] Seven years later, Ortiz-Monisterio et al developed the monobloc (MB) osteotomy to advance the orbits and midface as one unit[75] (Figs 54.4, 54.5). The procedure was combined with frontal bone repositioning to correct the Crouzon deformity.

Two years later, Van der Meulen described the 'medial faciotomy' for the correction of midline facial clefting.[80] By splitting the monobloc osteotomy vertically in the midline, he moved the two halves of the face together to correct the orbital hypertelorism. Tessier refined the vertical splitting and reshaping of the monobloc segment to correct the midface hypoplasia and associated orbital hypertelorism and the lack of midface curvature observed in Apert syndrome patients; this improved the midface deformity in all three facial dimensions through a procedure now known as facial bipartition (FB)[65] (Fig. 54.6).

The decision to complete a monobloc, facial bipartition, or a Le Fort III osteotomy to manage the horizontal, transverse, and vertical midface deficiencies will depend on the morphology of the patient's midface and anterior cranial vault.[22,79] If the supraorbital ridge with its overlying eyebrow sits in good position when viewed from the sagittal plane with adequate depth to the upper orbits, there is a normal arc of rotation to the midface–forehead, and the root of the nose is not too wide (orbital hypertelorism) then there is no need for further reconstruction of this region. In such patients, the total midface deficiency may be effectively managed through a Le Fort III osteotomy. If the supraorbital ridge and anterior cranial base are both deficient in the sagittal plane along with the zygomas, nose, lower orbits and maxilla then a monobloc osteotomy is indicated. Since the degree of horizontal deficiency at the orbits and the maxillary dentition are rarely uniform, further segmentalization of the midface complex at the Le Fort I level is also required. This may be carried out simultaneously with the 'total midface' procedure but, depending on the patient's age and other factors, is generally undertaken later as part of the overall staged reconstruction. If orbital hypertelorism and midface flattening with loss of the normal facial curvature is present the monobloc unit is split vertically in the midline (facial bipartition), a wedge of interorbital (nasal and ethmoidal) bone is removed, and the orbits are repositioned medially while the maxillary posterior arch is widened. In Apert syndrome, facial bipartition osteotomies permit more complete correction of the abnormal craniofacial skeleton. A more normal arc of rotation to the midface complex is achieved with the midline split, which further reduces the stigmata of the preoperative Apert 'flat and wide' facial appearance. Both the medial and lateral orbital rims are shifted to the midline while the posterior maxillary arch width is increased. Bipartitioning of the monobloc complex is less often required for the Crouzon midface deformity.

A common error is an attempt by the surgeon to simultaneously adjust the orbits and idealize the occlusion by using the Le Fort III, monobloc or facial bipartition in isolation without completing a separate Le Fort I osteotomy.[22,24,81] Rarely is it possible to normalize the orbits and occlusion without additional horizontal segmentalization of the total midface complex. If Le Fort I segmentalization of the total midface complex is not carried out and the surgeon attempts to achieve a positive overbite and overjet

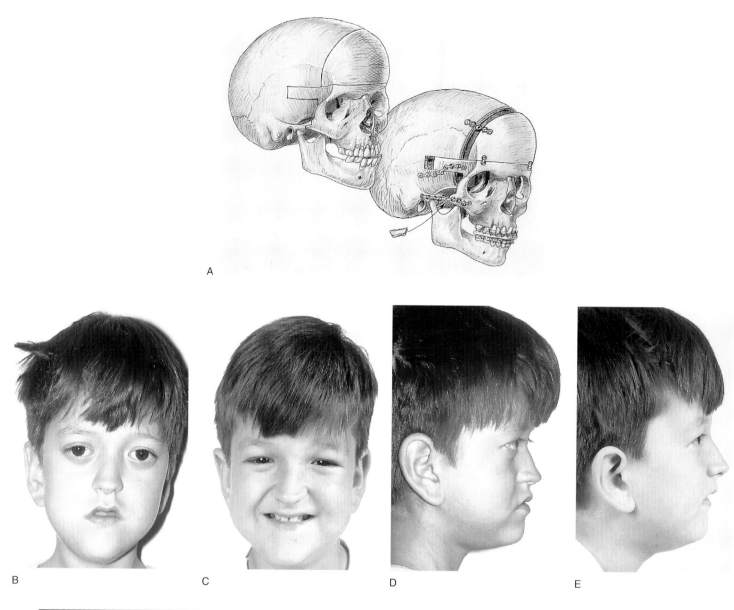

Fig. 54.4 An 8-year-old boy born with Crouzon syndrome who underwent first-stage cranial vault and orbital reshaping at 6 months of age is shown before and after anterior cranial vault and monobloc osteotomies with reshaping and advancement. **(A)** Illustration of craniofacial morphology before and after anterior cranial vault and monobloc osteotomies with advancement. Osteotomy locations indicated. Stabilization with cranial bone grafts and titanium miniplates and screws. **(B)** Preoperative frontal view. **(C)** Frontal view after reconstruction. **(D)** Preoperative profile view. **(E)** Profile view after reconstruction. **(F)** Two-dimensional axial CT scans. View through orbits before and after reconstruction indicating increased intraorbital depth with decreasing proptosis achieved. (From Posnick)[22]

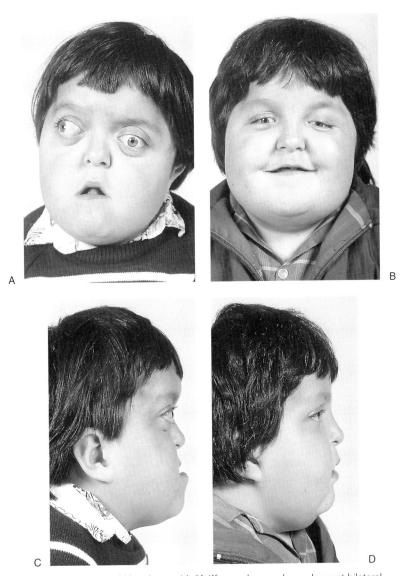

Fig. 54.5 A 7-year-old boy born with Pfeiffer syndrome who underwent bilateral canthal advancements through an intracranial approach at 3 months of age. He later required placement of a ventriculo-peritoneal shunt. He presents now for total cranial vault and monobloc osteotomy with reshaping and advancement. **(A)** Preoperative frontal view. **(B)** Frontal view 1 year after reconstruction. **(C)** Preoperative lateral view. **(D)** Lateral view 1 year after reconstruction. (From Posnick)[22]

at the incisors, enophthalmos will frequently be the result. The author's preference is to complete the separate Le Fort I osteotomy, often in conjunction with a genioplasty combined with orthodontic treatment planned for the time of skeletal maturity.

Problems specific to the Le Fort III osteotomy when its indications are less than ideal include unesthetic step-offs in the lateral orbital rims that occur when even a moderate advancement is carried out. These step-offs are often impossible to modify effectively later on. With the Le Fort III osteotomy, the ideal orbital depth is more difficult to judge, and either residual proptosis or enophthalmos is more likely to occur. Simultaneous correction of orbital hypertelorism cannot be achieved with a Le Fort III procedure. Excessive lengthening of the nose, accompanied by flattening of the nasofrontal angle, will also occur if a Le Fort III osteotomy is selected when the skeletal morphology would indicate a monobloc or facial bipartition procedure.

Total midface deficiency may be effectively managed as early as 5–7 years of age. The author's preference is to wait until the maxillary permanent 1st molars and central incisors

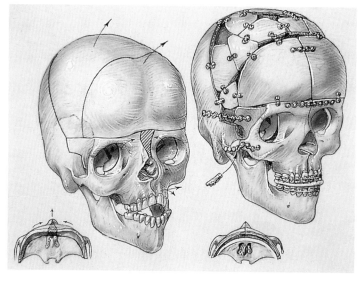

A

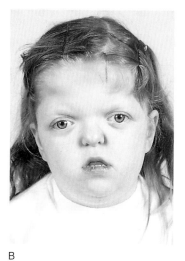

B

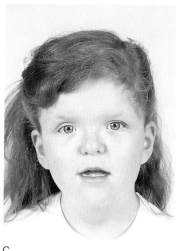

C

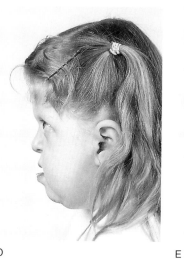

D

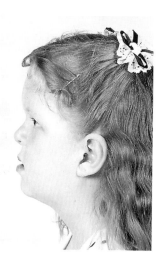

E

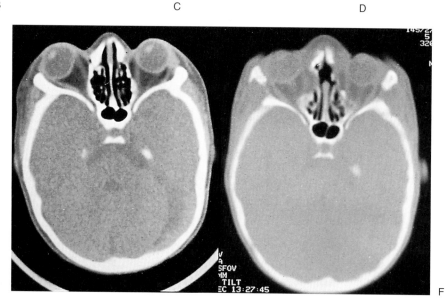

F

Fig. 54.6 A 5-year-old girl with Apert syndrome who underwent bicoronal suture release and cranio-orbital osteotomies with reshaping and advancement at 6 months of age. She presents now for cranial vault and facial bipartition osteotomies to reshape the skull and midface. **(A)** Illustration of preoperative craniofacial morphology, planned and completed osteotomies with reshaping. Stabilization is achieved with cranial bone grafts and titanium miniplate fixation. **(B)** Preoperative frontal view. **(C)** Frontal view 2 years after reconstruction. **(D)** Preoperative lateral view. **(E)** Lateral view 2 years after reconstruction. **(F)** Pre- and postoperative axial sliced CT scans through mid-orbits, demonstrating improvement in orbital hypertelorism and orbital depth with decrease in eye proptosis. (From Posnick)[22]

are fully erupted (closer to 7 years of age) (Figs 54.4–6). By this age, the cranial vault and orbits have attained approximately 85–90% of their adult size.[78] When the procedure is carried out at or after this age, the reconstructive result in the cranio-orbital region is permanent once healing has occurred. It is expected that routine orthognathic surgery will be necessary at the time of skeletal maturity to achieve an ideal occlusion, facial profile and smile.

Psychosocial considerations are important variables to consider when selecting the time frame for the elective total midface procedure. The procedure carried out at 5–7 years of age allows the child to start school with a real chance for satisfactory self-esteem.

MANAGEMENT OF THE ORTHOGNATHIC DEFORMITY IN ADOLESCENTS

The mandible has a normal basic growth pattern in the craniofacial dysostosis syndromes. The maxilla does not have the same growth potential and, as a result, an Angle class III malocclusion with anterior open bite often results. A Le Fort I osteotomy (horizontal advancement, transverse widening and vertical lengthening) is frequently required in combination with a genioplasty (vertical reduction and horizontal advancement) to further correct the lower face deformity. Bilateral sagittal split osteotomies of the mandible may also be required for correction of secondary growth disturbances and minor discrepancies. The elective jaw surgery is carried out in conjunction with orthodontic treatment planned for completion at 'early' skeletal maturity (approximately age 13–15 years in females and 15–17 years in males). Stabilization is achieved with both miniplates and screws and autogenous bone grafts.

CONCLUSION

Staged surgical procedures performed at intervals to coincide with facial growth, visceral function and psychosocial development constitute the current approach to the correction of the craniofacial deformities associated with the craniofacial dysostosis syndromes. Recognition by the surgeon and the patient's family of the need for a staged reconstructive approach serves to clarify the goals of treatment. This approach also allows the surgeon to take advantage of known differences in craniofacial growth patterns between normal and affected children and between the different bones within the craniofacial skeleton. By continuing to define our rationale for the timing and extent of surgical intervention, then evaluating the functional and morphologic results in an objective way, we will move into the twenty first century making further advances for patients affected by these disorders.

REFERENCES

1. Virchow R 1881 Uber den Cretinismus, nametlich in Franken und uber pathologische Schadelforamen. Ver Phys Med Cesselsch Wurzburg 2:230
2. Apert E 1906 De l'acrocephalosyndactlie. Bulletins et Memoires Societe Medicale des Hopitaux de Paris 23:1310
3. Crouzon O 1912 Dysostose cranio-faciale herediataire. Bulletins et Memoires Societe Medicale des Hopitaux de Paris 33:545
4. Cohen MM Jr 1975 An etiologic and nosologic overview of craniosynostosis syndromes. Birth Defects 11:137
5. Gorlin RJ, Cohen MM Jr, Levin LS 1990 Syndromes of the head and neck, Ch 14, 3rd edn. Oxford University Press, New York
6. Cohen MM Jr 1986 Craniosynostosis: diagnosis, evaluation and management. Raven Press, New York
7. Muenke M, Gripp KW, McDonald DM et al 1997 A unique point mutation in the fibroblast growth factor Receptor 3 gene (FGFR3) defines a new craniosynostosis syndrome. American Journal of Human Genetics 60:555
8. Cohen MM et al 1977 Genetic perspectives on craniosynostosis and syndromes with craniosynostosis. Journal of Neurosurgery 47:886
9. David DJ, Sheen R 1990 Surgical correction of Crouzon syndrome. Plastic and Reconstructive Surgery 85:344
10. Friede H, Lilja J, Lauritzen C et al 1986 Skull morphology after early craniotomy in patients with premature synostosis of the coronal suture. Cleft Palate Journal 23(suppl 1):1
11. Hogeman KE, Willmar K 1974 On Le Fort III osteotomy for Crouzon's disease in children: Report of a four year follow-up in one patient. Scandinavian Journal of Plastic and Reconstructive Surgery 8:169
12. Kolar JC, Munro IR, Farkas LG 1988 Patterns of dysmorphology in Crouzon syndrome: An anthropometric study. Cleft Palate Journal 25:235
13. Kreiborg S 1981 Craniofacial growth in plagiocephaly and Crouzon syndrome. Scandinavian Journal of Plastic and Reconstructive Surgery 15:187
14. Lauritzen C, Lilja J, Jarlstedt J 1986 Airway obstruction and sleep apnea in children with craniofacial anomalies. Plastic and Reconstructive Surgery 77:1
15. McCarthy JG, Epstein FJ, Wood-Smith D 1990 Craniosynostosis. In: McCarthy JG (ed) Plastic surgery, Vol 4. Saunders, Philadelphia pp 3013–3053
16. Kreiborg S, Bjork A 1982 Description of a dry skull with Crouzon syndrome. Scandinavian Journal of Plastic and Reconstructive Surgery 16:245
17. Kreiborg S 1981 Crouzon syndrome. A clinical and roentgencephalometric study. Scandinavian Journal of Plastic and Reconstructive Surgery (suppl) 18:1
18. Bjork A 1955 Cranial base development. American Journal of Orthodontics 41:198
19. Carr M, Posnick J, Armstrong D et al 1992 Cranio-orbito-zygomatic measurements from standard CT scans in unoperated Crouzon and Apert infants: Comparison with normal controls. Cleft Palate–Craniofacial Journal 29:129
20. Moss ML 1959 The pathogenesis of premature cranial synostosis in man. Acta Anatomica 37:351
21. Norgaard JO, Kvinnsland S 1979 Influence of submucous septal resection on facial growth in the rat. Plastic and Reconstructive Surgery 64:84
22. Posnick JC 1991 Craniofacial dysostosis: Staging of reconstruction

and management of the midface deformity. Neurosurgery Clinics of North America 2(3):638–702

23. Posnick JC, Lin KY, Jhawar BJ et al 1993 Crouzon syndrome: Quantitative assessment of presenting deformity and surgical results based on CT scans. Plastic and Reconstructive Surgery 92:1027–1037

24. Posnick JC 1992 Craniofacial dysostosis: Management of the midface deformity. In: Bell WH (ed) Orthognathic and reconstructive surgery. Saunders, Philadelphia, pp 1839–1887

25. Richtsmeier JT, Grausz HM, Morris GR et al 1991 Growth of the cranial base in craniosynostosis. Cleft Palate–Craniofacial Journal 28:55

26. Rune B, Selvik G, Kreiborg S et al 1979 Motion of bones and volume changes in the neurocranium after craniectomy in Crouzon's disease. A roentgen steremetric study. Journal of Neurosurgery 50:494

27. Sarnet BG 1978 Differential craniofacial skeletal changes after postnatal experimental surgery in young and adult animals. Annals of Plastic Surgery 1:131

28. Seeger JF, Gabrielsen TO 1971 Premature closure of the frontosphenoidal suture in synostosis of the coronal suture. Radiology 101:631

29. Bu BH, Kaban LB, Vargervik K 1989 Effect of LeFort III osteotomy on mandibular growth in patients with Crouzon and Apert syndrome. Journal of Oral and Maxillofacial Surgery 47:666

30. Cohen MM Jr 1979 Craniostenoses and syndromes with craniosynostosis. Incidence, genetics, penetrance, variability and new syndrome updating. Birth Defects 15:13–63

31. Cohen MM Jr, Gorlin RJ, Berkman MD et al 1971 Facial variability in the Apert type acrocephalosyndactyly. Birth Defects 7:143–146

32. Kreiborg S, Cohen MM Jr 1991 The infant Apert skull. Neurosurgery Clinics of North America 2(3):551–554

33. Ousterhout DK, Melsen B 1982 Cranial base deformity in Apert's syndrome. Plastic and Reconstructive Surgery 69:254

34. Stewart RE, Dixon G, Cohen A 1977 The pathogenesis of premature craniosynostosis in acrocephalosyndactyly (Apert syndrome): A reconsideration. Plastic and Reconstructive Surgery 59:699

35. Cohen MM Jr 1980 Perspectives on craniosynostosis. Western Journal of Medicine 132:508

36. Cohen MM Jr 1989 Agenesis of the corpus callosum and limbic malformations revisited (letter). Archives of Neurology 46:1270

37. Cohen MM Jr, Kreiborg S 1990 The central nervous system in the Apert syndrome. American Journal of Medical Genetics 35:36

38. Cohen MM Jr, Kreiborg S 1991 Agenesis of the corpus callosum. Its associated anomalies and syndromes with special reference to the Apert syndrome. Neurosurgery Clinics of North America 2:565

39. Renier D, Sainte-Rose C, Marchac D et al 1982 Intracranial pressure in craniosynostosis. Journal of Neurosurgery 57:370

40. Renier D 1989 Intracranial pressure in craniosynostosis: Pre and postoperative recordings – correlation with functional results. In: Persing JA, Edgerton MT, Jane JA (eds) Scientific foundations and surgical treatment of craniosynostosis. Williams & Wilkins, Baltimore, pp 263–269

41. Gault DT, Renier D, Marchac D et al 1990 Intracranial volume in children with craniosynostosis. Journal of Craniofacial Surgery 1:1

42. Posnick JC, Bite U, Nakano P et al 1992 Indirect intracranial volume measurements using CT scans: Clinical applications for craniosynostosis. Plastic and Reconstructive Surgery 89:1

43. Fishman MA, Hogan GR, Dodge PR 1971 The concurrence of hydrocephalus and craniosynostosis. Journal of Neurosurgery 34:621

44. Golabi M, Edwards MSB, Ousterhout DK 1987 Craniosynostosis and hydrocephalus. Neurosurgery 21:63

45. Murovic JA, Posnick JC, Drake JM et al 1993 Hydrocephalus in Apert syndrome: A retrospective review. Pediatric Neurosurgery 19:151–155

46. Farkas LG, Posnick JC 1992 Growth and development of regional units in the head and face based on anthropometric measurements. Cleft Palate–Craniofacial Journal 29(04):301

47. Farkas LG, Posnick JC, Hreczko T 1992 Growth patterns of the face: A morphometric study. Cleft Palate–Craniofacial Journal 29(04):308

48. Farkas LG, Posnick JC, Hreczko T 1992 Anthropometric growth study of the head. Cleft Palate–Craniofacial Journal 29(04):303

49. Farkas LG, Posnick JC, Hreczko T et al 1992 Growth patterns in the orbital region: A morphometric study. Cleft Palate–Craniofacial Journal 29(04):315

50. Kaban LB, Conover M, Mulliken J 1986 Midface position after LeFort III advancement: A long-term follow-up study. Cleft Palate Journal 23(suppl 1):75

51. Posnick JC, Goldstein JA, Waitzman A 1993 Surgical correction of the Treacher-Collins malar deficiency with quantitative CT scan analysis of long-term results. Plastic and Reconstructive Surgery 92:12

52. Posnick JC, Lin KY, Chen P et al 1993 Sagittal synostosis: Quantitative assessment of presenting deformity and surgical results based on CT Scans. Plastic and Reconstructive Surgery 92:1015–1024

53. Posnick JC, Lin KY, Chen P et al 1994 Metopic synostosis: Quantitative assessment of presenting deformity and surgical results based on CT scans. Plastic and Reconstructive Surgery 93:16

54. Posnick JC, Lin KY, Jhawar BJ et al 1994 Apert syndrome: Quantitative assessment of presenting deformity and surgical results after first-stage reconstruction by CT scan. Plastic and Reconstructive Surgery 93:489–487

55. Waitzman AA, Posnick JC, Armstrong D et al 1992 Craniofacial skeletal measurements based on computed tomography: Part 1. Accuracy and reproducibility. Cleft Palate–Craniofacial Journal 29:112

56. Waitzman AA, Posnick JC, Armstrong D et al 1992 Craniofacial skeletal measurements based on computed tomography. Part 2. Normal values and growth trends. Cleft Palate–Craniofacial Journal 29:118

57. Lannelongue M 1890 De la craniectomie dans la microcephalie. Compte-Rendu Academie des Sciences 110:1382

58. Lane LC 1892 Pioneer craniectomy for relief of mental imbecility due to premature sutural closure and microcephalus. Journal of the American Medical Association 18:49

59. Tessier P 1967 Osteotomies totales de la face. Syndrome de Crouzon, syndrome d'Apert: Oxcephalies, scaphocephalies, turricephalies. Annales de Chirurgie Plastique 12:273

60. Tessier P 1969 Dysostoses cranio-faciales (syndromes de Crouzon et d'Apert). Osteotomies totales de la face. In: Transactions of the Fourth International Congress of Plastic and Reconstructive Surgery, Amsterdam, p 774

61. Tessier P 1971 Relationship of craniostenoses to craniofacial dysostosis and to faciosynosis: a study with therapeutic implications. Plastic and Reconstructive Surgery 48:224

62. Tessier P 1982 Autogenous bone grafts taken from the calvarium for facial and cranial applications. Clinics in Plastic Surgery 9:531

63. Tessier P 1971 Total osteotomy of the middle third of the face for faciostenosis or for sequelae of the LeFort III fractures. Plastic and Reconstructive Surgery 48:533

64. Tessier P 1976 Recent improvement in the treatment of facial and cranial deformities in Crouzon's disease and Apert's syndrome. In: Symposium of plastic surgery of the orbital region. Mosby, St Louis, p 271

65. Tessier P 1985 Apert's syndrome: Acrocephalosyndactyly type I. In: Caronni EP (ed) Craniofacial surgery. Little Brown, Boston, p 280

66. Tessier P 1971 The definitive plastic surgical treatment of the severe facial deformities of craniofacial dysostosis: Crouzon and Apert's diseases. Plastic and Reconstructive Surgery 48:419

67. Hoffman HJ, Mohr G 1976 Lateral canthal advancement of the

cranio-orbital margin: A new corrective technique in the treatment of coronal synostosis. Journal of Neurosurgery 45:376

68. Whitaker LA, Schut L, Kerr LP 1977 Early surgery for isolated craniofacial dysostosis. Plastic and Reconstructive Surgery 60:575

69. Marchac D, Renier D 1979 'Le front flottant'. Traitement precoce des facio-craniostenoses. Annales de Chirurgie Plastique 24:121–126

70. Epstein F, McCarthy J 1981 Neonatal craniofacial surgery. Scandinavian Journal of Plastic and Reconstructive Surgery 15:217

71. McCarthy JG, Epstein F, Sadove M et al 1984 Early surgery for craniofacial synostosis an 8 year experience. Plastic and Reconstructive Surgery 73:521

72. McCarthy JG, Cutting CB 1990 The timing of surgical intervention in craniofacial anomalies. Clinics in Plastic Surgery 17(1):161

73. Posnick JC 1992 Craniosynostosis: Surgical management in infancy. In: Bell WH (ed) Orthognathic and reconstructive surgery. Saunders, Philadelphia

74. Siddiqi S, Rutka JT, Posnick JC, Hoffman HJ, Humphreys RP, Drake JM 1995 Detection and management of intracranial hypertension following early repair of complex craniosynostosis syndromes. Neurosurgery 36:703–709

75. Ortiz-Monasterio F, Fuente del Campo A, Carillo A 1978 Advancement of the orbits and the midface in one piece, combined with frontal repositioning for the correction of Crouzon's deformities. Plastic and Reconstructive Surgery 61:507

76. Ortiz-Monasterio F, Fuente del Campo A 1985 Refinements on the bloc orbitofacial advancement. In: Caronni EP (ed) Craniofacial surgery. Little Brown, Boston, pp 263–274

77. Posnick JC, Al-Qattan MM, Armstrong D 1996 Monobloc and facial bipartition osteotomies for reconstruction of craniofacial malformations: A study of extradural dead space and morbidity. Plastic and Reconstructive Surgery 77:1118–1135

78. Posnick JC, Waitzman A, Armstrong D, Pron G 1996 Monobloc and facial bipartition osteotomies: Quantitative assessment of presenting deformity and surgical results based on computed tomography scans. Journal of Oral and Maxillofacial Surgery 53:358–367

79. Posnick JC 1995 Craniofacial dysostosis syndromes: A staged reconstructive approach. In: Turvey, Vig, Fonseca (eds) 1995 Facial clefts and craniosynostosis: Principles and management, Ch 26. Saunders, Philadelphia, pp 630–685

80. Van der Meulen JCH 1979 Medical faciotomy. British Journal of Plastic Surgery 32:339

81. Wolfe SA, Morrison G, Page LK et al 1993 The monobloc frontofacial advancement: Do the pluses outweigh the minuses? Plastic and Reconstructive Surgery 91:977

Surgical treatment of craniosynostosis

55

JOACHIM MÜHLING

INTRODUCTION

Craniosynostosis is premature fusion of the craniofacial sutures. Virchow[1] recognized that a premature synostosis would impede the development of the bone perpendicular to the affected suture, resulting at the same time in increased expansion in the direction of the afflicted suture. Analysis of the face and skull deformities which develop according to this rule thus allows us to identify the affected suture.

This disease should be considered as a dynamic process. During growth, an imbalance between the volume of the cranial capsule and the growing brain develops, thus increasing intracranial pressure. This condition is called craniostenosis. Inhibition of growth caused by the premature synostosis is not restricted to the neurocranium but also has an adverse effect on the development of the viscerocranium,[2] thus causing esthetic impairments, which can be more or less distinct, as well as functional disorders.

PATHOGENESIS

The osteocranium develops in the area of the base through ossification of the chondral preformed chondrocranium and in the area of the calvaria through desmal ossification.[3] Osteogenesis is controlled by genetically determined hormonal mechanisms. In addition, the hydrostatic pressure of the cranial volume is a critical stimulus for the growth of the neurocranium. External influences such as the effects of positioning and gravity also influence the form of the skull. The brain grows the most in the first years of life and reaches approximately 80% of the adult volume at the age of 3. As the growth of the brain decreases, so does the activity of the osteogenous matrix, and this is reflected in an increasing interdigitation of the sutures. The cranial sutures are not active growth regions, the calvaria grows through bone deposition on the outside and bone resorption on the inside.

The neuro- and viscerocranium are to be regarded as a closed anatomic unit. Disorders in one system of sutures principally affect other systems so that the cranial capsule, base and facial bone mutually influence each other in their growth. The cranial base, as the linking part, is therefore of major importance.

Today, in general the growth of the skull is a process that is influenced by multiple factors, and is subject to endogenous genetic monitoring as well as exogenous influences. Thus we have to assume that the pathogenesis of premature synostosis is the result of diverse disorders[4,5] including genetic defects, metabolic malfunctions and insufficient growth of the brain.

The most common genetic syndromes – Crouzon,[2] Apert,[6] Saethre–Chotzen,[7] Chotzen[8] and Pfeiffer[9] – are inherited in an autosomal dominant manner with a high penetration and very different expressivity. The cause of the synostosis of a single suture remains unclear, though the occasionally observed hereditary case is an argument in favor of participating genetic factors.

SYMPTOMS

Premature fusion of one or more sutures and subsequent pathologic growth of the skull lead to various degrees of functional impairment and proportional asymmetries of the neuro- and viscerocranium. Functional impairment is caused either directly by the pathologic growth pattern or indirectly by the increased intracranial pressure.

The typical cranial deformities result from the inhibition

of growth perpendicular to the afflicted suture with a simultaneously increased expansion of the bone in the direction of the suture. The prognosis depends on whether the disease is restricted to the sutures of the calvaria or whether it also affects the sutures of the cranial base. If the cranial base is affected, severe growth inhibition in the neuro- as well as the viscerocranium is to be expected, with a more unfavorable growth pattern and an even higher intracranial pressure. The dynamic nature of the growth pattern means that these symptoms may be expected to increase during further development (Fig. 55.1).

As a consequence of the increasing disproportion between the volume of the cranial capsule and the growing brain, the intracranial pressure rises (Fig. 55.2); depending on the affected sutures, this pressure can be local or generalized. Less severe cases of synostosis can however be observed which are accompanied only by a growth inhibition without any clinical or radiologic sign of increased intracranial pressure. Irritation of brain tissue, impairment of the circulation of the cerebrospinal fluid, and impairment of the cerebral blood circulation can be a consequence of increased pressure.

Headaches are among the most common neurologic symptoms. As a consequence of the increased intracranial pressure, infants show restlessness, sleep disorders, frequent crying, vomiting, feeding difficulties and failure to develop. Occasionally mental retardation can be observed. The optic nerve is especially at risk. The chronically increased intra-

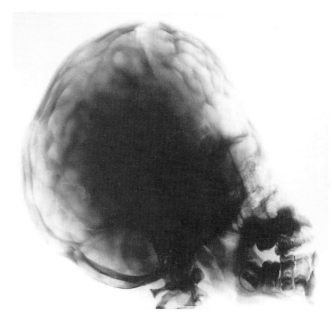

Fig. 55.2 'Cloudy skull' or 'copper beaten' caused by severely increased intracranial pressure.

cranial pressure can result in impairment of vision and, in extreme cases, atrophy of the optic nerve and blindness.

The most obvious result of growth impairment of the skull is exophthalmos caused by insufficient depth of the orbit. In severe cases, closure of the eyelid is no longer possible, thereby raising the risk of corneal erosion with subsequent impairment of vision. Craniosynostosis is frequently accompanied by dystophia of the orbits in the sense of hyper- or hypotelorism, resulting in possible interference with binocular vision. Blepharoptosis and blepharophimosis, occurring in the Saethre–Chotzen syndrome, can cause severe impairments.

The growth inhibition of the viscerocranium has considerable effects on the stomatognathic system (Fig. 55.3).

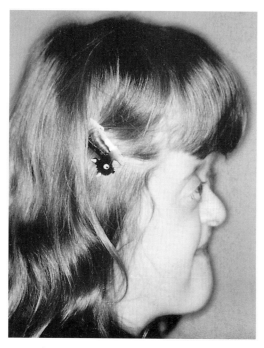

Fig. 55.1 Craniosynostosis in a case of Apert syndrome with midface hypoplasia, bulbar protrusion and pseudoprognathism.

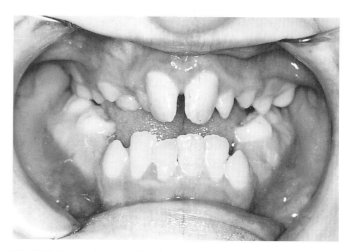

Fig. 55.3 Narrow jaw, dental malposition and narrowly spaced teeth in a case of midface hypoplasia.

The premature synostosis interferes with the anterio-caudal rotation of the maxillary bone resulting in a hypoplasia of the whole midface. This causes an obstruction in the naso-pharyngeal area with stenoses of the respiratory tract resulting in chronic infections and insufficient ventilation of the middle ear. Mouth breathing also accelerates teeth decay and loss. According to the severity of the condition there may be an open bite in the front connected with dental malposition. This is caused by the lack of space in the maxillary arch. The lower jaw is not affected, thus rendering the clinical appearance of a pseudomandibular prognathism. A genuine prognathic lower jaw can, however, develop during further growth. Maxillary hypoplasia also promotes rhinolalia clausa. It is not uncommon for palatal clefts to occur along with craniosynostosis.

Impairment of the facial appearance can also have an influence on the psychological development of the child. There may be concomitant extracranial malformations; for example syndactyly can occur in connection with cranio-facial dysmorphia, especially in certain syndromes.

CLASSIFICATION

The physiologic morphology of the neuro- and viscero-cranium displays considerable variation, however, from this natural variety we can define extreme deviations as patho-logic. In 1851, Virchow[1] distinguished nine deformities of the skull which he described as a result of the premature fusion of cranial sutures. This classification based on the shape of the skull has prevailed over classification according to the sutures affected or etiologic aspects.

For the purposes of surgical therapy only 5 skull forms are distinguished, according to Marchac & Renier:[10]

- trigonocephaly
- plagiocephaly
- oxycephaly
- brachycephaly
- scaphocephaly.

However, combinations of these forms are possible according to the sutures affected.

The site of the cranial suture synostosis determines the malformation of the neuro- and viscerocranium. These cranial anomalies can differ in severity and, furthermore, combinations are possible. Syndrome characterizations have gained prevalence in the clinical vernacular, particularly for those diseases that are accompanied by further malformations. Classification according to syndrome is of no relevance for surgical therapy, since the correction of the craniostenosis

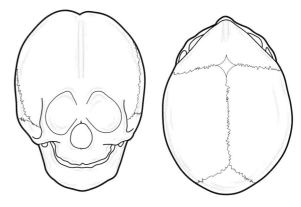

Fig. 55.4 Growth pattern of trigonocephaly.

is determined solely by the external appearance, neverthe-less, it does enable certain conclusions to be drawn as to the prognosis and likelihood of hereditary transmission.

TRIGONOCEPHALY

A trigonocephalic deformity (Fig. 55.4) is created by the premature ossification of the metopic suture. In most cases, this kind of malformation is identifiable at birth. Synostosis results in a bulging of the mid-forehead area which can be observed as a prominent bone ridge in some patients. At the same time, the frontolateral region is flattened. The forehead as a whole is narrow, whereas the occipital region appears to be broadened. The eyes are positioned close together in hypotelorism. The olfactory groove is deeply retracted between the upward reaching orbits. Midface growth is rarely affected and it is mainly the region of the frontal lobes that is restricted.

PLAGIOCEPHALY

A plagiocephalic deformity (Fig. 55.5) derives from an un-ilateral synostosis of a coronal suture or a lambdoid suture.

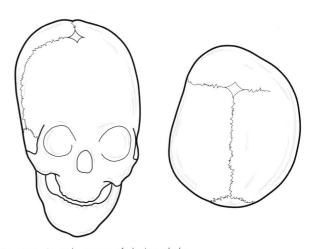

Fig. 55.5 Growth pattern of plagiocephaly.

Growth inhibition leads to flattening of the forehead on the affected side. The shortening of the skull in the sagittal direction reaches as far as the occipital region. The wing of the sphenoid bone is thickened and reaches quite far upwards. At the same time the anterior base of the skull is shortened on the affected side. On the inner surface of the calvaria finger printing – a sign of a local restriction of the brain – can be found.

The orbital funnel is flattened in the supraorbital region. The facial axis deviates to the unaffected side, thus the axis of the eyes is inclined towards this side while the occlusal plane drops to the affected side. Occlusion, however, is not disturbed.

OXYCEPHALY

An oxycephalic deformity (Fig. 55.6) is caused by a bilateral synostosis of the coronal suture. Growth inhibition perpendicular to the afflicted suture and expansion in the direction of the affected suture results in a flat and high forehead. The calvaria is shortened in the sagittal and broadened in the transverse plane. Since the cranial base is not involved, the anterio-caudal rotation of the maxilla is not restricted. Only the orbital funnels show a supraorbital growth inhibition, so that the typical bulbar protrusion is limited to this supraorbital region. The nasofrontal angle is flattened and the intracranial pressure is severely raised in most cases. The sphenoid wings are heavily thickened and reach far cranially. Finger printing can generally be found.

BRACHYCEPHALY

Brachycephaly (Fig. 55.7) results from the premature ossification of the coronal sutures and the simultaneous fusion of sutures of the cranial base. Growth of the sphenoid complex is inhibited in toto. Thus, in contrast to the previous

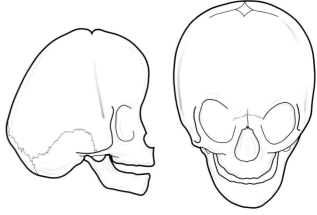

Fig. 55.7 Growth pattern of brachycephaly.

deformities, the malformation is not mainly restricted to the neurocranium, but has severe effects on the viscerocranium including the stomatognathic system. In addition, the sutures of the facial skeleton can be affected.

The sagittal extension of the skull and cranial base is reduced. Growth inhibition of the skull base prevents the calvaria from extending cranially in a tower-like fashion as is the case with an oxycephalic deformity. The growth pressure of the brain therefore leads to a compensatory protrusion of the frontal and temporal regions. The skull is short, broad, and round. The orbits are heavily flattened resulting in exorbitism. The frontolateral region is retracted; together with a simultaneous protrusion of the temporal region, this can cause the appearance of a cloverleaf skull in extreme cases. The interorbital distance is increased in hypertelorism. The whole maxilla is hypoplastic and the rotation of the upper jaw results in a circular open bite. As mandibular growth is unrestricted, the clinical picture of pseudomandibular prognathism and possibly true prognathism develops. The cranial base declines steeply in the dorsal direction. The olfactory lamina is often distinctly broadened.

SCAPHOCEPHALY

The scaphocephalic deformity (Fig. 55.8) is the most common form of craniosynostosis and develops from the premature synostosis of the sagittal suture. Growth inhibition perpendicular to the affected suture leads to a reduced extension of the skull in the transverse plane. This is compensated by increased growth in the sagittal direction. The clinical appearance is characterized by a long narrow skull with a high forehead. An osseous bulge in the area of the sagittal suture is frequently noticeable and in most cases a scaphocephalic deformity is clearly identifiable at birth.

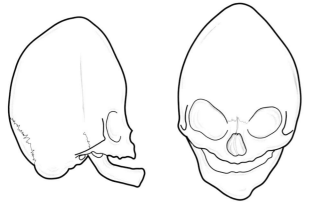

Fig. 55.6 Growth pattern of oxycephaly.

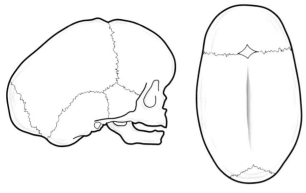

Fig. 55.8 Growth pattern of scaphocephaly.

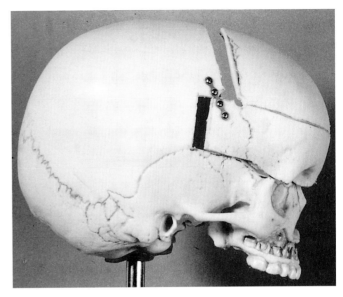

Fig. 55.9 Standardized fronto-orbital advancement.

SURGICAL TECHNIQUES

STANDARDIZED FRONTO-ORBITAL ADVANCEMENT

The standardized fronto-orbital advancement is best suited for surgical therapy.[11] It is based on the tongue-in-groove technique developed by Tessier[12] and on the early bilateral advancement introduced by Marchac.[10] This technique is based on the osteotomy, removal, modeling and displacing of the fronto-orbital region.

Osteotomy lines are placed along the cranial sutures and reaching as far as the cranial base thus eliminating the restrictive influence. The intracranial volume can be increased by repositioning the bone segments. By individually shaping and repositioning the fronto-orbital bone segments, the deformity can be corrected and further development of the skull can be guided in a more favorable direction (Fig. 55.9).

Surgical access for the fronto-orbital advancement is gained through a bicoronal incision. The incision should be made in the hair-bearing scalp approximately at the level of the coronal sutures so that a receding hairline in later life will not reveal visible scars. Careful hemostasis is required in order to keep blood loss to a minimum due to the increased collateral circulation.

First, the cutaneous flap of the galea is detached from the periosteum approximately as far as the supraorbital bulge. The flap is then dissected laterally above the temporal fascia on both sides. It is now possible to transect and detach the periosteum along the coronal sutures and the border of the temporal muscle. It remains frontally flapped, allowing for the possibility of using it for covering or filling defects. The separate dissection of galea and periosteum has the advantage that the cutaneous flap is rendered more flexible, allowing it to yield to the advancement.

While the periosteum is being detached heavy bleeding from the emissaries of the bone may occur, especially in cases with pronounced intracranial pressure, necessitating the use of bone wax. Bone perforations caused by the increased intracranial pressure may also complicate the preparation.

The next step is to detach the anterior portions of the temporal muscle subperiosteally from the temporal fossa. The osseous nasal pyramid is exposed past the nasofrontal suture. The eye capsule can now be detached from the orbital funnel. The base of the palpebral ligament has to be detached past the zygomaticofrontal suture as far as the lateral infraorbital border. In most cases the supraorbital nerve can be preserved since it lies inside an osseous groove. In rare cases it is surrounded by an osseous duct in the anterior region which requires widening with the aid of a small Luer's forceps.

After this preparation the osteotomy lines are marked (Fig. 55.10). The line runs from the nasofrontal suture into the orbital funnel and from there along the roof of the orbit to the zygomaticofrontal suture. The osteotomy curves from this point on, up to the coronal sutures, creating a retention form in the parietal region (tongue-and-groove technique). Proceeding alongside the coronal suture the opposite side is reached, where the operation is continued in the same manner. This fronto-orbital osseous area is then divided into a frontal and an orbital bone segment by performing a horizontal osteotomy. The horizontal osteotomy line runs right under the bulge of the forehead, allowing the surgeon to shape the orbital bone segment. This standardized osteotomy is applicable to surgery for all pathologic forms of the skull.

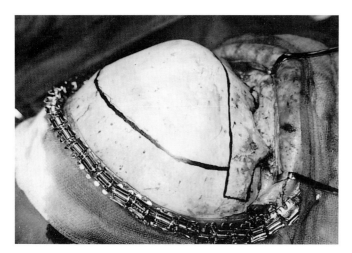

Fig. 55.10 Operative site with osteotomy lines marked.

The next step is to remove the frontal bone segment. For this procedure several holes have to be drilled using the trephine. With the aid of different raspatories the dura can be undermined and detached from the bone alongside the lines of the osteotomy. Next the osteotomy is made with the craniotome circling the frontal bone segment. After completely detaching the remaining adherent dura, this segment is removed. The preparation is frequently complicated by the fiinger printing which occasionally causes spicula. It is not always possible to avoid injuries to the dura.

There is now clear access to the intracranial region. Next, the frontal lobes and the anterior pole of the temporal lobes are epidurally detached from the bone. In order to achieve a clear view of the rhinobase, it is important to detach the connective tissue of the falx cerebri completely from the foramen caecum. The base of the olfactory strands can then be exposed. The next step is to osteotomize the orbital bone segment with a motorized microsaw. Our experience shows that it is more beneficial to perform the extracranial bone cuts first. The osteotomy starts in the orbital funnel and continues along the zygomaticofrontal suture to the parietal area. Since the tip of the saw has to reach as far as the intracranial region, it is important to protect the brain with spatulas. The nasofrontal suture is also opened extracranially. The blade of the saw is directed at a slight slant to ensure that the tip of the saw penetrates the cranial base, but not the nasal roof.

The osteotomy is then completed intracranially with the microsaw by transecting the sphenoid wing and the orbital roof. In the area of the sphenoid wing in particular it is important to make the incision sufficiently deep to overlap with the extracranial osteotomy, thereby leaving no osseous connections. During the osteotomy of the sphenoid wing and the orbital roof, the bulb has to be protected with a spatula to ensure that the eye capsule is not damaged by

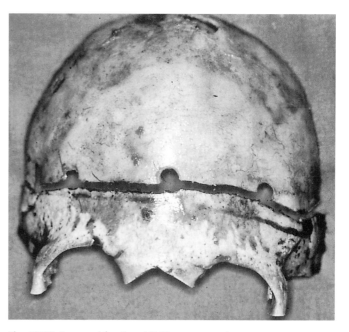

Fig. 55.11 Removed fronto-orbital bone segments.

the tip of the saw. In order to prevent premature reossification the stumps of the sphenoid wing are bluntly dissected with the Luer's forceps (Fig. 55.11).

In the second phase of the procedure the fronto-orbital bone segments are molded according to the type of deformity and repositioned. The plastic molding of the bone segments becomes increasingly difficult as the patient gets older. Whereas it is possible to shape the bone segments of children up to 6 months in the form of a greenstick fracture, special techniques have to be applied in older children and adults. In cases of brittle bones, the shaping of the orbital segment is possible only after a bone incision, such as a wedge-shaped bone excision. In addition, suitable molding and bending instruments may be used which are based on the principle of shaping the bone through 'crashing' it, causing microfractures. The new shape of the orbital segment is stabilized with wire sutures or microplates.

The orbital segment is then repositioned with an advancement. The extent of the osseous displacement is determined by the degree of the deformity and by the individual appearance. As a matter of principle, the malformation should be slightly overcompensated. Additionally, the orbital segment is slanted slightly in the ventral direction according to the type of deformity. Stabilization of the bone fragments in their exact position is of utmost importance for securing the result of the operation during the postsurgical phase when tension of the cutaneous galea flap and the formation of edema are to be anticipated. For this purpose, miniplates are fixed in the retention area. The miniplates have to be removed after three months through a small incision in the region of the old scar otherwise they could end up in the intracranial area due to the appositional bone growth. The last step is to adapt the frontal bone segment to the newly formed orbital segment, thereby creating an esthetic bulging of the forehead. For this purpose the frontal bone segment has to be shaped with special instruments according to the type of deformity. Once the frontal bone segments are adapted exactly to the orbital segment with the aid of shaping and bending instruments, they are fixed with wire sutures or microplates. The advancement results in a wide opening of the affected sutures without having to perform a craniectomy (Fig. 55.12), and the need for additional bone resection and the use of silicone foil is avoided. The intracranial pressure decreases immediately after surgery, since the previously confined brain can now expand.

The dissected temporal muscle is reattached to the bone with absorbable sutures. After insertion of a drainage tube the periostal flap is retracted, thereby covering the bone gaps. The brain will fill the newly formed space within 2–3 weeks.

After the cutaneous galea flap has been repositioned the wound is closed. This fronto-orbital advancement is applicable to all forms of deformities, with individual shaping and positioning of the bone segments according to the type of malformation. The only exception is the scaphocephalic deformity; in this case early linear craniectomy is still used because it results in a harmonious reshaping of the skull while simultaneously decreasing the intracranial pressure.

FRONTO-ORBITAL ADVANCEMENT WITH LINEAR CRANIECTOMY

In cases of extremely pronounced craniostenosis with severely increased intracranial pressure, as for example in pansyno-stosis, it is possible to combine the fronto-orbital advancement with a linear craniectomy in the occipital region[13] (Fig. 55.13). An active increase in the intracranial volume can be achieved through this procedure. Also, the growing brain puts pressure on the restricted occipital skull cap, thus molding it and achieving an additional decrease in pressure.

After the standardized advancement has been performed, a bone strip of approximately 1 cm is resected parallel to the sagittal suture. At the posterior fontanel, the craniectomy curves along the lambdoid suture and the squamous suture, back to the coronal suture. It ends just before the coronal suture, leaving a bone bridge of approximately 2 cm for fixation. The procedure is carried out in the same manner on the opposite side. In the area of the posterior fontanel the craniectomy is extended across the center line and connected with the linear craniectomy on the opposite side. This technique leaves a bone strip of around 2 cm above the sagittal sinus for protection purposes.

After the surgery, the brain expands into the space created by the advancement and the remaining need for expansion

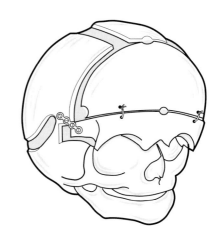

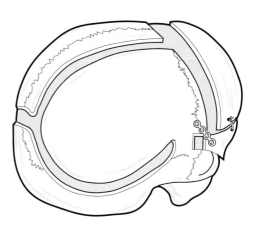

Fig. 55.13 Fronto-orbital advancement combined with a linear craniectomy.

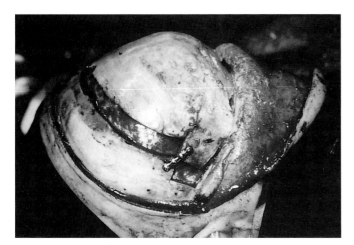

Fig. 55.12 Repositioned and advanced fronto-orbital bone segments; fixation with miniplates in the tongue-in-groove area.

is met by stretching of the rear parts of the skull. In older children, it is sufficient to open the calvaria without an additional craniectomy to avoid incomplete reossification.

FRONTO-ORBITAL ADVANCEMENT WITH TOTAL CRANIECTOMY

In infants with extreme pansynostosis and corresponding deformities of the fronto-parieto-occipital region, surgery is indicated at a very early stage. In such cases it is recommended that fronto-orbital advancement be combined with a total craniectomy according to Powiertowski & Matlosz[14] (Fig. 55.14).

The parietal bone is completely resected on both sides up to the temporosquamous suture and the lambdoid suture. The extensive bone defect is left to secondary reossification. At the same time, a fronto-orbital advancement is performed. This results in an extension of the cranial base and an opening of the base sutures. To ensure a satisfactory esthetic result, the fronto-orbital region should not be left to secondary reossification. Once a total craniectomy in the occipital area has been performed, it is possible to correct distinct malformations in this region without a great deal of effort. After the first 6 months of life, however, the potential for reossification decreases significantly; this technique is therefore not recommended after this age since it then carries the risk of incomplete skull ossification.

FRONTO-ORBITAL ADVANCEMENT WITH LE FORT III OSTEOTOMY

In extreme cases of distinct midface hypoplasia as well as a pronounced protrusion of the bulb, a Le Fort III osteotomy

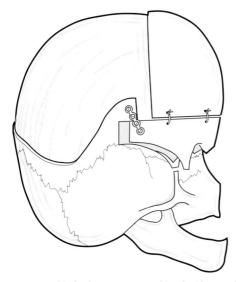

Fig. 55.14 Fronto-orbital advancement combined with a total craniectomy.

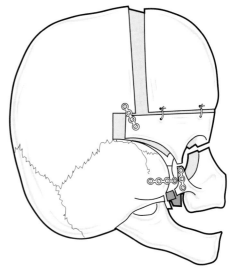

Fig. 55.15 Fronto-orbito-maxillary advancement.

in addition to the fronto-orbital advancement is needed (Fig. 55.15). This type of surgery can be performed in one session in older children and adults. However, there should be a waiting period of about 2–4 months when the procedure has to be performed at separate times since this considerably decreases the operational risk.

Surgical access is achieved through the use of a coronal incision. After the fronto-orbital advancement the same access is used to completely remove the soft tissues in the area of the maxilla as well as of the nose. The eye capsule is circumferentially detached from the osseous orbital funnel. The nasolacrimal duct and the inferior orbital fissure are exposed and the intranasal mucosa is detached via the bony aperture of the nose. The medial part of the temporal muscle is dissected from the temporal fossa. Subperiostial dissection along the back wall of the maxillary sinus ends at the pterygoid process. The remaining soft tissues are dissected from the upper jaw with an intraoral incision. The osteotomy in the region of the zygomaticofrontal suture can then be performed with the microsaw and extends to the inferior orbital fissure. The zygomatic arch is transected at the base of the zygomatic bone. The nasal pyramid is osteotomized along the nasofrontal suture including the osseous nasal septum. The incision is extended into the lamina papyraceus and the medial wall of the orbit. The floor of the orbit is osteotomized up to the inferior orbital fissure behind the nasolacrimal duct by bluntly depressing it with the chisel. This avoids injury to the infraorbital nerve. Finally the upper jaw is detached from the pterygoid process on both sides with the chisel.

The upper jaw is then held with the Gilles forceps and mobilized through down-fracture as well as rotating movements. After dissection of the remaining adherent soft tissues the midface can be shifted into the required position. It is fixed to the lateral orbital margin and the area of the glabella with miniplates. The resulting defects in the area of the zygomatic arch and between the pterygoid process and maxilla are reconstructed through osteoplasty. An exact adjustment of the occlusion, as can be obtained by the Le Fort I osteotomy, is not always possible. Sometimes postsurgical orthodontic treatment or Le Fort I osteotomy is necessary. Using this technique of 'fronto-orbito-maxillary advancement' pronounced malformations can be corrected and separate and individual adjustment of the forehead and the midface is possible. Although the 'fronto-orbito-maxillary advancement' should be reserved for the treatment of older patients, it can also be performed on small children when the condition is life-threatening, however it must be remembered that after surgery the midface will develop only slightly from the adjusted position and thus the Le Fort III osteotomy will have to be repeated later. When children have surgery at an early stage, the fronto-orbital advancement is performed within the first year of life followed by Le Fort III osteotomy at the age of 10. At this point the dental germs have reached a more favorable position in the upper jaw thereby minimizing the risk of injury; also, growth of the skull is almost complete and the adjusted position should be permanent.

OCCIPITAL ADVANCEMENT

In cases of isolated lambdoid suture synostoses the skull deformity is predominantly restricted to the occipital region. The skull is shortened in the sagittal and broadened in the transverse plane. The brain is increasingly confined in the occipital region. Surgery consists of an occipital osteotomy[15] with a coronal incision identical to that used for a fronto-orbital advancement. First, an occipital bone segment is removed. Then a bone strip is osteotomized below the bone segment in a tongue-in-groove technique. Brisk bleeding from the bone and the sagittal sinus must be expected.

The bone strip may be shaped in various ways. After the osteotomy the caudal segment can be shifted in the dorsal direction; if necessary it can also be slanted or rotated laterally. In some cases additional shaping is necessary. Again, the fixation is performed in the tongue-in-groove area with mini- or microplates. The occipital bone segment is subsequently adjusted to the form of the caudal segment and fixed with wire or plate osteosynthesis. By repositioning the occipital region in the manner described the intracranial volume can be increased and the synostosis opened. The skull is extended in the sagittal plane (Fig. 55.16).

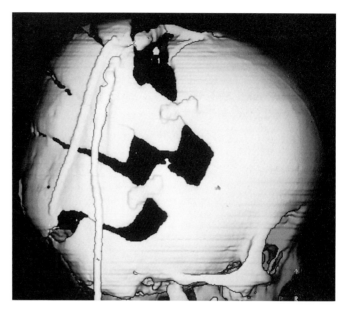

Fig. 55.16 3D CT after occipital advancement.

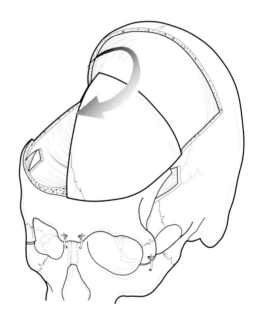

Fig. 55.17 Reshaping of the calvaria.

RESHAPING OF THE CALVARIA

In rare cases it is necessary to reshape the calvaria completely[16] (Fig. 55.17). This requires the osteotomy of the calvaria into several parts depending on the form of the malformation. Various techniques are described for this procedure. Often an acceptable skull form can be achieved by exchanging various spindle-shaped bone segments. If necessary the bone segments must be reduced to even smaller pieces. Fixation of the bone segments in their new position is achieved through microplates or wire sutures.

SPECIAL TECHNIQUES

Since older children have a reduced potential for reossification, bone gaps resulting from the advancement have to be closed. For the purpose of osteoplastic reconstruction the calvaria can be split. First the inner compact layer is separated from the outer one through the spongy layer with the saw. The curvature of the calvaria means that the final part of the osteotomy has to be completed with the chisel. The inner part of the calvaria can be used for the osteoplasty while the outer compact layer is repositioned in its original site. It is not always possible to apply this technique, especially in patients who suffer from a very high intracranial pressure, since their skull cap is often thinned. In such cases reconstruction has to be performed using free autologous bone transplants from the ribs or the iliac crest, or with homologous bone.

SURGICAL PROBLEMS AND COMPLICATIONS

Surgical problems must be anticipated, for example in cases with a very high intracranial pressure. The calvarial bone can be thinned and even partly resorbed as a result of the pressure. When dissecting the bone there is the danger of injury to the dura.

'Finger printing' sometimes results in sharp edges or spicula which further complicate the separation of the dura (Fig. 55.18), especially since the dura is often already thinning and under tension. The dura may also adhere to the bone in children who suffer from chronically increased intracranial pressure. Injury to the dura cannot always be prevented in spite of the most careful preparation. The drainage of cerebral fluid caused by an injury to the dura may even partly facilitate the preparation since it reduces the strain on the dura. Injuries to the dura must be repaired, however, in order to avoid a CSF fistula requiring extensive postoperative treatment.

In the anterior region of the falx cerebri the bone may bulge into the intercerebral cleft, thereby creating a razor-sharp bony edge; this can cause an injury to the sagittal sinus which may result in severe blood loss. Heavy hypertrophy of the sphenoid wing complicates the preparation of the anterior temporal pole. In such cases it is advisable to be quite generous in the resection of the sphenoid wing, thereby creating a better view of the region around the temporal pole.

In older children difficulties with the osteotomy may arise if the frontal sinus is already formed and there is the possible risk of an ascending infection. An opened frontal sinus should therefore be de-epithelialized and plastically covered.

As far as the blood vessels are concerned, the subdural venous complexes are sometimes heavily congested (Fig. 55.19) and can pose a risk during preparation since they can easily be injured in a similar way to the sagittal sinus. The middle meningeal artery may tear during exposure of the temporal pole because it is often quite difficult to separate it from the connective tissue of the sphenosquamous suture.

Heavy blood loss can also be caused by congested cutaneous veins which may appear because of the pronounced collateral circulation commonly associated with chronically increased intracranial pressure. Hemorrhagic shock can be avoided by careful presurgical planning and early intervention by substituting the exact amount of the blood lost.

In cases of very high intracranial pressure a life-threatening constriction of the brainstem can occur. Another possi-

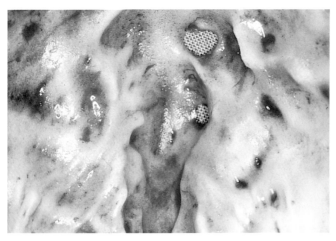

Fig. 55.18 Finger printing and bone perforations caused by severely increased intracranial pressure.

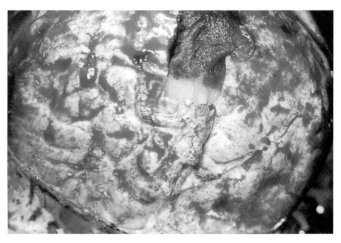

Fig. 55.19 Congested venous complexes resulting from severely increased intracranial pressure.

bility is massive bulging of the brain into the trepanation defect resulting in dangerous central shock. This situation can be controlled by an immediate generous decompressing craniectomy, however, at the first sign of its developing conservative measures should be taken to reduce the pressure on the brain.

Infections are quite rare since a broad-spectrum antibiotic is always administered before surgery. Other possible sources of infection, for example an opened frontal sinus during surgery, also need to be eliminated or dealt with.

It is remarkable how often subperiostial hematomas appear after a slight skull contusion in the operative region, usually within the first few months after surgery. These are no cause for worry and usually do not require treatment.

A serious complication is epidural postoperative bleeding. It is quite difficult to diagnose this complication because of physiologic bleeding into the epidural cavity, furthermore monitoring of the pupillary reaction is complicated by the puffiness of the eyelid and neurologic assessment is made difficult by postsurgical sedation. Cerebral dysfunction may result.

Detachment of the temporal muscle from the temporal fossa can cause trismus of the mandible postsurgically. In rare cases the temporal muscle has to be surgically separated from the muscular process.

With careful preparation there is only a very slight danger of injury to the nasolacrimal duct. The Le Fort III osteotomy in particular can cause mucosal tears in the area of the thin cribriform plate due to detachment of the intranasal mucosa and to the advancement, resulting in a permanent rhinorrhea.

The maxillary advancement is primarily aimed at correcting the exophthalmos. Thus, a frontal open bite can persist after the surgery and require orthodontic treatment or a second operation.

Tears of the eye capsule cannot always be avoided during periorbital dissection causing a fat prolapse. Although dysfunction rarely results, tears in the eye capsule should be treated appropriately.

Complications during craniofacial operations cannot always be avoided because of functional and anatomic peculiarities, however they can be kept to a minimum by careful planning and execution of the surgery.

Surgical complications are reported in 5–10% of all craniofacial operations and are responsible for an operational mortality rate of 2%. This corresponds to earlier figures for linear craniectomy, an operation which intervenes less dramatically. It is our permanent goal to further reduce the risks of surgery and early recognition of typical danger signs is an important prerequisite for this goal. The above mentioned figures are based on the early experiences in craniofacial surgery and have since been considerably reduced. Increased blood loss, postsurgical bleeding, infections and persisting CSF fistulae are the main operative risks.

Minor injuries to the dura are a common complication and occur in about 30–60% of all operations. These are due to gaps in the calvaria as well as a pathologically altered inner table of the skull.

POSTOPERATIVE CARE

Patients can generally be extubated immediately after a craniofacial operation. However, they should remain in intensive care for 24 hours after the surgery. At this stage neurologic check-ups are important to ensure the early detection of a subdural or epidural postsurgical haemorrhage. The large operative area and the length of the operation dictate the need for prophylactic antibiotics during surgery. Swelling of the soft tissues can be expected and measures should be taken to decrease this. The wound is often under a lot of strain because of the advancement and the postsurgical swelling, requiring careful observation. In small children the permanent plates from the osteosynthesis should be removed after 3–6 months. Regular check-ups should follow every 6–12 months, depending on the severity of the deformity. During postsurgical examinations further growth of the skull and the intracranial pressure are closely monitored.

REFERENCES

1. Virchow R 1851 Über den Cretinismus, namentlich in Franken und über pathologische Schädelformen. Verh Phys Med Ges Würzburg 2:230–271
2. Crouzon, O 1912 Dysostose cranio-faciale héréditaire. Bulletins et Memoires de Societe Medicale des Hopitaux de Paris 33:545–555
3. Lang J 1985 Praktische Anatomie. Begr. von T von Lanz, W. Wachsmuth. Bd 1/1 Kopf Teil A übergeordnete Systeme. Springer, Berlin
4. Cohen MM 1986 Perspectives on craniosynostosis. In: Cohen MM (ed) Craniosynostosis: Diagnosis, evaluation and management. Raven Press, New York, pp 21–57
5. Cohen MM 1986 Syndromes with craniosynostosis. In: Cohen MM (ed) Craniosynostosis: Diagnosis, evaluation and management. Raven Press, New York, pp 59–80
6. Apert E 1906 De Pacrocéphalosyndactylie. Bulletins et Memoires de Societe Medicale des Hopitaux de Paris 23:1310–1330
7. Saethre H 1931 Ein Beitrag zum Turmschädelproblem (Pathogenese, Erblichkeit und Symptomatologie). Zeitschrift Nervenheilk 117:533–555
8. Chotzen F 1932 Eine eigenartige familiäre Entwicklungsstörung (Akrocephalosyndaktylie, Dysostosis craniofacialis und Hypertelorismus). Monatsschrift Kinderheilk 55:97–122
9. Pfeiffer RA 1964 Dominant erbliche Akrocephalosyndaktylie. Zeitschrift Kinderheilk 90:301–319

10. Marchac D, Renier D 1982 Craniofacial surgery for craniosynostosis. Little Brown, Boston
11. Mühling J, Reuther J, Sörensen N 1987 Prämature Schdelnahtsynsotsen. Neue Wege der Chirurgischen Behandlung Klinikarzt 16:724
12. Tessier P 1967 Osteotomies totales de la face: syndrome de Crouzon, syndrome d' Apert; oxycéphalies, scapocéphalies, turricéphalies. Annales de Chirurgie Plastique 12:273
13. Mühling J, Reuther J, Sörensen NJ 1987 Therapie for severe Craniostenoses. In: Marchac D (ed) Craniofacial surgery. Springer, Berlin, p 88
14. Powiertowski H, Matlosz Z 1965 The treatment of craniostenosis by a method of extensive resection of the vault of the skull. Proceedings of the 3rd Congress of Neurological Surgeons Excerpta Medica International Congress Series 110:834
15. Zöller J 1997 Das occipitale Advancement. Mund-, Kiefer- und Gesichtschirurgie (in press)
16. Whitaker LA, Salyer KE, Munro IR, Jackson IT 1982 Atlas of craniofacial surgery. Mosby, St Louis

Fibrous dysplasia

56

IAN T. JACKSON/HENRY G. BONE/HEMEN JAJU

INTRODUCTION

Fibrous dysplasia was first described by von Recklinghausen in 1891.[1] It was recognized to be a developmental deformity of bone resulting from an abnormal proliferation of bone-forming mesenchyme.[2] The pathogenesis of this condition is not completely understood although trauma and endocrine disturbance were postulated in the past. More recently the molecular basis has been identified (see below). There are various classifications: in the clinical arena, the simple one of monostotic and polyostotic prevails, with a subtype of Albright syndrome.[3,4] In the latter condition there is sexual precocity, café-au-lait patches, early closure of epiphyses and endocrine abnormalities. A further subtype, cherubism, is familial and presents early in life.[5] The differential diagnosis is Paget's disease and meningioma. There is frequently confusion when the sphenoid wing is involved; on CT scan the appearance of fibrous dysplasia and meningioma in this region is very similar (Fig. 56.1),[6] but MRI scan can be helpful in differentiating one from the other. The diagnosis is often not confirmed until surgery is performed and the histology obtained.

The radiologists have a different classification and refer to fibrous dysplasia as either Pagetoid, sclerotic or cystic – the appearance varying with the relative amounts of fibrous and osseous material.[7] The Pagetoid type, which comprises 56%, shows alternating lucency and density. The sclerotic variety, which occurs in 23%, shows homogenous density. The cystic form constitutes 21%; it is a single oval or round lesion with well-defined margins. The radiologic classification is much closer to what is found in practice as it describes the spectrum of the condition.

PATHOGENESIS

The affected cells have one of several activating mutations of the G_s-alpha protein. This somatic mutation is present

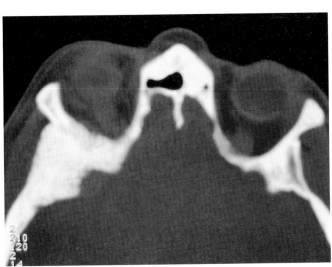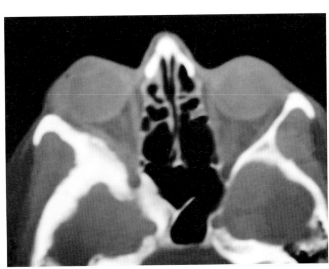

Fig. 56.1 Orbital CT scans showing **(A)** a meningioma of the lateral orbital wall and sphenoid, **(B)** fibrous dysplasia of the lateral orbital wall and sphenoid. As can be seen, the CT scans of these two disease processes are very similar and can easily cause diagnostic confusion.

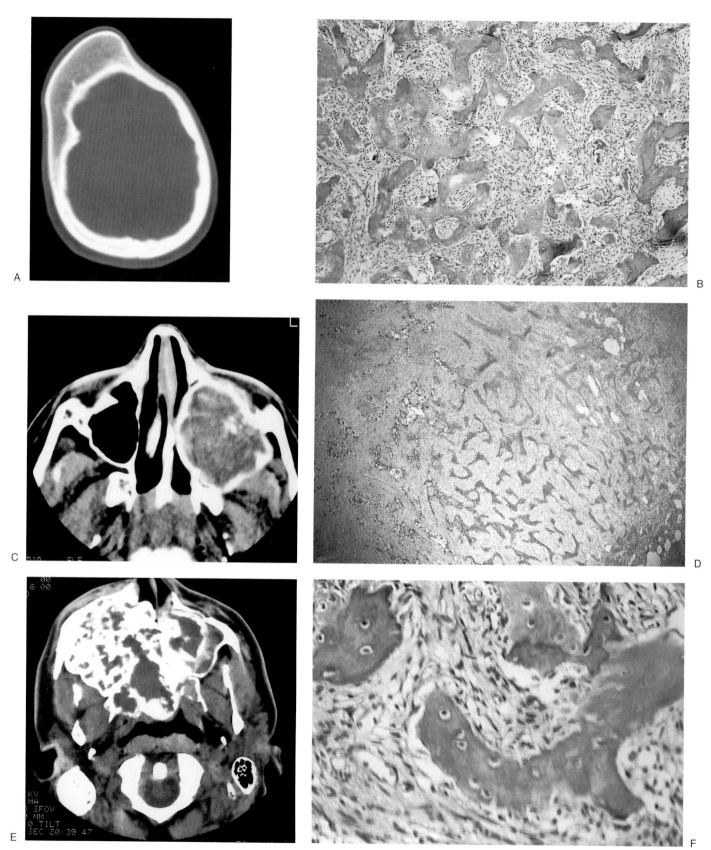

Fig. 56.2 Radiologic and histologic appearance of fibrous dysplasia. **(A,B)** Sclerotic: Frontal skull involvement showing uniform density. Histology shows more bone than fibrous stroma. **(C,D)** Fibro-osseous: involvement of the left maxillary antrum showing a radiologic pattern of bone and fibrous tissue. The histology shows the typical 'Chinese figures' arrangement of the bony spicules. **(E,F)** Fibrovascular: Radiologically there are large areas of soft tissue which are very vascular clinically. Histology shows many vessels in the fibrous stroma.

in all affected tissues in McCune–Albright syndrome, and in the dysplastic bone cells in fibrous dysplasia of bone.[8–11] Apparently this activation of the receptor–'second messenger' apparatus results in both a proliferative signal to the dysplastic cells and stimulation of the release of one or more cytokines, which cause apparently normal osteoclasts to congregate at the interface with adjacent normal bone and to initiate dysfunctional bone resorption at the margin. This creates a space within the adjacent normal bone into which the proliferating dysplastic tissue can expand. In this respect, dysplastic tissue expands much in the same way as osseous metastases of malignant tumors.

SUGGESTED CLASSIFICATION

Fibrous dysplasia ranges from fibrous to osseous, and can thus be classified in the following manner:

1. Sclerotic
2. Fibro-osseous
   a. Vascular
   b. Cystic
3. Fibrovascular

The **sclerotic** form (Fig. 56.2A,B) is composed of avascular homogeneous bone which may be soft or hard, and corresponds to the sclerotic variety mentioned above. This may be localized or widespread in one area or several areas.

The most frequent type, which can be designated as **fibro-osseous** (Fig. 56.2C,D), consists of a mass or masses of bone and soft tissue. Irregular spicules of osteoid are surrounded by a collagenous matrix and uniform spindle-shaped fibroblasts representing a disordered arrest of bone maturation at the woven bone stage.[12] This proliferation increases the bone mass, the relative volumes of which vary considerably. The vascularity of the lesion is variable and bleeding is often a problem at the time of surgery. This condition is often infiltrative, involving large areas of the facial skeleton and the skull base. It may present as a single mass or multiple lesions. The cystic type is probably just a variety of this type with fibrous tissue predominating.

The third type is almost purely comprised of fibrous and vascular tissue and may be described as **fibrovascular** (Fig. 56.2E,F). Although any facial area may be involved, it usually occurs in the maxillary antrum as a space occupying lesion. The walls of the antrum may or may not be involved.

The congenital variety, cherubism, may be homogenous, but more frequently the bone resembles a honeycomb. The multilocular spaces in the bone are filled with soft tissue which is usually fairly avascular.

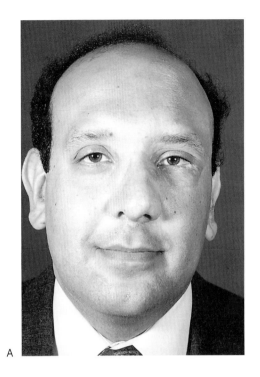

A

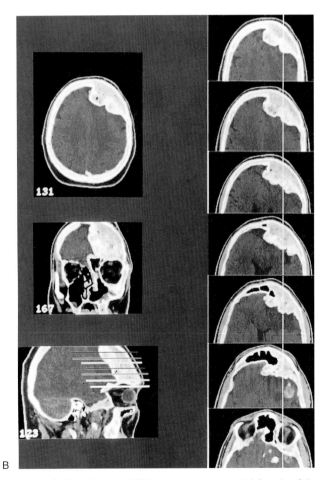

B

Fig. 56.3 Skull involvement. **(A)** There is some external deformity of the skull. **(B)** On CT scan the significant fibrous dysplasia can be seen extending into the cranial cavity.

DISTRIBUTION AND CLINICAL FEATURES OF THE DISEASE

In the head and neck area any portion of the craniofacial skeleton can be involved. It has been reported that the ethmoids and orbits are most frequently involved.[13,14] This in fact is not the case; these anatomic regions are at the skull base level, i.e. junction of maxilla and cranium, and are usually part of a wider involvement. The apparent frequency may well be related to the particular surgeon's area of specialization. Moore, an ophthalmologist, examined 48 cases and found 29 in the frontal area, 19 in the sphenoid sinus, and 13 in the ethmoid sinus.[15] The maxilla is more frequently involved than the mandible.[16]

Skull (Fig. 56.3). Involvement of the skull is frequent; this may be monostotic or polyostotic. The presentation may be that of masses or a single mass under the scalp or frontal skin. More significant, however, are pressure effects when the mass protrudes intracranially. Some patients have had limb paresis or frank paralysis, others deteriorating vision. When the skull base is involved, as in the anterior and middle cranial fossae, the sphenoid wing, orbital roof and cribriform plates are favorite sites. In aggressive forms, especially the fibro-osseous and fibrovascular, the skull

base, nasal cavity, orbits and maxilla may be involved. As a result of this, any of the cranial nerves may be compressed; the 2nd, 3rd, 4th, 6th and 7th nerves are the most frequently affected. The most significant situation is when compression results in varying levels of deafness, deteriorating vision, and eventual blindness.

Orbit (Fig. 56.4). The lesion may involve any or all of the walls of the orbit. The eye may be displaced vertically, horizontally, or anteroposteriorly. This can lead to double vision, deteriorating vision, or blindness. The latter results from optic canal involvement with compression of the optic nerve. Proptosis results from sphenoid or ethmoid disease and can lead to ophthalmoplegia and blindness. Occasionally there may be pain in the eye.

Ethmoid sinuses (Fig. 56.5). This is a frequently involved area but it is in conjunction with the lesion being present in the medial wall of the orbit and/or the anterior skull base. There may be nasal obstruction or eye displacement. A few patients have complained of pain.

Maxilla (Fig. 56.6). Involvement of the maxilla with fibrous dysplasia is very frequent[16] and may be generalized or localized. As mentioned previously, the lesion may

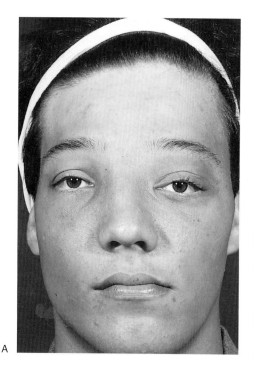

A

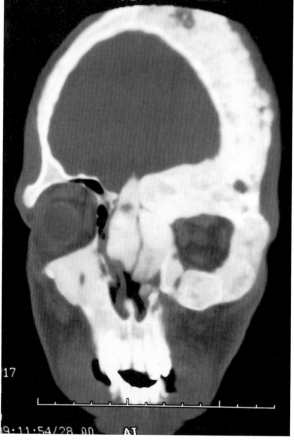

B

Fig. 56.4 Orbital involvement. **(A)** Proptosis and inferior displacement of the left eye. **(B)** The significant cranio-orbital involvement with fibrous dysplasia causing the eye displacement.

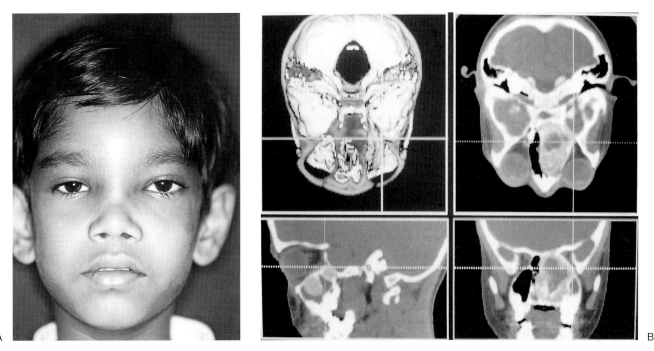

A   B

Fig. 56.5 Ethmoid sinus involvement. There is slight swelling over the frontal area **(A)** but the CT scan **(B)** shows an area of fibrous dysplasia in the left ethmoid sinus.

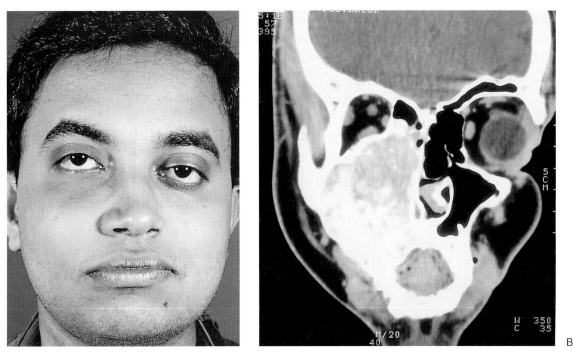

A   B

Fig. 56.6 Involvement of maxilla. **(A)** Right maxilla is enlarged producing a swelling of the right cheek. **(B)** CT scan shows the complete filling of the maxillary sinus with fibrous dysplasia.

involve the maxillary antrum, forming almost a cast of the cavity. In other cases the involvement may be more generalized and be either of the sclerotic type or the mixed fibro-osseous variety. Such a distribution is seen in cherubism and it is from the resulting deformity that the condition gets its name. The maxilla can grow to large proportions.

Frequently the alveolus alone, in toto or in part, is involved to a varying degree; the dentition may be poor and the occlusion disordered. Palatal involvement occurs but is asymptomatic. The orbit can be affected with resulting proptosis, diplopia, and rarely blindness. Infraorbital nerve compression may cause anesthesia in the nerve distribution.

Mandible (Fig. 56.7). Any area of the mandible can be involved in a solitary or a multiple fashion. The sclerotic variety is most common and can cause considerable deformity.

Many myths have sprung up about this condition. The usual one, especially in the past, was that the condition would cease to progress after adolescence. In the authors' experience this has rarely, if ever, occurred. The most dramatic situation was to see a patient in whom an acrylic plate for skull reconstruction placed after resection at the age of 18 was encased in recurrent fibrous dysplasia at the age of 36. Another case was that of a 45-year-old doctor experiencing increasing weakness of his right arm because fibrous dysplasia was pressing on his left fissure of Rolandi.

It was also taught at one time that the involved area is relatively avascular; this may be true for the sclerotic type but not for the mixed type, either fibro-osseous or fibrovascular. Frequently these lesions are very vascular; such a case was encountered in which, after midface and skull base resection, the bleeding was almost uncontrollable and multiple transfusion were required.

Malignant transformation is possible. This may be associated with radiation treatment with the lesion being slowly transformed into an osteogenic sarcoma. There have

also been cases where this change has been spontaneous without irradiation.[17,18] The overall incidence is 1%. In this situation the pathology is usually far advanced, mainly because of a delay in diagnosis.[19] The clue to malignant transformation is a change in the pattern of growth – it becomes more rapid, more invasive, and there may be associated pain.[20]

TREATMENT

General principles

The extent of involvement should be carefully evaluated and treatment planned accordingly. The factors to be considered in treatment planning are functional disability, danger to function, neurologic symptoms, and esthetic problems. Following this, the patient may be reassessed, or have medical or surgical treatment, or a combination of these two. Dental and ophthalmic consultation and treatment may be necessary.

Treatment need not always be active; if the condition is minor or the patient does not wish treatment, careful observation is acceptable. In this situation the possible behavior of the lesion must be discussed with the patient and he should be strongly advised to report if any worrisome change occurs, particularly relating to vision. The advised follow-up is discussed under Orbital Apex Involvement (p. 13). It is most distressing, as happened on one occasion, that a patient after a preoperative assessment became blind in the elevator when going to the

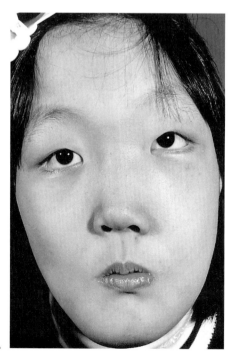

A

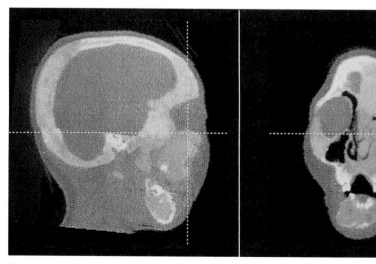

B

Fig. 56.7 Fibrous dysplasia of the mandible. **(A)** The patient shows facial asymmetry at all levels because of extensive involvement with fibrous dysplasia. **(B)** In addition to much of the facial skeleton being involved, the mandible also has areas of fibrous dysplastic change.

ophthalmologist for a consultation. In such a situation immediate surgery may be indicated or, as in a case of sudden bilateral blindness in an Albright syndrome girl, aged 19, massive doses of steroids may be given. Fortunately, this patient recovered her sight.

Surgical treatment

This consists of contouring and/or resection with bony reconstructon. Extensive or slowly growing lesions are contoured with a contouring bur. Softer lesions can be contoured with a scalpel, and liposuction has also been used.[21] Localized involvement can be treated by excision and reconstruction with bone grafts, usually split cranial bone. The diseased bone can be used after autoclaving[22] but it is very friable.

Medical management

Practical medical therapy is directed at the control of expansion of the lesions into the adjacent normal bone. There is no known treatment for the activating mutation per se, but effective therapy is available for the control of the activity of the osteoclasts which erode the normal bone at the margin. Various agents have been tried, but the only one which has been demonstrated to be consistently effective is the aminobisphosphonate, (pamidronate). It is recognized as effective for Paget's disease of bone, which is primarily a disease of osteoclasts, and also for control of hypercalcemia of malignancy and of osseous metastases, which involve osteoclasts in much the same way as fibrous dysplasia. Bisphosphonates are pyrophosphate analogs in which the linking oxygen is replaced by a carbon atom, rendering the structure highly resistant to hydrolysis. The activity is determined by side chains. The bisphosphonate structure has a high affinity for the exposed hydroxyapatite of bone mineral which is being 'excavated' by osteoclasts. When the osteoclast attempts to resorb an area of bone covered by the drug, the agent is taken up into the cell where it inactivates vital functions including acid secretion, thereby arresting the bone-resorbing activity. The high affinity for bone mineral and the resistance to metabolism result in a very long half-life in bone (several months to a year for pamidronate).

Pamidronate has been evaluated in two moderately sized series[23–25] and a number of individual cases and small series; it appears to reliably arrest invasion of fibrous dysplasia into adjacent normal bone as long as the regimen is maintained. It has no apparent effect on the growth of dysplastic tissue where there is no boundary with bone. The drug is administered as an intravenous infusion. A series consists of three doses of 60 mg (or 1 mg/kg in children) each, given at intervals of one day to one week. The series is repeated every six months, or more frequently if the biochemical effects do not appear to be maintained for the six months when surgery of fibrous dysplasia is planned, to schedule pre- and postoperative infusions. Serial biochemical markers of bone turnover and careful serial CT studies are important guides to assessing the response to treatment. For the time being at least, it is best for the treatment to be conducted under the direction of a physician who is experienced in the use of pamidronate and its effects. Other, orally administered bisphosphonates are becoming available, however they have not been systematically evaluated in fibrous dysplasia of bone and their use of fibrous dysplasia is not encouraged outside of clinical trials, especially in children.

Congenital type (Fig. 56.8)

Surgery presents a considerable challenge and is only done when the cherubism is very obvious and disfiguring. If the condition is of the sclerotic type simple contouring is advised. On occasion the bone can be soft and it will be possible to contour it with a scalpel. On other occasions a contouring drill is used.

When there is honeycombed bone filled with fibrous tissue a resection is required to improve on the facial contours. Often many teeth of the primary and secondary dentition may have to be sacrificed. In one case the soft tissue was rather gelatinous and much of it could be removed using the liposuction machine and the large cannula.[21]

No matter how much contouring is performed initially, further surgery will be necessary at a later date. This may take the form of osteotomies and dental rehabilitation.

Maxillary (Fig. 56.9)

If the alveolus alone is involved, observation may be all that is required. In many cases, however, the alveolus will be managed by contouring, taking special care to maintain the dentition. When the maxillary antrum is involved the approach is by a buccal sulcus incision and removal of the anterior surface of the maxilla. At this point it is usually possible to dissect and deliver the dysplastic material as a perfect cast of the antrum. Recurrence is possible after this but tends to happen infrequently.

When the lesion is more aggressive or recurrent and extends outwith the confines of the antrum to involve the true maxilla and cause significant deformity, the treatment is different. The palate, which is rarely affected, is main-

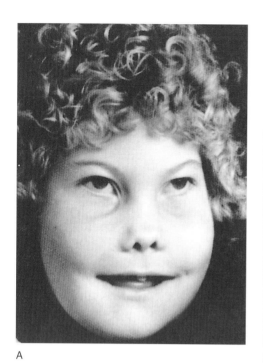

A

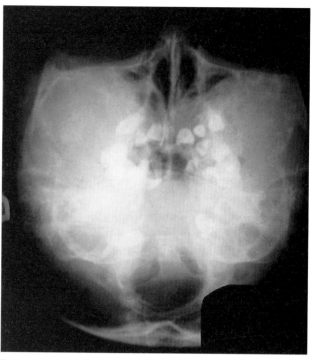

B

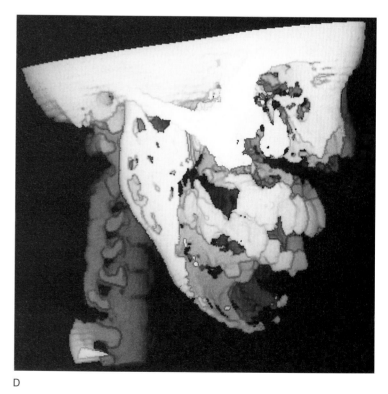

C

D

Fig. 56.8 Cherubism. **(A)** Typical appearance of congenital fibrous dysplasia – cherubism. **(B)** AP facial radiograph shows typical features of cherubism. **(C)** 3-D CT scan shows the honeycombed appearance of the maxilla and mandible. This was resected on several occasions. **(D)** The end result of treatment on 3-D CT scan.

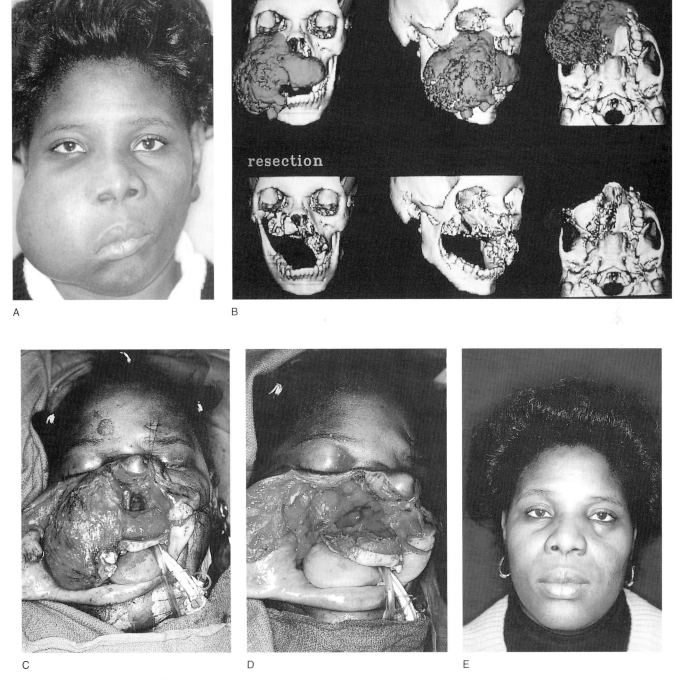

Fig. 56.9 Fibrous dysplasia of maxilla. **(A)** Patient showing involvement on right side. **(B)** CT scan shows the extensive replacement of the maxilla and upper alveolus with fibrous dysplasia. **(C)** Exposure. **(D)** Defect following resection. **(E)** Postoperative result.

tained intact but the remainder of the maxilla is resected. Medial and lateral buttresses are left to stabilize the palate, and the floor of the orbit is not sacrificed. The infraorbital nerve is totally freed by resection of the inferior portion of its foramen and osseous canal. The approach to this is intraoral whenever possible; on some occasions the Weber–Ferguson incision without the extension under the lower eyelid margin is used.

Recurrence is possible following this type of treatment, but does not occur as frequently as one might expect. On some occasions, and this is extremely rare, it may be necessary to perform a hemimaxillectomy. This is accomplished in the standard fashion and may require a Weber–Ferguson approach as described above. Rehabilitation should be with a dental prosthesis. A complex reconstruction is not advised in recurrent cases since further recurrence is possible.

In bilateral cases, if the tissue is sclerotic it should be contoured as a first line of treatment. If there is recurrence, resection with or without reconstruction is advised.[26,27]

Orbit (Fig. 56.10)

The orbit may be involved independently but this is rare. It is usually associated with ethmoid, skull base or sphenoid wing disease, although any of its seven bones can be involved.

A case of bilateral isolated orbital floor involvement presented in which the fibrous dysplasia was growing upwards from the orbital floor like a series of stalagmites. This necessitated a coronal flap approach with lateral wall osteotomies to allow an adequate approach to the orbital floor and complete removal of the formations. There was

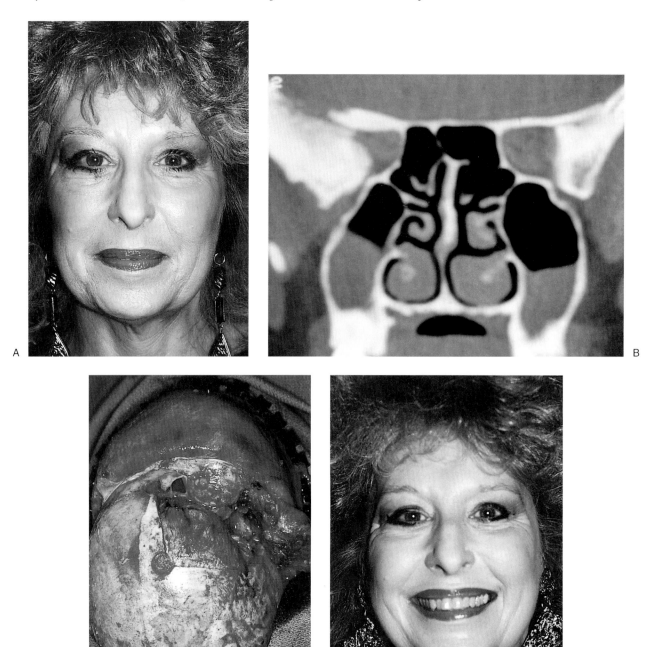

Fig. 56.10 Fibrous dysplasia of orbit. **(A)** Preoperative clinical appearance showing slight proptosis of right eye. **(B)** CT scan showing involvement of sphenoid wing. This involved the posterior orbit and lateral wall of the right orbit. **(C)** Resection of lesion using frontotemporal supraorbital approach. **(D)** Postoperative result.

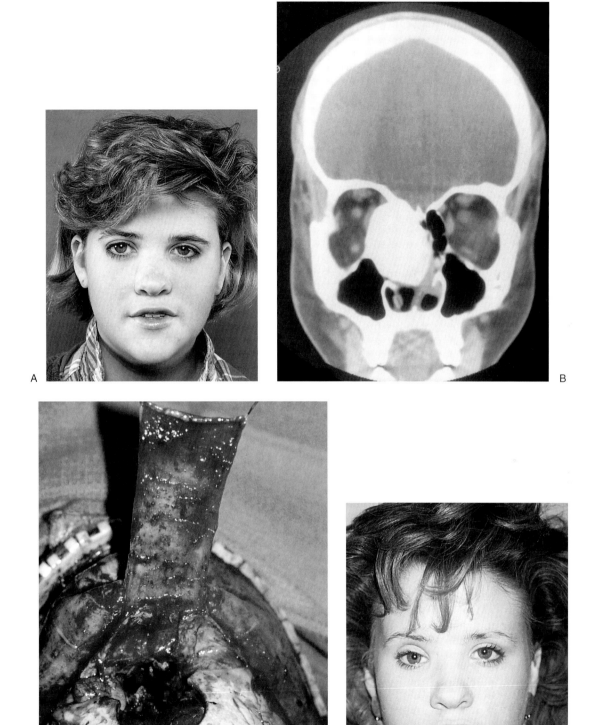

Fig. 56.11 Fibrous dysplasia of ethmoids. **(A)** Preoperative appearance of patient complaining of severe right-sided fronto-orbital headaches. **(B)** Coronal CT scan shows fibrous dysplasia of right orbit and ethmoid sinus. **(C)** Appearance at surgery following resection. Galeal frontalis flap ready to be placed into anterior skull base. **(D)** Postoperative result.

no recurrence of these lesions. Medial and lateral wall involvement and also that of the roof and apex will be discussed in relation to the other neighboring sites of involvement. Surgery in this area is frequent.[28]

Ethmoid (Fig. 56.11)

This, anatomically, consists of ethmoid, anterior skull base and medial orbital wall. The approach is intra- and extra-cranial. Using a coronal scalp flap, the frontosupraorbital and nasal areas are exposed. An osteotomy of the glabellar area is performed, either with a trephine of the appropriate size or a Midas Rex drill. The entry into the skull is made as small as possible but is also compatible with adequate exposure. If there are any problems such as ascending infection, only a small amount of bone would be lost. After the craniotomy bone is removed, the glabella inferior to this in continuity with the nasal bones is removed en bloc.

This approach gives excellent exposure to the nasal cavity and the central anterior skull base. Dissection and retraction of the orbital contents exposes the medial orbital wall. It is now possible to remove the affected areas as a block resection. This having been done, the defect is reconstructed with split cranial bone grafts which are wired or plated into position.[29–31] If resection is not possible the bone is contoured.

In order to protect these bone grafts from exposure in the nasal cavity and to close the floor of the anterior cranial fossa, a galeofrontalis myoperiosteal flap is used.[32] This vascular flap covers the medial wall bone graft on the side of the nasal cavity and is then sutured through drill holes in the anterior cranial fossa. It effectively separates the

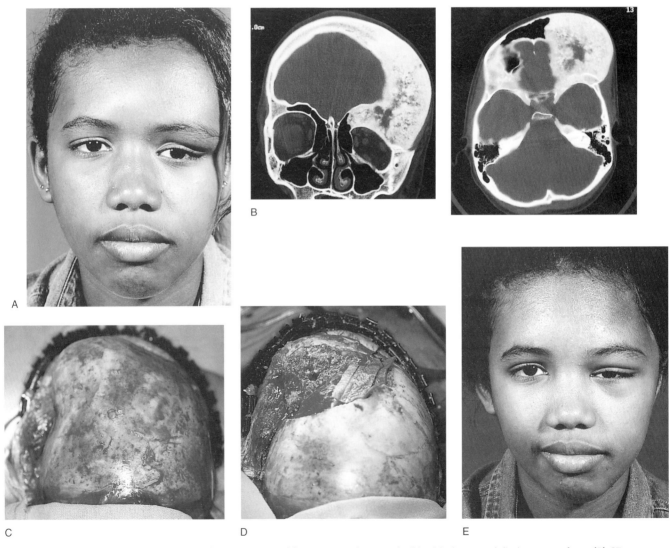

Fig. 56.12 Frontotemporo-orbital involvement. **(A)** Involvement of frontotemporal area and orbit with downward displacement of eye. **(B)** CT scan showing the involvement of the temporal area with the distortion of the orbit and the maxilla. Coronal (i) and occipital (ii) scans. **(C)** The appearance of the frontal area prior to removal of bone. **(D)** Frontal bone removed; the thickness of the involved portion of bone can be seen very readily. **(E)** Postoperative result.

nasal cavity from the extradural space. The removed bony segments are then plated back in position.

In these cases recurrence of fibrous dysplasia should not occur; this is a true tumor resection.

Frontotemporo-orbital involvement (Fig. 56.12)

When there is frontotemporo-orbital involvement there may be displacement of the eye downwards, with or without proptosis. With this involvement a craniotomy is performed and, if possible, all the involved areas are resected. This will result in a significant cranio-orbital defect which can be reconstructed using split cranial bone grafts secured with plates and screws. This usually gives a good cosmetic result. Autoclaved involved bone can also be used for reconstruction. Occasionally some double vision may persist, with or without enophthalmos. Irregularities in the frontal area may emerge later and can be treated if the patient wishes. This usually consists of a coronal flap approach and contouring with methyl methacrylate[33] or hydroxyapatite bone cement.

Sphenoid wing involvement (Fig. 56.1)

This is the condition which can be difficult to differentiate from meningioma when a CT scan is used.[6] MRI scan is more useful in that the meningioma tends to 'light up' more when the sphenoid is involved. Fibrous dysplasia affects the lateral wall of the orbit thus there may be proptosis, medial displacement of the globe and diplopia. Vision may begin to deteriorate if the enlargement continues.

Management is by a temporal or frontotemporal craniotomy which allows access to the sphenoid wing. Dissection of the temporalis muscle exposes the lateral wall of the orbit and the temporal bone. It is usually necessary to resect the temporal bone, the greater wing of the sphenoid, and the lateral orbital wall. This complex three-dimensional area is then reconstructed with split cranial bone grafts. The result of this procedure is gratifying; recurrence is very rare, but there may be enophthalmos and some residual diplopia.[26]

Orbital apex involvement (Fig. 56.13)

This is a very significant situation since blindness will occur if the involved area continues to enlarge. Blindness is sudden and irreversible. When there is involvement in this area, visual fields should be monitored regularly together with CT scans. A peripheral scotoma may be the first sign of optic nerve compression. The cause of blindness is

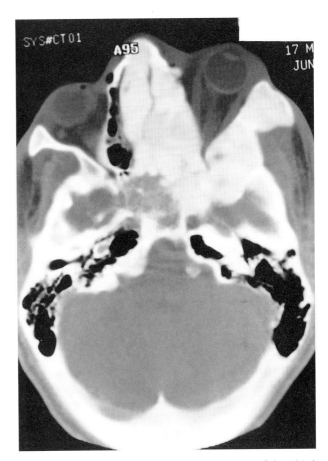

Fig. 56.13 Axial CT scan showing extensive involvement of the orbital apex; the same patient shown in Fig. 56.4. This was completely resected; decompression of the optic nerve resulting in improvement in vision.

ischemia of the optic nerve. In order to prevent this or to attempt to treat it, a coronal flap and a bilateral frontal craniotomy is performed. The frontal lobe is retracted in order to get to the area of the optic nerve entrance to the orbital apex. This is a difficult dissection since the internal carotid is also in this region.

The decussation of the optic nerves is located and the bone on the roof of the optic nerve canal is removed.[26] This is performed cautiously, protecting the nerve with a fine dissector as the roof is removed with a combination of drills and fine bone rongeurs. The anterior ring may be the most significant but the posterior intracranial portion must also be decompressed. A postoperative course of steroids is recommended. The dreaded complication of this procedure is blindness.

In some cases an anterior approach is indicated; it has been found that there is compression anterior to the canal in some cases, and this area must be decompressed. It has also been suggested that a frontal approach, as described previously, with removal of the nasal skeleton and an approach to the nerve through its medial wall can be satisfactory and safe. We have no experience with this but others find it to be a satisfactory method of nerve decompression, when indicated. It certainly reduces the amount of brain manipulation, and may reduce the risk of carotid artery damage.

Cranial involvement (Fig. 56.3)

This may be extensive with external deformity or, more significantly, with intracranial extension. In the latter situation there may be limb paresis or frank paralysis.

Shaving using a coronal approach may be satisfactory in the external protrusion type. However, not infrequently there may be recurrence requiring more radical measures, i.e. craniectomy and reconstruction.[33] A CT scan will reveal the offending area when there is a recurrence or when there are signs and symptoms of intracranial pressure. The treatment is coronal flap exposure with resection of the involved region and reconstruction with split cranial bone grafts. This usually gives a good cosmetic result and in most cases there will be reversal of paralysis.

Split rib grafts can be used if there is not enough cranial bone available. An alternative is alloplastic material, e.g. metal or acrylic. A less reliable but accepted method is to use a craniotome to generate bone dust. This dust is then placed on a layer of Surgicel which covers the skull defect; a further layer of Surgicel is then applied on top of the cranial bone dust. This will frequently, but not always, form a solid sheet of bone which follows the cranial contours.[30]

Skull base involvement (Fig. 56.14)

The involvement may be widespread, e.g. both maxillae, nasal cavity, anterior skull base, with an extension into the sphenoid and clival areas. The most difficult situation is when the fibrous dysplasia is of the fibro-osseous or fibro-vascular type.

The approach can be by a combined intra- and extra-cranial route. The simplest method of dealing with the face portion is to use a Weber–Ferguson incision. Bilateral exposure is gained by an osteotomy of the base of the nose with retraction of the nose on the contralateral face flap. In this way good exposure is obtained and a total or subtotal resection can be accomplished.[34] A total resection is preferred but is not always possible, thus only a partial resection and contouring may be possible.

In this situation reconstruction is limited by the amount of vascular cover which can be obtained. The most significant areas of the face should be reconstructed, e.g. the nose and other important areas of the craniofacial skeleton with cranial bone grafts, and the central anterior cranial base defects with the well-vascularized galeal frontalis myofascial periosteal flap. Bone replacement is not necessary in this region. In some situations a microvascular free tissue transfer may be necessary. Occasionally in the postoperative

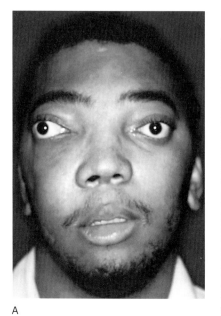

A

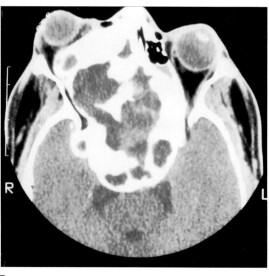

B

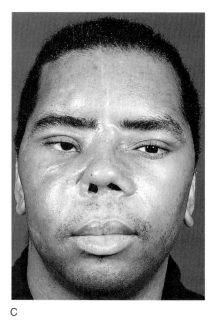

C

Fig. 56.14 Fibrous dysplasia of skull base. **(A)** Preoperative appearance. Note significant bilateral proptosis. **(B)** Axial scan showing the central involvement of the skull base with fibrous dysplasia. **(C)** Appearance after a facial split procedure and resection of the fibrous dysplasia. Note considerable improvement in eye position and also in appearance.

phase it may be necessary to remove portions of bone which become exposed and are devascularized.

RECURRENCE OF FIBROUS DYSPLASIA

This is unpredictable. It would be expected that simple shaving would always result in recurrence but strangely enough this does not always happen.

In the congenital type initial complete excision is not possible and there may be later growth requiring further surgery. In the mixed bony and soft tissue type aggressive behavior and resulting high recurrence rates are frequently seen.

There are cases of all types in which total resection is impossible. In this situation there may be various outcomes. Growth may be arrested by the surgery. Slow recurrence may occur or there may be almost accelerated growth with difficulty in gaining control. In this variety, pressure sequelae such as blindness, airway blockage or deafness may occur.

OCCURRENCE OF MALIGNANCY

This has rarely been reported as a de novo event.[17–20] The usual history is that of a recurrence of fibrous dysplasia treated with radiation; many years later there appears to be a recurrence which causes pain, grows rapidly and, on biopsy, is shown to be an osteogenic sarcoma. When this occurs the lesion is frequently very aggressive and the only hope is radical resection of the involved area with reconstruction. Unfortunately, the recurrence rate is high and there are few long-term survivors when this situation occurs.

CONCLUSION

Advances in craniomaxillofacial surgery have enabled progress to be made in the treatment of head and neck fibrous dysplasia. The involved area can be radically resected and reconstructed, and frequently the disease is eliminated. Unfortunately, this is not always the case; the lesion may be too extensive to resect and, in addition, it may involve significant functional areas. There may be recurrence in an inaccessible area. It may be that medical treatment will be effective in this situation.

At this moment in time, surgical resection is more possible than it was in the past. Reconstruction is more satisfactory because of developments in this area, e.g. vascularized local flaps, cranial bone grafts, free tissue transfer.

In summary, aggressive management of this ill understood condition has led to a better outlook for our patients.

REFERENCES

1. von Recklinghausen FD 1891 Die fibrose oder deformierende ostitis die osteomalacie und die osteoplastische carcinose in ihren gegensitigen Beziehungen. Rudolf Virchow Festschrift, Berlin
2. Lichtenstein L 1938 Polyostotic fibrous dysplasia. Archives of Surgery 36:874–898
3. Albright F et al 1937 Syndrome characterized by osteitis fibrosa disseminata, areas of pigmentation and endocrine dysfunction with precocious puberty in females: A report of five cases. New England Journal of Medicine 216:727
4. Albright F, Scoville B, Sulkowitch HW 1938 Syndrome characterized by osteitis fibrosa disseminata, areas of pigmentation and a gonadal dysfunction. Further observations including a report of two more cases. Endocrinology 22:411
5. Jones WA 1933 Familial multilocular cystic disease of the jaws. American Journal of Cancer 17:946
6. Hansen-Knarhoi M, Poole MD 1994 Preoperative difficulties in differentiating intraosseous meningiomas and fibrous dysplasia around the orbital apex. Journal of Cranio-Maxillo-Facial Surgery 22:226–230
7. Fries JW 1957 The roentgen features of fibrous dysplasia of the skull and facial bones: A critical analysis of thirty-nine pathologically proven cases. American Journal of Roentgenology 77:71
8. Weinstein LS, Shenker A, Gejman PV, Merino MJ, Friedman E, Spiegel AM 1991 Activating mutations of the stimulatory G protein in the McCune-Albright syndrome [see comments]. New England Journal of Medicine 325(24):1688–1695. Comment in New England Journal of Medicine 1991, 12; 325 (24):1738–1740
9. Shenker A, Weinstein LS, Moran A et al 1993 Severe endocrine and nonendocrine manifestations of the McCune-Albright syndrome associated with activating mutations of stimulatory G protein GS. Journal of Pediatrics 123(4):509–518
10. Shenker A, Weinstein LS, Sweet DE, Spiegel AM 1994 An activating Gs alpha mutation is present in fibrous dysplasia of bone in the McCune-Albright syndrome. Journal of Clinical Endocrinology and Metabolism 79(3):750–755
11. Shenker A, Chanson P, Weinstein LS, Chi P, Spiegel AM, Lomri A, Marie PJ 1995 Osteoblastic cells derived from isolated lesions of fibrous dysplasia contain activating somatic mutations of the Gs alpha gene. Human Molecular Genetics 4(9):1675–1676
12. Jacobiec FA, Rootman J 1979 Secondary and metastatic tumors of the orbit. In: Jones IS, Jacobiec FA (eds) Diseases of the orbit. Harper Row, Philadelphia
13. Georgiade N, Masters F, Horton C, Pickrell K 1955 Ossifying fibroma (fibrous dysplasia) of the facial bones in children and adolescents. Journal of Pediatrics 46:36
14. Leeds N, Seaman WB 1962 Fibrous dysplasia of the skull and its differential diagnosis. A clinical and roentgenographic study of 46 cases. Radiology 78:570
15. Moore RT 1969 Fibrous dysplasia of the orbit. Survey of Ophthalmology 13(6):321–334
16. Eversole LR 1972 Fibrous dysplasia: A nosologic problem in the diagnosis of fibro-osseous lesions of the jaws (review). Journal of Oral Pathology 1(5):189–220
17. Ruggieri P, Sim FH, Bond JR, Unni KK 1994 Malignancies in fibrous dysplasia. Cancer 73:1411–1424
18. Cheng MH, Chen YR 1997 Malignant fibrous histiocytoma degeneration in a patient with facial fibrous dysplasia. Annals of Plastic Surgery 39:638–642
19. Gross CW, Montgomery WW 1967 Fibrous dysplasia and malignant degeneration. Archives of Otolaryngology 85:653
20. Ramsey HE, Strong EW, Frazell EL 1968 Fibrous dysplasia of the craniofacial bones. American Journal of Surgery 116:542–547

21. Dubin B, Jackson IT 1990 The use of liposuction to contour cherubism (Ideas & Innovations). Plastic and Reconstructive Surgery 86(5):996–998

22. Lauritzen C, Alberius P, Santanelli F, Vallfors B, Lilja J, Stephensen H 1991 Repositioning of craniofacial tumorous bone after autoclaving. Scandinavian Journal of Plastic and Reconstructive Surgery and Hand Surgery 25(2):161–165

23. Liens D, Delmas PD, Meunier PJ 1994 Long-term effects of intravenous pamidronate in fibrous dysplasia of bone. Lancet 343(8903):953–954

24. Chapurlat RD, Delmas PD, Liens D, Meunier PJ 1997 Long-term effects of intravenous pamidronate in fibrous dysplasia of bone. Journal of Bone and Mineral Research 12(10):1746–1752

25. Bone HG 1996 Experience with pamidronate treatment of fibrous dysplasia of bone. Calcified Tissue International 59(3):221

26. Munro IR, Chen YR 1981 Radical treatment of fronto-orbital fibrous dysplasia: The chain-link fence. Plastic and Reconstructive Surgery 67(6):719

27. Jackson IT, Hide TAH, Gomuwka PK, Laws ER Jr, Langford K 1982 Treatment of cranio-orbital fibrous dysplasia. Journal of Maxillofacial Surgery 10:138–141

28. Moore AT, Buncic JR, Munro IR 1985 Fibrous dysplasia of the orbit in childhood: Clinical features and management. Ophthalmology 92:12–20

29. Jackson IT, Adham M, Bite U, Marx R 1987 Update on cranial bone grafts in craniofacial surgery. Annals of Plastic Surgery 18:37–40

30. Jackson IT 1992 Calvarial bone for head & neck reconstruction. In: Jackson IT, Sommerlad B (eds) Recent advances in plastic surgery 4. Churchill Livingstone, London

31. Jackson IT 1994 Principles of Craniomaxillofacial Surgery. In: Cohen M (ed) Mastery of surgery: Plastic and reconstructive surgery. Little, Brown, Boston, Ch 13, pp 135–168

32. Jackson IT, Adham MN, Marsh WR 1986 Use of the galeal frontalis myofascial flap in craniofacial surgery. Plastic and Reconstructive Surgery 77:905–910

33. Jackson IT 1986 Transcranial orbitectomy. In: Smith BC, Della Rocca RC, Nesi FA, Lisman RD (eds) Ophthalmic plastic and reconstructive surgery, Vol 2. CV Mosby, St. Louis, Ch 58, pp 1100–1123

34. Jackson IT, Webster HR 1994 Craniofacial tumors. In: Vander Kolk C (ed) Clinics in plastic surgery, Vol 21, No 3. WB Saunders, Philadelphia

Surgical complications of craniofacial surgery

J. KERWIN WILLIAMS/MICHAEL T. LONGAKER

INTRODUCTION

It is difficult to review the complete scope of complications that occur in craniofacial surgery without discussing individual syndromes and operative techniques. As this chapter is part of a comprehensive textbook, an adequate review of specific complications will have been accomplished under the respective topics. Therefore, the goal of this chapter is limited to reiterating the general principles of preoperative and perioperative management in the craniofacial patient that may prevent complications, and reviewing the types and rates of complications that have been reported from several major craniofacial centers. The discussion will also include reoperation rates seen in patients with non-syndromic and syndromic craniosynostosis. Complications encountered in craniofacial surgery will be divided into four general categories: preoperative, intraoperative, immediately postoperative (includes the initial hospitalization period) and the late postoperative period. Potential complications reflecting the natural course of a specific disorder will not be included.

PREOPERATIVE COMPLICATIONS

Surgical complications may be defined as an undesirable result following intervention, and may be either directly or indirectly related to the procedure. Included are complications that arise prior to the surgery because of an error in judgement during the critical preoperative decision-making period. Four areas of consideration must be addressed in order to make an accurate assessment whether or not to proceed with surgical intervention. As with any decision regarding surgical treatment, correct patient selection is

crucial. Both the functional and the esthetic goals of the procedure must be addressed, and there should be mutual agreement between the patient or family and the surgeon regarding these goals. This process is greatly facilitated by the active involvement of the patient throughout the presurgical planning, if their age permits.

Equally important is parent selection – a unique component of pediatric craniofacial surgery and often the most difficult to correctly assess preoperatively. The parents may be young and inexperienced in the management of high-stress issues. Financial concerns are frequently present, and one or both parents may have guilt or frustration about their child's condition. 'Parental preventive medicine' can follow in which every possible treatment option is pursued. Frequently, the pressures on parents are overwhelming and a marriage becomes dysfunctional. In each case it is important that the physician decides whether to inform, guide or lead the parents and patient in the decision process.

The timing of the procedure is the second component of adequate presurgical planning. Numerous articles have outlined treatment plans for craniofacial procedures, including the correction of craniosynostosis and midface advancements.[1-4] As a general rule, long-term results in craniofacial surgery are better achieved when the procedure is done at a later age, but psychological and functional requirements must be considered and may dictate early surgical intervention. Significant deformities are usually addressed prior to school age. Evidence of increased intracranial pressure or significant deformity secondary to craniosynostoses dictate surgery within the first year of life. Airway compromise and corneal exposure may also necessitate early surgical intervention.

Scheduled procedures often need to be postponed if the patient presents with a viral or bacterial infection involving the upper respiratory system. Respiratory infections in the pediatric age group are common and cancellations have been reported in 10–15% of patients in recent reviews.[5,6] Every pediatric patient should be seen shortly before the procedure to exclude a recent onset of illness.

Selection of the correct procedure is the third critical component in the decision process. A craniofacial disorder may manifest in varying degrees of severity, and each case should be assessed individually to determine the extent of surgery required. Options and details of the surgical technique are discussed elsewhere in this book.

Patient and parent education is the final component of the preoperative evaluation. Incorrect or unreasonable expectations may undermine an appropriate procedure on the right patient at the correct time. It is very difficult to correct the discontent of a parent or legal guardian with poor perceptions of the result. A general agreement on the expected results, locations of incisions and subsequent postoperative scars, and an outline of the immediate and extended postoperative course, should be well understood by all involved prior to surgery.

INTRAOPERATIVE COMPLICATIONS

Intraoperative complications may be categorized as either directly or indirectly related to the surgical procedure. Indirect complications can be related to the age and size of the pediatric patient, or develop from uncommon systemic abnormalities. Complications directly associated with surgical technique occur at either the primary site of the procedure or the secondary donor site.

INDIRECT COMPLICATIONS: SIZE AND AGE

Unlike adult patients, infants and children have very limited reserves. The body surface area of an infant is significantly increased compared to overall body size. Because of this increased exposure to the environment loss of heat may occur, leading to a dramatic drop in the core body temperature. Warming blankets, overhead lights and an elevated room temperature should be used to maintain an appropriate core body temperature. Warmed fluid replacements may also be given if necessary.

Overall blood volume in the very young patient is also decreased (usually calculated as 80 ml/kg), and sudden decompensation may occur in the operating room if blood loss is not replaced adequately. Blood loss is variable and reflects the complexity of the deformity (Table 57.1). Transfusion requirements during craniofacial surgery have been reported from 15% to nearly 250% of the patient's estimated red blood cell volume.[5,7] Eaton and associates[8]

Table 57.1 Intraoperative blood loss is listed as a function of the skull deformation. Mean (SD) percentage of estimated red cell volume lost and type of skull deformity. From Meyer et al,[7] with permission

Type of synostosis	During operation	After operation	Total
Oxycephaly	49.1 (22.9)	–3.7 (16.8)*	45.4 (36.9)
Plagiocephaly	59.0 (37.4)	27.7 (41.7)	86.7 (56.2)
Trigonocephaly	92.4 (49.7)	11.7 (16.6)	104.1 (49.2)
Brachycephaly	105.3 (48.45)	25.5 (56.5)	130.9 (69.1)
Scaphocephaly	92.1 (65.2)	35.9 (38.4)	121.7 (78.2)
Complex	198.5 (165)	44.5 (97.6)	243.1 (259.4)

reported postoperative transfusions in 15–50% of patients, and overtransfusion in 36%. The craniofacial surgeon should frequently communicate with the anesthesiologist regarding ongoing blood loss and characterize it as acute or chronic (insidious). It is the policy in some centers to have blood in the operating room or being infused at the start of an intracranial procedure. This conservative approach can be defended because the scalp incision and coronal flap are associated with substantial blood loss. The disastrous consequences of 'falling behind' on replacing lost blood during craniofacial procedures highlight the importance of communication between the surgeon and anesthesiologist during craniofacial surgery.

Special attention must be given to the airway in the pediatric patient. Because the diameter of the airway and the distance between the vocal cords and the carina are greatly decreased compared to the adult patient, manipulations of the head can dislodge the tube and quickly lead to decompensation. Furthermore, in a patient with a craniofacial anomaly, microagnathia, limited oral excursion and malposition of the larynx may complicate reintubation. To avoid this situation, the intubation tube must be adequately secured to an unobstructive region of the face once correct placement has been confirmed. If an endotracheal tube is used this may be accomplished with circum-mandibular wires. Alternatively, the endotracheal tube may be sutured to the first or second upper or lower molars. Nasotracheal tubes can be anchored to the membranous septum. One should be aware of the possibility that surgical tape used to secure the tube may become loose during lengthy procedures and lead to an unexpected extubation. During any craniofacial procedure the surgeon should always be prepared for an emergency tracheotomy.

INDIRECT COMPLICATIONS: SYSTEMIC ABNORMALITIES

Intraoperative systemic complications may not be directly related to surgical technique, but can cause a rapid deterioration of the patient. In most cases a high index of suspicion is required because these complications are not commonly seen. Air embolism has been well documented for procedures requiring an intracranial route, especially if the integrity of the sagittal sinus is compromised.[9,10] The traditional treatment of choice is immediate placement of the patient in a left lateral decubitus position and percutaneous aspiration of the air. Alternatively, central venous catheters may assist in removing the air from the right ventricle. Cerebral vascular accidents and myocardial infarctions are always a potential complication, but their risk is minimized in the pediatric population unless there are congenital cardiac abnormalities.

Coagulopathies may be life-threatening for the patient and should be considered if over 40–50% of total blood volume is transfused. In large craniofacial operations this magnitude of transfusion is not uncommon, and the associated coagulopathy must be anticipated. Other causes, such as a blood transfusion reaction and decreased core body temperature, may also lead to coagulopathies and must also be considered.

Finally, large craniofacial cases require significant amounts of fluid replacement and can lead to intraoperative metabolic abnormalities. Blood transfusions may produce hyperkalemia and metabolic acidosis as a result of cell lysis. A metabolic acidosis may also develop from hypovolemia and poor perfusion. This acid–base disturbance should be corrected with appropriate fluid replacements. Respiratory acidosis has also been reported from the use of an adult ventilatory circuit in a pediatric patient, because of the increased ventilatory dead space and accumulation of carbon dioxide.

DIRECT COMPLICATIONS: PRIMARY SURGICAL SITE

Complications associated with specific surgical procedures are described in more detail in other chapters. In general, technical complications occur at either the primary surgical site or a donor site. The overall mortality rate following craniofacial procedures has been reported to be from 0.1% to 1.6%.[11–13] Mortality increases to 2.2–2.3% in patients undergoing transcranial procedures. Causes of death include intraoperative hemorrhage with inadequate replacement of blood volume, acute respiratory obstruction and severe postsurgical infection (brain abscesses).

Globe

Many craniofacial procedures involve extensive dissection around the globe, either within the orbit or around the cornea. Protection of the globe is paramount and should always be addressed in craniofacial procedures.

The cornea may become irritated from skin preparation solutions or by direct trauma. Any soap-based skin cleansing solution (e.g. chlorhexidine) may cause significant irritation to the cornea (because of the decrease in the pH of the solution) and should not be used near the orbits. Betadine preparation solution (not betadine scrub solution) and benzalkonium are safe and used routinely for antisepsis of the skin around the orbits. Balanced salt solution should be used liberally to irrigate the eyes. The cornea may be protected from direct injury by careful placement of adequately sized corneal protectors and/or tarsorrhaphy stitches to the upper and lower lids. The orbit and globe should always be part of the surgical field and not covered with sheets, to prevent inadvertent pressure on the eye by the surgeon or an assistant. Finally, manipulation of the bone with a saw or burr should be done on a separate workstation if possible. If the bone work must be completed in situ, the patient's eyes should be protected by a towel or sheet to prevent bone dust injuring the cornea.

Dissection around the orbits requires careful retraction with malleable instruments and manipulation of the periorbita. Extreme pressure or traction on the globe will not only cause ischemia of the conical structures but may elicit an oculocardiac response, with bradycardia and hypotension. This response is usually corrected with an immediate release of pressure on the globe. Direct damage to the globe may be caused by dissecting instruments, especially in secondary procedures, and protection for the globe should always be provided when completing orbital osteotomies. As always, hemostasis should be meticulous to prevent hemorrhage, an orbital compartment syndrome and subsequent ischemia of the optic nerve.

The optic nerve is located inferolateral to the anterior and posterior ethmoidal vessels (approximately 15 mm from the latter and 20 mm from the former) (Fig. 57.1). The

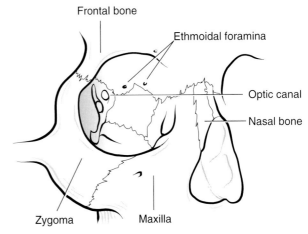

Fig. 57.1 The orbital anatomy. Note the relationship of the ethmoidal foramina to the optic foramen.

optic foramen is located superomedially at the apex of the orbit. In the normal adult the distance to the optic foramen from the inferior orbital rim is 35–40 mm and 40 mm from the superior orbital rim. Dissection of the periorbita is usually accomplished without visualizing the optic nerve, but the surgeon should always be aware of the potential for an aberrant location of the optic nerve secondary to abnormal anatomy.

In a six-center review of craniofacial complications Whitaker and associates[13] reported loss of vision in one patient and decreased visual acuity in a second. One patient with blindness following surgery regained full visual function after an emergency decompression of the periorbita. Other reviews have reported vision loss in 0.5–1.0% of patients following craniofacial surgery.[5,6]

Dura

The intimate association between the skull and the underlying dura makes careful elevation of bone flaps and subcranial dissection imperative. Neurosurgical support is very useful for cranial osteotomies following the initial frontal craniotomy and visualization of the anterior and middle cranial fossa (sphenoid ridge) during frontal bar advancement. Secondary transcranial procedures may involve dissection around cranial defects that could lead to compromise of the dura and cerebral spinal fluid (CSF) leaks if the defect is not recognized.

Dural tears were recognized in 10% of patients in one review, but no subsequent postoperative CSF leaks were reported.[5] In a second review the majority of the dural leaks closed spontaneously within 48 hours in most patients (cessation of CSF leaks), but three patients required a dural 'patch' for persistent drainage.[13] Dural tears should be repaired appropriately when identified. Postoperatively, large CSF leaks may require a lumbar drain for several days.

Facial nerve

Knowledge of the course of the facial nerve is required for any procedure in the region of the face and neck. Traditional craniofacial approaches use tissue planes deep to the level of the frontal branch of the facial nerve. Exposure of the zygomatic arch can be completed in the avascular plane between the superficial and deep layers of the deep temporal fascia. The dissection is completed without cautery. Alternatively, the zygomatic arch may be approached anterior to posterior in the subperiosteal plane from the lateral orbital rim. It is at the zygomatic arch where the facial nerve is least protected by the soft tissues. Damage to the frontal branch of the facial nerve may produce ptosis, brow asymmetry and an inability to wrinkle the forehead. Frontal nerve palsy has been reported, but the occurrence is rare (0.3–0.5%).[13,14] A neuropraxia of the frontal branch is often seen following extensive dissection and retraction. The symptoms usually improve in 6–8 weeks, therefore facial nerve dysfunction should undergo several months of observation prior to treatment.

Other nerves at risk during craniofacial exposure include the supraorbital (which often requires release from its foramina), the supratrochlear and the infraorbital.

Major blood vessels

Blood loss from major craniofacial procedures is usually insidious following osteotomies and large areas of bleeding surfaces. However, major blood vessels may also be injured, causing acute exsanguination. A transcranial approach can involve dissection or elevation of the bone over the midline sagittal sinus. Careful neurosurgical techniques of hemostasis can usually resolve the bleeding. If the bleeding is unmanageable, the sinus may be ligated in the anterior region of the sinus up to one-third of its length, with limited risk of focal injury to the brain parenchyma. The craniofacial surgeon should also be aware of the middle meningeal artery when dissecting around the sphenoid ridge. Finally, damage to these vessels may occur during rigid fixation if the screws are not carefully placed.

Major arteries of the midfacial skeleton are usually located in poorly accessible regions. A subperiosteal dissection in the midface should protect against damage to the sphenopalatine vessels. If excessive bleeding does occur from these vessels during exposure for Le Fort osteotomies, options may be limited and include extensive packing and, if necessary, abortion of the procedure until the blood loss is controlled and the patient adequately resuscitated. Emergency embolization by an interventional radiologist may also be considered if the bleeding is not controlled. Likewise, dissection in the temporal fossa within the soft tissue may lead to injury of the internal maxillary artery and deep temporal vessels. Packing may again be required if visibility is poor. Proximal control can be obtained via the external carotid artery in severe cases.

Dentition

It is recognized that osteotomies of the midface in children may disrupt normal tooth development. Browne and associates[15] demonstrated pulp damage in 31% of maxillary tooth pulps examined after a Le Fort I osteotomy. Subsequent studies appeared to show a transient deleterious effect on the tooth pulp, but little long-term change in development or viability.[16,17] Grayson and associates[18] did identify misplaced or damaged maxillary molars, with failure to erupt, in 30% of patients following Le Fort I osteotomies. Because of the potential derangement of tooth eruption, most authors recommend that procedures on the midface involving Le Fort osteotomies be completed after the age of 5 or 6.

DIRECT COMPLICATIONS: DONOR SITE

A second surgical site is often required for harvesting bone and cartilage, and can be associated with significant morbidity. Split thickness calvarial bone grafts are commonly used to supplement the facial skeleton. The greatest thickness of calvarial bone occurs in the parietal bone and mid-occipital regions (8–10 mm in adults and 3–5 mm in children).[19,20] When harvesting split thickness calvarial bone in situ, the integrity of the inner layer of cortical bone should be maintained to protect the dura. Complications have been reported, especially when the surgeon is unfamiliar with harvesting techniques.[21] Obtaining split thickness bone may be difficult in patients under 3 years old (inadequate development of diploe) or in those with a history of elevated intracranial pressure, in whom the bone is often abnormally thin and the potential for hemorrhage is increased.[22]

Rib grafts may also be used, either whole or split. Overall complication rates have ranged from 12% to 30%.[13,23] Significant resorption has been observed if the graft is not rigidly fixed, and rib grafts are especially susceptible to resorption in the zygomatic arch region.[6,24] Rib grafts are usually unacceptable for reconstruction of the forehead region because of the likelihood of producing a 'washboard' appearance. Inadvertent splinting of the ipsilateral chest secondary to pain following rib harvesting can induce hypoxemia in some young children. There have been reports of secondary brain edema because of hypoxemia following rib graft harvesting in major craniofacial procedures.[24] The incidence of pneumothorax when rib harvesting has been reported to be from 5% to 30%,[13] but increases significantly with the harvest of larger amounts of cartilage. Finally, functionally significant thoracic defects have been described following rib harvesting.[25]

The iliac crest has traditionally been a source of large amounts of bone. Cancellous bone is usually abundant and resorption appears to be less in craniofacial operations using corticocancellous iliac grafts than with rib grafts. Postoperative pain may be significant and can persist for months. A deformity of the anterior iliac crest may occur, as well as abdominal hernias and numbness in the distribution of the lateral femoral cutaneous nerve. Most of these complications can be avoided by a properly placed posterior skin incision and dissection in a subperiosteal plane.[26] No evidence of asymmetry from growth abnormalities of the harvested side has been shown, but disturbance of the cartilaginous cap can be minimized in young patients by a medial approach through the inner table of the crest.

IMMEDIATE POSTOPERATIVE COMPLICATIONS

INFECTION

Infection is the most common postoperative complication in craniofacial surgery. The bone and soft tissues of the face are very well vascularized and allow for extensive exposure of the facial skeleton, but several unique characteristics of craniofacial technique and exposure increase the potential for infection. These include devascularization of the facial skeleton through subperiosteal exposure and osteotomies, the need for transfusions, and the proximity of the operative site to areas of contamination, including the sinuses and the oral cavity.

Overall complication rates secondary to infection have been reported between 0.55 and 4.5%[12,13] (Table 57.2). Transcranial involvement increases the risk of infection (up to 29% in two reviews). David and associates[27] also reported infective complications in 6.5% of patients who underwent transcranial procedures: 70% of the infections in this review occurred after reoperation and 73% were in adults.

A recent review of infection rates following transcranial procedures at two major craniofacial centers revealed a decrease in the overall infection rate, from 6.2% previously reported by Whitaker and associates[13] to 2.5%.[28] Comparisons were also made between the two centers with regard to hair shaving, length of procedure (5.9 h vs 7.1 h) and the type of prophylactic antibiotic used (third-generation vs first-generation cephalosporins). No differences in infection rates were seen: 85% of the patients with infection had reoperative procedures and no infection was seen in patients under 13 months of age.

The most common Gram-positive organisms identified with craniofacial infections were either *Staphylococcus* or *Streptococcus* species. *Pseudomonas* species were the most common Gram-negative organism reported.[28]

From a review of infection rates at various craniofacial centers, several consistent risk factors for infection have emerged. Reoperations to the midface and cranial vault lead to a higher infection rate. This is probably related to three factors. First, the facial skeleton is further devascu-

Table 57.2 Postoperative infection following craniofacial surgery

Reference	Infection rates (%)			Infection (%)		Common organism
	Overall	Extracranial	Transcranial	In redo	In adults	
Whitaker et al[13]	4.4	2.3	6.2	—	—	Mixed flora
Wolfe et al[12]	1.2	—	1.7	—	—	*Staphylococcus* sp. *Pseudomonas* sp.
David et al[27]	—	—	6.5	70	73	*Staphylococcus* sp. *Streptococcus* sp. *Pseudomonas* sp. *Klebsiella* sp.
Fearon et al[28]	—	—	2.5	85	100	*Pseudomonas* sp. *Candida albicans*

*No infections were seen in patients under 13 years of age.

larized as a result of secondary and tertiary dissections and osteotomies. Therefore, the antibiotic load delivered to the bone is decreased. Repeat osteotomies also increase the risk of sequestration and avascular necrosis.[29] Secondly, the difficulty of a second procedure may increase the length of the operation and hence the risk of infection. Finally, second procedures are usually undertaken in older patients with better-developed sinus cavities. The sinuses, which contain colonized organisms, are often in the region of the osteotomy and therefore contaminate the surgical site. Limited bone debridement, intravenous antibiotics and continuous irrigation in selected cases have proven to be effective in the treatment of most postoperative infections[28] (Fig. 57.2).

MONOBLOC FACIAL ADVANCEMENT

In 1969, Tessier completed the first monobloc facial advancement.[30] The procedure was first cited in the literature in 1974 by Converse and associates.[31] However, the concept was 'reintroduced' in 1978 by Ortiz-Monasterio,[32] in a description of seven patients who underwent this procedure with minimal complications. The technique incorporates both midface advancement and transcranial vault remodeling/frontal bar advancement. Following the advancement, the nasal cavity and sinuses are exposed to the newly expanded intracranial dead space. Because of this, controversy exists regarding the potential infection and bone loss following the procedure.

In a series of 32 patients who underwent a successful monobloc advancement, one patient experienced a postoperative infection (3.1%) and there was one non-infectious complication[30] (Table 57.3). Patients were grouped into two categories. Monobloc advancements were accomplished in patients less than 2 years old who required correction of severe exophthalmos and presented with significant nasal obstruction. The second group of patients (3–14 years old)

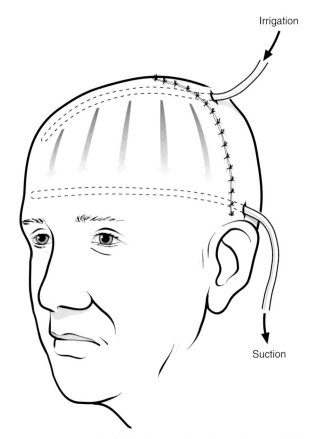

Irrigation

Suction

Fig. 57.2 Most craniofacial infections may be adequately treated with placement of an irrigation system. (Reproduced with permission from Fearon et al[28])

Table 57.3 Complications following monobloc frontofacial advancement

Reference	n	Overall (%)	Infection (%)	Non-infectious (%)	Death (%)
Wolfe[30]	32	2 (6.3)	1 (3.1)	1 (3.1)	0 (0.0)
Whitaker[60]	10	10 (100.0)	5 (50.0)	5 (50.0)	0 (0.0)
Kawamoto[34] (1997)	26	18 (69.1)	1 (3.8)	17 (65.3)	0 (0.0)

underwent the procedure for dysmorphism of the upper and midfacial regions. In the author's opinion, the most significant event in decreasing the rate of infection was the quick expansion of the brain into the newly created dead space. It was felt that this expansion is either delayed or not achieved in older patients, therefore patients over 14 did not undergo monobloc advancement.

Whitaker and associates reported a major infection rate of 20% and an overall complication rate of 100% in a review of monobloc procedures in 10 patients.[33] This was compared to 20 patients with extracranial Le Fort II advancements, of which only one experienced a transient infection. Non-infectious complications were comparable in both groups. Because of these findings, it was recommended that a staged procedure be performed for patients requiring correction of both frontal and midfacial regions. Finally, in a recent review of 26 patients undergoing monobloc advancement Benhaim and Kawamoto reported an overall complication rate of 69.1% but an infection rate of only 3.8% (one patient). Under specific guidelines outlined by the authors, the procedure was felt to be effective and safe. No deaths were reported in any of the previous reviews.[34]

Proponents of the monobloc procedure feel that the postoperative results, when combined with a facial bipartition, are excellent and address deficiencies in multiple regions of the face with a single procedure.[12] It has been questioned whether the results of monobloc advancement can be obtained using a staged procedure, which might possibly be safer.[33]

NON-INFECTIOUS COMPLICATIONS

Complications other than infection may also be seen in the postoperative period. In a recent review of 204 patients treated for non-syndromic craniosynostoses, seven patients developed SIADH (Syndrome of Inappropriate ADH secretion) (four in the sagittal vault remodeling group). Other complications included severe chemosis, urethritis and tear duct obstruction (Table 57.4).[14] Oh and associates[35] reviewed their 10-year experience. including 57 consecutive craniofacial surgeries. Non-infectious complications included loss of vision and persistent CSF leaks (Table 57.5). An increase in the length of the surgery was the only corollary to higher complication rates. CSF leaks and facial nerve paralysis may be first recognized in the immediate postoperative period. Metabolic abnormalities, including coagulopathies and hypovolemia, may also be present and should be corrected.

DELAYED POSTOPERATIVE COMPLICATIONS

RECURRENT INTRACRANIAL HYPERTENSION

Extended or delayed postoperative complications are seen after the initial postoperative hospitalization period and may present several years following the procedure. Included are patients who present with evidence of recurrent intracranial hypertension after corrective surgery.[36] Patients should

Table 57.4 Complications following treatment for craniosynostosis

Diagnosis	n	Perioperative (%)	Description	Postoperative (%)	Description
Non-syndromic					
Unicoronal	26	0 (0)		2 (8)	wound infection, frontal branch paresis
Bicoronal	15	2 (13)	CSF leak, urethritis (1)	0 (0)	
Metopic	51	8 (16)	Conjunctival chemosis Fever, SIADH (2) Hyponatremia, RSV	1 (2)	ICP
Sagittal	102	9 (9)	Hypovolemia (4) SIADH (5)	0 (0)	
Multiple	10	1 (10)	Hypovolemia	1 (10)	tear duct obstruction
Total	204	20 (9.8)		4 (2.0)	
Syndromic					
Syndromic	23	16 (70)	Tracheostomy (2) CSF (2) Abscess (2) SIADH (4) Hematoma RSV Pressure ulcer UTI	2 (9)	Subdural fluid CSF leak

Table 57.5 Complications are categorized according to the diagnosis. The diagnoses were divided into Tessier's five major categories as follows: group 1, orbital hypotelorism and hypertelorism; group 2, craniofacial dysostosis; group 3, facial clefts; group 4, trauma; group 5, tumors. (From Oh et al,[35] with permission)

Complication	Group 1 (n = 3)	Group 2 (n = 29)	Group 3 (n = 1)	Group 4 (n = 1)	Group 5 (n = 16)	Total
Type I: disastrous or life-threatening						
Death (from meningitis)	1	–	–	–	–	1
Immediate postoperative cardiac arrest	–	–	–	–	1	1
Type II: major complications						
Near-total unilateral visual loss	–	–	–	–	2	2
Persistent CSF leak	–	1	–	–	–	1
Type III: minor complications						
Hematoma/seroma	–	6	–	–	4	10
Wound infection	–	5	–	–	2	7
Temporary ocular motor disturbances	–	1	1	–	4	6
Bony defect	–	2	–	–	1	3
Atelectasis	–	2[a]	–	–	1	3
Laryngeal edema	–	1	–	–	2	3
URI/pneumonia	–	3	–	–	–	3
Keratoconjunctivitis	–	2	–	–	1	3
Temporary injury to frontal branch VII	–	–	–	–	3	3
Temporary SIADH	–	1	–	–	–	1
Temporary CSF leak	–	–	–	–	1	1
Temporary injury to supraorbital nerve	–	–	–	–	1	1
Urticaria	–	1	–	–	–	1
Intubation granuloma	–	–	–	–	1	1
Acute renal failure	–	1[b]	–	–	–	1
Total	1	28	1	0	26	56

[a]One patient had a pre-existing respiratory disease
[b]Pre-existing renal disease
CSF, cerebrospinal fluid; URI, upper respiratory infection; SIADH, syndrome of inappropriate antidiuretic hormone

be followed at regular intervals in a multidisciplinary craniofacial clinic for several years postoperatively. Symptoms suspicious of elevated intracranial pressure should be evaluated by ophthalmologic, neurologic and radiographic examinations. Evidence of recurrent intracranial hypertension requires a secondary cranial vault remodeling.

RIGID FIXATION

The use of rigid fixation in the craniofacial skeleton has dramatically improved outcomes and decreased morbidity and the length of the surgical procedures. Complications have been limited to palpation of the plates and screws in thin-skinned areas, occasional extrusion through the skin, and infrequent reports of infection secondary to the foreign material.[37–42] Recently, two issues emerged with the use of rigid fixation in the patient with a growing craniofacial skeleton (less than 3 years old).

The phenomenon of passive or false migration of plates and screws in the infant skull was initially reported in 1994.[43,44] Subsequent studies confirmed the translocation of plates and screws from extracranial to intracalvarial and intracranial positions. Papay and associates[45] reported a 35% incidence of plate migration in patients who underwent secondary cranial vault remodeling. Goldberg and associates[46] also demonstrated internalization of plates and screws in 14 of 27 pediatric patients evaluated by CT (average follow-up 25 months). In less than 36 months, 14% of all plates placed in this patient population showed evidence of internalization (7.5% intracalvarially, 6.6% intracranially); 80% of all migrations occurred in the temporal region, and syndromic patients demonstrated higher translocation rates than the non-syndromic group. Vander Kolk[47] also reported migration of 27.7% of plates on CT scans in 50 consecutive patients who underwent craniofacial procedures (greater than 1 year follow-up). Thirteen of the plates were found to be intracranial and eight were located in the frontal/temporal region. It is apparent that internalization of the miniplates occurs in patients with growing skulls. The preponderance of migration in the temporal region may reflect the unique growth patterns of this region of the skull in this dysmorphic patient population. Finally, no significant complications have been reported from translocation of the plates into the cranium. The recent development and clinical use of absorbable plates and screws may reduce concern about transcranial plate migration.

The second area of interest in the use of rigid fixation has been the potential inhibition of facial growth in children. Numerous animal studies have been performed using rigid fixation of cranial vault sutures and the frontonasal sutures. Evidence of regional growth restrictions was consistently found using either rigid or stainless steel wire fixation.[48–50] Furthermore, rigid fixation of the cranial vault that did not involve sutures also resulted in local growth restrictions.[51]

The impact of these findings on the treatment of patients with craniofacial disorders is unclear. Growth abnormalities independent of surgical procedures in this patient population are common, and often severe. The inhibition of potential normal growth after corrective procedures compared to a control group of patients with surgery is difficult to determine. Furthermore, overcorrection of the deformity is usually attempted in order to eliminate the need for a second procedure, and thereby decrease the need for further growth of the involved skeleton. Finally, most surgeons use a combination of rigid fixation, resorbable plates and resorbable sutures to accomplish the reconstruction. This may also minimize any possible inhibition of growth following surgery.

Nevertheless, the recent introduction of resorbable plates and screws means that the use of permanent fixation materials can be avoided.[52] Complications using resorbable materials have been very few,[53–56] and applications have included pediatric craniofacial surgery and the repair of traumatic midfacial and calvarial injuries.[57,58] In the largest series to date, no complications were noted after use in 100 patients.[59] Four patients required removal of the plates between 9 and 18 months, secondary to palpation. Most studies support the safe use of the resorbable plating system for craniofacial procedures. Long-term follow-up studies of outcome results are not yet available.

REOPERATION RATES

The rate of reoperation is an important outcome variable in the surgical treatment of craniosynostosis. Although quantitative changes in craniofacial shape and remodeling are critical to understanding operative results, the decision to reoperate on a particular child is determined primarily from subjective measures of outcome, most commonly esthetic appearance. Longitudinal studies of reoperation rates from a variety of centers are beginning to appear in the literature.[60–64] In a recent review, a prospective statistical study of reoperation rates was completed in the treatment of 167 consecutive children with non-syndromic and syndromic craniosynostosis over a 6-year period.[14] Mean

length of follow-up was 2.8 years. Fronto-orbital remodeling with a floating forehead was completed at 4–6 months of age for non-syndromic synostoses other than sagittal synostoses. Strip craniectomies were limited to sagittal synostoses with mild to moderate deformities. Total cranial vault remodeling was completed for severe scaphocephaly if the patient was older than 7 weeks. Patients with syndromic craniosynostoses underwent fronto-orbital advancement and cranial reshaping at 4–6 months unless increased cranial pressure required decompression.

Reoperation equal to or exceeding the magnitude of the original procedure occurred in 7% of cases. Total reoperation rates for syndromic and non-syndromic synostoses were 27.3% and 5.9%, respectively. Five of the 12 reoperative cases (41.6%) were completed for significant relapse as demonstrated clinically and radiographically (Table 57.3). The highest reoperative rate in non-syndromic children was found in bicoronal synostosis. In children with single synostoses, reoperative rates were highest with sagittal suture fusion requiring total vault remodeling (6.45%). Reoperative rates in metopic fusion were 2.86%, with an average follow-up of 42 months. The differences in reoperative rates for the various single suture synostoses were not found to be statistically significant.

Multiple regression analysis revealed that females and children with syndromic synostoses were more likely to require reoperation (Table 57.6). The reason for the increased odds ratio associated with females is unknown. The age of the patient at the time of the procedure did not appear to have an effect on reoperation rates: a 1-year increase in age at operation was not statistically significant after controlling for diagnostic group, nor was the effect of an increase in estimated blood loss (100 ml increments). Similarly, length of hospital stay, length of surgery, intensive care

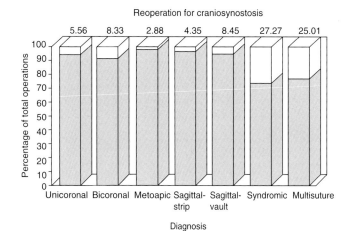

Fig. 57.3 Reoperation rates for craniosynostosis categorized by diagnosis. (From Williams et al.[14] with permission).

Table 57.6 Multivariate analysis of total reoperation rates. (From Williams et al,[14] with permission)

Control variable	Syndromic vs. non-syndromic	Sagittal vault vs. other	Only control variable (*P* value)
None	6.0	1.1	–
Female gender	5.9	1.3	3.9 (0.04)
Age at surgery (1 yr)	9.7	0.7	0.6 (0.19)
Blood loss (each 100 units)	6.4	0.4	1.1 (0.31)
Length of stay (days)	1.3	0.5	1.2 (0.07)
Length of surgery (each 100 min)	5.2	0.5	1.3 (0.53)
Months of follow-up	5.7	1.1	1.1 (0.74)
Any ICU stay	9.1	1.7	0.6 (0.59)
Any transfusion	6.3	0.5	2.3 (0.46)
Any complications	4.2	0.9	5.7
Early complications	4.4	0.8	2.4
Late complications	5.0	1.4	6.2

The odds ratio for each variable is given independent of other variables and controlling for diagnostic group. For example, the risk of total reoperation for a female patient is 3.9 times higher than for a male patient. The variable is independent of the diagnosis (6.0 vs 5.9). On the contrary, the risk of total reoperation as the length of stay increases is marginal (1.1), but is directly related to the diagnosis (6.0 vs 1.3).

unit admission and the amount of transfusion were not statistically significant after controlling for diagnostic category.

Whitaker's classification (Table 57.7) of clinical results after craniofacial procedures includes category III (CIII), requiring major bone grafting or other osteotomies, and category IV (CIV) requiring duplication of the previous craniofacial procedure.[60] Whitaker and associates showed a CIV reoperation rate of 3% for asymmetrical lesions (isolated synostosis) and 64% for the symmetrical lesions (95% in Apert syndrome). Excluding strip craniectomies, McCarthy had a 6.7% reoperation rate for isolated synostosis and 28.3% for syndromic deformities.[61,62] Again, the highest reoperation rate was found in Apert syndrome (37.5%). Finally, Wall and associates[64] demonstrated a reoperation rate of 5.1% for single suture synostosis and 10.8% for syndromic cases. Similar surgical approaches were utilized in each of the aforementioned studies. Other studies demonstrated similar differences in the reoperation rate between the two groups, but were not comparable in surgical technique.[60,63]

In most studies no differences were seen in reoperation rates for the treatment of single suture stenosis as related to age;[65,66] recommendations for primary intervention range from 2 to 18 months.[60–62] Wall and associates[64] showed an increased reoperation rate of 20% in non-syndromic synostosis when primary treatment was at less than 6 months of age, compared to 5.6% in patients older than 6 months. In syndromic disorders, patients under 6 months had a 30.2% reoperation rate, compared to 9.1% in those over 6 months (40.9 months follow-up). Other reviews have shown no relationship between age and reoperation rates.

In summary, adequate presurgical planning and adherence to correct craniofacial techniques will yield acceptably low complication rates. The standard of care (e.g. maintaining acceptable complication rates) in craniofacial surgery is best accomplished in centers that maintain a high volume and experience. The surgeon should never underestimate the value of an intimate knowledge of the anatomic relationships between the various facial structures.

Table 57.7 Whitaker's classification of outcome following craniofacial surgery (From Whitaker LA, Bartlett SP 1987 The craniofacial dysostoses: guidelines for management of the symmetric and asymmetric deformities. Clinics in Plastic Surgery 14:73–81, with permission)

Category I:	No refinements or surgical revisions considered
Category II:	Soft-tissue or lesser bone-contouring revisions desirable or performed
Category III:	Major alternative osteotomies or bone-grafting procedures needed or performed
Category IV:	Major craniofacial procedure duplicating or exceeding in extent original surgery needed or performed

REFERENCES

1. McCarthy JG, Cutting CB 1990 The timing of surgical intervention in craniofacial anomalies. Clinics in Plastic Surgery 17:161
2. Posnick JC 1992 Craniosynostosis: surgical management in infancy. In: Bell WH (ed) Orthognathic and reconstructive surgery. WB Saunders, Philadelphia, pp 1889–1931
3. McCarthy JG, Epstein F, Sadove M et al 1984 Early surgery for craniofacial synostosis. An 8-year experience. Plastic and Reconstructive Surgery 73:521
4. Whitaker LA, Schut L, Kerr LP 1977 Early surgery for isolated craniofacial dysostosis. Plastic and Reconstructive Surgery 60:575
5. Harrop CW, Avery BS, Marks SM, Putnam GD 1996

Craniosynostosis in babies: complications and management of 40 cases. British Journal of Oral and Maxillofacial Surgery 34:158

6. Goodrich JT, Hall CD 1995 Evaluation and management of complications in craniofacial surgery. In: Goodrich JT, Hall CD (eds) Craniofacial anomalies: growth and development from a surgical perspective. Thieme Medical Publishers, New York, p194

7. Meyer, P, Renier D, Arnard E et al 1993 Blood loss during repair of craniosynostosis British Journal of Anaesthesia. 71:854–857

8. Eaton AC, Marsh JL, Pilgram TK 1995 Transfusion requirements for craniosynotosis surgery in infants. Plastic and Reconstructive Surgery 95:277–283

9. Phillips RL, Mullken JB 1988 Venous air embolism during a craniofacial procedure. Plastic and Reconstructive Surgery 82:155

10. Cannell DM, Hopkins LN 1990 Superior sagittal sinus laceration complicating an autogenous calvarial bone graft harvest: report of a case. Journal of Oral and Maxillofacial Surgery 48:741

11. Tessier P 1981 Complications of major craniofacial surgery. In: Tessier P, Rougier J, Hervouet F, Woiller M, Lekieffre M, Derome P (eds) Plastic surgery of the orbit and eyelids (translated by S.A. Wolfe). Masson, New York, p 254

12. Wolfe SA 1989 Complications. In: Wolfe SA, Berkowitz S (eds) Plastic surgery of the facial skeleton. Little, Brown, Boston, p 763

13. Whitaker LA, Munro IR, Salyer KE, Jackson IT, Ortiz-Monasterio F, Marchac D 1979 Combined report of problems and complications in 793 craniofacial operations Plastic and Reconstructive Surgery 64:198

14. Williams JK, Cohen SR, Burstein FD et al 1997 A longitudinal statistical study of reoperation rates in craniosynostosis. Plastic and Reconstructive Surgery 100:305

15. Browne RM, Brady CL, Frame JW 1990 Tooth pulp changes following Le Fort I maxillary osteotomy in a primate model. British Journal of Oral and Maxillofacial Surgery 28:1

16. Di S, Bell W H, Mannai C et al 1988 Long-term evaluation of human teeth after Le Fort I osteotomy: a histologic and developmental study. Oral Surgery Oral Medicine Oral Pathology 65:379

17. Andreasen JO, Paulsen HU, Yu Z, Bayer T, Schwartz O 1990 A long-term study of 370 autotransplanted premolars. Part II, tooth survival and pulp healing subsequent to transplantation. European Journal of Orthodontics 12:14

18. Grayson BH, et al

19. Cavalcante D, Casanova R, Psillakis JM 1984 Anatomical study of calvarial thickness. Paper presented at the XXI Brazilian Plastic Surgery Meeting, November 1984, Rio de Janeiro, Brazil

20. Pensler J, McCarthy JG 1985 The calvarial donor site: an anatomic study in cadavers. Plastic and Reconstructive Surgery 75:648

21. Kline RM, Wolfe SA 1995 Complications associated with the harvesting of ranial bone grafts. Plastic and Reconstructive Surgery 95:5

22. Koenig WJ, Donovan JM, Pensler JM 1995 Cranial bone grafting in children. Plastic and Reconstructive Surgery 95:1

23. Salyer KE, Taylor DP 1987 Bone grafts in craniofacial surgery. Clinics in Plastic Surgery 14:27

24. Habal MB 1992 Craniofacial surgery. In: Habal MB, Reddi AH (eds) Bone grafts and bone substitutes. WB Saunders, Philadelphia, p 316

25. Thompson HG, Kim TY, Ein SH 1995 Residual problems in chest donor sites after microtia reconstruction: a long term study. Plastic and Reconstructive Surgery 95:761

26. Crockford DA, Converse JM 1997 The ilium as a source of bone grafts in children. Plastic and Reconstructive Surgery

27. David DJ, Cooter RD 1987 Craniofacial infection in10 years of transcranial surgery. Plastic and Reconstructive Surgery 80:213

28. Fadron JA, Yu J, Bartlett SP et al 1977 Infections in craniofacial surgery: a combined report of 567 procedures from two centers. Plastic and Reconstructive Surgery 100:862

29. Zellin Z, Alberus P, Lunde A 1997 Repeat bone repositioning in the growing rabbit calvarium hampers bone segment incorporation. Plastic and Reconstructive Surgery 100:619–626

30. Wolfe AS, Morrison G, Page LK et al 1989 The monobloc frontofacial advancement. Do the pluses outweigh the minuses? Plastic and Reconstructive Surgery 91:977–987

31. Firmin F, Coccaro PJ, Converse JM 1974 Cephalometric analysis in diagnosis and treatment of craniofacial synostoses. Plastic and Reconstructive Surgery 54:300

32. Ortiz-Monasterio F, Fuente del Campo A, Carrillo A 1978 Advancement of the orbits and the midface in one piece, combined with frontal repositioning for the correction of Crouzon deformities. Plastic and Reconstructive Surgery 61:507

33. Fearon JA, Whitaker LA 1993 Complications with facial advancement: a comparison between the Le Fort III and monobloc advancements. Plastic and Reconstructive Surgery 91:990–995

34. Benhaim P, Longaker MT, Kawamoto HK 1997 Monobloc frontofacial advancement: The UCLA experience 1988–1996. VII Congress of the International Society of Craniofacial Surgery, Santa Fe, NM, USA, pp81–82

35. Oh AK, Kim S, Wang KC et al 1997 Complications of pediatric craniofacial surgery in the orient: analysis of a 10 year experience. Journal of Craniofacial Surgery 8:340

36. Cohen SR, Dauser RC, Newman MH et al 1993 Surgical techniques of cranial vault expansion for increases in intracranial pressure in older children. Journal of Craniofacial Surgery 4:167

37. Sadove AM, Eppley BL 1991 Microfixation techniques in pediatric craniomaxillofacial surgery. Annals of Plastic Surgery 27:36

38. Eppley BL, Sadove AM 1991 Application of microfixation techniques in reconstructive maxillofacial surgery. Journal of Oral and Maxillofacial Surgery 49:683

39. Bartlett SP, Delozier JB 1992 Controversies in the management of peiatric facial fractures. Clinics in Plastic Surgery 19:245

40. Francel TJ, Birely BC, Ringelman PR, Manson PN 1992 The fate of plates and screws in facial fracture reconstruction. Plastic and Reconstructive Surgery 90:568

41. Marshall MA, Chikylio SA, Figueroa AA, Cohen M 1991 Long-term effects of rigid fixation on the growing craniomaxillofacial skeleton. Journal of Craniofacial Surgery 2:63

42. Zachariades N, Papademetriou I, Rallis G 1993 Complications associated with rigid internal fixation of facial bone fractures. Journal of Oral and Maxillofacial Surgery 51:275

43. Yu JY, Goldberg Ds, Bartlett SP et al 1994 A critical review of microfixation in pediatric craniofacial surgery: the passive intracranial translocation of microplates and screws. Presented at the 80th Annual Clinical Congress of the American College of Surgeons, Chicago

44. Yu JY, Goldberg DS, Bartlett SP et al 1994 The long term positional stability of microfixation on the growing swine craniofacial skeleton. Presented at the Annual Meeting of the American Society of Plastic and Reconstructive Surgeons, San Diego

45. Papay FA, Hardy S, Morales L et al 1995 'False' migration of rigid fixation appliances in pediatric craniofacial surgery. Journal of Craniofacial Surgery 6:309

46. Goldberg DS, Bartlett SP, Yu JC et al 1995 Critical review of microfixation in pediatric craniofacial surgery. Journal of Craniofacial Surgery 6:301

47. Vander Kolk C, Mofid MM, Robertson B et al 1997 New observations on plate and screw fixation and cranial growth. Presented at the International Society of Craniofacial Surgery, Sante Fe, New Mexico

48. Polley JW, Figueroa A, Hung KF et al 1995 Effect of rigid microfixation on the craniomaxillofacial skeleton. Journal of Craniofacial Surgery 6:132

49. Marschall MA, Chikylio SA, Figueroa AA et al 1991 Long-term effects of rigid fixation on the growing craniomaxillofacial skeleton. Journal of Craniofacial Surgery 2:63

50. Yaremchuk MJ 1994 Experimental studies addressing rigid fixation in craniofacial surgery. Clinics in Plastic Surgery 21:517

51. Wong L, Dufresne CR, Richtsmeier JT et al 1991 The effect of rigid fixation on growth or the neurocranium. Plastic and Recosntructive Surgery 88:395

52. Pietraz WS, Sarver D, Verstynen ML 1997 Bioabsorbable polymer science for the practicing surgeon. Journal of Craniofacial Surgery 8:87

53. Kumar AV, Staffenberg DA, Petronio JA et al 1997 Bioabsorbable plates and screws in pediatric craniofacial surgery: a review of 22 cases. Journal of Craniofacial Surgery 8:97

54. Montag ME, Morales L, Daane S 1997 Bioabsorbables: their use in pediatric craniofacial surgery. Journal of Craniofacial Surgery 8:100

55. Goldstein JA 1997 A preventable complication of lactosorb craniomaxillofacial fixation. Journal of Craniofacial Surgery 8:151

56. Pensler JM 1997 Role of resorbable plates and screws in craniofacial surgery. Journal of Craniofacial Surgery 8:129

57. Tatum SA, Kellman RM, Freije JE 1997 Maxillofacial fixation with absorbable miniplates: computed tomographic follow-up. Journal of Craniofacial Surgery 8:135

58. Eppley BL 1997 Potential for guided bone regeneration and bone graft fixation with resorbable membranes in pediatric craniofacial surgery. Journal of Craniofacial Surgery 8:116

59. Eppley BL, Sadove AM, Havlik RJ 1997 Resorbable plate fixation in pediatric craniofacial surgery. Plastic and Reconstructive Surgery 100:1

60. Whitaker LA, Barlett, Schut L, Bruce D 1987 Craniosynostosis: an analysis of the timing, treatment and complications in 164 consecutive patients. Plastic and Reconstructive Surgery 80:195

61. McCarthy JG, Glasberb SB, Cutting CB et al 1995 Twenty-year experience with early surgery for craniosynostosis: I Isolated craniofacial synostosis results and unsolved problems. Plastic and Reconstructive Surgery 96:272

62. McCarthy JG, Glasberg SB, Cutting CB et al 1995 Twenty-year experience with early surgery for craniosynostosis: II The craniofacial synostosis syndromes and pansynostosis – results and unsolved problems. Plastic and Reconstructive surgery 96:284

63. Colak A, Tahta K, Bertan V et al 1992 Craniosynostosis: a review of 143 surgically treated cases. Turkish Journal of Pediatrics 34:231

64. Wall SA, Goldin JH, Hockley AD, Wake MJC, Poole MD, Briggs M 1994 Fronto-orbital reoperation in craniosynostosis. British Journal of Plastic Surgery 47:180

65. Di Rocco C, Marchese E, Velardi F 1992 Craniosynostosis: surgical treatment during the first year of life. Journal of Neurosurgical Sciences 36:129

66. Prevot M, Renier D, Niarchac D 1993 Lack of ossification after cranioplasty for craniosynostosis: a review of relevant factors in 592 consecutive patients. Journal of Craniofacial Surgery 4:247

Hemifacial microsomia: the disorder and its surgical management

58

GERALD J. KEARNS/BONNIE L. PADWA/LEONARD B. KABAN

INTRODUCTION

Hemifacial microsomia (HFM) is a progressive, asymmetric craniofacial malformation, variably affecting structures derived from the first and second pharyngeal arches. It is characterized by structural abnormalities of the orbit, maxilla, mandible, external and middle ear, cranial nerves and facial soft tissues. Associated anomalies include ear tags (40%), epibulbar dermoids (20%), and macrostomia (61%).[1] The term HFM was first used by Gorlin Pindborg in 1964,[2] however the features of this condition were well recognized prior to that time. Other descriptive names assigned to the constellation of clinical features seen in HFM include: first and second branchial arch deformity,[3] oculoauriculovertebral spectrum,[4] oculoauriculovertebral dysplasia,[5] otomandibular dysostosis,[6] lateral facial dysplasia,[7] and unilateral craniofacial microsomia.[8] Goldenhar syndrome[9] was considered to be a variant of HFM, characterized by additional anomalies of the ribs and vertebrae and the presence of epibulbar dermoids. The multitude of labels assigned to what is essentially the same condition indicates an incomplete understanding of the genetics, etiology, pathogenesis and, ultimately, the management of HFM. The authors recommend the use of the term 'hemifacial microsomia', which was suggested by Mulliken[10] because of its 'brevity, clarity and euphony'.

EPIDEMIOLOGY

HFM is the second most common craniofacial anomaly after cleft lip and palate.[11,12] The reported incidence ranges from 1 in 3500[13] to 1 in 26,500 live births[14] because of the variable definition and confusion in terminology. How-ever, the most frequently reported incidence is 1 in 5600 live births.[3] Males and females are affected equally, with no difference in the predominant side (left versus right), and 16% of cases are bilateral. The hallmark of HFM, whether unilateral or bilateral, is asymmetry. This is in contrast to Treacher Collins syndrome which is a symmetrical deformity.

ETIOLOGY

The etiology of HFM is not well understood, but the wide spectrum of clinical manifestations suggests that it may be variable and heterogenous. Teratogenic agents such as thalidomide,[3] primidone[15] and retinoic acid[16] have been associated with congenital first and second arch defects in humans. HFM is probably not an inherited condition and most reported cases are isolated and sporadic. However, multiple occurrences in families have also been reported[3,17] and both discordance[18,19] and concordance[20,21] have occurred in monozygotic twins. The importance of the sporadic nature of HFM is evident when genetic counseling is provided to patients and families.

PATHOGENESIS

The mechanism by which HFM develops in humans is unknown. There are two pathogenic theories, one involving the vascular system[13] and the other neuroectodermal cell migration.[22] The 'stapedial artery hematoma' theory was proposed by Poswillo.[13] In 1973, he described an animal phenocopy of HFM in mice following the administration of triazene to the pregnant mother. Hemorrhage from the

917

developing stapedial artery produced a hematoma in the region of the first and second pharyngeal arches. The size of the hematoma and resultant tissue destruction determined the extent and variability of the deformity. This explanation may be applicable to humans as it provides an adequate explanation for the variability of HFM. Furthermore, in the human condition, cervicofacial hematoma may occur as a result of a variety of causes including hypoxia, hypertension, administration of anticoagulants[13] or anomalous development of the carotid artery system.[23]

Johnson,[22] using an animal model, found that thalidomide and retinoic acid exposure produced malformations similar to HFM in humans. Accutane (13-cis retinoic acid) is known to kill neural crest cells and interfere with cell migration. It has also produced a malformation similar to Treacher Collins syndrome in a mouse model due to its toxic effects on ganglionic placodal cells.[24] Neural crest cells within the mesenchyme are known to populate the pharyngeal arches. It is hypothesized that neural crest cell migration and distribution may be altered by retinoic acid, leading to abnormalities in the tissues derived from the pharyngeal arches. Inadvertent intrauterine exposure to isotretinoin has occurred: 25% of these children have craniofacial, cardiovascular and/or thymic anomalies.

CLINICAL FEATURES

SKELETAL DEFECTS

Asymmetric mandibular growth is the earliest skeletal manifestation of HFM and is responsible for the progressive deformity of the facial skeleton. The mandible is short, narrow and retrusive at birth and may become more asymmetrical with time as the growth of the normal mandible outpaces that of the affected side. The spectrum of mandibular malformation ranges from a small but normally shaped ramus and temporomandibular joint (TMJ) to complete absence of these structures. The midface (nose, maxilla, zygomas and orbits) normally grows down and forward away from the cranial base. In patients with HFM, the temporal bone abnormalities, mandibular hypoplasia and neuromuscular deficits inhibit normal downward (vertical) growth of the maxilla and midface on the affected side. This prevents separation of the piriform rim and maxillary alveolus from the orbit, resulting in a shortened maxilla with a canted occlusal plane (upwards on the affected side); in some cases the orbit is inferiorly displaced.[11,12,25]

The end-stage untreated skeletal malformation of HFM shows considerable variation. The mandible consists of a short, medially displaced or absent ramus. If present, the ramus and body may be flat in contour, and the chin is deviated towards the affected side. A line drawn between the mandibular dental and skeletal midlines is at an angle to the facial midline, so that the upper end (dental) points towards the normal side and the lower end (skeletal) points towards the affected side. There may be dental compensations for the skeletal discrepancy, so that the occlusal abnormality is less severe than the skeletal asymmetry.

SOFT-TISSUE DEFECTS

The contour deficiency in HFM is a combination of skeletal and soft-tissue hypoplasia. Skeletal correction may change the overall facial contour, and the soft-tissue deficiency must be re-evaluated after a symmetrical framework is established. The soft-tissue abnormalities involve first and second pharyngeal arch structures – ear, facial nerve, muscles, subcutaneous tissues and associated structures of the face. The soft-tissue defects in HFM are assessed by clinical examination as well as review of frontal, lateral, oblique and submental photographs, computed tomographs (CT scans), and electromyographic (EMG) studies.[26] There is usually a decrease in the bulk of subcutaneous fat as well as muscles of mastication and facial expression. Patients may have macrostomia, and skin tags may be present along a line from the tragus of the ear to the commissure of the mouth. Cranial nerve function, particularly that of the 7th nerve and rarely the 5th nerve, may be compromised.[27,28] Finally, soft palate function may also be abnormal.[29]

Skin tags are vestigial rests of epithelium which lie along a line from the tragus of the ear to the commissure of the lips (junction between the first and second pharyngeal arches). The tags are frequently associated with cartilaginous remnants and sinus tracts that may form inclusion cysts if obstructed.

Macrostomia was noted in 61% of patients with HFM by Vento et al in their series of 154 patients from Boston Children's Hospital.[1] This abnormality results from a failure of fusion of the maxillary and mandibular processes producing a cleft of the skin and underlying orbicularis oris muscle. Repair of the muscle is the most critical aspect of correction; the skin may be closed in a straight line.

External ear deformities are classified using the system described by Meurman,[30] and modified by Marx:[31]

– **Grade I:** mild hypoplasia, with obvious malformation, but with all structures present

- **Grade II:** atresia of the external auditory canal, with a vertically orientated cartilaginous remnant
- **Grade III:** absent auricle, the lobular remnant is anteriorly and inferiorly displaced.

Pruzansky[32] reported a moderate correlation between the degree of ear and severity of skeletal deformity. However, this was not confirmed by Murray et al.[12] They correlated the severity of external ear deformity with the presence of facial nerve deficit. There was no relationship between mandibular or soft-tissue hypoplasia and 7th nerve weakness.[11,12] Brent[33] reported that approximately 50% of children with microtia do not have an obvious skeletal deformity.

Patients with Grade II or III ear deformity, and some with Grade I, have hearing loss which must be carefully assessed. Hearing loss is usually conductive, resulting from hypoplasia of the ear ossicles which are derivatives of the first and second pharyngeal arches.[12] Computed tomographic (CT) scans of the temporal bone are used to define the presence or absence of the middle ear structures and also to determine if reconstruction of a canal and tympanic membrane is feasible. Reconstruction of the external ear is always a high priority in the management of these patients. The decreased anteroposterior dimension of the upper face and the absence of an adequate platform (i.e. temporal bone cavity) are factors which affect the ability to reconstruct the ear. The position and quality of the soft-tissue remnant also influence surgical construction.

Muscle deficits. The temporalis and pterygomasseteric muscle groups may be deficient in HFM. The severity of this deficit often correlates with the severity of the bony deformity. Absence of the temporalis muscle is usually associated with an absent coronoid process; a similar relationship exists between the pterygomasseteric muscles and the ramus of the mandible. Correction of the skeletal abnormality in HFM frequently accentuates the soft-tissue deficiency. Rotating the maxillomandibular complex and enlarging the affected side produces a stretching and attenuation of the soft tissues. Thus, while skeletal correction improves the dental occlusion and skeletal symmetry, it may accentuate the existing soft-tissue discrepancy.

Cranial nerve abnormalities. More than 25% of patients with HFM have cranial nerve abnormalities, usually consisting of facial nerve weakness and/or deviation of the soft palate towards the affected side in function. The most common facial nerve weakness is in the marginal mandibular branch, followed by the branch to the frontalis muscle. Rarely, there may be complete facial nerve involvement or a sensory deficit in the trigeminal nerve distribution.[27,28]

Soft palate function. The etiology of the soft palate deviation in HFM patients has been debated. Dellon[34] has suggested that the levator palatini muscle is innervated by a proximal branch of the facial nerve and that loss of this innervation due to facial nerve weakness may lead to palatal deviation. Shprintzen[35] failed to show any correlation between palatal deviation and cranial nerve involvement in HFM, suggesting that palatal deviation is due to hypoplasia of the palatal and pharyngeal muscles. The palatal deviation may, in fact, be due to a combination of structural asymmetry, cranial nerve weakness and muscle hypoplasia. Hypoplasia of the lateral pterygoid muscle ranges from mild to complete absence of the muscle and correlates with the severity of the skeletal defect. Muscle hypoplasia, short mandibular ramus, abnormal location of the TMJ, or absence of joint structures results in deviation of the mandible to the affected side on opening.

CLASSIFICATION OF HEMIFACIAL MICROSOMIA

Classification of HFM facilitates diagnosis, treatment planning, data evaluation and communication between healthcare specialists. It may also predict prognosis. The wide spectrum of anomalies in HFM makes standardized classification a difficult task. Most authors agree that the mandibular and TMJ abnormalities should be the cornerstone of any classification. Pruzansky proposed the original classification based on the degree of mandibular and TMJ deformity.[32] He described three types of HFM:

- **Type I:** a miniature mandible and TMJ, all structures present but hypoplastic
- **Type II:** characterized by a small abnormally shaped ramus and an underdeveloped displaced TMJ
- **Type III:** absence of the mandibular ramus and glenoid fossa.

Pruzansky's description of the deformity was limited by its failure to: (a) account for the relative position of the condyle and TMJ, and (b) include associated anomalies seen as part of the variable spectrum of HFM. Converse[36] grouped patients based on the extent of microtia and mandibular deformity. Harvold and colleagues[37] divided the mandibular deformity into five types and focused on muscle function in each category. The orbital, ear and nerve involvement were not included. Lauritzen et al[38] suggested a classification based on skeletal pathology as a guide to operative strategy for the midface and mandible, without including ear or nerve involvement. David et al[39] developed the SAT (**S**keletal, **A**uricular, soft **T**issue) classification modeled on the TNM classification of tumors. There are five mandibular types based on the Pruzansky schema, with two additional mandibular categories that include orbital involvement. The S category includes both mandibular and orbital deformity, the A category classifies the ear deformity, and the T category defines both soft-tissue and cranial nerve involvement.

At Boston Children's Hospital, Swanson & Murray[40] used a classification system based on the mandibular and TMJ deformity which was similar to Pruzansky's. Swanson & Murray's classification was subsequently amended by Kaban et al,[28] with the separation of type II into subgroups A and B, based on the relative position of the condyle and TMJ (Fig. 58.1).

- **Type IIA:** The glenoid fossa is in an acceptable functional position in reference to the opposite TMJ. The joint is adequately positioned for symmetrical opening of the mandible and, therefore, does not require TMJ construction.
- **Type IIB:** the TMJ is abnormal in form and location, being medial and anterior. TMJ and ramus construction are necessary.

Functionally, types I, IIA and some IIB are similar because they have a functional TMJ. Most types IIB and type III have an inadequate TMJ.

The Kaban classification addresses the cornerstone of the deformity (i.e. the mandibular and TMJ skeletal defect),

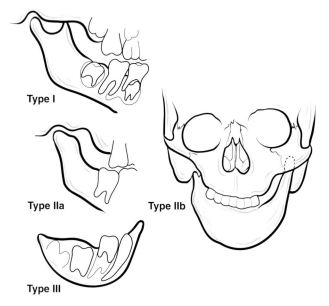

Fig. 58.1 Diagrammatic representation of skeletal classification of hemifacial microsomia. Note that the temporomandibular joint in type IIb is medially, inferiorly, and anteriorly displaced so as to be operationally equivalent to type III.

predicts progression, and guides treatment. It has been incorporated into the comprehensive OMENS classification for HFM.[1] This is a nosologic system devised to include the other skeletal and soft-tissue abnormalities that comprise the craniofacial spectrum of HFM. Each letter of the acronym OMENS represents one of the manifestations of the condition: **O**rbit, **M**andible, **E**ar, **N**erve, **S**oft tissue. Each category is graded from 0 (no abnormality) to 3 (most severe abnormality). A total OMENS score can be calculated for each patient, as the sum of the individual categories.

Cousley[41] compared the OMENS and SAT systems in 50 patients with HFM in the Australian Craniofacial Unit and reported that the OMENS system was more refined due to its differentiation between soft-tissue and nerve defects and between mandibular and orbital skeletal deformity. He also suggested that the OMENS system would be strengthened by the inclusion of noncraniofacial anomalies.[41] Cohen[42] also recommended that an expanded classification of HFM was needed to encompass the extracraniofacial features associated with the condition.

The OMENS Plus classification was proposed by Horgan et al.[43] In a study of 121 patients with HFM, these authors reported that 67 patients (55.4%) had at least one extracraniofacial anomaly, and many patients had more than one. Associated malformations occurring in more than 10–15% of patients[43] were found in the skeletal, cardiac and central nervous systems. Malformations were also found in the pulmonary, renal and gastrointestinal systems. Patients with higher OMENS scores were more likely to have extracraniofacial anomalies. The mean OMENS score for those without associated anomalies was 5.5 ± 3.1 versus a mean score of 6.7 ± 3.1 for those with associated anomalies. Therefore, the higher the OMENS score, the more diligent should be the search for extracraniofacial features of the condition.

PRACTICAL CLASSIFICATION

The classification presented is based on the presence or absence of critical structures and not on the degree of deformity in terms of size or shape.

Type I

Skeletal

All components of the mandible are present but hypoplastic to a variable degree. The TMJ has reduced cartilage and joint space. Hinge movement is normal but there is reduced translation with mandibular opening.

Muscles

The masticatory muscles are all present but small with inclusions of fatty tissue, as seen on CT scans.[26,44] The patterns of muscle use are within normal variation.

Type IIA

Skeletal

The joint is morphologically abnormal. The condylar process is cone shaped and located medial and anterior to the normal position. The coronoid process and gonial angle are well developed. The articulation of the TMJ allows hinge motion but no translation.

Muscles

All masticatory muscles are present but hypoplastic. The contraction of the lateral pterygoid does not advance the affected side of the mandible because of the abnormal position of the condyle.

Type IIB

Skeletal

There is no articulation between the condyle and temporal bone. The coronoid process is present and variable in size. There may be a small bony extension at the posterior border of the mandibular ramus representing a rudimentary condylar process.

Muscles

There are variable deficiencies of the pterygoid and masseter muscles. There is no attachment of the lateral pterygoid to the mandible. The temporalis muscle is small but palpable and attached to the coronoid process.

Type III

Skeletal

There is complete absence of the mandibular ramus including the condylar and coronoid processes.

Muscle

The masticatory muscles are markedly hypoplastic; the lateral pterygoid and temporalis remnants are not attached to the mandibular structures.

NORMAL MANDIBULAR GROWTH

The precise mechanism of mandibular growth is controversial but there are two main theories:

1. the functional matrix theory,[45] which affirms that bony mandibular development occurs in response to functional forces imposed by functioning muscles
2. the condylar growth center theory,[46] which suggests that mandibular growth is due to activity in a growth center located in the mandibular condyle, similar to long bone growth at the epiphyseal plates.

The functional matrix theory suggests that activity in the mandibular condyle is a passive adaptation in response to mandibular growth and that it is not the site of active growth. In reality, probably a combination of the two processes results in mandibular growth.

In the embryonic mandible, bone formation starts in association with Meckel's cartilage and is related to the developing tooth buds. The bony areas expand, coalesce, and form the bony mandible. The neuromuscular and vascular networks are established before bone formation commences and are likely prerequisites for bone formation. During the early stages of development, the mandibular structures are carried forward by the growing Meckel's cartilage. The muscles of mastication become attached to or included in the developing bone.

The posterior muscles extending into the temporal region provide an environment for the development of the mandibular ramus, coronoid and condylar processes. The TMJ develops in association with the lateral pterygoid muscle and then takes over the propulsive action previously provided by the growing Meckel's cartilage. The new propulsive mechanism continues postnatally throughout the growth period and functions by sensorimotor feedback, primarily through the joint structures.[47] It appears that periodic proliferation of the condylar cartilage towards the glenoid fossa leads to activity in the lateral pterygoid muscle which advances the condyle. The mandibular ramus, body and coronoid process also remodel in response to the functional forces applied to them via the muscles of mastication. The control of mandibular growth therefore appears to occur via a combination of condylar growth and bony adaptation secondary to the functional forces exerted by normal muscle activity. In patients with HFM, the structures essential for mandibular growth (mandibular condyle and muscles of mastication) are either absent or deficient. Impaired mandibular growth is, therefore, always present, varying in degree according to the primary tissue deficiencies.

MANDIBULAR GROWTH IN HEMIFACIAL MICROSOMIA

Type I

In the mildest form of HFM the condylar cartilage is diminutive and the disk may be absent. This is determined radiographically by a clear cortical margin on the condylar head and a reduced joint space. The shape of the condylar head is normal but small, and movements are mildly restricted, with normal rotation but reduced translation. The glenoid fossa is shallow or absent, however joint function is adequate and asymptomatic. The affected side of the mandible grows less than the normal side – first, because the contribution to mandibular growth attributed to condylar cartilage proliferation is inadequate, and second due to the deficiency in the muscles of mastication. Fatty and glandular tissues may also be reduced contributing to facial asymmetry. If the masseter and medial pterygoid are hypoplastic, the gonial area is reduced and positioned more medially than the unaffected side. There may or may not be associated 7th nerve impairment.

Type IIA

The condylar process lacks a defined head and neck and is medial and anterior to the normal position. It may have an articulation at the anterior slope of the temporal bone. The muscles of mastication are present, but hypoplastic to a variable extent. The patterns of use are relatively normal. The gonial angle is usually well developed and the coronoid and temporalis muscle are similarly present and well developed. During mouth opening, the mandibular asymmetry becomes more evident – the TMJ on the affected side does not translate forward because contraction of the lateral pterygoid muscle does not advance the mandible. Excessive movement of the contralateral joint is common and leads to occasional clicking of the TMJ in patients with both type I and IIA HFM.

Type IIB

Type IIB is characterized by absence of the glenoid fossa and condylar process of the mandible. The coronoid process is present but attenuated in length. The lateral pterygoid is either absent or not attached to the mandible. The medial pterygoid and masseter muscles are involved to a variable extent and the gonial angle development is dependent on the bulk of the pterygomasseteric sling. The skeletal deformity is severe because the condyle is absent and the muscles of mastication are poorly developed. Because there is no glenoid fossa, slope, eminence, and lateral pterygoid function, the body of the mandible and developing dentition is not disoccluded from the maxilla on the affected side. Consequently, the downward and forward growth of the maxilla is inhibited, leading to a canting of the maxillary occlusal plane and the piriform rim. This can also be seen in type IIA and to a lesser extent in type I HFM.

Type III

The most severe form of HFM is characterized by the absence of both the condylar and coronoid processes of the mandible, which results in the complete absence of the mandibular ramus. The muscles of mastication exist only in rudimentary form. The bony development of the body of the mandible is limited to the alveolar bone surrounding the tooth buds as they form. The affected side may not be attached by muscles to the temporal region and the zygomatic arch, causing an excessive freedom of mandibular movement. The mandible may be easily manipulated to an advanced and lowered position, however such a position cannot be maintained because of the absence of the bony and muscular structures. Paradoxically, maxillary vertical development may be less impaired under these circumstances due to the freedom of mandibular movement and lack of occlusal contact between the maxillary and mandibular teeth.

TREATMENT OF HEMIFACIAL MICROSOMIA

Accurate classification of the skeletal and soft-tissue defect is critical in developing the correct treatment protocol for patients with HFM. Table 58.1 provides a summary of general assessment principles by age and skeletal type. Treatment concepts will be discussed under two headings, based on the protocols used at the Boston Children's and Massachusetts General Hospitals, as follows:

1. treatment of the growing child
2. treatment of the 'end-stage' skeletal defect in nongrowing patients.

TREATMENT OF THE GROWING CHILD

The theoretical basis for surgical correction of craniofacial malformations in the growing child is that early correction provides a more normal functional matrix for completion of craniofacial skeletal growth. In theory, this strategy:

1. optimizes growth potential by placing structures in a more anatomic position, thus improving function

Table 58.1 General assessment principles by age and skeletal type[66]

Skeletal type	Deciduous	Mixed	Permanent
Type I	Skin tag removal	Functional appliance Mandibular elongation osteotomy/distraction Create posterior open-bite	Pre-surgical orthodontics Bimaxillary surgery
Type IIA	As above	As above Functional appliance Mandibular distraction	As above
Type IIB	As above	Construction of ramus, condyle, glenoid fossa Create posterior open-bite Level occlusal plane	Presurgical orthodontics Bimaxillary surgery Construct TMJ
Type III	As above	Construction of ramus, condyle, glenoid fossa Create posterior open-bite Level occlusal plane	As above

2. minimizes secondary deformity and distortion by releasing restricted growth of adjacent skeletal structures
3. improves appearance, body image and socialization of the child.

The premise for surgical correction of HFM in the child is the observation that facial asymmetry in patients with HFM is progressive. Furthermore, the rate of progression of the asymmetry is related to the severity of the mandibular deformity.[11,40,48] Investigators who believe that the deformity changes in proportion to the growing child rather than becoming progressively worse contend that the mandibular asymmetry should be addressed in adolescence.[49,50] The concept of interceptive surgical treatment for growing children with HFM is therefore a controversial topic[49] which will be discussed at a later stage in this chapter. The authors advocate interceptive surgical treatment for children with HFM, based on the concept that HFM is a progressive complex malformation and not a fixed anatomic deformity. It is against this background that guidelines are suggested for the management of the growing child with HFM.

The goal of treatment of HFM in childhood is improved function and optimal facial symmetry and esthetics when craniofacial growth is complete. Treatment is directed towards:

1. increasing the size of the underdeveloped and malformed mandible and related soft tissues
2. creating an articulation between the mandible and the temporal bone when missing
3. promoting maxillary growth and thus correcting secondary deformities of the maxilla
4. establishing a functional occlusion and esthetic appearance of the face and dentition.

The treatment approach is dictated by mandibular skeletal type (I, IIA, IIB, III), midface deformity (cant of the maxillary occlusal plane and piriform rims), age (chronologic, dental, skeletal), and psychosocial adjustment of the child. Treatment must proceed in a stepwise manner, conforming to a predictable sequence of biologic development, and characterized by several sequential phases consisting of:

- presurgical jaw orthopedic treatment when indicated
- mandibular surgery including joint reconstruction, if necessary
- immediate postsurgical functional appliance therapy to support graft remodeling and regenerate consolidation
- maxillary correction when necessary
- final orthodontic treatment
- soft-tissue augmentation.[11,12,26,51–53]

Presurgical orthodontic treatment

Impaired mandibular growth may be the result of absent or reduced condylar cartilage proliferation and reduced protrusive action of the condyle due to the absolute or relative absence of lateral pterygoid muscle function on the condylar head. A functional orthodontic appliance that enhances the neuromuscular environment, promotes mandibular and maxillary growth, and expands the soft-tissue envelope on the affected side may be used in young patients with HFM. The appliance is a removable acrylic orthodontic activator with guide planes and shields that is constructed to hold the affected side of the mandible in a lowered and protrusive position. The appliance stimulates bone apposition in the ramus–condyle unit and coronoid process by substituting for the normal translatory and protrusive motion produced by the lateral pterygoid muscle. The degree of deformity and patient compliance greatly affect the outcome of functional appliance therapy. Response to functional appliance therapy has been shown to be beneficial in patients with type I HFM (Fig. 58.2A–F).

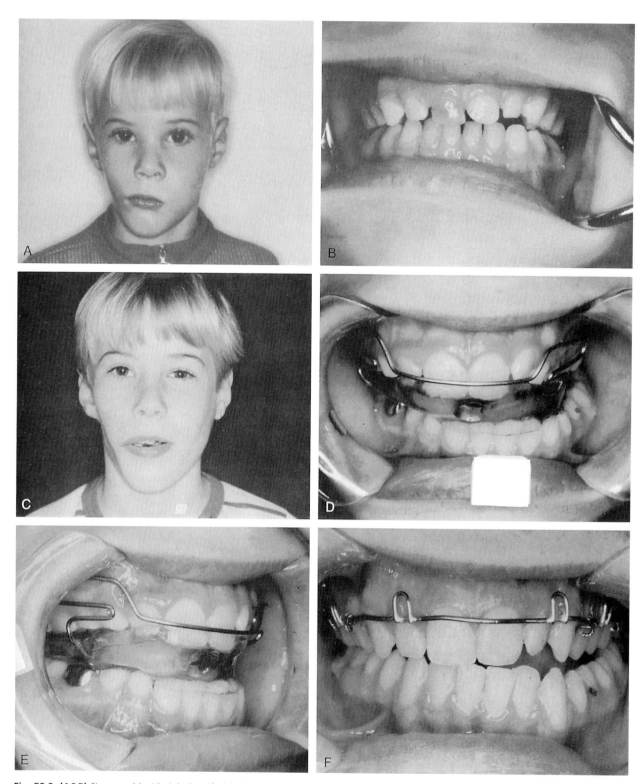

Fig. 58.2 (A&B) Six-year-old with right hemifacial microsomia. **(C, D)** and **(E)** A functional appliance is in place holding the affected side down and forward. The acrylic is removed below the maxillary posterior teeth on the affected side, allowing further vertical dentoalveolar development. The appliance serves as a biteblock for the teeth on the contralateral side, inhibiting vertical development. **(F)** The maxillary occlusal plane has improved, resulting in an open-bite on the contralateral side. The lower dental midline is now further over to the contralateral side, indicating more length increase of the mandible on the affected than on the contralateral side. A surgical arch bar has been placed on the maxillary teeth, and one will also be placed on the mandibular teeth in preparation for the mandibular surgery. Maxillary surgery can be avoided owing to favorable response to functional appliance treatment.[66]

A study of 15 type I HFM patients showed that, during treatment with a functional appliance, the affected side increased in size more than the unaffected side in 4 children, by an amount equal to the unaffected side in 4 children, and slightly less than the unaffected side in 7 children. There was, however, no significant mean difference between groups in the growth of the two sides in the sample.[51] A similar response was reported by Melsen et al.[54]

If the response to functional appliance therapy is good, then it may be possible to avoid surgical lengthening of the mandibular ramus on the affected side in patients with type I, provided the angulation of the maxillary occlusal plane is acceptable. If the inclination is severe, it will be necessary to elongate the mandible on the affected side, either at the time of eruption of the maxillary first permanent molars or close to the time of eruption of the premolars. The open-bite thus created can be closed by active orthodontic extrusion of maxillary teeth. The need for a Le Fort I osteotomy to level the occlusal plane is usually avoided. In type IIA HFM, a similar presurgical treatment phase may be beneficial.[52,54] Advocates of presurgical orthopedic therapy are of the opinion that, even when a functional appliance does not avoid the need for mandibular lengthening procedures, the appliance produces a soft-tissue environment which has a reduced tendency for postoperative skeletal relapse.

Orthodontic treatment

In patients with HFM there may be delayed tooth eruption and dental irregularities on the affected side, and crowding of the dentition is common.[17] Orthodontic treatment in childhood focuses on control of tooth eruption and prevention or correction of dentoalveolar adaptations to the asymmetric position of the maxilla and mandible. The orthodontist should be actively involved in the treatment of children with HFM throughout their growth period.

Surgical correction of mandibular deformity

Operative correction of the mandibular skeletal defect is indicated in certain children. If mandibular lengthening and creation of an open-bite on the affected side is carried out during the mixed dentition, vertical growth of the midface will minimize the secondary deformity of maxillary occlusal plane canting and often prevent the need for a Le Fort I osteotomy.

In type I and IIA patients, the mandible is elongated and rotated to the correct midline. The mandible can be elongated using either conventional orthognathic surgical methods or gradually elongated using the technique of distraction osteogenesis. Conventional techniques include a vertical ramus osteotomy, often combined with a coronoidectomy on the affected side or an inverted L osteotomy, leaving the condyle on the affected side in position. The proximal and distal fragments are secured using plate and screw fixation. A compensatory releasing subcondylar osteotomy may be required on the unaffected side to allow the mandible to sit passively in the new position without excessive torquing of the condyle on the unaffected side; this is usually not required in young children. With both conventional osteotomies and distraction osteogenesis no surgery is performed on the maxilla in a growing child; an open-bite is created on the affected side that is maintained and regulated to allow for eruption of teeth and vertical growth of the maxilla, thus leveling the maxillary occlusal plane.[11,12,27,28] The open-bite is first maintained with a bite block for 3–6 months. Then, eruption of the maxillary teeth is begun by gradually reducing the maxillary side of the bite block to permit inferior growth of the maxilla over the next 1–2 years. Finally, the open-bite closure is completed by active orthodontic movement of the maxillary teeth, thus leveling the maxillary occlusal plane (Fig. 58.3A-I).

In type IIB and type III patients, the mandible is elongated and rotated, either by distraction osteogenesis if there is sufficient bone and a TMJ or by construction of a mandibular ramus and TMJ using a costochondral graft. The new TMJ is constructed to be symmetric with the opposite joint, as lateral and posterior as possible. Creation of an open-bite and orthodontic control of maxillary growth and eruption of maxillary teeth is otherwise the same as for type I and IIA patients (Fig. 58.4). Following construction of a ramus–condyle unit, these patients have now been converted to a type IIA deformity. Their long-term prognosis depends on symmetric growth between the normal side and the constructed ramus–condyle unit. These patients must therefore be followed closely for recurrent progressive asymmetry and treated if necessary with either a functional appliance or secondary lengthening procedure if there is evidence of significant asymmetric mandibular growth.

The results of treatment of HFM in growing children have been reviewed and reported at the Boston Children's Hospital.[11,27] Twenty patients were studied and classified as type I or IIA (group 1, n = 10) and type IIB or III (group 2, n = 10). All patients were treated using the protocol described above. The average follow up was 50.9 months (group 1) and 45 months (group 2). In all children the midface grew vertically to close the surgically created open-bite and the maxillary occlusal plane was leveled without an osteotomy. Of the patients with type I or IIA (group 1), followed to completion of growth (n = 9/10), none required a maxillary osteotomy or a second procedure to lengthen the mandible. Of the patients with type IIB or III

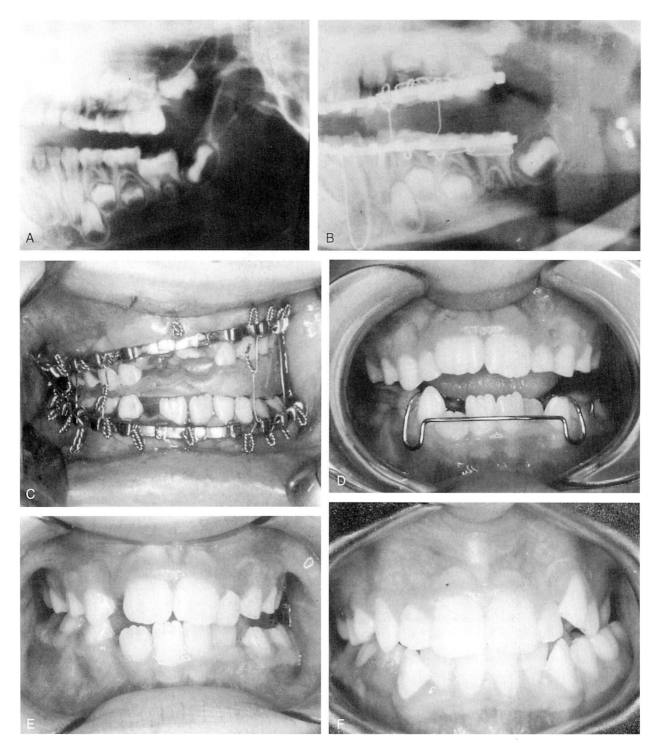

Fig. 58.3 Correction of HFM in a growing child with type IIA mandible. **(A)** Panoramic radiograph demonstrates a short, abnormally shaped ramus and a very narrow sigmoid notch with slight elongation of the coronoid process. **(B)** Immediate postoperative panorex after vertical lengthening of the mandibular ramus. A vertical osteotomy was performed. Coronoidectomy was also done at this time. The mandible was lengthened and an open-bite was created at the time of the surgery. **(C)** Immediate postoperative photograph demonstrating the surgically created open bite. Note the diversion of maxillary and mandibular arch bars, which demonstrates the tilting of the maxillary occlusal plane and the postoperative leveling of the mandibular occlusal plane. **(D and E)** These views demonstrate progressive closure of the open-bite over an 18-month period postoperatively. **(F)** Intraoral photograph of the same patient 5 years postoperatively demonstrates coincident maxillary and mandibular dental midlines and a level occlusal plane. The patient will have conventional orthodontic treatment for crowding and the slight maxillary width discrepancy.[66]

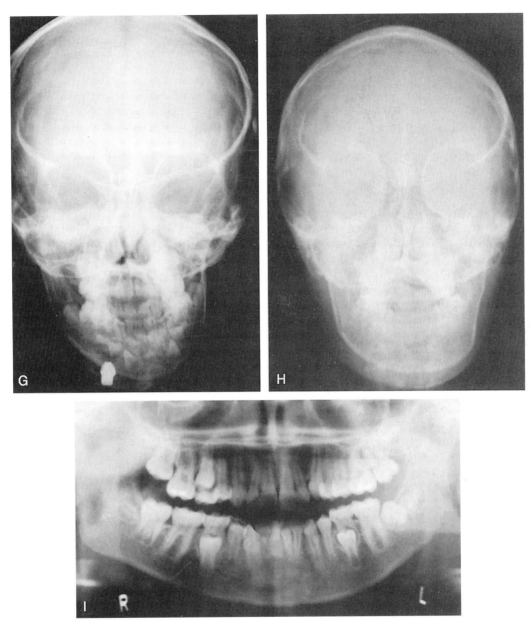

Fig. 58.3(contd) Preoperative **(G)** and 5-year postoperative **(H)** AP cephalograms and 5-year postoperative panoramic views **(I)** demonstrating mandibular symmetry and remodeling of the angle of the mandible. (Fig. 58.3 is partially reproduced with permission from Kaban LB: Pediatric Oral and Maxillofacial Surgery, pp 284–286. Philadelphia: WB Saunders, 1990.)

(group 2), operated on during the deciduous dentition (below age 5 years) and followed to growth completion, none required a maxillary osteotomy but 4 required a second mandibular elongation procedure in the late mixed dentition or the early teen years.

Padwa et al[55] at Boston Children's Hospital retrospectively studied midfacial growth in patients (n = 33) with type IIB and III HFM after early correction of the deformity as outlined in the above protocol. Patients who had symmetric growth of the constructed ramus and condyle (42%) had leveling of the intergonial angle and occlusal plane. Patients whose constructed ramus grew, but at an unequal rate to the normal side (42%), remained asymmetric with some improvement in but not complete leveling of the maxillary occlusal plane. Those who had poor growth of the graft (16%) had an increase in the maxillary and mandibular deformities (increase in occlusal cant and intergonial angle) (Tables 58.2, 58.3).

Vargervik & Ousterhout[5] at the University of California, San Francisco, reported continued growth of the lengthened mandible in the majority of 10 patients with HFM operated on early and followed until growth was completed. In 3 of

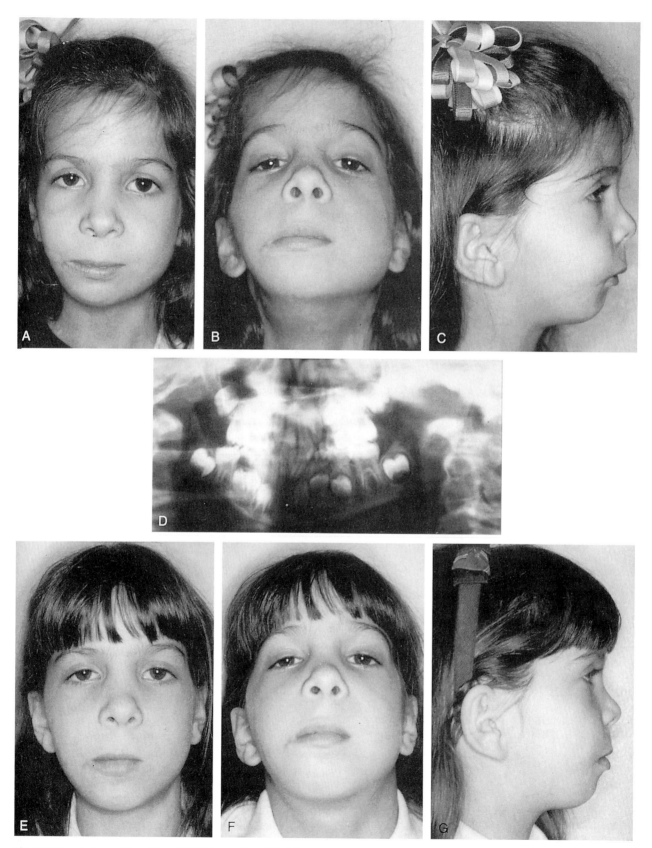

Fig. 58.4 Surgical correction of type III HFM in growing child. **(A)** Preoperative frontal photograph of a 6-year-old child with type III HFM with congenital absence of the ramus of the mandible. **(B)** Submental photograph shows the marked deviation of the chin point and the contour deficit of the right face. **(C)** Lateral photograph. **(D)** Preoperative panoramic radiograph demonstrating the absence of right mandibular ramus. Frontal **(E)**, submental **(F)**, and lateral **(G)** photographs 1 year postoperatively. Note the marked improvement in the symmetry of the face with the chin point being in the midline and marked improvement of the contour. Intraoral photographs with splint

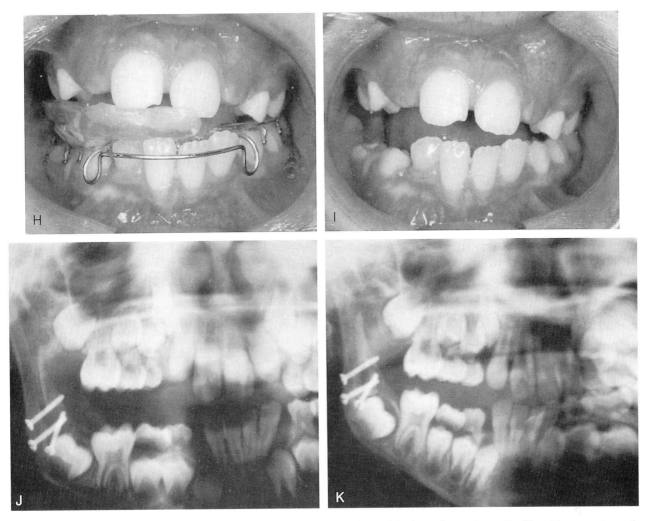

Fig. 58.4(contd) **(H)** and without splint **(I)** demonstrating the surgically created open-bite. Immediate postoperative **(J)** and 1-year postoperative **(K)** panoramic radiographs showing the constructed ramus, the surgically created open-bite with progressive closure, and the remodeling of the constructed ramus.[66]

Table 58.2 Growth of the ramus and condyle[55]

Occlusal Cant (degrees)	Pre-operative Mandibular Ratio	Post-operative Mandibular Ratio	Pre-operative Intergonial Angle	Post-operative Intergonial Angle
<5	0.74	1.0	5.4	2.0
≥5–<8	0.79	0.97	6.8	4.6
≥8	0.70	0.91	7.0	6.5

Table 58.3 Growth of the midface[55]

Occlusal Cant (degrees)	Pre-operative Occlusal Cant	Post-operative Occlusal Cant	Pre-operative Piriform Angle	Post-operative Piriform Angle
<5	4.8	2.1	6.8	7.0
≥5–<8	5.7	6.7	11.2	11.2
≥8	4.8	10.8	8.1	14.5

their patients, however, growth of the affected side did not keep pace with the normal side and facial asymmetry recurred, requiring a second mandibular lengthening procedure that also involved a maxillary osteotomy.

In summary, the midface hypoplasia that is a progressive secondary deformation due to the restriction of midface growth by the small mandible and underdeveloped muscu-lature can be intercepted or corrected. Elongation of the mandible and creation of an open-bite on the affected side, in growing children with HFM, decreases and may eliminate the need for bimaxillary orthognathic surgery in adult-hood.[12,27,28,51] However, the patient's and family's ability to cooperate in using the occlusal appliance must be con-sidered in deciding whether to proceed with early surgical therapy. If this aspect of the protocol cannot be successfully carried out, early treatment is doomed to failure. Under these circumstances, it is prudent to delay intervention. If this window of opportunity closes, it is appropriate to wait until growth has completed and to correct the 'end-stage' deformity at that time.

The role of mandibular distraction in patients with HFM

Distraction osteogenesis is a unique method for bone lengthening, utilizing natural healing mechanisms to generate new bone. The concept of distraction is not new – the original descriptions of the technique date to the last century. However, Ilizarov is recognized as the innovator of modern techniques of bone distraction.[56] The concept described by Ilizarov was adapted, initially for mandibular distraction,[57] and later for distraction of other facial bones.[58] The technique involves the creation of an osteotomy (corticotomy), followed by the placement of a distraction device fixed to the bone on either side of the osteotomy. Following a latency period the distraction device is used to gradually separate the bone fragments. Soft- and hard-tissue formation results from the tension stress effect created by the distraction. Upon completion of distraction, the device is used for fixation during the period of consolidation of the regenerate. In addition to generation of new bone, gradual distraction produces simultaneous soft-tissue expansion which creates a more stable environment for bony elongation.[59,60]

Mandibular lengthening, using the technique of distraction osteogenesis, is of benefit to patients with HFM,[57] particularly in types I and IIA and in some cases of type IIB where there is a functional ramus and condyle. Distraction osteogenesis is not indicated in patients who require construction of a ramus and condyle (i.e. most type IIB and all type III). The standard procedure is the creation of a mandibular ramus osteotomy from an intraoral approach on the lateral and anterior aspect of the mandibular ramus. The location of the osteotomy is determined by the mandibular movement necessary to correct the asymmetry. A horizontal osteotomy superior to the mandibular angle allows vertical distraction of the ascending ramus. A vertical osteotomy anterior to the gonial angle, in the body of the mandible, permits anterior mandibular elongation. A distraction device is fixed to the lateral aspect of the ramus and is secured to the bone on either side of the osteotomy. Numerous distraction devices are commercially available, all permitting a gradual separation of the bone fragments. The ideal device is technically easy to apply to the lateral mandible, completely buried (avoiding the cutaneous pin

tracks associated with transcutaneously placed pins and externally located devices), and easily removed following the period of distraction and retention.

A latency period follows the placement of the distraction device. Ilizarov recommends a 5-day period to permit soft-tissue healing.[56] Following the latency period elongation proceeds at a rate of 1 mm per day, lengthening the distraction device by 0.5 mm twice a day. Distraction continues until the desired end result is obtained. This is based on preoperative radiographic assessment of the magnitude of distraction that will correct mandibular asymmetry and adequately open the bite on the affected side allowing leveling of the maxillary occlusal plane. In addition, the amount of distraction is also influenced by clinical assessment during the distraction period. During the first 3–4 days of distraction the condyle is being fully seated in the glenoid fossa and as a result mandibular lengthening may not occur in the first several days. This should be taken into account when calculating the duration of distraction for these patients. The orthodontic appliance which will maintain the open-bite created on the affected side should be fitted on the final day of distraction to prevent any relapse in the open-bite. The distraction period is then followed by a period of retention to allow the regenerate to consolidate. The retention period recommended is double the period of distraction. Following this the distraction device is removed.

Radiographs (panoramic, PA, lateral cephalograms) are taken immediately after placement of the distraction device and again prior to removal of the device. It may be necessary to confirm the position of the bony fragments radiographically during the period of distraction.

Lengthening of the mandible in HFM may affect the position of the TMJ on the contralateral side, however the gradual process of lengthening by distraction appears to be well tolerated. The contralateral TMJ presumably adapts to the minor alteration in position. Nevertheless, these patients should be closely followed for any symptoms of TMJ pathology, particularly affecting the contralateral TMJ.

Mandibular elongation using the technique of distraction osteogenesis has a number of advantages. Interceptive mandibular lengthening occurs with minimal morbidity. The disadvantages of conventional orthognathic techniques, including the need for bone grafting, maxillomandibular fixation, prolonged surgery and postoperative stays, are avoided. Perhaps the most important benefit of distraction osteogenesis is the soft-tissue expansion which occurs simultaneously with bone lengthening.[60] This provides a soft-tissue environment which may permit greater long-term skeletal stability. However, a successful result depends on a clear understanding of the goals of early treatment, correct patient selection, and attention to detail.

Pitfalls with early treatment of skeletal deformity

In the growing child with HFM, a common cause for treatment failure and controversy is a lack of understanding of the rationale and goals of early treatment. The first goal is to surgically create an open-bite on the affected side by elongation and rotation of the mandible to the midline. This open-bite must be maintained and controlled to permit leveling of the occlusal plane by vertical maxillary growth on the affected side. The ultimate goals are to achieve and maintain facial symmetry and improved function at the completion of growth.

The treatment protocol must be applied correctly and at an appropriate age to achieve a successful outcome. A child with HFM must be in the mixed dentition to benefit from early management. Success depends on the potential for vertical growth of the midface and maxillary dentoalveolus as the deciduous teeth are shed and the permanent teeth erupt. The protocol is not applicable after the permanent teeth have erupted because vertical midfacial and dento-alveolar growth is essentially complete by this time. Therefore, orthodontically controlled eruption of the permanent teeth into the surgically created open-bite space will not be accompanied by vertical growth; the teeth will simply extrude.

The open-bite must be maintained by an orthodontic appliance (occlusal bite block) for a period of 3–6 months while the distracted, osteotomized or constructed ramus heals. If the ramus has been lengthened by distraction, the appliance should be fitted on the final day of distraction and worn throughout the period of retention. If the ramus has been lengthened by conventional osteotomy or ramus construction then the appliance should be fitted as soon as possible following the removal of maxillomandibular fixation. The maxillary teeth can be allowed to erupt by a combination of passive movement and orthodontic forces, thereby leveling the occlusal plane. If the open-bite is not maintained during this crucial period, it closes rapidly by a combination of supra-eruption of the maxillary and mandibular teeth and resorption and deformation of the lengthened ramus under the compressive forces of occlusion. The desired effect of early treatment will be lost (Fig. 58.6).

Surgical correction of soft-tissue defects

The correction of soft-tissue abnormalities associated with HFM should be coordinated with the management of skeletal problems. Frequently, small procedures to correct minor but obvious abnormalities may alleviate parents' concerns in the first year of life.

Skin tags are often removed in the first year of life. These are small vestigial remnants of epithelial tissue that may also include subcutaneous cartilaginous remnants and sinus tracts. They lie along the cleft between the first and second branchial arches, hence they can be in the pre-auricular area or on the cheek. Great care must be taken with the removal of deep cartilaginous structures because the facial nerve may be quite superficial in small children and can be injured during deep dissection. Sinus tracts can be injected with dyes (e.g. methylene blue) and complete removal of the stained tissue is necessary to avoid subsequent cyst formation.

Macrostomia, which is seen in up to 61% of patients with HFM,[1] results from failure of fusion of the maxillary and mandibular processes of the first and second branchial arches. Macrostomia is corrected in the first year of life and requires correction of the defect in the orbicularis oris muscle.

Parents frequently focus on correction of the external ear deformity which, indeed, may be the most obvious defect in the neonatal period. Surgeons must resist pressure to proceed with early ear construction, as it can result in a misplaced auricular framework, and once positioned can be exceedingly difficult to relocate. If the constructed ear is anterior to the correct position for the proposed glenoid fossa and TMJ then the auricular framework must be removed. The ideal age for ear construction is after 6 years because the ear is then 90% of adult size and there is usually adequate autogenous costal cartilage available. This is also a stage when body image is becoming important for young children. The precise timing must be individualized, taking into account the relative sizes of the ear and rib cartilage, as well as the child's emotional development.[53]

Autogenous construction, although technically demanding, is considered to be the ideal method of external ear construction.[61] The constructed ear becomes part of 'self' and the framework has the potential for growth.[62] Furthermore, there is no requirement for prosthetic support or long-term maintenance, and once constructed the autogenous ear has a small chance of late complications.[61] There is, however, a role for an osseointegrated implant retained alloplastic ear prosthesis, particularly in the case of failed autogenous construction. Finally, adhesive retained ear prostheses may be useful on an interim basis while patients await definitive ear construction.

Autogenous ear construction is a staged procedure, usually involving at least two surgical procedures over approximately 12–18 months to achieve a definitive result. The technique has been described by Tanzer[63] and subsequently refined by Brent (see Ch. 84).[33,64,65] At the initial stage cartilage is harvested from the synchondrosis of the contralateral sixth and seventh ribs and used as a framework; the cartilage of the eighth rib is attached to provide a helical

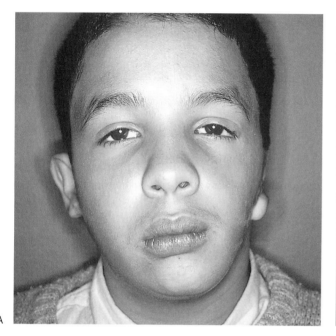

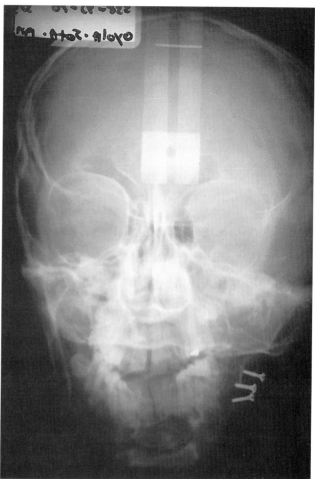

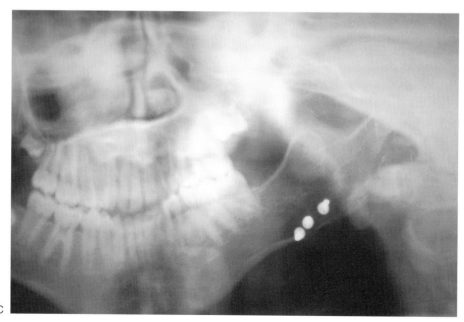

Fig. 58.6 (A) Frontal preoperative photograph shows marked deviation of chin point to left and short left mandibular ramus 3 years after costochondral graft construction. Preoperative radiographs **(B)** posteroanterior (PA) cephalogram demonstrates mandibular asymmetry with short left ramus, deviation of chin point to left, and cant of occlusal plane up on left. Three screws were provided for costochondral graft which was initially used in this patient. **(C)** Panoramic radiograph reveals costochondral graft construction of left ramus and condyle with screws for fixation.

rim. The ear framework is carved with exaggeration of the antihelical fold and concha to approximate the appearance of a normal ear. The framework is positioned as symmetrically as possible with the contralateral ear. On the affected side the vestigial cartilaginous remnants are removed and a thin skin flap elevated to cover the framework. The adherence of the flap is maintained by the use of suction drains and pressure dressings for several days. If there is inadequate skin coverage, two options are available; tissue expansion or the use of a temporoparietal fascial flap to provide adequate coverage for the framework, with skin graft closure over the fascia. Subsequent stages are separated by 4–6 months and consist of derotation of the lobule, separation of the framework from the base with a skin graft placed posteriorly and, finally, construction of a tragus.[66]

Patients with true anotia have no lobule or cartilaginous remnant and thus represent the most severe deformity. The use of a prosthetic ear may be indicated in these cases, particularly because of the associated soft-tissue deficit. An adhesive retained prosthesis may be used during growth and later replaced with an osseointegrated implant retained prosthesis. When an implant retained prosthesis is considered, it should be remembered that this will significantly compromise any subsequent attempt at autogenous external ear construction.

TREATMENT OF THE 'END-STAGE' SKELETAL DEFECT IN NONGROWING PATIENTS

Adolescents and adults with end-stage HFM are treated with standard orthognathic surgical methods, involving presurgical orthodontics and bimaxillary orthognathic surgery. In patients with type IIB and III HFM, construction of the ramus–condyle unit on the affected side is necessary.

Orthodontic management

In nongrowing patients, the dentoalveolar compensations to the skeletal asymmetry must be corrected and the arches coordinated before corrective jaw surgery is carried out. The principles of surgical treatment are similar to those that apply to any jaw asymmetry requiring orthognathic surgical correction.

Surgical correction of skeletal defects

Surgical correction of the 'end-stage' deformity consists of an operation to level the maxillary occlusal plane and piriform apertures, correct the mandibular asymmetry, construct a ramus–condyle unit if necessary and place the TMJ

in the correct position. Maxillary and mandibular transverse abnormalities can be corrected orthodontically or surgically. In the sagittal plane, the maxilla and mandible are mobilized and repositioned in a position dictated by their relationship to the cranial base. Skeletal contour defects are corrected using onlay bone grafts; soft-tissue and ear defects are usually corrected after skeletal symmetry has been achieved (Fig. 58.5).

Type I and IIA

In patients type I and IIA HFM, the first step in the treatment of the 'end-stage' deformity is to correctly position the maxilla, using a Le Fort I level osteotomy stabilized with plate and screw fixation. The preoperative planning is based on clinical examination and analysis of photographs, dental models, and lateral and anteroposterior cephalograms.

Correction of the maxillary position in the vertical plane requires a leveling of the maxillary occlusal plane. It is critical to choose the correct fulcrum for maxillary repositioning. Three clinical situations arise as follows:

1. Vertical maxillary excess (on the unaffected side). If there is vertical maxillary excess on the unaffected side, the fulcrum of rotation of the maxilla is on the affected (short) side. The occlusal plane is leveled by shortening the unaffected side.

2. Normal vertical maxillary position (on the unaffected side). If the maxillary vertical length is normal, the fulcrum of rotation is at the midline. The occlusal plane is leveled by lengthening the affected side and shortening the unaffected side.

3. Vertical maxillary deficiency (on the unaffected side). If there is vertical maxillary deficiency on the unaffected side, the fulcrum of rotation is on the abnormal side. The occlusal plane is leveled by differential maxillary elongation, with greater lengthening of the unaffected.

The need for maxillary repositioning in the sagittal plane is based on the relationship of the maxilla to the cranial base; this is corrected if necessary at the time of Le Fort I osteotomy. Maxillary transverse discrepancies can be corrected, if present, using preoperative orthodontics or at the time of Le Fort I osteotomy with a multipiece osteotomy. Once the maxilla is repositioned, bilateral mandibular osteotomies are required to rotate the mandible into the correct relationship with the maxilla. Depending on the anatomy and the magnitude of the malformation, the osteotomies

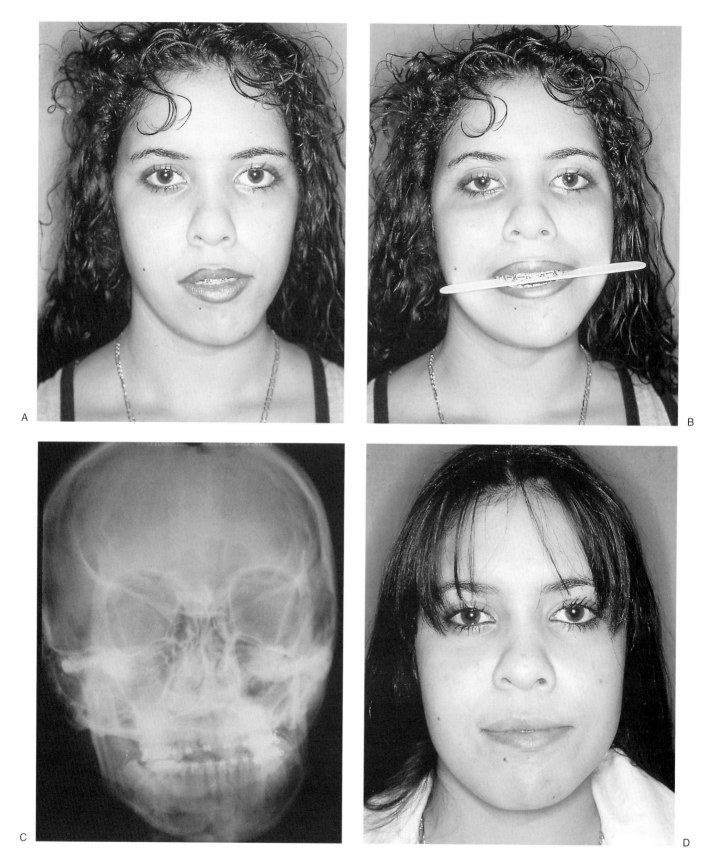

Fig. 58.5(A,B) Preoperative frontal photographs of seventeen year old with 'end stage' left predominant Type IIA mandibular deformity. Note mandibular asymmetry and deviated chin point. Left commissure and alar base canted; occlusal tilt demonstrated by throat stick. **(C)** Preoperative posteroanterior (PA) cephalogram demonstrates mandibular asymmetry: shortened left mandibular ramus, deviated chin point, and canted occlusal and piriform planes.

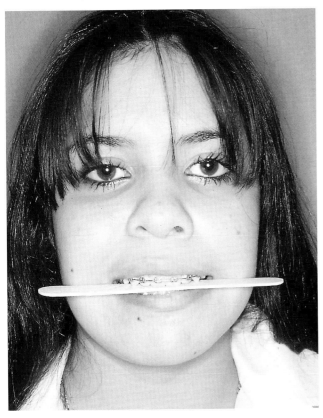 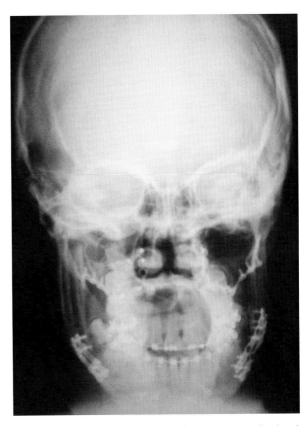

E

F

Fig. 58.5(D,E)(contd) One year postoperative: facial asymmetry improved with chin point in midline and minimal cant of commissure, occlusal and piriform planes. **(F)** Postoperative PA cephalogram documents mandibular symmetry and level occlusal and piriform planes.

may be combined with bone grafts. Bony contour deficiencies may be augmented with onlay bone grafts or autogenous material secured with plate and screw fixation. It is important to note that correction of skeletal asymmetry can often exacerbate the soft-tissue deficiency, which must then be addressed as a final stage in reconstruction for these patients.

Type IIB and III

Those patients with type IIB and III HFM often require construction of a ramus–condyle unit with the TMJ in the correct location. In patients with type III deformity the mandibular ramus and TMJ are missing. In those with type IIB HFM, the existing mandibular ramus is often extremely hypoplastic and abnormally positioned and therefore usually must be replaced.[12,28,53]

The initial step in planning the surgical correction of the end-stage deformity is to locate the correct position for the TMJ on the affected side. On an anteroposterior cephalogram (AP Ceph) the true vertical midline is drawn from the crista galli through the upper part of the nasal septum. The nasal septum may often be asymmetric in position. The vertical line is drawn as a perpendicular to a horizontal line joining the right and left frontozygomatic sutures. The distances from the affected and unaffected TMJ to the midline are measured perpendicular to the true vertical midline. The distance from the TMJs to the true horizontal, at the level of the supraorbital rims, is also measured. These horizontal and vertical measurements determine the amount of horizontal and vertical displacement of the affected TMJ.

At operation, the facial midline is drawn from the mid-forehead through the glabella and dorsum of the nose. The distance from the true midline at the glabella to the tragus of the ear is measured on the affected and unaffected sides of the face. The distance from the lateral canthus, on the affected and unaffected sides, to the tragus is measured. The correct location of the constructed TMJ is determined by these measurements.

Correction of the maxillary position for patients with type IIB and III HFM requires the same planning and operation on the maxilla as described above, followed by mandibular osteotomies to rotate the mandible into the correct relationship with the maxilla. A mandibular ramus is then constructed on the affected side using a costochondral graft. The TMJ is constructed using full thickness rib or iliac crest, secured lateral to the zygomatic arch remnant. A glenoid fossa may be hollowed out of this graft and lined with a temporalis muscle and fascia flap if present.[12,28,53]

A role for bimaxillary distraction in 'end-stage' HFM

In selected cases, the technique of bimaxillary distraction

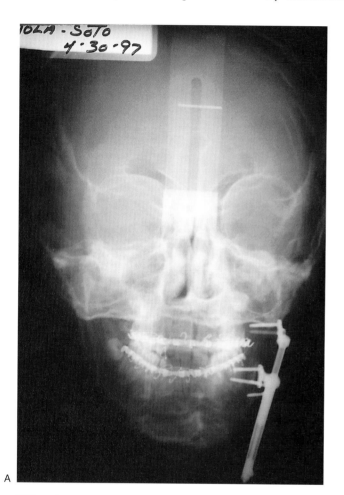

A

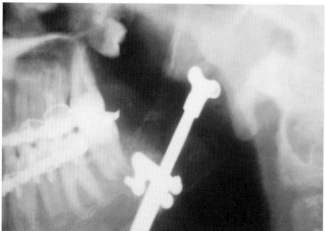

B

Fig. 58.7 Post-distraction/fixation radiographs: **(A)** PA cephalogram shows elongated left ramus, midline chin point, and level occlusal plant. **(B)** Panoramic radiograph demonstrates callus formation in distraction gap.

osteogenesis may be used to correct the 'end-stage' deformity in HFM. The treatment concept involves a gradual elongation of the maxilla on the affected side in harmony with elongation of the short mandibular ramus. However, there are a number of prerequisites for consideration of such a treatment option. First, an adequate mandibular ramus and TMJ must be present on the affected side to permit distraction of the distal fragment following corticotomy. This may confine the treatment technique to types 1 and IIA HFM. An exception would be a patient with type IIB or III HFM, with a previously constructed mandibular ramus and TMJ which had been of inadequate length initially or had relapsed postoperatively. Second, the vertical position of the maxilla on the normal side must be esthetically acceptable, because the technique of bimaxillary distraction osteogenesis does not permit alteration of the maxillary vertical dimension on the unaffected side. Third, the maxillary dental midline must be in an acceptable position relative to the facial midline. Similarly, the technique does not permit repositioning of the maxillary dental midline. Finally, the presence of an intact and periodontally sound dentition is necessary to permit the use of maxillomandibular fixation which must be tightened at regular intervals during the periods of distraction and retention (Figs 58.7–58.9).

The technique involves a limited Le Fort I level osteotomy

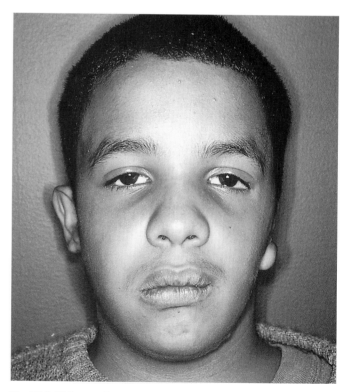

Fig. 58.8 Eight month postoperative frontal photograph demonstrates symmetric facial appearance with chin point midline, level alar base and oral commisure.

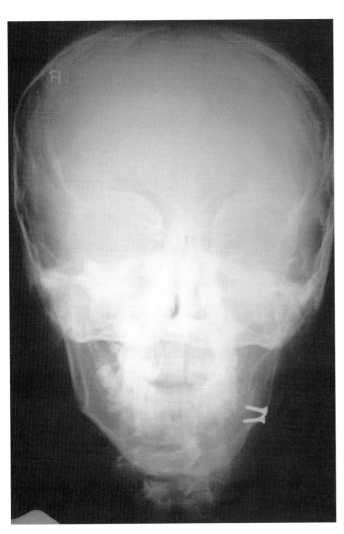

Fig. 58.9 Eight month postoperative PA cephalogram shows stable result with improved symmetry of ramus, midline chin point, and level occlusal plane. Note augmented contour of left ramus.

which includes osteotomies of the anterior and lateral maxillary and lateral nasal walls. The osteotomies are combined with pterygomaxillary dysjunction. The nasal septum is undisturbed and provides stability to the maxilla during distraction. The soft-tissue dissection is confined to the lateral aspects of the maxillary sulcus, tuberosities and pterygoid regions. The anterior soft-tissue pedicle in the maxillary incisor region is left undisturbed. The mandibular ramus is approached in a standard fashion, and a corticotomy made on the lateral and anterior ramus. The direction of the corticotomy is planned, based on the preoperative radiographs and the direction of distraction required. The distraction device is fixed to the lateral aspect of the mandible and the patient placed in maxillomandibular fixation. A period of latency follows and the maxillomandibular complex is then gradually distracted, lengthening the mandible and maxilla on the affected side. The period of distraction is followed by a period of retention. The overall effect permits leveling of the maxillary occlusal plane, elongation of the shortened mandibular ramus, and correction of the chin point.

The advantages offered by bimaxillary distraction are avoidance of major orthognathic surgery and the donor site morbidity associated with bone grafting. The surgical procedure involves a decreased initial operating room time and a reduced postoperative hospital stay. The use of this technique, however, demands considerable cooperation and understanding on the part of the patient during the distraction and fixation period and, depending on the particular distractor used, a second general anesthetic may be required to remove the device.

SURGICAL CORRECTION OF SOFT-TISSUE HYPOPLASIA

Correction of soft-tissue contour is one of the final steps in surgical reconstruction of HFM, and it must follow skeletal correction. Minor soft-tissue defects can be corrected with dermal grafts, which can be harvested from the abdomen or buttocks. The use of the buttocks as the donor site leaves a relatively inconspicuous scar and adequate graft thickness. A study compared dermal grafts to microvascular transfers and found that smaller defects were adequately corrected using free dermis whereas larger defects were better managed using microvascular tissue transfer.[67] A variety of donor sites have been proposed for microvascular tissue transfer, the primary distinction being between muscle flaps and de-epithelialized skin and subcutaneous flaps. If muscle is used the serratus anterior or radial forearm are those most commonly chosen; the main problem with muscle transfer is the unpredictable degree of atrophy which occurs following denervation. The use of de-epithelialized flaps is more reliable in this regard and also permits later adjustment using liposuction if overcorrection has occurred. It has, however, been noted in patients with HFM that the recipient vessels on the affected side may be anomalous.[68] The surgeon must therefore be alert to the possibility of technical difficulties associated with free microvascular tissue transfer in patients with HFM (Figs 58.10–58.12).

FACIAL NERVE PALSY

Complete facial nerve palsy in HFM is rare. The primary consideration in infancy is competent eye closure, without which exposure keratitis, corneal ulcerations, and blindness may occur. An active Bell's phenomenon, which involves upward rotation of the globe with eye closure may be adequate to protect the eye; failing this the use of eye patches

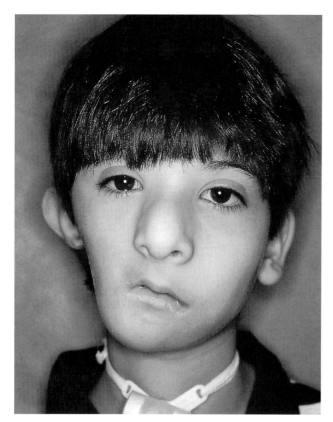

Fig. 58.10 Frontal photograph of 10-year-old boy with right predominant hemifacial microsomia. Note severe mandibular deformity with chin point deviated to right and cant of commissure and piriform plane.

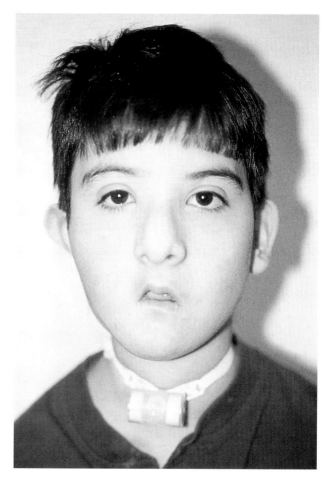

Fig. 58.12 One year-post distraction – a free scapular microvascular tissue transfer augmented the soft tissues. A one year follow up frontal photograph shows improved facial symmetry.

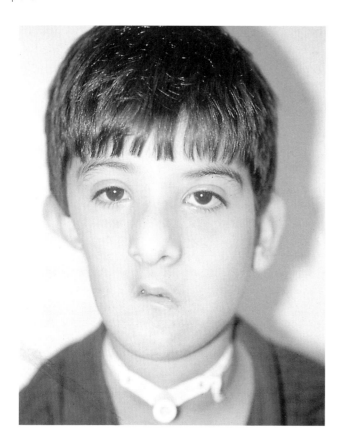

and lubricants may be necessary. In older patients, the use of a gold weight in the upper eyelid is a useful adjunctive procedure.

Correction of paralysis of the buccal and marginal mandibular branches of the facial nerve is more difficult. An asymmetric smile is often of considerable concern to patients and their families, and the atrophy of soft tissue associated with facial nerve paralysis serves to exacerbate the already existing deformity. In children with complete paralysis, the best reconstructive approach is a staged reconstruction with cross facial nerve grafting from the opposite side followed several months later by free microneurovascular transfer of muscle. The serratus anterior, pectoralis minor and gracilis have been used successfully for this purpose. The best results for this type of treatment are seen in children, in whom

Fig. 58.11 One year post right mandibular elongation by distraction. Note improved mandibular asymmetry with chin point to midline and leveling of commissure and piriform cants. Soft tissue deficiency of the right cheek remains.

muscle transfers can produce mimetic movement of the commissures of the mouth and upper lip. Transfer of the muscles of mastication in the presence of facial nerve paralysis can provide support but does not offer the possibility of coordinated movement with function. Static facial slings (e.g. tensor fasciae latae) are only indicated when patients are not candidates for alternative procedures.[69] Patients with marginal mandibular weakness and an asymmetric smile can have botulinum toxin injection of the normal depressor labialis to improve symmetry.

PROGRESSION OF FACIAL ASYMMETRY IN HFM

The subject of progression of facial deformity in HFM is controversial: there are two opposing theories. Clinicians who believe that the deformity changes in proportion to the growing child, rather than becoming progressively worse, contend that the mandibular asymmetry should be addressed in adolescence following completion of growth.[49,50] The contrasting view is that HFM is a progressive malformation[53] with the mandibular asymmetry becoming worse with age because the hypoplastic mandible restricts vertical growth of the midface leading to the secondary deformities associated with 'end-stage' HFM (vertically short maxilla, tilted occlusal plane, short mandible, deviated chin point).[28] The subject of the progressive nature of HFM is therefore central to the debate concerning early versus late treatment of the condition.

Craniofacial surgeons initially concentrated on the correction of 'end-stage' deformities in older children and adults. Advances in anesthetic and surgical techniques and also in the understanding of the pathogenesis of craniofacial anomalies encouraged surgeons to operate on certain deformities during growth. The hypothesis was that operative correction in a child would provide a more normal functional matrix within which the craniofacial skeleton could complete growth, however studies of early correction of midfacial hypoplasia in syndromic craniosynostoses showed disappointing results.[70,71] Despite the stability of midface advancement, the patients developed recurrent class III malocclusion due to inadequate midface growth relative to normal mandibular growth. This experience, however, is in marked contrast to the data reported for growing children with HFM.[28,55] These studies from Boston Children's Hospital documented that repair of mandibular hypoplasia in children with HFM produced improved growth, reduction of secondary deformity and improvement in body image development.

Further evidence supporting the progressive nature of facial asymmetry in HFM is provided by a number of clinical studies. Swanson and Murray[40] noted that patients with type II and III mandibular deformities developed a more significant end-stage asymmetry than those with type I. Kaban et al[11] followed 40 patients longitudinally; it was noted that the earliest skeletal manifestation of HFM was mandibular asymmetry – most patients had a level maxillary occlusal plane and piriform rim angle in infancy. Asymmetry became worse with growth as the normal side grew disproportionately larger than the affected side. This clinical observation was the basis of the protocol devised for the early treatment of HFM.

In a study of 36 patients with type IIB and III HFM, Padwa et al provided data regarding the progressive nature of HFM based on cephalometric analysis of PA cephalograms.[55] Patients underwent construction of the mandibular ramus and condyle on the affected side with costochondral grafts at a mean age of 6 years. The preoperative mean occlusal plane angle was 4.8 and 5.7 degrees for type IIB and III patients respectively. In those patients who had successful construction of the ramus–condyle unit (symmetrical growth both sides), the mean occlusal cant at follow up was 2 degrees. The maxilla grew vertically, thus leveling the occlusal plane. In those patients in whom the constructed ramus–condyle unit did not grow symmetrically with the unaffected side, the mean occlusal cant was 11 degrees (Tables 58.2, 58.3). The authors concluded that, without a growing ramus–condyle unit, asymmetry was progressive as evidenced by the increasing occlusal plane cant.

In a further study at Boston Children's Hospital of 67 unoperated HFM patients, a progression of facial asymmetry was noted based on an assessment of the piriform rim, maxillary occlusal plane and intergonial angles from PA cephalograms. The angles measured all showed a gradual increase with both growth and severity of the original skeletal deformity.[48] This provides further evidence that HFM is a progressive deformity (Fig. 58.13, Table 58.4).

The group at Chicago[49] have sought to provide evidence that HFM is not a progressive deformity, thus supporting the concept that patients should not be surgically treated until completion of growth. They studied 26 unoperated patients with HFM, using cephalometric measurements on standard PA cephalograms to record evidence of progression of facial asymmetry with growth. The authors' conclusions were that the mandibular asymmetry in HFM is not progressive in nature. However, careful assessment of the data would support the interpretation that there was a gradual increase in vertical mandibular asymmetry, both with growth and with the severity of the skeletal type, based on a gradually increasing intergonial angle and vertical gonial height from the initial to final radiographs.

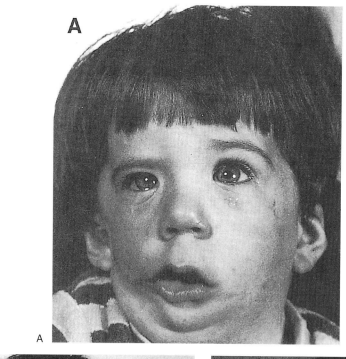

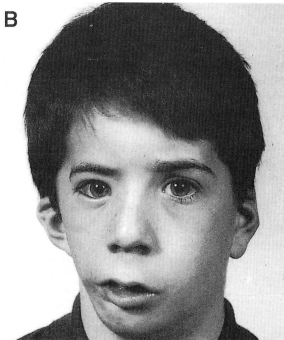

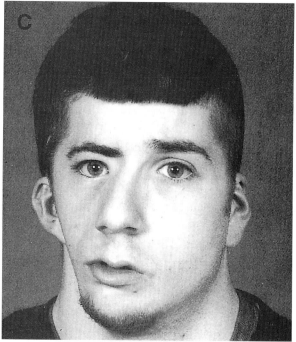

Fig. 58.13 Frontal photographs of a patient with type III HFM at **(A)** age 2, **(B)** age 12, and **(C)** age 21 illustrating the progressive increase of the cant of the alar base and labial commissures as well as progressive deviation of the chin to the right side.

In summary, the evidence available at present appears to support the hypothesis that facial asymmetry in HFM is indeed progressive in nature, and that the progression correlates with the mandibular skeletal type. If the progressive nature of the deformity is accepted then it would support early correction of all skeletal types of HFM in order to optimize growth and prevent the secondary distortion and worsening of facial asymmetry.

SUMMARY

The etiology, pathogenesis, classification, clinical features and treatment of HFM have been discussed. Emphasis has been placed on the importance of understanding the contrasting approaches to the management of the growing patient and the nongrowing patient. The purpose of treat-

Table 58.4 Progression of facial asymmetry in HFM[54]

	Group 1 (n = 38) (Type I, IIa)	Group II (n = 29) (Type IIB, III)
Deciduous dentition (<6 yr)		
Piriform rim angle	7.0° ± 3.6°	9.5° ± 3.5°
Maximal occlusal plane angle	4.3° ± 3.0°	6.2° ± 4.3°
Intergonial angle	4.4° ± 2.4°	5.3° ± 3.8°
Mean age (yr)	4.1 ± 0.9	3.4 ± 1.4
Mixed dentition (≥6 <13 yr)		
Piriform rim angle	7.7° ± 3.8°	11.7° ± 4.7°
Maximal occlusal plane angle	5.0° ± 3.5°	7.6° ± 3.8°
Intergonial angle	4.3° ± 2.8°	8.0° ± 3.4°
Mean age (yr)	8.6 ± 2.3	8.0 ± 1.7
Permanent dentition (≥13 yr)		
Piriform rim angle	8.4° ± 3.0°	
Maximal occlusal plane angle	6.6° ± 4.5°	
Intergonial angle	6.1° ± 3.6°	
Mean age (yr)	20.9 ± 8.9	

ment in the growing child is to enhance the growth potential of the mandible, to decrease or prevent secondary deformities in the facial skeletal structures, and to improve body image development by early intervention. In the adult patient with 'end-stage' deformity, accurate three-dimensional analysis and planning, taking into account both skeletal and soft-tissue defects, is critical for achievement of a satisfactory esthetic and functional outcome.

The role of mandibular and bimaxillary distraction osteogenesis has also been discussed relative to the management of HFM in the growing and nongrowing patient respectively. The reader is referred to Chapter 60 where the subject of distraction osteogenesis – including the historical perspectives, scientific background, and future directions for clinical and basic scientific research – is discussed in detail. The controversial issue of the progression of facial asymmetry in HFM has also been discussed, including a review of the evidence in favor of and against this hypothesis. The authors support the hypothesis that the deformity in HFM is progressive and therefore advocate interceptive surgical treatment for the growing child, as outlined in the treatment protocol, but accept that there are other investigators who hold an opposing opinion and advise against interceptive treatment, preferring to correct the 'end-stage' deformity when growth is complete.

The esthetic and functional end result of the treatment of HFM is difficult to quantitate accurately as it involves many features, some of which are difficult to assess and some of which are not related to the original anomaly. The final form of the structures depends upon the musculature, other soft tissues and orofacial functions and can be predicted only in association with the assessment of function and neuromuscular characteristics.

REFERENCES

1. Vento AR, LaBrie RA, Mulliken JB 1991 The OMENS Classification of hemifacial microsomia. Cleft Palate Craniofacial Journal 28:68–77
2. Gorlin RJ, Pindborg J 1964 Syndromes of the head and neck, 1st edn. McGraw-Hill, New York, pp. 261–265, 419–425
3. Grabb WC 1965 The first and second branchial arch syndrome. Plastic and Reconstructive Surgery 36:485–508
4. Cohen MM, Rollnick BR, Kaye CI 1989 Oculoauriculovertebral spectrum: an updated critique. Cleft Palate Journal 26:276–286
5. Gorlin RJ, Jue KL, Jacobson NP, Goldschmidt E 1963 Oculoauriculovertebral dysplasia. Journal of Pediatrics 63:991–999
6. Francois JJ, Haustrate L 1954 Anomalies colobomateuses du globe oculaire et syndrome du premier arc. Annales d'Oculistique 187:340–368
7. Ross RB 1975 Lateral facial dysplasia (first and second branchial arch syndrome: hemifacial microsomia). Birth Defects 11:51–59
8. Grayson BH, Boral S, Eisig S et al 1983 Unilateral craniofacial microsomia. I. Mandibular analysis. American Journal of Orthodortics 84:225
9. Goldenhar M 1952 Associations malformatives de l'oeil et de l'oreille, en particulier le syndrome dermoid epibulbaire-appendices auriculaires-fistula auris congenita et ses relations avec la dysostose mandibilo-faciale. Journal de Genetiques Humaines 1:243–282
10. Mulliken JB 1989 Preface. Cleft Palate Journal 26:275
11. Kaban LB, Mulliken JB, Murray JE 1981 Three dimensional approach to analysis and treatment of hemifacial microsomia. Cleft Palate Journal 18:90–99
12. Murray JE, Kaban LB, Mulliken JB 1984 Analysis and treatment of hemifacial microsomia. Plastic and Reconstructive Surgery 74:186–199
13. Poswillo DE 1973 The pathogenesis of first and second branchial arch syndrome. Oral Surgery 35:302–328
14. Melnick M 1980 The etiology of external ear malformations and its relation to abnormalities of the middle ear, inner ear and other organ systems. Birth Defects 16:303
15. Gustavson EE, Chen H 1985 Goldenhar syndrome, anterior encephalocele and aquaductal stenosis following fetal primidone exposure. Teratology 32:13
16. Lammer EJ, Chen DT, Hoar RM et al 1985 Retinoic acid embryopathy. New England Journal of Medicine 313:837–841
17. Cohen MM 1971 Variability versus 'incidental findings' in the first and second branchial arch syndrome: unilateral variants with anopthalmia. Birth Defects 7:103
18. Boles DJ, Bodurtha J, Nance WE 1987 Goldenhar complex in discordant monozygotic twins: A case report and review of the literature. American Journal of Medical Genetics 28:103
19. Stoll C, Roth MP, Dott B, Bigel T 1984 Discordance for skeletal and cardiac defect in monozygotic twins. Acta Geneticae Medicae et Gemellologicae 33:501
20. Rollnick BR 1988 Oculovertebral anomaly: Variability and causal heterogeneity. American Journal of Medical Genetics (suppl) 4:41
21. Ryan CA, Finer NN, Ives E 1988 Discordance of signs in monozygotic twins concordant for the Goldenhar anomaly. American Journal of Medical Genetics 29:755
22. Johnson MC, Bronsky PT 1991 Animal models for human craniofacial malformations. Journal of Craniofacial Genetics and Developmental Biology 11:227–291
23. Soltan HC, Homes LB 1986 Familial occurence of malformations possibly attributable to vascular abnormalities. Journal of Pediatrics 109:112–114
24. Johnson MC, Bronsky PT 1995 Prenatal craniofacial development: new insights on normal and abnormal mechanisms. Critical Reviews in Oral Biology and Medicine 6:25–79
25. Murray JE, Kaban LB, Mulliken JB, Evans CA 1985 Analysis and treatment of hemifacial microsomia. In: Caronni EP (ed) Craniofacial surgery. Little, Brown, Boston, pp 377–390

26. Vargervik K, Miller AJ 1984 Neuromuscular patterns in hemifacial microsomia. American Journal of Orthodontics 86:33–42
27. Kaban LB, Moses ML, Mulliken JB 1986 Correction of hemifacial microsomia in the growing child: a follow up study. Cleft Palate Journal 23 (suppl 1):50–52
28. Kaban LB, Moses ML, Mulliken JB 1988 Surgical correction of hemifacial microsomia in the growing child. Plastic and Reconstructive Surgery 82:9–19
29. Luce EA, McGibbon B, Hoopes JE 1977 Velopharyngeal insufficiency in hemifacial microsomia. Plastic and Reconstructive Surgery 60:602–606
30. Meurman Y 1957 Congenital microtia and meatal atresia. Archives of Otolaryngology 66:443
31. Marx H 1926 Die missbildungen des ohres: sekundare ohrmissbildungen. In: Henke F, Lubarsch O (eds) Handbuch des speziellen pathologischen anatomie und histologie. Springer-Verlag, Berlin, p 697
32. Pruzansky S 1969 Not all dwarfed mandibles are alike. Birth Defects 1:120–129
33. Brent B 1992 Auricular repair with autogenous rib grafts: Two decades of experience with 600 cases. Plastic and Reconstructive Surgery 90:355
34. Dellon AL, Claybaugh GJ, Hoopes JE 1983 Hemipalatal palsy and microtia. Annals of Plastic Surgery 10:475–479
35. Shprintzen RJ, Croft CB, Berkman MD, Rakoff SJ 1980 Velopharyngeal insufficiency in the facio-auriculo-vertebral malformation. Cleft Palate Journal 17:132–137
36. Converse JM, Coccaro PJ, Becker MH, Wood-Smith D 1979 Clinical aspects of craniofacial microsomia. In: Converse JM, McCarthy JG, Wood-Smith D (eds) Symposium on diagnosis and treatment of craniofacial anomalies. CV Mosby, St Louis, pp 461–475
37. Cherici G 1983 Radiological assessment of facial asymmetry. In: Harvold EP, Vargervik K, Cherici G (eds) Treatment of hemifacial microsomia. Alan Liss, New York, pp 74–87
38. Lauritzen C, Munro IR, Ross RB 1985 Classification and treatment of hemifacial microsomia. Scandinavian Journal of Plastic and Reconstructive Surgery 19:33–39
39. David DJ, Mahatumarat C, Cooter RD 1987 Hemifacial microsomia: a multisystem classification. Plastic and Reconstructive Surgery 80:525–533
40. Swanson LT, Murray JE 1978 Asymmetries of the lower part of the face. In: Whitaker LA, Randall P (eds) Symposium on reconstruction of jaw deformities. CV Mosby, St Louis, pp 171–196
41. Cousley RR 1993 A comparison of two classification systems for hemifacial microsomia. British Journal of Oral and Maxillofacial Surgery 31:78–82
42. Cohen MM 1991 A critique of the OMENS classification of hemifacial microsomia. Cleft Palate–Craniofacial Journal 28:77
43. Horgan JE, Padwa BL, LaBrie RA, Mulliken JB 1995 OMENS Plus: Analysis of craniofacial and extracraniofacial anomalies in hemifacial microsomia. Cleft Palate Craniofacial Journal 32:405–412
44. Marsh JL, Baca D, Vannier MW 1989 Facial musculoskeletal asymmetry in hemifacial microsomia. Cleft Palate Journal 26:292–302
45. Moss ML, Rankow RM 1968 The role of the functional matrix in mandibular growth. Angle Orthodontics 28:95
46. Ware WH, Brown SL 1981 Growth center transplantation to replace mandibular condyles. Journal of Maxillofacial Surgery 9:50
47. Storey A 1976 Temporomandibular joint receptor. In: Anderson OJ, Matthews B (eds) Mastication. John Wright, Bristol, p 50
48. Kaban LB, Padwa BL, Mulliken JB 1998 Surgical correction of mandibular correction of mandibular hypoplasia in hemifacial microsomia: The case for treatment in early childhood. Journal of Oral and Maxillofacial Surgery 56:628–638
49. Polley JW, Figueroa AA, Liou EJ, Cohen MM 1997 Longitudinal analysis of mandibular asymmetry in hemifacial microsomia. Plastic and Reconstructive Surgery 99:328–339
50. Rune B, Selvik G, Sarnas KV, Jacobsson S 1981 Growth in hemifacial microsomia studied with the aid of roentgen stereophotogrammetry and metallic implants. Cleft Palate Journal 18:128
51. Vargervik K, Ousterhout D 1986 Factors affecting long-term results in hemifacial mircosomia. Cleft Palate Journal 23 (suppl 1): 53–68
52. Harvold EP, Vargerik K, Cherici G (eds) 1983 Treatment of hemifacial microsomia. Alan Liss, New York
53. Mulliken JB, Kaban LB 1987 Analysis and treatment of hemifacial microsomia in childhood. Clinics in Plastic Surgery 14:91–100
54. Melsen B, Bjerregaard J, Bundgaard M 1986 The effect of functional appliances on a pathologic growth pattern of the condyle. American Journal of Orthodontics 90:503–512
55. Padwa BL, Mulliken JB, Maghen BA, Kaban LB 1998 Midfacial growth after costochondral graft construction of the mandibular ramus in hemifacial microsomia. Journal of Oral and Maxillofacial Surgery 56:122–127
56. Ilizarov GA 1990 Clinical application of the tension-stress effect for limb lengthening. Clinical Orthopaedics and Related Research 250:8–26
57. McCarthy JG, Schreiber J, Krp N et al 1992 Lengthening of the human mandible by gradual distraction. Plastic and Reconstructive Surgery 89:1
58. Chin M, Toth BA 1996 Distraction osteogenesis in maxillofacial surgery using internal devices: review of five cases. Journal of Oral and Maxillofacial Surgery 54:45
59. McCarthy JG 1994 The role of distraction osteogenesis in the reconstruction of the mandible in unilateral craniofacial microsomia. Clinics in Plastic Surgery 21:625
60. Molina F, Ortiz-Monasterio F 1995 Mandibular elongation and remodelling by distraction: a farewell to major osteotomies. Plastic and Reconstructive Surgery 94:825–840
61. Wilkes GH, Wolfaardt JF 1994 Osseointegrated alloplastic versus autogenous ear reconstruction: criteria for treatment selection. Plastic and Reconstructive Surgery 93:967–979
62. Thompson HG, Winslow J 1989 Microtia reconstruction: Does the cartilage framework grow. Plastic and Reconstructive Surgery 84:908
63. Tanzer RC 1971 The total reconstruction of the auricle. The evolution of a plan of treatment. Plastic and Reconstructive Surgery 47:523
64. Brent B 1980 The correction of microtia with autogenous cartilage grafts. 1. The classic deformity. Plastic and Reconstructive Surgery 66:1
65. Brent B, Byrd HS 1983 Secondary ear reconstruction with cartilage grafts covered by axial, random and free flaps of temporoparietal fascia. Plastic and Reconstructive Surgery 72:141
66. Vargervik K, Hoffman WY, Kaban LB 1996 Comprehensive surgical and orthodontic management of hemifacial microsomia. In: Turvey TA, Vig KWL, Fonseca RJ (eds) Facial clefts and craniosynostosis: Principles and management. WB Saunders, Philadelphia, pp 537–564
67. Mordick TG, Larossa D, Whitaker L 1992 Soft tissue reconstruction of the face: a comparison of dermal fat grafting and vascularized tissue transfer. Annals of Plastic Surgery 29:390
68. Huntsman WT, Lineweaver W, Ousterhout DK 1992 Recipient vessels for microvascular transplants in patients with hemifacial microsomia. Journal of Craniofacial Surgery 3:187
69. Hoffman WY 1992 Reanimation of the paralysed face. Otolaryngology Clinics of North America 25:649
70. Kaban LB, West B, Conover M, Will L, Mulliken JB, Murray JE 1984 Midface position after Le Fort III advancement. Plastic and Reconstructive Surgery 73:758
71. McCarthy JG, Epstein F, Sandove M et al 1984 Early surgery for craniofacial synostosis: An 8 year experience. Plastic and Reconstructive Surgery 73:521

Treacher Collins syndrome

59

DAVID A. KOPPEL/KHURSHEED F. MOOS

INTRODUCTION

From ancient times patients with this syndrome were identified in a recognizable form in the new world: there are pre-Columbian terracotta carvings of the typical facies of Treacher Collins syndrome, and the familial incidence had been recorded from AD 600 to 1000. The first description in the modern era was probably that of Thomson, the Professor of Physiology in the University of Edinburgh in 1846.[1,2] Other early descriptions were by Toynbee in 1847[3] and Berry[4] in 1889. E. Treacher Collins, an ophthalmic surgeon at Moorfields Hospital in London, described a case in 1900,[5] and it was from his description that the syndrome was named. Franceschetti[6] published extensively on the topic and labeled the condition 'mandibulofacial dysostosis'. He and his co-workers reviewed and consolidated many of the previous reports and classified them into several groups: complete, incomplete, abortive, unilateral and atypical. It is probable that their classification includes several cases of Nager syndrome and hemifacial microsomia – this may be why the pedigrees that they presented do not, in most cases, clearly demonstrate the pattern of genetic transmission. However, as a result of this extensive review and the importance of their contribution the condition is also known in Europe as Franceschetti–Zwahlen–Klein syndrome. Tessier describes the condition as the constellation of clefts 6, 7 and 8. Van der Meulen classifies the condition as zygo-auromandibular dysplasia.

This autosomal dominant condition has panfacial effects that are both functional and cosmetic. The management of children with this syndrome and their families requires a multidisciplinary approach to minimize or correct those functional problems and to address the craniofacial deformities.

GENETICS AND PATHOGENESIS

The condition is autosomal dominant with a variable degree of penetrance and expression. It occurs with a frequency of approximately 1/50 000 live births; between 50 and 60% of cases have no family history and are therefore mutations *de novo*. The range of presentation is wide, from mild cases with no functional deficit and minimal deformity, to severe cases that die in the perinatal period as a result of airway compromise.

The condition has been described as one of the first and second branchial arch syndromes, and it has been postulated that it is caused by a failure of migration of neural crest cells or alternatively a disorder of cell differentiation.[7] More recent work has indicated that the syndrome results from disordered development of the first and second branchial ectodermal placodes rather than from a primary neural crest cell disorder. A murine model of Treacher Collins syndrome supports this theory in that retinoic acid induces the syndrome (or at least a murine analog) when mice are exposed 9–9.5 days post fertilization.[8,9] The gene for Treacher Collins syndrome has been identified and named *Treacle*, and it has been localized to chromosome 5q32–33.1; to date five different mutations have been identified although no mutation to phenotype correlations have been identified. All five identified mutations result in premature termination in the as yet unknown protein.[10–13]

The connection between the genotype and the phenotype is not yet understood – as discussed above a murine model of Treacher Collins syndrome can be produced by exposing pregnant mice to retinoic acid. Experiments on rats indicate that the lack of development of the zygomatic arches results in a compensatory growth accounting for the hyper-projection and clockwise rotation of the maxilla.[14]

This may be an indication for early reconstruction of the malars to prevent or minimize further undesirable growth of the maxilla.

CLINICAL FEATURES

The typical facies of Treacher Collins syndrome usually make diagnosis easy. The palpebral fissures are downward sloping (antimongoloid), the malars are poorly developed or absent, the mandible is retrusive and there is also retrogenia (Fig. 59.1).

SKULL

The anterior cranial length is shorter with some increase in the posterior cranial length, and the overall cranial length is normal or reduced as compared with controls. The mastoid processes are often not pneumatized and may be sclerotic. The degree of underdevelopment or absence of the malar bone is variable and tends to be fairly symmetrical. The defect in malar development may be predominantly lateral, predominantly medial or a combination of the two (Fig. 59.2). This malar hypoplasia causes the orbit to be shallow and to be rotated inferolaterally with a resulting oval shape. The cranial base angle is high, resulting in an anteroposterior narrowing of the pharyngeal space. The cranial base length is normal; however the anterior cranial base is shortened with a compensatory increase in posterior length.[15,16]

NOSE AND FACIAL SOFT TISSUES

The frontonasal angle is high and the hypoplastic malars make the nose appear more prominent. The nasal root width

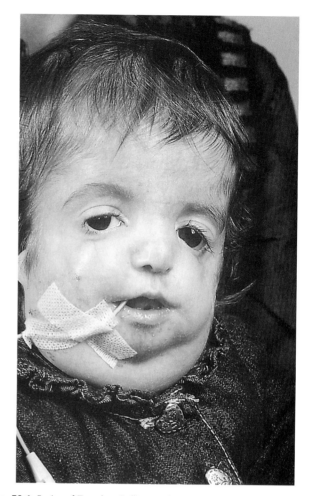

Fig. 59.1 Facies of Treacher Collins syndrome.

is increased but in fact the nose is usually of normal or even optimal size.[17] In approximately 25% of cases a tongue of hairbearing skin extends down on to the cheeks from the temporal region. The skin overlying the hypoplastic malars is often thin with minimal subcutaneous tissue.

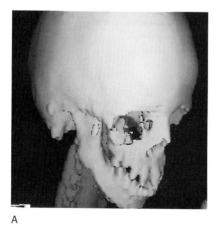
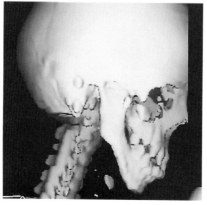
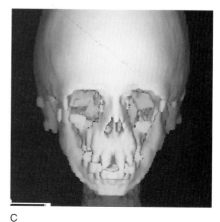

A   B   C

Fig. 59.2 (A–C) 3D reconstructions of CT scans of typical patient showing malar deficiency. (See also Figs 59.4 and 59.7.)

OPHTHALMIC FEATURES

Almost all patients in reported series have some ocular and adnexal problems. The antimongoloid slant of the palpebral fissures and the rudimentary, inferiorly placed lateral canthal ligaments are almost uniform. True colobomata are present in about 25% of cases, and pseudocolobomata occur in about 50% of cases – they tend to be in the lateral third of the lower eyelid. There is also typically a lack of eyelashes in the outer third of the lower lid. Refractive errors are very common, and amblyopia is not uncommon. Various other less common ophthalmic conditions have also been reported including Duane syndrome, lacrimal duct atresia, cataracts, microphthalmos, anophthalmos and other forms of strabismus.[18]

EAR AND HEARING

The pinna can present with a variety of different abnormalities, in form, size and position. There is usually slight asymmetry in the condition. The pinna may be relatively normal in size and shape, ranging to the presence of small ear tags with one or more (blind-ending) fistulae. The pinna, whatever the degree of deformity, tends to be anteriorly and inferiorly displaced, as well as having a crumpled appearance.

The external auditory meatus ranges in deformity from being patent to having a complete bony occlusion. In the majority of cases there is a degree of soft-tissue stenosis at the very least.

The middle ear is virtually always hypoplastic with the attic being mostly affected. The ossicular chain is often abnormal and again the severity is variable; the chain is frequently displaced anterolaterally.[19]

The inner ear is usually normal with some shortening and anterior displacement of the descending portion of the facial nerve.

A more detailed classification of the ear abnormalities is given by Altman (1955)[20] as modified by Cremers and Teunissen (1991),[21] which classifies the abnormalities into major and minor. As a general rule the severity of the middle ear abnormalities is reflected in the severity of pinna abnormalities.

MANDIBLE

The mandible is hypoplastic in the ascending ramus, body and in the projection of the chin. There is a marked antegonial notch with an obtuse gonial angle and a tendency for the chin to rotate inferiorly. This gives the mandible a bowed appearance. The pattern of bowing is different from that seen in other conditions such as Still's disease, and these differences have been quantified. The muscular attachment of the pterygomasseteric sling is abnormal – often with the masseter originating posteriorly from the base of the skull with the zygomatic arch remnant to insert on the posterior aspect of the mandible, seeming to fuse with the medial pterygoid muscle.

MAXILLA

The maxilla tends to have a high arched palate or cleft (30%). The posterior dental height is low with a degree of maxillary hyperprojection. This hyperprojection is, in some cases, rather more apparent than real and it is difficult to be sure from the published studies if the abnormality lies in the maxilla or the cranial base. There may be an associated choanal atresia which, if present, compounds the airway problems, especially in the neonatal period. The skeletal relationship of the jaws often results in a class II anterior open-bite. The teeth usually develop normally and are of normal size. However, the narrow arches and the small abnormally shaped mandible often lead to severe dental crowding.

MENTAL DEVELOPMENT

Learning difficulties have been reported but these are more likely to be related to deafness and delay in speech development.

DIAGNOSIS

If there is a positive family history diagnosis can usually be made easily on clinical grounds alone and be confirmed with genetic studies. In sporadic cases the most common differential diagnosis is Nager syndrome.[22] The latter syndrome is autosomal recessive and associated with preaxial limb abnormalities. Prenatal diagnosis is now possible in cases with a positive family history; a detailed ultrasound scan can also identify the extent of deformity.[23] The drawback of prenatal diagnosis is that, at present, this is only made relatively late in pregnancy so that if a termination is to be considered the decision obviously becomes more difficult.

MANAGEMENT

As with all craniofacial anomalies, the management of these patients and their parents should have specific goals and aim to maximize the child's potential. The overall treatment plan should be problem orientated but also flexible enough to meet the patient's and parents' desires and needs. Soon after the child's birth the craniofacial team should be involved; initially this involvement may only be in supportive role but on occasions airway or feeding problems may necessitate early surgical intervention.

The overall plan in the uncomplicated case should follow the outline given below:

Perinatal period
Airway support if necessary, including tracheostomy
Feeding support
Assessment of severity of condition
Exclusion of other abnormalities
General psychologic and practical support for the parents and family
Introduction to the craniofacial team
Introduction to a support group
Genetic advice

0–3 months
Formal hearing assessment
Provision of bone conducting hearing aid
Growth and development monitoring
Management of cleft palate following normal protocols
Ophthalmic assessment

3 months – 5 years
Growth and development monitoring
Airway support if necessary
Feeding support if necessary
Monitor hearing and speech development
Routine dental care and assessment
Consider early mandibular surgery if persistent airway problems

5 Years – cessation of growth
Consider mandibular lengthening
Malar reconstruction
Consider bone anchored hearing aid
Eyelid surgery
Orthodontics
Ear reconstruction
Rhinoplasty

After cessation of growth
Orthognathic surgery
Genetic counseling

In the perinatal period the priority for the care of these patients is airway management, feeding support, and confirmation of the diagnosis with the exclusion of other abnormalities. It is obviously a distressing and worrying time for the parents and families and it is necessary to be able to offer appropriate support and counseling. The craniofacial team should be introduced to the patient and parents at this time so that an early rapport is developed.

Feeding support, if necessary, is given in the perinatal period via a nasogastric tube; this can be continued at home should the need arise.

Early airway assessment is mandatory; this is essentially a clinical assessment, at least in the first few hours and days. If airway embarrassment is present a diagnosis must be made and if necessary a surgical airway secured. Choanal atresia and mandibular hypoplasia are the common causes but there may be tracheomalacia, hence the necessity for an early expert assessment.

In the first few months after birth a formal hearing assessment (with brainstem evoked potential) should be carried out and, if necessary, a bone conducting hearing aid provided to facilitate speech development. During this period the patient's airway should be regularly assessed as sleep apnea can lead to irreversible pulmonary hypertension. The child's growth and development should be closely monitored and the parents given the level of support and practical help that they need.

If there is a cleft palate, this is dealt with in the normal way using accepted protocols, and the timing of surgical repair is only modified if the patient's general condition precludes repair at the optimal time. (Details of the protocols for the repair of the cleft palate are given elsewhere in this book.)

Aside from management of the airway and the provision of a bone conducting hearing aid, the timing of surgical intervention can be tailored to suit the individual patient. Authorities differ in the suggested optimal time for the various interventions and the outlines given below should not be regarded as hard and fast rules. There is evidence that the degree of deformity does not change with growth and development, and the facial profile (as measured by the angle of convexity) neither worsens nor improves with time. Although there is some evidence (extrapolated from an animal study) that the absence of the zygomatic arches allows hyperprojection of the maxilla there is no evidence that early malar reconstruction modifies later maxillary development.

MANDIBULAR LENGTHENING

In the majority of uncomplicated cases this is probably best delayed until growth has been completed. Early distraction osteogenesis (age 12 or younger) should be reserved for patients with significant airway compromise (i.e. tracheostomy dependent or moderate to severe sleep apnea). In these selected cases bilateral mandibular distraction.[24] (Fig. 59.3)

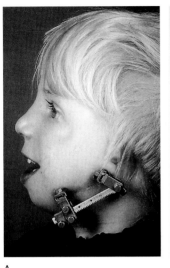
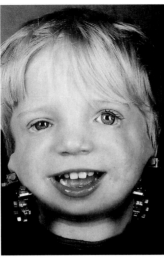

A   B

Fig. 59.3 (A,B) Distraction devices in place during the fixation period. The child underwent distraction at the age of 20 months because of severe sleep apnea. This intervention avoided the necessity for a tracheostomy.

may be life saving if it allows decannulation, however the technique, unless intraoral distracters are used, does lead to scarring of the skin. There is also risk to the developing tooth germs and the inferior dental neurovascular bundle. The younger (and smaller) the mandible, the more technically demanding is the procedure, and there is a greater risk of complications. If distraction is used in the period prior to the cessation of growth it is probable that further mandibular surgery will be required.

Technique for distraction osteogenesis

Once the treatment has been agreed, the patient and parents must be carefully counseled as to the nature of the therapy, its risks and complications. For the treatment to be successful, a high degree of cooperation and commitment from the patient and parents is necessary. The distraction devices must be turned on a daily basis, kept clean to prevent infection, and protected from trauma. The procedure must be carefully planned, taking into account the amount of lengthening, the site of lengthening (i.e. mandibular body, ramus or a combination), and the final desired occlusion. The design of the distraction device and the desired site of lengthening determine the ideal site for the placement of the pins, the site and the angulation of the corticotomy cut. This planning is carried out following clinical and radiographic assessments, and it is also helpful to have orthodontic input at this stage. Dental models, a mandibular model or a CT derived stereolithographic model are also of practical use.

Surgical procedure

This is carried out under general anesthesia. The medial and lateral surfaces of the mandible are exposed transorally and the inferior dental neurovascular bundle is protected medially, the corticotomy cut is marked and the superior pins for the distraction device are placed transcutaneously. The skin entry points for the superior pins should be caudal to the point of bone entry to minimize scarring. The corticotomy is completed, paying special attention to the posterior border of the mandible. The lower pins are then inserted, again pulling the skin, this time in a cranial direction. The intraoral wounds are closed with a resorbable (absorbable) suture. In the postoperative period a fluid diet is commenced and distraction is started on approximately day 5 – 1 mm per day is an acceptable amount. The patient should continue on a semisolid diet and the distraction devices are removed 3–4 weeks following the completion of distraction. It is useful to obtain a radiograph after 3 days of distraction to ensure even distraction with no 'hinging' across the corticotomy. If hinging does occur, the corticotomy should be reopened under general anesthesia to facilitate the planned distraction. It is possible to perform an advancement genioplasty and a suprahyoid muscle release at the same time to maximize the mandibular advancement (Fig. 59.4).

Postcondylar grafts

An alternative approach that has been used in the past is the placement of postcondylar grafts. This is carried out at around 10 years of age. This technique, by the insertion behind the mandibular condyle extracapsularly, of either an alloplastic material or cartilage harvested from the iliac crest, advances the mandible; over the first postoperative year a new glenoid fossa develops, giving a mandibular advancement of approximately 10–15 mm.

Ramus osteotomies

The mandible may also be lengthened by the use of ramus osteotomies. The most useful technique is the inverted L osteotomy which allows lengthening of the deficient ascending ramus and advancement of the mandible, as well as recontouring of the mandibular angle. It is carried out via an extraoral incision which facilitates release of the aberrant pterygomasseteric sling, the placement of an interpositional cortico-cancellous bone graft (usually Iliac crest) and the use of internal fixation devices. The mandibular angle can also be augmented. The results are stable and larger movements are possible, especially in lengthening the ramus, than

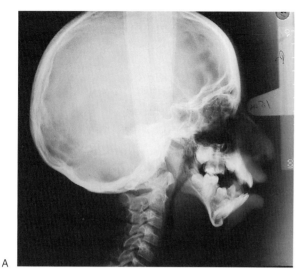

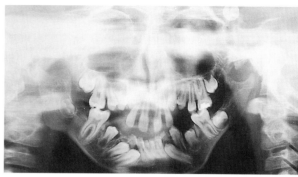

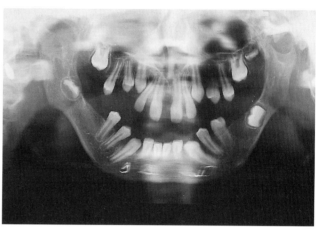

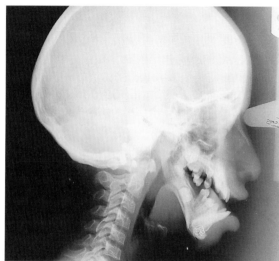

Fig. 59.4 (A–D) Lateral cephalograms and rotational tomograms before and after mandibular distraction. Note the bone anchored hearing aid and ear prostheses. Also an advancement genioplasty has been performed. (Same patient as Figs 59.2 and 59.7.)

with a sagittal split osteotomy (Fig. 59.5). The major disadvantage is the scar; however, with well placed incisions and careful suturing the scar can be relatively inconspicuous. The timing of this type of mandibular surgery is variable. In those cases where mandibular lengthening by distraction osteogenesis or postcondylar grafting is not performed, the inverted L osteotomy may be used early (i.e. age 8–14 years). In the vast majority of cases who have had mandibular lengthening, by whichever technique, before the cessation of growth, revisional surgery is usually required. The inverted L osteotomy may be used for this revisional surgery (even if the original surgery utilized an inverted L osteotomy) and should be integrated into the overall orthognathic treatment plan.

Body osteotomies and segmental procedures

A variety of procedures have been described for mandibular lengthening and may be applied to patients with Treacher Collins syndrome. These procedures are difficult to perform in the presence of a developing dentition and do not address the lack of ramus height. Where the dental occlusion is close to normal the use of alveolar segmental procedures may be helpful in preventing any restriction of mandibular advancement.

GENIOPLASTY

An advancement genioplasty can be performed both to improve the airway, as an early procedure, and as a part of the overall orthognathic treatment plan to maximize the effect of the mandibular advancement. There may be a degree of macrogenia in some cases, requiring a vertical reduction in association with the advancement. If the genioplasty is combined with a mandibular lengthening procedure for severe airway embarrassment, a suprahyoid myotomy may also be utilized to maximize the mandibular advancement. In some cases a double sliding genioplasty can be used, however the

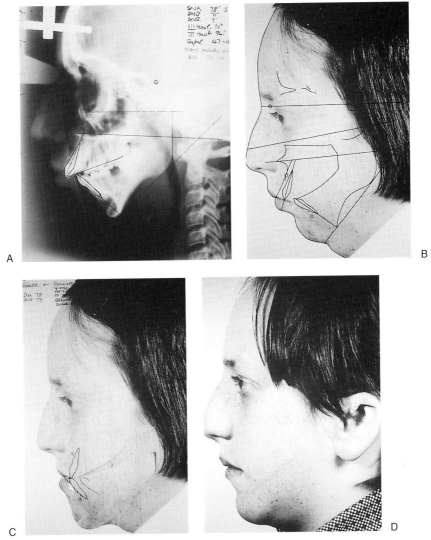

Fig. 59.5 (A–D) Relatively mild case demonstrating correction with a sagittal split osteotomy, illustrations showing preoperative cephalogram **(A)**, photocephalometric planning **(B,C)**, and postoperative appearance **(D)**.

anterior teeth should have erupted to allow enough depth for this to be performed.

MALAR RECONSTRUCTION

This can be carried out from about the age of 8 years, however the exact timing depends on the wishes of the patient and parents. There does not appear to be a surgical advantage in early reconstruction and the child's social, psychologic and educational development are paramount in deciding the time for malar reconstruction. Our preferred method for initial malar reconstruction is the use of outer table calvarial bone grafts fixed in place with screws and/or plates.

The surgical planning is facilitated by the use of 3D reconstructed CT scans (Fig. 59.2); a stereolithographic model may also be useful. The CT scans give information on the cleft deformity and also about the thickness of the calvarium in the area for the donor site. If the bone is seen to be too thin for harvesting an outer table calvarial graft, a craniotomy can be performed and the bone split on a side table. The donor site is chosen for the bone thickness and curvature; the 3D CT facilitates this planning. If a single layer of calvarial bone is not thick enough for the desired contour of the reconstructed malar, it can be layered and fixed with screws and/or plates.

The donor site and the areas to be reconstructed are approached with a bicoronal skin incision. If the malar deficiency has an anterior component, a lower eyelid, infra-orbital or transconjunctival incision is also necessary. (The choice of incision depends on the extent and form of the eyelid deformity.) An intraoral buccal sulcus approach may also be helpful.

The malar is reconstructed with a combination of onlay and inlay grafts to produce a normal bony contour (Fig. 59.6). A small amount of overcorrection is necessary to compensate for any resorption and the thinned soft tissue. In some cases the soft tissue can be augmented with the use of bilateral pericranial flaps folded on themselves and layered over the bone grafts.

At the same time as malar reconstruction it is desirable to refine the shape of the orbit and reposition the lateral canthus (Fig. 59.6C). Using the exposure afforded by the bicoronal flap the orbit may be recontoured to give a more normal shape; a crescent of bone is taken from the supero-lateral orbital rim (using a fine oscillating saw or burr) and repositioned as an overlay just above the site from which it was detached. The bone may be fixed with fine screws or a wire, this helps in giving the orbit a more normal shape. A lateral canthopexy is also carried out to reattach the canthus in a more superior position and to correct the antimongo-loid slant. It is advisable to overcorrect the canthopexy to allow for slight relapse. For the canthopexy 0.35 mm stain-less steel wire is used to suspend the attachment and adja-cent periorbita to a small hole drilled in the superolateral orbital rim.

In some cases which have undergone early malar recon-struction it may be necessary to carry out further malar osteotomies to optimize their position. This should be

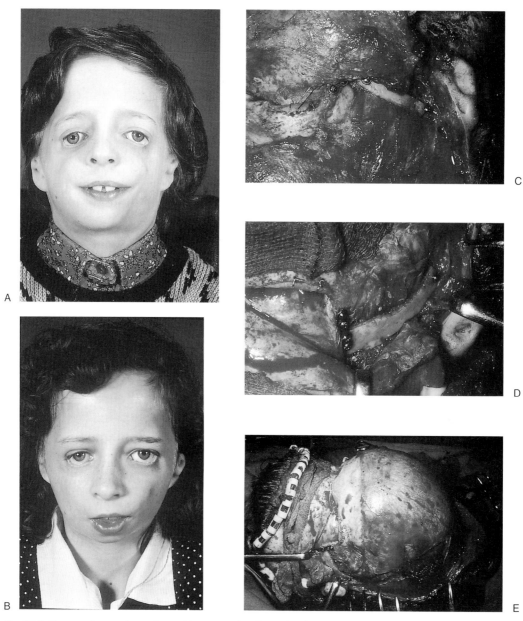

Fig. 59.6 Preoperative, postoperative and intraoperative views of malar reconstruction with calvarial bone graft.

deferred until the cessation of growth, when a conventional malar osteotomy may be performed. If reoperation is necessary, however, the quantity of bone should be assessed preoperatively with 3D CT scans as further bone grafting may be necessary.

Other strategies for malar reconstruction[25,26] have included rib grafts, which, though easier than cranial bone to manipulate and contour, tend to be more prone to resorption and also necessitate a distant donor site.

In cases where malar reconstruction is performed simultaneously with mandibular ramus surgery, there is a slight risk of ankylosis developing; this risk is heightened if intermaxillary fixation is used. For this reason our preferred practice is to perform such procedures separately.

ORTHOGNATHIC SURGERY

At the completion of growth the definitive orthognathic surgery should be performed. The planning for this should follow conventional lines and be preceded by orthodontic treatment where appropriate. The overall facial form depends on many factors, particularly the effects of the previous surgery, but bimaxillary surgery is the norm. Although some experts advocate a modified Le Fort II osteotomy,[27] a Le Fort I osteotomy is often satisfactory in repositioning the maxilla. In these cases the maxilla is downgrafted posteriorly and the mandibular ramus lengthened and the mandible advanced with an inverted L osteotomy. An advancement genioplasty is usually necessary and its extent may be determined by standard orthognathic planning techniques. There is no significant additional difficulty other than the necessity for the removal of metalwork if the same procedures have to be repeated. An alternative mandibular osteotomy in mild cases is the sagittal split advancement although for the reasons already discussed the inverted L is preferred (Fig. 59.5).

PINNA RECONSTRUCTION

The degree of pinna deformity is variable and thus the amount of surgery required varies. In those cases where the pinna is vestigial, grossly deformed or severely malpositioned the current options are for a staged autologous reconstruction or excision and the provision of an osseointegrated supported prosthesis. The timing of such surgery is again a matter for discussion between the parents, patient and craniofacial team. At present the osseointegrated prosthesis gives the most predictable results (Fig. 59.7) and obviates the necessity for a cartilage (usually costochondral) donor site. It should be noted that the transcutaneous implants supporting the prosthesis require meticulous hygiene and therefore the patient and family must be able to look after

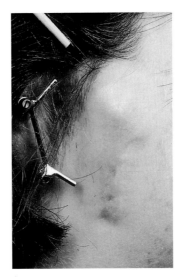 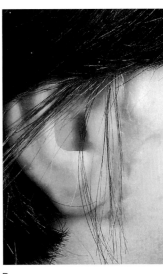

A   B

Fig. 59.7 (A,B) Ear reconstruction with bone supported prosthesis.

the implants and prosthesis. It is the degree of cooperation that usually determines the timing of the ear reconstruction. The previous provision of a bone anchored hearing aid is often a good pointer to the extent of patient cooperation.

EAR SURGERY

Surgery to the external meatus, to correct the stenosis, and middle ear surgery should be limited to those cases where the deformity is minimal. This is usually assessed by high resolution CT scanning and in general should be limited to those cases with minimal stenosis and an inner ear with a good prognosis. Expert otologic input is mandatory.[28]

EYELID SURGERY

The timing and type of eyelid surgery is determined by the extent of the deformity. In general the longer this is delayed the better the results, however early surgery is indicated if corneal ulceration is a problem. For this reason, and the assessment of other ocular problems, early and regular ophthalmic review is necessary.

ORTHODONTICS AND DENTAL CARE

As soon as the primary dentition starts to erupt it is necessary to institute good dental hygiene and care to develop good lifelong habits. This ensures that the dentition is optimal for the provision of orthodontic treatment and eventually for orthognathic surgery. The teeth are usually normal but crowding is a common problem; interventional extractions as guided by the orthodontist may be necessary. The orthodontic treatment plan should be integrated into the overall surgical plan to minimize unnecessary treatment and maximize gain. Unnecessary or ill timed treatment often demoralizes the patients and parents and makes further treatment difficult.

MANAGEMENT OF SLEEP APNEA

Obstructive sleep apnea may be a problem also in the older child. Poor school performance may be a pointer to the diagnosis but this should be confirmed with formal sleep studies. In mild cases tonsillectomy and adenoidectomy may be helpful. For the more severe cases with marked retropositioning of the jaws a bimaxillary advancement is often curative. For intermediate cases continuous positive airway pressure support with a custom-made mask should be tried.

SUMMARY

The care of the patient and family requires a skilled multi-disciplinary team working together with common aims. Initial care is geared towards airway and feeding management, later hearing and development are priorities, and finally the craniofacial reconstruction becomes the priority. The treatment plan must clearly reflect each individual's needs and desires to optimize the end result. Although various specialists are often able to provide individual items of treatment or operations, an integrated team approach is the best setting for the care of these patients.

REFERENCES

1. Thomson A 1846 Notice of several cases of malformation of the external ear, together with experiments on the state of hearing in such persons (part 1). Monthly Journal of Medical Science 7: 420–425
2. Thomson A 1847 Notice of several cases of malformation of the external ear, together with experiments on the state of hearing in such persons (part 2). Monthly Journal of Medical Science 10: 729–738
3. Toynbee J 1847 Description of a congenital malformation in the ears of a child. Monthly Journal of Medical Science 10: 738–742
4. Berry GA 1889 Note on a congenital defect (coloboma ?) of the lower lid. Royal London Ophthalmic Hospital Report 12: 255–257
5. Treacher Collins E 1900 Cases with symmetrical congenital notches in the outer part of each lid and defective development of the malar bones. Transactions of the Ophthalmological Society UK 20: 190–192
6. Franceschetti A, Klein D 1949 Mandibulo-facial dysostosis: new hereditary syndrome. Acta Ophthalmologica 27: 143–224
7. Poswillo D 1988 The aetiology and pathogenesis of craniofacial deformity. Development 103 (suppl): 207–212
8. Johnston MC, Bronsky PT 1995 Prenatal craniofacial development: new insights on normal and abnormal mechanisms. Corrected and republished article originally printed in Critical Reviews in Oral Biology and Medicine 6 (1): 25–79
9. Slavkin HC 1995 Molecular biology experimental strategies for craniofacial – oral – dental dysmorphology. Connective Tissue Research 32 (1–4): 233–239
10. Dixon M J 1996 Treacher Collins syndrome. Human Molecular Genetics 5 Spec No 1391–1396
11. Edwards SJ, Fowlie A, Cust MP, Liu DT, Young ID, Dixon MJ 1996 Prenatal diagnosis in Treacher Collins syndrome using combined linkage analysis and ultrasound imaging. Journal of Medical Genetics 33 (7): 603–606
12. Marres HA, Cremers CW, Dixon MJ, Huygen PL, Joosten FB 1995 The Treacher Collins syndrome. A clinical, radiological and genetic linkage study on two pedigrees. Archives of Otolaryngology – Head and Neck Surgery 121 (5): 509–514
13. Dixon MJ 1995 Treacher Collins syndrome. Journal of Medical Genetics 32 (10): 806–808
14. Fuente del Campo A, Martinez Elizondo M, Melloni Magnelli L, Salazar Valadez A, Saavedra Ontiveros D 1995 Craniofacial development in rats with early resection of the zygomatic arch. Plastic and Reconstructive Surgery 95 (3): 486–495
15. Posnick JC, al-Qattan MM, Moffat SM, Armstrong D 1995 Cranio-orbitozygomatic measurements from standard CT scans in unoperated Treacher Collins syndrome patients: comparison with normal controls. Cleft Palate–Craniofacial Journal 32 (1): 20–24
16. Bhatia S, Block MS, Hoffman DR, Lancaster D, Greene CL 1996 Radiocephalometric evaluation of a family with mandibulofacial dysostosis. American Journal of Orthodontics and Dentofacial Orthopedics 110 (6): 618–623
17. Farkas LG, Posnick JC 1989 Detailed morphometry of the nose in patients with Treacher Collins syndrome. Annals of Plastic Surgery 22 (3): 211–219
18. Hertle RW, Ziylan S, Katowitz JA 1993 Ophthalmic features and visual prognosis in the Treacher Collins syndrome. British Journal of Ophthalmology 77 (10): 642–645
19. Taylor DJ, Phelps PD 1993 Imaging of ear deformities in Treacher Collins syndrome. Clinical Otolaryngology 18 (4): 263–267
20. Altman F 1955 Congenital atresia of the ear in man and animals. Annals of Otology, Rhinology and Laryngology 64: 824–858
21. Cremers CWRJ, Teunissen E 1991 The impact of a syndromal diagnosis on surgery for congenital minor ear anomalies. International Journal of Pediatric Otorhinolaryngology 22: 59–74
22. Jackson IT, Bauer B, Saleh J, Sullivan C, Argenta LC 1989 A significant feature of Nager's syndrome: palatal agenesis. Plastic and Reconstructive Surgery 84 (2): 219–226
23. Meizner I, Carmi R, Katz M 1991 Prenatal ultrasonic diagnosis of mandibulofacial dysostosis (Treacher Collins syndrome). Journal of Clinical Ultrasound 19 (2): 124–127
24. Moore MH, Guzman-Stein G, Proudman TW, Abbott AH, Netherway DJ, David DJ 1994 Mandibular lengthening by distraction for airway obstruction in Treacher Collins syndrome. Journal of Craniofacial Surgery 5 (1): 22–25
25. Papacharalambous SK, Anastasoff KI 1993 Natural coral skeleton used as onlay graft for contour augmentation of the face. A preliminary report. International Journal of Oral and Maxillofacial Surgery 22 (5): 260–264
26. Musolas A, Columbini E, Michelena J 1991 Vascularised full-thickness parietal bone grafts in maxillofacial reconstruction: the role of the galea and superficial temporal vessels. Plastic and Reconstructive Surgery 87 (2): 261–267
27. Tulasne JF, Tessier PL 1986 Results of the Tessier integral procedure for correction of Treacher Collins syndrome. Cleft Palate Journal 23(suppl 1): 40–49
28. Marres HA, Cremers CW, Marres EH 1995 Treacher Collins syndrome. Management of major and minor anomalies of the ear. Revue de Laryngologie Otologie Rhinologie 116 (2): 105–108

Osteodistraction: the present and the future

60

J. KERWIN WILLIAMS/JOSEPH G. McCARTHY

Paradigms may be defined as a set of rules or regulations established in the context of previous experiences and study. In turn, new problems can be evaluated and solved within the framework of the paradigm with some degree of predictable success. With the insight that can only come from clinical experience, Joseph Murray, the plastic surgeon Nobel Laureate, illustrated two major paradigm shifts in the practice of surgery. Early surgical procedures were developed as a means of removal or *extirpation* (tumors, compromised extremities, etc.). With the development of immunosuppressive treatment and microvascular techniques, the era of *transplantation* (reconstruction/replacement) was instituted. In recent years, the practice of surgery has been altered by an increased understanding and manipulation of biologic systems, for example induction of the native tissue. Distraction osteogenesis of the craniofacial skeleton serves as an example of this most recent paradigm shift. As we enter the era of *inductive surgery*, a decrease in the magnitude of the surgical procedure, the associated morbidity and the length of hospitalization will result.

Distraction osteogenesis is a technique of applying stress to a site of surgically produced bone disruption. The mechanical forces are directed predominantly away from the above site and the technique takes advantage of the regenerative capacity of bone by creating and maintaining an active site of bone formation. This technique extends the healing activity of bone above its normal levels by increasing vascularity and recruiting osteoblasts.[1–3]

HISTORY

Distraction osteogenesis was developed predominantly as a treatment modality for problems of the axial skeleton (endochondral long bones of the extremities). The technique was initially utilized for correction of limb-length discrepancies at the beginning of the twentieth century.[4,5] Described as 'skeletal distraction', casts were repeatedly cut and advanced using large bedside frames (Fig. 60.1). The technique was eventually modified by the use of large pins in the fracture fragments[6,7] and the first controlled distraction system incorporated a screw device between cut casts at the osteotomy site.[8] Allan also recognized the importance of maintaining blood supply to the bone and the effects of distraction on the adjacent soft tissue. In the 1970s, smaller, self-contained external fixators were developed to distract bone while allowing the patient to be mobile.[9] The healing process was radiographically and surgically evaluated, with the consequences that bone grafting and plating of the osteotomy site were almost routine following distraction. The most recent advancements in endochondral bone distraction were introduced by Ilizarov, who popularized the technique.[10,11] The biologic response to distraction was studied and these reports provided the basis for technical guidelines, which are generally accepted today. Ilizarov should be considered the originator of the modern techniques of clinical distraction.

As interest in endochondral bone distraction increased, the technique was adopted for use in the membranous bone of the mandible. Initial canine experiments were performed by Snyder et al[12] and Michieli & Mioth[13] that demonstrated the effectiveness of this technique, but it was not until the papers from New York University[14,15] that clinical interest was generated in mandibular distraction. Histologic evaluation demonstrated similar biologic patterns during bone formation in mandibular distraction compared to endochondral distraction. Subsequently, the effectiveness of distraction in patients with mandibular deficiencies was established,[16] and confirmed by others.[17]

953

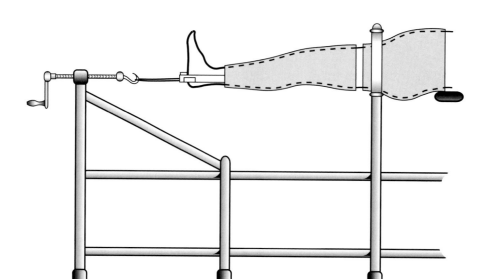

Fig. 60.1 Diagram of Codivilla's method of distraction described in 1905. The traction was applied to the cast which was transferred to the bone via the skin. (Reproduced from Moseley[61] with permission.)

BIOLOGY OF DISTRACTION

Studies of the biologic processes involved in the formation of bone through distraction have been conducted in endochondral and membranous bone.[15,18–23] Bone formation, in general, may be through a cartilaginous intermediate as seen in the axial skeleton (endochondral ossification) or from recruitment and differentiation of primitive mesenchymal cells (membranous ossification) as seen in the formation of the craniofacial skeleton.[14] Osteogenesis associated with distraction occurs primarily by the latter method, even when applied in the axial skeleton. With disruption of the cortex, migration of inflammatory cells and hematoma formation occur. As distraction progresses, a marked vascular response is observed along with the appearance of mesenchymal cells and the synthesis of type I collagen. A fibrovascular bridge is formed and the collagen fibrils increase in density and become oriented along the axis of distraction. Mineralization appears at days 10–14 at the edge of the bony disruption, while a central 'zone of fibrous tissue' is maintained. Bony spicules eventually replace the collagen bundles and the gap is gradually closed after the cessation of distraction.[15,24]

The molecular pathways involved in distraction-type bone healing have been studied in a preliminary manner. A number of growth factors have been implicated in the regulation of bone synthesis.[19,20,25] In a rat animal model of mandibular distraction,[25] bone morphogenic proteins (BMPs), insulin-like growth factors I and II (IGFs), members of the transforming growth factor family (TGFbs) and basic fibroblast growth factor (BFGF) have been the most well characterized. The expression of these factors is increased as noted during fracture healing and they stimulate osteoblast proliferation and bone formation. BMPs are unique in their effects on uncommitted precursor cells, as demonstrated by ectopic bone formation. This group of growth factors also promotes chemotaxis, mitosis, differentiation and extracellulr matrix formation, and may in the future provide a suitable therapeutic stimulus for accelerating bone formation during distraction and promoting more rapid consolidation of the distraction zone.

Animal studies have been associated with the study of distraction from inception.[26] Traditionally large animal models have been used to study the morphologic, biomechanical and technical aspects of distraction. While these models may more closely approximate human growth characteristics, extensive animal research at a molecular level is hampered by high costs, protracted growth rates, lack of available molecular reagents and difficulty of controlling experimental variables. The recent development of a rat model[25] for membranous bone distraction provides an expeditious method for acquiring regenerate bone and allows the use of established techniques that have been applied extensively in a murine model.

MANDIBULAR DISTRACTION

The mandible has an intimate association with several basic functions (breathing, eating, speaking). Its prominence in the facial skeleton as well as its unique shape (the only U-shaped bone) has made it a major focus of therapeutic attention in the patient with a dysmorphic facial appearance. It is also the closest in form to the axial bones and has, therefore, served as the ideal component of the craniofacial skeleton for transition from distraction of endochondral to membranous bone. Because of these reasons, the predominant clinical experience in distraction on the craniofacial skeleton has been the correction of the deficient mandible.

Any surgical intervention of the mandible must be discussed in the context of potential growth. Traditional surgery of the non-growing mandible (beyond 15–17 years old) has been guided by the necessity to produce a functional occlusion. In this patient group occlusion is usually obtainable with intraoral mandibular osteotomies. Following preoperative orthodontic therapy, surgical advancement of the tooth-bearing segment(s) of the mandible allows positioning into the desired dental occlusion and fixation within the operating room. The ability of distraction to provide predictable and precise movements necessary to obtain satisfactory occlusion is limited. Therefore, presently, distraction is most useful for the younger patient in whom the treatment goals are directed towards an increase in the volume and position of the mandible rather than towards achieving a definitive acceptable occlusion. In fact, the occlusion may often be worse following distraction but can usually be corrected with facial growth and orthodontic intervention.

Candidates for extraoral mandibular distraction should still meet the requirements initially stated by McCarthy:[27]

1. The patients must show that they would require a traditional surgical reconstructive technique that would employ an external incision.
2. The mandibular deficiency would require an osteotomy with bone grafting as part of the reconstruction.
3. The mandibular skeletal pathology should be moderate to severe.

The timing of the surgery is often dictated by a combination of the severity of the deficiency, the parents' goals and the need to reduce psychosocial handicaps that may be present. The youngest patient to undergo distraction at our institution was 18 months of age. However, the majority of patients have undergone mandibular distraction between the age of 2 and 8 years.

PREOPERATIVE EVALUATION AND PLANNING

The patient should first be examined with the head in a 'neutral' position, a goal often rendered difficult because of craniofacial asymmetry and head tilt. Forehead, orbital,

zygomatic and external ear position and relationships should also be noted by viewing the patient from the bird's eye and submental vertex positions. In patients with unilateral craniofacial microsomia, the position of the oral commissure should be documented and the distance between it and the external auditory canal (or ear remnant) recorded; the quality and thickness of the cheek soft tissue should also be observed. The position and contour of the chin (pogonion), inferior border and angle of the mandible (gonion) are, likewise, recorded. The location of the external ear is noted and it is graded according to the classification of Meurman.[28]

The intraoral examination documents the status of the occlusion and the presence or absence of crossbites. It is important to relate the intraoral pathology to the extraoral skeletal and soft-tissue abnormalities. The occlusal plane/cant should be related to the transorbital plane, a determination later facilitated by examination of the posteroanterior cephalogram, which also allows analysis of the transmeatal (horizontal) and midsagittal (vertical) planes (Fig. 60.2).

The functional clinical examination should include documentation of mandibular excursions, including maximum interincisal opening and lateral deviation, because a transient limitation to opening can be observed at the end of distraction. It is, therefore, important to know what the original

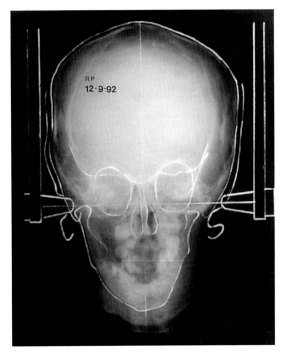

Fig. 60.2 Posteroanterior cephalogram of a patient with unilateral craniofacial microsomia. Note that the ear rod is positioned in the ear canal on the unaffected side but is placed on the calvaria on the affected side. However, the midsagittal plane is perpendicular and the lateral borders of the orbital rims are likewise parallel to the lateral verticle plane (Reproduced from Distraction of the Craniofacial Skeleton, McCarthy JG (ed), Springer, New York, 1999).

interincisal opening was as an objective goal for post-treatment physical therapy. The role of the temporomandibular joint and its actual function prior to distraction are also documented. The motor (muscles of mastication and facial expression) and sensory (infraorbital, inferior alveolar) nerve, function is likewise recorded.

Craniofacial pathology and asymmetry should be documented by facial photographs (frontal, laterals, obliques, submental), lateral and posteroanterior cephalograms, a panoramic roentgenogram (panorex), a three-dimensional (3D) CT scan (serial axial cuts from menton to cranial vertex); sedation is usually required in the younger patient.

In patients with unilateral craniofacial microsomia and microtia with meatal stenosis, particular attention must be paid to placing the head in the correct vertical or midsagittal plane when obtaining the cephalograms. The ear rod is positioned in the ear canal on the unaffected side but is placed on the calvaria on the affected side. The midsagittal plane is perpendicular and the lateral borders of the orbital rims are symmetrically positioned in relation to the lateral borders of the calvarium. This type of precise documentation must be carried out routinely in the preoperative period. The record of any discrepancy should be applied postoperatively. The lateral cephalogram is taken with the same protocol. The cephalograms still provide a significant advantage over CT scans, in that the clinician can obtain serial records in a relatively simple manner and evaluate long-term growth and developmental changes. The lateral and posteroanterior cephalograms, combined with a panoramic radiograph, are invaluable if they are produced accurately and they allow classification of the mandible according to the system proposed by Pruzansky[29] and modified by Kaban et al[30] (Fig. 60.3).

The panorex is extremely valuable in documenting the size and shape of the condyle, ramus and body, as well as the position of partially erupted teeth and tooth follicles and the potential site for the osteotomy. The 3D CT scan reproduces the skeletal pathology in detail and also gives a baseline study for postdistraction documentation of the increase in bone volume and change in mandibular morphology.

The diagnostic records also include dental study models, which can be mounted by a facebow to an articulator, yet respecting the anatomic deformity in the external auditory canal. In this way a fairly accurate set of 3D records of the pre-existing occlusion can be obtained preoperatively. Another important role of pretreatment study models is the construction of postdistraction orthodonic treatment appliances.

It was recognized early in the clinical study that in treatment planning there are several structural or architectural goals:

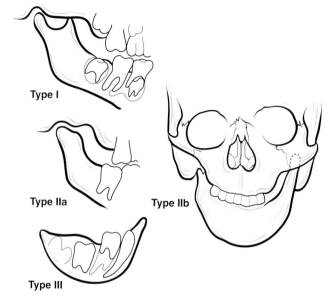

Fig. 60.3 Pruzansky classifications of the mandible[30]

1. Increasing the vertical dimension of the hypoplastic mandibular ramus.
2. Re-establishing the transverse position of the ramus (bigonial distance) to improve cheek contour.
3. Increasing the projection or anteroposterior dimension of the mandibular body and symphysis.
4. Improving the dentoalveolar relations.
5. 'Leveling' the occlusal plane in the unilateral distraction case.
6. Correcting any asymmetry of the oral commissure (in the unilateral case).
7. Increasing ('overcorrecting' in the growing patient) chin projection in bilateral cases.
8. 'Overcorrecting' chin point (movement to the contralateral side) in unilateral cases.

A retrospective review[31] of the clinical records has demonstrated that the postdistraction shape of the neomandible is dependent on the *trajectory* or movement in space of the distraction device, which, in turn, reflects the positioning of the distraction device on the mandible at the time of surgery (the *vector* of distraction). There are three vectors: the *vertical* which is perpendicular to the long axis of the body of the mandible, the *horizontal* which is best described as parallel to the inferior border of the body or parallel to the occlusal plane and the *oblique* which bisects these two positions (Fig. 60.4). This study has demonstrated that the vertical vector is most effective in lengthening the hypoplastic ramus in the vertical plane. It results in the greatest amount of posterior open-bite, and corrects a severe occlusal cant in the unilateral patient with deficient

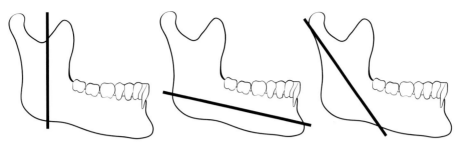

Fig. 60.4 Vectors of distraction. The vertical vector is perpendicular to the inferior border of the ramus, the horizontal vector is parallel to the inferior border of the body or parallel to the occlusal plane and the oblique vector is intermediary between the previous vectors. The vectors represent the position of the long axis of the distraction device which, in turn, is determined by the positions of the pins in the mandible.

vertical ramus height. Vertically placed distraction devices will also drive the pogonion toward the mid-sagittal plane. The devices are placed in a horizontal vector when there is a marked overjet or micrognathia with mandibular retrusion, as usually seen in bilateral mandibular deficiencies. The horizontal placement is most effective at thrusting the mandible in an anterior direction to correct a sagittal deficiency. The *oblique* vector represents a bisector of the vertical and horizontal vectors and is best used when one wants to maintain the general morphology of the mandible but increase the vertical dimension of the ramus and the anteroposterior dimension of the body. The introduction of multiplanar distraction devices, however, allows manipulation of the vector during the phase of active distraction.

SURGICAL TECHNIQUE

The buccal surface of the hypoplastic ramus is approached via either an *intraoral* or a *transcutaneous* (*extraoral*) incision (modified Risdon) (Fig. 60.5). The initial cases were carried out through an extraoral incision but, as clinical experience has accumulated, the intraoral approach, occasionally supplemented with a small 1.5-cm transcutaneous incision to improve visualization in the severely hypoplastic mandible, has been used almost exclusively. In either incision a dilute solution of xylocaine and adrenaline is injected over the oblique line and buccal surface of the ramus.

In the intraoral approach, an incision is made over the oblique line and the buccal surface is widely exposed in a subperiosteal plane. In the transcutaneous approach, a 3-cm incision is made in the skin lines of the submandibular fold at a position along the angle and inferior border of the mandible (at a somewhat higher position than the Risdon incision). Care is taken to identify and preserve the marginal mandibular nerve after the platysma muscle is incised. The masseter muscle is sharply dissected off the buccal aspect of the mandible in a subperiosteal plane.

Selection of the pin-hole sites requires careful attention to planning, because they dictate positioning of the device (i.e. the vector of distraction) (Fig. 60.6). Avoid drilling unerupted tooth follicles and also be sure that the pins project sufficiently above the skin so that the distraction device clears the cheek skin or any auricular remnant. In general, the most cephalic drill holes should be placed first

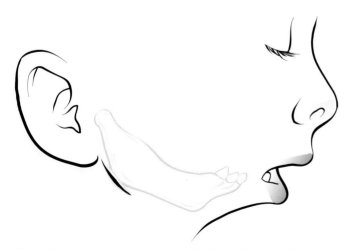

Fig. 60.5 The transcutaneous (extraoral) incision. A 2- to 3-cm incision is made at the angle of the mandible in the skin lines. Access is provided to the buccal surface of the mandible in a subperiosteal plane. (Reproduced from McCarthy[62] with permission.)

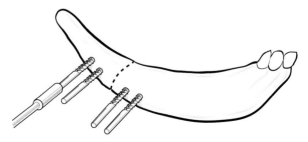

Fig. 60.6 Selection of drill holes determines the position of the distraction device and the vector. The distance between the drill holes is illustrated. The interrupted line indicates the site of the projected osteotomy. (Reproduced from McCarthy[62] with permission.)

because they are usually the technically most difficult because of the limited size of that portion of the affected mandible. The positions of the four drill holes dictate the orientation of the device and, thus, the vector of distraction. In the four-pin device, the skin and soft tissue are pinched between the two pairs of pins to reduce the length of the resulting scar and the skin is also retracted in a superior direction so that the pins penetrate the skin in the submandibular fold and the resulting scar will fall in the latter, relatively camouflaged, site.

After the drill holes have been completed, 50-mm self-drilling half pins are inserted. The recent development of self-drilling pins obviates the need for separate drill holes. The distraction device is then attached.

It is technically best to complete the osteotomy after the device has been applied and tightened. Alternatively, it can be removed and reapplied in its previously set position after completion of the osteotomy. The osteotomy can be performed in a variety of ways. A mechanical reciprocating saw (Fig. 60.7), supplemented by saline irrigation, can be used to interrupt the buccal surface (cortex), as well as the superior and inferior cortical borders of the affected mandible; the area of the lingula and path of the inferior alveolar nerve are thus spared. The osteotomy is completed by inserting and rotating an osteotome to demonstrate ('greenstick') separation of the bony segments. There is obviously disruption, albeit limited, of the periosteum and endosteum with the act of the osteotomy; the term 'corticotomy' has, therefore, been abandoned (Fig. 60.8).

The wound is irrigated with saline and, if the transcutaneous approach is employed, the platysma muscle is approximated with interrupted 4–0 chromic catgut sutures and the skin margins are approximated with interrupted 6–0 nylon or vicryl sutures. In the intraoral approach, the wound is closed with a single layer of interrupted 3–0 chromic catgut sutures.

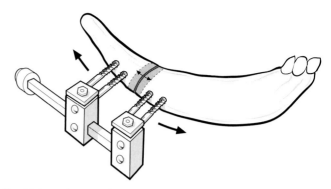

Fig. 60.8 Application of the distraction device and confirmation of the osteotomy. The distraction has begun in the direction of the arrows with the formation of bone regenerate at the distraction site. (Reproduced from McCarthy[61] with permission.)

POSTOPERATIVE PERIOD

Photographs and cephalograms are also obtained on the day following insertion of the pins and distraction device. The mandible is maintained in fixation for 5–7 days (*lag phase*) before activation of the device is commenced (*activation phase*) at the rate of 1 mm per day (0.5 mm twice a day). In the child under 6 years of age, a rate of 1.5 mm per day (0.5 mm three times a day) is preferred to avoid premature consolidation at the distraction site.

The progress of distraction is monitored by documenting changes in the relationships of the anterior maxillary and mandibular occlusion and the position or level of the occlusal plane, oral commissure and chin point. In general, and especially in the growing child, the deformity is overcorrected or activation is continued until the above parameters are exceeded beyond the 'normal' range.

After the completion of activation, the device is maintained in position for approximately 8 weeks (*fixation* or *consolidation* phase). The device is not removed until there is radiographic evidence of a cortical outline or mineralization of the regenerate portion of the mandible (neomandible). Upon removal of the pins and distraction device (performed as an outpatient procedure), photographs, lateral and posteroanterior cephalograms, panorex and 3D CT scan of the mandible are obtained.

In the unilateral series, if at the time of device removal there is a resulting leveling of the mandibular occlusal plane with a resulting posterior open-bite, a bite plate (worn on the mandibular dentition) is constructed by the orthodontist to maintain the space in order to allow eventual but gradual eruption of the maxillary teeth into the open-bite. Over the subsequent months the posterior portion of the prosthesis is serially reduced in size under the most terminal and distal maxillary molar to allow the latter to erupt down to

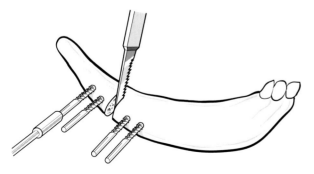

Fig. 60.7 The osteotomy is performed with a small reciprocating saw. The osteotomy is 90% completed before the distraction device is applied. The osteotomy is then completed. (Reproduced from McCarthy[61] with permission.)

the postdistraction occlusal plane, bringing with it the dento-alveolar process. Upon completion of hypereruption of the tooth, the occlusal plate is reduced under the more anterior pairs of teeth until the entire maxillary occlusal plane is leveled. In the younger patient (under 3 years of age), the maxillary teeth quickly fill the space and the above orthodontic maneuver is often not necessary.

Two case reports 60.9 and 60.10 are presented in the accompanying boxes.

CASE REPORT 60.1 (Fig. 60.9)

S.B. was a 4.5-year-old boy diagnosed with right craniofacial microsomia manifest by mild to moderate underdevelopment of the right face and partial weakness in the distribution of the right marginal mandibular branch (Fig. 60.9). The maxilla and the mandible (Pruzansky I) were involved with an associated complex microtia of the right ear. The second mandibular molar tooth bud was deliberately removed at 3.5 years of age in anticipation of bone distraction (21 mm). At 6 months post distraction, the patient demonstrated a slight anterior crossbite (2–3 mm) as well as a slight occlusal cant upward. The bigonial distance had increased significantly. Correction of the chin point to the midline was also achieved.

CASE REPORT 60.2 (Fig. 60.10)

J.C. was a 4-year-old girl with right craniofacial microsomia (Pruzansky IIa) with an ipsilateral microtia (Fig. 60.10). The microsomia was characterized by a significant mandibular deviation to the right with a right-sided crossbite and an overjet. The chin was also moderately retrusive. She underwent unilateral distraction of the right mandible to 25 mm (vertical vector). After distraction, the chin and midincisor line were positioned at the midline with marked increase in the volume of the right mandible and a right lateral open-bite. She subsequently underwent autogenous rib graft reconstruction (staged) of the right ear.

LONG-TERM STUDIES

In a preliminary longitudinal study,[31] 10 patients with unilateral craniofacial microsomia and bilateral micrognathia, who underwent correction of their mandibular deficiency by distraction techniques, were evaluated by clinical and cephalometric examination. The period of postdistraction follow-up ranged from 12 to 70 months. Five patients underwent unilateral mandibular distraction and five patients underwent bilateral distraction with an extraoral device.

Preoperative, post-treatment and annual radiographs (panoramic, posteroanterior and lateral cephalograms) were obtained and studied.

In the period of observation following distraction, the 10 mandibles showed cephalometric and clinical evidence of growth. In the five unilateral cases, the unoperated side grew in a pattern that would be expected for the unaffected side of a mandible with unilateral craniofacial microsomia. The distracted side, however, grew with a variable response (Fig. 60.11). Growth occurred at the site of the bone regenerate as well as in the adjacent body, ramus and the condylar head. No evidence of relapse was noted in any patient. The growth response of the operated side was variable and appeared to be dependent on the genetic program of the native bone and the surrounding soft-tissue matrix. Morphologic and volumetric improvements were maintained long term, with continued growth of the condyle without evidence of deformational changes.[32] The unoperated sites, including the body and condyle, also showed evidence of growth throughout the study period.

Comparison of lateral cephalograms revealed that a clockwise rotation of the mandible occurred with the passage of time (Fig. 60.12). Clockwise mandibular rotation occurred secondary to the expected vertical growth of the maxillary dentoalveolus, as the children passed from the primary to the mixed and finally the permanent states of dentition. Tooth development and eruption occurred with no evidence of delay.

In seven of 10 patients, the mandibles maintained their postdistraction morphology while demonstrating growth during the study period. Conversely, in three of the 10 patients, mandibular morphology was altered during distraction but returned to the predistraction shape with the passage of time. These three patients had undergone bilateral distraction, two of whom carried the diagnosis of Nager syndrome. These patients had their distraction devices placed horizontally with temporary loss of the gonial angle postdistraction. Within 2 years, the mandibles demonstrated growth but remodeled to assume the pre-expansion shape with restitution of the gonial angle.

All asymmetric mandibles (unilateral distraction) were expanded until the pogonion or chin point was translocated beyond the midsagittal plane. The overcorrected chin position was noted to decrease over time as the relative growth rate of the affected and unaffected sides of the mandible in patients with unilateral craniofacial microsomia was unequal. The overcorrected mandibles were noted to change from a Class III incisor relationship to an edge-to-edge relationship over time, a finding attributed to the clockwise rotation of the mandible, as previously discussed, as well as the re-expression of the syndrome-specific growth pattern of the affected and unaffected mandibular rami.

ADVANTAGES/DISADVANTAGES

For patients undergoing surgical reconstruction of the hypoplastic mandible by the distraction technique, the length of

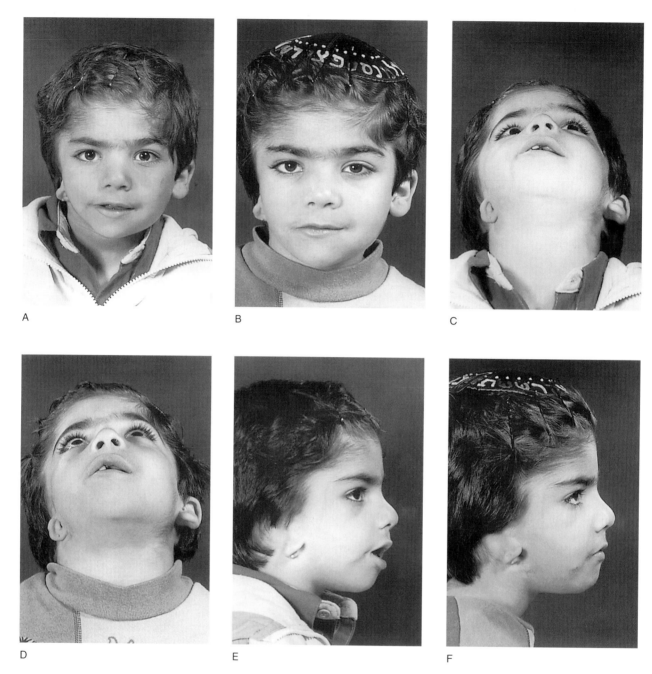

Fig. 60.9 Case 60.1. A 4½-year-old male with right craniofacial microsomia (Pruzansky I) who underwent unilateral mandibular distraction (21 mm). **(A)** Preoperative frontal view. The chin is deviated to the affected side and there is a slight occlusal cant. **(B)** Postoperative frontal view 9 months after completion of distraction. The chin is deviated to the opposite side and there is an overcorrection of the occlusal plane. **(C)** Preoperative submental view. **(D)** Postoperative submental view. Note the improvement in cheek contour on the affected side. **(E)** Preoperative right profile. **(F)** Postoperative right profile. Note the increased sagittal thrust of the mandible and the increased distance between the oral commissure and the ear remnant. The scar is well placed.

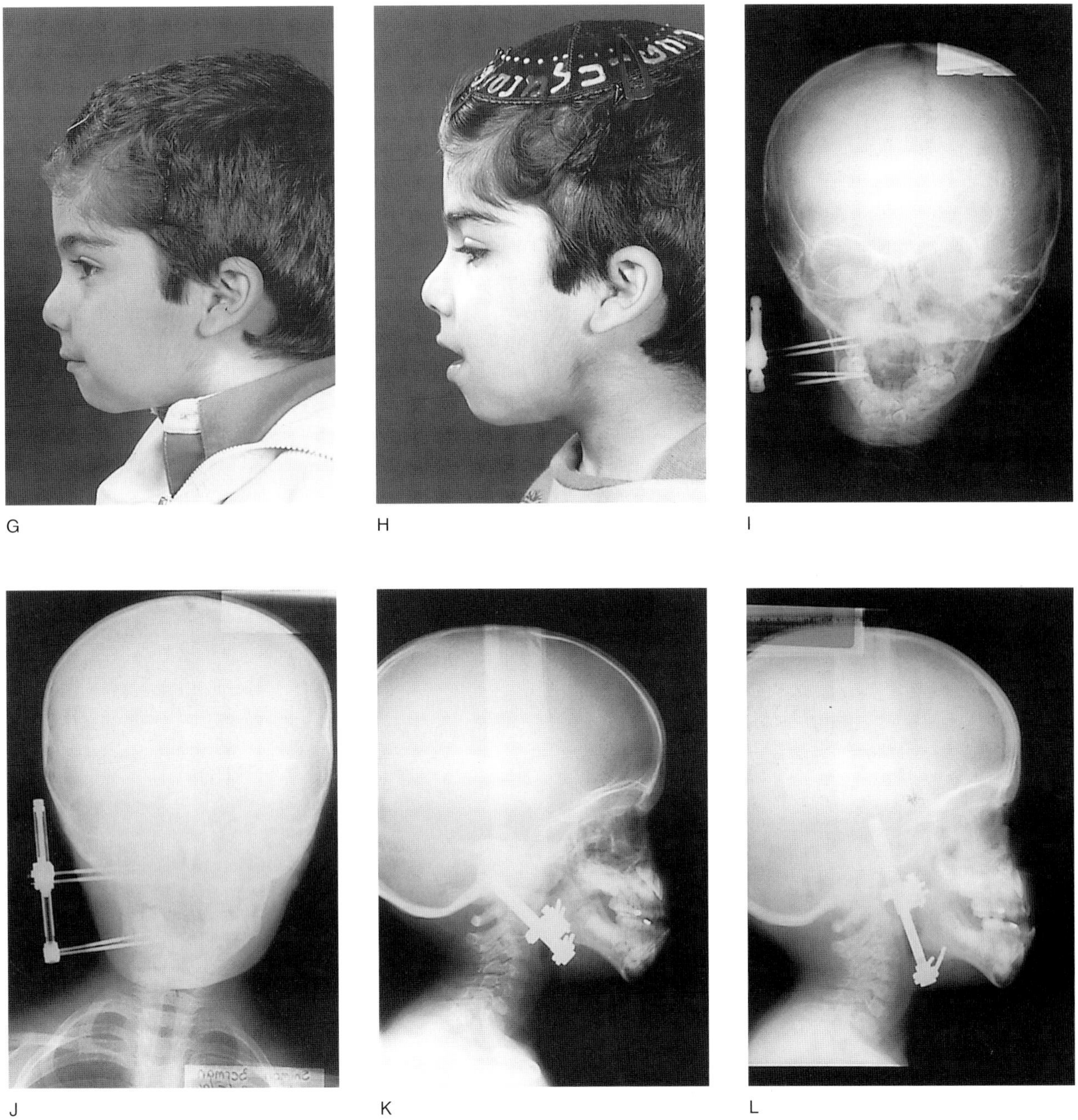

Fig. 60.9(cont'd) **(G)** Preoperative left profile. **(H)** Postoperative left profile. **(I)** Predistraction posteroanterior cephalogram. **(J)** Postdistraction posteroanterior cephalogram. Note the increased vertical dimension of the right mandibular ramus, the restoration of the gonial angle, and the improved chin position. The volume and quality of the regenerate in the right ramus should be noted. **(K)** Predistraction lateral cephalogram (oblique vector). **(L)** Postdistraction lateral cephalogram. Note the sagittal thrust of the mandible in an 'overcorrected' position. (Reproduced from Distraction of the Craniofacial Skeleton, McCarthy J.G. (ed), Springer, New York, 1999)

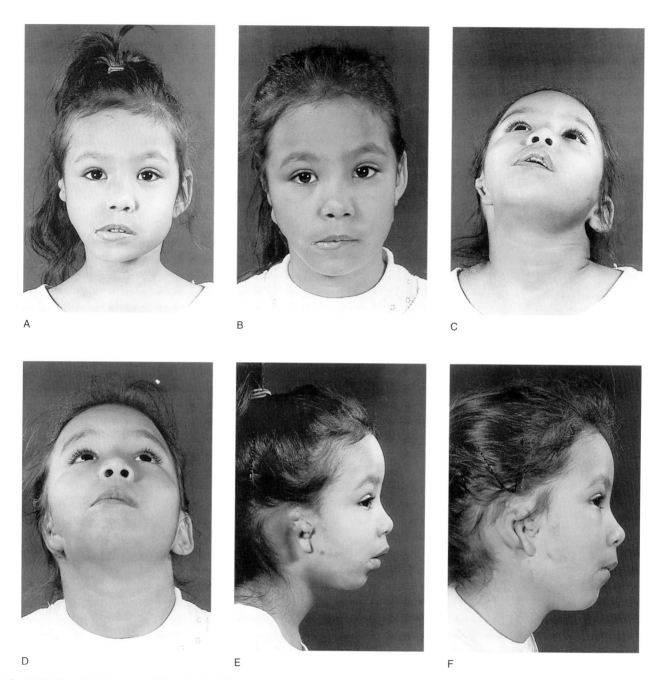

Fig. 60.10 Case 60.2. A 4-year-old female with right craniofacial microsomia (Pruzansky IIa) who underwent unilateral distraction of the hemimandible (25 mm). **(A)** Preoperative frontal view showing chin deviation and hypoplasia of the affected cheek. She has a marginal mandibular (VII) palsy on the contralateral (left) side. **(B)** Postoperative frontal view. **(C)** Preoperative submental view. **(D)** Postoperative submental view showing improved chin position and increased cheek fullness on the affected side. **(E)** Preoperative right profile. **(F)** Postoperative right profile showing increased sagittal thrust of the mandible. Staged auricular reconstruction has commenced.

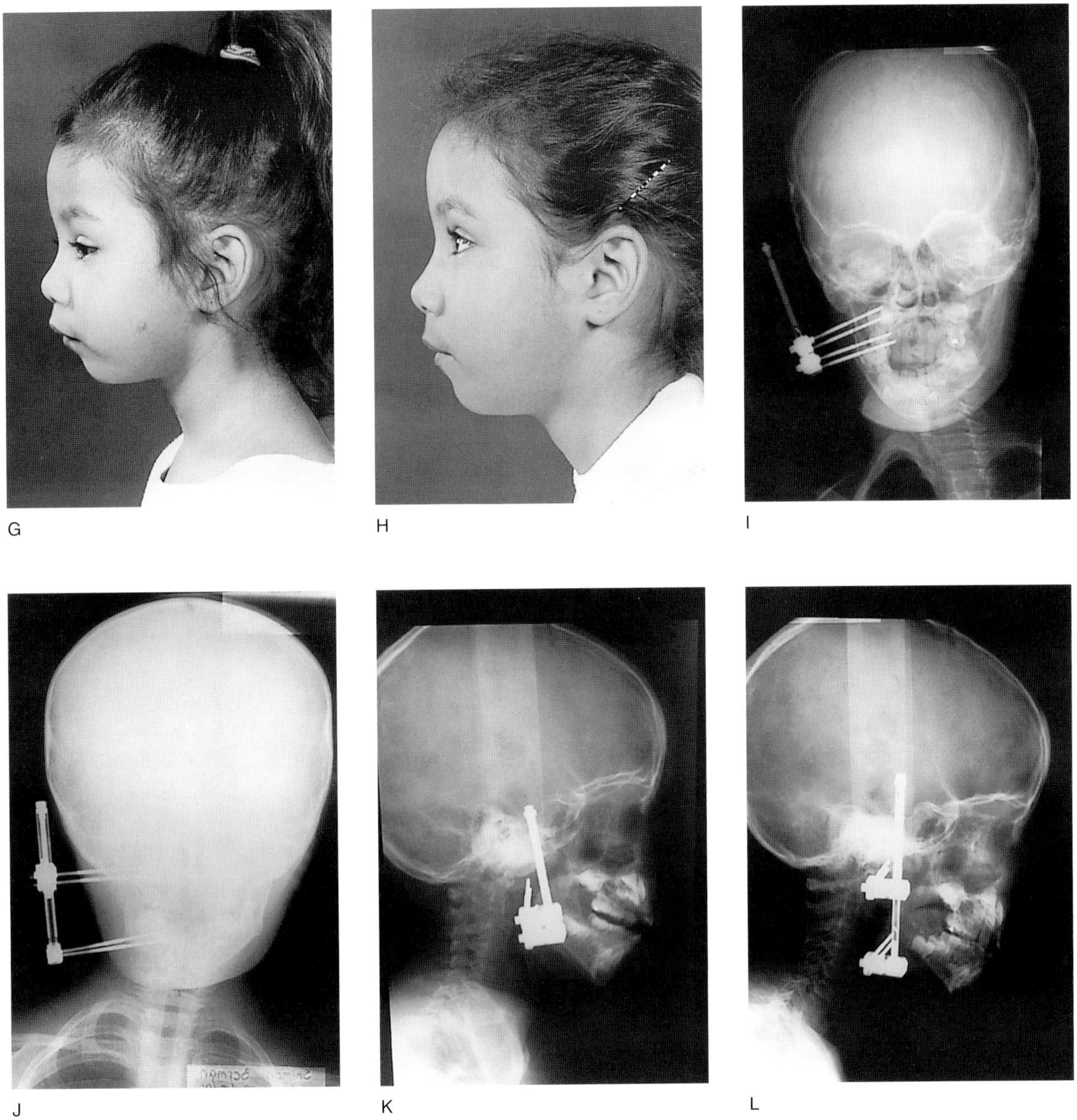

Fig. 60.10(cont'd) **(G)** Preoperative left profile. **(H)** Postoperative left profile. **(I)** Predistraction posteranterior cephalogram. **(J)** Postdistraction posteroanterior cephalogram. Note the increased vertical dimension of the right mandibular ramus. **(K)** Predistraction lateral cephalogram (vertical vector). **(L)** Postdistraction lateral cephalogram. (Reproduced from Distraction of the Craniofacial Skeleton, McCarthy J.G. (ed), Springer, New York, 1999.)

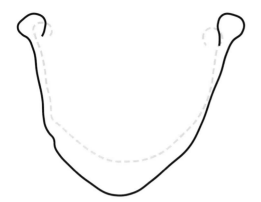

Fig. 60.11 Supplement tracings from a posteroanterior cephalogram. The dotted line indicates the contour of the mandible approximately 1 year after right-sided distraction. The solid line represents the contour 5 years later. Note that there was growth on the distracted side at the site of the bone regenerate as well as in the adjacent body, ramus and condylar head of the mandible. The chin point has remained in the midsagittal plane. (Reproduced from Distraction of the Craniofacial Skeleton, McCarthy J.G. (ed), Springer, New York, 1999.)

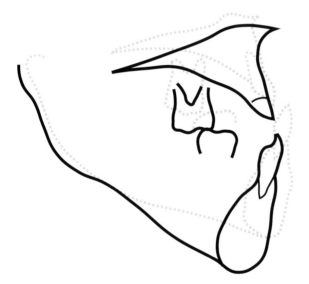

Fig. 60.12 Serial lateral cephalograms of a patient who underwent bilateral distraction for the correction of the developmental micrognathia. The lighter lines illustrate the position of the mandible immediately following distraction and the darker lines are the contour almost 2 years later. Note that there has been clockwise mandibular rotation secondary to the expected vertical growth of the maxillary dentoalveolus. (Reproduced from Distraction of the Craniofacial Skeleton, McCarthy J.G. (ed), Springer, New York, 1999.)

hospitalization and operating time have been drastically reduced; distraction can even be performed on an outpatient or ambulatory basis. The technique, which can be applied at a younger age, has obviated the need for blood transfusion and autogenous bone grafting, as often required in traditional orthognathic surgical procedures. It also allows the augmentation of hypoplastic mandibles that are not amenable to traditional orthognathic mandibular advancement procedures.

A benefit which should also be emphasized is that there is gradual distraction not only of the bony skeleton but also of the associated soft tissues, such as the muscles of mastication, subcutaneous tissue and skin ('functional matrix'). Because of the expansion of the associated soft tissues and muscles, there is a resulting *multidirectional* enlargement of the mandible characterized, for example, by an increase in the bigonial distance, an increase in the vertical dimension of the chin and the creation of a gonial angle. The secondary expansive effect on the soft tissues and muscles is also reflected in the fact that there is minimal, if any, evidence of clinical relapse. This is in contrast to the dental/skeletal relapse observed following traditional orthognathic advancement procedures to reconstruct the hypoplastic ramus in unilateral craniofacial microsomia and to advance the mandible (i.e. sagittal split osteotomy) in developmental micrognathia. Another factor contributing to the absence of relapse is the *gradual* (1 mm/day) rate at which the advancement/distraction is achieved.

Another advantage of the technique is that it can be applied as early as 2 years of age because the technique is relatively simple and because bone grafts are not required to augment the hypoplastic ramus and body.

There has also been concern about the effects of mandibular distraction on the temporomandibular joints. In one patient undergoing unilateral distraction, there was nocturnal temporomandibular joint (TMJ) pain on the affected side (presumably secondary to bruxism). This was relieved when an occlusal splint was constructed and worn. Serial radiographic studies[32] conducted on this series of patients showed that the hypoplastic condylar segment improved in size and in orientation and assumed a more anatomic radiographic appearance. A concomitant canine laboratory study[33] of changes in the TMJs following unilateral mandibular distraction showed that there was a transient posterior condylar flattening of the ipsilateral condyle and posterosuperior flattening of the contralateral condyle. There was histologic evidence of subchondral degeneration followed by repair and remodeling, the latter resulting in a correction of the condylar flattening.

There are disadvantages of the distraction technique. The most obvious is residual cutaneous scarring but, with careful placement of the incision, the scar can lie in the lines of minimal tension in the submandibular fold. The intraoral approach for the osteotomy/pin insertion has, however, evolved as the approach of choice because of reduction in the size of the scar. It can be anticipated that there will be further miniaturization of current intraoral devices. Despite these advances, intraoral devices cannot yet be applied effectively to the severely hypoplastic mandible and are restricted to repair of only moderate-minimal mandibular deficiencies.

There has also been concern about injury to the inferior alveolar nerve, a potential complication with all mandibular osteotomies. Questioning of our older patients has failed to detect any postoperative evidence of change in sensation of the lower lip. The presence of a fully functional inferior alveolar nerve in the hypoplastic mandible of patients in unilateral craniofacial microsomia is unknown. The Mexico City technique (buccal corticotomy without disruption of the lingual cortex) represents an effort to maintain the integrity of the inferior alveolar nerve, and its authors have noted that another benefit of this technique is a bowing out of the gonial angle. Our technique, described above, makes every effort to avoid injury to the mandibular canal, and the osteotomy (lingual aspect) is completed by 'greenstick fracture'.

The total treatment time approaches 3 months for reconstruction of the hypoplastic mandible by distraction, a length of treatment similar to that of traditional orthognathic mandibular surgery with intermaxillary fixation *before* the development of rigid skeletal fixation. However, it must be stressed that this criticism is more than offset by the reduced period of hospitalization and operating time and by the facts that there is no discomfort when the device is in place and the child is able to eat a regular (soft) diet during the period of treatment. It cannot be overemphasized that deglutition and distraction of the muscles of mastication have a positive influence on the resulting morphology of the bony regenerate.

MANDIBLE DISTRACTION FOR OBSTRUCTIVE SLEEP APNEA

The cause of sleep apnea may originate from a dysfunctional respiratory center in the nervous system (central etiology) or may be associated with structural abnormalities along the entire airway (peripheral etiology). This is usually recognized as an insidious process; the sequelae of chronic sleep apnea include daytime somnolence, impairment in weight gain, hemodynamic changes including cor pulmonale and pulmonary hypertension, and learning disabilities. A subgroup of patients has a mechanical cause of apnea during the neonatal period secondary to mandibular hypoplasia and inadequate tongue projection. If the airway obstruction is severe, surgical intervention is often indicated.

A tracheotomy is an effective method of treating severe cases of obstructive sleep apnea.[34] However, chronic tracheotomies are associated with numerous complications, including recurrent bronchitis, tracheomalacia, increased work of breathing and sudden death.[35,36] Longstanding tracheotomies may also interrupt family life, delay the development of communication skills, handicap social interaction and increase the cost of health care to the patient.

A retrospective review of tracheotomy-dependent patients with mandibular deficiencies who underwent mandibular distraction has been completed.[37] Lateral cephalograms were used to determine facial areas by a modified technique initially described by Imai and associates.[38,39] Changes in position of the hyoid bone secondary to distraction were also documented.

Four patients with severe mandibular deficiencies requiring a tracheotomy at infancy underwent bilateral mandibular distraction (Table 60.1). All of the patients were successfully decannulated within 5.5 months of device removal (average 3.75 months, range 1.5–5.5 months). The area of the lower face after bilateral distraction, as outlined by the profilogram, increased by an average of 26.9% from preoperative values (12.2%–53.5%). Advancement of the hyoid bone along the axis of the mandibular body after distraction was observed in all patients and averaged 14.5 mm (8–25 mm) (Fig. 60.13).

Other reviews have supported the use of distraction for obstructive sleep apnea in patients with mandibular deficiency. In a review of 18 patients with cerebral palsy and upper airway obstruction,[40] 15 of the patients with recommendations for tracheotomy were spared the procedure following multiple surgical interventions, including two patients who underwent mandibular distraction. In another review, distraction of the midface was also found to be effective in resolving sleep apnea in four patients who underwent intraoperative advancement combined with postoperative distraction.[41]

Table 60.1 Patient review

Patient	Diagnosis	Age at distraction	Decannulation after distraction	Amount of distraction	Change in area of lower (%) face	Hyoid advancement (mm)
1	Treacher Collins syndrome	3.0 y	4.5 months	L-17, R-15	23.6	8
2	Nager syndrome	3.2 y	3.5 months	L-21, R-21	12.2	13
3	Treacher Collins syndrome	2.5 y	1.5 months	L-27, R-27	53.5	25
4	Treacher Collins syndrome	2.2 y	5.5 months	L-20, R-20	18.1	12
Mean		2.7 y	3.8 months	L-21.3, R-20.8	26.9%	14.5 mm

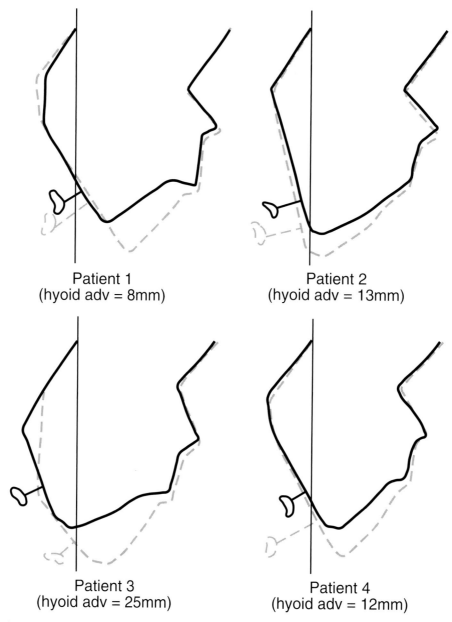

Patient 1
(hyoid adv = 8mm)

Patient 2
(hyoid adv = 13mm)

Patient 3
(hyoid adv = 25mm)

Patient 4
(hyoid adv = 12mm)

Fig. 60.13 Predistraction (solid line) and postdistraction (interrupted line) profilograms are superimposed on sella–nasion landmarks. Note the advancement of the hyoid bone along the axis of the mandibular body, and an increase in the dimensions of the lower face.

DISTRACTION OF OTHER COMPONENTS OF THE CRANIOFACIAL SKELETON

MAXILLARY DISTRACTION

The technique of maxillary distraction predates mandibular distraction in that orthodontists have traditionally used 'expansion' techniques for the treatment of palatal collapse. Anterior distraction of the maxilla has recently been introduced for patients with scar tissue acquired from previous repair of a cleft lip or palate.[42–44]

Polley & Figueroa[44] introduced the rigid external device (RED) system for advancement of the retruded maxillary segment secondary to postsurgical scarring. The device may be secured to the skull by screws (similar to external neurosurgical devices) and attached by a joiner arm to splints. The splints are placed on the upper dentition prior to device application (Fig. 60.14). Distraction of the hypoplastic maxilla is completed following Le Fort I osteotomies. Effective maxillary advancement has been demonstrated using the RED system but long-term results are not available (Fig. 60.15).

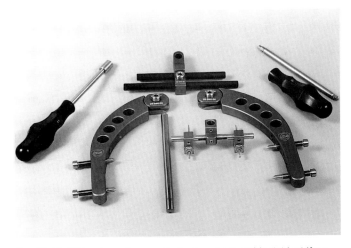

Fig. 60.14 RED system: disassembled external adjustable rigid midface distraction. (Reproduced from Polley & Figueroa[44] with permission.)

Ortiz-Monasterio has described a technique of combined maxillary–mandibular distraction for patients with hemifacial microsomia.[45] Seven adult patients with mandibular defi-

ciencies underwent device placement on the mandible combined with an incomplete Le Fort I osteotomy. After establishment of intermaxillary fixation on postoperative day 5, the mandible was simultaneously distracted along with the maxilla. The occlusion was preserved and the distance from the inferior orbital rim to the occlusal plane was increased on the affected side. A 95–100% correction of the deformity was reported in all patients.

MIDFACE

As a natural evolution from mandibular and maxillary distraction, the technique has been applied for the Le Fort III type of midface advancements. Traditional methods of treatment for the syndromic patient with midface hypoplasia have included a Le Fort III osteotomy and intraoperative advancement with interposition bone grafts at 5–6 years of age.[46] Although this approach has been generally effective, patients usually require bone grafts, blood transfusions,

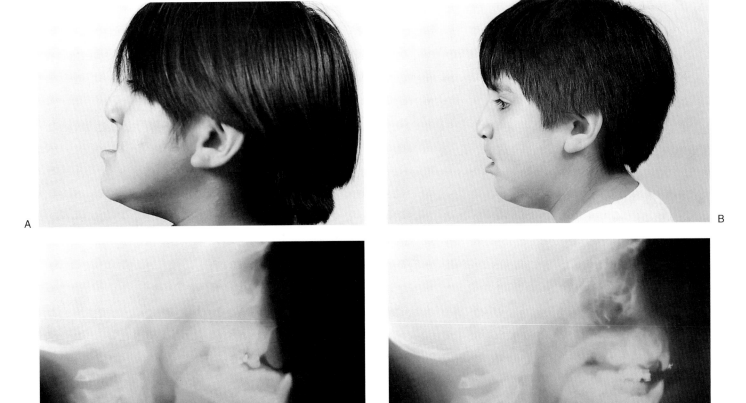

Fig. 60.15 A 9-year-old patient with severe maxillary deficiency secondary to bilateral cleft lip and palate deformity. He underwent a three piece Le Fort I maxillary osteotomy and maxillary distraction osteognesis RED. **(A)** Preoperative lateral photograph. **(B)** Postoperative lateral photograph. **(C)** Preoperative lateral cephalogram. **(D)** Postoperative lateral cephalogram. (Reproduced from Polley & Figueroa[44] with permission.)

skeletal fixation and extended stays in the intensive care unit. Furthermore, the resistance of the overlying soft tissues and the use of bone grafts promote relapse of the facial advancement in some of the patients. The elements of distraction (decreased intervention, soft-tissue expansion, gradual formation of vascularized regenerate bone) are useful in countering the complications associated with a traditional surgical advancement. The introduction of several types of 'internal' subcutaneous distraction devices has provided additional stimulus for application of this technique for midface hypoplasia.

Distraction of the midface was successfully completed in the canine model using external devices.[47,48] Midface advancement, characterized by a Class II dental occlusion and enophthalmos, was accomplished in canines with patent facial sutures (immature canines) without the need for midfacial osteotomies (Fig. 60.16). Advancement of the midface

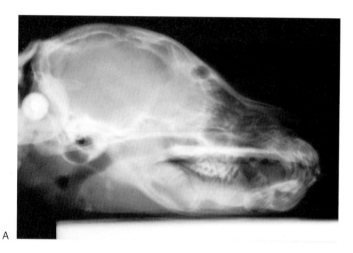

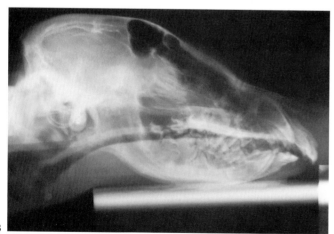

Fig. 60.16 Midface distraction in the immature canine is demonstrated by lateral cephalograms. **(A)** Preoperative. **(B)** Postdistraction. Note the widening of the nasofrontal and zygomaticotemporal suture and the development of a class II malocclusion. (Reproduced from Staffenberg et al[47] with permission.)

was limited when performed in mature canines without an osteotomy. However, following osteotomies of the naso-frontal and medial orbital regions, significant midface advancement with distraction was also obtained.

Several recent articles have described the successful clinical use of distraction for the midface. Cohen described a miniature subcutaneous device employed in two patients with midface hypoplasia.[49] Following midface osteotomies, both patients underwent successful correction of the midface deficiency. Chin and colleagues reported their experience with nine patients who underwent midface distraction.[41] The technique was modified to include an intraoperative advancement combined with postoperative distraction, elimination of a latency period and consolidation for 6 months. The average advancement was 20 mm (16–30 mm) and all midface advancements were found to be clinically stable. Despite early success with this procedure, a prospective study comparing traditional surgical advancement to distraction in respect to cost, length of hospitalization, blood transfusion and long-term follow-up has not yet been completed. In addition, a lower relapse rate would be expected following distraction when compared to conventional intraoperative advancement, but this has also not been studied.

ZYGOMA/ORBIT/CRANIAL VAULT

The most effective demonstration of zygomatic advancement has been in the NYU canine model by Glat and associates (Fig. 60.17).[50] Clinical application of distraction to other areas of the craniofacial skeleton has been limited. Isolated orbital distraction in patients prior to placement of a prosthesis has been anectodally reported.[40] Similarly, the clinical distraction of the zygoma in patients with Treacher Collins syndrome has been described.[17] In neither case has there been a clinical series documenting the effectiveness of the techniques.

Cranial vault distraction has also been demonstrated predominantly in animal models.[51,52] do Amaral and colleagues reported a series of seven patients with craniosynostosis who underwent cranial vault (fronto-orbital) distraction.[53] The mean age was 8 years, and all the patients were diagnosed with either Apert's or Crouzon syndrome. Three patients underwent a coronal craniectomy and gradual distraction. The remaining four patients completed distraction following monobloc frontofacial disjunction. The authors concluded that the monobloc osteotomy followed by distraction was effective in correcting the exorbitism and airway compromise and in improving the esthetics of the midface.

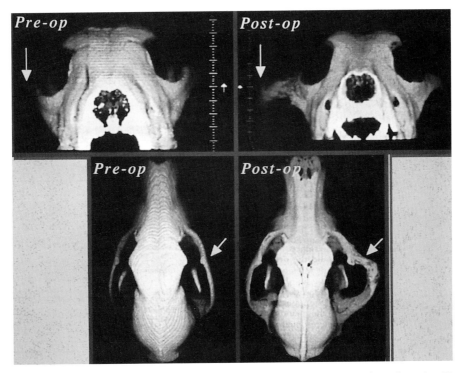

Fig. 60.17 Unilateral distraction of the zygoma was completed. Preoperative and postdistraction 3D CT scans demonstrate the changes following distraction of the zygoma away from the midline. Preoperative 3D-CT scan: Upper panel: anterior views. Lower panel: vertex views.[50]

THE FUTURE

Two major differences exist between the use of distraction devices on the axial bones and their application on the craniofacial skeleton. First, the deficiency of the craniofacial skeleton is recognized in three dimensions and successful reconstruction must address the 'breadth and width' of the defect. Second, the face is the one area of the human body that is predominantly exposed to the world. These differences have encouraged widespread adoption of craniofacial distraction techniques and have emphasized the need for the development of new devices and technical refinements.

MULTIPLANAR DISTRACTION DEVICES

With the accumulation of clinical experience in mandibular distraction, the limitations of uniplanar distraction for the 3D reconstruction of the deficient mandible have been demonstrated, for example the precise correction of malocclusion (open bite) or the increase in bigonial distance. Several devices have been developed to produce multiplanar distraction of the mandible. Pensler and colleagues described an external device with a ball and socket joint that provides the ability to achieve linear and angular translation of the mandible.[54] Manipulation during distraction, however, is based on clinical examination of the structural changes and is restricted to increasing the linear distraction and manually manipulating the regenerate at a secondary procedure in the operating room. Klein & Howaldt introduced a bidirectional device with an angulation joint, which allows rotation along the sagittal plane.[55] Similarly, Molina described a distraction device, which also provides angulation and distraction in two planes.[17] Vertical and horizontal deficiencies may be addressed with these devices, but adjustments in the angulation is limited during the distraction process. In addition, the latter devices require two osteotomies (three bone segments and the risk of avascular necrosis of the intervening segment) and three sets of pin sites. This may be difficult in patients with significant mandibular deficiencies and may run the risk of tooth injury in pin placement.

A multiplanar device was recently developed by the authors that permits controlled manipulation of the bone regenerate three dimensionally in space during the period of device activation in order to achieve satisfactory interdental relationships and to decrease facial asymmetry. It is an extraoral device with the ability to distract the deficient mandible in

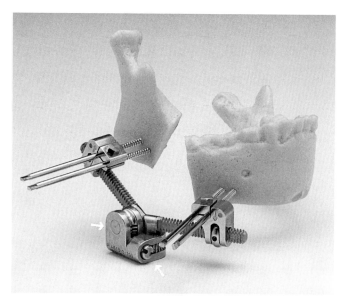

Fig. 60.18 The multiplanar device is displayed. The two separate housing gears are designated by arrows. Note the 'open housing' of the limb rods.

three planes: sagittal (z-axis), vertical (y-axis) and transverse (x-axis) (Fig. 60.18). The central housing contains two gears each positioned in a different plane. This design allows the arms to pivot in two perpendicular planes: angular (vertical or y-axis) and varus-valgus transversal (or x-axis). Two threaded rods extend from the central unit at 180 degrees to provide linear or sagittal distraction.

The ability to distract in three planes allows the surgeon to customize and contour the dimensions of the distraction process by directing the trajectory of translation of the regenerate bone. Distraction along the various planes can be carried out simultaneously. Successful use of the device requires that sagittal distraction initiates the process (10 mm) to provide sufficient bony regenerate and to avoid creating a hinge point at which premature bony consolidation could occur; it is then continued throughout the secondary movements (either angular or transverse).

The multiplanar distraction device has also demonstrated other advantages. Because the rotational points for multiplanar distraction are located at a single point on the device, only a single osteotomy and two pin sites are required. Therefore, smaller amounts of bone stock are needed for osteotomy placement, pin insertion and device application, a distinct advantage in the hypoplastic mandible. In addition, control of the trajectory of the regenerate bone is possible during the distraction process because manipulation in the various planes is independent of each other and may be adjusted individually. Finally, the size of the device is comparable to that of the unidirectional devices.

It must be emphasized, however, that linear distraction

(sagittal plane) remains the key maneuver and often totally satisfies the reconstruction requirements. In addition, there is some loss of linear gain when simultaneous angular or transverse distraction is employed.

INTERNAL DEVICES

The desire for minimal scarring in the facial region has led to the development of several intraoral or buried 'internal' devices. The devices contain percutaneous ports for distraction, which may be placed at a remote site or intraorally in the buccal sulcus intraorally. Intraoral devices were initially developed and used in the canine model (Fig. 60.19).[56] The devices were placed through a buccal incision and attached by pins to the mandible. The distraction port was placed in the buccal sulcus. The device was effective in elongating the mandible without the need for a cutaneous incision. There was no evidence of associated infection.

Cohen and colleagues introduced a modular device of plates and screws that can disperse the force of the distraction over a wider region of the skeleton (Fig. 60.20). A coaxial port can be placed behind the hairline (midface distraction) or exited intraorally (mandibular distraction). The thickness of the plates and screws may also be varied.

Several smaller intraoral devices have recently been developed with dual rod guides and plate-like bases for direct application to the bone. These include the Guererro-Bell and Diner[57,58] distraction devices (Leibinger-Howmedica) and the smallest intraoral device currently available (from KLS Martin) (Fig. 60.21). The devices are smaller than the traditional external devices and have extended ports on universal joints for remote placement. The smallest of these can distract only to 10 mm, but most devices have a choice of 10, 20 and 30 mm distraction lengths.

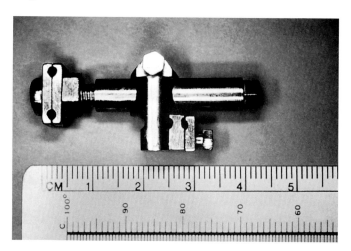

Fig. 60.19 The McCarthy 'intraoral device'. Note the housing unit containing the distraction rod.

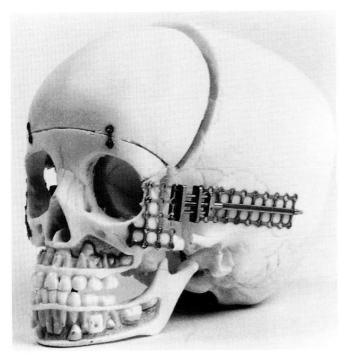

Fig. 60.20 Placement of the subcutaneous device is demonstrated on a model. (Reproduced from Cohen SR et al[42] with permission.)

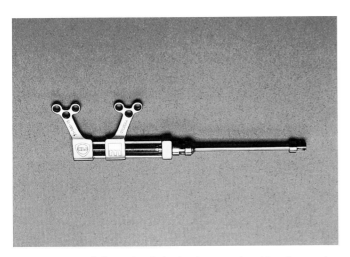

Fig. 60.21 A small distraction device has been produced for placement underneath the buccal mucosa in patients with hypoplastic mandibles. The port may be exposed percutaneously or in the buccal sulcus (KLS Martin Inc.).

Intraoral devices provide the opportunity for distraction while minimizing external scars. The major limitation remains the availability of sufficient bone stock (especially in the mandible) for adequate purchase of the device. This is especially true for patients with severe mandibular deficiencies (Pruzansky type II). Furthermore, gaining access to the severe hypoplastic mandible usually requires an external approach despite the availability of internal devices. Finally, current internal devices provide distraction in a single plane without the ability to manipulate the regenerate bone in multiple planes, as is available in some external devices.

ENDOSCOPY AND DISTRACTION

Endoscopy has provided a technique of minimal access for traditional surgical procedures. The application of this technique in craniofacial surgery has been limited by the difficulty in maintaining an optical space, and the need to remove bone and blood while performing the osteotomy. Cadaveric studies have demonstrated the ability to access and complete a Le Fort III osteotomy using minimal incisions.[59] Reports of clinical application have been limited to the cranial vault for correction of sagittal synostosis.[60]

A canine model of midface distraction that incorporates endoscopic equipment for the performance of the midface osteotomies has been recently established.[48] Combined with the development of new instrumentation, the procedure has been used to complete the osteotomies and successfully distract the midface. The combination of the two procedures is inherently appealing and should find wider application in the future.[61,62]

REFERENCES

1. Aronson J 1994 Temporal and spatial increases in blood flow during distraction osteogenesis. Clinical Orthopaedics and Related Research 301:124–131
2. Grundnes O, Reikeras O 1992 Blood flow and mechanical properties of healing bone. Femoral osteotomies studies in rats. Acta Orthopaedica Scandinavica 63:487–491
3. Mosheiff R, Cordey J, Rhan BA, Parren SM et al 1996 The vascular supply to bone in distraction osteogenesis: An experimental study. Journal of Bone Joint Surgery 78:497–498
4. Codivilla A 1905 On the means of lengthening in the lower limbs, the muscles and tissues which are shortened through deformity. American Journal of Orthopedic Surgery 2:353
5. Magnuson P 1913 Lengthening of shortened bones of the leg by operation. Ivory screw with removal heads as a means of holding the two bone fragments. Surgery, Gynecology and Obstetrics 16:63
6. Abbot LC 1932 Lengthening of the lower extremities. California and Western Medicine 36:6
7. Carrell W 1929 Leg lengthening. Southern Medical Journal 22:216
8. Allan FG 1948 Bone lengthening. Journal of Bone and Joint Surgery 30:490
9. Wagner H 1971 Operative Beinvertangerung. (Surgical leg prolongation.) Chirurgie 42:260
10. Ilizarov GA 1988 The principles of the Ilizarov method. Bulletin of the Hospital for Joint Diseases Orthopaedic Institute 48:1–9
11. Ilizarov GA 1990 Clinical application of the tension-stress effect for limb lengthening. Clinical Orthopedics 250:268
12. Synder DC, Levine GA, Swanson HM, Browne EZ Jr 1973 Mandibular lengthening by gradual distraction. Preliminary report. Plastic and Reconstructive Surgery 51:506–508
13. Michieli S, Mioth B 1977 Lengthening of mandible body by gradual

surgical orthodontic distraction. Journal of Oral Surgery 35:187–192

14. Karp NS, Thorne CH, McCarthy JG, Sissons HA 1990 Bone lengthening in the craniofacial skeleton. Annals of Plastic Surgery 24:231–237

15. Karp NS, McCarthy JG, Schreiber JS et al 1992 Membranous bone lengthening: a serial histological study. Annals of Plastic Surgery 29:2–7

16. McCarthy JG, Schreiber J, Karp N, Thorne CH, Grayson BH 1992 Lengthening the human mandible by gradual distraction. Plastic and Reconstructive Surgery 89:1–8

17. Molina F, Ortiz Monasterio F 1995 Mandibular elongation and remodeling by distraction: a farewell to major osteotomies. Plastic and Reconstructive Surgery 96:825

18. Nakamura E, Mizuta H, Otsuka Y, Mizumoto Y, Takagi K 1995 Leg lengthening and glycosaminoglycans in the rabbit knee. Acta Orthopaedica Scandinavica 66:33–37

19. Miura Y, Fitzsimmons JS, Commissi CN, Gallay SH, O'Driscoll SW 1994 Enhancement of periosteal chondrogenesis in vitro. Clinical Orthopaedics and Related Research 301:271–280

20. Oni OOA 1995 Protine immunohistochemistry as a means of unravelling the mysteries of fracture repair. International Journal of Care of the Injured 26:523–525

21. Hughes SS, Hicks DG, O'Keefe RJ et al 1995 Shared phenotypic expression of osteoblasts and chondrocytes in fracture callus. Journal of Bone and Mineral Research 10:533–544

22. Leung KS, Fung KP, Liu PPL, Lee KM 1995 Bone-specific alkaline phosphatase activities in plasma and callus during callotasis in rabbits. Life Sciences 57:637–643

23. Grundes O, Reikeras O 1993 The role of hematoma and periosteal sealing for fracture healing in rats. Acta Orthopaedica Scandinavica 64:47–49

24. Aronson J, Harrison BH, Steward CL, Harp JH 1989 The histology of distraction osteogenesis using different external fixators. Clinical Orthopaedics and Related Research 2441:106–116

25. Rowe NM, Mehrara BJ, Oudziak ME et al 1998 Rat mandibular distraction osteogenesis: Part I: histologic and radiographic analysis. Journal of Craniofacial Surgery (in press)

26. Magnuson P 1908 Lengthening shortened bones of the leg by operation. University of Pennsylvania Medical Bulletin XXI:103

27. McCarthy JG 1994 The role of distraction osteogenesis in the reconstruction of the mandible in unilateral craniofacial microsomia. Clinics in Plastic Surgery 21:625–631

28. Meurmann Y 1957 Congenital microtia and meatal atresia. Archives of Otolaryngology 66:443–446

29. Pruzansky S 1969 Not all dwarfed mandibles are alike. Birth Defects. 5:120–124

30. Kaban LB, Moses MH, Mulliken JB 1988 Surgical correction of hemifacial microsomia in the growing child. Plastic and Reconstructive Surgery 82:9–19

31. Grayson BH, McCormack S, Santiago PE, McCarthy JM 1997 Vector of device placement and trajectory of mandibular distraction. Journal of Craniofacial Surgery 8: 473–480

32. McCormack SU, McCarthy JG, Grayson BH, Staffenberg DA, McCormack SA 1995 Effects of mandibular distraction on the temporomandibular joint: Part II, clinical study. Journal of Craniofacial Surgery 6:358–363

33. McCormack SU, McCarthy JG, Grayson GH et al 1995 Effects of mandibular distraction on the temporomandibular joint: Part 1, canine study. Journal of Craniofacial Surgery 6:348–357

34. Lauritzen C, Lilja J, Jaristedt J 1996 Airway obstruction and sleep apnea in children with craniofacial anomalies. Plastic and Reconstructive Surgery 77:1–5

35. Conway WA, Victor LO, Magilligan DG et al 1981 Adverse effects of tracheostomy for sleep apnea. Journal of the American Medical Association 246:347–350

36. Sasaki CT, Masatoshi H, Koss N 1979 Tracheostomy related subglotic stenosis: bacteriologic pathogenesis. Laryngoscope 89:857–865

37. Williams JK, Maull DM, Grayson BH, McCarthy JG 1998 Early intervention with bilateral mandibular distraction for tracheostomy dependent patients. Plastic and Reconstructive Surgery (in press)

38. Imai K, Tajima S, Tanaka Y 1993 Measurement of the intraoral space and its relationship to apnea attacks during sleep in craniofacial synostosis patients. Japanese Journal of Plastic and Reconstructive Surgery 36:177–182

39. Imai K, Tajima S, Kakitsuba N 1994 A pre- and postoperative assessment of the pharyngeal air space in craniomaxillofacial anomalies and its relationship to the obstructive sleep apnea syndrome. Japanese Journal of Plastic and Reconstructive Surgery 37:223

40. Cohen SR, Lefaivre JF, Burstein FD et al 1997 Surgical treatment of obstructive sleep apnea in neurologically compromised patients. Plastic and Reconstructive Surgery 99:638–646

41. Chin M, Toth BA 1997 LeFort III advancement with gradual distraction using internal devices. Plastic and Reconstructive Surgery 100:819–830

42. Cohen SR, Burnstein FD, Steward MB, Rathburn MA 1997 Maxillary-midface distraction in children with cleft lip and palate: a preliminary report. Plastic and Reconstructive Surgery 99:1421–1428

43. Yamamoto H, Sawaki Y, Ohkubo H, Ueda M 1997 Maxillary advancement by distraction osteogenesis using osseointegrated implants. Journal of Craniomaxillofacial Surgery 25:186–191

44. Polley JW, Figueroa AA 1997 Management of severe maxillary deficiency in childhood and adolescence through distraction osteogenesis with an external, adjustable, rigid distraction device. Journal of Craniofacial Surgery 8:181–185

45. Ortiz Monasterio F, Molina F, Andrade L et al 1997 Stimultaneous mandibular and maxillary distraction in hemifacial microsomia in adults: Avoiding occlusal disasters. Plastic and Reconstructive Surgery 100:852–861

46. McCarthy JG, LaTrenta GS, Breitbart AS et al 1990 The LeFort III advancement osteotomy in the child under 7 years of age. Plastic and Reconstructive Surgery 86:633–646

47. Staffenberg DA, Wood RJ, McCarthy JG et al 1995 Midface distraction advancement in the canine without osteotomies. Annals of Plastic Surgery 34:512–517

48. Levine JP, Rowe NM, Bradley JP et al 1998 The combination of endoscopy and distraction osteogenesis in the development of a canine midface advancement model. Journal of Craniofacial Surgery 5:423–32

49. Cohen SR, Rutrick RE, Burnstein FD 1995 Distraction osteogenesis of the human craniofacial skeleton: initial experience with new distraction system. Journal of Craniofacial Surgery 6:368–374

50. Glat PM, Staffenberg DA, Karp NS et al 1994 Multidimensional distraction osteogenesis: the canine zygoma. Plastic and Reconstructive Surgery 94:753–758

51. Remmier D, McCoy FJ, O'Neil D et al 1992 Osseous expansion of the cranial vault by craniostasis. Plastic and Reconstructive Surgery 89:767–797

52. Lalikos JF, Tschakaloff A, Mooney MP et al 1995 Internal calvarial bone distraction in rabbits with experimental coronal suture immobilization: Effects of overdistraction. Plastic Reconstructive Surgery 96:689–698

53. doAmaral CM, DiDomizio G, Tiziani V et al 1997 Gradual bone distraction in craniosynostosis. Preliminary results in seven cases. Scandinavian Journal of Plastic and Reconstructive Hand Surgery 31:25–37

54. Pensler JM, Goldberg DP, Lindell B, Carroll NC 1995 Skeletal distraction of the hypoplastic mandible. Annals of Plastic Surgery 34:130–137

55. Klein C, Howaldt HP 1996 Correction of mandibular hypoplasia by means of bidirectional callus distraction. Journal of Craniofacial Surgery 7:258–266

56. McCarthy JG, Steffenberg DA, Wood RS et al 1995 Introduction of an intraoral bone lengthening device. Plastic and Reconstructive Surgery 96:978–981

57. Guerroro CA, Bell WH, Contasti GI 1997 Mandibular widening by intraoral distraction. Osteogenesis 35:383–392

58. Diner PA, Kollar E, Martinez M, Vasquez MP 1997 Submerged intraoral device for mandibular lengthening. Journal of Craniofacial Surgery 25:114–123

59. Wood R, Staffenberg D, Harris S et al 1996 Endoscopic LeFort III Osteotomy. In: Marchac D (ed) Craniofacial Surgery VI. Monduzzi Editore, Bologna, pp 257–258

60. Vicanni F, Zukowski M 1996 Endoscopic assisted craniofacial surgery. In: Marchac D (ed) Craniofacial Surgery VI. Monduzzi Editore, Bologna, pp 259–260

61. Moseley CF 1991 Leg lengthening. The historical perspective. Orthopedic Clinics of North America 22:556

62. McCarthy JG 1997 Craniofacial microsomia: Grabb & Smith's plastic surgery. Little Brown, Boston

Reanimation in congenital disorders

HARRY J. BUNCKE Jr

INTRODUCTION

Congenital facial paralysis, or facial paralysis at birth, may be partial or complete, idiopathic in nature or secondary to birth trauma, tumors or other intrauterine environmental anomalies. Early diagnosis is important and complex, and best performed by pediatric otolaryngologists familiar with and skilled in the various diagnostic tests and studies. If the paralysis is traumatic in nature early decompression of the facial nerve may be indicated, the idiopathic type, which may be partial, complete, unilateral or bilateral, supranuclear or infranuclear in location, does not require early intervention.[1]

Other conditions that may be associated with facial paralysis – again, unilateral, bilateral partial or complete, upper face or lower face – are Möbius syndrome, pseudo-Möbius syndrome,[2] hemifacial microsomia,[3] hypoplasia of the depressor anguli oris (DAOM) syndrome, also known as Cayler's syndrome, or asymmetrical crying facies, and CULLP syndrome, or congenital unilateral lower lip palsy, which has a strong hereditary pattern and has been documented in five generations.[4] Hereditary congenital facial paralysis is an unusual condition that also has a strong hereditary pattern, and the side of paralysis may be handed down from generation to generation.[5] Johnson–McMillen syndrome is a rare autosomal dominant condition associated with facial paralysis and multiple truncal café-au-lait spots, hyposmia, poor growth and development, microtia and mental retardation.[6] Certain cranial bone congenital anomalies are associated with facial paralysis secondary to pressure on the facial nerve at various areas throughout its course. Cranial diaphyseal dysplasia involves thickening of all the cranial bones, with facial paralysis, blindness, mental retardation, seizures and, usually, death by the second or third decade.[7] Another condition, dominant osteopetrosis, involves hyperostosis of the petrous bones with secondary cranial palsies of nerves II, III and VII. This is an autosomal dominant condition compatible with normal life expectancy.[8] Hyperostosis corticalis generalisata involves hyperostosis of the mandible and cranial base, with facial paralysis, blindness and deafness, again compatible with normal life expectancy and an autosomal recessive condition.[9]

There are other complex syndromes where facial paralysis may play a part and the multiple deformities may be present in various degrees of intensity. Treacher–Collins syndrome, or mandibulofacial dysostosis, also known as Franceschetti–Lwalen–Kline syndrome, is an autosomal dominant deformity of the first and second branchial arches.[10] It is usually bilateral, and probably secondary to vascular anomalies in the first 5 weeks of gestation. The deformity can be produced in mice by teratogenic high doses of vitamin A. The main features are antimongoloid obliquity of the palpebral fissures, notched lower eyelids, coloboma of the iris, ovoid orbital apertures, micrognathia, hypoplasia of the malar and mandibular bones, large mouth, irregular teeth and malocclusion, deformities of the external (and occasionally the inner ear), deafness, preauricular sinuses, dwarfism, cardiac and skeletal defects and abnormalities of the upper airway, and varying degrees of facial paralysis. The 'CHARGE' syndrome is a complex autosomal dominant deformity in which the mnemonic stands for *Coloboma*, *Heart* disease, *Atresia* choanal, *Retardation* of mental and skeletal growth, *Genital* hypoplasia and *Ear* deformities.[11] Each of these features can vary from minimal to severe. These children are usually normal at birth, but fall behind as they enter infancy and childhood. The prognosis is better than reported in the literature if early feeding problems are addressed. Cleft lip and palate and pectus carinatum may also be present. OAVS, oculo-auriculo-vertebral spectrum, can also be associated with the CHARGE syndrome, adding torticollis, plagiocephaly and heminostril deformities.[12] FSH,

fascio-scapulo-humeral dystrophy, is an autosomal dominant condition associated with weakness of the face and
shoulder muscles and the legs, plus hearing loss.[13] In some
severe cases it is slowly progressive, but in most intelligence and lifespan are normal. CBPS, congenital bilateral
perisylvian syndrome, involves weakness of the facial and
pharyngeal muscles and muscles of mastication, of variable
severity. There can be dysarthria to no intelligible speech,
mental retardation and epilepsy. On MRI there are bilateral
perisylvian cortical macrogyria.[14] Microtia with atresia can
be associated with partial to complete facial paralysis,
depending upon the deformities of the middle ear that
produce malposition of the facial nerve. It is seen after
thalidomide ingestion, rubella and intrauterine infections,
and has an increased frequency in Navajo Indians. It is more
common on the right side than the left, and one in six cases
is bilateral.[15] Melkersson syndrome is a familial, often bilateral
paralysis associated with angioneurotic facial edema and
lingua plicata (furrowing in the tongue).[16]

Möbius syndrome, mentioned earlier, is also known as
congenital oculofacial paralysis or congenital facial diplegia.
The full-blown syndrome involves bilateral facial paralysis,
paralysis of the lateral rectus, or 6th abducens nerve, tongue
hypoplasia, mental retardation, and absence of the pectoral
muscles, syndactyly and brachydactyly. It is a heterogeneic
entity which can affect the nervous system in many ways.[17]

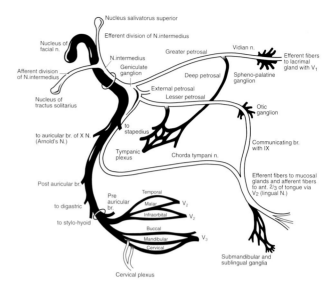

Fig. 61.1 Communications of the facial nerve with cranial nerves V
(trigeminal and divisions of V_1, V_2, V_3), IX (glossopharyngeal), and X
(vagus) and with the cervical plexus (greater auricular and transverse
cervical branches). (Modified with permission from Gray's *Anatomy*.) The
anatomical course of the facial nerve is depicted from its nucleus in the
pons, where it curves around the nucleus of the 6th nerve, then joins the
8th nerve to exit the internal auditory meatus, goes through the
geniculate ganglion and then through the fallopian aqueduct in the
mastoid bone, where it finally exits the styloid foramen. The location of
the facial nerve involvement can be discerned by various clinical
symptoms and tests. (Reproduced with permission from Mackinnon and
Dellon.[29])

DIFFERENTIAL DIAGNOSIS OF FACIAL PARALYSIS

Direct biopsy of the facial muscles is useful for differentiating between congenital facial paralysis and neonatal
trauma, particularly when it is long-standing. This was first
used by Duchenne in 1868. In complete paralysis, most
people feel that the facial muscles atrophy and disappear
after a year or so.[18]

There are a variety of tests, some simple and some
elaborate, based on various physiological responses, plus
electrophysiological methods for diagnosing congenital
facial paralysis. These are designed to locate the site of the
lesion and the degree of involvement, evaluate the need for
early decompression, and follow the recovery, spontaneous
or postsurgical (Fig. 61.1).

METHODS

Three of the most popular neurophysiological tests are MST,
ENG and EMG.[1] The MST, or maximum stimulation test,
is used after 48–72 hours, as all nerve injuries will respond

to direct stimulation for this period of time. The test should
be repeated daily to give some indication of the direction
of degeneration or regeneration. This test is based on the
concept that a motor nerve will conduct in response to an
electrical stimulus distal to the lesion, even though the
muscles will not respond volitionally. The test is performed
by stimulating the major branches of the nerve of the
forehead, eye, upper lip and lower lip, and comparing the
response with the normal side. The stimulus is usually about
5 amps, or higher if tolerated by the patient. In a first-
degree lesion the contraction of the paralyzed side is equal
to that of the normal side in spite of the absence of volitional response. In a second-degree lesion an increased intensity is needed to produce a response comparable to or less
than the normal side, and this indicates axonal damage.
With a third-degree lesion there is no response on maximal
stimulation, indicating severe axonal injury and degeneration. First and second degrees indicate some element of
neurapraxia, whereas a third degree indicates neurotmesis.
If the second-degree response seems to be improving, surgical
intervention is postponed. However, if there is a decrease,
surgical intervention and decompression are necessary.

Electroneurography (ENG), which evaluates the proportion of denervated fibers, is performed on the 4th, 7th and 10th days. Recordings of summated muscle action potentials are integrated and averaged, giving a numerical value which expresses the number of fibers blocked and denervated. The facial nerve is stimulated at the mastoid area at just below the painful threshold, and recordings are made in the nasolabial fold.

EMG studies are particularly helpful in peripheral paralysis. Recording electrodes in a normal muscle at rest are silent. Motor action potentials appear on volition or with stimulation of the peripheral trunk. With denervation, fibrillation potentials appear within 10–12 days of paralysis. Reappearance of motor action potentials is the first sign of regeneration and precedes the return of volitional response.

LOCATION OF LESION

If facial paralysis is due to a central lesion, the frontalis branch of the facial nerve still works because it has bilateral cortical input. There is loss of voluntary control of the rest of the branches, but there is emotional response, such as with laughing, and preservation of muscle tone, probably because the extrapyramidal system is spared. Bell's phenomenon is also not present. Lesions of the nucleus of the facial nerve in the pons or brainstem, where cranial nerve VII curves around the nucleus of cranial nerve VI, usually result in a peripheral paralysis of both nerves, resulting in facial paralysis and loss of the ability of the involved eye to rotate to the paralyzed side.

From the cerebellopontine angle to the internal auditory canal the facial nerve is covered with only a thin film of glia as it lies next to the 8th nerve and on the sensory intermedius nerve. In this area the 7th nerve is vulnerable to surgical trauma, but can tolerate a fair amount of stretching produced by an expanding neurilemmoma in the 8th nerve before the facial muscle weakness is noted. The sensory intermedius nerve is less tolerant, and loss of taste and salivation may precede facial paralysis.

Decreased or absent lacrimation places a lesion at or proximal to the geniculate ganglion, where the greater petrosal nerve to the lacrimal gland comes off.[19] Rapid onset of facial paralysis in 3–10 days is a poor prognostic sign, as is loss of tearing. In such cases 90% have poor recovery of facial nerve function. Evidence of spontaneous recovery in the first 2 weeks portends a full recovery, even with decreased salivation and electrical tests.[20]

If lacrimation is present but the stapedius muscle reflex is gone and taste is gone, which comes through the chorda tympani, the lesion is distal to the geniculate ganglion. If these three tests are normal, then the lesion is in the bony canal of the mastoid.

Various tests to measure salivary flow by cannulating the parotid, sublingual and submaxillary glands have been described. On stimulation with a sour taste, such as lemon or pickle, a 25% decrease compared to the normal side indicates a poor prognosis and surgical decompression should be considered. Reduction in salivary flow is an early sign of potential denervation.[19]

The blink reflex is an interesting test similar to the corneal reflex. Stimulation of the supraorbital nerve with a reflex hammer produces a bilateral blinking contracture of the orbicularis oculi which can be recorded with surface or needle electrodes. It has two components, R1 and R2. R1 is an oligosynaptic response which appears only on the side stimulated and is a subclinical contraction, but can be recorded and has a 10–12 second latency. The R2 reflex involves clinical closure and occurs bilaterally at 20–45 ms latency. Early return of a blink reflex within 2 weeks of facial paralysis carries a better prognosis for recovery and reflects the status of the entire facial nerve.[21] Terzis has used this reflex in a rat model to demonstrate that cross-temporal facial nerve grafting from one orbicularis to the other in a two-stage procedure can be considered when motor end-plates are still present on the paralyzed side.[22]

Early diagnosis of the cause of facial paralysis in the newborn is extremely important, as traumatic defects should be corrected immediately, whereas congenital or idiopathic problems can be treated with less urgency. In the newborn the mastoid process is poorly developed and the facial nerve is almost subcutaneous, where it is vulnerable to injury in utero from pressures from forceps or from the sacral prominence of the mother. Compression on the side of the face, particularly in the mandibular area, may produce individual branch temporary paralysis. If there is improvement, it is safe to follow the paralysis. Without early improvement decompression should be considered. The isolated paralysis of the marginal mandibular nerve may be confused with other congenital facial paralysis, such as asymmetrical crying facies. However, the pressure type usually clears and no specific treatment is needed.[23]

There is no general agreement on whether or not idiopathic congenital facial paralysis can be treated early by decompression and/or nerve grafting. Anatomic studies of neonatal specimens with facial paralysis have shown that there are postnuclear lesions in the facial nerve where it seems normal, only to become a thread at the geniculate ganglion, an area where it is surgically accessible. Terzis has confirmed these anatomical findings on 24 such dissections (Terzis 1997, personal communication). With MRI and gadolinium MRI studies, the anatomic course and thickness of the facial nerve can be traced quite accurately. Such studies are particularly helpful in patients with traumatic or obscure causes for facial paralysis.

The surgical management of lesions to the facial nerve in the mastoid canal and the temporal bone requires the skills of a neuro-otologist or pediatric ENT specialist with expertise in this area.

hypertrophy and become functional with cross-facial nerve grafts to these areas. Earl Owen of Sydney, Australia, has performed over 100 cross-facial nerve grafts in children for partial congenital paralysis, with very worthwhile results (Owen 1997, personal communication). After 2.5–3.5 years, most people feel that the best results can achieved with a cross-facial nerve graft as a preliminary procedure, followed by a functional muscle transplant after the nerve has regenerated across the face to the paralyzed side[24] (Figs 61.2, 61.3).

SURGICAL MANAGEMENT OF CONGENITAL FACIAL PARALYSIS

There are some who feel that with incomplete paralysis some of the facial muscles may still be present and may

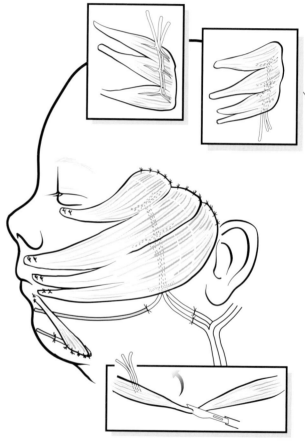

Fig. 61.3 Second stage: functional neuromuscular microvascular transplant of the serratus anterior. The lower three slips of the serratus muscle, VII, VIII and IX, are on the superficial surface on the chest (upper left). The neurovascular bundles then lie on the deeper surface when the muscle is rotated 180 degrees (upper right). The IX slip is passed across the lower lid to the inner canthal area. The VIII slip is split, with one slip going to the columella and the other portion to the outer third of the upper lip. The VII slip is sutured to the corner of the mouth. The nerve from the serratus is anastomosed to the cross-facial nerve graft, which is picked up in the preauricular area. The artery and vein from the serratus are anastomosed to the anterior facial vessels as they cross the mandible. The cross-facial nerve graft passed under the chin is anastomosed to the nerve supply to the anterior belly of the digastric muscle, which is cut and mobilized 160 degrees on its vascular pedicle so that it parallels the direction of the depressor triangularis of the lower lip.

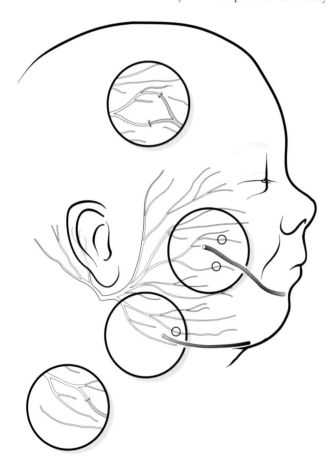

Fig. 61.2 First stage: cross-facial nerve graft. One cable of the superficial peroneal nerve is passed across the upper lip and anastomosed to branches to the zygomatic and risorius area of the normal side (depicted in the upper circle). The second cable of the superficial peroneal nerve is smaller. It is passed under the chin and anastomosed to branches of the marginal mandibular nerve on the normal side.

The three areas of concern are eye closure and protection of the globe, oral continence, and spontaneous animation. May has pointed out that most children up to age 5 seldom have problems with eye closure even in the presence of decreased tearing and reduced blinking.[1] However, the lower lid tends to sag and tears not carried to the medial punctum spill over the lower lid down the cheek. During the second stage of the cross-facial functional muscle transplant, the lower lid can be tightened up and brought into good contact with the globe, with the ninth slip of the functional muscle transplant across the lower lid to the medial canthal area. Turndown of the anterior 2 cm of the temporalis muscle with fascial extensions into the upper and lower lid causes lid movement with chewing, which is often unacceptable to patients. We no longer perform this

transfer in children. Satisfactory upper lid closure can be accomplished by inserting a gold weight into the upper eyelid, so that with spontaneous relaxation of the levator, which occurs with blinking, the lid closes passively when the patient is sitting or semirecumbent. Using test weights (MedDev Corp., Palo Alto, CA) one can accurately determine the size of the lid weight necessary by placing the test weights on the skin of the upper eyelid, held in place with tincture of benzoin. The child then blinks and one assesses the degree of closure. A videotape of the act will help the patient and family see the degree of lid closure accomplished with the particular lid weight (Fig. 61.4). However, the weights in place are not inconspicuous and some patients request their removal. Various types of spring have been devised which reproduce the passive blink reflex, but

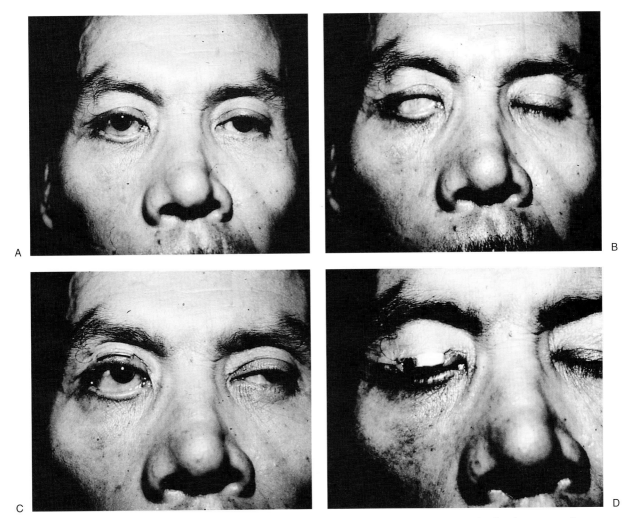

Fig. 61.4 (A) Preoperatively this patient was unable to close the right eye. **(B)** Fortunately, because of Bell's phenomenon (in which the globe rotates upward), the cornea was protected during sleep. **(C)** With the test weight stuck to the upper lid with tincture of benzoin. The levator palpebrae superioris muscle reflexively relaxes on closing the eyelids. **(D)** Gravity closure is achieved. (Reproduced with permission from Buncke HJ, Buncke GM 1995 Secondary procedures in facial reanimation. In: Grotting JC (ed) Reoperative aesthetic and reconstructive plastic surgery. Quality Medical Publishing, St. Louis, p. 635.)

problems with fixation and erosion through the skin and conjunctiva are not uncommon.

In the management of the upper lip, several factors must be taken into account. The philtrum is pulled to the normal side by the relatively overactive normal muscles, which results in stretching of the lip on the paralyzed side. The degree of sagging of the modiolus of the corner of the mouth in children is not as great as that in adults with facial paralysis, but must still be addressed. We now prefer during the first stage to place fascial strips to bring the philtrum to the midline and raise the corner of the mouth, so that when the functional muscle is placed during the second operation the muscle does not stretch out. As the placement of the fascia in the first stage and the muscle in the second stage requires considerable dissection in the upper lip area, we prefer to put the cross-facial nerve graft across the lower lip, where it is not exposed to possible damage.

The functional muscle transplant is inserted during the second stage, superficial to the previous fascial sheet, to the philtrum, the upper lip and the angle of the mouth.

The problem with the lower lip is the loss of the downward and outward contraction of the triangularis and lip depressor muscles. Edgerton attempted to correct this by advancing the anterior belly of the digastric with a fascial strip to the lower lip.[25] Connolly and Baker turned the anterior belly, sectioning the tendon at the pulley and rotating the muscle 180 degrees, tunneling it to the lateral portion of the lower lip.[26] Unfortunately, both of these transfers pull the lip downward rather than downward and outward. In addition, the digastric is supplied by cranial nerve V, so that it does not contract spontaneously with 7th nerve animation. We have found with cadaver sections that the anterior belly of the digastric and its tendon and part of the tendon of the posterior belly can be mobilized entirely on the neurovascular pedicle, which comes in on the deep surface of the muscle from lateral to medial. The muscle and its tendon on this pedicle then can be rotated 160 degrees, placing the muscle belly along the lower border of the mandible and the tendon obliquely into the lower lip, exactly paralleling the contraction of the depressor triangularis. The muscle can then be converted to a 7th nerve muscle, with a second cross-facial nerve graft passed under the chin, anastomosed to the mandibular branch on the normal side.

We no longer use the sural nerve as our cross-facial nerve graft for several reasons:

- Its intrafascicular pattern is not consistent and there is a great deal of crossover, so that the fascicular bundles at the proximal end cannot be compared to the fascicular bundles at the distal end.

- It is a difficult dissection for the harvesting team when the patient is in a supine or face-up position.
- The superficial peroneal nerve has a much more dependable fascicular bundle pattern throughout the distal 25 cm of its length. The area of anesthesia created by the use of the superficial peroneal nerve is on the dorsal lateral surface of the foot, decreases in size with time, and is less critical than the sensory defect produced by using the sural nerve, which sometimes supplies the lateral part of the side of the foot and plantar skin.

We prefer to use the lower three slips of the serratus muscle as our functional transplant for complete facial paralysis, and the gracilis muscle for incomplete paralysis. The three slips of the serratus can be separated into three separate neurovascular pedicles.[27] Meuli-Simmen, one of our Research Fellows, did several cadaver dissections and injection studies documenting the regional distribution of the neurovascular pedicles. She also performed the same dissections using the sheep serratus, which has a similar anatomic pattern. She was able to separate these three fascicles in the sheep serratus and stimulate each bundle separately through the proximal nerve.[28] McKenna and Dillon have done the same thing with the latissimus, separating it into two independent neurovascular islands so that they can be set differentially into the upper lip.[29] Manktelow has also used this technique to isolate a portion of the gracilis muscle on a single neurovascular pedicle, rather than using the entire muscle.[30] Terzis prefers the pectoralis minor muscle, which also has a segmental nerve supply from the medial and lateral pectoral nerves.[31]

POSTOPERATIVE CARE

We feel that the venous Doppler initially described and popularized by Schwarz, and recently modified, offers the most reliable way to continually monitor circulation to microvascular transplants and replants.[32,33] With early detection of vascular problems we have been able to salvage a much higher percentage of take-backs than we did when using the fluoroscan or external Doppler.

All elective microvascular transplant patients receive aspirin for its platelet-stabilizing effect, 3 mg/kg preoperatively, beginning 7 days prior to surgery and continuing for a month afterwards. Low-molecular weight dextran is begun intraoperatively as soon as the microvascular repairs are begun, and is continued for 5 days postoperatively. The dose of 25 ml/h for adults is modulated to the child's weight. Aspirin is discontinued in children if they develop any signs of a cold in the postoperative period because of the rare occurrence of Reye's syndrome.[34]

With continuous monitoring of the venous outflow signal we are able to detect instantaneously any complications, and patients are immediately brought back to the operating room for exploration of the wounds. In some cases the signal is lost because the Doppler probe is dislodged, but it is well worth confirmation to be sure that there are no venous or arterial problems. Most patients stay in the hospital for 6–10 days after the functional muscle transplant, depending on their progress. They are usually in the hospital for 3–5 days after the first procedure.

We use percutaneous muscle stimulation with DC current in the early postoperative period, and continue this until we have evidence of voluntary muscle contraction, when the nerve stimulus is then shifted from direct to alternating current. There are no fixed protocols for the frequency, time or duration of such muscle stimulation, but it is our impression and that of others that muscle bulk is better preserved and reinnervation hastened.[35] Weak voluntary and spontaneous contractions start to appear in 3–6 months, and become stronger over 3–4 months.

Our problem in more cases has been overactivity of the muscle, rather than underactivity. Also, muscle bulk is difficult to predict. After transplantation we always anticipate atrophy anywhere between 40 and 50%. Again this varies from patient to patient. It is not unusual to go back secondarily to debulk the muscle, particularly in the malar area, as this is the greatest area of fullness. As the nerve and blood supply to the microvascular transplant are on the deep surface, this type of muscle thinning can be achieved without fear of denervating or devascularizing the transplant. It is also possible to tighten the transplant or move the angle of pull secondarily by detaching it from its temporal insertion. We have on occasion lengthened muscles in the nasolabial area in a V–Y fashion, and in some of our early patients had to return for removal of the muscle slips we had placed into the upper eyelid, which were in fact deforming eye closure rather than assisting it.

Our goal in reconstruction for facial paralysis is to restore spontaneous function and animation. If we can fool the scanning reflex, we feel that the operation has been successful. The scanning reflex is a primordial one present in all creatures, down to the level of the salamander. In a fraction of a second the animal scans the horizon as it comes out of its hole, instinctively searching for abnormal activity or structures. If everything appears normal, the animal proceeds with its activity. We use this scanning reflex each time we look at someone. If nothing fixes our gaze, the scanning reflex has been satisfied. There are a variety of complicated techniques for measuring functional results after facial paralysis, but perfection is impossible. Most patients who receive some degree of spontaneous activity and return of facial symmetry and smile are appreciative of the improvement, even though it may be 50%, 70% or 80% (Figs. 61.5–61.9).

OPERATIVE SEQUENCE

FIRST-STAGE OPERATION

Before operation the position of the nasolabial fold is carefully marked to mimic the fold on the normal side at rest and with smiling. The patient is placed supine, face up, with a nasotracheal intubation tube exiting over the forehead to leave the entire lower face, mouth, chin and submental area free.

1. Two teams work simultaneously, a surgeon and assistant on the face and a surgeon and assistant harvesting the nerve grafts on the lower extremity.
2. The facial team begins by infiltrating the entire normal side of the face with 1/200 000 adrenaline and saline using a 25 gauge, long spinal needle, starting in the temporal area and doing down to the cheek and nasolabial fold, across the upper lip and across and underneath the chin.
3. The skin incision starts in the temporal area and goes down to the level of the outer canthus, curving backwards into the preauricular region, inside the tragus, down to the earlobe and then down under the chin, with a Risdon extension in the submental fold.
4. The skin flap is raised out to the outer canthal area anterior to the parotid, and down in the submental area. These skin flaps are held forward by placing 3/0 silk sutures underneath to roll them forward, thereby exposing the anterior parotid area.
5. Donor nerve branches are then dissected out sharply, paralleling the course of the nerves, selecting and stimulating a branch to the angle of the mouth, the zygomatic area and under the chin for the marginal mandibular. A small battery-powered stimulator is used to isolate the proper branches, which are then marked with loops of 3/0 silk and knotted loosely, but not clamped, to prevent traction damage to the nerve branches.
6. The nerve harvesting team, usually on the opposite lower extremity, works under tourniquet control developing the superficial peroneal nerve on the dorsum of the foot at the level of the lateral malleolus. One or two

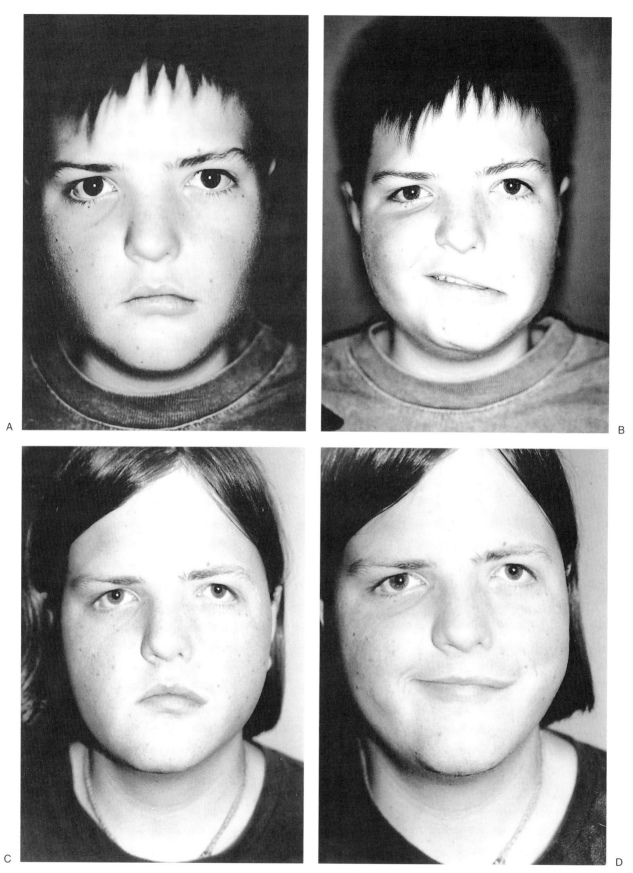

Fig. 61.5 Congenital facial paralysis. **(A)** At rest. This child seldom smiled because he realized he was different. His teachers and classmates thought he was sullen and withdrawn. **(B)** Marked assymetry on smiling. **(C)** Four years postoperatively, at rest. The muscle transplant has decreased in size about 50%. **(D)** Postoperative, smiling. The nasolabial scar is acceptable and the symmetry, though not perfect, fools the scanning reflex (see text).

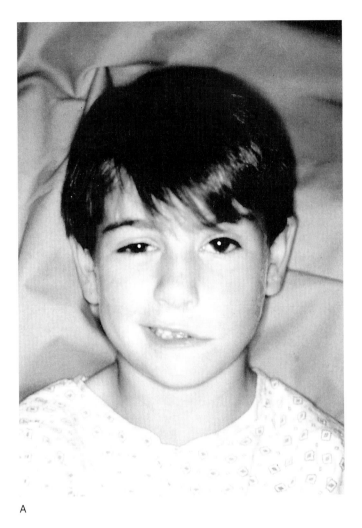

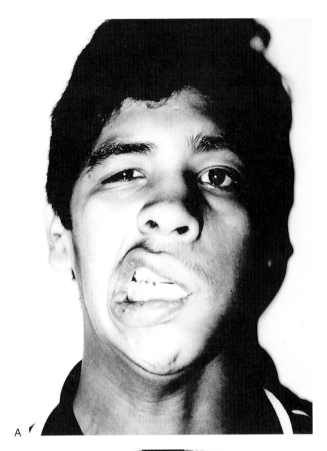

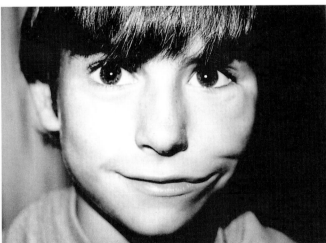

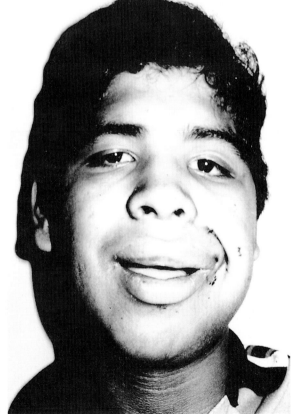

Fig. 61.6 (A) Preoperative, smiling. **(B)** Postoperative, smiling. The nasolabial fold is too far lateral, but the stigma of facial paralysis has been eliminated. (Reproduced with permission from Buncke HJ.[27])

Fig. 61.7 (A) Incomplete congenital facial paralysis, patient grimacing. **(B)** Early postoperative after muscle transplant. The nasolabial fold is overcorrected. (Reproduced with permission from Buncke HJ.[27])

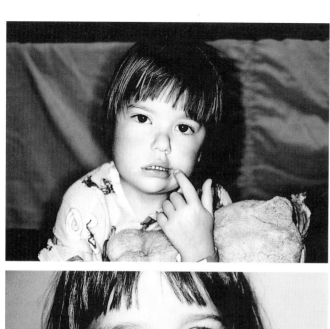

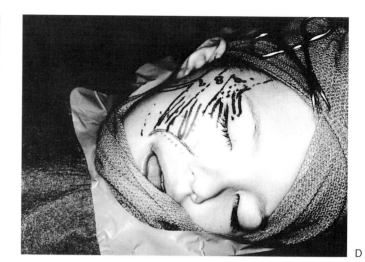

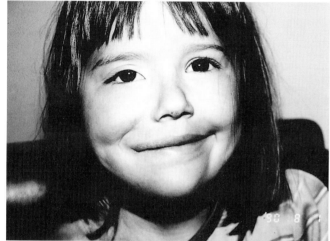

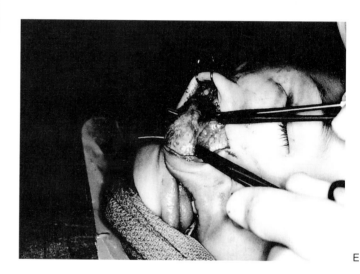

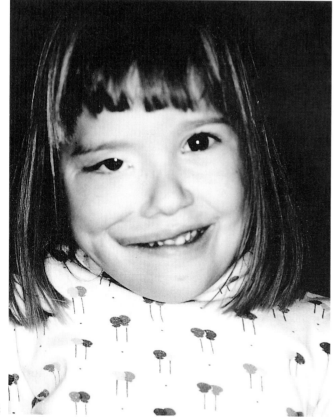

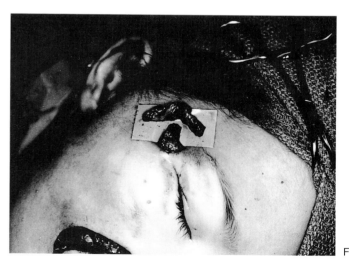

Fig. 61.8 (A) Even at an early age, this child suppressed her asymmetrical smile. A cross-facial nerve graft and a free microneurovascular transplant of the serratus anterior muscle were performed. **(B)** Early postoperatively the slips to the angle of the mouth and upper lip were working and the eye was not distorted. **(C)** Two months later, however, the slips to the mouth and eyelids were overactive. **(D)** A secondary procedure was planned to lengthen the muscle insertions. **(E)** A well-defined slip to the mouth was isolated for V–Y lengthening. **(F)** The slips to the eyelids were isolated and split for V–Y lengthening.

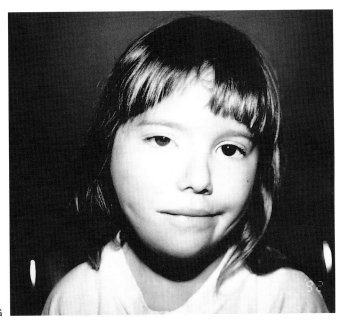

G

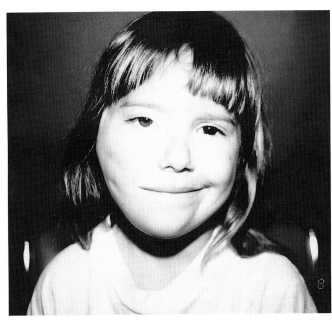

H

Fig. 61.8 (contd) **(G)** One year after the muscle-lengthening procedure, the appearance of the smile and the eye has improved. **(H)** However, the nasolabial fold has been lost due to overcorrection. (Reproduced with permission from Buncke HJ, Buncke GM 1995 Secondary procedures in facial reanimation. In: Grotting JC (ed). Reoperative aesthetic and reconstructive plastic surgery. Quality Medical Publishing, St. Louis, pp. 638–640)

branches can usually be palpated against the underlying tarsal bones. Through a small incision the branch is isolated, transected and then carefully dissected proximally using a 5 mm external vein stripper. Once resistance is felt, a second incision is made at this level through which the other major branch many be identified. Traction placed on the branch delineates the distal course of the branch. The branch is mobilized proximally through a second incision. Both branches are then brought out through the upper incision and the dissection is carried proximally, again using the external vein stripper around both branches.

7. The superficial peroneal nerve goes deeply in the intermuscular septum in the midportion of the calf. At this level a linear incision is made along the intermuscular septum proximally for 10–12 cm to permit further, deeper dissection of the superficial peroneal nerve, and also to expose a large area of fascia over the muscles of the anterior compartment; 25 cm of the nerve are mobilized. The proximal end is marked with a purple dye (purple for 'proximal'). A piece of fascial strip 10–12 cm long and 3–4 cm wide is excised over the muscles of the anterior compartment. A large fascial defect is better tolerated than a small one as far as muscle herniation is concerned.

8. The leg wound is closed and a bulky dressing applied and held in place with a circumferential Ace bandage prior to lowering the tourniquet.

9. The nerve graft and the fascial graft are transferred to the facial team and placed in moist saline sponges, carefully identified and stored on the back table.

10. The facial team now creates a long subcutaneous tunnel across the upper lip and under the chin. An incision is made on the paralyzed side in the preauricular area, of adequate length to join the tunnel across the lip.

11. The superficial peroneal nerve is then split into its two major fascicles. This can be done in situ before it is cut in the leg, or on the back table under loupe magnification. The epineurium is carefully opened, which permits the fascicles to separate. Very few, small interfascicular branches will be encountered. The two separate nerve grafts are then ready to be placed through the cross-facial nerve tunnels.

12. A 14 Fr catheter with a stylet is passed across the lower lip, starting on the normal side and ending on the paralyzed side. The funnel end of the catheter is trimmed down and the end of the catheter coming out of the paralyzed side is trimmed at the flap edge. The nerve graft is then sucked through the catheter by placing the purple-marked proximal end into the funnel on the normal side with a stream of irrigation solution, and suction on the other end of the catheter. The graft is grasped with a clamp at the distal end on the normal side to prevent it being sucked completely through the tubing. Once the end of the nerve appears on the paralyzed side it is grasped with a clamp and the catheter

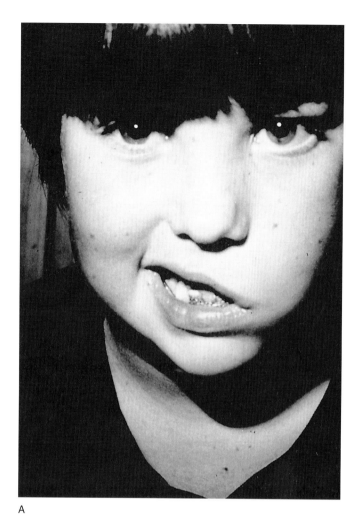

A

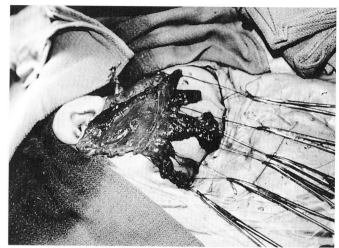

B

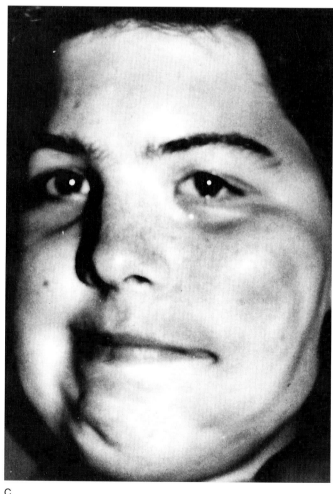

C

gradually removed, leaving the cross-facial nerve graft comfortably in its tunnel. In a similar fashion, the second cross-facial nerve graft is passed through the submental tunnel, coming out through the small incision in the submandibular area on the paralyzed side.

13. The microneural repairs are performed to the zygomatic branch and the risorius branch to the cross-facial nerve graft across the upper lip, and the mandibular branch to the graft under the chin.

14. The incision on the normal side is partially closed and the head turned to expose the paralyzed side.

15. The end of the nerve graft across the upper lip is marked with a hemoclip and sutured to the preauricular area. The end of the nerve graft under the chin is marked in a similar fashion in the submandibular wound.

16. The nasolabial incision is made in the premarked line and the incision on the paralyzed side is carried up into the temporal area. A tunnel is created from the temporal area and zygomatic area obliquely across the cheek, to the nasolabial incision, wide enough to accommodate the fascial sheet. The upper half of the

Fig. 61.9 **(A)** Asymmetry on smiling. **(B)** Serratus slips split, laid out over cheek. We no longer put a slip into the upper lid. **(C)** Postoperative, smiling. The nasolabial fold is not deep enough; however, appearance is acceptable and the stigma of facial paralysis has been removed. (Reproduced with permission from Buncke HJ[27])

fascia extends to the filtral ridge on the paralyzed side. Passage is facilitated by using a long K wire with a hole in the end to bridge from the nasolabial incision to the base of the columella and the junction of the filtrum and lip mucosa. The upper half of the fascial slip is then pulled through the tunnel with these sutures, which are tied over xeroform boluses. The lower half of the fascial sheet is sutured to the outer third of the lip and the angle of the mouth. The upper end of the fascial slip is secured under tension to the fascia over the zygomatic arch.

17. The head is then placed in the midline and all facial wounds on both sides closed. A 0.25 Penrose drain is brought out of the preauricular region bilaterally, and a large bulky dressing similar to a facelift dressing is applied and held in place with mesh gauze. In older patients, where redundancy of the cheek and prolapse of the mouth are much more severe, a McLaughlin procedure is done to stabilize the corner of the mouth and the upper lip, rather than the fascial slip. Occasionally, older patients are happy with the improvement at rest and with the activity produced by the 5th nerve contraction created by the McLaughlin procedure, and choose not to go on to the second-stage functional muscle transplant.

SECOND-STAGE OPERATION

Again a two-team approach is used, a surgeon and assistant working on the face and a surgeon and assistant working in the donor muscle area. The patient is placed in a one-half-lateral position with the paralyzed side up if the serratus muscle is to be used, or in the supine position if the gracilis muscle is to be used.

1. The facial team opens the paralyzed side of the face through the previous incisions carrying them up into the temporal area, out to the level of the outer canthus and down under the chin to the previous submandibular incision. The ends of the cross-facial nerve grafts marked with the hemoclips in the preauricular and submental areas are identified, as are the anterior facial artery and vein. The nerve grafts are mobilized for about 2 cm and a biopsy is taken of the distal end of the nerve with the hemoclip and submitted for frozen section evaluation of the fascicular bundle density. One can obtain an impression of the quality of nerve regeneration by the appearance of the nerve graft, which will have a firm body and axial vessels on its surface. On transection of the graft with a razor blade flake, the pouting fascicular bundles can be readily identified under the microscope. This pattern was described many years ago by Raymond Villan of Paris (personal communication 1975) as 'les yeux d'escargot.'

2. The nasolabial incision is reopened, this time creating a narrow dermal flange based medially. Tunnels to the philtral ridge and the entire side of the cheek to the corner of the mouth and upper lip are carefully developed superficial to the previously placed fascial strip, or McLaughlin transfer. A wide tunnel is also created across the cheek and lower eyelid to the medial canthal area.

3. The muscle harvesting team, working simultaneously, harvests the serratus muscle through an incision paralleling the anterior axillary fold down to the seventh rib, where it is curved anteriorly, paralleling the submammary fold. The anterior edge of the latissimus is elevated and the underlying oblique fibers of the lower three slips of the serratus identified. The ninth, eighth and seventh slips are elevated anteriorly, where they insert into the lateral rib cage, and posteriorly to the angle of the scapula. The thoracodorsal vessels are identified and the branch to the serratus carefully dissected off the upper slips of the serratus down to the upper border of the seventh slip. This is a tedious dissection and there are many branches going from the vascular bundle to the underlying proximal slips. The lateral thoracic nerve of Bell lies deep to the vessels on the fascia of the sixth, fifth and fourth slips, anterior to the artery and vein. Occasionally there is an abnormal blood supply to the serratus coming directly from the axillary vessels paralleling the anterior thoracic vessels.[36] Wherever their source, these vessels enter the lower slips of the serratus at the junction of the middle and posterior third. The lower border of the ninth slip is cleared and the deeper surface of the ninth, eighth and seventh slips easily developed. The seventh slip is separated from the sixth slip, carefully protecting the neurovascular pedicle as it enters and spreads out over the lower slips. The lateral thoracic nerve has a separate fascicular bundle going to these three slips, which can be split off from the fibers going to the more proximal slips. In this fashion a nerve pedicle of 2–3 cm can be developed which will facilitate the microneural repair to the cross-facial nerve graft. However, the closer the nerve repair is made to the muscle, the sooner the muscle will be reinnervated. In a similar fashion, the vascular pedicle can be extended proximally by tying off the branch to the latissimus and developing the thoracodorsal artery and vein proximally. However, a long pedicle is seldom necessary, as the anterior facial vessels will be found just as they cross the lower border of the mandible. If the gracilis muscle is to be used as a functional muscle transplant the dissection

is simpler, as it is performed at a distance from the facial team.

4. The facial team continues repairing the bed for the microvascular transplant. A submandibular incision is carried medially almost to the midline, so that the anterior belly of the digastric muscle can be exposed from its mandibular insertion to the pulley at the hyoid bone. The muscle belly is shaved off the undersurface of the mandible and the tendon cut proximal to the pulley, thus mobilizing the muscle and its tendon on its neurovascular pedicle, which enters the deep side of the muscle from lateral to medial. The vessels pass laterally deep to the submandibular gland and can be mobilized for a centimeter or two. The nerve that joins the mylohyoid nerve back to the inferior alveolar nerve can be separated under the chin to provide a longer nerve pedicle. A short incision is then made at the mucosal–cutaneous junction of the lower lip, about a centimeter medial to the angle of the mouth. A subcutaneous tunnel is then created from the submandibular wound in a superficial plane so that the cross-facial nerve graft running under the lower lip lies deep to this tunnel. The tendon of the digastric muscle is then rotated so that the muscle belly will now lie laterally and the tendon can be passed through the tunnel to the lower lip, adjusting the muscle so that it parallels the oblique inferior direction of the depressor triangularis. The short nerve pedicle can now be brought below the muscle and anastomosed to the cross-facial nerve graft in the submandibular area. This very small nerve is usually half the size of the cross-facial nerve graft. Under the microscope, a fascicle the same size as the small nerve can be dissected out of the cross-facial nerve graft and an end-to-end repair performed with 10/0 or 11/0 sutures. The extra fascicles can be split off and used to directly neurotize the muscle.

5. The muscle transplant is then handed to the facial team and the inset commenced. The anterior slips of the muscle should be inserted and stabilized first, so that the muscle can be folded forward, and then the microneural repairs performed on the deep surface. The ninth slip is passed across the lower lid to the medial canthal area and secured here with tie-over sutures and xeroform gauze boluses. The eighth slip is split so that half of it goes across the upper lip to the columella above the fascia, again passing it with long needles. The other half of the eight is secured to the outer third of the upper lip. The seventh slip is secured to the angle of the mouth into the previous fascial slip. The muscle is then folded medially and the neurovascular bundle brought down, anastomosing the artery and vein of the serratus or thoracodorsal system to the anterior facial vessels and the cross-facial nerve to the nerve to the serratus. The nerve from the serratus may be half the size of the fascicular bundles in the cross-facial nerve graft, and again these extra fascicles are directly neurotized to the serratus slips. A 1 mm venous Doppler is placed around the anterior facial vein on the cardiac side of the anastomosis, held in place with a small cuff of Vicryl mesh. The lead is carefully sutured along its course to the postauricular region, where it is sutured and stapled to the skin to prevent traction or withdrawal with movement of the head and dressing changes. The venous Doppler thus provides a continuous monitor of circulation. A small drain is brought out through the preauricular incision just below the lobe and a bulky dressing applied, held in place with elastic mesh.

Patients are followed in the ICU ward for 1–2 days and are immediately returned to surgery for re-exploration if the Doppler signal is lost. Most patients leave hospital in 6–8 days.

SUMMARY

Congenital facial paralysis may be idiopathic or associated with a wide variety of syndromes. Early diagnosis is important, to rule out birth trauma from forceps or other mechanisms which require early surgical decompression of the nerve. Elective reconstruction can be considered at $3\frac{1}{2}$ years of age or earlier, depending upon the size of the child. A step-by-step outline of the two-stage cross-facial functional muscle transplant is presented.

REFERENCES

1. May M 1990 Facial paralysis in children. In: Bluestone CD, Stool SE (eds) Pediatric otolaryngology, 2nd edn. W.B. Saunders, Philadelphia, pp 401–419
2. Sudarshan A, Goldie WD 1985 The spectrum of congenital facial diplegia (Moebius syndrome). Pediatric Neurology 1:180–184
3. Ysunza A, Inigo F, Ortiz-Monasterio F, Drucker-Colin R 1996 Recovery of congenital facial palsy in patients with hemifacial microsomia subjected to sural to facial nerve grafts is enhanced by electric field stimulation. Archives of Medical Research 27:7–13
4. Holmich LR, Medgyesi S 1994 Congenital hereditary paresis of ramus marginalis nervus facialis in five generations. Annals of Plastic Surgery 33:96–99
5. Nicolai JP, Bos MY, ter Haar BG 1986 Hereditary congenital facial paralysis. Scandinavian Journal of Plastic and Reconstructive Surgery 20:37–39
6. Hennekam RC, Holtus FJ 1993 Johnson–McMillin syndrome: report of another family (Review). American Journal of Medical Genetics 47:714–716
7. Spranger JW 1973 Craniodiaphyseal dysplasia. In: Bergsma D (ed) Birth defects: atlas and compendium. Williams and Wilkins, Baltimore, p. 309

8. Rimoin DL, Hollister DW 1973 Dominant osteopetrosis. In: Bergsma D (ed) Birth defects: atlas and compendium. Williams and Wilkins, Baltimore, p. 348

9. Spranger JW. 1973 Hyperostosis corticalis generalisata. In: Bergsma D (ed) Birth defects: atlas and compendium. Williams and Wilkins, Baltimore, p 502

10. Sailez HF, Gratz KW, Locher MC 1994 Mandibular dysostosis. In: Cohen M (ed) Mastery of plastic and reconstructive surgery. Little Brown, Boston, pp 527–535

11. Kaplan LC 1989 The CHARGE association: choanal atresia and multiple congenital anomalies (Review). Otolaryngology Clinics of North America 22:661–672

12. Van Meter TD, Weaver DD 1996 Oculo-auriculo-vertebral spectrum and the CHARGE association: clinical evidence for a common pathogenetic mechanism. Clinical Dysmorphology 5:187–196

13. Meyerson MD, Lewis E, Ill K 1984 Facioscapulohumeral muscular dystrophy and accompanying hearing loss. Archives of Otolaryngology 110:261–266

14. Kuzniecky R, Andermann F, Guerrini R 1993 Congenital bilateral perisylvian syndrome: study of 31 patients. The CBPS Multicenter Collaborative Study. Lancet 341:608–612

15. Bergstrom L 1973 Microtia–atresia. In: Bergsma D (ed) Birth defects: atlas and compendium. Williams and Wilkins, Baltimore, pp. 619–620

16. Inigo F, Ysunza A, Rojo P, Trigos I 1994 Recovery of facial palsy after crossed facial nerve grafts. British Journal of Plastic Surgery 47:312–317

17. Haslam RHA 1973 Congenital facial diplegia. In: Bergsma D (ed) Birth defects: atlas and compendium. Williams and Wilkins, Baltimore, pp 287–288

18. Belal A 1985 Myobiopsy in facial palsy. In: Portmann M (ed) Facial nerve. Proceedings of the Fifth International Symposium on the Facial Nerve, Bordeaux, France, 3–6 September 1984. Masson New York, pp. 194–197

19. May M, Hardin WB, Sullivan J, Wette R 1976 Natural history of Bell's palsy: the salivary flow test and other prognostic indicators. Laryngoscope 86:704–712

20. May M, Hardin WB 1978 Facial palsy: interpretation of neurologic findings. Laryngoscope 88:1352–1362

21. Lu Z, Tang X 1996 Blink reflex: normal values and its findings on peripheral facial paralysis. Chinese Medical Journal 109:308–312

22. Terrell GS, Terzis JK 1994 An experimental model to study the blink reflex. Journal of Reconstructive Microsurgery 10:175–183

23. Devars F 1990 Facial paralysis in children. In: Castro D (ed) Facial nerve. Proceedings of the Sixth International Symposium on the Facial Nerve, Rio de Janeiro, Brazil, 2–5 October 1988. Kugler, Amsterdam, pp. 159–163

24. Harii K, Ohmori K, Torii S 1976 Free gracilis transplantation, with microneurovascular anastomosis for the treatment of facial paralysis. A preliminary report. Plastic and Reconstructive Surgery 57:133–143

25. Edgerton MT 1965 Digastric muscle transfer to correct deformity of the lower lip resulting from paralysis of the facial nerve. Presented at the Annual Meeting of the American Society for Plastic and Reconstructive Surgery, Philadelphia, October 1965

26. Conley J, Baker DC, Selfe RW 1982 Paralysis of the mandibular branch of the facial nerve. Plastic and Reconstructive Surgery 70:569–577

27. Buncke HJ, Whitney TM, Milliken RG 1991 Facial paralysis. In: Buncke HJ (ed) Microsurgery: transplantation–replantation. An atlas text. Lea and Febiger, Philadelphia, pp 487–506

28. Meuli-Simmen C, Yingling CD, Adzick NS, Buncke HJ 1995 Selective neural control of individual serratus muscle slips for facial palsy reconstruction. In: Frey M, Giovanoli P (eds) Proceedings of the Fourth International Muscle Symposium. Universitätsspital Zürich, Zurich, pp 198–201

29. Mackinnon SE, Dellon LA 1988 Surgery of the peripheral nerve. Thieme, New York, pp 113–115

30. Manktelow RT, McKee NH, Vettese T 1980 Anatomical study of pectoralis major muscle as related to functioning free muscle transplantation. Plastic and Reconstructive Surgery 65:610–615

31. Terzis JK, Manktelow RT 1982 Pectoralis minor: a new concept in facial reanimation. Plastic Surgery Forum. American Society of Plastic and Reconstructive Surgeons, Chicago

32. Swartz WM, Jones NJ, Cherup L, Klein A 1988 Direct monitoring of microvascular anastomoses with the 20-mHZ ultrasonic Doppler probe: an experimental and clinical study. Plastic and Reconstructive Surgery 81:149–161

33. Kind GM, Buncke GM, Newlin L, Siko PP, Buntic RF, Buncke HJ 1996 Implantable, adsorbable Doppler probe monitoring of microvascular tissue transplants. Plastic Surgery Forum. 65th Annual Scientific Meeting of the American Society of Plastic and Reconstructive Surgeons, Plastic Surgery Educational Foundation and American Society of Maxillofacial Surgeons, Chicago, pp 179–181

34. Quam DA 1995 Recognizing a case of Reye's syndrome. Review. American Family Physician 50:1491–1496

35. Nemoto K, Williams HB 1988 The effects of electrical stimulation on denervated muscle using implantable electrodes. Journal of Reconstructive Microsurgery 4:251–255, 257

36. Goldberg JA, Lineaweaver WC, Buncke HJ 1990 An aberrant independent origin of the serratus anterior pedicle. Annals of Plastic Surgery 25:487–490

Etiology, prevalence, growth and trends in cleft lip, alveolus and palate

62

KARSTEN K. H. GUNDLACH

EMBRYOGENESIS

The embryogenesis of the face is well known and clear cut. Most textbooks on embryology state that in humans the neural tube closes at its cranial end during the 4th week of gestation. At the same time placodes are formed by thickened ectoderm (olfactory placode, optic lens placode, otic placode, etc.), and the neural crest cells become identifiable and start to migrate to the front. By these developments the frontonasal prominence (forming the medial and the lateral nasal prominences), the nasal pits, the so-called branchial or visceral arches (forming among others the maxillary and the mandibular prominences) and the stomodeum are outlined with the buccopharyngeal membrane closing the foregut, i.e. the anterior end of the gut, the pharynx. The stomodeum, the primitive oral cavity, is thus encircled by both the mandibular prominences below, both the maxillary ones in the upper lateral and both the medial nasal ones in the upper central area.

Development of the face is controlled by two organizing centers. The prosencephalic organizer is located at the rostral end of the chorda dorsalis and induces formation of the upper third of the face. The rhombencephalic organizer is located caudally to the former and induces formation of the middle and the caudal third of the face.[1] The border between these two territories was named the diacephalic border.[2] Various growth factors are then produced that induce formation of 'growth centers'. A defect in one of these organizers or poor cooperation among two organizers or growth centers will result in typical facial malformations, like frontonasal dysplasia or Berry–Treacher Collins–Franceschetti mandibulofacial dysostosis. (Some authors consider these to be defined as clefts. However, the terms used here are still used internationally by syndromologists.)

The next step is merging of the two mandibular prominences in the midline. The indentation between these prominences is leveled out due to the influx of neural crest cells. The angle between mandibular and maxillary prominences later transforms into the angle of the mouth. The maxillary prominence merges with the medial nasal prominence. Here two epithelial linings touch each other, with Hochstetter's epithelial membrane resulting. This situation does not last for very long, and is resolved by programmed death of the ectodermal cells (Fig. 62.1). The neural crest cells from both sides of this epithelial wall are intermingled with each other and thus the upper lip is formed. The area of this line of fusion is located at the site of the philtral columns that border the premaxillary lip portion on either side. A deficit in neural crest cells, or a failure of these to reach their destination, will result in typical facial malformations, such as hemifacial microsomia* or the various forms of median pseudocleft of the upper lip. Delayed apoptosis of the epithelial cells results in the classical lateral clefts of lip with/without cleft palate.

Particular genes express proteins at particular regions, which in turn leads to various 'gene expression patterns'. Mutation of a specific gene may thus interfere with a specific step in the formation of the face and result in a typical type of malformation. An example of this is the well-known Demarquay–van der Woude syndrome (see Fig. 62.5) in which the relevant gene is located on the long arm of chromosome 1. This gene was thought to have some relation to the transforming growth factor alpha (TGFA), which is expressed in the palatal shelves at the time of palatal fusion and is found significantly often in patients with clefts. How-

---

*According to Poswillo, hemifacial microsomia in laboratory animals can be explained by maldevelopment of the primitive stapedial artery leading to a hematoma, which in turn results in a tissue deficit.[5] The small amount of neural crest cells surviving are unable to sculpt perfect auricle, tympanon, mandible, parotid gland and masticatory muscles.

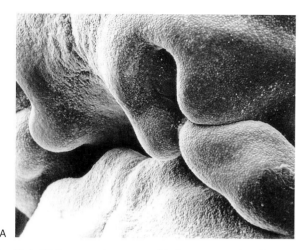
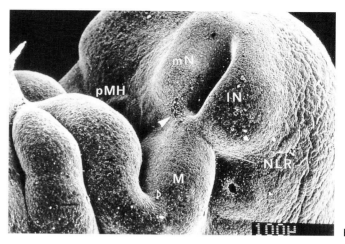

Fig. 62.1 **(A)** Human embryo, stage 17: Crown–Trump length = 11. 7 mm. (Reproduced from Hinrichsen 1991[3] with permission.) **(B)** Rat embryo. pMH, stomodeum; mN, medial nasal; lN, lateral nasal swelling; M, maxillary swelling; NLR, nasolacrimal fold. (Reproduced from Mangold 1982[4] with permission.)

ever, there is still no evidence for any kind of linkage among the two.[6] Transforming growth factor beta 3 is now focused on as a candidate for explaining human cleft palate.[7] Lidral et al[7a] have just published data indicating that TGF beta 3 is not a common cause of cleft palate only. They suggest that there may also be links to cleft lip.

The stomodeum is formed on the 28th day when the buccopharyngeal membrane perforates. The medial nasal 'processus' and the maxillary 'processus' unite around day 32, and by merging of these bipartition of the nasal and oral cavities commences. In the 7th week the perpendicular palatal shelves change their orientation and become horizontal. In the 8th week (around the 52nd day) the palatal shelves fuse like a zipper, starting in the region of the naso-palatine nerve and ending in merging of both soft palate swellings with formation of the uvula (Fig. 62.2).[8] Various

mechanisms are involved in these fusion processes, apoptotic cell death is only one of them. In cases of defective fusion of the two facial swellings, namely the maxillary and the medial nasal swelling, a cleft of the lip (alveolus and palate) will result. In cases of non-fusion of the palatal shelves, an isolated cleft palate will result. Non-merging of the posterior parts of the palate will result in a cleft velum.

CLASSIFICATION, MORPHOLOGY AND ETIOLOGY

Facial clefting is one of the most common malformations in man. There are many attempts to *classify* clefts of the face. Three will be mentioned here in detail.

I.   G. Sanvenero-Rosselli published the Report of the Subcommittee on Nomenclature and Classification of the Lateral Clefts of Lip, Alveolus and Palate as proposed in 1967.[10] This classification was then approved by the delegates at the Fourth Congress of the International Confederation for Plastic Surgery in Rome, 1967.

1. Clefts of anterior (primary) palate:
   a. Lip: right and/or left.
   b. Alveolus : right and/or left.
2. Clefts of anterior and posterior (primary and secondary) palate:
   a. Lip: right and/or left.
   b. Alveolus: right and/or left.
   c. Hard palate: right and/or left.
   d. Soft palate: medial*.

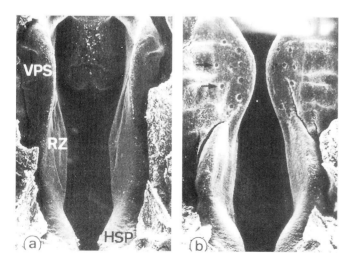

Fig. 62.2 Rat fetus: **(A)** day 15; **(B)** day 16. VPS, vertical palatal shelves; RZ, remodeling zone; HSP, horizontal soft palatal shelves. (Reproduced from Schüpbach 1983[9] with permission.)

---

*Should be 'median'.

3. Clefts of posterior (secondary) palate:
   a. Hard palate: right and/or left.
   b. Soft palate: median*.

Finally there was a fourth group, named 'rare clefts'.

II. In 1968 Gerhard Pfeifer described three areas of the head into which he divided the human face and in which malformations may be found.[11] These areas are identical with the spheres of influence of both the major organizing centers and the border zone between them. He used the terms posterolateral area (rhombencephalic organizer), diacephalic border and frontonasal area (prosencephalic organizer). He located the clefts of lip (alveolus) and/or palate in the diacephalic region (Fig. 62.3).

III. In 1976 Paul Tessier published his anatomic classification of facial clefts.[12] He described 14 different types of clefting which he defined according to their location in relation to eye and orbit. Clefts of lip (alveolus) and/or palate were numbered 1, 2 or 3 (Fig. 62.4).

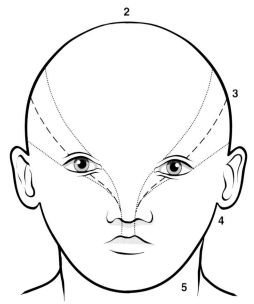

Fig. 62.3 Pfeifer's morphogenetic classification of craniofacial anomalies:[2] 1, generalized malformations; 2, malformations in the frontonasal region; 3, malformations in the diacephalic border; 4, malformations in the posterolateral region; 5, malformations in the neck. (Reproduced from Pfeifer[2] with permission.)

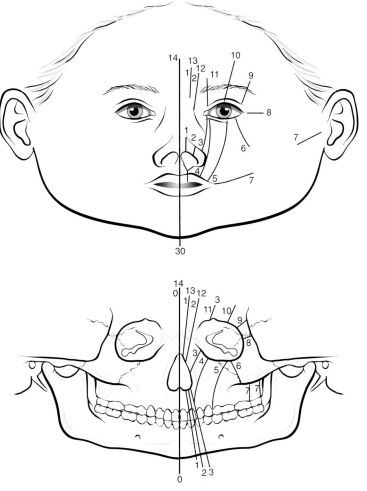

Fig. 62.4 Tessier's classification of facial, craniofacial and laterofacial clefts. (Reproduced from Tessier[12] with permission.)

Apart from classifying malformations according to embryology and etiology (chromosomal, monogenic (enzymatic or structural), environmental, unknown yet), there is also a pathogenetic method of classification. Here the following terms are used:

- Deformation: abnormal shape due to mechanical forces (e.g. due to oligohydramnion).
- Disruption: abnormal shape due to extrinsic breakdown (e.g. due to amniotic bands).
- Dysplasia: abnormal shape due to abnormal tissue (e.g. due to collagen abnormalities).
- Malformation: abnormal shape due to poor morphogenesis (e.g. clefts of lip and/or palate).

This pathogenetic classification, however, is not used widely in surgical departments.

It is important to note that there is a wide variety of facial clefts. The most common forms of these are so-called lateral cleft lip (alveolus and palate) on the one hand and isolated palatal cleft on the other. According to Pfeifer, they are both located in the border zone between the frontonasal and the posterolateral areas.[11] However, they are different malformations because they develop:

- in different embryological units (primary and secondary palate);
- at different times in embryonic life (lip approximately 6th to 7th week, palate approximately 9th to 10th week);
- by disturbance of different mechanisms (perforation and dissolution of Hochstetter's epithelial wall versus zipper-like fusion of the palatal shelves); and are
- inherited as different traits.[13]

It should be noted, however, that clefts of lip *and* palate are both a part of the cleft lip problem. It is understood that clefting of the (secondary) palate in these cases is just a consequence of non-fusion of the primary palate: the latter results in a wide distance between the elevated palatal shelves, which in turn inhibits fusion as they just do not contact each other.

There is a wide variety of cleft forms among the two types just mentioned. Without trying to offer a complete list, a spectrum is given to demonstrate the range of various kinds of clefts, stretching from the almost invisible to the most impressive forms. There are three so-called morphologic orders:

1. a. Unilateral subcutaneous clefting of the orbicularis oris muscle with lowered nasal sill and floor.
   b. Notching of the vermilion.
   c. Partial clefting of lip, two lateral deciduous incisors.

   d. Complete cleft of lip with nasal floor and alveolus still intact.
   e. Complete cleft of lip plus notching of alveolus.
   f. Complete cleft of lip and alveolus, one lateral incisor – palate fused.
   g. Complete cleft of lip and alveolus plus partial cleft of soft palate.
   h. Complete cleft of lip, alveolus and soft palate.
   i. Complete cleft of lip, alveolus and soft palate, partial cleft of hard palate.
   j. Unilateral complete cleft of lip, alveolus and palate, no lateral incisor.
2. As bilateral clefts may be symmetric or asymmetric, there are again a huge number of combinations to be seen.
3. a. Bifid uvula, no speech problems.
   b. Submucous cleft of soft palate with bifid uvula and bifid posterior nasal spine.
   c. Partially cleft soft palate.
   d. Completely cleft soft palate.
   e. Cleft soft palate with partially cleft hard palate.
   f. Complete cleft of palate with V-shaped commissure in the area of the incisive foramen.
   g. Complete cleft of palate with U-shaped commissure.

The existence of such a variety, namely of these quasi-continuous morphologic orders, is one argument for today's theory of the multifactorial *etiology* of clefting.

Genetic factors and exogenous factors are known to be of relevance. For the genetic factors there is a multitude of monogenic cleft syndromes that are either sex-chromosomal or autosomal, dominantly or recessively inherited.[14] Among the dominant syndromes are:

- Demarquay–van der Woude's syndrome (clefts of lip and/or palate and lip pits; Fig. 62.5).

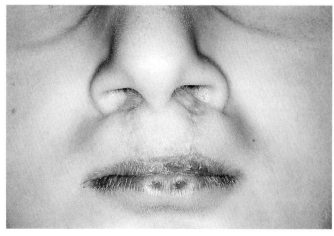

Fig. 62.5 16-year-old girl with (operated) bilateral cleft lip, alveolus and palate and symmetrical pits in the lower lip.

- Popliteal pterygium syndrome (clefts of lip (and palate), popliteal pterygia and other abnormalities).
- EEC syndrome (Ectrodactyly of hands and/or feet, Ectodermal dysplasia with sparse blond hair, oligodontia, etc. and Cleft lip (and palate)); however, heterogeneity for this syndrome may exist.
- Clefting of lip (and palate) with ankyloblepharon filiforme ad natum.
- Oral-facial-digital syndrome I (dominant X-linked inheritance, dystopia canthorum, hypoplastic alar cartilages, median (!) cleft lip and cleft palate, multiple intraoral frenula, lobed tongue, digital abnormalities).
- Velocardiofacial syndrome (typical facies with prominent nose, cleft palate and cardiovascular anomalies like ventriculo-septal defect, and medial displacement of the internal carotid artery).

In addition, there is an interesting article on cleft palate with autosomal recessive transmission in dogs (Brittany Spaniels) that appeared in the *Cleft Palate Journal* in 1994.[15]

Although various authors still believe in the multifactorial theory of etiology (see below), some now favor some kind of mendelian pattern of inheritance (single gene, reduced penetrance). Therefore scientists are working hard on finding specific genes, and a number of these have been suggested in the relevant scientific literature up to now. One of those in non-syndromic cases is located on the long arm of chromosome 17 (17q21–24) and is important for clefting.[7] In syndromic cases, however, as in the Demarquay–van der Woude syndrome, the relevant gene appears to be located on the long arm of chromosome 1.[6] One of the genes relevant for the velocardiofacial cleft syndrome (as well as for Di George's syndrome!) is located on the long arm of chromosome 22.[16] A group in Iceland was able to locate the gene for cleft palate in combination with ankyloglosson on the X chromosome.[17]

It has already been mentioned that cleft lip (alveolus and palate) is a different trait than isolated cleft palate.[13] It is also known from genetic studies that the risk of recurrence of the cleft in a subsequent child increases with each additional affected relative in the family history.[18] This proves the importance of genetic factors in the etiology of cleft lip and/or palate.

Apart from genetically induced clefts, there are also malformation syndromes that are known to be caused by drugs, i.e. environmental factors. Some of these syndromes may include clefting,[14,18] for example:

- Isotretinoin (etretinate or retinol (vitamin A)) embryopathy (among others: cleft palate and possibly cleft lip as well).
- Aminopterin (folic acid deficiency) – induced embryopathy (some times with cleft palate associated with a striking micrognathia).
- Fetal alcohol syndrome (among others: cleft palate).
- Fetal trimethadione syndrome (among others: cleft lip and palate).

It is also known from animal experiments that clefts can be produced by many different teratogens. These animals most often have a multitude of additional malformations. One of those teratogens is cyclophosphamide,[19] a cytostatic drug that is derived from mustard gas. This poison gas was found by Taher to have raised the rate of incidence of clefts in the Iranian population following the war between Iran and Iraq.[20] Finally, it is known that cleft patients most often exhibit many more anomalies than just clefts.[21] All these facts are strong indicators for exogenous agents as important (co)factors for cleft formation.

It is now believed that in the average cleft patient several factors – both genetic and environmental – have come together and acted in concert to produce this malformation. In other words clefting is most likely to be of multifactorial etiology,[8] it is not a single-gene disease!

INCIDENCE AND RECURRENCE RATES

In *genetic counseling* parents afraid of having a (another) child with a cleft ask for figures on the risk of such an event. However, the risk of having a child with a cleft lip and/or palate varies from family to family, from region to region, and from continent to continent.

Differentiation has to be made between:

1. Recurrence rate, i.e. the chance of a relapse or recurrence of a specific disorder in a person or – in the case of malformation – in a family.
2. Incidence, i.e. the number of new cases with a specific disorder at a given time in a certain population.
3. Incidence rate, i.e. the number of persons having a specific disorder per time unit in relation to the number of persons exposed to the risk of getting this disorder.
4. Prevalence, i.e. the number of all cases with a disorder at a given time in a certain population.

Interestingly, prevalence and incidence vary among races. Clefting occurs much more often in Orientals than in whites and in whites more often than in blacks. Apparently prevalence is lowest in Africa and highest among Amerindians. When looking at all the data available, the development of clefting can be compared with the history of man.

Approximately 6 million years ago the first ancestor of man started to walk on two feet instead of four. Australopithecus was living in East Africa 4 million years ago.[22] Hominids must have then left this place[23] and emigrated into Europe and Asia 2 million years ago,[24] as the oldest mandible of *Homo erectus* found in Dmanisi, Georgia, Europe was dated back to 1.8 million years. The oldest human fossil found in China dates back approximately 800 000 years. However, this is only today's theory and has nothing to do with human racial differences as we see them today. Fifty and more years ago scientists thought the cradle of man was located in Indonesia (Java) and in 50 years from now we will certainly know more.

From the scientific medical literature we can learn about incidence rates of clefts in various countries (Table 62.1).

The data in Table 62.1 were calculated for all clefts taken together. This overall tendency is similar in some subgroups: for example, the prevalence of bifid uvula is low in blacks (1 : 300),[33] intermediate in Danish Caucasians (1 : 90)[37] and high in Amerindians (1 : 10).[33] However, all these figures on prevalence and incidence should be interpreted with reservations. In some studies all live births have been taken into consideration, in others stillbirths might have been included. We also know that genes can be pooled in small populations, in so-called isolates like the Barí Indians of Western Venezuela.[38] This may be an important reason for the high incidence rates in American Indians. It is also known that in prehistoric times – and in some countries even in the twentieth century – children with overt malformations were not allowed to live (infanticide) or to have children themselves. This is another reason why the figures cited have to be looked at with the utmost caution.[39] The interpretation offered here is just one way of looking at the data

that have been published by many authorities over past decades. It may be possible that scientists using current methods for investigating genetic markers in genes thought to be important for clefting and for linkage analyses will help to shed light on this problem.[7,7a,8]

If a major group of genes is found, then the multifactorial inheritance model may have to be rejected. However, the model is to be favored. This goes along with the so-called threshold theory according to Falconer & Carter, as illustrated in my paper published in 1986,[40] which has been elaborated even more by Tolarova:[32] In a given population only a small portion of individuals is affected with a cleft. In a subpopulation with a genetic background for clefting this proportion of affected persons is greater, they have been 'pushed across the threshold'. The same holds true for a subpopulation that has been exposed to an environmental factor leading to cleft formation (Fig. 62.6).

This, on the other hand, is the theoretical background for the many attempts to *prevent clefting*. Many groups of scientists have developed drug regimens – mostly based on high doses of water-soluble vitamins and folic acid – that are prescribed to women in early pregnancy. It is felt by many that these regimens are successful in an interesting percentage of cases treated.[32,40]

All these ideas come to mind when genetic counseling is asked for. But there is another important fact: the rates of incidence have been rising gradually over the past decades as doctors have become more and more aware of microforms and surgeons have taken more and more care of minor manifestations as well. It has taken a diligent researcher, Poul Fogh-Andersen, who was chairman of the single cleft center in Copenhagen, Denmark to consider this further. In his years in office he looked at the numbers of cases he had treated. He noted that apparently the incidence of all patients with a cleft born in that country has risen from

Table 62.1 Rates of incidence of clefts of lip and/or palate in various regions of the world

Race and region	Approximate incidence
Blacks in	
South Africa	1 : 3000[25]
Nigeria	1 : 2700[26]
Blacks in	
New York City, USA	1 : 1700[27]
New Orleans, USA	1 : 1550[28]
Caucasians in	
Latvia	1 : 740[29]
France	1 : 680[30]
Rostock, Germany	1 : 640[31]
Bohemia	1 : 550[32]
Orientals in Japan	1 : 425[33]
American Indians in	
British Columbia	1 : 340[34]
Montana	1 : 280[35,36]

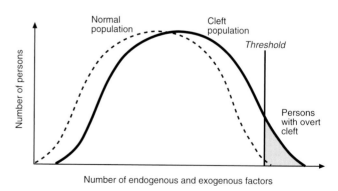

Falconer's Model

Fig. 62.6 Falconer's threshold model. (Reproduced from Gundlach et al[40] with permission.)

1.31 out of 1000 live births in the period 1938–42 up to 1.78 in the years 1968–72. Later on, this figure rose to over 2.0, not only in Denmark but also in other European countries.[13] Today one out of 500 live births in Central Europe produces a baby with a cleft. This figure will rise even more, because better surgery will help more people to look better. This will increase their chances to mate and have children with a cleft. In addition, cleft prevention will mask gene carriers: persons without a cleft who would have had one if their parents had not had such preventive treatment will not be aware of the risk of having a child of their own with a cleft. These persons may 'suddenly' have a baby with a cleft themselves.

In calculating the *recurrence rates*, one first has to rule out all (known) syndromes with genetic inheritance.[41] After ruling out all (known) exogenous teratogens, tables may be used that come out of pooled data. This will be adequate in the vast majority of families, as only in a small fraction of cases a known syndrome will be recognizable. Variations of these tables have been published[8,33,42] and are used by geneticists for this purpose. For information and demonstration a small one taken from Tolarova's data on the Bohemian population[42] is presented here. In this table ranges are listed rather than exact figures, as various factors have to be taken into consideration such as sex and subtype of clefting. In Caucasians cleft palate is more often found in females (with the exception that bifid uvula is found more frequently in males). Boys have a higher risk of being afflicted with a cleft lip (alveolus and/or palate), with the exception that a partially cleft lip is encountered more often in females. The risk of recurrence is higher in the case of a bilateral cleft rather than a unilateral cleft in the family (Table 62.2). In contrast, palatal extension of a cleft lip seems to be of no statistical significance with regard to the recurrence rate.

GROWTH AND DEVELOPMENT

All members of a cleft team aim at the best outcome for every patient they are taking care of. Therefore they have to find answers to the following questions:

- What is 'the best' outcome?
- When and where should therapy be started?
- How should therapy be carried out?

The answer to the first question was given by Gerhard Pfeifer. The best outcome for an individual probably is to have no visible stigma of facial clefting any more and, at the same time, to still carry typical markers that are found in his or her family. However, outcome studies are initiated throughout the world now, and these will give us important clues to help to tackle the other two problems. To this end it has to be taken into consideration:

- What are the conditions to start with.
- What are the forces to work with.

Once we know these we may start to influence the growth and development of soft and hard tissues of the oral and maxillofacial region ourselves.

When deciding on the conditions to start with, it has been mentioned before that the primary palate develops in early embryonal life by obliteration ('merging') of the facial ectodermal grooves that are found between the so-called first branchial arch with its maxillary process and the central globular mass with its nasal processus. The epithelial wall of Hochstetter is deteriorating, breaks down and the primary palate is formed. If these mechanisms are disturbed, a so-called primary cleft of lip (and alveolus) will result. If, however, formation of the primary palate starts correctly but then is held up and a tearing of tissue occurs, a so-called secondary cleft of lip (and alveolus) will result. The secondary palate develops in a different manner a little time later. The palatine processes of the maxillary processes form the palatal shelves, assume a horizontal orientation, and come in contact with each other and the nasal septum. Both these shelves, and the septum fuse, starting in the area of the nasopalatine foramen. Failure of contact or of programmed epithelial cell death will result in a so-called primary cleft palate, while tearing of tissue that had already fused will result in a so-called secondary cleft.

The further development of these structures depends on *the amount of tissue* available. This will have to be taken into consideration when making treatment plans; for example

Table 62.2 Risk of recurrence of a cleft (in the case of one cleft in the family already)

Cleft type	Risk for a subsequent sibling (%)	Risk for a subsequent child (%)	Risk for another relative (%)
Cleft lip (with or without cleft alveolus and/or cleft palate)*	1–8	2–17	0.4–1.2
Isolated cleft palate†	1.7–2.7	0.8–8.6	0.3–1.0

According to Tolarova:[42]
*There is a higher risk for male offspring;
  there is a higher risk for bilateral cases;
  palatal extension of cleft lip is *not* indicating a higher risk.
–There is a higher risk for female offspring.

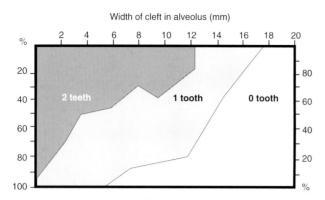

Fig. 62.7 Absolute and relative frequency of double, single and missing anlagen of teeth in relation to the width of the cleft alveolus. (Reproduced from Ehmann et al[43] with permission.)

in the area of the *alveolar cleft* there may be no lateral incisor (especially wide clefts), just one lateral incisor (medium-sized clefting of the alveolus) or even two lateral incisors (in narrow clefts of the alveolus – most often in combination with an only partially cleft lip; Fig. 62.7).[43] Where there is no mesectoderm, no anlage of a tooth will develop out of the labio-dento-gingival lamina; and where there is no tooth bud alveolar bone will not develop. These findings are important at the time of planning orthodontic alignment, when bone is to be transplanted and/or when dental implants are considered.

Otto Kriens has noted that the *bony palate* is shorter in complete palatal clefts than in partially cleft palates pre-operatively, and is wider in complete clefts of the palate than in clefts of the soft palate only.[44] These facts have to be taken into consideration in designing palatoplasty.

Facial development and growth then takes place after primary and secondary palates have fused and is influenced by all those factors that have been called 'functional matrix' by Moss some time ago.[45] Here eruption of teeth, the forces of the tongue and of the muscles of mastication, patency of the nasal airways, function (and scarring after an operation!) of the cheeks and lips when speaking, eating and swallowing as well as at rest, and in addition the forces of the velopharyngeal muscles when breathing, speaking and swallowing, seem to exert an influence. After all cranio-facial bones are of intramembranous and not cartilagenous origin, they are more dependent on external influences than the long bones. The fact that all functions mentioned before are able to control the growth of the maxillofacial skeleton probably is the reason why orthodontists can work so efficiently in the way they do! Important examples of this are the Hotz plate and the so-called 'Funktions-Kieferorthopädie' (functional orthodontics); Delaire's ideas on reconstruction of facial musculature is also based on these thoughts. However, experience has taught us that

growth of the face in children is not predictable in all dimensions nor in all individuals.

When considering the factors to work with there are variations among the patients we take care of that vex the cleft team again and again. However, some information has been gathered during the last 100 years, especially by evaluating adults with a cleft who have never been operated upon, or who have never been treated at all. There have also been papers published in which large numbers of patients collected from more than just one center were analysed and interesting data presented. The facts produced from this type of research are described in detail below.

INTRINSIC GROWTH VARIATIONS

1. There may be a different shape and angulation of the anterior skull base in cleft patients, but this has not been found by all authors.[46]

2. There is a close relationship between the type and degree of the cleft of the primary palate on the one hand and the arrangement of the muscle bundles in the upper lip on the other side. In microforms the natural anatomy is almost unaltered and the muscular bundles 'flow' around the indentation. However the larger and wider the cleft the more often the muscle arrangement and orientation of bundles is deteriorating. The muscle fibers also often end directly at the border of the cleft, the number of insertions at the cleft margins increases and the remaining muscle fibers in the subnasal skin bridge decrease (Fig. 62.8).[47]

3. It has already been mentioned that in narrow alveolar clefts there is more alveolar bone available containing more teeth (e.g. two lateral incisors, Fig. 62.7) than in wide alveolar clefts. Wide clefts have only little alveolar bone and sometimes not even a single lateral incisor.[43]

4. The most impressive characteristic to be found in the

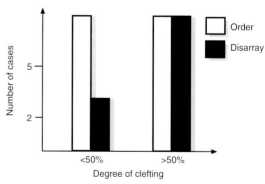

Fig. 62.8 Ratio of derangement of muscle fibers found in the skin bridge of incompletely cleft lips. (Reproduced from Gundlach & Pfeifer[47] with permission.)

faces of patients with a cleft is midfacial retrusion. This is, in part, a negative result of surgical closure (see below), but convincing data have been presented that there is already a tissue deficit in these patients *before* treatment commences. Painstaking measurements carried out by Kriens on plaster casts taken of palates in newborns prior to any kind of therapy revealed that the hard palate is shorter in babies with completely cleft palates only and in patients with unilateral clefts of lip, alveolus and palate than in newborns without clefting.[44] This was corroborated when measuring the distance between anterior and posterior nasal spines on lateral cephalograms, or when it was realized that the anterior nasal spine was located more posteriorly in cases with unilateral clefts of lip, alveolus and palate.[46,48] This tissue deficiency is definitely intrinsic, and so is the poor vertical development of the posterior maxilla. Grabowski (by measuring the distance between sella and posterior nasal spine),[46] Ross (who calipered the inferior point of the pterygomaxillary fissure where it meets the maxillary plane and the sella as well as the 'registration point' at the sphenoid bone),[48] as well as others, have clearly documented this in all kinds of palatal clefting.

5. In complete unilateral clefts of lip, alveolus and palate, there is also an asymmetry of the anterior maxilla, tilting of the premaxilla cranially, dislocation of the septum to the contralateral side with deviation (bulging) to the cleft side, and flaring of the ala on the cleft side with ipsilateral depression of the nose tip while the columella is stretched to the non-cleft side.[49] Most of these features are thought to be due to unbalanced pull of the various anterior facial muscles.

6. There is a well-defined muscular derangement in the cleft soft palate. In non-cleft vela the anterior portion is amuscular and the tensor tendon ends in the horizontal anterior velar aponeurosis. In the posterior portion of the velum the muscle fibers belonging to levator and palato-pharyngeus interdigitate[50] and insert into the aponeurosis. In cleft palates, however, the tensor tendon attaches in a right angle to the vertically oriented velopharyngeal fascia and the velar aponeurosis is only of minimal size. It has dwindled to just a narrow attachment area at the vertical velopharyngeal fascia and is located laterally but medial to the hamulus and posterior to the palatine bone. It was found to be also vertically oriented rather than horizontally. The cleft velar muscles thus have almost lost their entire attachment area and are inserting into the nasal and oral mucosa instead. The displacement of the fascial structures just described causes most of the shortness of the velar halves.[44]

7. The mandible of the average cleft patient also has a different shape when compared to non-cleft individuals. The ramus and body are shorter than average and vertical or clockwise growth, i.e. posterior rotation of the mandible, is typical for the average patient with a cleft palate. This is true for various human races: North German Caucasians,[46] unoperated adult cleft patients in Sri Lanka ('... the mandibles appear to be smaller and retropositioned. In addition, there is an increased Frankfort mandibular plane angle and an increased gonial angle.'),[51] in Japan[52] and in Brazil.[53] Da Silva et al[53] compared 91 unoperated cleft patients with 113 operated patients and stated that 'surgery did not induce significant changes in the mandibular growth' in all three types of clefting analyzed (complete unilateral cleft of lip and alveolus, complete cleft of unilateral lip, alveolus and palate, isolated cleft palate).

EXTRINSIC GROWTH VARIATIONS

1. Presurgical orthodontic therapy using removable plates like the Hotz-type treatment has no long-lasting effect on facial growth and development.[48] While Ross stated in 1987[48] that even rapid reposition of the protruding premaxilla appears to exert no long-term influence on growth of the maxilla, Mølsted commented in her findings from the Six-Center International Study as follows: 'The rather poor treatment outcome ... could in part be attributed to the use of extraoral strapping'.[54] This was in contrast to repositioning of the premaxilla using pinned orthopedic plates resulting in retrusion of the midface later on.[55,56]

2. In unoperated cases an excellent sagittal midface development has been noted, while lip repair inhibited maxillary growth.[48] Some authors even think that cleft lip surgery influences dentofacial morphology more than palatal closure[57] Here especially scars resulting from wide (and unnecessary) incisions in the upper vestibulum and undermining of soft tissue lateral to the piriform aperture is detrimental. Minimal manipulation of soft tissue – as is typical for the wave line procedure – seems to be best.[47]

3. It is also well known that repair of the alveolar cleft in infancy has undesirable effects, especially when bone grafts are used.[48,58] Anterior crossbite, reduced length of the maxilla and lower height of the midface resulting in both poor facial vertical proportions and a more acute nasolabial angle are the results of primary osteoplasty. Gingivoperiosteoplasty also has negative effects on the sagittal growth of the maxilla when performed in infants.[55] 'There are grounds for supposing, therefore, that the early bone grafting and (active) orthopedics is responsible ... for ... lower ranking' of certain participating centers in the Six-Center International Study.[59]

All data available today indicate that soft-tissue repair of the alveolar cleft and/or osteoplasty of the alveolus should be postponed to the 10th year of life, i.e. prior to eruption of the lateral incisor or the canine adjacent to the cleft.[60]

4. Palatoplasty and veloplasty, however, are the treatment modalities that affect maxillary and midfacial growth most.[46,48] Forward translation of the whole midfacial complex is impeded. This is true for *all* types of palatal repair, as stated by Ross in 1987.[48] Mølsted et al have corroborated this by not finding any statistically significant difference among the cephalometric data when comparing different techniques in the six European centers.[54] Therefore the depth of the pharynx in cleft patients is of smaller dimensions, a finding well known in persons with long faces (dolichoprosopy) when compared to those with broad faces (brachyprosopy). An increased tendency to mouthbreathe, snoring and symptoms typical for adenoid hypertrophy are a result of this.[61]

In addition posterior maxillary height is reduced not only as a result of intrinsic factors but also any type of palatal repair. The latter, however, does not seem to be of clinical importance.[48]

There are two more important findings that stand out. It should not be overseen or forgotten that:

a. When analyzing and comparing long-term results in patients with unilateral clefts of the lip, alveolus and palate from 13 different cleft centers (all of which adhering to different treatment protocols), Ross noted that the facial profile was excellent in those patients (from Marburg) in whom the hard palate had not been closed surgically before the age of 16.[48] There are definite advantages in midfacial growth when the hard palate is closed late![62]

b. It is well known that early repair of the hard palate leads to severe crossbite. 'Although orthodontists can repair constriction of the dental arch, it is much better if the surgeon does not produce a palate that has to be repaired in any case'.[62,63]

5. It is also known that agressive primary veloplasty using rubber bands and not handling the soft tissue diligently will result in a short hard palate, a short (and possibly also rigid) soft palate and a high percentage of velopharyngeal incompetence.[62]

6. Finally, pharyngeal flap procedures have been accused of leading to growth disturbances. These flaps are intended to reduce velopharyngeal incompetence. They work by reducing the nasopharyngeal air space and increasing upper airway resistance. The result is an increasing prevalence of mouthbreathing.[64] In keeping with the classical orthodontic theories on maxillary and mandibular adaptation to airway obstruction,[65] this may help in shaping the upper and lower

jaws and in positioning the mandible to those patterns that are so typical for cleft patients.[66]

The most important research finding is the following (and last) fact that the regional surgeon who is specializing in a restricted area of surgery is much more experienced and more successful in his anatomic field than any 'generalist'.[67] This has been noticed by those authors who have edited the two most important multicenter studies on treatment outcome in patients with clefts of lip, alveolus and palate:

Experienced surgeons with soft hands and gentleness in the manipulation of soft tissue are probably the key to success.[48]

The centers where surgery was performed by operators with high personal case loads ranked highest in quality of result whereas centers with large numbers of low volume operators ranked lowest.[59]

TRENDS IN CLEFT LIP AND PALATE

Various information is encountered when discussing clefts with colleagues, listening to papers on this subject presented at scientific meetings or reading articles in the journals and newpapers. These deal with new (or not so new) trends in research, diagnosis and treatment of clefts. This chapter has therefore tried to define six major fields of interest that seem to be in current debate, namely:

1. prevention
2. preterm diagnosis
3. early repair
4. perfection of surgical techniques
5. better psychological support
6. improvement of analytic armamentarium.

All these trends will be mentioned and their aims described in short, without giving any references to authors, groups or projects. Some of the fields of interest are dealt with in more detail in one or more of the following chapters of this book, while others are only listed as possible foci for research in the near future.

1. The prevention of clefting has been attempted for many years by using vitamin B, as it has been shown that spina bifida can be successfully prevented in this way. Now as prevention of spina bifida by applying folic acid appears to be even more successful this has also been tried to prevent clefting. However, prospective double-blind clinical trials in approximately 60 000 pregnancies are necessary in order

to achieve enough data on babies with a cleft for statistical analysis. The ethical problems of a mass screening of these dimensions have also not yet been solved.

2. Preterm diagnosis has been aimed at for many years. Three possibilities are discussed apart from genetic counseling:

a. genome analysis;

b. amniotic enzyme analysis;

c. prenatal ultrasound screening.

All of these methods have been applied with a certain degree of success in amniotic fluid tests and with a high degree of success when using sonography. However, early diagnosis may lead to a high abortion rate and this ethical problem has also to be tackled.

3. Early surgery versus staged repair of cleft lip and palate has been discussed frequently over the last decades. Four trends are seen:

a. surgery of clefts in utero;

b. neonatal cleft lip and/or neonatal cleft palate repair;

c. one-stage closure of clefts of the lip, alveolus and palate in the first year of life;

d. early nose correction at the time of labioplasty.

While intrauterine and neonatal surgery is still in an experimental phase, one-stage repair before 1 year of age is once more a 'hot' topic among cleft surgeons. However, as long as no valid long-term results in large groups of patients are published, it seems untimely to form a final opinion on this matter for the time being.

4. The perfection of surgical techniques is, and will be, an ever-lasting research project. Six major topics are presently under discussion:

a. Scar free repair of soft-tissue clefts. This may be a spin-off from the attempts of intrauterine repair; this is aimed at avoiding to denude the maxillary and palatal bone as well as by covering surgically created tissue defects with so-called biologic dressing materials.

b. Avoiding major stress on soft-tissue scars by presurgical orthodontic appliances (e.g. McNeil, Hotz, Latham).

c. Trying to close the bony alveolar cleft without a bone transplant by applying gingivoperiosteoplasty, guided tissue regeneration techniques and bone morphogenetic proteins.

d. Completing the dentition by inserting dental implants.

e. Achieving harmonious facial profiles by protraction of the maxilla, by applying distraction osteogenesis instead of major maxillary advancement procedures in patients with midface retrusion. This technique has also been proposed for closing the alveolar cleft.

f. Discrimination between different techniques of pharyngoplasties according to preoperative endoscopic findings. However, internationally accepted, easily identifiable and solid predictors have to be defined first.

5. It is generally felt that there is a demand for better psychological help, emotional support and professional advice to parents and affected persons. However, funding for this type of help is a major obstacle that has not yet been solved.

6. The development of internationally applicable standards for reporting and for yardsticks for objective evaluation of preoperative and postoperative functional and aesthetic findings in cleft patients has been unanimously asked for. Only then will we be prepared to start international prospective multicenter trials and outcome studies on a random basis, to evaluate the various surgical methods still in use.

It has also been realized that our knowledge on the neuromuscular function of lip and palate, of neuromotor skills, as well as of sensory nerve sensitivity in the affected person is not at all satisfactory. More knowledge is needed in order to investigate better the problems that affected patients are afflicted with.

REFERENCES

1. Sperber GH 1989 Craniofacial embryology, 4th edn. Butterworth, Guildford

2. Gundlach KKH, Pfeifer G 1981 Classification of facial malformations. International Journal of Oral Surgery 10 (suppl 1):267–272

3. Hinrichsen K 1991 Early development and morphology of the human head. In: Pfeifer G (ed) Craniofacial abnormalities and clefts of the lip, alveolus and palate. Thieme, Stuttgart

4. Mangold U 1982 Die Bildung der Nase und des primitiven Gaumens bei Ratten. In: Pfeifer G (ed) Lippen-Kiefer-Gaumenspalten. Thieme, Stuttgart

5. Poswillo D 1973 The pathogenesis of the first and second branchial arch syndrome. Oral Surgery, Oral Medicine and Oral Pathology 35:302–328

6. Sander A, Moser H, Grimm T, Liechti-Gallati S, Malipiero U, Raveh J 1994 Gen-Lokalisation des van der Woude Syndroms. Deutsche Zeitschrift Mund-Kiefer-Gesichtschirurgie 18:184–189

7. Wyszinski DF, Beaty TH, Maestri NE 1996 Genetics of nonsyndromic oral clefts revisited. Cleft Palate Craniofacial Journal 33:406–417

7a.Lidral AC, Romitti P, Basart A, Doetschman T, et al 1998 Genetic analysis of candidate genes for nonsyndromic lip and cleft palate. ACPA Annual Meeting, April, 20–25, Baltimore, Md, Abstract 6.

8. Greene RM, Pratt RM 1976 Developmental aspects of secondary palate formation. Journal of Embryology and Experimental Morphology 36:225–245

9. Schüpbach PM 1983 Experimental induction of an incomplete hard palate cleft in the rat. Oral Surgery, Oral Medicine and Oral Pathology 55:2–9

10. Report of the Subcommittee on Nomenclature and Classification of Clefts of Lip, Alveolus and Palate and Proposals for Further Activities 1969. In: Sanvenero-Rosselli G (ed) Transactions of the Fourth International Congress on Plastic and Reconstructive Surgery in Rome, October 1967. Excerpta Medica Foundation, Amsterdam

11. Pfeifer G 1968 Angeborene Fehlbildungen des Gesichtes, der Kiefer

und der Mundhöhle. In: Opitz H, Schmid F (eds) Handbuch der Kinderheilkunde, vol 9. Springer, Berlin

12. Tessier P 1976 Anatomical classification of facial, cranio-facial and latero-facial clefts. Journal of Maxillofacial Surgery 4:69–92

13. Fogh-Andersen P 1982 Ätiologie und Epidemiologie der Lippen-Kiefer-Gaumenspalten. In: Pfeifer G (ed) Lippen-Kiefer-Gaumenspalten. Thieme, Stuttgart

14. Cohen MM 1978 Syndromes with cleft lip and cleft palate. Cleft Palate Journal 15:306–328

15. Richtsmeier JT, Sack GH Jr, Grausz HM, Cork LC 1994 Cleft palate with autosomal recessive transmission in Brittany Spaniels. Cleft Palate Craniofacial Journal 31:364–371

16. Driscoll DA, Salvin J, Sellinger B et al 1993 Prevalence of 22q 11 microdeletion in Di George and velocardiofacial syndromes: implications for genetic counselling and prenatal diagnosis. Journal of Medical Genetics 30:813–817

17. Moore GE, Ivens A, Chambers J et al 1987 Linkage of an X-chromosome cleft palate gene. Nature 326:91–92

18. Gorlin RJ, Cohen MM Jr, Levin LS 1990 Syndromes of the head and neck, 3rd edn. University Press, New York

19. Gundlach KKH 1982 Mißbildungen des Kiefergelenkes – Experimentelle und klinische Untersuchungen. Hanser, München

20. Taher AAY 1992 Cleft lip and palate in Tehran. Cleft Palate Craniofacial Journal 29:15–16

21. Pelz L, Amling A 1996 Informative morphogenetic and phenogenetic variants in children with cleft lip/cleft palate. American Journal of Medical Genetics 63:305–309

22. Leakey RE, Lewin R 1977 Origins. Rainbird, London

23. Pilbeam D 1984 The descent of hominoids and hominids. Scientific American 250(3):84–96

24. Gabunia L, Vekua A 1995 A plio-pleistocene hominid from Dmanisi, East Georgia, Caucasus. Nature 373 (9 February):509–512

25. Morrison G 1985 The incidence of cleft lip and palate in the Western Cape. South African Medical Journal 68:576–577

26. Iregbulem LM 1982 The incidence of cleft lip and palate in Nigeria. Cleft Palate Journal 19:201–205

27. Erhardt CL, Nelson FG 1964 Reported congenital malformations in New York City 1958–1959. American Journal of Public Health 54:1489–1506

28. Longenecker CG, Ryan RF, Vincent RW 1965 Cleft lip and cleft palate. Incidence at a large charity hospital. Plastic and Reconstructive Surgery 35:548–551

29. Akota I, Barkane B, Grasmanis N, Purina G, Sokolova L 1995 The incidence of cleft lip and palate in connection with other congenital malformations in Latvia. Rostock Medizin Beiträge 3:97–102

30. Briard ML, Bonaiti-Pellie C, Feingold J, Pavy B, Kaplan J, Bois E 1974 A genetic and epidemiological approach of cleft lip and palate. Annales de Chirurgie Plastique 19:87–95

31. Neumann H-J 1996 Entstehung, Prävention und klinisches Bild der Lippen-, Kiefer-Gaumenspalten. In: Andrä A, Neumann H-J (eds) Lippen-, Kiefer-Gaumenspalten. Einhorn, Reinbek

32. Tolarova M 1991 Etiology of clefts of lip and/or palate: 23 years of genetic follow-up in 3660 individual cases. In: Pfeifer G (ed) Craniofacial abnormalities and clefts of the lip, alveolus and palate. Thieme, Stuttgart

33. Gorlin RJ 1970 Developmental anomalies of the face and oral structures. In: Gorlin RJ, Goldman HM (eds) Thoma's oral pathology, vol 1. CV Mosby, St Louis

34. Miller JR 1963 The use of registries and vital statistics in the study of congenital malformations. In: International Medical Congress (ed) Second International Conference on Congenital Malformations, New York

35. Tretsven VE 1963 Incidence of cleft lip and palate in Montana Indians. Journal of Speech and Hearing Disorders 28:52–57

36. Bardanoue VT 1969 Cleft palate in Montana, a ten year report. Cleft Palate Journal 6:213–220

37. Lindemann G, Riis B, Sewerin I 1977 Prevalence of cleft uvula among 2737 Danes. Cleft Palate Journal 14:226–229

38. Ballew C, Beckerman SJ, Lizzeralde R 1993 High prevalence of cleft lip among the Bari Indians of Western Venezuela. Cleft Palate Craniofacial Journal 30:411–413

39. Vanderas AP 1987 Incidence of cleft lip, cleft palate, and cleft lip and palate among races: a review. Cleft Palate Journal 24:216–225

40. Gundlach KKH, Abou Tara N, von Kreybig T 1986 Tierexperimentelle Ergebnisse zur Entstehung und Prävention von Gesichtsspalten und anderen kraniofazialen Anomalien. Fortschritte der Kieferorthopadie 47:356–361

41. Cohen MM Jr, Bankier A 1991 Syndrome delineation involving orofacial clefting. Cleft Palate Craniofacial Journal 28:119–120

42. Tolarova M 1990 Genetic aspects and classification. In: Bardach J, Morris HL (eds) Multidisciplinary management of cleft lip and palate. Saunders, Philadelphia

43. Ehmann G, Pfeifer G, Gundlach KKH 1976 Morphological findings in unoperated cleft lips and palates. Cleft Palate Journal 13:262–272

44. Kriens OB 1997 Update on intravelar veloplasty. Advances in Plastic and Reconstructive Surgery 13:1–24

45. Moss ML 1959 Embryology, growth, and malformations of the temporomandibular joint. In: Schwartz L (ed) Disorders of the temporomandibular joint. Saunders, Philadelphia

46. Grabowski R 1996 Wachstum und Entwicklung des Gesichtsschädels unter den Bedingungen einer Spaltbildung aus kieferorthopädischer Sicht. In: Andrä A, Neumann H-J (eds) Lippen-, Kiefer-, Gaumenspalten. Einhorn, Reinbek

47. Gundlach KKH, Pfeifer G 1979 The arrangement of muscle fibres in cleft lips. Journal of Maxillofacial Surgery 7:109–116

48. Ross RB 1987 Treatment variables affecting facial growth in complete unilateral cleft lip and palate. Cleft Palate Journal 24:5–77

49. Latham RA 1969 The pathogenesis of the skeletal deformity associated with unilateral cleft lip and palate. Cleft Palate Journal 6:404–414

50. Dickson DR 1972 Normal and cleft palate anatomy. Cleft Palate Journal 9:280–290

51. Mars M 1991 In: Commentary on the three preceding articles. Cleft Palate Craniofacial Journal 28:47

52. Yoshida H, Nakamura A, Michi K-I, Go-Ming W, Kan L, Wei-Liu Q 1992 Cephalometric analysis of maxillo-facial morphology in unoperated cleft palate patients. Cleft Palate Craniofacial Journal 29:419–424

53. Da Silva OG Jr, Corrêa Normando AD, Capelozza L Jr 1992 Mandibular morphology and spatial position in patients with clefts: intrinsic or iatrogenic? Cleft Palate Craniofacial Journal 29:369–375

54. Mølsted K, Asher-McDade C, Brattström V et al 1992 A six-center international study of treatment outcome in patients with clefts of the lip and palate: Part 2. Craniofacial form and soft tissue profile. Cleft Palate Craniofacial Journal 29:398–404

55. Henkel K-O 1996 An analysis of primary gingivoperiosteoplasty in alveolar cleft repair. Abstract of the prize-winning paper. Journal of Cranio-Maxillofacial Surgery 24:53

56. Roberts-Harry D, Semb G, Hathorn I, Killingback N 1996 Facial growth in patients with unilateral clefts of the lip and palate: a two-center study. Cleft Palate Craniofacial Journal 33:489–493

57. Capelozza Filho L, Correa Normando AD, Da Silva Filho OG 1996 Isolated influences of lip and palate surgery on facial growth: comparison of operated and unoperated male adults with UCLP. Cleft Palate Craniofacial Journal 33:51–56

58. Rehrmann A, Koberg W, Koch H 1973 Die Auswirkungen der Osteoplastik auf das Wachstum des Oberkiefers – Erhebungen der Ergebnisse mit Hilfe der elektronischen Datenverarbeitung. Fortschritte der Kiefer-Gesichts-chirurgie 16/17:102–108

59. Shaw WC, Dahl E, Asher-McDade C et al 1992 A six-center international study of treatment outcome in patients with clefts of the

lip and palate: Part 5. General discussion and conclusions. Cleft Palate Craniofacial Journal 29:413–418

60. Scheuer H, Hasund A, Pfeifer G 1991 Changes in facial morphology in patients with unilateral clefts – a cephalometric study. In: Pfeifer G (ed) Craniofacial abnormalities and clefts of the lip, alveolus and palate. 4th Hamburg International Symposium. Thieme, Stuttgart

61. Quick CA, Gundlach KKH 1978 Adenoid facies. Laryngoscope 88:327–333

62. Bardach J, Morris HL, Olin WH 1984 Late results of primary veloplasty: the Marburg project. Plastic Reconstructive Surgery 73:207–215

63. Gundlach KKH, Behlfelt K, Pfeifer G 1991 The maxillary arch in 8- and 16-year-old patients with complete unilateral clefts treated according to the Hamburg regimen. In: Pfeifer G (ed) Craniofacial abnormalities and clefts of the lip, alveolus and palate. 4th Hamburg International Symposium. Thieme, Stuttgart

64. Hairfield MA, Warren DW, Seaton DL 1988 Prevalence of mouth breathing in cleft lip and palate. Cleft Palate Journal 25:135–138

65. Subtelny JD, Pineda Nieto R 1978 A longitudinal study of maxillary growth following pharyngeal flap surgery. Cleft Palate Journal 15:118–131

66. Semb G, Shaw WC 1996 Facial growth in orofacial clefting disorders. In: Turvey TA, Vig KWL, Fonseca RJ (eds) Facial clefts and craniosynostosis. Saunders, Philadelphia

67. Boyes JH 1975 The regional surgeon – a new kind of specialist. Plastic and Reconstructive Surgery 56:199–201

Primary repair of the lip and palate using the Delaire philosophy

63

ROBERTO BRUSATI/NICOLA MANNUCCI

The treatment of complex congenital malformations such as cleft lip and palate, which not only compromise the appearance but also impair functions such as phonation, mastication, respiration, lingual posture and the growth of the maxillomandibulary complex, must be based on a sound knowledge of the anatomy, physiology and growth of the involved regions, as well as of the pathologic anatomy characteristic of the deformity itself.

All of these aspects have long been studied by Delaire, who has published a large number of articles,[1-12] and constructed a 'philosophy' concerning the significance and interrelationships of the various structures from which he derived a rationale for the treatment of cleft lip and palate deformities. His therapeutic approach is thoroughly logical and consequential and, although it has not all been scientifically supported by experimental data, his philosophy is highly attractive and the results obtained from its application seem to be particularly valid from a clinical point of view.

For these reasons, and albeit with the inevitable personal modifications developed during more than ten years' experience in applying the philosophy, we think that Delaire's primary uni- and bilateral cheilorhinoplasty procedures are particularly good, as is his secondary gingivoalveoloplasty procedure during the course of the surgical repair of the hard palate. This last, like the repair of the soft palate during the course of cheilorhinoplasty, has been considerably modified by us but always in accordance with the basic principles underlined by Delaire.

In order to allow readers to understand Delaire's logic to the full, it is necessary to begin by considering the normal and pathologic anatomy of the muscles and structures involved in the deformity, and the role that some structures (the nasal septum, musculature, tongue) and some functions (dental occlusion, nasal respiration) play in maxillary and particularly premaxillary growth.

NORMAL ANATOMY AND PHYSIOLOGY OF THE LABIONASOGENAL MUSCULATURE AND THE MEDIAL SEPTUM OF THE UPPER LIP

In relation to upper lip reconstructive surgery, a rather simplistic view is taken of upper lip anatomy, and the orbicularis oris muscle is generally referred to as if it were a single horizontal muscle whose only function was to compress the upper and lower lips by means of synergistic, concentric contractions. In reality, the upper lip contains three muscle formations (a horizontal band or the internal orbicularis, oblique bands or the external orbicularis, and incisal bands), and involves numerous other muscle terminations which will be described later, all of which form part of a system of three closely interconnected sphincteric rings extending from the upper part of the face to the chin (Fig. 63.1).

UPPER RING

The upper ring consists of a large number of muscles on both sides: the transversus nasi, the levator labii superioris alaeque nasi, the levator labii superioris, the zygomaticus minor, and the levator anguli oris (caninus), the lower insertions of which participate in the anatomy and physiology of the upper lip.

Transversus nasi

This originates at the level of the nasal dorsum near the midline, and then runs downwards superficially to the lateral part of the triangular cartilage. Its fibers intermingle with those of the levator labii superioris alaeque nasi and the

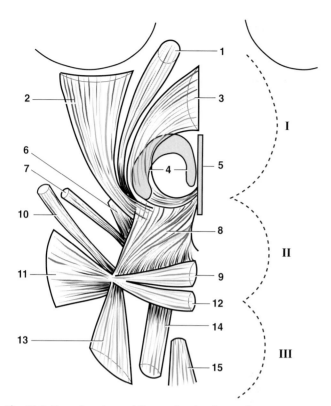

Fig. 63.1 Normal anatomy of the nasal and oral musculature: I upper ring; II middle ring; III lower ring. 1. Levator labii superioris alaeque nasi; 2. levator labii superioris; 3. transversus nasi; 4. alar cartilage; 5. nasal septum; 6. levator anguli oris (caninus); 7. zygomaticus minor; 8. external orbicularis labii superioris; 9. internal orbicularis labii superioris; 10. zygomaticus major; 11. buccinatorius; 12. orbicularis inferior; 13. triangularis labii; 14. quadratus labii; 15. mentalis.

levator labii superioris to form a true modiolus laterally to the nasal alae in the nasogenal sulcus, and then pass medially and horizontally under the floor of the nares until they insert themselves into the incisal crest and the base of the nasal septum at the level of the nasal spine, and superficially into the skin of the nasolabial groove and the vestibule of the nares. During its course, this muscle adheres to the periosteum of the lateral border of the pyriform aperture and, at the level of the floor of the nares, is in continuity with the depressor septi muscle that arises from the incisal fossa and then inserts itself medially into the septum and laterally into the posterior part of the nasal alae.

It needs to be borne in mind that the anatomic dissection and identification of these terminations may be difficult and give rise to erroneous interpretations, to the extent that, in their anatomic studies, equally authoritative authors[13] have localized the lower insertion of the transversus nasi to the incisal fossa. This last finding, together with clinical observations of the morphology of the nares during cleft lip surgery, was to become the basis of one of our and

Talmant's[14] modifications to Delaire's cheilorhinoplasty technique.

Levator labii superioris

This muscle originates from the lower margin of the orbit, above the infraorbital foramen, and runs downwards superficially to the caninus muscle (levator anguli oris) and below the levator labii superioris alaeque nasi, until it reaches the lateral modiolus of the nasal alae. Some deep fibers run to the mucosa of the vestibular fornix to assure their synchronous raising with that of the lips.

Levator anguli oris (*m. caninus*)

Beginning in the canine fossa, this runs laterally and deeply to the levator labii superioris, and is inferiorly inserted in the outer border of the external orbicularis.

Levator labii superioris alaeque nasi

Originating in the upper part of the frontal process of the maxilla, this runs downwards superficially to the lateral portion of the transversus nasi, where it divides into two fascicles. The first becomes inserted into the skin and cartilage of the most lateral part of the nasal alae, where it intermingles with the other muscular insertions in the lateronasal modiolus. The second runs medially in front of the fibers of the transversus nasi and enters the most anterior part of the nasal vestibule, where it intermingles with the fibers of the transversus nasi, the depressor septi and the oblique bands of the external orbicularis, thus terminating partially in the nasal spine and partially in the anteroinferior part of the septum.

Zygomaticus minor

This muscle originates at the surface of the zygoma, from where it runs downwards and medially until it fuses with the lateral fibers of the external orbicularis superficially to the insertion of the caninus muscle, between the insertion of the zygomaticus major into the commissural modiolus and the insertion of the levator labii muscles.

MIDDLE RING

The middle ring, which represents the oral sphincter, fundamentally consists of the upper and lower lip orbicularis oris muscle. In the upper lip, the orbicularis oris is made up of three strata on each side (horizontal bands or the internal orbicularis, oblique bands or the external orbicularis, and incisal bands), to which should be added the myrtiformis. The terminations of the nasogenal muscles that intermingle with the musculature of the upper lip itself have been described in the above analysis of the muscles of the first ring. We shall now consider the individual components of the muscles that are intrinsic to the upper lip.

Internal orbicularis labii superioris

This is the most well known component, characterized by the horizontal course of fibers extending from one commissure to the other, where they intermingle with the fibers of the lower lip orbicularis oris and of the buccinatorius. They run the thickness of the upper lip just below the depression of the philtrum and are superficially inserted to the mucocutaneous junction, giving them the prominence of the so-called 'white roll'.

External orbicularis labii superioris

The more medial fibers run almost vertically, superficially to those of the internal orbicularis, and determine the presence of the philtral crests. The other fibers fan out from the nasal spine, the lower part of the columella and the threshold of the nares, and then run downwards and laterally in the direction of the commissures. At this point, they intermingle with the fibers of the depressor anguli oris, buccinatorius, risorius, platysma and triangularis. As already described, they also intermingle with the fibers of the levator anguli oris, the zygomaticus major and minor, the levator labii superioris alaeque nasi, the transversus nasi and the depressor septi. Superficially, the fibers are inserted into the labial dermis and in correspondence with the mucocutaneous rim.

Incisal fibers

The incisal fibers lie deeper than the oblique fibers and are inserted medially into the external border of the myrtiformis fossa, from where they run downwards and laterally toward the commissures in the same way as the oblique fibers of the external orbicularis.

Myrtiformis

This is a small muscle inserted into the myrtiformis fossa, which is on the vestibular aspect of the premaxilla in correspondence with the apex of the lateral incisor, and runs upwards to insert itself in the proximity of the most anterior part of the floor of the nares, where it intermingles with the fibers of the transversus nasi.

As far as the labii superioris is concerned, which is less involved in our present subject, it is sufficient to remember that its muscular scaffold is based on the horizontal fibers of the lower orbicularis muscle, which intermingle with those of the buccinatorius, the caninus and the zygomaticus major at the level of the commissures.

LOWER RING

The lower ring has an incomplete circumference, and consists of the previously described orbicularis inferior, the triangularis labii and the quadratus labii inferioris. Whereas the fibers of the triangularis labii begin in the lower mandibular border lateral to the chin and then extend upwards until they intermingle with the orbicularis oris of the upper lip, those of the quadratus labii inferioris originate more medially (but still in the chin region) and insert themselves in the inferior orbicularis.

PHYSIOLOGY OF THE THREE MUSCLE RINGS: EFFECTS ON SKELETAL GROWTH

The organization of the perioral and perinasal muscles (described above in the form of three annular sphincters going from the root of the nose to the chin) means that their anatomy and function greatly affect the growth of the underlying skeleton. The integrity of the first ring (which is of course disrupted in the case of a cleft lip) is fundamental for sustaining and allowing the normal function of the other two. The cartilaginous nasal septum, by means of all of the tendinous terminations reaching its anteroinferior border, supports and draws forward the upper and middle rings as it grows; through them, it stimulates the periosteum of the anterior part of the maxilla and thus ensures the harmonious growth of the latter. Labial motility, in addition to modeling directly the underlying dentoalveolar structure by means of the median septum also acts synergistically with Latham's ligament in positively influencing the fan-shaped growth of the premaxilla (see below). The lower ring acts by modeling the dentoalveolar complex and the chin portion of the mandible, both vertically and transversely.

GROWTH OF THE PREMAXILLA

The premaxilla is the anterior portion of the maxilla; it consists of two equal and symmetrical parts which are separated along the midline by means of one suture and joined to the rest of the maxilla by means of a transverse suture that extends from the canine alveolus to the nasopalatine canal.

At the level of the vestibular cortex corresponding to the canine this suture is soon obliterated but, starting at 6–7 years of age, it gradually closes from the outside in, and from the nasal floor to the oral cavity, though evidence of this sutural structure remains visible in adults.

This part of the maxilla grows under the influence of various mechanisms including lingual pressure, the development of the teeth, occlusal forces, and the force transmitted by the median nasal system and the nasolabial muscles. The growth is characterized by three elements: a principally fan-shaped movement (Fig. 63.2) with the rotation of each hemipremaxilla around a vertical axis located at the level of the canines; vestibular apposition; and a transverse translation of the whole of each hemimaxilla. Of particular interest in terms of the pathology under consideration here is the role of the median septal system and the musculature.

The median septal system is a fibrous septum that extends vertically from the septal cartilage (where it was described by Latham[15] as a septo-premaxillary ligament) to the median frenulum of the upper lip. Superficially, it goes from the deep fascia of the dermis and has its deep insertion throughout the length of the median suture, penetrating deeply where the suture is particularly wide (the alveolar process). This system therefore transmits to the premaxilla not only the traction forces developed by the anterior growth of the septum, but also those originating during the movements of protruding or laterally stretching the lips.

Perhaps the main role in the transverse and anterior growth of the premaxilla is played by the nasolabial muscles which, by their insertion in the incisal crest and nasal spine, exert a transverse traction. Furthermore, the insertion of these muscles into the cartilaginous septum means that the anterior growth of the latter provides constant functional stimulation to the vestibular aspect of the premaxilla by

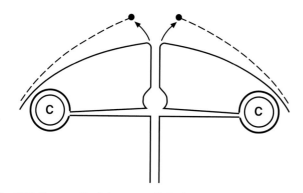

Fig. 63.2 The growth of the premaxilla is characterized by a fan-shaped movement with rotation of each hemipremaxilla around a vertical axis located at the level of the cuspids. C = cuspid.

means of a musculoperiosteal tent and consequent periosteal apposition.

PATHOLOGIC ANATOMY OF LABIOMAXILLOPALATINE CLEFTS

The anatomopathologic pictures of cleft lip and palate vary greatly, depending upon the particular type of deformity under examination. For this reason, we shall analyze unilateral and bilateral clefts separately, bearing in mind further differences in the clinical picture according to whether the cleft is limited to the primary palate (lip and maxilla up to the nasopalatine canal) or also involves the secondary palate (lips, maxilla, and the hard and soft palate). In particular, we shall analyze the nasolabial musculature, the nose, the skin, the mucosa, the skeleton, and the hard and soft palate.

TOTAL UNILATERAL CLEFT

Alterations in nasolabial musculature

The lack of fusion of the maxillary and nasal (internal and external) processes prevents the laterally derived vascular, nervous and muscular elements from reaching the midline. Consequently, all of the muscle groups that normally insert themselves into the nasal spine, septum and the external aspect of the premaxilla become massed on the lateral border of the cleft.

The behavior of the musculature on the cleft border is a subject of controversy in the literature. According to some authors,[16] the muscle fibers run parallel to the border of the cleft and are inserted into the base of the nasal alae and the columella; according to others,[17] the borders of the cleft are characterized by a chaotic massing of muscle fibers that is irreconcilable with the normal muscle strata, and by their disordered insertion into the cleft border dermis without any evidence of fascicles parallel to the cleft itself. This absence of a central insertion leads to disequilibrium of the first and second muscle rings, whose effects on the nose and maxilla will be considered below (Fig. 63.3).

Nasal abnormalities

The base of the nasal septum, and therefore the columella, are deviated toward the contralateral side of the cleft as a result of the unbalanced traction of the muscles inserted into the nasal spine and anterior part of the maxilla on the healthy side, and of the lateralization of the main maxillary stump. Conversely, the tip of the nose is deviated toward the same side as the cleft and is characterized by a diastasis

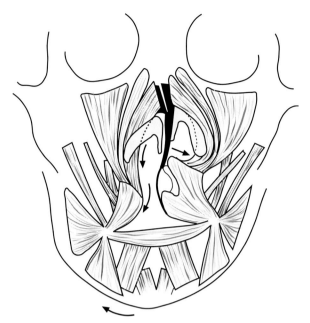

Fig. 63.3 The lack of correct insertion of the nasolabial muscles leads to disequilibrium of the first and second muscle rings with stretching, rotation and displacement of alar cartilage, septonasal contralateral deviation, premaxillary contralateral deviation, lowering of oral commissurae of the cleft side and mental deviation toward the cleft side.

between the domes of the alar cartilages. In particular, the alar cartilage of the affected side is ptotic, stretched and rotated, and there is a simultaneous lowering of the ipsilateral triangular cartilage; the foot of the medial crus and the dome are also lowered (Fig. 63.4). The cartilaginous structures are deformed and dislocated (but not hypoplastic)

because of the direct action of the musculature inserted into the nasal ala and the deformation of the underlying maxillary skeleton, which is hypoplastic and drawn backwards to the level of the pyriform aperture.

Mucocutaneous abnormalities

It is essential that these are delineated, because they provide the basis for identifying the fundamental elements necessary for cleft repair. On both the internal and external stumps of the cleft, it is important to differentiate the skin of the nasal floor from that of the lip. The former has a fine-grained appearance whereas the latter is more flat; furthermore, the lip skin on the external stump can be distinguished by the cutaneous retraction associated with the insertion of the muscles, whereas the skin of the nasal floor is flatter. The two components of the external stump can be easily distinguished by drawing a perpendicular line from the base of the nasal ala to the mucocutaneous border; as far as the internal stump is concerned, it is first necessary to identify the base of the columella on the cleft side (the same distance as that from the upper internal angle of the naris to the base of the healthy side), and then trace a line perpendicular to that of the mucocutaneous border (Fig. 63.5). As already mentioned, the lip skin is retracted as a result of the action of the underlying muscles: on the internal stump it therefore usually shows a vertical contraction, whereas on the external stump it shows a concentric contraction with the raising of the skin. The mucocutaneous rim (white roll), which consists of the cutaneous insertion of the fibers of the external orbicularis, tends to decrease in size on the

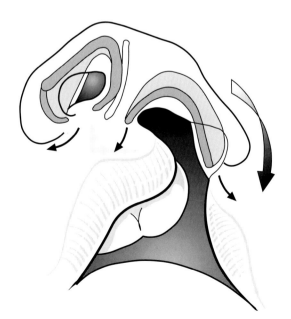

Fig. 63.4 Nasal deformities. Alar displacement of the cleft side with downward rotation of the dome and luxation from triangular cartilage; the nasal septum and healthy cartilage are displaced contralaterally.

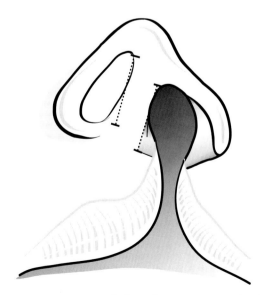

Fig. 63.5 A line drawn perpendicular to the mucocutaneous border from the alar and columellar base allows the differentiation of the skin of the nasal floor from that of the lip.

internal stump to just beyond the midline; on the external stump, after the point of maximum lip thickness (corresponding to what will become the lateral point of Cupid's bow), it tends to disappear within the space of 2–3 mm. The mucosa lining the borders of the cleft is also different from the normal 'dry' mucosa making up the vermilion; it is a mucosa that Veau[18] called sterile and is better removed. It is not particularly easy to differentiate it from the normal vermilion, but this can be done by tracing a perpendicular line on the large and small stumps to the edge of the cutaneous mucosa at those points identified as the peaks of Cupid's bow.

Skeletal abnormalities

There are profound differences in the skeletal abnormalities encountered when treating an exclusively cleft lip (in which skeletal alterations are virtually absent), a cleft of the lip and primary palate (up to the level of the nasopalatine canal) and a total cleft involving the lip and the primary and secondary palate (hard and soft palate). Here, it is necessary to distinguish the positional, morphologic and developmental abnormalities of the main and small stumps.

The most typical situation is that of a complete cleft lip and palate. The main stump is rotated outward from a fulcrum located in the pterygoid region as a result of the simultaneous action of the pressure of the tongue and traction of the musculature of the healthy side, which is not counterbalanced by that of the cleft side. The anterior part of the alveolar arch presents a less accentuated curve, with hypoplasia of the alveolomaxillary portion of the premaxilla, which lies between the cleft and the median suture. This is due not only to the absence of the transmission of mechanical stresses on this part of the premaxilla, but also to the frequent agenesis of the lateral incisor. The small stump shows signs of lack of development and malpositioning. The malpositioning may be due to its outward rotation as a result of the interposition of the tongue in the cleft, or to the collapse of the small stump with a narrow cleft, particularly in the anterior part of the hard palate. The lack of development is particularly accentuated vertically, mainly in the most anterior part of the small stump, but its anteroposterior dimensions are also reduced. These alterations in the maxillary stumps are normally accompanied by an increase in the transverse diameter of the maxillary tuberosities and pterygoid processes because of the non-fusion of the palatine muscles along the midline. Finally, as a result of the lateral shift of the main stump, both the bony and cartilaginous parts of the nasal septum are stretched toward the healthy side, with a convex curvature of the lower part toward the cleft side.

Musculomucosal hard and soft palate alterations

A hard and soft palate cleft leads to a complete disturbance of the musculature, which not only fails to complete the palatine muscle ring at the midline but also, like the musculature present on the borders of lip clefts, modifies the direction of its fibers and gives rise to abnormal insertions. Different interpretations have been made of the pathological anatomy of the levator palati. Kriens[19] considers that all of the fibers of this muscle are parallel to the border of the cleft and inserted into the posterior border of the palatine laminae (Fig. 63.6) but Pigott[20] considers that this disposition is only apparent and is due to the lateral collapse of the hemivelum whereas, in reality, alongside the more anterior fibers inserted into the posterior part of the cleft, the majority insert themselves perpendicularly into the border of the cleft itself. Obviously, this difference in interpretation leads to two completely different reparative procedures.

According to Delaire,[11] it is particularly important to differentiate three types of fibromucosa on the hard palate. Gingival fibromucosa lines the cervical region of the teeth, extending apically for some millimeters to cover part of the alveolar process, thus making a significant contribution to its vertical growth. The maxillary fibromucosa, which is rich in vessels and nerves, is particularly important for the

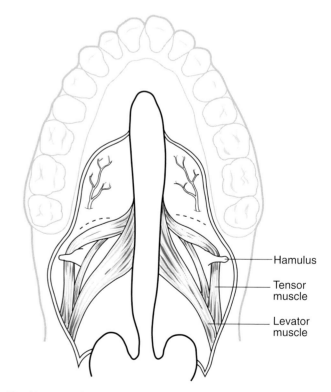

Hamulus

Tensor muscle

Levator muscle

Fig. 63.6 According to Kriens, the levator muscles are oriented longitudinally in cleft cases and insert on the posterior edge of the palatal bone and along the bony cleft margins.

vertical and transverse growth of the palate as a whole. The fibromucosa of the palatine laminae is particularly thin at the center and gradually thickens as it approaches the maxillary fibromucosa; it allows the lowering of the palatine laminae which, during the course of their growth, undergo reabsorption on the nasal side and apposition on the oral side.

The lateral stumps are characterized by a reduction in the fibromucosa of the palatine lamina as a consequence of the underdevelopment of the laminae themselves, whereas the maxillary and gingival fibromucosa remain practically normal. It should also be noted, however, that the reduction in the fibromucosa of the palatine lamina is also caused by a contraction of the periosteum (which is effectively reduced), and its incision makes it possible to extend the fibromucosa to cover an almost normal width.

The large stump has the palatine lamina normally fused to the septum, which at its base is characterized by a convexity toward the cleft. The point of passage between the vomerine mucosa and the fibromucosa of the palatine lamina is therefore shifted toward the healthy side, and is not in its expected position when referring to the perpendicular portion of the septum.

TOTAL BILATERAL CLEFTS

Alterations in nasolabial musculature

The muscular abnormalities in the lateral stumps of complete bilateral clefts are similar to those found in unilateral cleft lip, but the situation is profoundly different at the level of the median tubercle which, for embryonic reasons, has no traces of muscle because the muscles, originating from the sides, migrate within the maxillary process and stops at the border of the cleft. Although it is seldom usable, in incomplete forms some musculature is partially present in the superior part of the median tubercle.

Nasal alterations

These are similar to those described for the affected side of a unilateral cleft, the only difference being that they are symmetrical. The bases of the nasal alae are broadened and withdrawn (as a result of hypoplasia and the backward position of the underlying skeleton, and also because the muscular insertions end at this level), and the domes of alar cartilages show diastasis and a downward rotation, with a dislocation of the relationship between the upper border of the alar cartilage and the lower border of the triangular cartilage. The foot of the medial crus is lowered toward the nasal spine; between the diastatic domes, the anterior border of the cartilaginous septum is positioned nearer the surface and can sometimes even be visible at the tip of the nose.

Mucocutaneous alterations

Once again, the lateral stumps are similar to those observed in the case of unilateral clefts, whereas the skin of the median tubercle is underdeveloped (particularly vertically) as a result of concentric retraction caused by the absence of the underlying muscular ring, which means that it is no longer subject to physiological downward stretching. The lowering of the bases of the alar cartilages is also accompanied by the downward migration of what should be the skin of the columella, which therefore joins that of the median tubercle and creates the typical shortness of the columella itself. The mucosa covering three quarters of the circumference of the prolabium is characterized by the absence of the vestibular fornix and, in complete forms, by the absence of the white roll (this may however be more or less present in incomplete forms). The white roll is in fact considered to be nothing more than the muscular insertion of the external orbicularis at the level of the mucocutaneous rim.

Skeletal abnormalities

The lateral stumps show the same alterations as those described for the small stumps of unilateral clefts, although there is a greater diastasis of the maxillary tuberosities. There is a form with an anterior collapse of the small stumps behind the protruding median tubercle, and other forms with externally rotated small stumps and broad clefts. Premaxillary alterations are highly pronounced: the premaxilla is particularly protuberant and rotated forwards (with its fulcrum at the level of the nasal spine) because of the absence of the muscular cingulum which should counterbalance the pressure of the tongue and the interposition of the lateral labial stumps. The transverse dimensions of the premaxilla are reduced because of the underactivity of the median suture, which does not undergo the musculoperiosteal traction leading to its activation. The frequent absence of lateral incisor germs also contributes toward the reduced volume of the premaxilla.

Musculomucosal hard and soft palate alterations

These are substantially the same as those described in the case of total unilateral clefts, the only difference being that there is not one main stump and a small stump but two small stumps and, centrally, the nasal septum and the premaxilla. The posterior part of the nasal septum is vertically underdeveloped and does not reach the level of the palatine processes, a situation that, as we shall see, has therapeutic implications. At the level of the premaxilla, the palatine fibromucosa takes on the form of a triangle with a posterior apex and is vascularized by nasopalatine vessels and an intraosseous network anastomosed to the soft parts of the vestibule. The palatine fibromucosa is continuous with the fibromucosa of the lateral aspects of the premaxilla and of the nasal septum with clear modifications in its appearance.

PREOPERATIVE ORTHOPEDIC TREATMENT

We have seen that the presence of a cleft, together with the consequent muscular imbalance and the interposition or pressure of the tongue, may cause severe alterations in the position of the stumps, and these alterations are different depending on whether the cleft is unilateral or bilateral.

Unilateral clefts are usually wide and have the tongue positioned inside them. In our view, this situation can be greatly improved by using a passive orthopedic plate as suggested by the Zurich Group.[21] The principle underlying this procedure, which should be implemented within the first days of life (if started later, after some weeks, it is less readily accepted by the baby), is to remove the dislocating pressure of the tongue on the maxillae while simultaneously allowing the growth of the stumps on their borders; this makes it possible to obtain a considerable reduction in the width of the cleft and therefore a better surgical situation, together with re-education of the tongue position.

In rare cases, the plate may be of the active type: that is, consisting of two parts (corresponding to the two stumps) with a posterior hinge and an anterior screw allowing their fan-shaped divarication. This type of plate is used when the cleft is narrow with the collapse of the anterior part of the small stump, which may even position itself behind the large stump. Any lip reconstruction under these conditions, with the consequent pressure on the stumps, would only perpetuate this state and lead to severe alterations in maxillary development.

The use of a plate is particularly important in the treatment of bilateral clefts, which present two different problems: the position of the lateral stumps and the position of the premaxilla.

In the most favorable situation, the lateral stumps may have an anterior diastasis that allows the retracting premaxilla to find its correct position. In these cases, the constructed plate is simply ground out in the central portion in order to allow the prominent premaxilla to move backward (this is described later). If the lateral stumps have collapsed, however, it is necessary to apply an active plate with a posterior hinge and anterior expansion screw in order to position the stumps correctly and thus permit the premaxilla to move backward.

As it is not contained by its muscular cingulum, and is under pressure from the growth of the septum and tongue, the premaxilla is usually very prominent and often deviated, which places limitations on tension-free lip repair. It is important to remember that the prominence of the premaxilla is not a consequence of a forward shifting of the premaxilla, but of a rotation around the nasal spine which, as demonstrated by Ross,[22] retains its correct anteroposterior position. It follows that there is no sense in moving the premaxilla in toto backward, with a distraction of the premaxilla along the septum (as happens when a Georgiade and Latham orthopedic device is used)[23]; it is much more correct to reduce the protrusion of the premaxilla by a rotatory movement having its hinge at the nasal spine. We use what in our opinion is the most simple and efficacious procedure for doing this: an appropriately cut strip of non-allergic tape goes from one cheek to the other and rests with moderate tension on the lower part of the premaxilla.

In rare cases we have found that a lack of parental collaboration has prevented us from moving the premaxilla significantly backward, and it is only in such cases that we have had recourse to lip adhesion in order to improve the position of the premaxilla before moving on to the definitive reconstruction of the lip and nose.

If the plate has aligned the stumps well, its use can be discontinued postoperatively as the restored muscle balance maintains the same orthopedic effect. We are also sparing in the use of orthodontic treatment of deciduous teeth, considering that it is indicated only in the presence of precontacts dislocating the mandible from the central condylar position, because this could lead to skeletal alterations.

REPAIR OF A TOTAL UNILATERAL CLEFT

Within the context of a large number of treatment protocols Delaire[1,6,10] opted for cheilorhinoplasty with soft palate surgery at 7 months, and hard palate surgery with gingivoalveoloplasty at 14–18 months. For the first intervention, it was considered ideal to wait for the incisors to emerge in order to avoid the inversion that frequently takes place if the operation is carried out before; this obviously did not apply in the case of incomplete forms, for which the surgical intervention could be brought forward to about the fourth month.

We agree with Delaire as far as the cheilorhinoplasty is concerned, but we prefer to repair the hard palate with gingivoalveoplasty at an age of 18–24 months if the palatal cleft is wide and it can be presumed that a real phonetic advantage can be gained from its early closure, and to postpone it until as late as three years if the cleft is narrow, because spontaneous bone apposition at the gingivoalveoplasty site may optimally occur even in patients aged 6–8 years.

REPAIR OF THE SOFT PALATE

The principle of good palatine reconstruction is to draw the velum backward (without doing the same to the palatine fibromucosa, because of the effects that this may have on maxillary growth), lengthening and prolonging it.

The first objective is reached by disconnecting the muscular insertions from the posterior bony borders of the palatine laminae, as well as from the area of the nasal floor that lies immediately behind them. Retrotuberal release incisions extended along the border between the fibromucosa of the palatine processes and the maxillary fibromucosa make it possible to create two small posteriorly pedicled flaps that are then sutured in the midline in order to cover the nasal floor; however, using a particular periosteal incision of the palatine fibromucosal flaps, we are able to obtain sufficient tension-free mobility, without any lateral release incision, to be able to withdraw the velum and simultaneously suture the flaps along the midline above the nasal floor. This has proved to be practicable in 80% of cases.[24]

The palate is lengthened by the careful reconstruction of the palatine musculature, and so we consider the use of Z-plasty according to Furlow[25] to be unphysiologic. In reconstructing the soft palate, we prefer to follow the principles of Pigott[20] in relation to the uvular muscle, beneath which we reconstruct the palatine levator muscle. When necessary (as in the case of a short palate) and feasible (for a cleft that is not too wide), we follow Delaire's[11] suggestion of using a series of small Z-plasties. The use of muscular reconstruction and Z-plasties makes it possible to obtain a true lengthening of the palate.

In order to obtain a tension-free muscle suture, we think that it is sometimes impossible to avoid fracturing one or both of the pterygoid hamuli; this is done without making any retrotuberal incision, but by using an appropriately positioned Trelat angular periosteal elevator that is subsequently gently pushed backwards. Extension of the palate can be obtained by means of the synthesis of the posterior palatine pillars and, in particular, of their musculature (the pharyngopalatini) as described by Sanvenero Rosselli.[26] After considerable experience in its use, we abandoned this technique some time ago because it did not seem to provide any particular functional advantages: the geniculum of the palate, which comes into contact with the posterior wall of the pharynx, is always represented by the posterior border

of the palatal levator muscle, and the synthesis of the palatine pillars sometimes pulls the palate downwards, possibly even hindering its raising during phonation (according to Pigott[20] the dynamic sphincter of Orticochea[27] sometimes improves velopharyngeal competence simply because of the fact that it sections the posterior palatine pillars!).

CHEILORHINOPLASTY

The objective of this operative phase is to restore the anatomy of the nose and lip in a manner that is as physiologic as possible by ensuring that the correct positioning of the various structures (particularly those of the nose) is the consequence of two principles: the wide-ranging release of the dislocated structures (above all the alar cartilage) and the careful reconstruction of the nasolabial muscles in such a way that they are responsible for the correct positioning of the released structures. It is certainly not the use of suspension or stitches or splints that will assure the quality of the result. Cleft lip surgery above all involves nasal surgery, and we shall see that, after the extended release, the reconstruction is first a rhinoplasty and then a cheiloplasty. The peculiarity of this procedure is the simple identification of some anatomic points without the need for measurements (which would have little meaning in relation to tissues that are retracted as a result of the cleft itself).

The objectives of the repair should be:

- symmetry of the nares both at the tip, with the raising of the ptotic dome, and at the base of the nasal alae, with floors at the same level
- a labial scar that is positioned in a way that is symmetrical with the contralateral crest of the philtrum
- a correctly reconstituted labial musculature, with good projection of the lip
- a continuous mucocutaneous line with the restoration of Cupid's bow
- a symmetrical red border
- a lip height that is the same on both the operated and the healthy side.

These objectives should be reached progressively, beginning from above (with the nose) and moving downwards (to the vermilion).

Drawing the cutaneous and mucosal incision lines

The drawing of the cutaneous incision line will vary depending on the extent of skin retraction and its distensibility, and the characteristics of the mucocutaneous rim.

The upper part of the drawing remains more or less constant but, as a result of the above-mentioned anatomic factors, the lower part may change even during the course of the operation itself. It is first of all necessary to identify the landmarks illustrated schematically in Figure 63.7.

The cutaneous incision is made on the inner stump, following an arcuate course that begins at 1 and passes medially to point 2, through point 3 before being continued to 4. From 2, it goes up along the mucocutaneous junction until it reaches the base of the alveolar process. The mucocutaneous border and the mucosa of the free side of the main stump is discarded. If the white roll is particularly accentuated, the mucocutaneous border is incised from 3 to C. On the small stump, an incision is made from 5 to 6 and then, providing the mucocutaneous line is not particularly pronounced, from 6 to 7 and from 7 to 8 (Fig. 63.8A); if it is pronounced, it is necessary to preserve that part of the white roll that runs from 7 to E in the form of a small triangular flap (Fig. 63.8B). Moving upwards, the incision is taken from 6, along the mucocutaneous border, until it reaches the base of the alveolar process of the small stump. The delimited mucosa of the free border of the small stump from these landmarks towards the skin can be preserved in the form of a flap pedicled to the alveolus for possible use in advancing the base of the nasal ala. As already stated, additional Z-plasties may be used to lengthen the lip after the reconstruction of the nose and the upper part of the lip musculature. Once the cutaneous incisions and the excision or preservation of the mucosa of the free border have been performed, the mucosa of the alveolar process of the small stump is incised from the border of the cleft to the molar region, maintaining a distance of at least 1 mm from the attached gingiva; this incision simultaneously involves the periosteum of the alveolar process. We have thus described the process for:

- recovering from both the internal and external stump the nasal skin that has 'migrated downwards' with the aim of reconstructing the nasal floor as effectively as possible

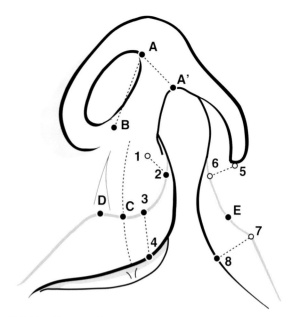

Fig. 63.7 Identification of landmarks before cheilorhinoplasty. A. The upper corner of the healthy nostril; A'. the upper corner of the cleft nostril; B. base of columella on the healthy side; C. the center line of the philtrum and of the future Cupid's bow; D. the peak of Cupid's bow on the healthy side; E. the end of the mucocutaneous rim on the small stump. 1. the landmark on the base of the columella on the cleft side, at a distance from the midline that is equal to the distance from the midline to B (the line B–1 will be parallel to the line A–A'); 2. the landmark at which the continuation of the line B–1 intersects the mucocutaneous line of the inner side; 3. the landmark on the mucocutaneous line, whose distance from the midline of the philtrum is just a little less than that of the distance C–D (in fact account must be taken of the transverse retraction of the skin); 4. the landmark on the border between the vermilion and the wet mucosa, identified by means of the line parallel to the midline of the lip drawn for landmark 3; 5. the base of the nasal ala on the cleft side; 6. the meeting on the mucocutaneous line of the perpendicular originating from landmark 5; 7. the landmark of greatest vermilion width on the cleft side, where the mucocutaneous rim begins to diminish (future lateral peak of Cupid's bow); 8. the point of passage between the vermilion and the wet mucosa on the perpendicular line to the mucocutaneous rim passing through landmark 7.

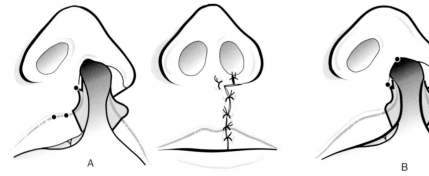

Fig. 63.8 The lower part of the skin incision varies according to the characteristics of the white roll: **(A)** incision without an evident white roll; **(B)** in a case of an evident white roll the insertion of the lateral white roll into the main stump is indicated.

- obtaining a scar location that is as similar as possible to the philtrum crest (although it may be necessary to perform a small Z-plasty in the lower part)
- reconstructing a good Cupid's bow and a normally shaped lip, with the elimination of the pathologic mucosa.

Finding the muscles on the sides of the cleft and their insertion zones

This is the decisive moment of the intervention insofar as its precise execution provides the possibility of making a correct muscular reconstruction. It is important to identify the muscle formations existing on both the external and internal stumps, as well as the insertions of the latter. The transversus nasi muscle can be found on the small stump, immediately beneath the nasal skin (above the line 5–6 – Fig. 63.7). This needs to be isolated on the prolongation of the line 5–6 to the base of the ala where, after the undermining of a few millimeters of skin, it is possible to find the levator labii superioris alaeque nasi muscle. Beneath the line 5–6, it is possible to identify the external orbicularis on the border of the cleft and, more deeply, the internal orbicularis whose lower part adheres to the vermilion. At the mucosal level, just a few millimeters of muscle should be identified, taking care not to detach the fibers of the levator labii superioris muscle at the base of the fornix; these fibers are inserted into the mucosa and will keep it well raised at the base of the fornix once the reconstruction has been completed. On the main stump, the extremity of the internal orbicularis is isolated from the mucosa, taking care not to involve the median frenulum. The periosteum of the vestibular surface of the premaxilla on the cleft side is laid bare, as is the nasal spine.

Subperiosteal undermining at the anterior part of the maxilla

In order to ensure tension-free suturing of the nasolabial musculature, the muscular insertions on the anterior face of the maxilla must be widely undermined. The most physiologic way of doing this is not supraperiosteally, as many authors have claimed, but subperiosteally, a procedure that does not seem to have any effect on facial growth.[28] The stressing and advancement of the periosteum even leads to new bone apposition on the external surface of the maxilla, which is underdeveloped precisely because of the collapse of the overlying musculature. Through the incision made in the fornix, the subperiosteal dissection has to be extended to the frontal branch of the maxilla, including its endonasal side, to the orbital rim (going around the infraorbital nerve), to the zygoma and as far as the maxillomalar buttress.

Subperichondral undermining and release of alar cartilage

In order to ensure that the reconstructed nasolabial muscular ring is in a condition to render the nasal deformities symmetrical, it is necessary to free the pathologic half of the nose completely from its connections with the healthy half. The pathologic alar cartilage must also be freed from its superficial cutaneous lining. This is done by reaching the lower border of the nasal septum at the level of the nasal spine, and then subperichondrally undermining all of the mucoperiosteum of the septum on the cleft side from its base as far as the tip of the nose and the nasal bones themselves. Subsequently, through incision 1–2 (Fig. 63.7), a pair of small blunt dissection scissors are used to dissociate the two medial crura, remaining exactly on the midline of the columella, reaching the tip and then extending the separation of skin from alar cartilage on the cleft side. The same undermining of the skin is performed on the dome of the healthy side and on the dorsum over the triangular cartilages of both sides. The freeing of the two halves of the nose is then completed by sectioning the midline connective bridges that separate the intercrural tunnel from the previously dissected septal subperichondral space. The base of the columella on the cleft side is then further released by means of submucosal dissection.

Reconstruction of the nasal floor, muscle, mucosa and skin

If necessary, the base of the ala is brought forward by means of an incision of the endonasal lining along the border of the pyriform aperture. Having positioned the small mucosal flap taken from the free border of the small stump (Muir[29] modified procedure), the nasal floor is reconstructed. We limit this to the anterior portion, without extending it to the alveolar cleft, so as not to find any scar at this level during subsequent surgery. The flaps are sutured from the deep layers towards the surface, initially limiting the suturing to the deeper parts. The mucosa is then sutured; if necessary, the mucosal flap can be mobilized by means of a small vertical incision in the most distal part of the previous incision made at the level of the fornix on the small stump. The mucosal suture begins posteriorly in the fornix and then runs medially to where the mucosal borders of the small and large stumps are sutured. In this phase, the suturing stops at the inferior third of the lip until it is completed (including the vermilion) at the end of the operation.

The next step is the most important phase of the intervention: the reconstruction of the muscles. This begins with the medial insertion of the transversus nasi which, after a small length has been isolated, is anchored in the original procedure to the base of the septum. In order to avoid excessive raising of the nasal floor and the base of the ala, and in agreement with Talmant,[30] we however prefer a lower anchorage on the periosteum of the premaxilla. Above this, the superficial and deep levator labii muscles, as well as the external orbicularis, are sutured to the nasal spine and the corresponding contralateral muscles. This is followed by suturing the internal orbicularis toward the vermilion. Precise juxtapositioning of the previously identified and tattooed landmarks of the mucocutaneous borders is essential. Two results are thus immediately obtained: the nares are made symmetrical, with correction of alar ptosis, and the upper lip is projected (taking on the shape of a ship's prow). The intervention is then completed with the suturing of the skin in the most superficial part of the nasal floor and the upper half of the lip. The lower half of the lip is carefully sutured subcutaneously, as is the landmark of the mucocutaneous border, regardless of whether the initial incision was linear or in the form of a small triangle containing the white roll. At this point, it is necessary to evaluate the symmetry of the lip: if it is symmetrical or only slightly short, the skin of the lower half can also be sutured; if it is too short, it is possible to perform a small Z-plasty just above the line of the mucocutaneous border. It is essential that, even after the Z-plasty, the lip is symmetrical or at most only slightly short. A lip reconstructed using a small Z-plasty, if it changes at all, will tend to increase in length,[31] and it is easier to perform a secondary correction of a short lip than one that is too long.

The intervention concludes with careful reconstruction of the vermilion. In order to ensure optimal continuity, the mucosal layer should be released for a few millimeters from the underlying orbicularis, after the muscle has been previously sutured using a few very thin nylon stitches (6–0), and carefully sutured. The final procedure is the completion of the suture of the internal mucosa of the lower third of the lip, which was excluded from the first phase of the intervention. After this, some transfixing stitches should be applied at the nasal ala and dome simply to reduce the hematoma between the external and endonasal skin (Fig. 63.9).

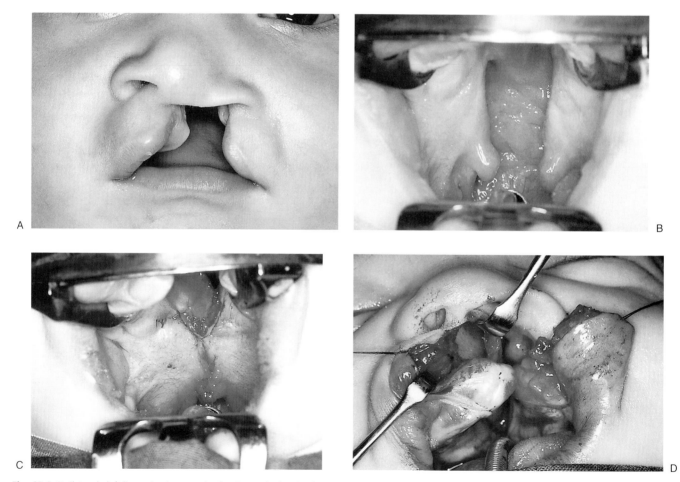

Fig. 63.9 Unilateral cleft lip and palate repaired at 5 months by simultaneous cheilorhinoplasty and soft palate repair. **(A)** Preoperative view, note lip and nose deformities and the width of the cleft; **(B)** preoperative view of the wide hard and soft palate cleft; **(C)** immediate postoperative view after soft palate repair without lateral release incisions; **(D)** intraoperative view showing wide nasal dissection (not the same case);

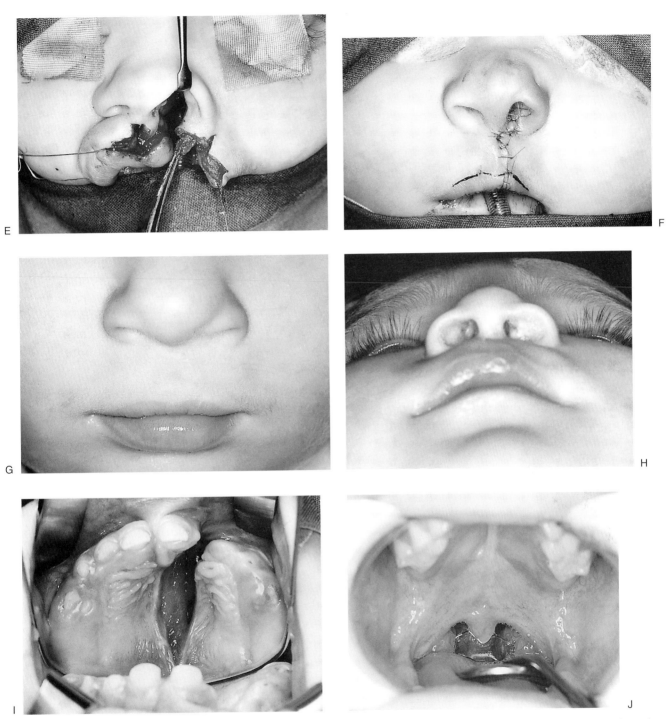

Fig. 63.9(contd) **(E)** intraoperative view showing the muscular preparation: note, on the lateral stump, the separation of the transversus nasi muscle from the orbicularis oris muscle (not the same case); **(F)** immediate postoperative view after lip and nose repair; note the reconstructed Cupid's bow; **(G,H)** lip and nose appearance two years after surgery; **(I)** residual hard palate and alveolar cleft before gingivoalveoloplasty; **(J)** soft palate appearance five years after surgery.

No medication or restraint (Logan's arch) is necessary because the reconstruction must be free of tension. We prefer to remove the stitches (including the transfixing stitches) on the fifth day with the patient under sedation. Feeding by breast, bottle or spoon can be resumed on the day of the operation without any problem. The baby is only required to wear rigid arm braces for a fortnight.

REPAIR OF A TOTAL BILATERAL CLEFT

In these cases, the timing of the intervention is partly determined by the position of the premaxilla and the small stumps: if these are favorably positioned, surgery is recommended from the fourth month. As already described in the case of total unilateral clefts, the operation begins with the repair of the soft palate, the only difference being that no attempt is made to reconstruct the nasal layer by means of vomerine flaps. The vomer is vertically underdeveloped in its posterior part, and reconstruction of the nasal layer by suturing it to the vomerine flaps would cause a high anchorage of the nasal floor and subsequently hampered maxillary growth (particularly vertically). We therefore prefer to suture the two nasal layers directly together below the intact vomer at the posterior part of the hard palate.

After completing soft palate reconstruction in the same way as for unilateral clefts, the next step is to reconstruct the lip, both sides of which are repaired during the same surgical session.

The objectives of the repair are:

- symmetrical nares
- the repositioning in the columella of the skin that has descended into the prolabium (which thus leads to lengthening of the columella)
- the symmetrical reconstruction of the lip and the vermilion, with a Cupid's bow, scars positioned along the crest of the philtrum, and the reinsertion of the underlying muscles.

These objectives are reached progressively, moving from above (nose) to below (vermilion), and from the deepest point (floor of the nose and mucosal layer) to the surface (skin).

In cases in which the columella is extremely short, we first lengthen it using the techniques of McComb[32] or Mulliken[33] (see articles for details). Although this differs from Delaire's philosophy, it is the only aspect of the reconstruction that differs for these particular cases from the procedure described below.

Drawing the cutaneous and mucosal incision lines

The upper part remains the same for both the premaxilla and the lateral stumps; the lower part may be approached in one of two different ways depending on the quantity of white roll on the lateral stumps.

The outline drawn (Fig. 63.10A,B) on the lateral stump is exactly the same as that used for unilateral clefts: a perpendicular line from the base of the ala to the mucocutaneous junction separates labial skin from the skin of the nasal floor, and a skin incision is made at this level. Having identified the point that will correspond to the tip of Cupid's bow, if there is little white roll, it is necessary to identify on the free border of the vermilion the point at which it begins to decrease in thickness, which is then joined by an incision that reaches the point on the mucocutaneous junction corresponding to the future tip of Cupid's bow. From here, following the mucocutaneous border, the incision is extended upwards until it reaches the base of the alveolar process, and the circumscribed mucosa is either removed or used to advance the nasal ala as described above for a unilateral cleft.

If the white roll is highly accentuated, from the point corresponding to the tip of the future Cupid's bow, the cutaneous incision is drawn from just above the white roll and along the mucocutaneous border as far as the base of the alveolar process, without eliminating anything during this phase.

The subsequent steps – identification of the nasolabial muscles, incision of the alveolar mucoperiosteum, and wide subperiosteal undermining on the anterolateral side of the maxilla – are exactly the same as those described for the treatment of a unilateral cleft.

In the prolabium, as in the lateral stump, there is a concentric cutaneous contraction due to the absence of muscle distension, and the descent of the skin of the columella into the prolabium itself. This means that it is necessary to identify where this border should be. Given that their anatomic characteristics are very similar, it can be considered that, in the dimension running from the upper inside angle of the nares to the future top of Cupid's bow on the skin of the prolabium, the upper half is columellar skin and the lower half labial skin.

Two symmetrical points (2) are therefore marked on the ideal extension of the lateral borders of the columella, and the points of the two peaks of Cupid's bow (3) are identified. These last points need to be closer to each other than may appear to be correct at first sight because the ensuing cutaneous distension caused by the musculature will separate them considerably. From point 2 to point 3 an incision is performed following a curve medially concave, then the

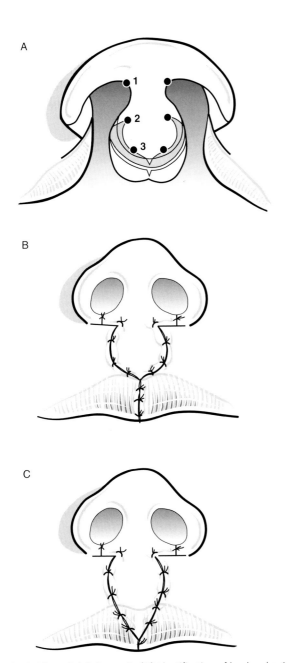

Fig. 63.10 Bilateral cleft lip repair. **(A)** Identification of landmarks: 1. upper corner of cleft nostril; 2. point marked on the ideal extension of the lateral borders of the columella (considering that in the dimension running from 1 to 3 the upper half is columellar skin, and the lower half is labial skin); 3. points of the two peaks of Cupid's bow; on the lateral stumps, as in a unilateral cleft, a perpendicular line from the base of the ala to the mucocutaneous border separates labial skin from the skin of the nasal floor. **(B)** The cleft repaired. **(C)** Unlike Delaire, if there is little white roll in the lateral stump, we prefer to descend with an incision from the two mucocutaneous points (3) to 4–5 mm inside the prolabial mucosa, thus circumscribing and preserving a mucosal triangle with a superior base that will constitute the center of the reconstructed lip.

skin delimited by the incisions takes on the shape of a shield, and the mucosa of the prolabium is in part eliminated and in part used to construct the premaxillary mucosal lining of the fornix. From point 2 another incision is made perpendicular to the mucocutaneous junction; once the junction is reached it is prolonged to the level of the bone.

Unlike Delaire, if there is little white roll in the lateral stump, we prefer to descend with an incision from the two mucocutaneous points (3) to 4–5 mm inside the prolabial mucosa, thus circumscribing and preserving a mucosal triangle with a superior base that will constitute the center of the reconstructed lip (Fig. 63.10C).

Whichever of these two approaches is used, the prolabial skin is lifted by cleaving it from the underlying periosteum. The nasal spine and lower border of the septal cartilage is reached, and these are exposed together with the lower border of the pyriform aperture. At this point, we also perform a certain degree of bilateral subperichondral and subperiosteal undermining of the septum in order to ensure good mobility when advancing and projecting the columella and the tip of the nose.

After having bilaterally reconstructed the posterior part of the anterior nasal floor and sutured the mucosal flaps of the lateral stumps at the level of the alveolar incision laterally and together on the midline, we move on to reconstruct the muscles. As in the case of a unilateral cleft lip, we first suture the transversus nasi muscle on both sides to the vestibular periosteum about halfway up the premaxilla; then, above this muscle, we suture the highest part of the external orbicularis of the two sides to the apex of the nasal spine, at the level of the septo-premaxillary ligament. Muscle suturing then continues in the direction of the vermilion until the border of the lip is reached. Given that this suture considerably narrows the distance between the skin sides of the two lateral stumps, it is worth separating the skin from the underlying musculature for a distance of a few millimeters in order to be able to position the cutaneous portion of the prolabium. After eliminating the subcutaneous excess that is usually present on the underside of the prolabial cutis, while taking care not to damage its vascularization by over-thinning, a median subcutaneous stitch is used to anchor the point separating the columellar and prolabial skin to the base of the septum (this leads to the redistribution of columellar skin in its natural location and also somewhat lengthens the columella itself). Proceeding equally on both sides, the anterior part of the nasal floor and the upper part of the skin suture are completed. There is often a vertical disproportion between the skin of the lateral segments and that of the prolabium, the latter seeming to be deficient as a result of the lack-of distension. In such situations, we never lengthen the prolabial skin, but prefer

incision is continued to the midline following a curve whose concave side is downward (and always remaining above the mucocutaneous border); at the midline, it meets the corresponding contralateral incision. In this way, the prolabial

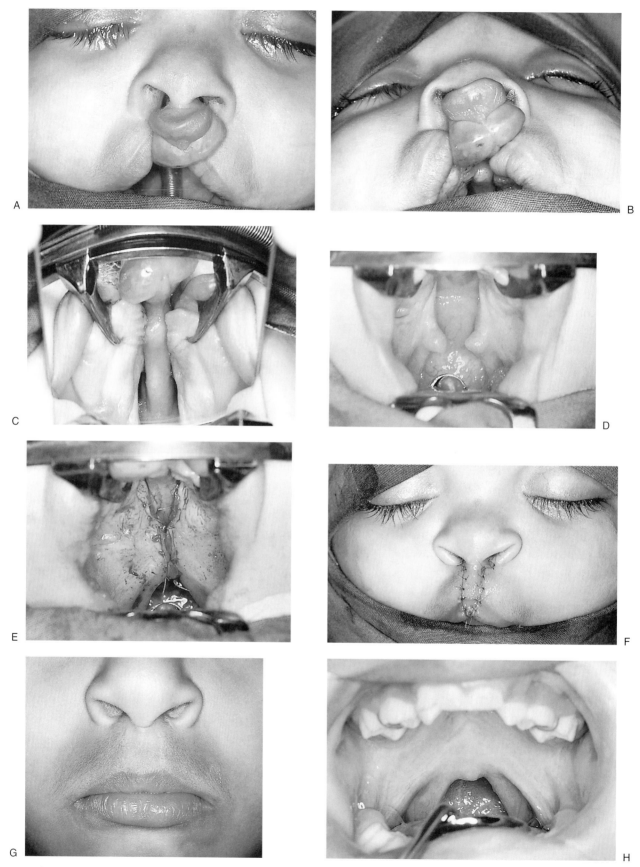

Fig. 63.11 Bilateral cleft lip and palate repaired at 6 months by simultaneous soft palate and lip plasty. **(A–D)** preoperative view; **(E,F)** postoperative view; **(G,H)** lip, nose and soft palate appearance five years after surgery.

to adapt the skin of the lateral stump to the skin of the prolabium (without any lateral skin resection) by first suturing the landmarks at the level of the mucocutaneous rim that were drawn at the beginning of the procedure for the purpose of reconstructing Cupid's bow. This obviously leads to some stretching of the skin of the prolabium and the presence of an excess of skin laterally. This is done whether the triangle of prolabial mucosa has been preserved (when the white roll is not very definite), or whether all of the prolabial mucosa has been sacrificed and it is intended to reconstruct Cupid's bow using the mucocutaneous rim of the lateral stumps.

Even in the case of marked underdevelopment of the prolabial skin, in our experience the action of the underlying muscular cingulum has always led to its vertical growth over time, thus making it possible to obtain a well-proportioned lip (there is nothing less esthetic or more difficult to correct than a bilateral lip with an exaggerated vertical dimension) (Fig. 63.11).

SPECIFIC PRIMARY PROCEDURES

LIP ADHESION

As already mentioned in our discussion on the preoperative orthopedic treatment of premaxillary protrusion, there are rare cases in which poor parental collaboration, or the fact that the child is first seen when he/she is already of a suitable age for the operation, means that the protrusion of the premaxilla is such as to advise against a primary lip repair as described above. The excessive tension to which the soft tissues would be subjected could lead to a greater risk of dehiscence, as well as poor quality muscle reconstruction and scarring.

In such cases recourse can be made to lip adhesion, which transforms a total cleft into a partial cleft, followed by an

orthopedic molding capable of ensuring that the premaxilla is subsequently displaced to a position which will allow a good definitive lip repair. Delaire[8] recommends the reconstruction of the transversus nasi muscle, the upper part of the lip and the nasal floor, without worrying about the correct reconstruction of Cupid's bow and the lower part of the lip (Fig. 63.12); this intervention would be performed at the age of 4–5 months together with the repair of the palate. About 10 months later, the anatomic situation should allow definitive lip repair at the same time as the repair of the residual cleft of the hard palate and gingivoalveoloplasty.

On the other hand, other authors prefer simply to suture the skin and mucosa of the upper half of the lip.[34] Even though there is no muscular cingulum to act on the premaxilla, we have obtained excellent results using this simpler and less invasive procedure which has enabled us to perform second-stage surgery on intact rather than scarred tissue (the inevitable result of the former procedure) and thus create an optimal muscular, mucosal and skin reconstruction.

PRIMARY LENGTHENING OF THE COLUMELLA

As we have seen, columellar repair using prolabial skin makes it possible to achieve a certain lengthening of the columella. When the columella is extremely short (or practically absent), however, we prefer to use more effective primary procedures. Given the anatomic observation that the shortness of the columella is caused only by the lateral migration of the alar domes, which are also twisted downwards and have therefore lost their correct relationship with the triangularis cartilage,[32] the rationale underlying our approach is that the correct positioning of the domes leads to normal length of the medial crus and good projection of the tip of the nose. This can obviously only be achieved after the extensive perialar release and muscular recon-

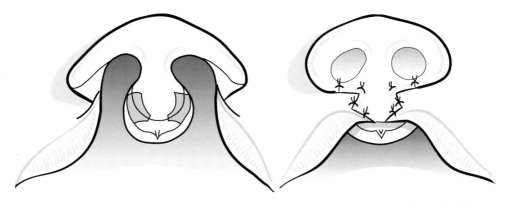

Fig. 63.12 Lip adhesion according to the Delaire concept of reinserting the transversus nasi muscle and reconstructing the upper part of the lip and the nasal floor.

struction described above in order to eliminate the cause of the dislocation of the cartilaginous domes. The access and strategy for releasing and repositioning the domes vary from author to author. McComb[32] prefers a V incision (to be Y sutured) at the tip of the nose, which allows the method to be performed exactly as necessary with a wide access; however, the considerable lengthening of the columella is obtained at the cost of a rather visible scar and a bulbous nasal tip. The intervention should preferably be performed at the same time as lip adhesion in order to avoid detaching the prolabium from the premaxilla and the consequent problems of premaxillary vascularization that this can involve.

Mulliken[33] obtains the same result using a marginal incision associated with a short midline cutaneous incision on the tip of the nose, an intervention that is performed at the same time as the definitive muscular and cutaneous reconstruction of the lip. The median scar is practically invisible, whereas the cutaneous excision that needs to be made at the upper angle of the nares can sometimes lead to a little residual asymmetry.

REPAIR OF THE HARD PALATE WITH GINGIVOALVEOLOPLASTY (GAP)

After the primary repair of the lip and soft palate, there still remains the problem of repairing the hard palate and alveolomaxillary cleft. As a result of the modeling action of the reconstructed anterior orofacial and posterior soft palate muscular cinguli, the residual cleft undergoes a gradual narrowing which, although it maintains the harmonious form of the alveolar arch, brings the alveolar borders of the cleft into contact with each other and, at the level of the palate, sometimes reduces the cleft to negligible proportions. But although the alveolar stumps are in contact with each other, there is still a gap (usually of a few millimeters) between the bone stumps underneath the alveolar mucoperiosteal lining. Nevertheless, premaxillary growth is optimized not only by muscle reconstruction, but also by the mucoperiosteal continuity of the nasal floor, the palate and the vestibular side of the alveolar process. The vertical and anteroposterior growth of the small stump is also favorably influenced by its connection to the main stump, with which it forms a single complex that is influenced by the growth of the nasal septum and by the harmoniously reconstructed functional matrix. The restoration of maxillary continuity finally allows the correct eruption and alignment of the deciduous teeth, making early orthodontics possible and stable, even in the case of those teeth erupting at the level of the cleft.

For all of these reasons, and starting with the experience of Millard[35,36] who performed his intervention during the course of labioplasty and therefore (because it was necessary to have the stumps in contact with each other) made use of an active and rather invasive preoperative orthopedic procedure, Delaire[10] perfected his GAP technique, which he performed at the time of the repair of the hard palate when the patients were aged 14–18 months.

From the point of view of the execution of the technique, the mucoperiosteal flaps that are prepared at the level of the alveolar flaps are practically identical[37] to those described by Boyne and Sands[38] for a secondary bone graft (Fig. 63.13). The cervical incision begins at the level of the central incisor and is extended laterally until it reaches the border of the cleft. It then passes around the mesial border of the cleft to the base of the fornix, from where it descends on the distal side of the cleft until reaching the neck of the canine or, if this has not yet erupted, the alveolar crest of the first molar. The cervical incision continues distally for at least 1 cm (in the neck of the second molar or, if this is absent, along the alveolar crest) until reaching the base of

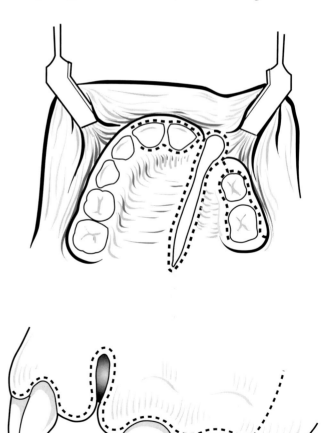

Fig. 63.13 Gingivoalveoloplasty (GAP). Gingival and mucosal incisions are shown on the palate (above) and vestibular (below) surfaces, extending along the cleft borders.

the fornix by means of a release incision. On the palatal side, the incision follows the borders of the cleft until it reaches the soft palate. After extensive subperiosteal undermining, during which the posterior border of the palatal process is skeletonized in order to be able to obtain the freedom for a further posterior dislocation of the soft palate by means of the subsequent median suture, the palatal and vestibular sides of the nasal plane are reconstructed.

Providing the incisions have been correctly positioned, there are never any problems in suturing the nasal plane apart from the difficulties of execution which, in the case of the narrowest clefts, may require the use of microsurgical instruments. The hermetic reconstruction of this plane is vital in order to achieve a good result. Given the narrowness of the cleft and the ogival shape of the palate, the suturing of the palatal plane can usually be carried out without any difficulty. In the majority of cases of broader clefts, the closure can be obtained without lateral release

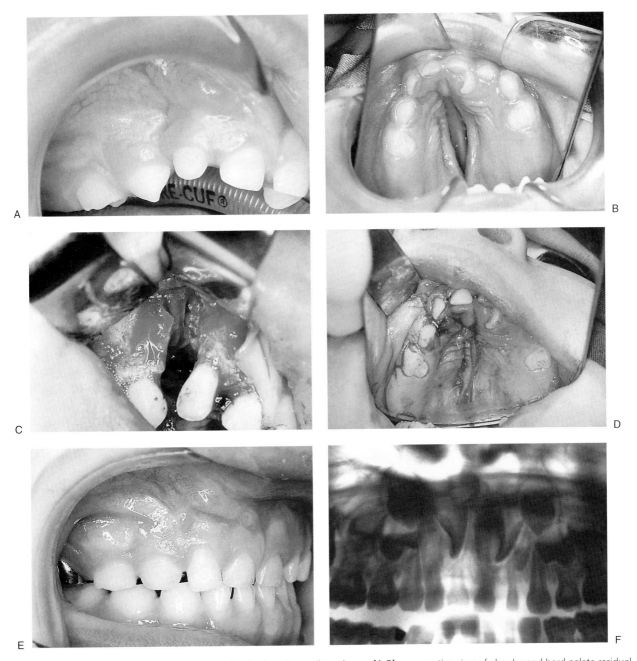

Fig. 63.14 Alveolar and hard palate closure by gingivoalveoloplasty in a unilateral case. **(A,B)** preoperative view of alveolar and hard palate residual cleft; **(C)** intraoperative view of alveolar cleft after closure of the nasal and mucoperiosteal flaps and before vestibular mucoperiosteal flap suture; **(D)** immediate postoperative view of hard palate and vestibular suture; **(E)** alveolar morphology three years after gingivoalveoloplasty; **(F)** panoramic X-ray: note the spontaneous bone obliteration of the right alveolar cleft from the floor of the nose to the alveolar margin.

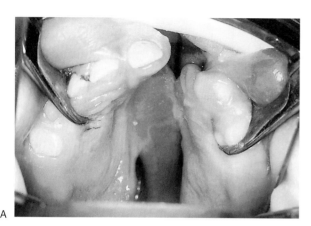
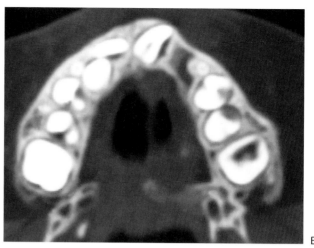

Fig. 63.15 Unilateral cleft lip and palate before and after treatment. **(A)** Preoperative view of alveolar and hard palate cleft; **(B)** CT scan: note the maxillary bone continuity and good thickness on the cleft side after gingivoalveoloplasty.

incisions by means of submucosal section of the fascia of the tensor of the palate and the periosteum.[24] This avoids the need for bare lateral surfaces whose secondary healing may have consequences for the growth (particularly transverse) of the maxilla and the alveolar arch. We only make a release incision when this procedure is not possible (in the case of a flat palate or a very broad residual cleft), and then if possible only on the main stump at the border between the maxillary and gingival fibromucosa.

The repair of the vestibular plane should be preceded by releasing the distal vestibular flap by a periosteal incision at the base of the flap in such a way as to allow it to be brought forward without any tension. This creates a pyramidal space between the above-mentioned mucoperiosteal planes by which the bony borders of the cleft are faced. The insertion of reabsorbable material (Surgicel, Spongostan, etc.) into this space has the sole purpose of keeping the nasal plane well elevated in order to obtain extensive vertical ossi-

fication in which the eruption of the permanent teeth can be as physiologic as possible (Figs 63.14 and 63.15).

The procedure is almost identical in the case of bilateral clefts, the difference being that the nasal plane is completed with septal mucoperiosteum only in its anterior third, in order not to anchor the nasal plane to the septum in the central and posterior part of the hard palate (which could have negative repercussions on the vertical growth of the maxilla), and the undermining of the vestibular periosteum of the premaxilla must be reduced to a minimum in order to maintain the adherence of broad surfaces of soft tissue to the vestibular face of the premaxilla and thus ensure its vascularization (Fig. 63.16).

At an optimal age for the beginning of phonation, the procedure ensures the definitive closure of the palate with the minimum of surgical insult (only subperiosteal undermining with no secondary healing), and also a precise and anatomic reconstruction of the mucoperiosteal functional

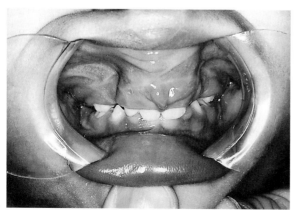
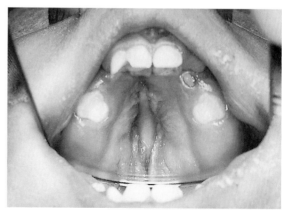

Fig. 63.16 Bilateral alveolar and hard palate cleft repair by simultaneous gingivoalveoloplasty. **(A,B)** Preoperative view;

matrix of the maxilla. This leads to the ossification of the alveolomaxillary cleft by means of excellent quality bone which, in the great majority of cases, does not require the secondary bone graft needed after primary procedures involving periosteal grafts or flaps.[39–41] These latter procedures in fact do not faithfully reconstruct the anatomy of the alveolar region, and the result is a modest quantity of bone that is usually insufficient for good tooth eruption. On the other hand, post-GAP ossification is of excellent quality in 95% of cases,[37] a finding that we have recently confirmed by means of CT investigations.[42]

The quality of the results from the point of view of mucoperiosteal morphology, and therefore ossification, is proportional to the width of the cleft, and so a good primary muscle reconstruction that harmonizes the relationships between the maxillary stumps is very important, particularly in bilateral cases.

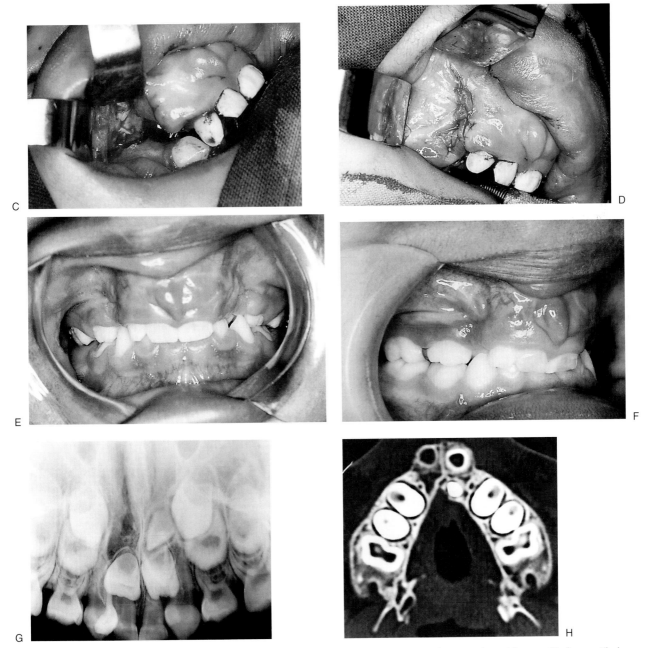

Fig. 63.16(cont'd) **(C)** intraoperative view of the right alveolar cleft after closure of the nasal and oral mucoperiosteal flaps and before vestibular mucoperiosteal flap suture; **(D)** immediate postoperative view of the right alveolar cleft repair; **(E,F)** dental occlusion and alveolar morphology four years after surgery; **(G,H)** status X-ray and CT scan showing good bone ossification at the alveolar clefts (both horizontally and vertically).

CLEFT PALATE

As is known, an isolated cleft palate is an entity in itself, and its treatment protocol is also different. The procedure itself depends on the width of the cleft. In the case of particularly wide clefts, especially in the anterior part (as can be seen in Robin syndrome), closure by means of the submucosal release procedure is impossible, and so we prefer to reconstruct the soft palate at an age of 6–8 months and postpone the repair of the hard palate until the patients are 14–18 months old or even older, depending on its gradual narrowing. It is known that the transposition of flaps, even with vast areas of healing by secondary intention, has practically no consequences on maxillary growth at an age of 10–12 years.

If the cleft is not particularly wide, however, Delaire[10] has developed a hard palate procedure that makes use of bi-pedicled flaps of only the fibromucosa of the palatal laminae, delimited by means of a mucoperiosteal incision that runs to the border between the maxillary fibromucosa and that of the palatal laminae. This requires two secondary healing areas whose location has practically no negative effect on maxillary growth. The procedure is best carried out at an age of 10–12 months.

We have never used this technique because, especially in the presence of a cleft that is not particularly wide, our own procedure of fibromucosal release[24] has always allowed us to obtain a tension-free midline suture of the palatal flaps without any lateral release incisions (the incidence of fistulae and dehiscence in our patients is 2%) and with a certain degree of posterior dislocation of the soft palate.

Soft palate cleft and submucous cleft (if identified early) is treated at an age of 10–12 months using the same procedure as that described for a complete labiomaxillopalatal cleft. Early treatment greatly reduces the frequency of functional problems.[43]

CLEFT LIP

A cleft lip, be it complete or incomplete, with or without a cleft of the primary palate, can be operated on at an age of four months insofar as the base of the maxilla is healthy or only fissured in its anterior portion, and is therefore capable of sustaining earlier muscle reconstruction.

The principles of the reconstruction are the same, with the identification of the areas of nasal skin that have slipped downwards. In the case of an incomplete cleft this skin is apparently excessive; however, not too much of this skin should be eliminated because, on the basis of the principles already described, after muscle reconstruction involving more or less wide-ranging subperiosteal undermining and primary rhinoplasty (depending upon whether or not there are also nasal deformities), the skin adjusts to the underlying muscle bed and any excess on the nasal floor normalizes in a short time.

Skeletal involvement may range from mild clefting (more evident on the nasal floor than at the alveolar level) to a complete alveolomaxillary cleft of the primary palate. In the former case, primary periosteoplasty is performed during the course of the reconstruction of the musculature and the nasal floor by raising the latter from the underlying fissured or depressed bone plane and inserting reabsorbable material in the periosteal pocket in order to keep the nasal plane raised. In the case of a complete cleft of the primary palate, providing the diastasis is not too accentuated, primary gingivoalveoloplasty according to the procedure described above is indicated. It is necessary to remember that the raising of the mucoperiosteal plane will be more difficult as a result of the underlying presence of unerupted tooth germs. On the other hand, if the cleft is very wide and the premaxilla is externally rotated, it is better to limit the initial intervention to cheilorhinoplasty and to schedule the gingivoalveoloplasty for when the patient is 14–18 months old and his/her anatomic condition is more favorable with the stumps in contact.

CONCLUSIONS

It seems to us to be important to summarize here the points that Delaire considers to be fundamental to his philosophy of the primary treatment of cleft lip and palates:

1. The dissection and identification of the nasolabial muscles on the external borders of the clefts.
2. The extended subperiosteal undermining of the anterior of the maxilla, the nasal pyramid, the malar body and the lower orbital border.
3. The subperichondral undermining of the nasal septum of the cleft side extending to the nasal bone.
4. The identification of the anterior border of the septum, nasal spine and septo-premaxillary ligament.
5. The separation of the crus medialis and the domes of the alar cartilages on the midline and their release from the overlying skin.
6. The reconstruction of the muscular planes of the nasal floor and the threshold of the nares, with the fixation

of the musculature to the septum and the septo-premaxillary ligament.

7. The reinsertion of the external orbicularis to the nasal septum and the contralateral musculature.

8. The reconstruction of the rest of the lip: mucosa, musculature and skin.

9. The two-stage closure of all wide palatal clefts (soft palate first).

10. The one-stage closure of narrow clefts using the fibromucosa of the palatal laminae.

11. The reconstruction of the anatomo-functional equilibrium of the palate by moving backwards and making a sphincter at the anterior part, lengthening the intermediate part (small Z-plasty) and extending the posterior part (bringing together the posterior palatal pillars).

12. Closure of the soft palate at 6 months and the hard palate at 14–16 months; hard palate repair can be postponed up to the age of 3 years if dislocation of the maxillary fibromucosa is needed.

13. The vomerine mucoperiosteum is not used in palate closure because this may cause a defect in the vertical development of the palate itself.

14. If the patient is first seen after the age of 12 years, even very broad clefts can be surgically treated by means of the mobilization of the entire palatal fibromucosa without interfering with maxillary growth.

REFERENCES

1. Delaire J 1975 La cheilo-rhino-plastie primaire pour fente labio-maxillaire congenitale unilaterale. Essai de schematisation d'une technique. Revue de Stomatologie 76:193–215
2. Delaire J 1976 Influence du voile du palais sur la statique linguale et la croissance mandibulaire. Deductions therapeutiques. Revue de Stomatologie 77:821–834
3. Delaire J, Feve JR, Chateau JP, Courtay D, Tulasne JF 1977 Anatomie et physiologie des muscles et du frein median de la levre superieure. Premiers resultats de l'electromyographie selective. Revue de Stomatologie 78:93–103
4. Delaire J, Chateau JP 1977 Comment le septum nasal influence-t-il la croissance premaxillaire et maxillaire. Deductions en chirurgie des fentes labio-maxillaires. Revue de Stomatologie 78:241–254
5. Delaire J 1978 The potential role of facial muscles in monitoring maxillary growth and morphogenesis. In: MacNamara monograph no. 8: Cranio growth series. Center for human growth and development, The University of Michigan, Ann Arbor, Michigan
6. Delaire J 1978 Theoretical principles and technique of functional closure of the lip and nasal aperture. Journal of Maxillofacial Surgery 6:109–116
7. Delaire J, Precious D 1985 Avoidance of the use of vomerine mucosa in primary surgical management of velopalatine clefts. Oral Surgery, Oral Medicine and Oral Pathology 60:589–597
8. Delaire J 1989 Le revetement cutaneo-muqueux dans les fentes labio-maxillaires. Deductions chirurgicales. In: Brunati S (ed) La

rehabilitation fonctionelle chirurgicale et orthopedique des fentes labio-maxillo-palatines congenitales. Tipografia Cesare Nani, Vol II. Lipomo, Como, Italy, pp 13–26
9. Delaire J, Precious D, Gordeeff A 1989 Interet des grands decollements sous-periostes dans la correction chirurgicale primaire des fentes labio-maxillaires. In: Brunati S (ed) La rehabilitation fonctionelle chirurgicale et orthopedique des fentes labio-maxillo-palatines congenitales. Tipografia Cesare Nani, Vol II. Lipomo, Como, Italy, pp 27–30
10. Delaire J 1989 Premiers resultats de la gingivo-periosto-plastie primaire (avec ou sans osteo-plastie). In: Brunati S (ed) La rehabilitation fonctionelle chirurgicale et orthopedique des fentes labio-maxillo-palatines congenitales. Tipografia Cesare Nani, Vol II. Lipomo, Como, Italy, pp 121–131
11. Delaire J, Mercier J, Gordeeff A, Bedhet N 1989 Les trois fibro-muqueuses palatines. Leur role dans la croissance du maxillaire. Deductions therapeutiques dans la chirurgie des divisions palatines. Revue de Stomatologie et de Chirurgie Maxillo-faciale 90:379–390
12. Delaire J 1991 Un exemple de chirurgie physiologique: la rehabilitation 'primaire' du premaxillaire dans le fentes labio-maxillaires. Revue d'Orthopedie Dento Faciale 25:453–475
13. Tajima S 1983 The importance of the musculus nasalis and the use of the cleft margin flap in the repair of complete unilateral cleft lip. Journal of Maxillofacial Surgery 11:64–70
14. Talmant JC 1993 Nasal malformations associated with unilateral cleft lip. Accurate diagnosis management. Scandinavian Journal of Plastic and Reconstructive Surgery and Hand Surgery 27:183–191
15. Latham RA 1969 The septopremaxillary ligament and maxillary development. Journal of Anatomy 104:584
16. Fara M 1977 The musculature of cleft lip and palate. In: Converse JM (ed) Reconstructive plastic surgery, Vol IV. Saunders, Philadelphia
17. Kernahan DA, Dado DV, Bauer BS 1984 The anatomy of the orbicularis oris muscle in unilateral cleft lip based on a three-dimensional histological reconstruction. Plastic and Reconstructive Surgery 73:875–879
18. Veau V 1931 Division palatine, anatomie, chirurgie, phonètique. Masson, Paris
19. Kriens O 1970 Fundamental anatomic findings for an intravelar veloplasty. Cleft Palate Journal 7:27
20. Pigott RW 1976 Objectives for cleft palate repair. Annals of Plastic Surgery 19:247
21. Hotz M, Gnoinski WM 1976 Comprehensive care of cleft lip and palate children at Zurich University: a preliminary report. American Journal of Orthodontics 70:481–504
22. Ross RB, Johnston MC 1972 Cleft lip and palate. Williams & Wilkins, Baltimore
23. Georgiade NG, Latham RA 1975 Maxillary arch alignment in the bilateral cleft lip and palate infant, using the pinned coaxial screw appliance. Plastic and Reconstructive Surgery 56:52
24. Brusati R, Mannucci N 1994 Repair of the cleft palate without lateral release incisions: results concerning 124 cases. Journal of Craniomaxillofacial Surgery 22:138–143
25. Furlow LT Jr 1986 Cleft palate repair by double opposing Z-plasty. Plastic and Reconstructive Surgery 78:724
26. Sanvenero Rosselli G 1973 Labiopalatoschisi. In: Filipo G (ed) Patologia otorinolaringoiatrica e cervico-facciale. UTET, Torino
27. Orticochea M 1983 A review of 236 cleft palate patients treated with dynamic muscle sphincter. Plastic and Reconstructive Surgery 71:180
28. Mannucci N, D'Orto O, Di Francesco A, Brusati R 1997 A comparison of the effect of supraperiosteal versus subperiosteal dissection on growing maxilla in rabbits: an experimental study. In: Lee ST (ed) Proceedings of the Eighth International Congress on Cleft Palate and Related Craniofacial Anomalies, Singapore
29. Muir J 1966 Repair of the cleft alveolus. British Journal of Plastic Surgery 19:30–36

30. Talmant JC 1995 Reflexions sur l'etiopathogenie des fentes labio-maxillo-palatines et l'evolution de leurs traitements. Annales de Chirurgie Plastique et Esthetique: 40:639–656

31. Brusati R, Mannucci N, Biglioli F, Di Francesco A 1996 Analysis on photographs of the growth of the cleft lip following a rotation-advancement flap repair: preliminary report. Journal of Craniomaxillofacial Surgery 24:140–144

32. McComb H 1990 Primary repair of the bilateral cleft lip nose: a 15-year review and a new treatment plan. Plastic and Reconstructive Surgery 86:882–889

33. Mulliken JB 1995 Bilateral complete cleft lip and nasal deformity: an anthropometric analysis of staged to synchronous repair. Plastic and Reconstructive Surgery 96:9–23

34. Randall P, Graham WP 1971 Lip adhesion in the repair of bilateral cleft lip. In: Grabb WC, Rosenstein SW, Bzoch KR (eds) Cleft lip and palate. Little Brown, Boston

35. Millard DR 1980 Cleft craft III. Little Brown, Boston, pp 263–298, 355–382

36. Millard DR, Latham RA 1990 Improved primary surgical and dental treatment of clefts. Plastic and Reconstructive Surgery 86:856–871

37. Brusati R, Mannucci N 1992 The early gingivoalveoloplasty. Preliminary results. Scandinavian Journal of Plastic and Reconstructive Surgery and Hand Surgery 26:65–70

38. Boyne PJ, Sands NR 1972 Secondary bone grafting of residual alveolar and palatal defects. Journal of Oral Surgery 30:87–92

39. Skoog T 1965 The use of periosteal flaps in the repair of cleft of the primary palate. Cleft Palate Journal 2:332

40. Rintala AE, Ranta R 1989 Periosteal flaps and grafts in primary cleft repair: a follow-up study. Plastic and Reconstructive Surgery 83:17

41. Stricker M, Chancholle AR, Flot F, Malka G, Montoya A 1977 La greffe periostee dans la reparation de la fente totale du palais primaire. Annales de Chirurgie Plastique 22:17

42. Brusati R, Mannucci N, Autelitano L 1996 Computed tomography evaluation of alveolar cleft treated by primary gingivo-alveolo-plasty. Journal of Craniomaxillofacial Surgery 24(suppl 1):22–23

43. Dorf DS, Curtin JW 1982 Early cleft palate repair and speech outcome. Plastic and Reconstructive Surgery 70:74

The traditional 'Millard' approach to lip and palate repair

64

MAURICE Y. MOMMAERTS

INTRODUCTION

The Millard unilateral cleft lip repair has become the most popular single procedure in cleft palate treatment in use today. This indicates its validity as a physiological procedure and reflects the marked influence Millard has asserted in the field of cleft surgery. Because of his total dedication to improving surgical outcome, he designed many concepts in cleft surgery, of which some were accepted while others were discarded after analysis. Some are still under evaluation. Millard was one of the early proponents of a lip adhesion as an orthopedic procedure to mold palatal segments to their normal geometric relationship. He was also among the first to advocate primary rhinoplasty without external incisions. His concept of using the 'island flap' for palatal closure was not successful. That procedure involved vast mucoperiosteal stripping at an early age which proved to be detrimental to transverse and anteroposterior maxillary growth. In 1983 he implemented an active redesigned presurgical orthodontic and primary gingivoperiosteoplasty regimen to obtain early esthetics, to close the floor of the nose, and to avoid secondary alveolar bone grafts.

In this chapter, a detailed overview of Millard's accomplishments and thought processes for primary cleft surgery is presented. It does not reflect the preference of the author and his cleft palate team, although a modification of the skin incision design and the alar shift procedure, and a similar lip adhesion are used in their treatment plan for unilateral clefts.

We are also thankful to Berkowitz for reporting some of his experience and supplying a few photographs of Millard's and his patients.

UNILATERAL CLEFT LIP REPAIR

The first rotation-advancement repair was executed in 1954 on a Korean boy with an incomplete cleft.[1] The technique was presented at the first International Congress of Plastic Surgery in Stockholm in August of 1955 and it was first published in its transactions in 1957.[2] It was soon adopted for complete clefts.[3] The rotation-advancement lip repair has been subject to some refinements, extensions and modifications during its forty years of existence. Most of them were introduced by the originator himself, according to his motto 'semper investigans, numquam perficiens'.

RATIONALE OF THE TECHNIQUE

The technique is based on flexibility in uniting the lip, guided by certain principles. The principles are Ambrose Paré's 'To restore to their place things which are displaced' and the Gillies 'Never throw anything away until you know you do not need it',[2] which became principles 14 ('Return what is normal to normal position and retain it there') and 18 ('Invoke a Scot's economy') in Millard's book *Principlization of Plastic Surgery*.[4] The flexibility of the technique is reflected in the advice to 'cut-as-you-go' and the adaptability to the individual pathomorphology of the affected area.

Millard viewed a cleft lip 'as if nature had left out a portion and she had allowed distortion of what remained'.[5,6] Thus, the medial lip element which was rotated out of its distorted position needed to be retained by an advancement flap from the lateral lip element, hence the 'rotation-advancement' was born. A minimal amount of tissue is discarded.

FUNDAMENTAL ACTIONS OF THE SURGICAL TECHNIQUE

1. Rotation. The main component of the lip on the non-cleft side has two thirds to three quarters of a cupid's bow, a median tubercle in the vermilion, and one column of the philtrum and its associated dimple. All of this is rotated down into the normal position.

2. Advancement. An advancement flap fills the gap and corrects the alar flare and the wide nostril.

The scar is maneuvered into hidden crevices, under the columella, and the lower part simulates a natural landmark, the philtrum column.

INCISION DESIGN

The curved incision in the medial cleft lip element, in its lower part a mirror image of the contralateral normal philtrum column, should cross the midline under the columella to allow the downward rotation of the cupid's bow by 2 to 10 mm and to allow the philtrum dimple component to come into normal position (flap A) (Fig. 64.1A). At the same time, it will lengthen the short side of the columella by freeing it from the lip. Millard stressed frequently that the common mistake is insufficient rotation, which leads to a cupid's bow sitting slightly askew and to a shorter cleft side. In 1964 he suggested the implementation of a 45 degree 'back-cut' of 1 to 2 mm, not passing beyond the

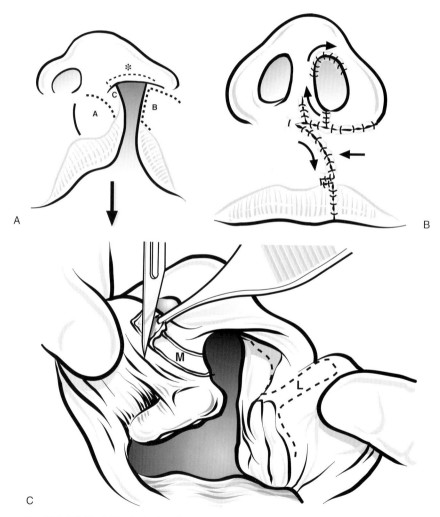

Fig. 64.1 **(A)** The Millard I design: the rotation flap A, the advancement flap B, and the nostril sill advancement flap C. A small rotation flap was used to correct the slumping alar margin. **(B)** The 1964–1968 refinements (Millard II design) depicted: a back-cut if 1 to 2 mm (x), rotation of the C-flap into the columella and a small rectangular 'white roll flap'. **(C)** The Millared III design: The M (medial) flap was used as oral layer in the anterior hard palate, and the L (lateral) flap to line the nasal vestibule after alar base release. The m-m medial muscle edge flap was used to bolster the high lateral muscle defect. Callipers were used to match lip flap segments. Nasal morphology benefited from a primary alar lift and a bolster of the denuded alar base flap into the columella.

normal philtrum column, to gain more rotation.[7] The back-cut lowers the horizontal scar into the lip, and the incision should therefore skirt the columella.[8] The rotation gap created by the back-cut was more than half closed by flap C being rotated into it, and half by flap B being advanced into it (Fig. 64.1B). In the 1968 article, the importance of maintaining the rotation with a 'key suture' of the tip of the advancement flap in the back-cut gap was emphasized.[9] Many surgeons still avoid the back-cut since it increases the gap and requires more tissue from the hypoplastic flap B to be advanced. This increases the amount of obliquity in the upper portion of the scar, and the chance of scar hypertrophy.[10] Mohler extends the marking at the medial side into the columellar base a specific distance and then utilizes a 90 degree back-cut, aiming to create a straight philtrum column instead of a curved one. Flap C is left long and fills the rotation gap completely.[10] This is an adaptation to variations of the normal.

The lateral cleft lip element provides an advancement flap (flap B) (Fig. 64.1a), whose tip fills the gap created by rotating flap A. The tip consists of tissue from Simonart's band in incomplete clefts, tissue from the nostril floor when available in wide complete clefts, or tissue advanced from under the alar base in a 'cut-as-you-go' fashion. This creates tension high in the lip which reduces a wide nostril floor and protrudes the lower portion of the lip, resulting in the semblance of a pout. The maxilla splints the tension and avoids distortions in the free border of the lip. The cleft edge on the cleft side is freshened a distance to match the length of the rotation incision on the opposite side. In the beginning this was also performed in a 'cut-as-you-go' fashion,[2,5] but soon the distances were measured with calipers,[3] and later wires were used to compare opposite sides.[11,12] A vermilion flap is turned off flap B to give the necessary length. The lower endpoint of the incision corresponds very closely to the point at which the 'white line' or mucocutaneous ridge disappears on the lateral side of the lip.[13]

Flap C was primarily destined to form the nostril sill and to absorb a part of the pull at the tightest point in the closure. It pulls the deviated columella and anterior septum into a straight position. In 1964, Millard advocated lengthening the cleft side of the columella by advancing flap C into the defect in the columellar base.[7] This defect becomes apparent when a hook is placed in the height of the nostril on the slumped side. This sliding advancement was later facilitated by a membranous septal incision.[14] Sliding one half of the columella onto the other seems to have originated with Ericksen in 1869,[15] and was perfected by Holdsworth with scissor dissection between the medial crura.[16] It can lengthen the columella by 2 to 4 mm and in

the meantime brings fullness at the columellar base.[8] Any excess length of flap C, usually only a small amount of tissue, can be excised so that flap C lies within the nasal vestibule and forms the medial part of the nostril sill.

A minute, 1 mm wide rectangular[7] or triangular[13,17,18] flap is raised at the end of the 'white line' on the lateral side of the lip element. This 'white roll flap' breaks up the basically straight line as it joins the vermilion, interrupting the vermilion red and the pink scar (Fig. 64.1B). It also slightly increases the length of the medial side.[13]

COMPARISON WITH CONTEMPORARY INCISION DESIGNS

The rotation-advancement design originated as a lop-sided Z-plasty, with its horizontal limb high in the lip, and its long leg curved to mimic a philtrum column. Millard stressed the importance of not crossing natural landmarks: 'Any scar that criss-crosses normal lines will pass if a good scar is achieved, but if a bad scar happens to develop then its unnatural position exaggerates its effect'.[3,6]

At that time, cleft surgeons tried to lengthen the cleft lip side with a flap from the lateral lip element into the lower part of the medial element like Tennison[19] and LeMesurier,[20] or into the upper and lower part like Trauner[21] and Skoog.[22] A Z-plasty in the lower part transsects the philtral column and creates side-to-side tightness, especially along the free border and most markedly in wide clefts. The introduction of a flap into the lower portion of the philtrum flattens the dimple whereas insertion of the flap high above this drops the philtrum without diminishing its dimple. *In the author's opinion, this is the most important asset of the rotation-advancement technique.*

Because the natural landmarks are preserved and only a little tissue is discarded, the technique lends itself to complete revision surgery, e.g. re-rotation if primary rotation was inadequate. This is not feasible with other techniques.

MILLARD I, II, III AND IV DESIGN

The design with the refinements – such as the advancement of the C-flap into the columella, the back-cut for the A-flap and the 'white roll flap' – published in 1964 and 1968, was coined the 'Millard II' by Musgrave.[23] In 1974 and 1976 Millard proposed saving the parings of the cleft sides, called the m (medial) and L (lateral) flaps.[11,12] The M-flap was used for oral closure of the anterior hard palate, or for lining the buccal sulcus. The L-flap, after Mir y Mir[24] and Muir[25] was used to fill the vestibular gap produced during the release of the alar base from the maxilla. The high lateral muscle defect in the tip of the advancement flap, sometimes noted as a secondary grooving in the upper aspect of the lateral lip element, was bolstered with a medial (m-m) or lateral (l-m) muscle edge flap. Millard started also to measure the distance from the commissure to the cupid's bow peak at the non-cleft side and to transfer this to the lateral lip element. The marking was a limiting point for the paring of the advancement flap. These adjuncts, together with a primary alar lift, a denuded alar base flap sutured to the septum and a preliminary lip adhesion, prompted him to label it the 'Millard III' method (Fig. 64.1C).[11]

In 1983, the concept of producing a horizontal nasal platform before the final lip and nose repair was optimized by introducing active orthopedics with a pinned screw appliance and a gingivoperiosteoplasty that permanently stabilizes the corrected segmental relationship.[26] The sequence of active orthopedics, gingivoperiosteoplasty and lip adhesion, followed at 6 to 8 months with rotation-advancement repair of the lip and primary correction of the nose with alar cartilage freeing and lifting, columella lengthening and alar base cinching, can be called the Millard IV method.

MOBILIZATION OF THE B-FLAP

Millard performed wide radical supraperiosteal undermining as far as the infraorbital foramen in all types of clefts, but to a degree found necessary by trial in each case.[2,3,5,18,27] This was aimed at dividing abnormal muscle attachments and allowing muscle approximation at the point of tension. In 1954 he started performing an incision around the alar base in wider complete clefts in order to have differentiated advancement of the B-flap and the alar base flap.[9,27,28] When he started with primary alar lifts, he found that sometimes a nasal mucosa incision was necessary along the piriform aperture to advance the B-flap and the ala, and to free the lateral crus.[9] The gap created was filled with the L-flap later on.[11]

Most surgeons place an incision in the labial sulcus extending to the area of the first molar tooth, and perform just enough dissection, in a supraperiosteal plane, of lip and cheek tissue from the maxilla, to obtain a tension-free closure.[13,29] Excessive tension and undermining may produce increased scarring in the lip that can unfavorably influence maxillary growth.[30,31]

ORBICULARIS ORIS MUSCLE

Nicolau[32] noted that the orbicularis oris consists of two layers of muscle fibers: one is inserted into the philtral ridges and skin, the other is a deeper layer that has little or no attachment to the skin. In an incomplete cleft lip, the muscles on the medial side of the cleft exhibit more hypoplasia and do not extend to the cleft margin to the degree that they do on the lateral side. This may explain why bulging of the orbicularis oris is more obvious in the lateral portion than on the medial side, where it is usually undetected.[33] In complete clefts, the superficial fibers of the orbicularis oris muscle may insert into the columella and septum medially and into the alar base laterally.[34,35]

From his first publications, Millard has always stressed careful muscle approximation.[2,5] The skin and mucosa along each side to be approximated are undermined several millimeters to facilitate separate and individual suturing of the muscle, mucosa, and skin. Wide undermining at the medial side is contraindicated since it will destroy the philtral dimple and column. The rotation component is not quite enough for horizontal muscle alignment; in wide incomplete clefts in particular, a deficiency in tissue bulk in the tip of the advancement flap can leave a groove. In 1974 and 1976, Millard proposed dividing the muscle transversely under the deficient area, rotating the caudal muscle fibers until they attain an horizontal position, and filling the muscular defect with a medial muscle (m-m) flap (Fig. 64.1C).[11,27] Leaving some muscle cranially in the B-flap and suturing it in the back-cut extension removes tension from the skin wound edges.

VERMILION

In the first publications, Millard stated that the vermilion of the cupid's bow on the medial cleft side tends to thin out. He proposed bolstering it with lateral lip vermilion, either as an onlay flap, as a central tongue into a dart, or as a posterior interdigitation (Fig. 64.2).[2,3,5] Millard gave up the medial mucosal overlaps because he experienced excess of vermilion in an unnatural position.[36] If the lateral lip element is weak in vermilion, then an interpolated mucosal pedicle from the medial cleft edge can be inserted laterally. If both are weak in vermilion then each will welcome the other's flap, at least in part.[3] When there is a shortness of vermilion a vertical V–Y type of advancement of the posterior mucosa, or a Z-plasty will even the line of the free border (Fig. 64.2).[3,7,9,13,18,37] Later on, Millard stated that lengthening of the vermilion by a vestibular Z-plasty is often unnecessary in the long run.[36] A small zigzag is sufficient.

Another guide for proper alignment of the vermilion is the 'red line' that divides the extraoral vermilion from the intraoral vermilion. Typically there is a distinct change in

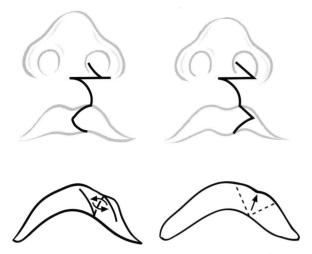

Fig. 64.2 Bolstering of medial or lateral deficient vermilion with a contralateral mucosal flap. A vestibular Z-plasty or a V–Y plasty to correct vertical shortness of the vermilion.

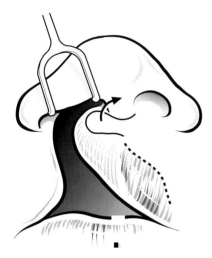

Fig. 64.3 Reichert's method of lengthening the medial lip segment with a rotation flap of the nostril sill. The vermilion tapers at the cleft edges and careful adaptation of the 'red line' is necessary to prevent a red spot in the vermilion that tends to crust when dried out.

color at this point. V–Y or Z-plasties can be used to match the 'red line'.

VESTIBULUM

After a lip adhesion procedure, M- and L-cleft edge flaps can be turned upwards on the alveolus to deepen the sulcus.[27] These flaps are superfluous in most cases.[31]

LENGTHENING THE VERTICAL AXIS

The problem of the lateral lip element

The lateral lip element varies in three areas:

1. the amount of tissue present medial to the alar base
2. the vertical height from the alar base to the presumed peak of the cupid's bow
3. the thickness of the lateral lip vermilion.[38]

The lateral lip element is short when compared with the non-cleft side. This shortness exists regardless of the severity of the cleft, and it involves the lateral vermilion, commonly deficient in bulk, as much as it does skin deficiency.[39]

In incomplete clefts, the lateral lip element can be longer, which can be treated with a high horizontal lentoid resection[38] or by patterning the upper margin of the B-flap.[18,12] In complete clefts, the lateral lip is always deficient in height. It is commonly presumed that attaining proper vertical height of the lateral lip is not a problem in the incomplete cleft lip. Millard recognized that the main problem of the rotation-advancement technique seemed to be a shortness in the vertical lip length, and the length from the nasal floor to the commissure.[9] Compared with other repair techniques, the Millard method tends to produce shorter lips.[40,41] Amaratunga measured a 13.9% shorter philtral edge height with Millard's method.[42]

Looking for solutions

Randall, as quoted by Millard (1976), stated in 1971 that there are three reasons for peaking of the cupid's bow at the cleft side:

1. not enough rotation and not enough lateral paring
2. straight scar contraction
3. orbicularis oris sweeping up.[43]

Not enough rotation

The failure to rotate adequately and to provide an advancement flap of sufficient length and width is quite common. This ends in the cupid's bow and the vermilion sitting askew. A back-cut was introduced to enable more rotation. The medial insertion of the white roll flap, meant to prevent the 'bleeding up' of the scar, also lengthens the medial element by bringing the cupid's bow peak down by 1.5 to 2 mm. Also Meyer,[44] Onizuka,[45] Lintilhac[46] and Bernstein[47] used an inset of a tiny Tennison flap, a triangle of less than 2.5 mm, to lengthen the medial side of the cleft instead of a small rectangular 'white roll flap'. Lengthening at the medial side with a rotation flap from the inner aspect of the columella was proposed by Reichert.[48] This, though, takes away valuable tissue from the columella (Fig. 64.3).

Not enough lateral paring

Millard reasoned initially that lateral paring to match the rotation incision would carry to good thick vermilion and would provide a turn-back flap of excess vermilion which can be dove-tailed across the cleft behind the lip or interdigitated to bolster the weak side of the cupid's bow.[2] Over-lifting of the lateral lip element with attenuation of the vermilion on the cleft side can occur when the advancement flap is deficient.[7] It was only in 1974 that Millard took account of the distance between the commissure and the cupid's bow peak at the non-cleft side as a limiting factor for the paring of the lateral lip element.[11] 'Digression of the lateral incision past the marking is rarely necessary and should be limited to 2 mm at most, in order to avoid excessive shortness of the distance between the peak of the Cupid's bow and the commissure on the cleft side.' (Figs. 64.4, 64.6C)[13,27] According to many, the small difference in the left and right distances from the commissure to the cupid's bow is insignificant and hardly noticeable.[31]

However, vermilion height was also seen to be short with Millard's method (compared to LeMesurier) (Fig. 64.4). This is because the narrow vermilion from the lateral element is brought to the middle, which is necessary in Millard's method in order to match philtral edge height. In LeMesurier's method, the quadrilateral flap brings down vermilion from the cleft edge which is thicker and therefore produces a more symmetric vermilion.[42] Millard accepts that his method produces an asymmetric, attenuated vermilion and he has designed a V–Y plasty as a secondary procedure to correct this problem.[3,7,18] The need for a V–Y procedure is usually avoided by a Z-plasty of posterior mucosa during the primary procedure.[7,9,18]

Another of Millard's 'tricks' is to make the cleft side concave, to match the convex medial side, but also to lengthen it a little by more paring (Fig. 64.5),[11,17] after the concept of Von Graefe's straight line closure.[49] Asensio is extending this concept by a Rose and Thompson like lengthening of flap B. This involves triangular paring and bringing in a quadrangular tip. The C-flap is turned underneath the alar base.[50,51] This means lateral lengthening at the expense of more horizontal scarring and midlip tension (Fig. 64.5).

Incorporation of as much nasal vestibular tissue as possible in the advancement tip is mandatory to gain height (Fig. 64.6C).[3,5–7,9]

Millard also proposes raising the upper horizontal incision to include a bit of alar base.[11,17] (Fig. 64.5) Arrunategui transplants a whole-thickness semilunar postauricular graft under the alar base to bring the ala up.[52]

Millard has also proposed trimming of the vermilion free border at the non-cleft side to match its counterpart.[7]

Straight scar contraction

The most common criticism reported is what is referred to as 'contracture of the scar'. Contracture occurs mainly in the long oblique line of the lop-sided 'Z'.[31] Lip scar hypertrophy, partial or total, occurred more frequently following rotation-advancement repair than after triangular repair.[53] Some report notching during the first weeks or months.[5,31] Millard says that if this is present one year after surgery it represents, in all probability, either failure to rotate enough or inadequate filling of the rotation gap.[3,7,18] While the softening continues for years, the straightening may take as long.[16] All literature on the subject agrees that the primary

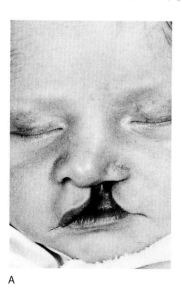 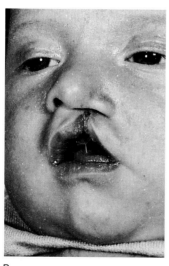 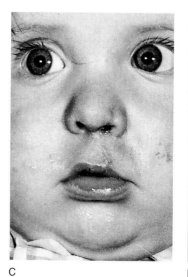 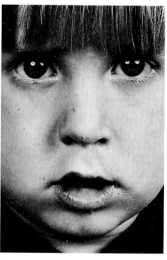

A   B   C   D

Fig. 64.4 Facial photographs of Millard III-type of lip repair. **(A)**: new-born with unilateral cleft lip and palate. **(B)**: after lip adhesion. **(C)**: at 8 months. **(D)**: at 4 years of age (patient operated by Dr Millard. Photographs courtesy of Dr Berkowitz).

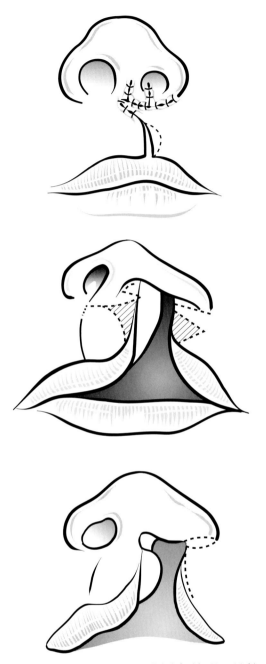

Fig. 64.5 Technique to lengthen the medial cleft side: Top: Making the cleft side incision more concave to match the rotation incision does also lengthen it. Middle: Asensio's technique of triangular paring of the cleft side. Bottom: incorporation of alar base into the advancement flap.

length, attained at the end of the procedure, will reappear.[38]

Orbicularis oris sweeping up

To prevent the orbicularis oris sweeping up, a lateral muscle flap can be placed into the medial vermilion. This can result in an off-center bulge.[43]

More on skin and muscle deficiency in the lateral lip element

In 1965 Cosman & Crikelair pointed out the absolute deficiency of tissue in the unilateral cleft lip of a roughly trapezoidal shape, with the magnitude of the defect greatest beneath the nostril floor rather than at the vermilion border of the lip.[54] (Fig. 64.7) The medial triangular defect is reconstructed with the Millard procedure, but not the lateral triangular defect. In complete clefts the advancement flap is stretched over the lateral and medial defect, pulling up the lateral lip element. In our opinion this is the main cause of the short lateral vertical axis.

We are looking for a solution for this problem. The muscular defect beneath the alar base is corrected with the Delaire musculo-aponeurotic reconstruction of the nasolabial muscles. A disadvantage of this is the increased height of the nostril floor. The rotation incision is also carried into the columella, to avoid the horizontal scar ending in the upper lip. The C-flap is shifted up into the columella, to lengthen both the columella and the vertical axis at the medial cleft side. The C-flap fills the gap created by the rotation incision almost completely. The B-flap is not used to contribute to the reconstruction of the medial triangular defect. Paring of the B-flap is based upon the width from the commissure to cupid's bow, the total height of the vermilion, and the position of the 'red line'. Extending the incision more laterally to obtain more height of the B-flap will inevitably lead to a stretched lateral vermilion, diminutive both in width and in height (Fig 64.4). The difference between the medial vermilion bulge and the lateral hypoplastic vermilion will be accentuated with smiling. Vermilion height can be partially corrected with V–Y roll down flaps, bringing out non-keratinized mucosa. The mismatch in the red line can be corrected with a Z-plasty or horizontal V–Y plasty. Vermilion width cannot be corrected, however, except with a lip switch technique.

Instead of pulling the B-flap up and over the lateral defect, it is rotated downward together with the underlying muscle fibers. When marking, rotating and advancing the B-flap, a triangular defect will become visible under the alar base, as predicted by Cosman & Crikelair,[54] and noted by Arrunategui (Fig. 64.6D).[8] This defect in the skin envelope can be filled with a nasolabial rotation flap. This is sound in principle: the tissue loss is replaced with tissue in kind (principle 15), borrowed from the cheek that can afford it (principle 19), with an acceptable scar in the donor area (principle 20) (Fig. 64.6).[4] The disadvantages are the horizontal scar, the dog ear, and the flattening of the alar-facial crease (Fig. 64.6G).

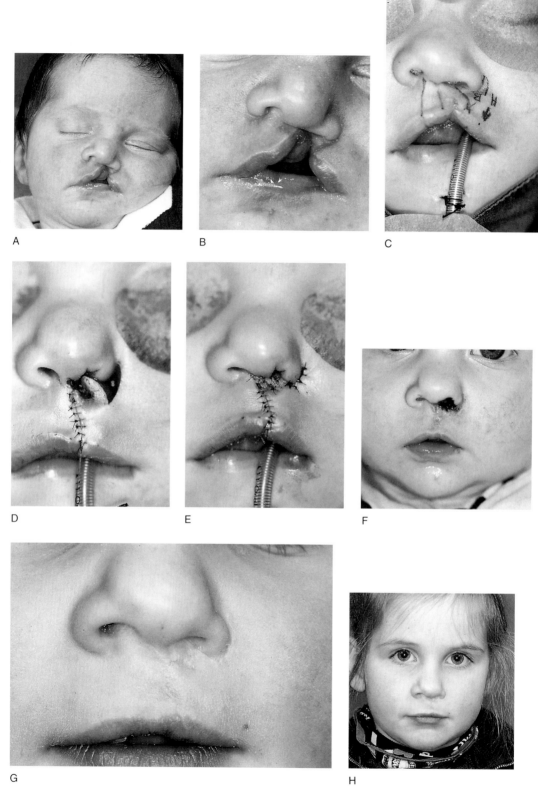

Fig. 64.6 Sequence of unilateral cleft lip repair with a nasolabial rotation flap. **(A)** & **(B)** Presurgical views. **(C)** At age 4 months, after lip adhesion at age 3 weeks and presurgical orthopedics with passive guidance plate. The right philtrum column is marked, the Mohler modification of the incision at the medial side, flap B extending into the nasal vestibule and the nasolabial flap. 'H' marks the end of the incision at the lateral side, that would achieve proper height. 'B' marks the end of the incision that would achieve proper width. The incision line marking ends 2 mm lateral to point 'B', in order to gain more height by taking some of the width. The discrepancy in this case is so big that a nasolabial flap was rotated to gain more height. **(D)** Rotation of the nasolabial skin flap in the upper part of the lip underneath the alar base and the nostril. The alar cartilage has been freed and advanced into the nasal tip. **(E)** After suturing, proper lateral lip height is accomplished. **(F)** Two weeks postoperatively. **(G)** & **(H)** Final lip appearance at age 3.5 years.

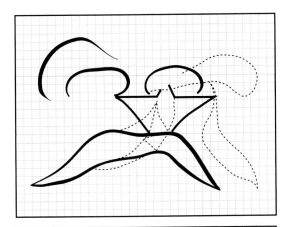

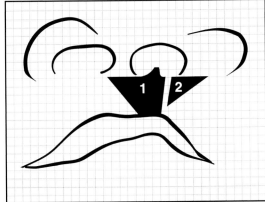

Fig. 64.7 Absolute deficiency in the medial and lateral cleft lip side according to Cosman and Crikelair (1965).

NOSE

The alar rim and the alar cartilages

The medial crus is inferiorly placed in the columella, and the cartilage is peripherally positioned along the alar margin. The lateral crus creates a spine in the vestibular web.[14]

Millard did not mobilize and reposition the alar cartilages in his first publications.[2,5] Berkeley's principle of primary repositioning of the alar cartilage with an external incision seemed sound to him, but not the incision.[3] The drooping alar arch was primarily corrected with a crescentic Kilner-like excision of skin and alar cartilage.[2,3,5] He took more skin, less lining, and least, if any, cartilage.[3] A medial nick in the lining layer can be used to allow its upward advancement of 1 or 2 mm with maintenance of an improved arch along the alar margin (Fig. 64.1A).[7] This technique was later reserved for minor nasal deformities.[9]

In 1964 Millard preferred to wait until early adulthood for the nasal work. He used a marginal incision to free the cartilage, lift and suture, and to bolster it with a free graft of normal alar cartilage.[3]

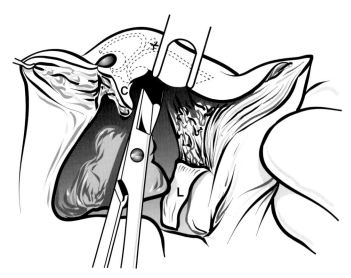

Fig. 64.8 The lateral vestibular incision is extended along the intercartilaginous line up to the membranous septum. The alar cartilage is freed from its skin cover and the chondromucosal flap is tied up to the opposite septum. The L-flap is used to prevent contracture.

Brown & McDowell[55] freed the slumped alar cartilage from the overlying skin and combined it with through-and-through mattress sutures tied externally, including skin on the uninvolved side. The alar correction was not always dramatic and was seldom permanent.[14,55] Wynn combined the through-and-through mattress suturing of the lateral crus to the lining and cover with medial through-and-through mattress suturing of both medial crura to their lining.[56] Millard preferred internal suspension and was inspired by Reynolds & Horton, who used suspension on either side of the dome to the opposite upper lateral cartilage.[57]

A full correction may require up to a 5 mm shift of the lateral crus in some cases, and it does not seem possible that this can be achieved with intact mucosa.[29] In the mid 60s Millard used marginal and intercartilaginous incisions to make a chondro-mucosal flap, tied to the opposite septum, taking up some slack in the vestibular lining. But he noticed scarring of the marginal incision and contracture, though this appeared to correct.[58] In 1974 he stopped using the marginal incision and extended the lateral freeing incision along the intercartilaginous line up to the nasal tip joining the membranous septal incision. Lateral ala release was obtained and contracture was prevented by an L-flap (Fig. 64.8).[11,13,25,27]

It is unclear if he used a secondary L-flap in the final lip repair, although one was used during the lip adhesion procedure.[14] Salyer uses the L-flap in 50% of his cases, but with little improvement.[31]

In 1982, Millard performed an alar lift at the age of five years, sometimes earlier.[14] The lateral cartilage was freed from its attachments and advanced and fixed through a marginal incision.[14] One Prolene 4/0 suture was used to lift the proposed new crus angle, then the tip of the medial crus was sutured to the septal tip to force a fixed arch for better contour.[14] This not only reduces the web, but allows the base of the flap of cartilage to shift up during the lift and partially fill the unnaturally deep alar crease. Sometimes Millard used bolstering, from the opposite cartilage or auricular cartilage.[14] Excess vestibular mucosa was trimmed. At one time, through-and-through sutures were tied over a rubber catheter to draw the free vestibular lining up against the repositioned alar cartilage for improved vestibular vault and airway.[14] Millard continued to use the same technique and the same sequence in 1986.[4] In 1989, he was using the 1974 approach[59] and in 1993 and 1996 he again showed a marginal and an intercartilaginous-membranous septum incision.[28,60] In the mid 80s, Millard started to correct the alar cartilage malposition at the time of the lip repair.[60] In his opinion, this was possible because the Latham appliance, the lip adhesion, and the gingivoperiosteoplasty had created a symmetrical bony platform.

Nostril sill, alar base and nasal floor

The perimeter of the cleft and normal ala do not differ much,[54] but the cleft alar base is flared, and the nostril floor can be very wide. Advancement of the B-flap can produce a relative tightening of the nostril. It adjusts in time with a gentle spread. If not, a later tuck by a wedge excision of the normal ala will even the alae.[3] A wedge excision of a wide nostril floor may also be indicated.[5] Some lateral alar drift was noted in certain cases, hence the alar base was cut free from the lateral lip element primarily and its tip was denuded of epithelium so that this freed component could be advanced beyond the advancement of the lateral lip flap and sutured to the septum at the nasal spine for a more permanent fixation.[4,11,14,60] This flap, denuded of epithelium, pulls the underlying nasalis muscle fibers to a more medial position.

Millard closes the nasal floor with a mucoperichondrial flap from the septal side and a mucoperiosteal one from the lateral nasal wall; these are mattress-sutured before the lip closure.[27]

Vestibular webbing, caused by greater rotation of the alar base medially, is correctable by a later Z-plasty.[13]

Septum

Before the combination coaxial orthopedic appliance and gingivoperiosteoplasty was used, Millard freed the deflected septum from its vomerian groove, straightened it by scoring

at the non-cleft side, and held it in place by suturing it to the upper edge of the lip muscle from the cleft side.[27] He preferred to do a corrective rhinoplasty at the age of 16 years.[4,11] When the septal deviation was not severe, he also postponed the septoplasty until that age.[4]

In the 80s, with the advent of the Latham appliance, Millard describes that the cant of the septal portion is remarkably corrected by the orthopedic appliance as it pivots in the vomerian groove and gradually assumes a vertical (upright) stance.[28,60]

Compared to other techniques

The alar flare and the wide nostril are only partly corrected with LeMesurier and Tennison's methods.[37,61] Compared to the latter method, major secondary nasal deformity surgery has been recommended less frequently in rotation-advancement repairs.[53,62] Until the mid 80s, Millard preferred to postpone the alar lift until the age of 4½ to 5 years, because he found the cartilages to be friable and severely adherent to the nasal lining, which itself is extremely thin.[60] For more than 10 years, Millard has now performed primary cheilorhinoplasties (Millard IV).

ALVEOLAR SEGMENT MOLDING PRIOR TO LIP REPAIR

The aberrant muscle forces in a complete unilateral cleft lip and palate pull the lateral palatal segments laterally, and the tongue pushes them apart.[64] Some believe that the small segment is not just smaller but is also retro-displaced within the face. Berkowitz has shown that the cleft segments in complete unilateral and bilateral clefts are not posterior but can be deficient in mass as well as distorted in their spatial relationship.[64] Segment molding will generally advance the smaller segment. Millard has always been an advocate of early segmental repositioning to be able to perform the lip and nose repair on top of a symmetrical supporting maxillary platform. This is according to principle 14 'Return what is normal to normal and retain it there'.[4,7] When primary bone grafting became 'en vogue', Millard for a short time placed rib grafts in certain cases of maxillary alveolar deficiency because he believed that this could be a partial remedy for the problem.[7,9] In the last 20 years he has found presurgical orthopedics to be of great value in aligning the cleft maxilla to correct the asymmetric foundation of the nose, but it was some time before the orthodontic opportunity was realized.[14] Once, confronted with a wide cleft of exceptional severity in a Jamaican girl, he began thinking of performing a lip adhesion as a preliminary procedure in establishing muscle continuity.[7]

Then, from 1963 on, he used a lip adhesion in very wide clefts in both unilateral and bilateral cleft lip and palate patients when the infant was 2 to 3 weeks old.[11] It was a simple first stage approximation of the superior one third of the lip cleft with two cleft edge hinge flaps. This was carried out high enough to avoid destruction of any natural landmarks. The lateral lip element was not undermined to avoid growth disturbances.[65] Partial union of the lip helps to mold the distorted maxilla and, if deemed necessary, better alignment could be achieved with orthodontia (McNeil type).[7] Occasionally during the lip adhesion procedure, Millard used an L-flap from the cleft edge, based above in the maxilla and transposed into the release of the vestibular lining along the piriform opening. This supplied extra lining in an area that has consistently shown shortness and webbing.[14]

Wanting to eliminate the need for secondary alveolar bone grafting, to close the nasal floor and to achieve early esthetics, Millard, in 1983, had Latham apply presurgical orthodontics; this was followed by gingivoperiosteoplasty and lip adhesion in all complete cleft lip and palate cases.[26,66] Presurgical orthopedics, as performed by Latham (Fig. 64.9), can achieve butt alignment of the alveolar segments to within 2–3 mm, so that the mucoperiosteum creates a periosteal tunnel across the cleft, allowing subsequent bone formation and eventual tooth eruption. This was not a simple modification of Skoog's procedure.[67] A lip adhesion was utilized at this time to avoid unnecessary tension on the periosteoplasty and to allow time for healing and bone migration. After several months of healing, the lip and nose were repaired. According to Millard and Berkowitz, late alveolar bone grafting has been rendered unnecesary in many but not in all of these cases.[28,68] Berkowitz, studying facial growth and dental development in these cases, found anterior crossbites to appear more often than usual.[64,69] The anterior bodily displacement of the smaller segment, coupled with the palatal movement of the premaxillary portion of the larger segment, obstructed the upper lateral incisor space (Fig. 64.10). This was associated with alveolar bone deficiency at the cleft area reducing intra-

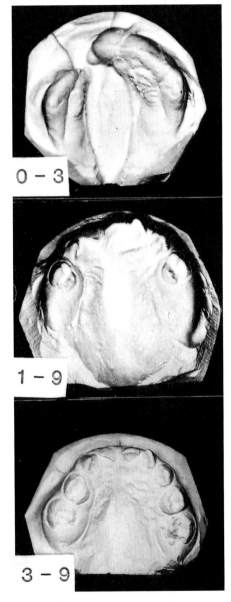

Fig. 64.10 Latham–Millard presurgical orthopedic treatment in unilateral cleft lip and palate. The cleft segment and premaxillary portion of the larger segment have been brought into contact. The remaining casts show the absence of a right lateral incisor space and the creation of an anterior crossbite. (Photographs courtesy of Dr Berkowitz)

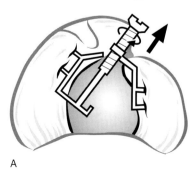
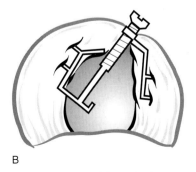

A   B

Fig. 64.9 Latham's coaxial screw appliance in unilateral complete cleft lip and palate.

arch length between the cuspids.[69] In 50% of the analyzed cases, Berkowitz found either a class II or class I relationship. The class II relationship could have been due to the anterior positioning of the smaller cleft segment. Others found that Latham maxillary orthopedic manipulation did not harm facial skeletal growth as judged before puberty.[70,71] Facial asymmetry and recession of the cleft alar base was less evident and was replaced by good lip and nose symmetry.[70] Delaire suggested a secondary gingivo-periosteoplasty, to be carried out during the repair of the hard palate.[72] Brusati and Mannucci found 100% bridging of bone in the tunnel of such a secondary gingivo-periosteoplasty.[73] Berkowitz found in a few cases only a 1–4 mm bar of bone across the gap after primary gingivo-periosteoplasty, which he speculates might be inadequate to permit proper tooth migration when the palatal segments do not make physical contact after orthopedics.[69] There was also a reduced possibility that bone migration across the cleft space would occur. In some cases bone bridging occurred in an ideal fashion, extending from the nasal aperture to the alveolar ridge.

TIMING OF UNILATERAL LIP REPAIR

Millard initially preferred to operate at the age of 3 months[3,5,7,18] because he believed that advancement of the B-flap was not a problem then and the slight tension no danger to dehiscence.[5] The tissues were more generous for approximation and the maxillary segments had at least 3 vital months to grow without lip restraint.[3,6,18] He would then do a minimal cleft repair at the age of 3–6 months.[6]

When lip adhesion was implemented, he performed this at 2–3 weeks, and the definitive lip closure 5–7 months later.[11]

Later he chose to repair only the incomplete clefts of the lip and palate at the age of 3–6 months. For complete clefts, he chose a lip adhesion at three weeks, and definitive closure at 6–8 months.[8]

In 1976 he presented a short-lived scheme of using soft palate adhesion with a Silastic prosthesis to prevent collapse, and superior lip adhesion with an L-flap during the adhesion procedure.[74]

BILATERAL CLEFT LIP REPAIR

As in unilateral cleft lip, the scars from the incisions and parings of the prolabial and lateral lip elements should mimic the philtrum columns. The alar flare is similarly corrected with de-epithelialized alar base flaps joined to each other near the nasal spine, called the 'alar cinch'.[60]

The need for bilateral columellar lengthening poses a problem of tissue replacement and of timing. In 1956, Millard used for the first time a 'forked flap'. The legs consisted of the vertical lip scars, and the fork was pedicled at the deficient columellar base. Both legs were joined in the midline and shifted cranially to shape the columella.

In 1960, the forked flap was designed as a delayed procedure in primary bilateral lip and nose correction. In 1966, Millard tried primary columellar lengthening with the forked flap, but discontinued this sequence after a modest series, mainly because of the resulting long lip and the precarious blood supply to the prolabium.[60,75]

From the mid 60s to the mid 80s, his standard approach was a two or three stage correction, depending upon the size of the prolabium.[60] When it was big, he banked forked flaps in a whisker position, to be used for columellar lengthening at a later stage (Fig. 64.11). This 'banking of the fork' concept was first described by Duffy in 1971[60] in order to avoid going back to the lip for tissue to increase columellar length. The orbicularis oris muscle was united primarily and the mucosa that could be spared from the prolabium was sutured over the raw area of the premaxilla to create lining for the posterior side of the vestibulum.[76] When the prolabium was small, he let a lip adhesion stretch it, and banked the fork flaps during the lip repair which was performed simultaneously with palatal closure.[28]

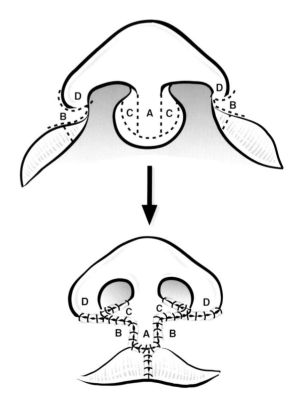

Fig. 64.11 Banking of the forked flap in whisker position at time of final lip closure.

The Latham presurgical orthopedics to bring the protruding premaxilla within the arch, in complete lip clefts combined with bilateral gingivoperiosteoplasties, allows for earlier correction of the nose. If the prolabium is small, a lip adhesion will stretch it for a year or two, after which it is 'banked' during palatal closure at approximately 18 months of age. If the prolabium is large, the fork is banked in 'whisker position' at the time of primary closure of the alveolar defects and the lip.

The columellar lengthening has always been performed at the age of 4,[28,60,77] at which time the alar cartilages have had ample time to develop.[28] Millard was performing an open rhinoplasty at that time, with dissection and suturing of the alar cartilages during the advancement of the forked flap.[60]

Millard has underscored that, in bilateral clefts of the lip, the prolabium – regardless of its size – should always be positioned to the vermilion border which is formed by the lateral lip elements.[78] The inferior prolabial vermilion was used to bolster the central neotuberculum.[76]

ALVEOLAR SEGMENTS

Lip adhesion does not position the premaxilla well enough for closure of the cleft.[66]

Latham's presurgical orthopedic procedure was introduced to retract the premaxilla after spreading the maxillary segments to achieve early ideal arch alignment.[28,79] It is speculated that early positioning of the alveolar segments and joining them with gingivoperiosteoplasties ensures that the retarded lateral segments will be carried forward by the septo-vomerine growth spurt.[28] Buckling of the premaxilla on the septum was generally not found.[70] Millard noted that, with active presurgical orthopedics, the premaxilla first slides backward, and then forward again.[66] Millard is hopeful that telescoping of the premaxilla on the septum will not cause synostosis of the premaxillary vomerine suture, which in turn would interfere with midfacial growth.

At 9 years of age, the midfaces became retrusive, while anterior crossbite, sometimes present at 6 years of age, was present in 50% of the cases at the age of 9, and the cases sometimes developed into anterior open bites.[80] Berkowitz's serial records of conservatively and presurgically treated cases have shown the importance of a functioning premaxillary vomerine suture for achieving good facial growth. For this reason Berkowitz does not favor the retraction of the premaxilla to reduce the anterior cleft space in the newborn period. He believes that the united lip positioned over the protruding premaxilla will slow down midfacial growth, allowing for positive changes to the facial profile.

PALATAL CLEFT REPAIR

SURGERY TO LENGTHEN THE VELUM AND CLOSE THE PALATAL CLEFT SPACE – THE ISLAND FLAP

Wardill[81] and Kilner[82] push-backs and von Langenbeck procedures[83] were commonly used techniques when Millard started in cleft surgery. The problem with the push-back techniques was that the nasal layer could not be lengthened, unless a raw area was left to scar. For this purpose, Millard developed the palatal island flap procedure.[84–86] Dividing the soft palate from the hard, and sandwiching a portion of palatal tissue provided lengthening of the nasal layer but it also enabled better medial mobilization, which in turn avoided pharyngeal flaps (Fig. 64.12).[85,87]

The island flap could be combined with a Wardill–Kilner push-back or a Dorrance flap.[84,85] Two flaps were used in wide clefts, one transverse for the nasal defect, one longitudinally for the oral defect.[84] Two flaps were also used to bridge wide nasal defects.[85] In 1977 Millard described use of the island flap in palatal defects secondary to ablative surgery.[88] In 1970 he presented two cases where the island flaps could not be taken and the nasal defect was closed with T-shaped pharyngeal flaps.[89]

At least 300 of these island flap push-back operations were carried out on patients at 1 year of age.[90] The 'island patch' caused a heavy transpalatal scar that after contracture narrowed the arch form, creating uncorrectable buccal crossbites (Fig. 64.13). It also interfered with midfacial development, resulting in a severe class III malocclusion.[64,91] It has been abandoned in cleft cases until the age of 7 because of these adverse effects.[92]

Lindsay compared V–Y push-backs with von Langenbeck procedures.[93] The speech results were similar, but less crossbite was noted with the von Langenbeck procedure

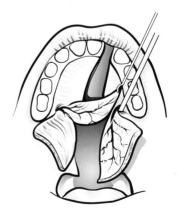

Fig. 64.12 Palatal island flap to reconstruct the defect in the nasal layer in a push-back procedure.

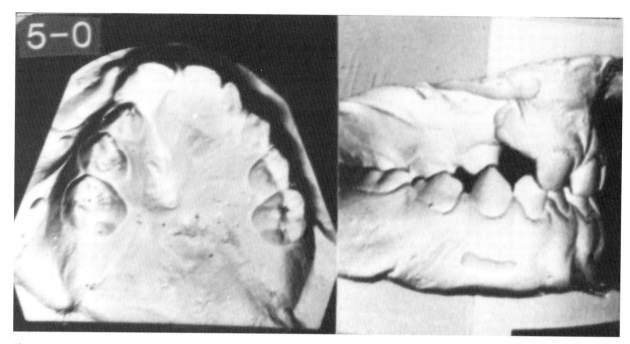

Fig. 64.13 Island flap combined with push-back procedure. When performing the 'pushback' a large denuded bone area is created anteriorly. The 'island' of mucoperiosteum is placed on the nasal surface of the velum to create a sandwich of mucoperiosteal tissue. This area ultimately becomes a transpalatal scar which narrows the palatal arch creating a posterior crossbite and interference with growth (courtesy of Dr. Berkowitz).

when performed at 18 months of age. This report, and the unfavorable growth results with the 'island' push-backs convinced Millard to return to von Langenbeck closures.[90] Lateral incisions were made at least 5 mm palatal to the buccal teeth, to prevent creating an hourglass shape and leaving little bone exposed[64,92] as suggested by Kremenak.[94] Millard freed the abnormal attachments of the levator muscle and joined them, after Braithwaite.[95] Some of the clefts experienced such good marginal growth that they could be closed with simple mucosal approximation.[64] In very wide clefts a vomer flap was utilized and joined to a conservatively undermined mucoperiosteal flap.[64,92]

A combination of the Wardill and von Langenbeck procedures was proposed in wide anterior clefts (after gingivoperiosteoplasty and anterior hard palate closure) and clefts with asymmetrical length.[90]

Between 1978 and 1988 151 cleft palates were reviewed; there were 99 von Langenbeck, 30 von Langenbeck and vomer flap, 9 palatal push-back and island flap, and 5 V–Y palatal push-back.[96]

ON UNILATERAL COMPLETE CLEFT LIP AND PALATE – ARE THE SEGMENTS DEFICIENT IN MASS AND/OR RETROPOSITIONED WITHIN THE FACE?

An important question regarding unilateral cleft palate is 'Is the little segment posteriorly positioned within the face

as a result of being detached from the vomer and having lost its growth impetus, or is it too small?'.[66] In 36 longitudinally followed cases of unilateral cleft palate that received the earlier non-orthopedic treatment, Millard and Berkowitz found 66% of the cases to have a cuspid crossbite only, 17% a complete crossbite, and 17% no crossbite. There were only a minimal number (5) of anterior crossbites. Most significantly, no class III malocclusion of the lesser or larger non-cleft segment was observed. This finding disproves McNeil's belief that the cleft segment needs to be brought forward using neonatal maxillary orthopedics.[64,92] In this series, a modified von Langenbeck procedure with a vomer flap between 18 and 24 months of age was utilized.

ON BILATERAL COMPLETE CLEFT LIP AND PALATE – TRANSVERSE AND ANTEROPOSTERIOR POSITION OF THE PALATAL SEGMENTS

Berkowitz states that the lateral palatal segments are not collapsed at birth. In complete palatal clefts the palatal segments are pulled laterally by the aberrant muscle systems, as well as being pushed outward by tongue action.[66] As already stated, the lateral palatal segments are not more posteriorly positioned relative to the mandible. These may grow to normal size and have normal occlusion as long as the surgery is within physiologic range.[64] Latham, on the other hand, believes that some segments are collapsed and some are expanded, but that control is needed.[66] His aim is to retract the protruding premaxilla and position it within the dental arch.

TIMING OF SURGERY

Millard simultaneously closes the soft and hard palate between the ages of $1\frac{1}{2}$ and $2\frac{1}{2}$ years.[86] Based on theoretical and anecdotal evidence that extensive surgery should not be performed during periods of rapid growth, many surgeons choose $1\frac{1}{2}$ to 2 years for closure as a compromise between speech and growth.

If the cleft space is wide, Millard prefers to wait following Berkowitz's suggestions until additional growth had narrowed the cleft dimensions. An obturator was used only if surgery had to be delayed until 3 years of age or later.[64,92]

The amount of scar tissue created is directly proportional to the area of bone denuded. Berkowitz strongly believes that there are occasions when the palate can successfully be closed at 1 year of age when the cleft space is very narrow, but that it should be postponed until a later age if necessary.[92]

REFERENCES

1. Millard DR Jr 1976 Cleft craft. Vol I. Little, Brown, Boston, pp 165–173
2. Millard DR Jr 1957 A primary camouflage of the unilateral harelook. In: Transactions of the International Congress of Plastic Surgeons. Williams & Wilkins, Baltimore, Md, pp 160–166
3. Millard DR Jr 1960 Complete unilateral clefts of the lip. Plastic and Reconstructive Surgery 25:595–605
4. Millard DR Jr 1986 Principlization of plastic surgery. Little, Brown, Boston
5. Millard DR Jr 1958 A radical rotation in single harelip. American Journal of Surgery 95:318–322
6. Millard DR Jr 1959 Preservation of natural landmarks in unilateral cleft lip. Journal of the American Medical Association 169:133–134
7. Millard DR Jr 1964 Refinements in rotation-advancement cleft lip technique. Plastic and Reconstructive Surgery 33: 26–38
8. Millard DR Jr 1976 Cleft craft. Vol I. Little, Brown, Boston, pp 217–228
9. Millard DR Jr 1968 Extensions of the rotation-advancement principle for wide unilateral cleft lips. Plastic and Reconstructive Surgery 42:535–544
10. Mohler LR 1987 Unilateral cleft lip repair. Plastic and Reconstructive Surgery 80:511–516
11. Millard DR Jr 1974 Further adjuncts in rotation and advancement. In: Georgiade NG, Hagerty RF, (eds) Symposium on management of cleft lip and palate and associated deformities. Mosby, St Louis, pp 67–71
12. Millard DR Jr 1976 Cleft craft. Vol I. Little, Brown, Boston, pp 313–333
13. Trier WC 1985 Repair of unilateral cleft lip: the rotation-advancement operation. Clinics in Plastic Surgery 12:573–594
14. Millard DR Jr 1982 Earlier correction of the unilateral cleft lip nose. Plastic and Reconstructive Surgery 70:64–73
15. Ericksen JE 1869 Operation for harelip on an infant aged ten days. Lancet 1:318
16. Holdsworth WG 1970 Cleft lip and palate, 4th edn. Heinemann, London
17. Millard DR Jr 1976 Cleft craft. Vol I. Little, Brown, Boston, pp 229–238
18. Millard DR 1971 Rotation-advancement in the repair of unilateral cleft lip. In: Grabb W C (ed) Cleft lip and palate. Little, Brown, Boston, pp 195–203
19. Tennison CW 1952 The repair of unilateral cleft lip by the stencil method. Plastic and Reconstructive Surgery 9:115–120
20. LeMesurier AB 1949 A method of cutting and suturing the lip in the treatment of complete unilateral clefts. Plastic and Reconstructive Surgery 4:1–12
21. Trauner R 1967 Results of cleft lip operations. Plastic and Reconstructive Surgery 40:209–219
22. Skoog T 1958 A design for the repair of unilateral cleft lips. American Journal of Surgery 95:223–225
23. Musgrave RH 1971 General aspects of the unilateral cleft lip repair. In: Grabb W C, Rosenstein S W, Bzoch KR (eds) Cleft lip and palate. Little, Brown, Boston, pp 175–194
24. Mir y Mir L 1957 Nasal deformity and single cleft lip. In: Transactions of the International Congress of Plastic Surgeons. Williams & Wilkins, Baltimore, Md, pp 171–174
25. Muir IFK 1966 Repair of the cleft alveolus. British Journal of Plastic Surgery 29:30–36
26. Latham R 1980 Presurgical maxillary orthopedics. In: Millard DR Jr (ed) Cleft craft. Vol III. Little, Brown, Boston, pp 284–298
27. Millard DR Jr 1976 Cleft craft. Vol I. Little, Brown, Boston, pp 449–524
28. Millard DR Jr 1994 Embryonic rationale for the primary correction of classical congenital clefts of the lip and palate. Annals of the Royal College of Surgeons of England 76:150–160
29. Pigott RW 1985 Alar leapfrog. A technique for repositioning the total alar cartilage at primary cleft lip repair. Clinics in Plastic Surgery 12:643–658
30. Bardach J, Mooney M, Giedrojc-Juraha Z L 1982 A comparative study of facial growth following cleft lip repair with or without soft-tissue undermining: an experimental study in rabbits. Plastic and Reconstructive Surgery 69:745–753
31. Bardach J, Salyer K E 1991 Unilateral cleft lip repair. In: Bardach J, Salyer KE (eds) Surgical techniques in cleft lip and palate. Mosby Year Book, St Louis, pp 1–57
32. Nicolau PJ 1983 The orbicularis oris muscle: a functional approach to its repair in the cleft lip. British Journal of Plastic Surgery 36:141–153
33. Fara M, Chlumska A, Hrivnakova J 1965 Musculus orbicularis oris in incomplete hare-lip. Acta Chirurgiae Plasticae (Prague) 7:125–132
34. Fara M 1971 The importance of folding down muscle stumps in the operation of unilateral clefts of the lip. Acta Chirurgiae Plasticae 13:162–169
35. Pennisi VR, Shadish WR, Klabunde EH 1969 Orbicularis oris muscle in the cleft lip repair. American Cleft Palate Journal 6:141–153
36. Millard DR Jr 1976 Cleft craft. Vol I. Little, Brown, Boston, pp 239–245
37. Joss GR, Rouillard L M 1962 A critical evaluation of the rotation-advancement (Millard) method for unilateral cleft lip repair. British Journal of Plastic Surgery 15:349–361
38. Pool R 1966 The configurations of the unilateral cleft lip, with reference to the rotation advancement repair. Plastic and Reconstructive Surgery 37:558–565
39. Witt PD, Hardesty RA 1993 Rotation-advancement repair of the unilateral cleft lip. Clinics in Plastic Surgery 20:633–645
40. Chowdri NA, Darzi MA, Ashraf MM 1990 A comparative study of

surgical results with rotation-advancement and triangular flap techniques in unilateral cleft lip. British Journal of Plastic Surgery 43:551–556

41. Williams HB 1968 A method of assessing cleft lip repairs: comparison of LeMesurier and Millard technique. Plastic and Reconstructive Surgery 41:103–107

42. Amaratunga NA 1988 A comparison of Millard's and LeMesurier's methods of repair of the complete unilateral cleft lip using a new symmetry index. Journal of Oral and Maxillofacial Surgery 46:353–356

43. Millard DR Jr 1976 Cleft craft. Vol I. Little, Brown, Boston, pp 245–250

44. Meyer R 1966 Discussion. In: Schuchardt K (ed) Treatment of patients with clefts of lip, alveolus and palate. Grune & Stratton, New York

45. Onizuka T 1966 My experience with cleft lip repair: Part I. On Millard's method. Japanese Journal of Plastic and Reconstructive Surgery 9:268–276

46. Lintilhac JP, Cochain JP 1966 Fentes et divisions labiales. Considérations sur la terminologie, la statistique au Maroc et l'évolution des techniques opératoires. Chirurgie Plastique Maroc-Médical Avril: 276–287

47. Bernstein K 1970 Modified operation for wide unilateral cleft lips. Archives of Otolaryngology 91:11–18

48. Reichert H 1983 Philtrum formation in cleft lip surgery. Annals of the Academy of Medicine 12:337–340

49. Lexer E 1904 Malformations, injuries and diseases of the face. Von Bergmann's System of practical surgery. Lea & Febiger, Philadelphia

50. Asensio OE 1971 Labio leporino y paladar heindido. Acta Odontologica Venezuelae 3:229–242

51. Asensio O 1974 A variation of the rotation-advancement operation for repair of wide unilateral cleft lips. Plastic and Reconstructive surgery 53:340–341

52. Millard DR Jr 1976 Cleft craft. Vol I. Little, Brown, Boston, pp 412–414

53. Holtmann B, Wray RC 1971 A randomized comparison of triangular rotation-advancement unilateral cleft lip repairs. Plastic and Reconstructive Surgery 2:172–178

54. Cosman B, Crikelair GF 1965 The shape of the unilateral cleft lip defect. Plastic and Reconstructive Surgery 35:484–493

55. Brown JB, McDowell F 1945 Simplified design for repair of single cleft lips. Surgical Gynecology and Obstetrics 80:12–26

56. Wynn SK 1972 Primary nostril reconstruction in complete cleft lips. Plastic and Reconstructive Surgery 49:56–60

57. Reynolds JR, Horton CE 1965 An alar lift procedure in cleft lip rhinoplasty. Plastic and Reconstructive Surgery 35:377–384

58. Millard DR Jr 1976 Cleft craft. Vol I. Little, Brown, Boston, pp 251–268

59. Millard DR Jr 1989 Personal communication

60. Millard DR Jr 1996 A rhinoplasty tetralogy. Corrective, secondary, congenital, reconstructive. Little, Brown, Boston, pp 334–344

61. Cutting CB, Bardach J, Pang R 1989 A comparative study of the skin envelope of the unilateral cleft lip nose subsequent to rotation-advancement and triangular flap lip repairs. Plastic and Reconstructive Surgery 84:409–417

62. Perko M 1987 Shape and function of the unilateral cleft nose in adolescents following modified Millard lip repair. Journal of Cranio-Maxillo-Facial Surgery 15:117–121

63. Horswell BB, Pospisil OA 1995 Nasal symmetry after primary cleft lip repair: comparison between Delaire cheilorhinoplasty and modified rotation-advancement. Journal of Oral and Maxillofacial Surgery 53:1025–1030

64. Berkowitz S 1989 Cleft lip and palate. In: Wolfe SA, Berkowitz S (eds) Plastic surgery of the facial skeleton. Little, Brown, Boston, pp 291–416

65. Walker JC, Collito MB, Mancusi-Ungaro A, Meyer R 1966 Physiologic considerations in cleft lip closure: the C-W technique. Plastic and Reconstructive Surgery 37:522–557

66. Millard Jr, Berkowitz S, Latham RA, Wolfe SA 1988 A discussion of presurgical orthodontics in patients with clefts. Cleft Palate Journal 25:403–412

67. Skoog T 1965 The use of periosteal flaps in the repair of cleft of the primary palate. Cleft Palate Journal 2:332–339

68. Millard DR Jr 1993 Introduction, clefts 1993. Clinics in Plastic Surgery 4:597–598

69. Berkowitz S 1996 Neonatal maxillary orthopedics. In: Berkowitz S (ed) Cleft lip and palate. Vol I. Singular Publishing, San Diego, pp 115–164

70. Spolyer JL, Jackson IT, Philips RJL, Sullivan WG, Clayman L, Vyas ST 1993 The Latham technique. Contemporary presurgical orthopedics for the complete oral cleft. Technique and preliminary evaluation. A bone marker study. Perspectives in Plastic Surgery. Outside Insights: 179–210

71. Wood RJ, Grayson BH, Cutting C 1997 Gingivoperiosteoplasty and midfacial growth. Cleft Palate Journal 34:17–20

72. Delaire J 1989 Premiers résultats de la gingivo-périosteoplastie primaire (avec ou sans ostéoplastie). In: II trattamento chirurgico ed orthodontico della labiopalatoschisi. La riconstruzione dell'equilibrio funzionale. ACPS Magenta, Milano, Vol II, p 121

73. Brusati R, Mannucci N 1992 The early gingivoalveoloplasty. Preliminary results. Scandinavian Journal of Plastic and Reconstructive Surgery and Hand Surgery 26:65–70

74. Millard DR Jr 1976 Cleft craft. Vol I. Little, Brown, Boston, p 448

75. Millard DR Jr 1977 Cleft craft. Vol II. Little, Brown, Boston, p 174

76. Millard DR Jr 1977 Cleft craft. Vol II. Little, Brown, Boston, pp 341–358

77. Millard DR Jr 1971 Closure of bilateral cleft lip and elongation of the columella by two operations in infancy. Plastic and Reconstructive Surgery 47:324–330

78. Millard DR Jr 1980 Cleft craft. Vol II. Little, Brown, Boston, p 240

79. Millard DR, Latham RA 1990 Improved primary surgical and dental treatment of clefts. Plastic and Reconstructive Surgery 86:856–871

80. Berkowitz S 1996 Lip and palatal surgery. In: Berkowitz S (ed) Cleft lip and palate. Vol I. Singular Publishing, San Diego, pp 65–102

81. Wardill MEM 1937 The technique of operation for cleft palate. British Journal of Surgery 25:117–130

82. Kilner TP 1937 Cleft lip and palate repair technique. St Thomas Hospital Report 2:37

83. von Langenbeck 1864 Weitere Erfahrungen im Gebiet der Uranoplastik mittels Ablösung des mucoperiostalen Gaumenüberzuges. Arch Klin Chir 4:1

84. Millard DR Jr 1966 A new use of the island flap in wide palate clefts. Plastic and Reconstructive Surgery 38:330–335

85. Millard DR 1963 The island flap in cleft palate surgery. Surgical Gynecology and Obstetrics 116:297–300

86. Millard DR Jr 1980 Cleft craft. Vol III. Little, Brown, Boston, pp 525–541

87. Millard DR Jr 1962 Wide and/or short cleft palate. Plastic and Reconstructive Surgery 29:40–57

88. Millard DR Jr, Seider HA 1977 The versatile palatal island flap: its use in soft palate reconstruction and nasopharyngeal and choanal atresia. British Journal of Plastic Surgery 30:300–305

89. Millard DR 1970 T-shaped pharyngeal flap. Plastic and Reconstructive Surgery 45:511–513

90. Millard DR Jr, Flynn W, Rao MP 1992 Combining the von Langenbeck and the Wardill–Kilner operations in certain clefts of the palate. Cleft Palate–Craniofacial Journal 29:85–86

91. Millard DR Jr 1980 Cleft craft. Vol III. Little, Brown, Boston, pp 587–600

92. Berkowitz S 1985 Timing cleft palate closure – age should not be the sole determinant. In: Cohen MM Jr, Rollnick BR (eds) Journal of Craniofacial Genetics and Developmental Biology 1 (suppl): 69–83

93. Lindsay WK 1971 von Langenbeck palatoraphy. In: Grabb WC, Rosenstein SW, Bzoch KR (eds.) Cleft lip and palate. Little, Brown, Boston, pp 393–403

94. Kremenak CR Jr, Huffman WC, Olin WH 1970 Maxillary growth inhibition by mucoperiosteal denudation of palatal shelf bone in non-cleft beagles. Cleft Palate Journal 7:817–825

95. Braithwaite F 1968 The importance of the levator muscle in cleft palate closure. British Journal of Plastic Surgery 21:60–62

96. Baker S, Millard DR 1993 Intraoperative suction test as a predictor of velopharyngeal competence. Cleft Palate–Craniofacial Journal 30:452–453

Alveolar bone grafting – how I do it

LEO F. A. STASSEN

65

INTRODUCTION

Management of the cleft patient has developed signifi-cantly over recent years. One of the major advances has been the development of a successful method to recon-struct the cleft alveolar (bony) defect with bone (secondary bone grafting) with few complications and no restriction of facial growth;[1] this method was popularized by Åbyholm in 1981.[2] Better methods should always be looked for: bone biology research is under way and it will be possible eventually to reconstruct the defect without the need for a bone graft using either bone morphogenetic protein[3] or alveolar osteodistraction.

The history of alveolar bone grafting is interesting; as long ago as 1901, von Eiselsberg used pedicled bone to fill the alveolus and, in 1908, Lexer tried using free bone grafts.[4] Surgeons in the past placed bone in the alveolar defect at the time of lip repair but unfortunately this bone grafting technique disturbed facial growth. Analysis of their results showed a significant restriction in facial growth,[5-7] and this technique was subsequently abandoned by cleft surgeons.

It is not surprising when one reviews the history that alveolar bone grafting has taken many years in some units to become the accepted norm; some antagonists have very strongly advocated no treatment, allowing the defect to be closed by juxtaposition of the lesser and greater segments. They believe that the interalveolar mucosa atrophies and degenerates, and that the alveolar bones then fuse. If this failed to occur, the defect could in any case be obturated with a prosthesis. Primary bone grafting with rib, by con-trast, seemed a major and barbaric procedure.[8]

The philosophy of seeking to reconstruct the bony defect has fortunately persisted. The ideal subject is an esthetically pleasing young person, who is dentally fit with a class I occlusion, and who has neither missing teeth nor oral fistulae and has normal speech.

ALVEOLAR BONE GRAFTING

Alveolar bone grafting can be classified as:

- primary (usually at same time as the lip repair – 0–2½ years)
- early secondary (2–5 years)
- secondary (6–13 years)
- late (> 13 years)
- grafting at the time of Le Fort I osteotomy
- revision grafting.

The alveolar bone defect can also be closed by segmental repositioning of the maxilla if teeth are not a considera-tion.[9,10]

Primary bone grafting is rarely undertaken but it still has its advocates.[11,12] Some surgeons believe that, with a func-tional lip and alveolar repair, primary bone grafting may still have a place, especially with our developing under-standing of the scarring mechanism and the development of bone morphogenic proteins. Most researchers have over recent years advocated secondary bone grafting and there is good evidence that grafting secondarily does not impair facial growth.[2]

The problems associated with an alveolar defect depend on its size and whether it is a unilateral or a bilateral cleft-ing condition (Fig. 65.1). The problems are both func-tional and esthetic. Patients may complain of :

- food/fluids coming out of their nose
- an inability to blow balloons or to suck a straw
- a persistent smell or discharge from their nose
- poor speech

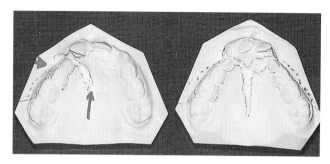

Fig. 65.1 Unilateral and bilateral clefts.

- an inability to clean their teeth in the cleft area
- decayed or deformed teeth in the cleft area
- missing or extra teeth in the area
- lack of bone support for teeth adjacent to the defect
- poor alignment of the teeth of the lesser and greater segments
- mobility and overgrowth of the premaxilla in the bilateral case
- lack of support for the alar base of the nose and lip in the unilateral case
- lack of support for the alar base, columella and lip in the bilateral case.

Of these, the last two are most important and are often overlooked.

The aims of treatment are:

1. to restore physiologic continuity of the dental arch to enable oral and dental health to be maintained (Fig. 65.2)
2. to provide bone for stability of the dental arch, premaxilla and adjacent teeth and to allow for eruption of unerupted permanent teeth (usually canines) (Fig. 65.3) or placement of a dental implant (Fig. 65.4)

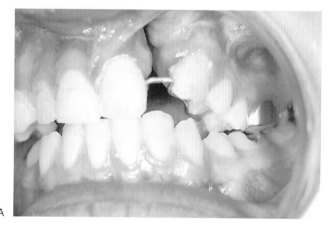

A

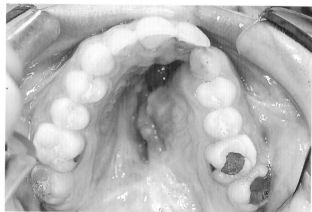

B

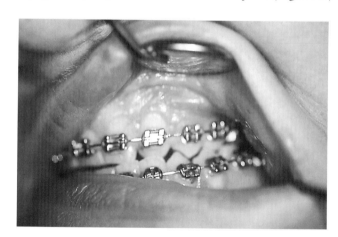

Fig. 65.3 Canine erupted through bone graft.

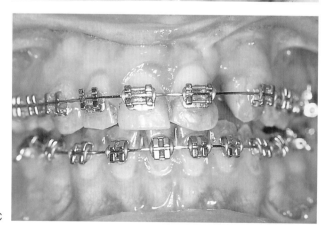

C

Fig. 65.2 **(A)** Alveolar defect; **(B)** palatal defect; **(C)** defect bone grafted.

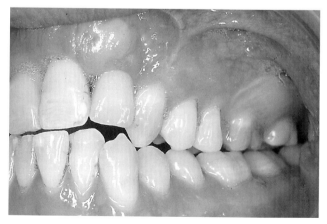

Fig. 65.4 Lateral incisor implanted in alveolar bone graft.

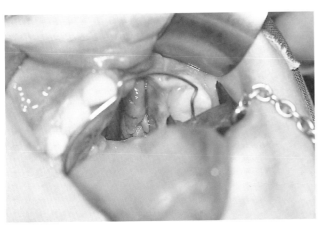

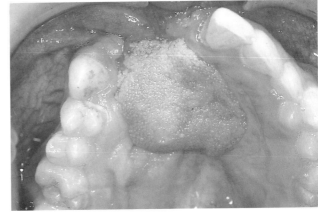

A   B

Fig. 65.5 (A) A large oronasal fistula. **(B)** Tongue flap in situ.

3. to allow for orthodontic alignment of the teeth
4. to provide support for the lip and nose and to close a persistent oronasal fistula (Fig. 65.5).

Treatment should cause minimal impairment of growth and development in the maxillofacial complex.

ASSESSMENT

The size of the alveolar defect is very variable and depends on many factors including the width of the original unilateral or bilateral embryological defect, the extent, type and success of primary lip and palate surgery, and naturally the patient's own growth potential. Clefts of the lip and palate have the most severe alveolar defects. Clefts of the lip, even minimal defects, are often accompanied by alveolar defects, and careful clinical and radiologic assessment of the alveolus is required. Patients with a cleft palate and no lip involvement do not have any alveolar defect.

Patients are regularly reviewed in the cleft clinic. When a patient's permanent first molars have erupted, he should be assessed by the orthodontist and maxillofacial surgeon to decide on the need and appropriate timing for an alveolar bone graft. The aim is to place bone to allow for the successful eruption of the permanent canine and to provide support for the lateral incisor, taking into consideration deformed, missing and supernumerary teeth. The ideal time for grafting is when the canine root is one third formed. Dixon[13] showed that the alveolar defect may interfere with the dental lamina and be associated with either a hypo- or a hyperplastic alveolar event. The canine teeth are usually found in the posterior margins of the residual alveolar defect or displaced superiorly along the bony defect. The lateral incisor can be on either side but usually is on the anterior aspect and often has little bony support. It is essential that the patient's oral hygiene and dental state are of the highest standard. Poor oral hygiene and dental care contribute to bone graft failure. Most studies[14,15] indicate that grafting is best carried out when the canine root is one third formed; there is now a tendency to do this earlier to obtain satisfactory bone support for the lateral incisor or even eruption of the lateral incisor if it is placed on the lateral segment. Care must be taken to ensure that the bone grafting is undertaken after the majority of maxillary growth is complete (8 years). Assessment is with models and radiographs (oral pantomogram, anterior occlusal through the cleft and periapicals) of teeth on either side of the cleft (Figs 65.1, 65.6). This enables the surgeon and orthodontist to outline the defect, assess the teeth, and agree which if any teeth (deciduous or supernumerary) should be removed at the time of grafting. Three-dimensional CT scanning of the defect is becoming important to assess the full defect, the volume of bone required and measuring of the eventual outcome. This allows a full understanding and visualization of a very difficult area. The radiation dose has been reduced by coning techniques. The anatomic dimensions of the defect are outlined by the model and CT scan.

PREPARATION FOR SURGERY

The surgeon must assess the health and the amount of

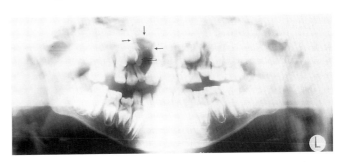

Fig. 65.6 Radiograph outlining alveolar defect supernumerary tooth (outline arrow), and teeth.

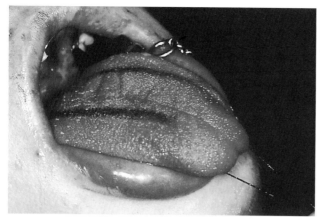 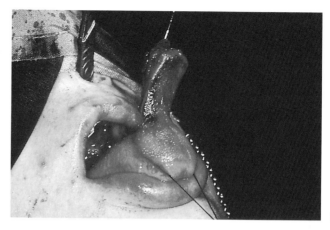

Fig. 65.7 (A) Tongue flap marked out. **(B)** Tongue flap raised.

available appropriate soft tissue. There is usually enough tissue for the nasal mucosal layer to be primarily closed. Occasionally the oral mucosal defect is too large for a satisfactory oral layer to be obtained, and in these cases the use of additional tissue such as rotation flaps, a tongue flap or free tissue transfer must be considered (Figs 65.5, 65.7). A tongue flap is my preferred option; it is usually placed after the orthodontic preparation and six months before the bone grafting is undertaken. The nasal layer is closed with palatal/nasal mucosa by elevating fairly wide flaps, and the oral layer is covered by the tongue flap. The tongue defect is minimal and there is no interference with speech.

The repaired cleft defect must be covered by keratinized epithelium or the tooth will not erupt and the periodontal state of the adjacent teeth will be jeopardized. Erupted teeth around the alveolar defect that require removal should be removed at least three months prior to the grafting procedure.

Orthodontic preparation includes assessment of the bite; if the incisors are locked, a removable appliance is used to free the bite. Dental arch expansion (or, really, de-rotation and alignment) is usually achieved with a Quadhelix; once it has been achieved, a passive palatal arch is placed to maintain the expansion and allow surgery to proceed. It is important to maintain expansion for at least three months after surgery while the graft stabilizes. This is particularly important in the bilateral case with a mobile premaxilla. The orthodontist and the surgeon have to decide whether they want to expand the dental arch and thereby the alveolar defect prior to or after bone grafting. It is my preferred option to have the dental arch expanded beforehand.

SURGERY

Surgery usually takes place under general anesthesia. The anesthetist is asked to place a naso-endotracheal tube in the unaffected nostril in the unilateral case; a laterally placed, reinforced oral tube is preferred in the bilateral cleft cases.

Alveolar bone grafting can be a bloody procedure and it is worthwhile trying to limit the blood loss. In the anesthetic room, local anesthetic – 2% lignocaine with 1:80 000 adrenaline or bupivacaine 0.25% with 1:100 000 adrenaline – is infiltrated, buccally and palatally and into the defect. The patient should also be head-up to help decrease bleeding. Prophylactic antibiotics are prescribed and continued for three days. I use intravenous benzylpenicillin for three doses and then oral penicillin.

The patient is draped, with the whole mouth and nose exposed. The area is cleaned with an aqueous chlorhexidine solution, particular attention being paid to the nose and alveolar defect. The site for donor cancellous bone graft harvesting is prepared. Bone graft may be harvested by a trephine technique from the iliac crest, anterior tibia and the olecranon process of the ulna. An open technique is unnecessary.[16] Calvarial bone has been used in the past but was found to be too dense and to delay eruption of the canine. Bone has been harvested from the chin but there is occasionally not enough bone;[17] and I used supporting mentalis/mucosal stay sutures to preserve the soft-tissue chin point support. Bone has been mixed with hydroxyapatite and other bone substitutes but again this has been found to be less satisfactory if eruption of teeth is required than autogenous cancellous bone alone.

Autogenous cancellous bone and marrow are still the gold standard[18] and are both inductive and conductive agents, especially when in contact with the connective tissue closely related to living bone – periosteum. It is for this reason that subperiosteal mucosal flaps are developed and mobilized to enable the mobilised periosteum to cover the bone graft in the alveolar defect.

After preparation, the alveolar defect is examined and probed (Fig. 65.8), the X-rays are re-examined (Fig. 65.9).

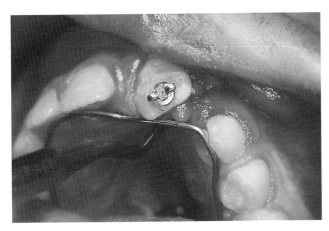

Fig. 65.8 Probing the alveolar defect.

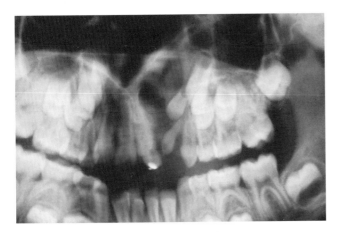

Fig. 65.9 Radiograph with supernumerary teeth.

An attempt is made to visualize the defect in three dimensions. This is the difficult part of the operation. The 3D CT scan makes it easier. How far should one dissect back into the palate? Should palatal fistulae be closed? It is my philosophy to close the alveolar defect and any palatal extension in one sitting. How much scar tissue should be excised to make room for bone? I excise as much as possible and leave enough tissue to allow a tension-free closure of the nasal layer. Will there be enough soft tissue to obtain closure? The blood supply of a cleft case is often compromised[19] and this should be taken into consideration when designing mucoperiosteal flaps. The flaps must have broad bases. If there is insufficient soft tissue to cover the palatal aspect, consider delaying the bone graft and bring in additional tissue (tongue).

Unilateral cleft

It is best to think of the alveolar defect as a pyramid with its base on the buccal aspect of the defect and its apex on the palate (Fig. 65.10). The aim, by making incisions along the cleft margins, is to turn the mucoperiosteal flaps covering the walls of the pyramid carefully and gently in on themselves to produce enough healthy tissue for a clean nasal closure. The palatal tissue is mobilized locally to enable palatal closure. Finally the labial and buccal tissues are mobilized subperiosteally off the lesser segment, the flap is incised in a full thickness manner posteriorly from the gingival margin for approximately 15 mm into the vestibule in an oblique and posterosuperior manner. The flap is turned out on itself and the periosteum incised as high up in the buccal vestibule as possible, avoiding the infraorbital nerve. The flap is then mobilized anteriorly to allow closure of the labial defect (base of the pyramid) and the interdental defect in a tension-free manner. This periosteal incision is best completed with a knife. The surgeon then carefully inspects the flap while trying to mobilize it anteriorly. If there is any particular area holding the flap back, it should be explored and the periosteum further incised. When dissection is complete, a finger is placed high up in the buccal sulcus and the flap mobilized even further. The labial mucosa over the premaxilla is minimally elevated.

The labial mucosa superior to the cleft defect needs to be separated into two mucosal/submucosal layers to produce an oral and a nasal layer. This is easily achieved with a sharp blade by keeping the mucosa under tension, visualizing the nasal defect, and keeping the blade parallel to an imaginary line joining the lateral pyriform aperture and the premaxillary labial segment.

The apex on the palate needs to be thought of as two layers and requires splitting to allow a separate nasal and oral closure. The nasal layer is mobilized from the alveolar defect and nasal walls. Sometimes there is an excess of intra-alveolar tissue, scar and mucosa; this must be excised to allow room for the complete alveolar defect to be packed with cancellous bone. The nasal layer is closed with interrupted resorbable sutures (Vicryl 4.0), everting the nasal mucosa into the nose. The needle is best shaped as a J to enable suturing in this narrow area and to avoid tearing of the thin friable nasal layer. Sutures are placed but not tied down until they are all in place. This gives room and flexibility to suture the nasal layer and to prevent tearing.

The palatal layer should be raised with a gingival incision. Although diagrams in textbooks show the palatal mucosa well rotated over the fistula, the reality is often very different. In a heavily scarred palate, it is almost impossible to rotate these flaps. In practice, closure is often only achieved by pulling the flaps away from the curvature of the palate. While this produces a tension-free closure it does increase the

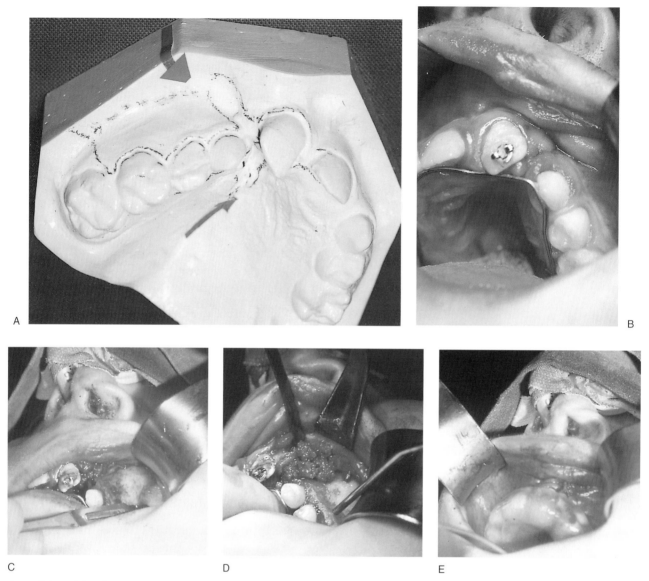

Fig. 65.10 **(A)** Model outlining incisions – broken line = subperiosteal incision; **(B)** alveolar defect; **(C)** buccal flap raised and incising periosteum; **(D)** bone graft in situ; **(E)** splint in situ.

buccal-palatal width of the defect. This requires advancement of the buccal mucosa. The palatal layer is closed with interrupted resorbable sutures, commencing anteriorly and working back onto the palate.

Cancellous bone is broken down into very small pieces (preferably with a bone mill) to allow overpacking of the alveolar defect/s. The flaps have been designed in such a way to ensure that the grafted bone is covered by attached gingiva. The oral labial wound is closed with interrupted sutures. The operation is planned so that the alveolar bone graft recipient site is prepared and ready to receive the bone graft as soon as it is harvested. This protects the osteogenic cells. The bone is placed and packed in the prepared alveolar bed. When the alveolar packing is complete the labial mucosa

is sutured to the palatal layer and the keratinized tissue from the labial and buccal flaps carried to cover the alveolus.

The wound is protected with a preformed blowdown splint. This splint is prepared from a plaster model which has been relieved in the peri-defect area to allow coverage without pressure on the wound edges. The technician covers the area of the alveolar defect and proposed flaps and suture lines with a layer of wax to ensure that there is no pressure. I place chlormycetin cream in the splint and over the wound.

Bilateral cleft

The bilateral cleft is a little more difficult and demands more thought and planning. There is an alveolar defect in the shape of a Y (Fig. 65.11A,B). There are three segments. The premaxilla has a very small bone stalk (Fig. 65.11C) and relatively poor blood supply. Its stripping must be minimal (Fig. 65.11D,E). It is particularly difficult to see the palatal aspect to define the nasal and palatal (oral) layer. Methods of fracture of the bone stalk have been advocated[20] to enable better visualization but I prefer not to risk the blood supply and use a beaver blade and careful dissection to obtain the two layers. Oral soft tissue is occasionally deficient and a more extensive palatal dissection is required to allow medial displacement of the lateral flaps and closure of the two medial defects. The labial tissue is occasionally deficient and must be well mobilized bilaterally (Fig. 65.11F) to allow keratinized tissue to be transferred over the alveolus to cover the oral layer.

It is often advocated that bilateral clefts should be grafted one side at a time to protect the blood supply to the premaxilla. I aim to do it in one procedure but warn the patient and family that it may require two procedures. The passive orthodontic palatal arch is kept in place to maintain stability, and in fact I use the arch to sling sutures over after suturing the mucosa to give the flap support (Fig. 65.11G).

POSTOPERATIVE CARE

The patient is returned to the ward to recover in a semi-prone position. The splint (Fig. 65.11H) remains in situ for 24 hours and the patient is allowed to eat and drink as soon as he or she wakes. The patient is discharged the following day with strict oral and splint hygiene instructions. The patient wears the splint continuously for one week, taking it out to wash it and the mouth after each meal. The splint is then worn only when eating for a further week; the patient can then discard the splint. The area is kept under close supervision by both the orthodontist and surgeon. The orthodontist commences further treatment if necessary after three months to move teeth as required into the defect and monitor eruption of the canine.

Teeth that erupt through the grafted bone further increase the bone stock and they seem to respond well to orthodontic or orthopedic forces and do not interfere with maxillary growth.

If there is deficiency of keratinized gingiva, the teeth will not erupt and sometimes it is necessary to widen the area of keratinized labial gingiva with a free graft as soon as the area has healed and before further orthodontic treatment.

COMPLICATIONS

Any surgical procedure has the potential for complications, especially a procedure performed under general anesthesia. The complications discussed here are those relating to the local and bone donor site areas: there may be bleeding, pain, wound breakdown at both sites, low grade infection if oral hygiene is not meticulous, bone sequestra, bone loss, bone resorption, residual fistula, loss of vestibular depth and gingival hyperplasia. Injury to adjacent teeth and external root resorption can also occur. External resorption is thought to be related to trauma to the periodontal membrane and drying of the root surface or osteoclastic activity of bone cells. All these complications can be reduced by attention to detail and meticulous surgery.

Donor site complications include pain, blood loss, scarring, contour abnormalities, neurologic complications such as lateral cutaneous nerve of the thigh dysesthesia, tibial plateau fractures and fractured instruments.

RESULTS

A successful bone graft with eruption of a canine is a very gratifying experience. In spite of the popularity and extensive description of alveolar bone grafting, not all procedures are successful; the success of the technique in each unit needs to be audited. This will lead to change and improvements in our methods. The success rate ranges from no improvement to partial improvement to ideal bone fill-in and satisfactory tooth support.

The literature is confusing on the importance of surgical trials. Logically, a surgeon who performs a procedure more and more often should get better and better at it.[21] A surgeon may find it difficult to compare techniques as he is likely to achieve better results with a technique with which he is familiar. Kalaaji et al in 1994 showed that surgical experience made no difference to the long-term results of bone grafting in patients with cleft lip and palate, although the same authors, in a paper in 1996, confirmed that experienced surgeons had significantly better results ($P < 0.05$) when wide clefts were considered; they also found less (but not significantly less) dehiscence and total resorption when experienced surgeons operated.[15,22] Ross, in 1987, studied 538 unilateral cleft lip and palate male patients and argued that it was the surgeon that was the most important variable and not the technique.[5] Rintala and Haapanen presented an exciting paper in 1993 analyzing 439 cleft patients; they showed that training was important but definitely not synonymous with skill, and that surgeons (8) working together in pairs could improve their results.[23] Cohen et al in 1996 reported the development of a simple teaching

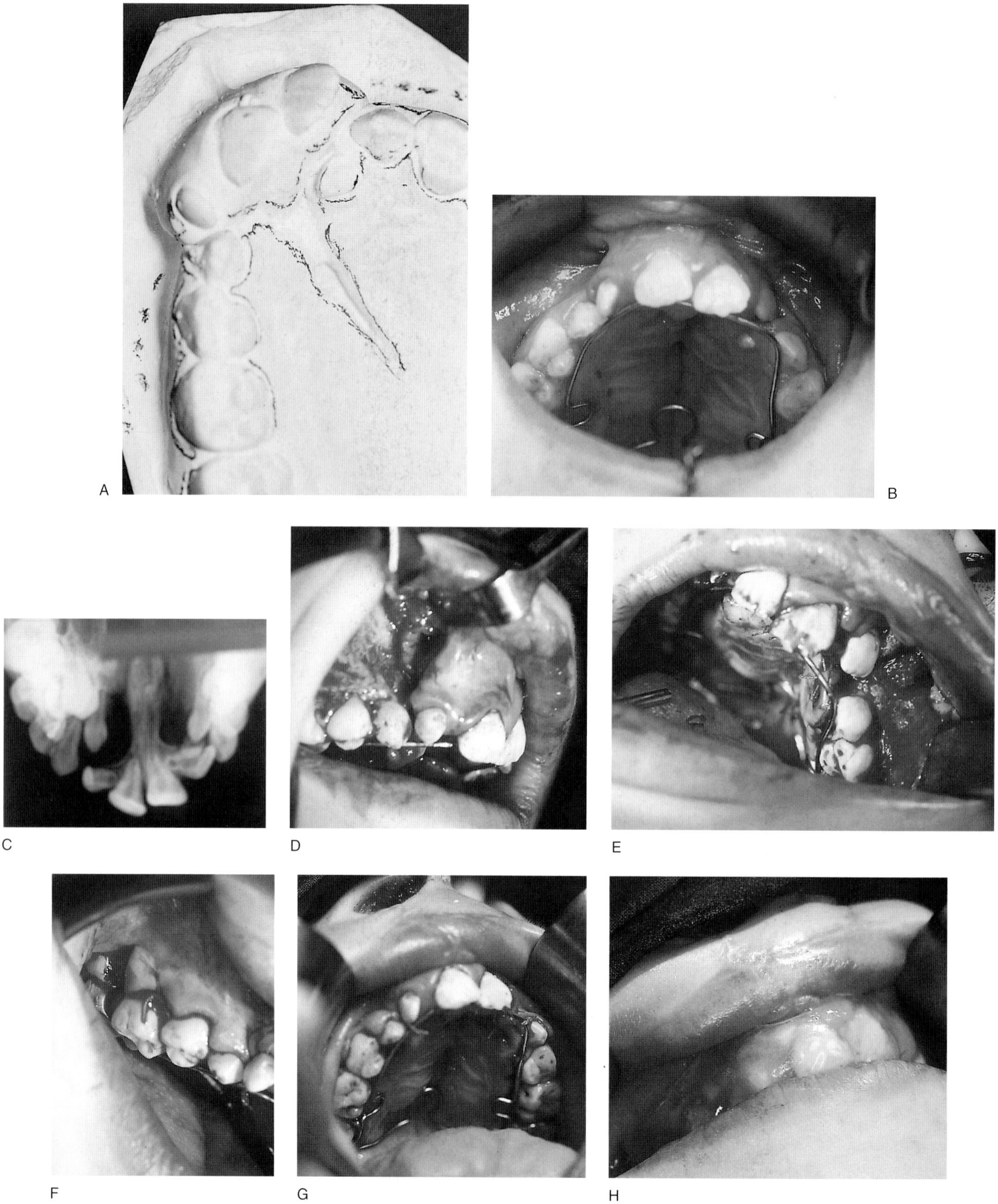

Fig. 65.11 **(A)** Model outlining incisions – broken line = subperiosteal incision; **(B)** alveolar defect (bilateral); **(C)** radiograph showing premaxilla bone support; **(D)** buccal flap raised and demonstrating premaxillary dissection; **(E)** palatal repair and extent of buccal dissection; **(F)** buccal flap posterior incision and final defect; **(G)** repair (bilateral cleft); **(H)** splint in situ.

model to aid the surgeon in conceptualizing the defect and the surgical steps required.[24]

Success is measured by:

1. closure of the fistula (95%)
2. eruption of the canine and bone support for adjacent teeth (95%)
3. assessing the bone architecture of the bone graft – a bone strut in 95% of cases.

Interdental alveolar bone height in the cleft area is different and can be judged in many ways.[25,26] It is usually assessed by reviewing radiographs (long cone periapicals or anterior occlusals):

Grade I: normal interdental alveolar height
Grade II: >75% normal interdental alveolar height
Grade III: 50–75% interdental alveolar height
Grade IV: <50% normal interdental alveolar height.

Success for this varies from 0–100% and is usually around 80%.

Alveolar bone grafting is an important development and a rewarding procedure to undertake. It is probably the most difficult of all the cleft procedures because of the three-dimensional conceptualization required and the tight confines of the alveolar defect in which surgery needs to be carried out. The maxillofacial surgeon needs to work closely with the orthodontist to define the optimal time for surgery; most revision nasal and lip surgery should be postponed until the alveolar bone grafting is complete.

REFERENCES

1. Boyne PJ, Sands NR 1972 Secondary bone grafting of residual alveolar and palatal clefts. Journal of Oral Surgery 30:87–92
2. Åbyholm FE, Bergland O, Semb G 1981 Secondary bone grafting of alveolar clefts. A surgical/orthodontic treatment enabling a non-prosthodontic rehabilitation in cleft lip and palate patients. Scandinavian Journal of Plastic and Reconstructive Surgery 15:127–140
3. Boyne PJ, Nath R, Nakamura A 1998 Human recombinant BMP-2 in osseous reconstruction of simulated cleft palate defects. British Journal of Maxillofacial Surgery 36(2):84–90
4. Koberg WR 1973 Present view of bone grafting in cleft palate (a review of the literature). Journal of Maxillofacial Surgery 1:185–193
5. Ross RB 1987 Treatment variables affecting facial growth in complete unilateral cleft lip and palate. Part 7: an overview of treatment and facial growth. Cleft Palate Journal 24:71–77
6. Suzuki A, Goto K, Nakamura N, Honda Y, Ohishi M, Tashiro H, Fujino H 1996 Cephalometric comparison of craniofacial morphology between primary bone grafted and nongrafted complete unilateral cleft lip and palate adults. Cleft Palate–Craniofacial Journal 33(5):429–435
7. Trotman C A, Long R E, Rosenstein S W, Murphy C, Johnston L E 1996 Comparison of facial form in primary alveolar bone-grafted and nongrafted unilateral cleft lip and palate patients: intercenter retrospective study. Cleft Palate–Craniofacial Journal 33(2):91–99
8. Pruzansky S 1964 Presurgical orthopaedics and bone grafting for infants with cleft lip and palate: a dissent. Cleft Palate Journal 1:164
9. Stoelinga PJW, van den Vijver RM, Leenen RJ, Soubry RJ, Blijdorp PA, Schoenars JHA 1987 The prevention of relapse after maxillary osteotomies in cleft palate patients. Journal of Cranio-Maxillo-Facial Surgery 15:326–331
10. Erbe M, Stoelinga PJW, Leenen RJ 1996 Long term results of segmental repositioning of the maxilla in cleft palate patients without previously grafted alveolo-palatal clefts. Journal of Cranio-Maxillo-Facial Surgery 24(2):109–117
11. Rosenstein SW, Monroe CW, Kernahan DA, Jacobson BN, Griffith BH, Bauer BS 1982 The case for early bone grafting in cleft lip and palate. Plastic and Reconstructive Surgery 70:297–309
12. Rosenstein SW, Dado DV, Kernahan DA, Griffith BH, Grasseschi M 1991 The case for early bone grafting in cleft lip and palate: a second report. Plastic and Reconstructive Surgery 87:644–654
13. Dixon DA, Edwards JRG, Newton J 1976 Orthodontically induced eruption of the permanent canine combined with alveolar cleft osteoplasty: a new procedure illustrated by a case with stereophotogrammetric reconstruction. Journal of Maxillofacial Surgery 4:61
14. Witsenburg B 1985 The reconstruction of anterior residual bone defects in patients with cleft lip, alveolus and palate. A review. Journal of Maxillofacial Surgery 13:197–208
15. Kalaaji A, Lilja J, Friede H, Elander A 1996 Bone grafting in the mixed and permanent dentition in cleft lip and palate patients: long term results and the role of the surgeon's experience. Journal of Cranio-Maxillo-Facial Surgery 24(1):29–35
16. Ilankovan V, Stronczek M, Telfer M, Peterson LJ, Stassen LFA, Ward-Booth P 1998 A prospective study of trephined bone grafts of the tibial shaft and iliac crest. British Journal of Maxillofacial Surgery 36:6
17. Bosker H, van Dijk L 1980 Het bottransplantaat uit de mandibula voor herstel van de gnatho-palatoschisis. Nederlands Tijdschrift voor Tandheelkunde 87:383
18. Ellis E III 1992 Biology of bone grafting: an overview. Selected Readings in Oral and Maxillofacial Surgery 2:1
19. Drommer R 1979 Selective angiographic studies prior to Le Fort 1 osteotomy in patients with cleft lip and palate. Journal of Maxillo-Facial Surgery 7:264–270
20. Banks P 1983 The surgical anatomy of secondary cleft lip and palate deformity and its significance in reconstruction. British Journal of Oral Surgery 21:78
21. Roberts C T, Semb G, Shaw W 1991 Strategies for the advancement of surgical methods in cleft lip and palate. Cleft Palate Cranio-Facial Journal 28:141–149
22. Kalaaji A, Lilja J, Friede H 1994 Bone grafting at the stage of mixed and permanent dentition in patients with clefts of the lip and primary palate. Plastic and Reconstructive Surgery 93:690–696
23. Rintala AE, Haapanen ML 1993 Correlation between speech results of CP-repair and the surgeon's training and skill. Personal communication and Abstract 446 7th International Congress on Cleft Palate and Related Cranio Facial Anomalies, Broadbeach, Australia
24. Cohen M, Polley JW, Figueroa A, Habakuk SW, Iwamoto C 1996 Teaching model for closure of oronasal fistula and bone grafting of the maxilla. Cleft Palate Cranio-Facial Journal 33(3): 198–201
25. Bergland O, Semb G, Åbyholm FE 1986 Elimination of the residual alveolar cleft by secondary bone grafting and subsequent orthodontic treatment. Cleft Palate Journal 23: 175–205
26. Long RE, Spangler BE, Yow M 1995 Cleft width and secondary alveolar bone graft success. Cleft Palate–Craniofacial Journal 32(5):420–427

Secondary surgery for cleft lip and palate

66

ANTHONY F. MARKUS/DAVID S. PRECIOUS

INTRODUCTION

That so much has been written by so many about secondary procedures in cleft surgery is testament not only to the complexity and variable expression of the cleft deformity itself but also to the need to find methods of primary surgery that will reduce, if not avoid, the adverse effects on all the structures and functions involved and affected. It must be the principal aim of the cleft surgeon to restore the deformed and displaced regional anatomy to as close to normality as possible, whether or not there exists true hypoplasia. Only in this way can one reasonably expect restoration of function and so enable optimal growth and development. Primary surgical methods encompassing these ideals should, theoretically, reduce the frequently observed sequelae of both the cleft deformity and surgery and so, in turn, the need for secondary surgery. In reality, given even the most favorable circumstances, secondary surgery will be required.

Ideally, secondary deformities of cleft lip and palate are therefore best managed by adopting a method of primary surgery that not only recognizes the inherent problems but prevents them from occurring. Veau[1] introduced the concept of embryological surgery: the surgeon must have a full understanding of all the anatomic elements involved in the cleft deformity, should seek to improve surgical methods where failure seems to be apparent, and must make every attempt to restore to normality all the tissues involved in the cleft and in particular the underlying musculature, rather than just confining activity to the overlying skin. This concept of 'embryological' surgery, embodied somewhat later by Millard,[2] is given credence in histochemical studies of embryos between 16 and 22 weeks[3] which not only demonstrate that the deformities of the nasal cartilages, the premaxilla and maxilla and the musculature are recognizable

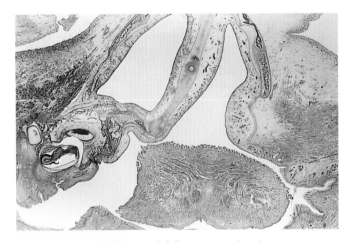

Fig. 66.1 22-week-old human cleft fetus – coronal section.

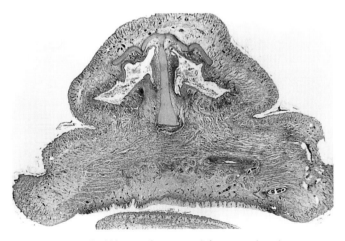

Fig. 66.2 22-week-old human fetus, non-cleft – coronal section.

at a very early stage in development (Figs 66.1 and 66.2) but also the very significant growth potential in the midline, compared to the non-cleft subject, of the nasal septal cartilages and the nasolabial muscles, confirming the belief of Delaire[4-6] that it is essential to restore the connection between these two anatomic units if growth in the cleft child is to proceed with any degree of normality. Delaire's[7–9] anatomic studies and subsequent development of a surgical technique confirmed the presence of a median cellular septum which establishes a functional connection between the lip and premaxilla in the midline, inserting into the interincisive suture and drawing together the anterior midline structures of the midface. Further studies by Joos[10,11] using magnetic resonance imaging confirmed the relationship of the anterior facial musculature to the underlying structures and further stressed the importance of early restoration of these structures if one is to reduce the need for multiple secondary procedures.

Other significant contributions to the correction of secondary deformities have been made by surgeons[12–16] emphasizing the importance of early correction of the lip–nose deformity, all of whom, like Delaire, adopt a radical approach to correction of the nasal cartilaginous deformity as part of their primary procedure. If this radical approach

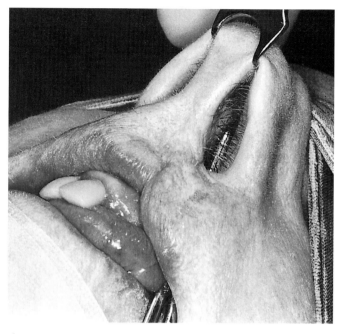

Fig. 66.4 Persistent oronasal Fistula (forceps from mouth to nostril).

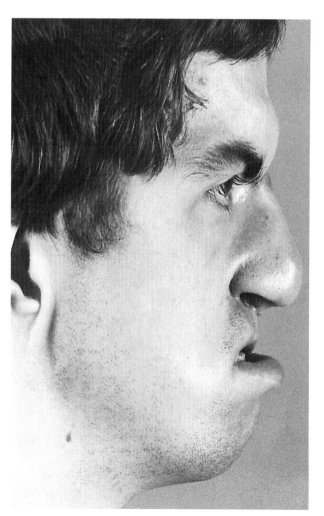

Fig. 66.3 Cleft and cleft surgery sequelae.

is adopted then not only are potential further interventions, in theory, reduced but also later corrections can be based on a sound anatomic foundation and do not compound an already incorrect previous repair. Questions must be asked about the effect of such radical and aggressive surgery on facial development, the number of secondary corrections that are required during the subsequent period of development and the nature of these corrections. Outcome studies to date do suggest that this approach is correct.[17–21]

Early indicators of dysfunction include obvious signs of failure of midfacial growth (Fig. 66.3), collapse or deviation of the nasal structures, and evidence of muscle dysfunction including an inability to protrude the upper lip, whether symmetrically or asymmetrically, persistent oronasal fistulae (Fig. 66.4), recurrent bouts of secretory otitis media and failure of normal speech and language development. All these complications of dysfunction are equally important and need to be corrected at the earliest possible opportunity. Clearly, the earlier secondary revisional procedures are carried out, the less will be the adverse effect on growth and development. However, even where growth has ceased, every opportunity to improve dysfunction should be taken. A complete revision of lip and nose repair, with the aim of restoring the anatomic structures that have been disrupted by the cleft and subsequent surgery should be carried out if the above-mentioned aims are to be achieved. Such 'interceptive surgery' has the potential to favorably transform outcomes and reduce the need for further major surgery.[21–24]

INDICATIONS AND OPPORTUNITIES FOR SURGICAL INTERVENTION

One is often reminded that growth and development is a long-term process, taking the better part of twenty years and that, therefore, it is not possible to assess the outcome of a particular surgical regime for the management of cleft lip and palate until this process has come to its natural end. This has not only been an excuse for failure to assess outcome at an early age, for example at five years, but it has also led to an approach whereby many major deficits and the resultant dysfunctions are not revised for fear of interference with growth. Instead a multiplicity of operations are carried out to correct deformities such as are seen from time to time at various ages. Many of these procedures will in themselves produce an immediate improvement in the situation with which they are attempting to remedy, but the improvements are short-lived as the underlying deformity and dysfunction have not been corrected. Indeed, these operations may be considered as compounding an already less than ideal situation, and the more that are carried out the more difficult it becomes to correct the underlying problem. It would seem logical, therefore, to correct the sequelae of cleft lip and palate, which comprise deformities directly due to the cleft itself as well as the deformities arising from the primary surgical technique employed and the resultant scar tissue, as early as possible.

EARLY SECONDARY ALVEOLAR BONE GRAFTING

Primary, early (within the first 18 months of life), autogenous bone grafting in reconstruction of clefts of the palate and alveolus has been demonstrated in most treatment centers to fall short of desired therapeutic results. Whatever the ultimate effect on facial growth and dental arch relationship,[25,26] even when the technique used avoids disruption of vomerine mucosa,[27] the quantity of bone present at the times of eruption of the maxillary permanent incisor and canine teeth is usually insufficient to permit these teeth to enjoy normal periodontal support and reach functional positions in the upper dental arch.

After conventional primary closure of a cleft lip, there is inevitable scar tissue, vestibular oronasal fistula, inadequate support for the ala of the nose, and absence of bone in the region of the future permanent lateral incisor and canine teeth. The goals of early secondary alveolar bone grafting, performed when the permanent central incisor adjacent to the cleft is about two-thirds erupted, are:

- closure of vestibular and palatal oronasal fistulae
- provision of bone of sufficient quantity and appropriate quality to ensure healthy periodontal support of the permanent central incisor and to allow eruption of the permanent lateral incisor (if present) and canine teeth
- provision of support for the lateral ala of the nose by establishing an adequate skeletal nasal base
- provision of suitable bony architecture of the premaxilla and the anterior face of the maxilla on the cleft side to support accurate muscle reconstruction
- establishment of a functional nasal airway on the cleft side.[28,29]

Success of secondary alveolar bone grafts is time dependent to the extent that certain critical events such as eruption of teeth have windows of limited duration. Alveolar bone grafts, however, can be successfully performed in adults. If the bone graft is performed prior to the eruption of the permanent canine tooth the result is almost always successful.[30,31] Criteria of success are:

- long-term preservation of alveolar bone
- eruption and periodontal health of the permanent central incisor, lateral incisor and canine teeth
- adequate width of the attached gingivae in the region of the cleft
- absence of exposed cementum on teeth adjacent to the cleft.

The graft material of choice is autogenous cancellous marrow of the ilium[32] (iliac crest bone graft), which is packed into the alveolar cleft defect, the soft-tissue margins of which are, concomitantly, surgically repaired. These soft-tissue margins are the palatal mucoperiosteum, the nasal mucosa, and the attached and unattached buccal, vestibular gingiva. The erupting tooth 'stimulates' alveolar and graft bone growth and in the vast majority of cases, in our clinical experience, the canine tooth spontaneously erupts through the graft to assume a functional final position in the maxillary dental arch. If the bone graft is delayed until 8 or 9 years of age, the maxillary incisor will already have erupted (at approximately 6 years of age) which carries the risk of periodontal bone loss and root resorption. For this and other reasons, the most appropriate time to perform alveolar bone grafting is at about 5–6 years of age. Alveolar bone is differentially responsive in such situations because it has a distinctive physiology, reflecting its separate developmental origin from the bone that constitutes the bulk of the mandible. Alveolar bone is derived from the dental primordium, the dental papilla; its affiliation is therefore with odontoblasts that deposit dentine. This affinity reflects the fact that alveolar bone is a derivative of the original vertebrate exoskeleton.[33] Alveolar bone is much more dependent upon mechanical stimuli for maintenance than is bone of the body of the mandible; it is lost very rapidly when teeth are removed with the loss of mechanical stimulation. Alveolar bone also turns over much more rapidly than does bone of the body of the mandible.

The mandibular symphysis can also be used as a donor site for bone grafting in maxillofacial clefts. The success of mandibular bone as a graft in this region may be partly explained by the common ectomesenchymal origin of both donor and recipient sites. Nevertheless, in the reconstruction of secondary alveolar clefts, anterior iliac crest bone is the most often chosen because of the ease with which an adequate quantity of cancellous bone can be obtained. In unilateral clefts we perform concomitant nasolabial muscle surgery at this age in order to establish midline symmetry of the face, maxilla, mandible and cranium.[34] In bilateral cases, we perform alveolar grafts prior to orthodontic arch expansion. It is not possible to perform simultaneous nasolabial muscle surgery because of the risk of vascular compromise to the premaxilla. Whether unilateral or bilateral, when appropriate grafting and soft-tissue procedures accomplish almost normal anatomic reconstruction of the cleft defect, there is usually significant improvement in growth, function and esthetics.

EARLY SECONDARY ALVEOLAR BONE GRAFTING: THE UNILATERAL DEFORMITY

Craniofacial development is both hierarchical and integrated, consequently there is no single basis for facial malformations. In cleft lip and palate, initial facial bone formation takes place at the direction and under the influence of asymmetric and distorted muscle forces. Several authors have recommended cleft treatment protocols using primary rib grafts in conjunction with other treatment modalities such as neonatal orthopedics because they state that teeth can erupt through the rib graft and that there is more favorable maxillary segment alignment, both of which contribute to a better overall conclusion.

We conducted a study to determine the need for early secondary alveolar bone grafts in patients who had previously undergone primary rib grafts. Outcomes of primary treatment of a group of 74 pediatric and adolescent cleft lip and palate patients who underwent early secondary alveolar grafting were assessed. The study population was restricted to 26 patients with unilateral total labiomaxillopalatine clefts who had undergone both primary rib grafts and early secondary alveolar bone grafts, for whom there were complete and excellent quality records. The mean age of the patients at the time of rib graft replacement was 7 months. The mean age of early secondary alveolar graft was 6.9 years. Parameters of assessment included presence or absence of vestibular oronasal fistula, palatal oronasal fistula, deviation of nasal septum to the non-cleft side, dental overjet, coincidence of the maxillary and mandibular dental and skeletal midlines, radiographic evidence of bone and actual bone stock at the time of the secondary surgery. Of the 26 patients, 93% had vestibular oronasal fistulae, 86% had palatal oronasal fistulae, and 71% had deviation of the nasal septum to the non-cleft side. Vestibular oronasal fistulae are not simply defects in the integrity of the oral mucosa which constitute a source of irritation to the patient. In fact, they represent clinical proof of insufficient reconstruction of the nasolabial muscles, a part of which is normally resident in the nostril sill and on the anterior part of the floor of the nose. Failure to reconstruct adequately the middle of the three interdependent muscle rings of the anterior face leads to global facial imbalance.

Even when the disruption in mucosal integrity appeared to be minimal, the underlying bony defect was significant and prevented the normal eruption of teeth. The presence of anterior palatal oronasal fistulae necessitated revision surgery in order to establish the palatal floor of the secondary graft. Deviation of the nasal septum to the non-cleft side represents asymmetry of the entire labial-septal-premaxillary traction system, the complexity of which can be appreciated in the Masson's trichrome stained sagittal section of a 22 week-old human non-cleft fetus (Fig. 66.5). We see this deformity in utero, in infants and adolescents and adults, until and unless the septo-premaxillary complex is directed by symmetrical function of the nasolabial muscles.

Five patients demonstrated class I incisor relationships, 7 patients had class II incisor relationships and 14 patients (>50%) had class III incisor relationships. No patient demonstrated maxillo-mandibular midline coincidence.

Whatever the effect of surgery on maxillofacial growth,

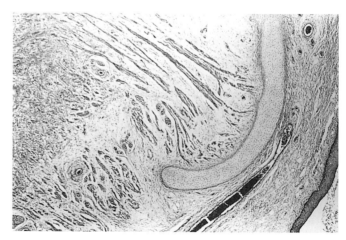

Fig. 66.5 22-week-old human fetus, non-cleft – sagittal section.

it is not the only factor which is at play during development. To assign solely to the surgical procedures either favorable or unfavorable attributes on the basis of observed cephalometric jaw relationships at a given age overlooks several other important factors, one of which is cranial predisposition to facial imbalance. When the anterior cranial angle is small and the sphenoidal angle is open or large, there is a tendency of the glenoid fossa to assume a more posterior position in the cranial base, thereby favoring a skeletal class III relationship. A class II relationship is favored when the anterior cranial angle is open and the sphenoidal angle is more acute.[35] Lack of coincidence of the maxillary and mandibular midlines which was seen in varying degrees of severity confirms that the non-cleft side, the so-called normal side is, in fact, not normal. When the entire premaxilla is deviated to the non-cleft side there is very frequently tooth size and arch length discrepancy in this region. Radiographic and actual evidence of alveolar bone was simply not present in over 90% of patients, 15 of the 16 patients showing no radiographic evidence of adequate bone stock to permit tooth eruption. Radiographs in one patient showed there was a small bony bridge across the cleft, but this too was inadequate to support tooth eruption. The radiographic findings were confirmed at surgery in that this persistent cleft defect was the rule rather than the exception.

Placement of particulate marrow secondary alveolar bone grafts was carried out in the conventional manner, concomitant with nasolabial muscle reconstruction when indicated. In our experience, in this group of patients, primary alveolar bone grafting did not eliminate the need for early secondary bone grafts.

EARLY SECONDARY ALVEOLAR BONE GRAFTING: THE BILATERAL DEFORMITY

The optimal time for performing alveolar bone grafting with concomitant closure of oronasal fistulae remains somewhat controversial, particularly with respect to bilateral cleft lip/palate deformities. Premaxillary osteotomy can improve the accuracy of alveolar bone graft surgery but there is concern that this maneuver significantly inhibits subsequent maxillary growth. In a recent retrospective study to evaluate treatment outcomes of a group of pediatric and adolescent cleft lip/cleft palate patients who had previously undergone bilateral alveolar bone grafts concomitant with premaxillary osteotomy, the study population included 18 patients with bilateral labiomaxillopalatine clefts. All patients underwent single-stage bilateral alveolar bone grafts, premaxillary osteotomy, closure of vestibular oronasal fistula and closure of palatal oronasal fistula. Follow-up times ranged from 29 months to 8 years. The following parameters were assessed: vestibular oronasal fistula, palatal oronasal fistula, radiographic evidence of bone in the cleft, and maxillary-mandibular incisor relationship. Conventional cephalometric analyses were avoided because of the inherent imperfections of superimposition techniques, inappropriate reliance on statistical norms, and failure to take into account the influence of cranial influence on facial development. Most operations were performed at approximately 5–6 years of age (range 5–11 years); 15 patients had no orthodontic expansion prior to the bone grafts, and 3 patients had only minimal pre-graft orthodontic expansion. Seventeen patients had complete closure of both vestibular and palatal oronasal fistulae; 1 patient, a juvenile diabetic, had failure of closure of the palatal oronasal fistula but the vestibular closures were successful. No alveolar bone graft failures occurred as assessed both clinically and radiographically. No premaxillary segments were lost and there was clinical evidence of acceptable vascular supply to both the buccal and palatal dentoalveolar soft tissues. In this investigation, premaxillary osteotomy was successfully carried out as part of the secondary bilateral alveolar bone graft procedure. It appears that the risk of loss of premaxillary segments is low. The effect of premaxillary osteotomy on subsequent maxillary growth should be considered in clinical terms of risk–benefit ratios as they pertain to the presence of adequate bone to support dental development and eruption of teeth and the ultimate need for orthognathic surgery.

SECONDARY MUSCULAR RECONSTRUCTION OF THE LIP AND NOSE

Typically, in secondary deformities of labiomaxillopalatine clefts one sees not only the stigmata of the initial deformity and the failure to obtain complete reconstruction of the deep structures but also the problems arising from scar patterns which vary among both techniques and operators. For these reasons it is absolutely indispensable to perform a very thorough examination in order to establish an accurate diagnosis on which specific treatment can be based.

The means by which the surgeon achieves the goals of secondary reconstruction of the nasolabial muscles include:

1. complete opening of the cleft
2. wide subperiosteal dissection, particularly of the facial aspect of the maxilla
3. repositioning of the nasal septum

4. reconstruction of the nasolabial muscles of the cleft side

5. reconstruction of the orbicularis oris muscle in two planes with sliding of the lateral side of the cleft under the medial side

6. repositioning of the alar cartilage using a unilateral marginal incision.

The design of the incision for reopening the cleft is essentially similar to those described for primary closure by Delaire[28,36,37] (Fig. 66.6).

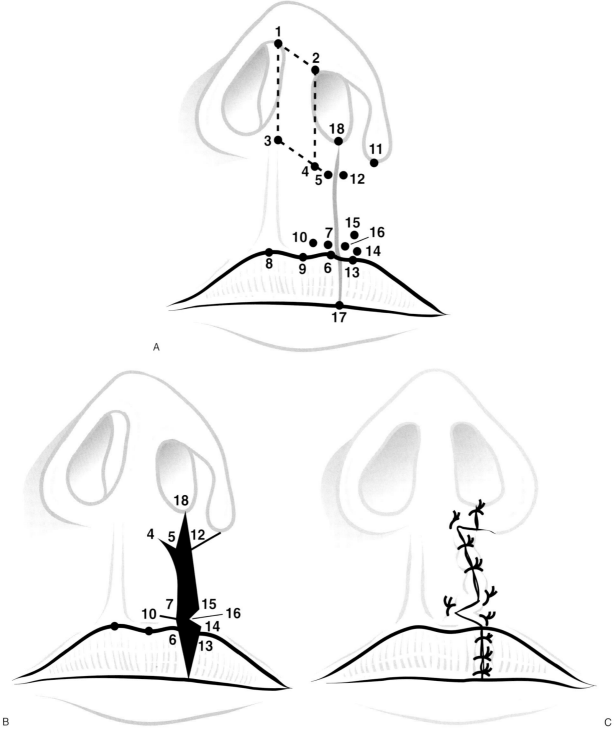

Fig. 66.6 Unilateral cleft lip: **(A)** landmarks for incision; **(B)** incision and area of excised scar; **(C)** final appearance.

In the unilateral cleft, on the non-cleft side, the following points are used:

1. superior internal angle of the nostril on the non-cleft side
2. superior internal angle on the cleft side
3. base of the columella on the non-cleft side
4. point situated at the base of the columella on the cleft side such that the distance 3–4 is the same as 1–2 and 2–4 is the same as 1–3
5. point on the medial aspect of the scar of the lip in the elongation of the line 3–4
6. as 5, on the medial aspect of the scar at the mucocutaneous junction
7. a point approximately 1 mm above 6
8. the peak of the cupid's bow on the non-cleft side
9. the base of the cupid's bow in line with the upper labial frenum and such that 8–9 equals 9–6
10. a point situated approximately 2 mm above the mucocutaneous junction at a distance medial to 7 which is related to the distance 4–6 and in essence is the difference in length between 4–6 and 3–8; in practice this point never crosses over the midline.

On the outer aspect of the repaired cleft:

11. the junction between the lower lateral cartilage and the skin of the lip
12. a point exactly opposite 5 on the medial side of the scar
13. a point on the mucocutaneous junction on the lateral margin of the scar
14. a point 1 mm or so above 13 such that 13–14 equals 6–7
15. a point situated above 14 at a distance equal to 7–10
16. the same length at 14–15 and 7–10 forming an equilateral triangle made up of the points 14–15–16
17. a point situated on the free margin of the upper lip below points 6 and 13
18. a point in the floor of the nose at the extremity of the scar.

The V–Y flap at the mucocutaneous junction, just above the white roll, may be avoided by using a curved incision as described by Pfeiffer.[38] Excellent lengthening of the scar can be achieved without making transverse incisions, so improving the potential esthetic as well as functional gain (Fig. 66.7).

In bilateral clefts, the procedure is also similar to the primary functional cheilorhinoplasty described by Delaire[28,37] utilizing incisions that are almost identical; it must be borne in mind, however, that the repair that is being revised may not primarily have re-established muscle continuity across

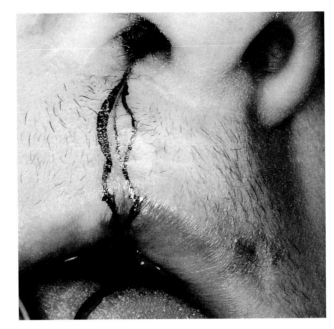

Fig. 66.7 Wavy line incision.

the midline and that the prolabial tissues are not only esthetically displeasing but non-functional. It is therefore necessary to raise a midline prolabial flap to identify all the nasolabial muscles and return them to their correct symmetrical position.

The design of the lateral incision is as already described for unilateral clefts. In the midline, the following points are recommended (Fig. 66.8):

- **Points 1 and 2**: at the base of the columella on both sides, at the inferior internal angle of the nares
- **Point 3**: the midpoint of a line joining points 1 and 2
- **Point 4**: on the mucocutaneous junction, in the midline of the upper lip
- **Points 5 and 6**: on a horizontal line which bisects the line 3–4 and being the inferior extension of lines drawn for continuity with the straightest part of the columella on either side such that the distance 5–6 equals the width of the columella
- **Points 7–7' and 8–8'**: on the line 5–6 which has been extended laterally and on each side of the residual scar
- **Points 9 and 10**: the most inferior points of the lower lateral cartilage where they meet the labial skin
- **Points 11 and 12**: on the lateral aspect of the residual scar, 1 mm above the mucocutaneous junction
- **Points 13 and 14**: at the upper extremity of the residual scar.

Having made the incisions according to this design and joining points 4–5 and 4–6 such that a shield shaped skin flap is produced, the residual scar can be excised and the

was used to free the nostril along the length of the pyriform aperture. This flap, which will restore bulk to the nasal vestibule, can be developed on the excision of labial mucosal scar tissue, extended as necessary to the neighboring tissues and then transposed into the nose as an island flap, based on a deep submucous and muscular pedicle. On the medial aspect of the cleft, the subperiosteal dissection is limited such that it leaves in place all fibrous connective tissue near the midline, the anterior nasal spine and the labial frenum which will serve as anchorage points to which the lateral muscular structures can be sutured. A unilateral interseptocolumellar incision is used to gain access to the cartilaginous nasal septum which can be widely exposed so as to treat the deformities by resecting only that tissue which is absolutely necessary to reposition the septum.

It is this part of the operation that is most important. The deep nasolabial musculature includes the transverse nasal muscle and the depressor septi muscle – these should be considered as one muscle group being fixed at two extremities: originating from the nasal bone above, the transverse nasal muscle descends on the triangular cartilage, skirts the nostril and continues with the depressor septi to insert on the premaxilla, from the apex of the lateral incisor tooth laterally to that of the canine and even the first premolar tooth. Medially, one can attach the fibers of the depressor of the tip of the nose which has its origin at the apex of the central incisor tooth and then passes towards the medial crus and the skin overlying the columella. From each head of the transverse and the depressor septi muscles some fibers are given off to form the sill of the nostril. There are connections of these muscles with the lateral expansion of the septo-premaxillary ligament and obvious relationships with the incisive crest and the anterior nasal spine.

It is probably impossible to surgically reconstruct the sill of the nostril in minute anatomic detail and reinsertion of this deep muscle group to the region of the anterior nasal spine is not devoid of pitfall because excessive ascension of the nasal sill and of the alar base will aggravate the eversion of the nostril and amplify the nostril defect. On the other hand, the role which the deep muscular layer plays in the stability of the nasal sill and alar base is important; therefore, these muscles ought to be sutured medially, as low as possible and extended across the midline, to the connective tissue overlying the maxilla which was preserved precisely for this purpose during the surgical exposure. If no appropriate support point for the suture is available, one can use the tissue of the frenum or the maxillary vestibule.

This descending deep layer will be crossed by the ascending layer of the orbicularis oris that will be widely undermined from the skin but left attached to its mucosa. In the

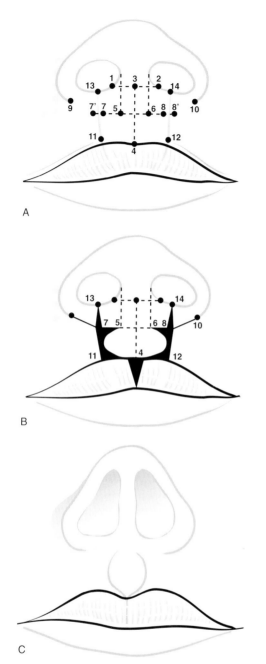

A

B

C

Fig. 66.8 Bilateral cleft lip: **(A)** landmarks for incision; **(B)** incision and area of excised scar; **(C)** final appearance.

prolabial skin elevated to expose the anterior nasal spine and anterior and inferior part of the nasal septum.

Wide subperiosteal undermining of the cleft side is carried out on the facial aspect of the maxilla up to and including the infraorbital rim, the pyriform aperture and the nasal bone. When the preoperative examination reveals a significant retraction of the external nasal vestibule with nostril defect rigidly adherent to the underlying maxilla, it is necessary to foresee the need for the contribution of a mucosal flap to fill in at the junction of the incision which

region immediately subjacent to the nostril, the labial fibers of the levator muscles are separated from the nasolabial bundle of the external portion of the orbicularis oris muscle. A solid, nonresorbable nylon suture is passed from the deep, superior part of the nasolabial bundle to the fibrous tissue at the base of the septum just below the anterior nasal spine. This stitch will fix the advancement of the lateral aspect of the cleft which is possible as a result of the wide undermining already carried out, thus permitting the lip to be superiorly repositioned and in turn correcting the ptosis that was part of the original deformity. In doing this it is necessary to avoid ascension and advancement that would permit the persistence of lateral vermilion ptosis. It is also necessary to avoid excessive repositioning which can give the appearance of hypoplasia of the vermilion.

By their crossing directions, these first two muscular points have a correcting effect on the vertical distension of the nasolabial region. This distension is usually not written about but can almost always be observed, even in the articles of the most famous surgeons, by an excess in height between the point of implantation of the nostril and the mucocutaneous line of the upper lip.

The orbicularis muscle is next reconstructed in two planes. In the deep plane the lateral head of the orbicularis oris muscle is taken across the midline to join the same muscular bundle of the non-cleft side. This act requires partial dissection of the median connective tissue septum of the upper lip. The deep plane includes part of the labial mucosa which is attached to the muscle which is carried deep, very high above and almost behind the labial frenum, so that this region is almost normal while at the same time avoiding excessive scarring with the maxilla. The suturing then progresses to the superficial plane, permitting further final control of the vertical length of the lip by pressure on the opposite medial crus or the ipsilateral superficial muscles of the nostril. The quality of this muscular suture is a determining factor in the prevention of secondary scar contracture and the achievement of fullness of the lip, particularly that of the philtrum and the nasolabial angle, owing to the importance of the muscular advancement and to the differences in tension between the deep and superficial planes of the orbicularis oris muscle.

The width of the nostril sill is controlled by suturing the superficial muscles of the nostril to the contralateral muscles in the midline under the flap. When the muscular reconstruction is complete, the skin approximation is already almost perfect and requires only a few finishing stitches (Figs 66.9 and 66.10).

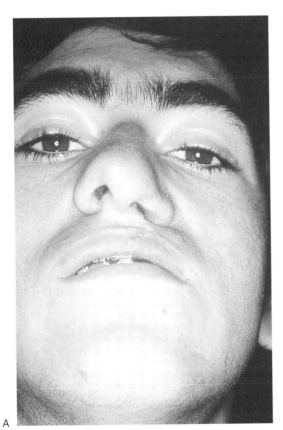 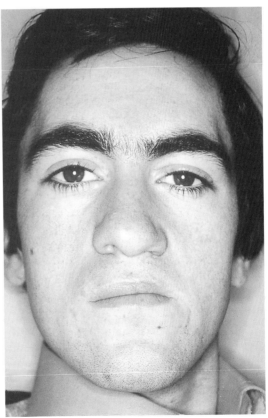

A   B

Fig. 66.9 Unilateral cleft lip: **(A)** preoperative appearance; **(B)** postoperative appearance.

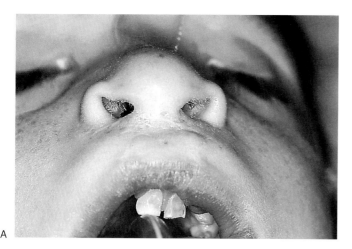 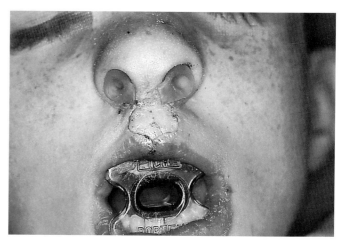

Fig. 66.10 Bilateral cleft lip: **(A)** preoperative appearance; **(B)** postoperative appearance.

SUMMARY

With the exception of those special cases of clefts associated with holoprosencephaly, where there exists true hypoplasia, the anomalies observed in labiomaxillary clefts result essentially from displacement, deformation and functional hypotrophy of the dentoskeletal elements and the covering soft tissues. This is particularly true with the maxillary bony segments, the dentoalveolar elements which they support, and the nasal cartilages. It is also true for the nasolabial muscles, which are all present on the cleft side but whose absence of normal insertions and the resultant dysfunctions are directly responsible for both supra- and subjacent anomalies. Displacement, deformation and functional hypotrophy also affect the mucocutaneous structures which border the labial clefts. This fact is less well known, but it has, nevertheless, great importance in the selection of incision design in the primary closure of cleft lip. The goal of primary closure is not only to re-establish normal insertions of all the nasolabial muscles but also to restore normal position of all of the other soft tissues including the mucocutaneous elements. Thus, one can only realize Veau's 'embryological surgery' by re-establishing at operation 'all of the anatomical and functional conditions which normally ought to have been present at the end of the embryonic stage'.

Conventional surgical wisdom, which holds that one should wait until growth has finished before undertaking surgical correction of the postoperative sequelae of primary cheiloplasty, carries with it many disadvantages. If, after primary surgery of the lip, oral-labial dysfunctions exist, they will exert their nefarious influences throughout growth and by themselves lead to long-term dentofacial imbalances, some of which can be considerable. These imbalances have significant influence on facial harmony and unless accurate,

symmetrical and functional reconstruction of the nasolabial muscles is achieved during primary surgery, not only will the existing dentoskeletal imbalances be exaggerated but other deformities will be caused during subsequent growth, among which the most important are nasal obstruction and mouth breathing, reduced translation of the maxilla, asymmetry of the nose and inability of the patient to project the upper lip, reduced growth of the premaxilla and excessive vertical height of the anterior mandible. Thus, no matter what the initial esthetic result of the primary surgery, it is essential that the clinician conduct the most rigorous surveillance of operated patients in order to maintain an index of suspicion, to identify and, indeed, to correct as early as possible, by the most appropriate means. These are secondary functional cheilorhinoplasty, functional genioplasty and orthognathic surgery, the goals of which are to improve nasal respiration, occlusion, labial and labiomental function and indirectly velar-lingual function and global facial harmony.

SECONDARY SURGERY FOR CLEFT PALATE

Without doubt, closure of the cleft palate has an effect on midfacial growth, speech and hearing and that effect is, of course, to some extent dependent on the severity of the cleft in terms of the hard- and soft-tissue deficit and whether or not it is associated with a cleft of the lip and/or alveolus. However, a critical review of the evidence, both clinical and experimental, in the literature does not substantiate the argument that palatoplasty is the major cause of failure of midfacial growth. Such ideas were promoted in particular by Graber[39] and Herfert[40] citing, amongst other factors, the use of mucoperiosteal flaps and early closure as the major culprits and reasoning for modifications in both technique and timing such as the use of mucosal rather than muco-periosteal flaps[41] and delayed closure of the hard palate.[42,43] The latter workers Witzel et al[43], however, ceased delayed closure of hard palate as they could show no long-term benefit. Ross[44] noted that the best skeletal relationships were, in fact, found in those patients in whom cleft palate repair had been completed before the age of 18 months. Evidence from the Sri Lankan studies[45] showed that normal growth could be expected in the adult with an unoperated cleft lip and palate but suggested that the palatal surgery was of more significance than lip surgery. In reality, closure of both lip and palate have, to some extent, an adverse effect on midfacial growth. Of great significance in cleft palate alone is the effect of repair on speech and hearing. It is, therefore, essential that the training and experience of the cleft surgeon is such that not only does he understand the deformity but is in a position to choose a primary surgical technique that will avoid adverse outcomes.

Bardach[46] suggests that a one-stage, two-flap palatoplasty has a minimal effect on midfacial growth and speech development and does not result in the production of significant palatal fistulae. This is in contrast to the two-stage method described by Delaire[47,48] which is completed by the age of 12–15 months. Delaire drew attention to the three distinct mucosal zones of the hard palate (Fig. 66.11) as well as the importance of restoring the muscle sphincter of the soft palate. He advocates avoidance of vomerine mucosal flaps in primary closure of the palate,[47] a topic which is the cause of much heated debate between those with whom this approach finds favor and those with whom it does not. There seem to be conflicting views within Scandinavia alone: Friede & Lilja[49] confirm Delaire's view that use of a vomerine flap results in a reduction in vertical height and anterior projection of the maxilla. Semb[50] provided equally forceful evidence that this flap does not have an adverse effect on growth of the midface, although in other studies, somewhat equivocally, she demonstrated its adverse effects on midfacial growth as well as maxillary symmetry.[51,52] Ross's assessment of the outcome of Malek's technique,[53,54] a method of palatal repair not dissimilar to Delaire's, showed excellent results when compared to the Toronto group.

Cleft palate repair may result in poor hearing, poor quality speech and failure of midfacial growth. All three adverse outcomes are intimately connected, with poor hearing being an indicator of soft palate dysfunction, and failure of speech and language development being, likewise, an indicator of dysfunction either from shortness of the soft palate and, therefore, velopharyngeal inadequacy, immobility of the soft palate, or the presence of fistulae, both anterior and

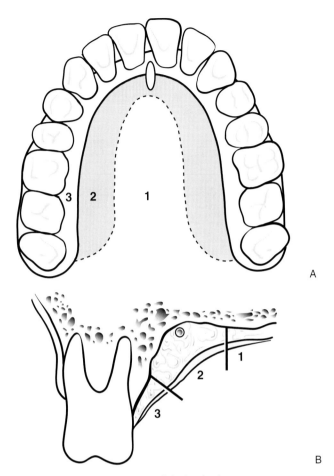

Fig. 66.11 The three mucosal zones of the hard palate.

posterior. Also of importance is the immobile scarred palate, with considerably reduced height of the palatal vault. This in turn displaces the tongue such that the anterior portion of the tongue applies pressure against the anterior part of the mandible and so favors the development of a class III dentoskeletal relationship.[55]

SECONDARY CORRECTION OF THE CLEFT PALATE DEFORMITY

The potential problems following primary cleft palate repair have already been outlined. Prior to any surgery their effect must be fully assessed; this assessment, primarily of function, must form part of the protocol for any well organized multidisciplinary cleft team. In particular, regular assessments must be made of hearing and speech and language development. Hearing assessment should commence prior to closure of the cleft palate at approximately six months of age and must include auditory brainstem response (ABR) and visual reinforced audiometry (VRA) to exclude sensorineural deficit, and tympanometry. Carefully structured assessments of speech and language development should be considered an essential part of the program of care and should include examination with the aerophonoscope[56,57] or anemometry, multiview videofluoroscopy and possibly nasoendoscopy. In this way, it is possible to assess the exact nature of the dysfunction and its site such that any operative procedure can be tailored accordingly and carried out at the optimum time. Sell[58] describes such a 'model of practice' – one which, if adhered to, would detect sooner rather than later the need for secondary surgery of both the palate and pharynx.

Closure of palatal fistulae

Palatal fistulae may occur in any position along the site of the original repair and, as already indicated, must be considered a functional complication related to the type of primary repair. Those that are symptomatic, or likely to become so, should be closed.[59–61] Closure of anterior palatal fistulae, in the complete cleft of lip and palate, should be considered as an essential component of the total revision and restoration of function already described. In those situations where the size is such that available local tissue is at a premium, either in the complete cleft or the isolated cleft of the palate, then tissue may need to be imported, for example from the tongue.

Revision of palatoplasty and velar lengthening

Inadequate movement of the entire soft palate but normal movement of the pharyngeal musculature implies incomplete, limited or, possibly, complete absence of restoration of muscle continuity at the time of primary surgery. Revision of the palatoplasty must be the procedure of choice. This approach has the additional benefit of lengthening the palatal soft tissues, so avoiding the adoption of inappropriate methods of surgical correction, such as the V–Y pushback,[62] which because of the large amount of resultant scar tissue will lead to further complications, in particular retropositioning of the maxilla, the creation of palatal fistulae, or the development of previously asymptomatic fistulae. Sommerlad,[63] in his study of re-repair of cleft palate, confirmed the benefits to be gained from revision of the primary palatoplasty. In such circumstances it is imperative that the soft palate musculature be restored to normal or as near normal as possible. This may be more or less difficult depending on the initial method of repair and width of the cleft, as well as the position of the resultant scar. Reconstruction of the normal anatomy of the soft palate will produce lengthening, to some extent dependent on the posterior extension of the incision along the palatoglossal fold.[48]

Island flap of the Uvula

In those situations where velopharyngeal inadequacy may be due to failure of movement of the posterior part of the soft palate, an island flap of the uvula is a simple and effective method of correcting the problem[48] (Fig. 66.12).

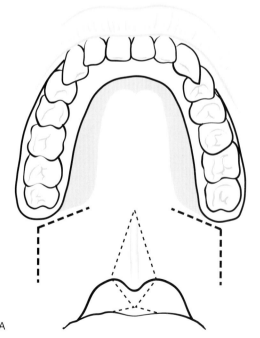
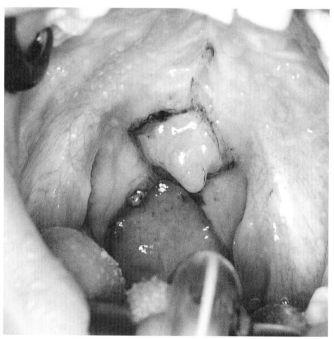

A B

Fig. 66.12 Island uvula flap: **(A)** outline for incision; **(B)** operative view.

PHARYNGEAL SURGERY

The indications for pharyngoplasty are clearly defined following careful multitechnique assessment. The most effective method of surgical management remains controversial. What is certain, however, is the need to work closely with the speech pathologist in deciding which of the many different approaches is appropriate and to develop a protocol which ensures a consistent approach to the specific anomaly. Despite the evidence that revision palatoplasty might be more appropriate in the first instance, pharyngeal surgery, with or without palatal lengthening, remains a popular first line method of managing velopharyngeal inadequacy. The techniques are described fully in other chapters but essentially are divided into two groups, depending on the abnormality found – posterior or lateral pharyngeal wall surgery. The indications for one or the other have been well outlined by Shprintzen,[64] the amount of lateral wall movement or lack of posterior wall movement being the decisive factors.

Posterior pharyngoplasty

The flap may be superiorly or inferiorly based; relative advantages and disadvantages remain a matter for continuing debate despite evidence that there is no effect on outcome.[65] There is no doubt that the superiorly based flap is currently more popular, with its base at the level of the tubercle of the atlas and its insertion into the soft palate at points determined in accordance with preoperative assessment of need (Fig. 66.13). However, the inferiorly based flap continues to be advocated by many, including Millard,[66] and by Delaire[67] with a modification that raises the level of the base of the flap more superiorly (Fig. 66.14). This modification overcomes the major concerns relating to the

A) Incisions

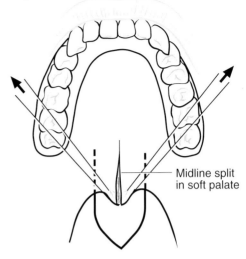

Midline split in soft palate

B) Insertion of flap into soft palate

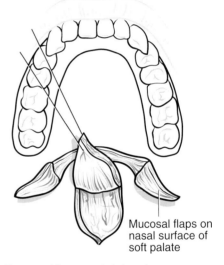

Mucosal flaps on nasal surface of soft palate

Fig. 66.13 Pharyngeal flap, superiorly based.

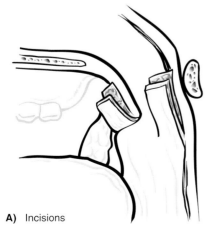

A) Incisions

A

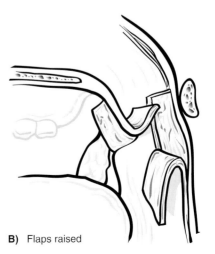

B) Flaps raised

B

Fig. 66.14 Pharyngeal flap, inferiorly based.

inferiorly based flap, these being an apparent limitation of length and downward pull of the flap.[68,69] Perhaps of greater importance in this debate is the width of the flap and the resulting lateral ports, a concern initially raised by Hogan[70] and confirmed by Shprintzen et al[64] and Witt & D'Antonio.[69]

Lateral pharyngoplasty

The concept of managing velopharyngeal inadequacy by creating a dynamic muscle sphincter rather than a pharyngeal flap to control the size of the pharyngeal orifice was initially described by Hynes.[71] Many modifications have since been described, including those by Orticochea[72] and Jackson,[73] whose method is most widely used nowadays. The sphincter is formed from the posterior tonsillar pillars, which are raised to include the palatopharyngeus, rotated and sutured end-to-end[74] (Fig. 66.15). This procedure is designed to reduce the size of the lateral ports and tighten the central area. While this approach has the appeal of maintaining neuromuscular function and is relatively easy to perform, very many variations have been incorporated, making it well nigh impossible to make valid assessments of published outcome studies and the value, or otherwise, of the technique.[70] It should, however, remain in the armamentarium of the cleft surgeon.

CONCLUSIONS

Of major importance in the management of cleft lip and palate is the adoption of a primary surgical approach that will minimize those sequelae commonly associated with surgery, an approach which will also promote function and, therefore, growth and development. With this in mind, this chapter has outlined and emphasized those procedures that will re-establish, at the earliest opportunity, a degree of normality. The multitudinous techniques used to correct individual aspects of the deformity, outside the context of the whole deformity, have been omitted in the belief that they represent an uncoordinated approach to cleft management, an approach that should be discouraged. Unless the foundations are correct, it is not possible to overcome the sequelae of both the cleft deformity and cleft surgery, and the abnormality will be ever increasingly compounded. Descriptions of these techniques are available in most texts on cleft management and, for the sake of completeness, we would recommend that the reader become familiar with them.

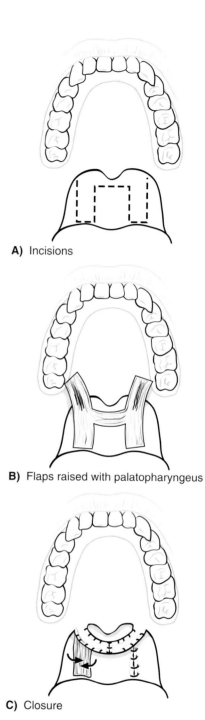

A) Incisions

B) Flaps raised with palatopharyngeus

C) Closure

Fig. 66.15 Sphincter pharyngoplasty.

ACKNOWLEDGMENTS

The authors are most grateful to the Departments of Medical Illustration at Dalhousie University and Poole Hospital. They would like to thank the Editor of the *British Journal of Oral and Maxillofacial Surgery* for permission to reproduce Figures 66.1–3.

REFERENCES

1. Veau V 1938 Bec-de-lièvre. Masson, Paris
2. Millard DR 1964 The unilateral cleft lip nose. Plastic and Reconstructive Surgery 34:169–175
3. Precious DS, Delaire J 1993 Clinical observations of cleft lip and palate. Oral Surgery, Oral Medicine, and Oral Pathology 75:141–151
4. Delaire J, Fevre JR, Chateau JP, Courtay D, Tulasne JF 1977 Anatomie et physiologie des muscles et de frein median de la levre superieure. Revue de Stomatologie et de Chirurgie Maxillofaciale 78:93–103
5. Chateau JP 1977 Etudes anatomiques du complexe musculaire naso-labiale. Incidences sur la chirurgie reconstructive des fentes labiales. Thèse Médecine, Nantes
6. Delaire J, Chateau JP 1977 Comment le septum nasale influence-t-il la croissance premaxillaire et maxillaire? Revue de Stomatologie et de Chirurgie Maxillofaciale 78:241–254
7. Delaire J 1971 Considerations sur la croissance faciale en particulier du maxillaire superieur. Revue de Stomatologie et de Chirurgie Maxillofaciale 72:57–76
8. Delaire J, Talmant JC, Billet J 1972 Evolution des techniques de cheilorhinoplastie pour fentes labiomaxillaires. Revue de Stomatologie et de Chirurgie Maxillofaciale 73:337–357
9. Delaire J 1975 La cheilorhinoplastie primaire pour fente labiomaxillaire congenitale unilaterale. Essai de schematisation d'une technique. Revue de Stomatologie et de Chirurgie Maxillofaciale 76:193–215
10. Joos U, Friedburg H 1987 Darstellung des Verlaufs der mimischen Muskulatur in der Kernspintomographie. Fortschritte der Mond, Kiefer-Gesichstchirurgie 32:125–127
11. Joos U 1987 The importance of muscular reconstruction in the treatment of cleft lip and palate. Scandinavian Journal of Plastic and Reconstructive Surgery 21:109–113
12. Anderl H 1997 Extensive primary nose repair in unilateral cleft lip. In: Abstracts of the Third International Congress on Cleft Palate and Related Craniofacial Anomalies, Toronto. p 150
13. McComb H 1985 Primary correction of unilateral cleft lip nasal deformity: a 10 year review. Plastic and Reconstructive Surgery 75:791–799
14. Salyer KE 1986 Primary correction of the unilateral cleft lip nose: a 15 year experience. Plastic and Reconstructive Surgery 77:558–568
15. Talmant JC 1984 Correction de la narine du bec-de-lièvre unilatéral. Ses grands principes. Annales de Chirurgie Plastique et Esthetique 29:123–132
16. Joos U 1989 Muscle reconstruction in primary cleft lip surgery. Journal of Craniomaxillofacial Surgery 17:8–10
17. Joos U 1995 Skeletal growth after muscular reconstruction for cleft lip, alveolus, and palate. British Journal of Oral and Maxillofacial Surgery 33:139–144
18. Horswell BB, Pospisil OA 1995 Nasal symmetry after primary cleft lip repair: comparison between Delaire cheilorhinoplasty and modified rotation-advancement. Journal of Oral and Maxillofacial Surgery 53:1025–1030
19. Markus AF, Precious DS 1997 Effect of primary surgery for cleft lip and palate on mid-facial growth. British Journal of Oral and Maxillofacial Surgery 35:6–10
20. Adcock S, Markus AF 1997 Mid-facial growth following functional cleft surgery. British Journal of Oral and Maxillofacial Surgery 35:1–5
21. Joos U 1997 Late outcomes of cleft surgery: a comparison between Delaire and other techniques. In: Abstracts of the Annual Scientific Conference of the Craniofacial Society of Great Britain, p 17
22. Delaire J 1979 La cheilorhinoplastie fonctionelle secondaire. Revue de Stomatologie et de Chirurgie Maxillofaciale 80:218–224
23. Talmant JC 1995 Reflections on the etiopathogenesis of cleft lip and palate and the development of their treatment. Annales de Chirurgie Plastique et Esthetique 40:639–656
24. Schendel SA, Delaire J 1981 Functional musculo-skeletal correction of secondary unilateral cleft lip deformities: combined lip-nose correction and Le Fort I osteotomy. Journal of Maxillofacial Surgery 9:108–116
25. Robertson NR, Jolleys A 1968 Effects of early bone grafting in complete clefts of the lip and palate. Plastic and Reconstructive Surgery 42:414–421
26. Jolleys A, Robertson NR 1972 A study of the effects of early bone grafting in complete clefts of the lip and palate: five year study. British Journal of Plastic Surgery 25:229–237
27. Rosenstein SW, Monroe CW, Kernahan DA, Jacobson BN, Griffith BH, Bauer BS 1982 The case for early bone grafting in cleft lip and cleft palate. Plastic and Reconstructive Surgery 70:297–309
28. Precious DS, Delaire J 1992 Surgical considerations in patients with cleft deformities. In: Bell WH (ed) Modern practice in orthognathic and reconstructive surgery. Vol 1. WB Saunders, Philadelphia, pp 391–425
29. Delaire J, Precious DS, Gordeff A 1985 Surgical considerations of mucocutaneous anomalies in cleft lip. In: Abstracts of the Fifth International Congress on Cleft Palate and Related Craniofacial Anomalies, Monaco
30. Bergland O, Semb G, Abyholm FE 1986 Elimination of the residual alveolar cleft by secondary bone grafting and subsequent orthodontic treatment. Cleft Palate Journal 23:175–205
31. Enemark H, Sindet-Pedersen S, Bundgaard M 1987 Long-term results after secondary bone grafting of alveolar clefts. Journal of Oral and Maxillofacial Surgery 45:913–919
32. Boyne PJ, Sands NR 1976 Combined orthodontic-surgical management of residual palato-alveolar cleft defects. American Journal of Orthodontics 70:20–37
33. Smith MM, Hall BK 1990 Development and evolutionary origins of vertebrate skeletogenic and odontogenic tissues. Biological Reviews of the Cambridge Philosophical Society 65:277–373
34. Delaire J, Precious DS 1986 Influence of the nasal septum on maxillonasal growth in patients with congenital labiomaxillary cleft. Cleft Palate Journal 23:270–277
35. Precious DS, Bosco D, Gooddday RH 1997 Cranial predisposition to dental/skeletal deformity in cleft and non-cleft patients. In: Abstracts of the Annual Scientific Conference of the Craniofacial Society of Great Britain, p 16
36. Delaire J 1978 Theoretical principles and technique of functional closure of the lip and nasal aperture. Journal of Maxillofacial Surgery 6:109–116
37. Markus AF, Delaire J 1993 Functional primary closure of cleft lip. British Journal of Oral and Maxillofacial Surgery 31:281–291
38. Pfeifer G, Schmitz R, Herwerth-Lenck M, Gundlach KKH 1991 Long-term results following primary lifting of the nose and labioplasty according to the wave-line procedure in unilateral complete clefts. In: Pfeifer G (ed) Craniofacial anomalies and clefts of the lip, alveolus and palate – Fourth Hamburg International Symposium. Thieme, New York, pp 239–246
39. Graber TM 1949 Craniofacial morphology in cleft palate and cleft lip deformities. Surgical Gynecology and Obstetrics 88:359–364
40. Herfert O 1958 Fundamental investigations into the problems related to cleft palate surgery. British Journal of Plastic Surgery 11:97–102
41. Perko MA 1979 Two-stage closure of cleft palate (progress report). Journal of Maxillofacial Surgery 7:46–80
42. Friede H, Johanson B 1977 A follow-up study of cleft children treated with vomer flap as part of a three-stage soft tissue surgical procedure. Facial morphology and dental occlusion. Scandinavian Journal of Plastic and Reconstructive Surgery 11:45–49
43. Witzel MA, Salyer KE, Ross RB 1984 Delayed hard palate closure: the philosophy revisited. Cleft Palate Journal 21:263–269

44. Ross RB 1987 Treatment variables affecting facial growth in complete unilateral cleft lip and palate. Part I : Treatment affecting growth. Cleft Palate Journal 24:5–23

45. Mars M, Houston WJB 1990 A preliminary study of facial growth and morphology in unoperated male unilateral cleft lip and palate subjects over 13 years of age. Cleft Palate Journal 27:7–10

46. Bardach J, Morris HL, Olin WH 1984 Late results of primary veloplasty: the Marburg Project. Plastic and Reconstructive Surgery 73:207–218

47. Delaire J, Precious DS 1985 Avoidance of the use of vomerine mucosa in primary surgical management of velopalatine clefts. Oral Surgery Oral Medicine, and Oral Pathology 60:589–597

48. Markus AF, Smith WP, Delaire J 1993 Primary closure of cleft palate: a functional approach. British Journal of Oral and Maxillofacial Surgery 31:71–77

49. Friede H, Lilja J 1994 Dentofacial morphology in adolescent or early adult patients with cleft lip and palate after a treatment regimen that included vomer flap surgery and pushback palatal repair. Scandinavian Journal of Plastic and Reconstructive Surgery and Hand Surgery 28:113–121

50. Semb G 1991 A study of facial growth in patients with unilateral cleft lip and palate treated by the Oslo CLP Team. Cleft Palate Craniofacial Journal 28:1–21

51. Semb G 1991 A study of facial growth in patients with bilateral cleft lip and palate treated by the Oslo CLP Team. Cleft Palate Craniofacial Journal 28:22–39

52. Molsted K, Dahl E, Brattström V, McWilliam J, Semb G 1993 A six-centre international study of treatment outcome in patients with clefts of the lip and palate: evaluation of maxillary asymmetry. Cleft Palate Craniofacial Journal 30:22–28

53. Ross RB 1995 Growth of the facial skeleton following the Malek repair for unilateral cleft lip and palate. Cleft Palate Craniofacial Journal 32:194–198

54. Malek R, Psaume J 1983 Nouvelle conception de la chronologie et de la technique chirurgicale du traitement des fentes labio-palatines. Resultats sur 220 cas. Annales de Chirurgie Plastique 28:237–247

55. Delaire J 1976 Influence du voile du palais sur la statique linguale et la croissance maxillofaciale. Revue de Stomatologie et de Chirurgie Maxillofaciale 77:821–834

56. Rineau G 1993 L'aerophonoscope. Observation des déperditions nasales dans les divisions palatines au moyen de l'aerophonoscope. Revue Glossa 34:4–14

57. Rousteau G, Peuvrel E, Bouric JM, Rineau G 1995 L'aerophonoscope: principes – intérêts. Etude préliminaire. Bulletin d'Audiophonologie – Annal Scientifique de Université de France-Compté 11:571–603

58. Sell D, Ma L 1996 A model of practice for the management of velopharyngeal dysfunction. British Journal of Oral and Maxillofacial Surgery 34:357–363

59. Abyholm FE, Borchgrevink HHC, Eskeland G 1979 Palatal fistulae following cleft palate surgery. Scandinavian Journal of Plastic and Reconstructive Surgery 13:295

60. Cohen SR, Kalinowski J, LaRossa D et al 1991 Cleft palate fistulae: A multivariate statistical analysis of prevalence, aetiology and surgical management. Plastic and Reconstructive Surgery 87:1041

61. Dufresne CR 1990 Oronasal and nasolabial fistulae. In: Bardach J, Morris HL (eds) Multi-disciplinary management of cleft lip and palate. WB Saunders, Philadelphia

62. Wardill WEM 1937 The technique of operation for cleft palate. British Journal of Surgery 21:117–130

63. Sommerlad BC, Henley M, Birch M, Harland K, Moiemen N, Boorman JG 1994 Cleft palate re-repair – a clinical and radiographic study of 32 consecutive cases. British Journal of Plastic Surgery 47:406–410

64. Shprintzen RJ, Lewin ML, Craft CB et al 1979 A comprehensive study of pharyngeal flap surgery: Tailor made flaps. Cleft Palate Journal 16:46

65. Whitaker LA, Randall P, Graham WP et al 1972 A prospective and randomised series comparing superiorly and inferiorly based posterior pharyngeal flaps. Cleft Palate Journal 9:304

66. Millard DR Jr 1980 Cleft Craft, III. The evolution of its surgery: alveolar and palatal deformities. Little, Brown, Boston, p 240

67. Delaire J, Tulasne J-F 1979 Technique de l'urano-staphylo-pharyngo-plastie a pedicule inferieur. Quelques details operatoires. Revue de Stomatologie et de Chirurgie Maxillofaciale 80(1):26–32

68. Trier WC 1985 The pharyngeal flap operation. Clinics in Plastic Surgery 12:697

69. Witt PD, D'Antonio LD 1993 Velopharyngeal insufficiency and secondary palatal management. A new look at an old problem. Clinics in Plastic Surgery 20:707–721

70. Hogan MV 1973 Clarification of the surgical goals in cleft palate speech and the introduction of lateral port control (LPC) pharyngeal flap. Cleft Palate Journal 10:331

71. Hynes W 1950 Observations on pharyngoplasty. British Journal of Plastic Surgery 20:244

72. Orticochea M 1970 Results of the dynamic muscle sphincter operation in cleft palates. British Journal of Plastic Surgery 23:128

73. Jackson IT 1985 Sphincter pharyngoplasty. Clinics in Plastic Surgery 12:711

74. Moss ALH, Pigott RW, Albery EH 1987 Hynes pharyngoplasty revisited. Plastic and Reconstructive Surgery 79:346

Management of cleft speech

67

ROSEMARY WATTS

INTRODUCTION

This chapter outlines principles in the management of speech in children with cleft lip and palate, emphasizing the role of the speech and language therapist working closely with other members of a comprehensive multidisciplinary cleft team. It briefly describes the vocal tract, explaining the production of speech sounds, and reviews the protocols of assessment that will enable effective diagnosis and management of cleft speech, and long-term followup.

MULTIDISCIPLINARY TEAM APPROACH

There is an increasing awareness of the need for specialists involved in the care of children with cleft lip and palate to work closely together and not in isolation.[1-6] This is essential not only from the clinician's point of view but also in view of the complex effects that clefts and cleft speech may have on a child's development, relationships, confidence and self-esteem.

In recent years speech and language therapists have worked towards gaining a key role in the cleft team; this has been advantageous not just for the speech and language therapist and other members of the team, but, primarily, for the child with a cleft. It has made involvement with the child from birth onwards much easier to achieve and has enabled meticulous monitoring of development of speech, language and communication skills.

The establishment of an effective care plan for cleft speech must be based initially on protocols that ensure assessment of a child's progress at key stages using agreed and realistic patterns of testing. This forms the foundation for future management and detailed discussion with other members of the team so that the most appropriate decisions can be made to achieve the best possible care. Each member of the team will visualize the way forward from a slightly dif-ferent perspective, an approach that is helpful in managing complex disorders. As the speech and language therapist needs to be aware of the key surgical, orthodontic and otological phases, likewise the surgeon, orthodontist and otologist must be aware of the critical stages of speech development. The concept of leaving one aspect of care to another specialist in the team without an understanding of that person's work is not an acceptable way of working, and all team members should be equally well informed. Each member of the team retains a distinct professional identity while participating in an holistic approach to the total management of every child, sharing expertise to develop greater understanding and knowledge between disciplines.

THE VOCAL TRACT

Control of the airstream within the vocal tract to realize speech is a complex procedure involving coordinated movements of the larynx, pharynx, nasal cavity and structures of the oral cavity. Air is pushed up from the lungs and is directed and controlled, according to the sound being produced, through the glottis and pharynx, and is shaped by the articulators to be released by the nasal or oral cavity depending on the target sound – e.g. /m/ /n/ /ng/ are released nasally, all other sounds in English are released orally.

In cleft palate, speech anomalies are caused by:

- insufficient intraoral pressure
- weak lip pressure
- abnormal tongue position
- velopharyngeal inadequacy
- abnormal neuromuscular function
- abnormal jaw relationships
- abnormal dentition
- hearing loss due to a conductive deficit
- hearing loss due to a sensorineural deficit.

The cleft palate may be further compounded by nasal obstruction, nasal septal deviation, narrowing of the overall dimension of the nasal aperture, turbinate hyperplasia, or hypertrophy of the tonsils and adenoids.

The structure most obviously directly affected by a cleft of the soft palate is the velopharyngeal sphincter. It should always be remembered that other functions within the entire vocal tract may be indirectly affected to various degrees, as a result of efforts by the child to control the air at alternative sites if the velopharyngeal sphincter is not functioning competently.[7]

Competent functioning of the velopharyngeal sphincter involves a number of factors, both direct and indirect. Some of the direct factors include the anatomy of the relevant parts involved – the pharyngeal walls, velum, tonsils, adenoid tissue – and the existence of any fistula. Indirect factors include hearing, articulatory development relevant to age, or possibly a learning disability.

The child born with a cleft is dependent upon the primary surgery to restore the anatomy, enabling the development of the normal function that produces good speech. However there are considerable difficulties in completely restoring the anatomic configuration to normality and therefore function. This may be due in part to true hypoplasia or malformation of the anatomico-functional units. For example, despite extensive research into the anatomy of the eustachian tube and its muscular attachments, it is still not known whether the basic deformity and therefore malfunction that leads potentially to an increased incidence of chronic secretory otitis media, is due to the presence of abnormal cartilage or to abnormal or absent muscle insertions.[8]

It is, therefore, essential that the choice of primary surgical technique pays particular attention to the meticulous restoration of all the elements involved in the cleft[9] and that consideration is given to timing of the repair.[10] Speech and language therapists have been advocating early repair of the palate for some time[11,12] to give the child the best possible opportunity of developing good speech without the need to establish compensatory articulations, e.g. backing voiceless plosives /p/ /t/ /k/ to pharyngeal /pˤ/ /tˤ/ /kˤ/ or glottal ʔ/ placement, or backing the alveolar voiceless fricative /s/ as velar or pharyngeal fricatives / x ħ/ respectively.

ASSESSMENT OF CLEFT SPEECH

PRINCIPLES OF ASSESSMENT

The type and timing of treatment of cleft speech disorders must be based on an effective understanding of the abnormality and the ability to make an accurate diagnosis. Any assessment must take into account normal development of speech, language and communication. Normal developmental immaturities need to be differentiated from articulatory errors related to the cleft. It could be a normal process for a child to use a velar plosive instead of an alveolar – e.g. /kæk/ for cat or gɒg for dog. This could also be a cleft type characteristic. It is important that any assessment incorporates both views and takes place in conjunction with an oral assessment. A speech and language therapist working with a cleft team has the advantage of a joint oral assessment with other members of the team.

STANDARDIZATION OF METHODS OF ASSESSMENT

Standardization of the approach to reaching an accurate diagnosis and therefore high quality treatment is an effective way of ensuring the best outcome. Every cleft center must have an overall management protocol within which each team member has an individual plan of action. In the United Kingdom, speech and language therapists have progressively, over the years, developed and agreed upon methods of assessment, initially producing the Great Ormond Street Speech Profile Assessment (GOS.SPASS)[13] for clinical assessment and subsequently the Cleft Audit Protocol for Speech (CAPS)[14] for audit purposes.

CAPS offers a series of sentences specially designed to assess all speech sounds in all positions. This, together with counting 1–20 and a sample of spontaneous speech, gives a recorded format producing a comprehensive record of these results, as well as offering the facility to group any speech disorders into those of anterior or posterior cause (Fig. 67.1). The majority of specialist cleft speech and language therapists follow the same protocol for the ages at which assessments take place, these being 18 months, 3 years, 5 years, 10 years, 15 years and 20 years. Contact before 18 months of age varies from center to center. The involvement of the speech and language therapist in the Dorset Cleft Center begins sometimes from birth and always within the first six months.

CLINICAL PROTOCOL USED IN THE DORSET CLEFT CENTRE

Birth to 6 months

The pediatric liaison health visitor, specialist pediatric nurse, or speech and language therapist – all trained in establishing early feeding patterns – give any necessary feeding advice. This advice always encourages as normal feeding as possible. Nonsyndromic babies use a Mead Johnson soft bottle and ordinary teat, sometimes with a cross. The majo-

CLEFT AUDIT PROTOCOL FOR SPEECH

Name:		Date:	Audit No:
Date of Birth:	Age:	Centre:	
Cleft Type:		Therapist:	

INTELLIGIBILITY RATING

0 = Normal
1 = Different from other children's speech, but not enough to cause comment
2 = Different enough to provoke comment but possible to understand most speech
3 = Only just intelligible to strangers
4 = Impossible to understand

NASALITY and NASAL AIRFLOW

HYPERNASAL RESONANCE	0	0–1	1	2	3
HYPONASAL RESONANCE	0	0–1	1	2	3
AUDIBLE NASAL EMISSION	0	0–1	1	2	3
NASAL TURBULENCE	0	0–1	1	2	3
GRIMACE	0	0–1	1	2	3

VOICE	0 = Normal	1 = Dysphonic	Comment:

CONSONANT PRODUCTION

	LABIAL			ALVEOLAR				POST AOLVEOLAR			VELAR	
INITIAL REALISATION												
CORRECT TARGET	p	b	f	n	t	d	s	ʃ	tʃ	dz	k	g
FINAL REALISATION												

CLEFT-TYPE CHARACTERISTICS (CTCs)

1. Lateralisation/lateral		6. Glottal	
2. Palatalisation/palatal		7. Active nasal fricative	
3. Backing to velar		8. Weak/Nasalised consonants	
4. Backing to uvular		9. Nasal realisations	
5. Pharyngeal		10. Absent pressure consonants	

SUMMARY OF SPEECH PATTERN

0 = No CTCs (cleft type characteristics)
1 = Anterior Oral CTCs
2 = Posterior Oral CTCs
3 = Non-oral CTCs
4 = Passive CTCs
5 = Developmental Errors
6 = Other

COMMENTS

Fig. 67.1 The Cleft Audit Protocol for Speech with the Cleft Palate Speech Assessment Audit Form key (with kind permission of author.)

CLEFT PALATE SPEECH ASSESSMENT AUDIT FORM
KEY

HYPERNASAL RESONANCE	0	=	Not present
	0–1	=	Mild and occasional
	1	=	Mild and consistent
	2	=	Moderate and consistent
	3	=	Severe and consistent
HYPONASAL RESONANCE	0	=	Not present
	0–1	=	Mild and occasional
	1	=	Mild and consistent
	2	=	Moderate and consistent
	3	=	Denasalised consonants
AUDIBLE NASAL EMISSION	0	=	Not present
	0–1	=	Mild and occasional
	1	=	Mild and consistent
	2	=	Moderate and consistent
	3	=	Severe and consistent
NASAL TURBULENCE	0	=	Not present
	0–1	=	Mild and occasional
	1	=	Mild and consistent
	2	=	Moderate and consistent
	3	=	Severe and consistent
GRIMACE	0	=	Not present
	1	=	Nasal flare
	2	=	Nasal grimace
	3	=	Facial grimace

SUMMARY OF SPEECH PATTERN — KEY

Group together the Cleft type characteristics from the boxes above thus:

0	=	No Cleft type characteristics
1	=	Boxes 1 and 2 (Palatalisation/Palatal + Lateralisation/Lateral)
2	=	Boxes 3 and 4 (Backing to velar + Backing to uvular)
3	=	Boxes 5 and 6 and 7 (Pharyngeal + Glottal + Active nasal fricative)
4	=	Boxes 8 and 9 and 10 (Weak nasal consonants + Nasal realisations + Absent pressure consonants)
5	=	Developmental errors
6	=	Other

Fig. 67.1 (Cont'd)

rity of the syndromic babies also cope with this. Severely micrognathic babies, if they are experiencing difficulties with breathing such that oxygen saturation levels cannot be maintained, are managed surgically, for example with a labio-glossopexy.[15] Presurgical orthodontics are not practiced, as it is not considered necessary for feeding and the effects of maxillary appliances on speech development are still unknown.

The close inter-relationship between oral and aural development necessitates a thorough audiologic assessment within the first three months, primarily to exclude sensori-neural deficit; the assessment includes auditory brainstem response or oto-acoustic emission. Tympanometric assessment is carried out immediately prior to the primary surgery at between 4 and 5 months. Should there be any question concerning the tympanic membrane function, grommets will be inserted at this operation.

The speech and language therapist gives the parents

information on the development of speech and language skills and appropriate advice on how to facilitate sound production. The more informed parents are about development of speech, the better equipped they will be to offer positive, appropriate and relaxed stimulation.[16]

6 to 18 months

Following the closure of the soft palate and lip, the baby is regularly reviewed by the cleft team to enable the monitoring of the completed surgery, the gradual reduction in width of any remaining hard palatal defect, and hearing and speech and language development. The parents may be encouraged to facilitate sounds that require little or no intraoral pressure, e.g. /m/ /w/ /n/ /j/ /l/, before the complete closure of the palate. Closure of the hard palate will be completed by 12–14 months of age.

At 18 months of age, the first formal assessment of speech sounds is made. Regular intervention continues if there is any indication that compensatory articulatory patterns are developing. The information is obtained through play; all sounds and sound sequences heard are recorded. Articulatory placements are assessed and any cleft type compensatory patterns investigated further. If velopharyngeal dysfunction is suspected to be the cause this also is assessed further according to the child's level of cooperation, as described below under Assessment of cleft speech and velopharyngeal function.

18 months to 3 years

Routine review by all members of the team continues on a regular basis. Referral to other disciplines is made as required.

At 3 years of age the first full formal assessment of speech is undertaken. The CAPS assessment is completed and renders a comprehensive record of all the child's speech, separating any articulatory inaccuracies into those of anterior or posterior cause. This assessment should be recorded on video as well as on high quality audio tape.

Direct intervention continues if there are any speech problems. If there is a suggestion of a velopharyngeal inadequacy this is further investigated. The child has probably already been assessed using the aerophonoscope (see below) and may even have been taken for multiview videofluoroscopy, if further information is required to clarify any persistent speech anomaly. A team discussion takes place with any relevant members to decide upon the best management – either speech therapy alone or surgical intervention followed by speech therapy.

3 to 5 years

During this period every effort is made to enable the child to enter school with intelligible speech. Routine reviews continue, any intervention required is undertaken by the relevant team members. At 5 years of age a further full routine assessment of speech is recorded on both video and audio tape.

5 to 10 years

Routine reviews and therapy continue if required, as during this period there may be other procedures that affect speech. Consideration may have to be given to any orthodontic or surgical interventions that could affect articulatory placements or interrupt therapy.

10 to 15 years

Routine reviews continue. When the child is 10 years of age, the speech and language therapist records a further full speech assessment. During this time there is greater emphasis on monitoring growth and development; surgical and orthodontic procedures that may affect speech may be performed. Speech is again assessed and recorded at 15 years.

15 years to 20 years

During this time, it may be decided whether or not orthognathic surgery is required. If maxillary advancement is necessary, presurgical and postsurgical speech assessments are essential. The speech and language therapist should also make a final assessment of speech at 20 years of age.

ASSESSMENT OF CLEFT SPEECH AND VELOPHARYNGEAL FUNCTION

There are 24 consonant sounds and an equal number of vowel sounds in 'normal' English speech.[17] Consonant sounds are categorized according to voice (depending on whether the vocal folds are vibrating or not), place (depending on where in the vocal tract they are articulated), and manner (depending on how the airstream is modified to produce a particular sound).

A phonetic and phonologic assessment should be obtained when assessing children's speech. While the original cause of a distortion or substitution in the phonetic development of a child with a cleft is anatomic or physiologic, the relationship between phonetic and phonologic acquisition has been demonstrated by Russell and Grunwell.[18] It is therefore important to address both systems. The medical model of assessment can account for any articulatory deficit caused by a structural or functional abnormality but cannot be used to analyze the deviant acquisition of the full phonologic system.

As already outlined, speech assessments should be video and audio recorded and detailed transcriptions completed, in this case using the Cleft Audit Protocol for Speech. Speech therapy intervention has to take into consideration both the phonetic and phonologic aspects shown to be needing correction and may therefore have to look to the psycholinguistic model for remediation, for example by assessing auditory discrimination of speech sounds.

Early intervention is valuable as part of a multidisciplinary preventative approach to the management of children with cleft lip and palate. Encouraging sounds that require little or no intraoral pressure before complete closure of the palate is a useful and helpful early intervention. Suggestions of ways to stimulate prelinguistic skills to encourage communication can be given to parents, together with details of early language development.

Assessments of babbling vocalizations have been made from 3 months and predictions suggested concerning those babies at risk of developing deviant speech patterns.[16,18] Input can be offered at an early stage by encouraging oral awareness and production of achievable sounds, so helping articulatory placements and capitalizing on the basic abilities to speak. Mousset and Trichet[19] recommended treatment at 15 months for children not producing voiceless plosives /p/ /t/ /k/; although this was a French paper it has equally valid applications in the English language.

Comprehensive perceptual and instrumental speech assessments on cleft patients at our unit are conducted at the ages of 18 months and 3, 5, 10 and 15 years. In the younger child, this consists of evaluating the sound system by monitoring phonetic vocabulary and carrying out a phonologic assessment of the sequencing of sounds. From 18 months onwards, resonance and nasal emission, receptive and expressive language, prosody (intonation patterns) and pragmatics (use of language) are all assessed, together with communication skills and intelligibility, and recorded as shown in Figure 67.1.

There is considerable variation in the terminology used to describe velopharyngeal anomalies. The terms incompetence, inadequacy and insufficiency have been used interchangeably to describe these disorders. Trost-Cardamone[20] suggested that the term 'velopharyngeal inadequacy' be used generically, using 'velopharyngeal insufficiency' where there is a lack of tissue and 'velopharyngeal incompetency' in those situations where function is inadequate. Loney and Bloem[21] and Bzoch[22] recommend the overall terms

velopharyngeal dysfunction (VPD) or velopharyngeal insufficiency to describe all disturbances of the mechanism arising from structural, functional, neurogenic and behavioral causes. Included in the general expression VPD are the terms:

— **velopharyngeal inadequacy**, which refers to a structural or anatomic deficiency
— **velopharyngeal incompetence**, which refers to an active or passive defect in neuromuscular function or neurogenic impairment
— **velopharyngeal mislearning (VPM)**, which refers to faulty articulatory behavior.[23]

Any velopharyngeal dysfunction will cause a defect of nasality which may present as a nasal emission of air (most easily detected on the production of voiceless plosives, fricatives and affricatives), hypernasality (excess resonance of the voice in the nasal cavity and perceived on the production of voiced consonants and vowels), hyponasality (when there is too little nasal resonance resulting in a 'blocked up' tone most noticeable on the release of nasal consonants). Mixed nasality may occur producing both 'hyper' and 'hypo' symptoms. A nasal snort may be heard, suggesting there is a minimal escape of air or resonance and nasal turbulence where there is a 'cul-de-sac' effect. Any of these characteristics may occur independently or in any combination.

Nasality and nasal air flow studies include hypernasal resonance, hyponasal resonance, audible nasal emission, nasal turbulence, and nasal grimace;[24,25] they are classified as shown in Figure 67.1.

With the exception of the three nasal consonants /m/ /n/ /ng/, there is complete closure of the velopharyngeal sphincter, although recently it has been suggested that for the high back vowel /a/ complete closure is not necessary. This mechanism ensures that there is appropriate oral pressure and tone during speech.

Assessment of any velopharyngeal dysfunction starts with the perceptual record of speech: this may show any of the distortions, substitutions or omissions of articulation already mentioned or purely an emission of nasal air or abnormal nasal resonance or a combination of these characteristics. These cleft characteristics are also categorized as errors of place, manner or voice.

Cleft speech type characteristics are assessed on the following scale (Fig. 67.1):

0: no cleft type characteristics
1: 1 and 2 (palatalization/palatal + lateralization/lateral)
2: 3 and 4 (backing to velar + backing to uvula)
3: 5, 6 and 7 (pharyngeal + glottal + active nasal fricative)

4: 8, 9 and 10 (weak nasal consonants + nasal realizations + absent pressure consonants)

5: developmental errors

6: other.

Further studies are required to render accurate information on the structure and function of the velopharyngeal sphincter and to enable decisions to be made about the most effective treatment and intervention. Many specialist instruments for airflow studies are available, the one used being largely dependent on personal preference. The investigations of choice for the direct visualization and diagnosis of the structural and functional characteristics of VPD are nasopharyngoscopy and multiview videofluoroscopy. In addition, a number of indirect techniques involving the assessment of nasal emission and nasal airflow have been described. These include the Czermak mirror test, the Sea-Scape monitor, the 'N' nasal indicator, the Exeter Nasal Anemometer, the Super Nasal Oral Ratiometry System (SNORS), the nasometer and the aerophonoscope.[7,26–31]

The aerophonoscope allows the simultaneous visualization of airflow from both nostrils and the mouth, as well as voice levels, and provides qualitative and quantitative information in a graphic form. The equipment also permits the recording and saving of speech assessment data, which can be reviewed subsequently and compared with other stored information as necessary. Its use has been described in the evaluation of velopharyngeal function before and after laser uvulopalatoplasty.[32] This method of assessing cleft palate speech has formed an important part of the overall speech assessment at our unit since 1993.[33]

The aerophonoscope apparatus consists of a handpiece connected to a computerized monitor or directly to a desktop or laptop computer (Fig. 67.2). The handpiece has three airflow sensors – one for each nostril and one for oral airflow – and an integrated microphone to record voice

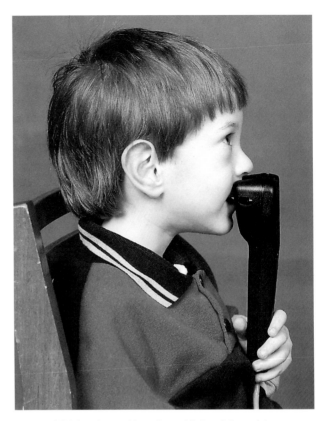

Fig. 67.3 Child showing position of portable handpiece of the aerophonoscope.

levels. During speech assessment, it is placed just below the nostrils and the lips to allow for precise detection and recording of nasal and oral airflow, and sound (Fig. 67.3). Different combinations of measurements may be chosen and the settings for each assessment are made on the monitor keyboard or computer, in a standard window and menu layout (Fig. 67.4). The monitor body houses a small computer that transforms the nasal emission data into a screen display, which can be printed or transferred to a PC or Mac database and saved. Alternatively, an internal or PCMIA card enables direct transfer to the desktop or laptop computer. The display shows the quality and magnitude of nasal emission in a simple two axis format and also provides information on the breathing pattern and voice. It is a reliable, user-friendly machine, able to measure and store comparative data, and also, by enabling bio-feedback, to act as a useful therapeutic tool.

These instruments offer detailed information concerning nasal emission of air and/or nasal resonance but further investigation is required to determine the precise cause to allow for correct diagnosis and decisions about management. It is therefore necessary to use multiview videofluoroscopy, nasopharyngoscopy or magnetic resonance imaging or any combination required to render accurate information on

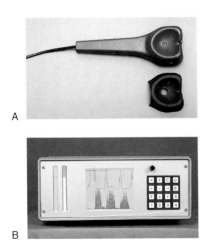

A

B

Fig. 67.2 Handpiece and computerized monitor of the aerophonoscope.

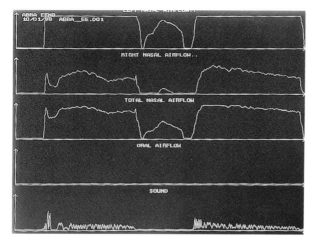

Fig. 67.4 Visualized computer reading of oral blowing showing nasal emission of air.

the structure and function of the velopharyngeal sphincter to determine the most effective intervention. Different information is obtained from nasopharyngoscopy and multiview videofluoroscopy,[34] making it advisable to administer both procedures in the management of cleft speech where possible. Sell and Ma, in a comprehensive outline of one model of practice, discuss some of the surprising factors uncovered by audit, one of which was that some non-cleft VPD groups, including submucous cleft, were not being routinely referred for both assessments. They have now changed their protocol.[35]

It is important that the speech and language therapist is present for these investigations and it is obviously beneficial if a team works regularly together. In our center, an otorhinolaryngologist and a radiologist form part of the team. This enables a good relationship to develop and has proved invaluable when taking children for these assessments.

This complete assessment procedure provides comprehensive information on the speech symptoms, the amount and sometimes variability of nasal emission of air and/or resonance, the anatomic structure, and the function of the velopharyngeal sphincter. Consistency of the nasal emission is an important factor when considering effective management, as speech therapy intervention should facilitate correction of phoneme specific disorders. There may be other inconsistencies, however, which cannot be corrected by speech therapy alone, e.g. a velopharyngeal dysfunction which is achieving a closure but is not able to maintain it to produce spontaneous speech. Where these assessments have demonstrated an insufficiency or incompetence, surgical intervention is probably indicated. Once a velopharyngeal inadequacy has been identified and the decision made about the most appropriate surgical intervention, this procedure

should be carried out as soon as possible to prevent misarticulations occurring.

CONCLUSION

Remedial articulatory or phonologic work should be addressed at the appropriate time in the child's development, always being aware of the cleft type and the developmental factor and allowing for the possibility of the co-occurrence of these two factors. Consideration must be given to intervention by other members of the multidisciplinary team. Robert Shprintzen[34] said that it is 'abnormal for a child to have to attend for speech therapy regularly over long periods of time', and children with clefts are sometimes expected to tolerate just that. Our philosophy of management would wholly endorse this – no child, let alone parent, is able to sustain full cooperation if the demands are too great and no limits are set.

It is still of prime importance to recall that the basis for the best speech outcomes lies in the primary surgical methods of repair that are employed, the timing of those repairs and the surgeon's understanding of the anatomy and physiology involved. The speech and language therapist should take advantage of early intervention; making an informed, correct diagnosis of a speech deficit as early as possible is vital for the most appropriate intervention at the optimum time to achieve the best outcome.

The management of children with a cleft should work towards intelligible speech that will not cause them any embarrassment when they enter school, while they are at school, or thereafter.

REFERENCES

1. American Association of Oral and Maxillofacial Surgeons 1995 Parameters of care for oral and maxillofacial surgery. Journal of Oral and Maxillofacial Surgery 53 (9) suppl 5:108–121
2. Parameters for the Evaluation and Treatment of Patients with Cleft Lip/Palate or Other Craniofacial Anomalies. Cleft Palate-Craniofacial Journal 30 (suppl 1)
3. Shaw WC, Williams AC, Sandy JR, Devlin HB 1996 Minimum standard for the management of cleft lip and palate: efforts to close the audit loop. Annals of the Royal College of Surgeons 78:110–114
4. Clinical Standards Advisory Group 1998 Cleft lip and palate. HMSO, London
5. Strauss RP, Ellis JHP 1996 Comprehensive team management. In: Turvey TA, Vig KWL, Fonseca RJ (eds) Facial clefts and craniosynostosis, principles and management. WB Saunders, Philadelphia, pp 130–142
6. Bardach J, Morris HL 1990 International review of management of cleft lip and palate. Multidisciplinary management of cleft lip and palate. WB Saunders, Philadephia, pp 1–98

7. Lohle E, Joos U, Goz G 1991 Phoniatric results following reconstruction of palatoglossus and palatopharyngeus muscles. In: Pfeifer G (ed) Craniofacial anomalies and clefts of the lip alveolus and palate – 4th Hamburg International Symposium. Thieme, New York, pp 393–395

8. Matsume S, Sando I, Takahashi H 1991 Abnormalities of the lateral cartilaginous lamina and lumen of the Eustachian tube in cleft palate. Annals of Otorhinolaryngology 100:909–913

9. Markus AF, Delaire J, Smith WP 1992 Facial balance in cleft lip and palate I. Normal development and cleft palate. British Journal of Oral Maxillofacial Surgery 30:287–295

10. Kemp-Fincham SI, Kuhen DP, Trost-Cardamone JE 1990 Speech development and the timing of primary palatoplasty. In: Bardach J, Morris HL (eds) Multidisciplinary management of cleft lip and palate. WB Saunders, Philadelphia, pp 736–745

11. Trost-Cardamone JE 1989 Speech in the first year of life: A perspective on early acquisition. In: Kernahan DA, Rosenstein SW (eds) Cleft lip and palate: a system of management. Williams & Wilkins, Baltimore

12. Harding A, Grunwell P 1993 Relationship between speech and timing of hard palate repair. In: Grunwell P (ed) Analysing cleft palate speech. Studies in disorders of communication. Whurr, London

13. Sell D, Harding A, Grunwell P 1994 A screening for cleft palate speech. Great Ormond Street Speech Assessment (GOS.SP.ASS). European Journal of Disorder of Communication 29:1–15

14. Harding A, Harland K, Razzell R 1996 Cleft audit protocol for speech.

15. Bedhet N, Mercier J, Gordeef A, Mouzard A, Delaire J 1990 Labioglossopexy in Pierre-Robin Syndrome: our experiences in 70 cases. Revue de Stomatologie et de Chirurgie Maxillofaciale 91:326–334

16. O'Gara MM, Logemann JA 1990 Early speech development in cleft palate babies. In: Bardach J, Morris HL (eds) Multidisciplinary management of cleft lip and palate. WB Saunders, Philadelphia, pp 717–721

17. Wyatt R, Sell D, Russell J, Harding A, Harland K, Albery E 1996 Cleft palate speech dissected: A review of current knowledge and analysis. British Journal of Plastic Surgery 49:143–149

18. Russell J, Grunwell P 1993 Speech development in children with cleft lip and palate. In: Grunwell P (ed) Analysing cleft palate speech: studies in disorders of communication. Whurr, London

19. Mousset MR, Trichet C 1985 Babbling and phonetic acquisitions after early complete surgical repair of cleft lip and palate. Paper presented at the Fifth International Congress on Cleft Palate and Related Craniofacial Abnormalities, Monte Carlo

20. Trost-Cardamone JE 1981 Differential diagnosis of velopharyngeal disorders. Communication Disorders: An Audio Journal of Continuing Education 6(7), July 1981

21. Loney RW, Bloem TJ 1987 Velopharyngeal dysfunction: recommendations for use of nomenclature. Cleft Palate Journal 24:334–335

22. Bzoch KR 1989 Etiological factors related to cleft palate speech. In: Bzoch KR (ed) Communicative disorders related to cleft lip and palate, 3rd edn. Little, Brown, Boston, pp 79–105

23. Trost-Cardamone JE 1989 Coming to terms with VPI: a response to Loney and Bloem. Cleft Palate Journal 26:68–70

24. Kummer AW, Curtic C, Wiggs M, Lee L, Strife JL 1992 Comparison of velopharyngeal gap size in patients with hypernasality, hypernasality with nasal emission and nasal emission or nasal turbulence (rustle) as the primary speech characteristic. Cleft Palate Craniofacial Journal 29:152–156

25. McWilliams BJ, Morris HL, Shelton RL 1990 Cleft palate speech, 2nd edn. CV Mosby, Chicago, pp 22–41

26. Stengelhofen J 1993 The nature and causes of communication problems in cleft palate. In: Stengelhofen J (ed) Cleft palate – nature and remediation of communication problems. Whurr, London, pp 10–134

27. Ellis RE 1979 The Exeter nasal anemometer. In: Ellis RE, Flack FC (eds) Diagnosis and treatment of palatoglossal malfunction. The College of Speech Therapists, London

28. Main A, Kelly SW, Manley MCG 1990 Instrumental assessment and treatment of hypernasality following maxillofacial surgery using SNORS: single case study. International Journal of Language and Communication Disorders (In press)

29. Rineau G 1993 L'aerophonoscope: Observation des deperditions nasales dans les divisions palatines au moyen de l'aerophonoscope. Revue Glossa 34:4–14

30. Delaire J 1995 Assessment of speech: the aerophonscope. Address to the Spring Meeting of the British Association of Oral and Maxillofacial Surgeons: focus session on developments in assessment of patients with cleft lip and palate

31. Rousteau G, Peuvrel E, Bourie JM, Rineau G 1995 L'aerophonoscope: principes-interets. Etude preliminaire. Bulletin d'Audiophonologie – Ann Sc Univ Fr Compte 11:571–603

32. Huet P, Sene JM, Rineau G, Mercier J, Legent F, Beauvillain C 1993 Evaluation of velopharyngeal function using the Aerophonoscope before and after surgery for snoring. Annales d'Oto-laryngologie et de Chirurgie Cervico-faciale 110:372–382 (French, English abstract)

33. Devani P, Watts R, Markus AF 1990 Speech outcomes in children with cleft palate: aerophonoscope assessment of nasal emission (In press)

34. Shprintzen R 1990 The conceptual framework for pharyngeal flap surgery. In: Bardach J, Morris HL (eds) Multidisciplinary management of cleft lip and palate. WB Saunders, Philadelphia, pp 806–809

35. Sell D, Ma L 1996 A model of practice for the management of velopharyngeal dysfunction. British Journal of Oral and Maxillofacial Surgery 34:357–363

Secondary palatal surgery and pharyngoplasty

68

JOHN G. BOORMAN/SHIVARAM BHARATHWAJ

Following primary cleft repair, a child enters a period of follow up during which hearing, speech and language development, dental eruption and growth are monitored. In many cases no further surgery will be required. In others, where there exists a significant maxillary bony cleft, a bone graft will be required and is usually carried out in the mixed dentition phase at around 9 years of age. Maxillary growth may be impaired in some repaired cleft lip and palate patients, and a maxillary osteotomy may be beneficial once growth is complete. These procedures are covered in other chapters. Here we consider other problems which may arise following palate repair and which may require treatment.

SYMPTOMS

The palate separates the oral and nasal cavities; the posterior part, the velum or soft palate, is a mobile mucosal flap containing muscle and glands which, together with the lateral and posterior pharyngeal walls, forms the velopharyngeal sphincter. This dynamic structure closes the nasal cavity from the oropharynx during swallowing, blowing, sucking, vomiting and, most critically, speech. The sphincter is open during normal nasal respiration. During eating, the palate prevents food gaining access to the nasal cavity. When the palate fails to serve these functions adequately, additional surgery or other treatment may be required. Inadequate function results either from a fistula through the palate providing a communication between nasal and oral cavities, or from failure of the sphincter, termed velopharyngeal dysfunction. The two may occur simultaneously, have some symptoms in common and, as will be discussed, the presence of a fistula may be deleterious to velopharyngeal function. It is therefore appropriate to consider the presentation and assessment together, before considering the treatment,

which is distinct for each condition but which may be combined in a single operation where appropriate.

The history from the patient or parents is important. Food coming down the nose, vomiting through the nose, inability to blow out candles or suck through a straw are all symptoms of palatal dysfunction, which may be apparent in the infant or young child before speech is fully developed. In speech, inappropriate air flow into or through the nasal cavity results in a 'nasal' quality to the speech, which will often have been noted by family or teacher. The hearing is very important to speech development and is frequently impaired in the young cleft patient due to the high prevalence of otitis media with effusion (OME; 'glue ear'). Any history of previous surgery is important, particularly adenoidectomy which should rarely, if ever, be performed in cleft palate. The loss of the adenoidal pad, the point at which the palate contacts the posterior pharyngeal wall, will exacerbate any tendency to velopharyngeal dysfunction.

EXAMINATION

Examination of the patient involves listening as well as looking. The 'nasal' quality to the speech is made up of hypernasal resonance, nasal emission of air which may be audible or inaudible, audible nasal friction or turbulence, weak oral consonants and frequently compensatory articulatory errors, for example glottal stops or pharyngeal fricatives. In addition, the extra strain placed on the larynx in an attempt to be understood may cause the patient to develop hoarseness of the voice. In the hospital or clinic situation, it is important to be aware that patients produce their 'best' speech – talking slowly and deliberately. In their more normal surroundings, when hurried or excited and talking more spontaneously, there is frequently a deterioration in speech. A thorough assessment of speech, particularly in the young child, is best carried out by the specialist speech and language therapist on a one-to-one basis and is time consuming.

In addition to these audible signs, the patient may have a nasal grimace, an abnormal movement of the external nose as part of the effort to prevent air escaping inappropriately through the nose.

Intraoral examination is important, although there is a limited amount of functional information to be obtained. Fistulae are usually, but not always, obvious. The length of the palate can be seen and its movement assessed when the patient says 'aaah'. In a non-cleft child, or in a well repaired cleft palate, the palate lifts and a dimple appears at around the junction of the anterior two thirds and posterior one third of the soft palate.[1] This is an indication of the locus of action of the palatal muscle sling, to which the most important contributor is the levator veli palatini with a contribution from palatopharyngeus. Any asymmetry of movement should be noted. The size of the tonsils should also be noted. Occasionally large tonsils may interfere with the velopharyngeal sphincter and closure.[2-4] While the length of the palate may be judged, it is impossible to visualize the normal point of contact of the velum with the posterior pharyngeal wall, as it occurs above the plane of the palate. Thus a palate which appears short may be long enough to achieve closure against the posterior pharyngeal wall, and vice versa, depending on the shape of the nasopharynx.

Occasionally, patients are seen who were thought to have merely a cleft of the lip and possibly primary palate with no involvement of the secondary palate, but who exhibit features of submucous cleft palate, i.e. bifid uvula, notching of the posterior border of the hard palate, and the translucent midline strip in the soft palate indicative of incomplete muscle sling.[5] A bifid uvula on its own, however, may occur in 1–2% of the normal population[6-9] and does not, in itself, imply a submucous cleft palate.

Some simple clinical tests may be employed to help in assessing function. A wisp of cotton wool held under the nostrils during phonation of oral consonants is disturbed if there is inappropriate nasal air flow. Similarly, a mirror held under the nostril mists up in the nasal airstream. When a fistula has been identified, it may be occluded on a temporary basis with cotton wool or chewing gum. If a change occurs in the speech, this shows that the fistula is the cause. If the speech remains the same, it indicates either that the fistula is not responsible or that it was not completely obturated. A plate may also be provided as a temporary measure to assess the importance of the fistula in the perceived speech disorder.

The frequency of velopharyngeal dysfunction (VPD) following cleft palate repair varies in reports in the litera-ture from 10% to as high as 50%. The cause of this large variation is not well established; methods used to assess speech vary considerably as do thresholds for diagnosing and treating VPD. Case mix, for example the number of syndromic cases, will vary, and the technique of primary palate repair itself may also be very important.

VELOCARDIOFACIAL SYNDROME

This complex syndrome is associated with a microdeletion on chromosome 22 in the 22q11 region and is sometimes termed 22q11 microdeletion syndrome. The syndrome has wide-ranging effects, among which are a characteristic facial appearance (Fig. 68.1), velopharyngeal dysfunction,

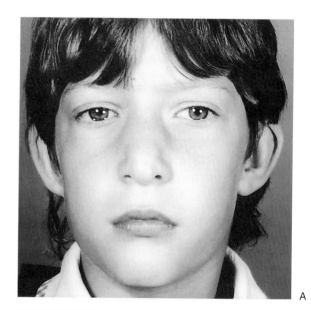

A

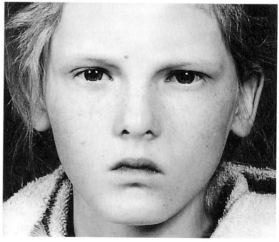

B

Fig. 68.1 (A,B) Facial appearance of two patients with velocardiofacial (22q11 microdeletion) syndrome.

and cardiac anomalies.[10,11] Expression of the features is variable, and while most cases do not have overt cleft palate, many do have a cleft of the secondary palate with no lip cleft, and occasionally VPD is seen in association with cleft lip and palate. In addition, specific learning difficulties and a relative lack of adenoidal tissue compound the problem. A detailed discussion of the syndrome is beyond the scope of this chapter, but one important feature of which the surgeon must be aware is that up to 15% of cases have an aberrant internal carotid artery which lies posterior to the pharynx and is at risk in pharyngoplasty. Aberrant vessels may produce visible pulsation on the posterior pharyngeal wall at nasoendoscopy, but magnetic resonance imaging is reported to be a more reliable indicator of such vessels and should be considered in appropriate cases.[3,10]

FISTULAE AND VELOPHARYNGEAL FUNCTION

The presence of a palatal fistula may also, in itself, have a deleterious effect on velopharyngeal function.[12,13] Henningsson and Isberg showed that velopharyngeal function improved in certain groups of patients with fistulae following non-surgical closure of the fistula but no procedure on the velopharyngeal sphincter. In the presence of both a fistula and velopharyngeal dysfunction, it is often appropriate to repair the fistula first prior to further investigation and management of the velopharyngeal dysfunction.[14]

INVESTIGATIONS

If there is any suspicion of velopharyngeal dysfunction, then the sphincter should be visualized to obtain further information, as discussed in the previous chapters. The sphincter is a three-dimensional structure and no single view provides adequate information. Thus videofluoroscopy and nasopharyngoscopy both have information to contribute. Unfortunately, children with palatal fistulae may not tolerate the instillation of local anesthetic to allow nasoendoscopy to be carried out, in which case reliance has to be placed on multiview videofluoroscopy. The combination of history, physical examination and investigations should allow a decision to be made about the extent of the problem and whether it is related to fistula or velopharyngeal dysfunction.

The timing of secondary palatal surgery has to be tailored to the patient's needs. In general there is agreement that the earlier a satisfactorily functioning velopharyngeal

sphincter can be established, the better will be the speech results.[15] On the other hand, earlier surgery on the palate carries a greater risk of growth interference. If, however, the regurgitation of food down the nose is causing the child to be the butt of excessive teasing and making life difficult at school, it seems unreasonable to the authors to withhold treatment for a palatal fistula and leave the child subject to more years of misery.

FISTULAE

A fistula between the oral and nasal cavities following primary repair of the cleft palate can occur at any site posterior to the alveolus. Fistulae immediately posterior to the alveolus may be the result of technical difficulty in achieving closure during primary surgery due to poor access and are discounted from discussion by many authors. The incidence of fistulae following primary repair varies widely, with figures quoted ranging from 18–34%.[16-20] Attempts to pinpoint causes are frustrated by the number of variables in the type and treatment of cleft palate. Nevertheless, several factors are known to influence occurrence of fistulae:[18-21]

- extent of the cleft
- type of repair
- operating surgeon
- width of the palatal cleft
- bilateral versus unilateral cleft lip and palate
- simultaneous repair of bilateral clefts
- cleft lip and palate versus cleft palate only.

Fistulae appear to increase in frequency as the severity of the cleft increases.[19] In the same study, a multivariate analysis of factors associated with cleft palate fistulae, the authors found that 43% of patients undergoing the Wardill type closure developed a fistula compared with 22%, 10% and 0% for von Langenbeck, Furlow and Dorrance style closures respectively. The surgeon performing the procedure was also found to be a significant predictor of outcome, after accounting for other variables. The width of the palate compared to the width of the cleft may be a critical factor above a particular ratio.[21] Closure of bilateral complete cleft lip and palate in one operation increased the fistula rate fourfold; this could possibly be explained by the damage to the blood supply of the vomerine flaps commonly used to close a wide defect.[18] Fistulae have been found to be more common in cleft lip and palate patients compared to those with isolated cleft palate.[18] It is tempting to postulate that small fistulae represent a failure of repair due to tension, ischemia or infection, with the larger ones resulting from significant loss of flaps used in the repair of the primary cleft. However, there may be several factors, yet to be elucidated, that may contribute to fistula formation.

An oronasal fistula is not necessarily symptomatic. The most common complaint is regurgitation of fluid to the nasal cavity. Other reported symptoms include packing of food in the fistulous track, causing mucosal inflammation and malodor[18] defective speech,[12] nasal catarrh[22] and hearing loss.[21] A small asymptomatic fistula may become symptomatic when it enlarges after orthodontic treatment to expand the alveolar arch.

Fistulae have been classified according to size,[16] and Schulz has described them as pinpoint, slit, oval and total dehiscence.[21] The size of a fistula on oral examination may however, differ from that seen from the nasal aspect endoscopically.[20] Most fistulae are small and slitlike; although larger fistulae are more likely to be symptomatic,[20] even small ones can occasionally cause symptoms.[23] The site of the fistula does not appear to determine whether speech will be affected.[20]

TIMING OF FISTULA REPAIR

The need for and timing of treatment must be assessed individually for each patient and is determined by several factors including the severity of symptoms, the need for other secondary procedures, and maxillary expansion. While there is no urgency for repair of the mildly symptomatic fistula in isolation, the child with persistent regurgitation of food or significant speech problems warrants early surgery. Insertion of a bone graft improves the success of closure in anterior fistula[24] and so it may be appropriate to postpone closure until bone grafting if possible, although there is a case for bringing this procedure forward in more severe cases.

Some symptomatic fistulae may well be managed by obturators which may also carry replacements for missing dental segments, but there are inherent problems.[22] An obturator may be useful as a temporary therapeutic measure if the child is considered not to be old enough for surgery.

PRINCIPLES OF FISTULA REPAIR

The plethora of techniques that have been described for closure of palatal fistulae attests to the fact that no single procedure is consistently satisfactory for all cases given the variation in the clinical situation and the inherent difficulty in achieving closure. The choice of procedure is governed by the location and size of the fistula, previous operations on the palate and of course the preference of the surgeon.

Certain principles, however, should guide the surgical approach:

- Avoid epithelial continuity between mouth and nose. Recurrence of a fistula may have less to do with the size of the defect than with the difficulty in removing the epithelial continuity between the oral and nasal cavities.[25]
- Avoid overlapping suture lines.
- Avoid devascularized tissue.
- The operation should ideally re-establish normal anatomy with a partition between the two cavities lined by epithelium on either side; however, closure with one sound epithelial layer (oral or nasal) may be better than two poorly vascularized layers.
- The addition of an interposing layer, usually of bone, between the two epithelial layers improves the chances of success.[24]
- Ensure optimal oral hygiene.

TECHNIQUES OF FISTULA REPAIR

Surgical procedures that have been described for closure of palatal fistula range from simple techniques utilizing a single-layer closure to more elaborate methods involving microsurgical transfer of tissue from distant sites.

For simple fistulae, a single flap of mucosa hinged onto one of the margins of the fistula attributed to Hynes[16] or two overlapping mucosal flaps hinged on either margin[26] may be sufficient for closure. This may not be appropriate for anterior palatal fistulae as the mucoperiosteum behind the alveolus may be difficult to dissect and mobilize.[27] A large variety of mucoperiosteal flaps based on the von Langenbeck flap have been used as sliding or transposition flaps to provide the oral lining to cover mucosal turnover flaps used as the nasal layer. The addition of bone grafts has been said to enhance the success of these flaps.[28] A further refinement has been the island palatal flap, first used for nasal lining of the defect left after a palatal pushback procedure,[29] that has been successfully used for closure of anterior fistulae.[27] This technique involves raising an island of palatal mucoperiosteum pedicled on the greater palatine vessels and advancing it to provide the oral layer for closure of the fistula. Suggested modifications include the use of a bilateral island flap as well as inclusion of some nasal lining in the advancing edge of the flap.[27] This flap had been used earlier for midpalate fistulae, and mobility is said to be aided by removing the medial part of the bony canal.[30]

The use of alveolar mucosal flaps to close the anterior portion of bone grafted fistulae[31] was followed by the successful use of combined buccal and palatal flaps after bone grafting large anterior fistulae.[32] The essentials of this procedure are accurate closure of the nasal and oral layers and the use of cancellous bone grafts to fill the space with a buccal flap for closure of the anterior defect. Buccal flaps have also been used as island flaps to cover wide anterior fistulae.[33] The fistula is closed in two layers with one or two hinge flaps from the margins of the defect to provide a nasal lining and an island flap from the labiobuccal mucosa based on a wide submucosal pedicle. An advantage of this technique may be the elevation of the alar base and the use of the bulky pedicle to fill the space between the nasal and oral linings.

Interpositional grafts

Grafts of autologous tissue other than bone, for example conchal cartilage[34] and dermis–fat,[35] have been used to separate the nasal and oral mucosal layers with good success rates. In the hard palate, which is by nature bony, bone is an obvious choice. In the primary palate, where there is an associated defect of the alveolus, a cancellous graft is ideal. In the bony secondary palate, where a lesser thickness of bone is necessary, the authors have used cortical bone, usually from the iliac crest, either combined with cancellous grafting of the alveolar defect or in isolation, with gratifying results (see Fig. 68.2). In fistulae with a significant depth from oral to nasal cavity, such as in the primary palate, the addition of this bone to fill the space effectively provides additional mucoperiosteal tissue from the fistula track to enable tension-free closure with no formal flap elevation from the hard palate. These techniques appear to have the advantage of minimizing dissection of the hard palate mucoperiosteum, which should help to minimize tissue loss through ischemia and in the long term, growth disturbances.

Tongue flaps

The tongue is an extremely well vascularized organ and has been used extensively for reconstruction of defects in the oral cavity including palatal fistulae.[36–38] The dorsal mucosal vasculature appears to consist mainly of horizontal ramifications of vessels which, although random laterally, assume a longitudinal orientation medially. This medial axiality, described as a constant feature, is the main basis for the reliability of dorsal mucosal flaps.[39] Although posteriorly based flaps are better perfused, the anteriorly based flap is better oriented to close more anterior defects and has been found to be quite reliable.

The flap width should be slightly greater than the defect and only 2–3 mm of muscle need be included in the mucosal flap to safely preserve the blood vessels. The procedure is outlined in the operative series shown in Figure 68.3. The procedure is done in two stages and the pedicle can be divided as early as 7 days postoperatively. Contrary to earlier teaching, intermaxillary fixation devices do not appear to be necessary and are seldom used.[40] Several modifications have been described; these are mainly related to the base of the flap and its width and site on the tongue[41–43] as well as attempts to use it to lengthen the palate.[44]

Success rates of 85–100% have been reported after the use of tongue flaps in fistula closures.[41,42,44,45] Complications are surprisingly infrequent and include hemorrhage, hematoma, dehiscence and flap necrosis, temporary loss of tongue sensation, taste, and changes in articulation and resonance.[37,44–47] While the tongue flap is not the operation of choice for the small fistula, it remains a reliable and simple technique for the management of the large fistula.

Extraoral flaps

Intraoral tissue is not adequate for the largest fistulae, and a variety of skin, muscle and fascial flaps have been described,

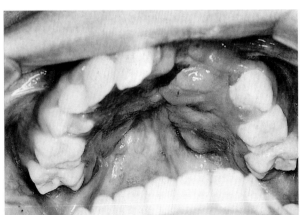

Fig. 68.2 **(A)** Preoperative view showing significant palatal fistula occupying the anterior half of the hard palate in continuity with an alveolar defect. **(B)** Postoperative view showing successful closure of the fistula four months following alveolar bone grafting with the use of additional cortical iliac crest bone for the hard palate.

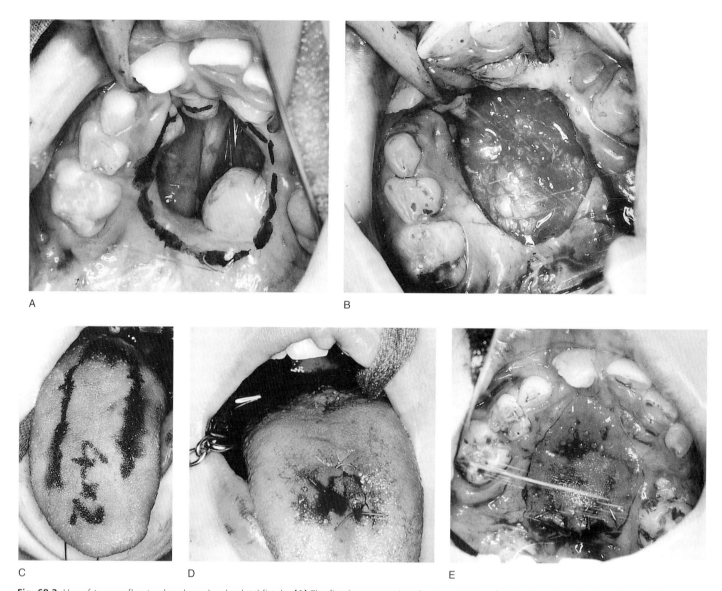

Fig. 68.3 Use of tongue flap to close large hard palatal fistula. **(A)** The fistula at operation showing incisions for the hinge flaps to close the nasal layer. **(B)** Nasal layer closure with hinge flaps completed. **(C)** An anteriorly based midline dorsal tongue flap is designed, 4 cm long by 2 cm wide. **(D)** The tongue donor site at the time of flap division. **(E)** Mirror view of hard palate showing successful closure of the fistula by the tongue flap. There were no postoperative problems with the tongue function following surgery.

although these are rarely required. Some of the distant skin flaps, which require microvascular transfer, may be combined with bone to fill in bony defects in the hard palate.[48–51]

Other techniques that have been used include the now historical tube pedicle[52] and, more recently, tissue expansion using custom-made implants,[53] both of which involve staged procedures and should rarely be required. Table 68.1 provides a summary of the authors' approach to selecting a technique for fistula closure.

SUCCESS RATE IN FISTULA CLOSURE

The success of fistula surgery in terms of eradication of the

fistula, as already mentioned, is disappointing[18,19,21] but a reduction in size may be adequate in many cases to eliminate symptoms or reduce them to an acceptable level. Reoperation is therefore not always necessary.[18] Reoperation, when needed, should follow the same principles as for the first attempt at closure.

VELOPHARYNGEAL DYSFUNCTION

Velopharyngeal dysfunction is caused by inadequate movement in the sphincter, preventing closure. In cleft palate

Table 68.1 Choice of operation for fistula closure. This table is intended as a guide only. The enormous variation in size, shape and position of the fistula, the patient's age, oral hygiene, fitness for operation and the extent and scarring of previous surgery must all be taken into consideration.

Asymptomatic (speech, eating, hearing)	Leave
Suitable age/site for bone graft	Bone graft (with alveolar bone graft if appropriate)
Too young for bone graft	Obturate if tolerated until old enough or consider dermis–fat graft
Secondary palate, child	Minimal scar procedure. Either single-layer repair or cartilage graft
Secondary palate, adult	Big robust flaps, 2 or 3 layer
Too big for local tissue or graft?	Tongue flap
Too big for tongue flap?	Extraoral flap

patients, this may be the result of inadequate palate function, although it may also occur in the presence of good palate function if the pharynx is unusually deep. Techniques developed to allow visualization of the sphincter or measurement of function have improved our understanding of the way the sphincter works and have allowed a more informed approach to treatment. Lateral videofluoroscopy shows the degree and speed of palatal lift, degree of posterior wall movement, presence or absence of a Passavant's ridge, and the anteroposterior extent of the defect. It also allows the tongue to be visualized, and thus identifies patients who use tongue movements to aid palatal lift. Nasoendoscopy allows the lateral wall movements to be seen, together with palate and posterior wall movement. Similar information may be obtained by using other videofluoroscopic views, although these are harder to interpret than the lateral view and the endoscopic image. Patterns of velopharyngeal valving vary between individuals and even for one individual on different occasions.[14] When closure is obtained by palate lift, the pattern is termed 'valvular' or 'coronal'. If lateral wall movement predominates, the pattern is termed 'sagittal'. A mixed picture is termed 'sphincteric' or 'circular'.

POSTERIOR PHARYNGEAL FLAP

The traditional and still popular operation for velopharyngeal dysfunction is the pharyngeal flap. This was described in the 19th century and consists of a flap of tissue taken from the posterior pharyngeal wall and sutured into the palate. It has the effect of providing a degree of obturation of the sphincter, such that the existing muscle activity provides adequate closure. The history of the technique has been reviewed elsewhere.[15,54,55] There are a number of

variations possible in the technique. The flap has been described based either superiorly or inferiorly, and there is no good evidence that one is more effective than the other. In a randomized prospective study of 35 patients undergoing posterior pharyngeal flaps, postoperative speech results were not significantly different,[15,56–58] and another study found little difference in the appearances of the two techniques postoperatively.[59] From a practical viewpoint, the superiorly based flap has advantages: based high on the posterior wall, it is relatively easy to obtain a good length of flap and suture it into any area of the soft palate. This places the flap within the velopharyngeal sphincter. The inferiorly based flap, in contrast, is effectively restricted in length and, as it is made longer, gets further away from the velum. In theory it might tether the velum inferiorly. A further problem is that the end to be sutured has usually been raised from the adenoidal pad, which is technically very difficult to suture securely as the stitches tend to cut out. If bleeding occurs from the donor site, access to visualize and control it is poor, and the flap may have to be undone.[55] One report has suggested a higher rate of dehiscence for the inferiorly based flap.[57]

It has recently been suggested[60] that the inferiorly based flap is more likely to include an axial blood vessel, which would allow it to be raised safely with a longer length/width ratio. We do not know, however, whether the concept of axiality and length/width ratio applies in the pharynx in the same way as in the skin, or whether the superior flap is compromised by a poor blood supply. The superiorly based flap tends to be preferred by most surgeons.

The pharyngeal flap has been said to negate velar movement[10] and relies for its effectiveness on lateral wall movement to close the two ports; the flap must be placed at the level of maximal lateral wall movement for the best results. Studies of operated patients using cineradiography,[59] multiview videofluoroscopy[61] and endoscopy[62] have stressed the importance of correct positioning and size of the flap.

The lateral port control flap[63] is a variant of the superiorly based pharyngeal flap in which catheters of set diameter are placed either side of the flap, with the aim of producing two ports, each with a cross-sectional area of less than 10 mm.[2] This approach is based on the results of acoustic and airflow studies which suggested that velopharyngeal competence was achieved with a total velopharyngeal port cross-sectional area of 20 mm^2 or less. More recently the endoscopic discovery that velopharyngeal dysfunction could be associated with small defects, as in the occult submucous cleft palate,[64] has cast doubt on the theory behind this approach, and it has not found wide acceptance.

A pharyngeal flap may be lined or unlined. If the flap is not lined, then it has a raw surface which will heal partly by contracture, the flap either tubing itself until mucosal healing has occurred, resulting in narrowing of the flap, or contraction of the raw surface may shorten the flap[59] and tether the palate, restricting movement rather as a guy rope prevents a tent from flapping. The lining flap is obtained by turning back a mucosal flap from the velum, from the nasal aspect for a superiorly based flap or from the oral aspect to line an inferiorly based flap.

The superiorly based flap may be inserted quite far anteriorly into the velum, and provide tissue to maintain a simultaneous pushback of the palate in the Honig pharyngoplasty.[65]

The use of nasoendoscopy to study patients who have undergone pharyngeal flap surgery shows that palatal lift may be impaired,[66] that closure of the sphincter after flap surgery is largely dependent on the movement of the lateral pharyngeal walls[62] and that the midline pharyngeal flap is not dynamic.[62,67] Thus the idea of tailoring the flap to the defect was proposed. In the presence of good lateral pharyngeal wall movement a relatively narrow flap will be adequate, but with lesser degrees of lateral pharyngeal wall activity a wider flap is needed. In the presence of asymmetry of the lateral pharyngeal wall movement, the flap may be raised to one side or other of the midline to complement the function. If there is no lateral pharyngeal wall function, the flap would have to obturate the velopharyngeal sphincter completely to eliminate velopharyngeal dysfunction. In Shprintzen's study[62] the outcome in a group of patients who had been selected for flap surgery of prescribed width based on nasoendoscopic appearances was compared with the outcome of a similar group of historical controls who underwent surgery prior to the use of endoscopy using flaps of various widths depending on the operating surgeon. It was concluded that tailoring the flap width produced better results.

SPHINCTER PHARYNGOPLASTY

An alternative type of pharyngoplasty consists of raising two superiorly based flaps containing both mucosa and muscle from the lateral walls of the pharynx and suturing them together onto the posterior pharyngeal wall. Hynes[68–71] was the first to do this, his flaps consisting of the entire width of the lateral pharyngeal walls and the underlying salpingopharyngeus muscle and palatopharyngeus. These two flaps were raised with the pedicle lying just below the eustachian orifice and were sutured side by side to one another into a mucosa-only incision on the posterior pharyngeal wall at this high level. The secondary defects were closed to narrow the oropharynx and obliterate the lateral pharyngeal recesses. To obtain access for this operation the velum was split in the midline, unless it was very short. This operation both narrowed the oropharynx and created a muscular ridge high on the posterior pharyngeal wall which was observed to contract actively, with the palate, to produce velopharyngeal closure in 15 of 36 reported cases.[69] Hynes commented that those patients with active movement achieved the best results, and hypothesized that damage to the blood or nerve supply had occurred in the others. He also noted that the adenoidal pad interfered with the high suturing of the flaps on the pharyngeal wall.

A similar approach was proposed by Orticochea,[72] who described a dynamic sphincter pharyngoplasty using flaps from the posterior tonsillar pillars with the underlying palatopharyngeus (PP) muscles which were sutured to each other and to a small inferiorly based flap on the posterior wall. He stressed that this flap should not be the full width of the pharynx to avoid a large scar which he thought would impair the sphincteric movement postoperatively.[73] He maintained that, provided the flaps were not dissected to a point higher than the apex of the tonsil, the nerve supply was preserved and the pharyngoplasty was capable of functioning as an additional sphincter. This upper limit of dissection in order to preserve function has been emphasized by others.[60,74] Active movement of the flaps has been reported after surgery and may not appear for up to 18 months according to one study.[74] This new sphincter is at a lower level in the pharynx than in the Hynes procedure. Hynes did in fact also describe the use of the posterior tonsillar pillar musculomucosal flaps as a secondary procedure in the 20% of his patients whose speech still exhibited cleft palate stigmata following his muscle flap pharyngoplasty. These secondary flaps were inset on top of the previously placed flaps to augment further the muscle ridge on the posterior wall.[71] He did not comment on the success of the maneuver, nor did he note whether movement was seen.

The operation was modified by Jackson, who inset the flaps onto a short superiorly based flap on the posterior wall.[75] Jackson later described the inset of the tonsillar pillar flaps merely into a transverse incision between the upper ends of the flaps.[76] The advantages claimed for this type of pharyngoplasty were that the palate did not have to be split nor its function interfered with and that it was quick to perform and easy to revise or use following a previous pharyngeal flap. He claimed no increase in middle ear problems and no obstructive sleep apnea following his sphincter pharyngoplasty, although many patients did snore postoperatively. The tonsillar pillar flaps may be overlapped and sutured side by side in the same manner as Hynes described.[77]

Interestingly, one study of 28 patients undergoing sphincter pharyngoplasty showed an increased degree of palate lift following surgery.[78] The authors postulated that the palatopharyngeus might be to some extent a levator antagonist, and that dividing these muscles in raising the flaps allows the levators to act unopposed. The degree of increase was not related to the speech results, nor to the method of sphincter pharyngoplasty (the Hynes, Orticochea and Jackson variants were all studied). We have observed a similar improvement in velar lift in some cases following sphincter pharyngoplasty. If the nerve supply has been preserved, insetting the palatopharyngeus muscles higher on the posterior pharyngeal wall will alter the vector of muscle action, and the muscle may thereby become a partial elevator of the palate rather than a depressor. The variability of these observations might be a result of inadvertent nerve or vascular damage in some cases.

POSTERIOR WALL AUGMENTATION

Another approach to velopharyngeal surgery is augmentation of the posterior wall. If it can be built up in the manner of a Passavant's ridge, the wall is brought forward to meet the lift of the palate. A sphincter type pharyngoplasty such as the Hynes, particularly with a high inset, might work in this way. More common is the idea of introducing a graft of some type of alloplastic material beneath the posterior wall. A variety of autologous tissues and implant materials such as cartilage, fat, and silicone have been used in the past.[79–81] The ideal alloplastic material is non-toxic, stable in position and shape following the procedure, and injectable, allowing surgery to be carried out endoscopically and tailored to the functional defect.[82] An ideal material has yet to be found; Teflon has been the most popular, while silicone and collagen have been used.[82,83] This type of approach works best for small velopharyngeal defects (less than 5 mm in anteroposterior dimension) and overcorrection is recommended. It may be used following a pharyngoplasty if velopharyngeal insufficiency persists with a small gap. The lack of more recent reports of this approach in the literature suggests either that it has not fulfilled its early promise or that surgeons are concerned about the safety of the materials used.

OTHER TECHNIQUES

A further approach is to increase the bulk of the velum to obliterate the velopharyngeal space. The use of superiorly based lateral pharyngeal wall flaps inset onto the nasal velar aspect was described by Moore and Sullivan.[84,85] Recently a flap from the oral aspect was transferred through the velum to augment the midline nasal aspect in selected cases.[86] These techniques have not found general acceptance.

A laterally based bipedicle chevron flap raised from the posterior pharyngeal wall and inset into the velum was recommended on the basis of anatomic studies of the pharyngeal nerve supply which is based laterally and is thus liable to be damaged in any vertically orientated flap.[67]

Bardach has described a pharyngoplasty based on the midline approximation of the posterior tonsillar pillars, which are sutured not to the posterior pharyngeal wall but to the velum and to each other, creating a single midline port with less restriction of the nasal airway. The success of the procedure was not reported.[87]

PALATE RE-REPAIR

All the above methods work largely by an obturation effect (apart possibly from the dynamic sphincter pharyngoplasty). There is always a balance to strike between the elimination of velopharyngeal incompetence and interference with the normal nasal airway, which is narrowed in the process. Such narrowing or overclosure may result in hyponasal resonance (as if the patient has a cold), catarrh, difficulty in nasal breathing, snoring and obstructive sleep apnea, or problems with subsequent maxillary osteotomy if required. Other reported problems are death, the need for a tracheostomy, serious hemorrhage, and neck stiffness.[57,59,76,86,88–91]

Ideally one wishes to obtain or maintain the greatest range of opening and closure of the sphincter. Many cleft patients with velopharyngeal dysfunction have not had an adequate muscle correction at the time of primary palatoplasty. The importance of muscle correction at the time of cleft palate repair has been stressed on anatomic and theoretical grounds by many authors,[1,76,92,93] and the term 'Intravelar veloplasty' was coined[93] to describe this muscle correction. A similar approach, that of re-repairing the palate, has been suggested to correct velopharyngeal dysfunction in cleft palate patients.[76,94] The operation might also be termed 'secondary intravelar veloplasty', and consists of opening the velum through a midline peroral approach, with careful and radical dissection of the abnormally inserted muscles. These are freed from attachments to the posterior edge of the hard palate as far laterally as the hamulus. They are then brought through between the nasal and oral mucosal layers to lie in the normal position in the posterior portion of the soft palate,[1] where they are sutured together in the midline to reconstitute the levator sling. The operation is carried out under the operating microscope to permit a more precise dissection.[94] The Furlow double reversing Z-plasty technique for primary veloplasty[95] has also been applied as a secondary procedure in 18 cleft patients with velopharyngeal dysfunction. Success was related to a velopharyngeal gap size less than or equal to 10 mm and the presence of better lateral wall movement as seen on preoperative investigation, but not to patient age or pattern of closure.[96] We have also used this approach for the past few years and found it to be very helpful. Palate re-repair has the advantage over pharyngoplasty of not producing nasal obstruction as there is no obturation of the sphincter involved.[94,96] In a recent study, two methods of palate re-repair (intravelar veloplasty and Furlow Z) were compared using measurements of velar movement on lateral videofluoroscopy recordings. Both procedures produced a significant improvement in velopharyngeal closure, but no significant differences between the two emerged.[97]

Fistulae can occur occasionally with either method of re-repair, and are likely to require closure. In cases where velopharyngeal dysfunction persists following re-repair, the improved range of palate movement may allow a less obturating pharyngoplasty to be carried out than would otherwise have been the case, with less risk of obstructive sequelae.

Palatal pushback procedures, such as the Honig operation alluded to above, are another approach to the treatment of velopharyngeal dysfunction. These have to a large extent been superseded by the Furlow approach to palatal lengthening which combines a muscle retropositioning and realignment with velar lengthening, but which avoids additional hard palate surgery and scarring which may be detrimental to maxillary arch form and growth. We have combined in one case a modified Furlow procedure with a midline pharyngeal flap, and produced velopharyngeal competence with an improved range of velar movement.

NON-SURGICAL TREATMENT

There are cleft patients with velopharyngeal dysfunction for whom surgery is not appropriate. Those with phoneme-specific velopharyngeal dysfunction (where the sphincter is competent for the majority of sounds but is incompetent for some sounds) exhibit an articulatory problem which is usually amenable to a short course of appropriate speech therapy. Some patients with intermittent incompetence may benefit from a speech bulb reduction programme or biofeedback therapy.[10] At the other end of the spectrum of severity are patients who have such poor velopharyngeal function or who already exhibit features of an inadequate nasal airway (e.g. severe catarrh, sleep apnea) that their problems would be made worse by pharyngoplasty. Many of these are syndromic patients. In this small group, con-

sideration should be given to the use of a prosthetic obturator. This is a dental plate built up posteriorly to extend into the velopharyngeal sphincter and fill any defects. Obturators are time-consuming to make and require collaboration between orthodontist, endoscopist, speech therapist and, not least, the patient for success. Not all patients will tolerate these appliances.

CHOICE OF OPERATION

How is the surgeon to choose an operative technique in those patients in whom the detailed multidisciplinary assessment indicates that surgery is the preferred alternative? The different procedures appear to produce comparable results. The difficulties in analyzing the success of operations are considerable. The goal is normal speech, which is both subjective and difficult to measure. The judgment of a lay person or panel may differ from that of the specialized therapist.[98] The influence of therapy on the results should be considered separately from that of any operation. Speech may still fall short of normality but yet be acceptable to the patient and/or family. Success is therefore often measured by a lack of further surgery, but this may represent disenchantment and disinterest rather than patient satisfaction.

Normal speech should exhibit normal resonance, being neither hyponasal nor hypernasal. In many patients this may be impossible to achieve. Few studies are randomized, nor they are assessed blindly, or by assessors who have had no involvement in the treatment program. These problems have been discussed elsewhere.[99]

There is no good evidence that one type of operation for velopharyngeal dysfunction is better than another. In a brief report on 85 patients following pharyngeal flap (75 patients) or sphincter pharyngoplasty (10 patients) no significant difference was found in the outcome.[58] No details are provided, however, as to why particular patients underwent one operation rather than the other, and there may be differences between the groups.

A retrospective analysis of 298 procedures[100] for velopharyngeal dysfunction over a 15-year period to determine whether one operation was better than another found similar success rates of 75–80% for sphincter pharyngoplasty, pharyngeal flap, and palate re-repair. Success rates were higher (81%) when endoscopy was used than when it was not (68%), and when preoperative movement either of palate, lateral walls, posterior walls or overall movement was greater. Patients with sphincteric closure patterns, i.e. with a significant degree of lateral wall movement, did better than those with a coronal movement pattern, whether treated by pharyngeal flap or sphincter pharyngoplasty.

TIMING OF SURGERY

While in general the speech results of surgery for velopharyngeal dysfunction are best when treatment is carried out early, the investigative techniques required for proper assessment cannot reliably be carried out in young children. A minimum age of approximately $4\frac{1}{2}$ years of age has been suggested[10] for reasons of adequate speech and language development, compliance and morbidity as well as the ability to cope with the investigations. We would carry out certain procedures, such as fistula closure or palate re-repair, at an earlier age on the basis of clinical examination, speech and language assessment and investigation where possible. If the child's articulation exhibits many glottal stops, the velopharyngeal sphincter is not used, and therapy to correct the articulation should be carried out first as velopharyngeal function may be better than it appears.[10] Similarly, velopharyngeal surgery should often be deferred until any fistulae have been closed, for reasons mentioned earlier.

TAILORING THE OPERATION

We have many options, all of which seem equivalent in terms of 'success'. Can we select patients who will do better with one type of operation than another on the basis of pre-operative assessment and investigation? Pigott[66] was the first to propose tailoring the surgical procedure to the extent of the defect as seen endoscopically. He used a type of posterior wall augmentation in 14 patients with good levator mobility, a superiorly based flap if palate movement was poor but length adequate (24 patients), and a Honig procedure when palate function and length were poor (5 patients). Posterior wall augmentation patients fared worse than the other two groups, despite probably starting with the smallest gaps and best movement.

More recently, the same group has reported on two further series of endoscopically selected operations for velopharyngeal dysfunction.[86,101] The operations used were mainly the Honig and sphincter pharyngoplasties, with some superiorly based flaps, posterior wall augmentation and, more recently, the fish flap transposed through the palate from the oral aspect to augment the nasal. The latter was not recommended. Results for cleft palate patients were

similar for the sphincter and Honig procedures, with 13/15 and 24/30 cases respectively having acceptable nasal resonance.

In a videofluoroscopic and endoscopic study of 120 patients undergoing pharyngeal flap surgery using three variations on the technique, Shprintzen et al[62] were able to show that different techniques produced different widths of pharyngeal flap. Following surgery, velopharyngeal closure was seen to be dependent solely on lateral wall movement. In the first group of 60 cases, operated prior to the use of endoscopy, the choice of operation depended on surgeon preference. In the second 60 patients, the technique to be used was decided after assessment of the degree of lateral pharyngeal wall movement, to produce a width of flap adequate to fill the midline defect, based on retrospective analysis of the first group. The study showed that tailoring the width produced both fewer persistent gaps seen endoscopically and improved speech results. This study, however, used historical controls, considered only superiorly based pharyngeal flaps and was not randomized.

In the Canniesburn study of 298 procedures,[100] numbers were too small in each group to relate the success rates of different procedures to the endoscopic appearances; overall, patients with better movement preoperatively did better than those with worse, and patients with sphincteric closure patterns better than those with valvular. Palate re-repair had similar success rates to pharyngoplasty.

The importance of tailoring the operation to the defect has been emphasized repeatedly.[14,76,77,86] The concept, while logically appealing, remains unproven.

The authors' approach to the selection of operation *in cleft patients* with velopharyngeal dysfunction (see Table 68.2) is to use pharyngoplasty as the final surgical option. Thus we would firstly carry out fistula closure or tonsillectomy where appropriate. If palate function is present but poor we prefer to carry out a palate re-repair before

Table 68.2 Choice of procedure for velopharyngeal dysfunction in cleft patients

Sphincter function	Procedure selected
Patient happy with speech	Leave alone
Phoneme-specific velopharyngeal dysfunction	Speech therapy
Normal/good palate function; gap <5 mm	Posterior wall augmentation
Palate function poor but improvable	Re-repair palate (Furlow)
Moderate gap; palate movement > lateral pharyngeal wall	Sphincter pharyngoplasty
Moderate gap; lateral pharyngeal wall movement > palate	Superior lined flap
Large gap; little movement	Sphincter pharyngoplasty
No movement; obstructive symptoms	Speech bulb/obturator

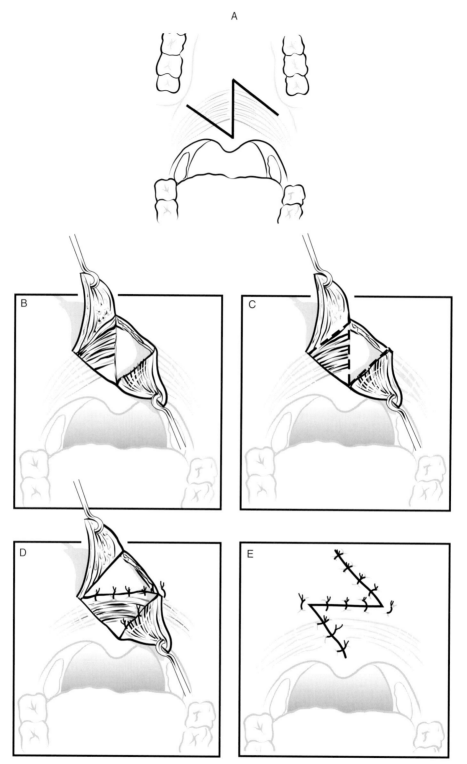

Fig. 68.4 The use of the Furlow double reversing Z-plasty method of palate repair as applied in a cleft patient with velopharyngeal dysfunction following primary repair. **(A)** The oral Z-plasty is outlined. The anteriorly based oral mucosal flap on the patient's right side is raised to include the mucosa and underlying glandular tissue only, leaving the muscle. The posteriorly based oral mucosal flap is raised to include the muscle running into it. **(B)** The two oral mucosal flaps are raised, that on the patient's left side with the muscle included. **(C)** The nasal Z-plasty is drawn with its common limb along the midline of the palate, but its two other limbs in the opposite orientation from the oral Z-plasty. Thus the posteriorly based nasal mucosal flap on the patient's right side will include the muscle which runs into it, while that on the patient's left side will be a mucosa-only flap. **(D)** The nasal mucosal flaps have been sutured together. Note the reorientation of the musculature in the posteriorly based nasal flap on the patient's right side, which now lies transversely. **(E)** The oral mucosal flap closure has been completed with overlapping of the muscles from each side.

embarking on a pharyngoplasty. Palatal lift is best seen on lateral videofluoroscopy. If the levator knee is not well formed and positioned, but anteriorly situated, rounded and the palate limited in stretch and/or lift, then we use the Furlow re-repair method, see Figure 68.4. If there is *no* active palate movement, function is unlikely to be improved by re-repair. Where palate function is judged so good as to be unimprovable, and the size of the anteroposterior defect is less than about 5 mm, posterior wall augmentation is employed, usually using autologous tissue. For cases with bigger defects, our inclination is to use a midline pharyngeal flap where lateral pharyngeal wall movement dominates, or a sphincter pharyngoplasty where there is a sphincteric or valvular pattern of closure. These techniques are shown in diagrammatic form in Figures 68.5 and 68.6. Having seen improved palate lift following sphincter pharyngoplasty, we sometimes also use it for small defects in place of a posterior wall augmentation. The sphincter pharyngoplasty is quicker to perform than a midline flap and does not involve opening the palate or interfering with palate function. In patients with little or no movement, or those who exhibit symptoms of nasal obstruction or poor airway control such as snoring or obstructive sleep apnea, non-surgical treatment should be tried.

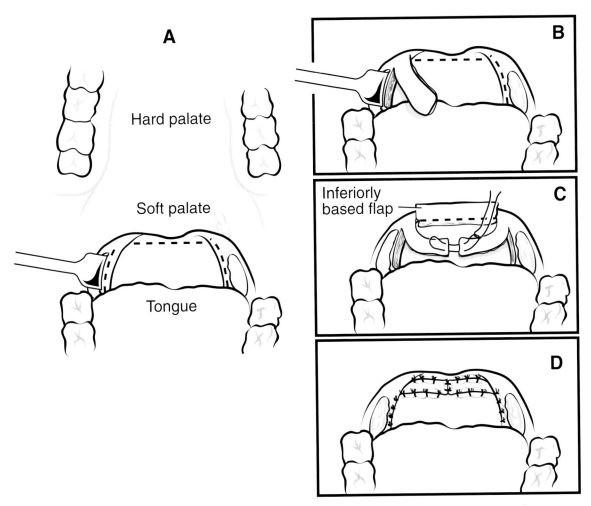

Fig. 68.5 The sphincter pharyngoplasty as performed by the authors. The palate is retracted by means of a suction catheter passed through the nose and sutured to the posterior free border of the palate to allow retraction. **(A)** Superiorly based flaps are illustrated and both posterior tonsillar pillars. The incision line is made immediately posterior to the tonsil and the section includes all the underlying musculature. The flap is transected as low as possible. **(B)** Illustrates the elevated flap of posterior tonsillar pillar and underlying musculature. **(C)** A broad, short, inferiorly based flap is raised on the posterior pharyngeal wall connecting the two flap donor sites and lying at the level of the base of the adenoids. The two posterior pillar flaps are sutured together in the midline. **(D)** The two flaps are then sutured to the inferiorly based flap and to its donor site on the posterior pharyngeal wall. **(E)** Following release of the traction stitch in the nose, the palate and uvula come to lie in front of the new pharyngoplasty.

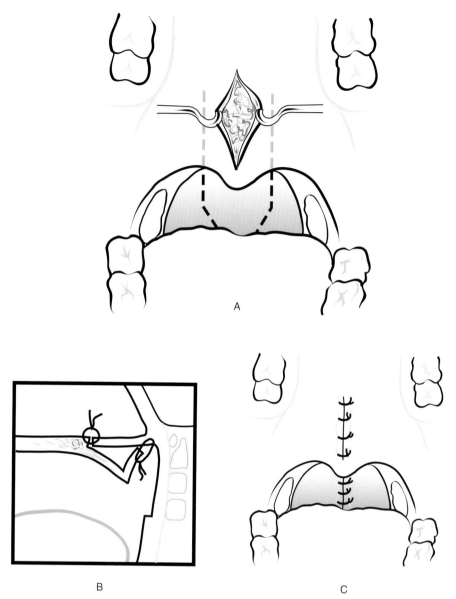

A

B

C

Fig. 68.6 The superiorly based lined pharyngeal flap operation. **(A)** The palate is split to gain access, usually by a midline incision. Retraction of the incision in the oral layer and underlying glands allows access to the nasal layer where a posteriorly based lining flap is raised, illustrated by dashed lines. The superiorly based posterior pharyngeal wall flap is also illustrated extending inferiorly as far as possible. **(B)** This lateral view illustrates the inset of the superiorly based posterior wall pharyngeal flap into the defect on the nasal aspect of the palate. The nasal lining flap from the palate is sutured to the base of the posterior wall flap. **(C)** The midline palatal incision is closed as is the donor site from the posterior pharyngeal flap.

FAILURE AND REDO SURGERY

The management of failed surgery has received less attention and the few published series are small.[102–106] Failure may be caused by poor choice of procedure, unpredictable effects of scarring, or breakdown. No procedure is immune from failure or complications. In the event of persistent symptoms following surgery for velopharyngeal dysfunction, thorough investigation including nasoendoscopy and video-fluoroscopy is mandatory if a further operation is contemplated. We would allow at least a year, to allow scarring to mature and the benefits of postoperative speech and language therapy to be fully realized, before deciding on treatment. After a failed palate re-repair, any appropriate pharyngoplasty may be used. Following a previous pharyngoplasty, the use of an additional superiorly based pharyngeal flap, Z-plasty closure of defects, or, sometimes, division of the previous flap have been recommended. A speech bulb may be helpful in certain cases after a sphincter pharyngoplasty, but has been said to be unsuitable after pharyngeal flap.[106]

CONCLUSION

The surgical options in the management of secondary palatal problems and velopharyngeal dysfunction are numerous, and the literature lacks prospective comparative series. There are no clear-cut best procedures. The use of sophisticated imaging and investigative techniques is important in making a correct and detailed diagnosis. While there is as yet no clear evidence that we can make the treatment fit the problem, it is only by using these techniques that our understanding of the velopharyngeal mechanism will increase until we are able to demonstrate the effectiveness of the procedures we employ. Our philosophy, where practicable, is to close fistulae and maximize palate function before embarking on pharyngoplasty.

REFERENCES

1. Boorman JG, Sommerlad BC 1985 Levator palati and palatal dimples: their anatomy, relationship and clinical significance. British Journal of Plastic Surgery 38:326–332
2. Shprintzen RJ, Sher AE, Croft CB 1987 Hypernasal speech caused by tonsillar hypertrophy. International Journal of Paediatric Otorhinolaryngology 14:45–56
3. MacKenzie-Stepner K, Witzel MA, Stringer DA, Laskin R 1987 Velopharyngeal insufficiency due to hypertrophic tonsils: a report of two cases. International Journal of Paediatric Otorhinolaryngology 14:57–63
4. Finkelstein Y, Nachmani A, Ophir D 1994 The functional role of the tonsils in speech. Archives of Otolaryngology 120:846–851
5. Calnan J 1954 Submucous cleft palate. British Journal of Plastic Surgery 6:264–282
6. Lindemann G, Riis B, Sewerin I 1977 Prevalence of cleft uvula among 2732 Danes. Cleft Palate Journal 14:226–229
7. Bagatin M 1985 Cleft uvula. Acta Chirurgiae Plasticae 27:202–206
8. Bagatin M 1985 Submucous cleft palate. Journal of Maxillofacial Surgery 13:37–38
9. Wharton P, Mowrer DE 1992 Prevalence of cleft uvula among school children in kindergarten through grade five. Cleft Palate–Craniofacial Journal 29:10–14
10. Shprintzen RJ 1995 The use of information obtained from speech and instrumental evaluations in treatment planning for velopharyngeal insufficiency. In:Shprintzen RJ, Bardach J (eds) Cleft palate speech management: a multidisciplinary approach. Mosby, St Louis
11. Shprintzen RJ, Goldberg RB, Yong D, Wolford L 1981 The velo-cardio-facial syndrome: a clinical and genetic analysis. Pediatrics 67:167–172
12. Henningsson G, Isberg A 1987 Influence of palatal fistulas on speech and resonance. Folia Phoniatrica et Logopedica 39:183–191
13. Isberg A, Henningsson G 1987 Influence of palatal fistula on velopharyngeal movements: a cineradiographic study. Plastic and Reconstructive Surgery 79:525–530
14. Witt PD, D'Antonio LL 1993 Velopharyngeal insufficiency and secondary palatal management. Cleft Palate Journal 20:707–721
15. Skoog T 1965 The pharyngeal flap operation in cleft palate. British Journal of Plastic Surgery 18:265–282
16. Reid DAC 1962 Fistulae in the hard palate following cleft palate surgery. British Journal of Plastic Surgery 15:377–384
17. Amaratunga NA 1988 Occurrence of oronasal fistulas in operated cleft palate patients. Journal of Oral and Maxillofacial Surgery 46:834–837
18. Abyholm FE, Borchegrevnik HHC, Eskeland G 1979 Palatal fistulae following cleft palate surgery. Scandinavian Journal of Plastic and Reconstructive Surgery 13:295–300
19. Cohen SR, Kalinowski J, LaRossa D, Randall P 1991 Cleft palate fistulas: A multivariate statistical analysis of prevalence, etiology, and surgical management. Plastic and Reconstructive Surgery 87:1041–1047
20. Karling J, Larson O, Henningsson G 1993 Oronasal fistulas in cleft palate patients and their influence on speech. Scandinavian Journal of Plastic and Reconstructive Surgery 27:193–210
21. Schulz RC 1986 Management and timing of cleft palate fistula repair. Plastic and Reconstructive Surgery 78:739–745
22. Lehman JA, Curtin P, Haas DC 1978 Closure of anterior palatal fistulae. Cleft Palate Journal 15(1):33–38
23. Morley M 1996 In: Cleft palate and speech: The assessment of speech, 6th edn. Livingstone, Edinburgh, pp 154–155
24. Schulz RC 1984 Free periosteal graft repair of maxillary clefts in adolescents. Plastic and Reconstructive Surgery 73:556–560
25. Rintala AE 1980 Surgical closure of palatal fistulae. Scandinavian Journal of Plastic and Reconstructive Surgery 14:235–238
26. Rintala AE 1971 A double overlapping hinge flap to close palatal fistula. Scandinavian Journal of Plastic and Reconstructive Surgery 5:91–95
27. Henderson HP 1982 The 'tadpole flap': an advancement flap for the closure of anterior palatal fistulae. British Journal of Plastic Surgery 35:163–166
28. Stal S, Spira M 1984 Secondary reconstructive procedures for patients with clefts. In: Serafin D, Georgiade NG (eds) Paediatric plastic surgery, Vol 1. Mosby, St Louis, p 352
29. Millard DR, Seider HA 1977 The versatile palatal island flap: its use in soft palate reconstruction and nasopharyngeal and choanal atresia. British Journal of Plastic Surgery 30:300–305
30. Hirshowitz B, Mahler D 1970 Two new surgical procedures for closure of palatal fistulae. Cleft Palate Journal 7:685–689
31. Stenstrom SJ, Thilander BL 1963 Bone grafting in secondary cases of cleft lip and palate. Plastic and Reconstructive Surgery 32:353–360
32. Jackson IT 1972 Closure of secondary palatal fistulae with intra oral tissue and bone grafting. British Journal of Plastic Surgery 25:93–105
33. Rintala AE 1979 Labiobuccal mucosal flap for closure of anterior palatal fistulae. Scandinavian Journal of Plastic and Reconstructive Surgery 13:480–482
34. Matsuo K, Kiyono M, Hirose T 1991 A simple technique for closure of a palatal fistula using a conchal cartilage graft. Plastic and Reconstructive Surgery 88:334–337
35. Vandeput JJ, Droogmans B, Tanner JC 1995 Closure of palatal fistulas using a dermis–fat graft. Plastic and Reconstructive Surgery 95:1105–1107
36. Klopp CT, Schurter M 1956 The surgical treatment of cancer of the soft palate and tonsil. Cancer 9:1239–1243
37. Guerrero-Santos J, Altamirano JT 1966 The use of lingual flaps in the repair of fistulas of the hard palate. Plastic and Reconstructive Surgery 38:123–128
38. Posnick JC, Getz SB 1987 Surgical closure of end stage palatal

fistulas using anteriorly based dorsal tongue flaps. Journal of Oral and Maxillofacial Surgery 45:907–912

39. Bracka A 1981 The blood supply of dorsal tongue flaps. British Journal of Plastic Surgery 34:379–384

40. Jackson IT 1972 Use of tongue flaps to resurface lip defects and close palatal fistulae in children. Plastic and Reconstructive Surgery 49:537–541

41. Carreirao S, Lessa S 1980 Tongue flaps and the closing of large fistulas of the hard palate. Annals of Plastic Surgery 4:182–190

42. Carlesso J, Mondolfi P, Flicki E 1980 Hemitongue flaps. Plastic and Reconstructive Surgery 66:574–577

43. Johnson PA, Banks P, Brown AE 1992 Use of the posteriorly based lateral tongue flap in the repair of palatal fistulae. International Journal of Oral and Maxillofacial Surgery 21:6–9

44. Pigott RW, Rieger FW, Moodie AF 1984 Tongue flap repair of cleft palate fistulae. British Journal of Plastic Surgery 37:285–293

45. Busic N, Bagain M, Boric V 1989 Tongue flaps in repair of large palatal defects. International Journal of Oral and Maxillofacial Surgery 18:291–293

46. Steinhauser EW 1982 Experience with dorsal tongue flaps for closure of defects of the hard palate. Journal of Oral and Maxillofacial Surgery 40:787–789

47. Kummer AW, Neale HW 1989 Changes in articulation and resonance after tongue flap closure of palatal fistulas: case reports. Cleft Palate Journal 26:51–55

48. Batchelor AG, Palmer JH 1990 A novel method of closing a palatal fistula: the free fascial flap. British Journal of Plastic Surgery 43:359–361

49. Chem RC, Franciosi LFN 1983 Dorsalis pedis free flap to close extensive palate fistulae. Microsurgery 4:35–49

50. Chen H, Ganos DL, Coessens BC, Kyutoku S, Noordhoff MS 1992 Free forearm flap for closure of difficult oronasal fistulas in cleft palate patients. Plastic and Reconstructive Surgery 90:757–762

51. Macleod AM, Morrison WA, McCann JJ, Thistlethwaite S, Vanderkolk CA, Ryan AD 1987 The free radial forearm flap with and without bone for closure of large palatal fistulae. British Journal of Plastic Surgery 40:391–395

52. Gillies HD, Evans AJ 1957 Experiences of the tube pedicle flap in cleft palate. Transactions of the International Society of Plastic Surgeons, First Congress. Williams & Wilkins, Baltimore, p 208

53. De Mey A, Malevez C, Lejour M 1990 Treatment of palatal fistula by expansion. British Journal of Plastic Surgery 43:362–364

54. Moran RE 1951 The pharyngeal flap operation as a speech aid. Plastic and Reconstructive Surgery 7:202–213

55. Trier WC 1985 The pharyngeal flap operation. Cleft Palate Journal 12:697–710

56. Whitaker LA, Randall P, Graham WP, Hamilton RW, Winchester R 1972 A prospective and randomised series comparing superiorly and inferiorly based posterior pharyngeal flaps. Cleft Palate Journal 9:304–311

57. Graham WP, Hamilton R, Randall P, Winchester R, Stool S 1973 Complications following posterior pharyngeal flap surgery. Cleft Palate Journal 10:176–180

58. Pensler JM, Reich DS 1991 A comparison of speech results after the pharyngeal flap and the dynamic sphincteroplasty procedures. Annals of Plastic Surgery 26:441–443

59. Owsley JQ, Blackfield HM 1965 The technique and complications of pharyngeal flap surgery. Plastic and Reconstructive Surgery 35:531–539

60. Mercer NSG, MacCarthy P 1995 The arterial basis of pharyngeal flaps. Plastic and Reconstructive Surgery 96:1026–1037

61. Skolnick ML, McCall GN 1972 Velopharyngeal incompetence following pharyngeal flap surgery: Videofluoroscopic study in multiple projections. Cleft Palate Journal 9:1–12

62. Shprintzen RJ, Lewin ML, Croft CB, Daniller AI, Argamaso RV,

63. Ship AG, Strauch B 1979 A comprehensive study of pharyngeal flap surgery: tailor made flaps. Cleft Palate Journal 16:46–55

63. Hogan VM 1975 A biased approach to the treatment of velopharyngeal incompetence. Clinics in Plastic Surgery 2:319–323

64. Croft CB, Shprintzen RJ, Daniller A, Lewin ML 1978 The occult submucous cleft palate and the musculus uvulae. Cleft Palate Journal 15:150–154

65. Honig CA 1967 The treatment of velopharyngeal insufficiency after palatal repair. Archivum Chirurgicum Nederlandicum 19:71–81

66. Pigott RW 1974 The results of nasopharyngoscopic assessment of pharyngoplasty. Scandinavian Journal of Plastic and Reconstructive Surgery 8:148–152

67. McCoy FJ, Zahorsky C 1972 A new approach to the elusive dynamic pharyngeal flap. Plastic and Reconstructive Surgery 49:160–164

68. Hynes W 1950 Pharyngoplasty by muscle transplantation. British Journal of Plastic Surgery 3:128–135

69. Hynes W 1953 The results of pharyngoplasty by muscle transplantation in 'failed cleft palate' cases, with special reference to the influence of the pharynx on voice production. Annals of the Royal College of Surgeons of England 13:17–35

70. Hynes W 1957 The examination of imperfect speech following cleft palate operations. British Journal of Plastic Surgery 10:114–121

71. Hynes W 1967 Observations on pharyngoplasty. British Journal of Plastic Surgery 20:244–256

72. Orticochea M 1968 Construction of a dynamic muscle sphincter in cleft palates. Plastic and Reconstructive Surgery 41:323–327

73. Orticochea M 1983 A review of 236 cleft palate patients treated with dynamic muscle sphincter. Plastic and Reconstructive Surgery 71:180–188

74. Lendrum J, Dhar BK 1984 The Orticochea dynamic pharyngoplasty. British Journal of Plastic Surgery 37:160–168

75. Jackson IT, Silverton JS 1977 The sphincter pharyngoplasty as a secondary procedure in cleft palates. Plastic and Reconstructive Surgery 59:518–524

76. Jackson IT 1985 Sphincter pharyngoplasty. Clinics in Plastic Surgery 12:711–717

77. Riski JE, Ruff GL, Georgiade GS, Barwick WJ, Edwards PD 1992 Evaluation of the sphincter pharyngoplasty. Cleft Palate Journal 29:254–261

78. Georgantopolou AA, Thatte MR, Razzell RE, Watson ACH 1996 The effect of sphincter pharyngoplasty on the range of velar movement. British Journal of Plastic Surgery 49:358–362

79. Blocksma R 1963 Correction of velopharyngeal insufficiency by silastic pharyngeal implant. Plastic and Reconstructive Surgery 31:268–274

80. Brauer RO 1973 Retropharyngeal implantation of silicone pillows for velopharyngeal incompetence. Plastic and Reconstructive Surgery 51:254–262

81. Denny AD, Marks SM, Oliff-Carneol S 1993 Correction of velopharyngeal insufficiency by pharyngeal augmentation using autogenous cartilage: a preliminary report. Cleft Palate Journal 30:46–54

82. Furlow LT, Williams WN, Eisenbach CR, Bzoch KR 1982 A long term study on treating velopharyngeal insufficiency by Teflon injection. Cleft Palate Journal 19:47–56

83. Trier WC 1983 Velopharyngeal incompetency in the absence of overt cleft palate – anatomical and surgical considerations. Cleft Palate Journal 20:209–217

84. Moore FT 1960 A new operation to cure nasopharyngeal incompetence. British Journal of Surgery 47:424–428

85. Sullivan DE 1961 Bilateral pharyngoplasty as an aid to velopharyngeal closure. Plastic and Reconstructive Surgery 27:31–39

86. Peat BG, Albery EH, Jones K, Pigott RW 1994 Tailoring

velopharyngeal surgery: the influence of aetiology and type of operation. Plastic and Reconstructive Surgery 93:948–953

87. Bardach J 1995 Secondary surgery for velopharyngeal insufficiency. In: Shprintzen RJ, Bardach J (eds) Cleft palate speech management: a multidisciplinary approach. Mosby, St Louis

88. Cox JB, Silverstein B 1961 Experiences with the posterior pharyngeal flap for correction of velopharyngeal incompetence. Plastic and Reconstructive Surgery 27:40–48

89. Riski JE, Georgiade NG, Serafin D, Barwick W, Georgiade GS, Riefkohl R 1987 The Orticochea pharyngoplasty and primary palatoplasty: an evaluation. Annals of Plastic Surgery 18:303–309

90. Spauwen RH, Ritsma RJ, Huffstadt BJ, Scutte HK, Brown IF 1988 The inferiorly based pharyngoplasty: effects on chronic otitis media with effusion. Cleft Palate Journal 25:26–32

91. Long RE, McNamara JA 1985 Facial growth following pharyngeal flap surgery: skeletal assessment on serial lateral cephalometric radiographs. American Journal of Orthodontics and Dentofacial Orthopedics 87:187–196

92. Braithwaite F, Maurice DG 1968 The importance of the levator muscle in cleft palate closure. British Journal of Plastic Surgery 21:60–62

93. Kriens OB 1970 Fundamental anatomic findings for an intravelar veloplasty. Cleft Palate Journal 7:27–36

94. Sommerlad BC, Henley M, Birch M, Harland K, Moieman N, Boorman JG 1994 Cleft palate re-repair – a clinical and radiological study of 32 consecutive cases. British Journal of Plastic Surgery 47:406–410

95. Furlow LT 1986 Cleft palate repair by double reversing Z-plasty. Plastic and Reconstructive Surgery 78:724–736

96. Chen PK-T, Wu J, Chen Y-R, Noordhoff MS 1994 Correction of secondary velopharyngeal insufficiency in cleft palate patients with the Furlow palatoplasty. Plastic and Reconstructive Surgery 94:933–941

97. Boorman JG, Sommerlad BC, Birch MJ, Fenn C, Pandya A 1997 Velar function following secondary palate repair by intravelar veloplasty versus Furlow. Presented at 8th International Congress on Cleft Palate, Singapore

98. Witt PD, Berry LA, Marsh JA, Grames LM, Pilgram TK 1996 Speech outcome following palatoplasty in primary school children: do lay peer observers agree with speech pathologists? Plastic and Reconstructive Surgery 98:958–970

99. Witt PD, D'Antonio LL, Zimmerman GJ, Marsh JL 1994 Sphincter pharyngoplasty: a preoperative and postoperative analysis of perceptual speech characteristics and endoscopic studies of velopharyngeal function. Plastic and Reconstructive Surgery 93:1154–1168

100. Boorman JG, Ray AK 1994 How to select an operation for velopharyngeal dysfunction. Presented at The Craniofacial Society of Great Britain, Cambridge

101. Albery EH, Bennett JA, Pigott RW, Simmons RM 1982 The results of figures 100 operations for velopharyngeal incompetence – selected on the findings of endoscopic and radiological examination. British Journal of Plastic Surgery 35:118–126

102. Barot LR, Cohen M, LaRossa D 1992 Surgical indications and techniques for posterior pharyngeal flap revision. Plastic and Reconstructive Surgery 90:774–778

103. Barone CM, Shprintzen RJ, Strauch B, Sablay LB, Argamasso RV 1994 Pharyngeal flap revisions: flap elevation from a scarred posterior pharynx. Plastic and Reconstructive Surgery 93:279–283

104. Owsley JQ, Creech BJ, Dedo HH 1972 Poor speech following the pharyngeal flap operation: etiology and treatment. Cleft Palate Journal 9:312–317

105. Friedman HI, Haines PC, Coston GN, Lett ED, Edgerton MT 1992 Augmentation of the failed pharyngeal flap. Plastic and Reconstructive Surgery 90:314–318

106. Ma L, James DR, Sell DA 1996 Failed pharyngoplasty and subsequent management. British Journal of Oral and Maxillofacial Surgery 34:348–356

Orthodontic role in clefts

69

KIRT EDWARD SIMMONS

INTRODUCTION

Cleft-affected patients can benefit greatly from orthodontic and/or craniofacial orthopedic treatment. Effective treatment of this type requires a specialized knowledge of these patients' unique features. This chapter will describe generalities, although each patient will have a unique presentation because of individual differences. For brevity, this chapter will deal only with the common clefting patterns:

- cleft lip only (CL), which may be unilateral or bilateral and which may or may not involve the maxillary alveolus;
- cleft palate only (CP);
- unilateral cleft lip and palate (UCLP);
- bilateral cleft lip and palate (BCLP).

Many different treatment techniques and philosophies are currently practiced in the complex care of these patients. This chapter will provide a general overview of these techniques and describe the role of orthodontic therapy.

Typical orthodontic treatment for these patients may involve long periods of time at various ages. Because of this, and the intense nature of orthodontic therapy, active treatment should be planned in stages rather than long term and continuous. Classically, the treatment stages to be considered relate to four developmental stages: infancy, primary dentition, mixed dentition and permanent dentition. A typical cleft lip and/or palate patient might undergo orthodontic treatment at one or more of these different developmental stages. Their potential orthodontic needs and treatment possibilities will be discussed for each stage.

INFANCY

Although at present controversial, orthopedic treatment in infancy was almost universally practiced in the past. This is easy to understand, given the significant distortion of the maxilla evident at birth in individuals with unrepaired unilateral or bilateral clefts of the lip and palate (Fig. 69.1). One approach to this problem was orthopedic alignment of the maxillary segments prior to primary bone grafting (i.e. bone grafting done at the time of lip and/or palate closure), so that the maxilla would have a normal shape postoperatively. Theoretically, surgical correction of the problem at this early age would allow normal function, growth and development.[1] This attractive philosophy had many followers until extensive early surgery, with its concomitant increased scarring, was shown to have potentially deleterious effects on future growth and development.[2,3] Furthermore, untreated cleft-affected adults demonstrated relatively normal development,[4] indicating that the scarring and tissue reaction from surgical procedures might account for many of the latter classic craniofacial effects ascribed to the clefting itself. Excessive maxillary distortion at the time of the initial surgical procedure may result in a difficult, and less ideal, lip repair unless the segments are more closely approximated. Bilaterally cleft infants present with multiple problems in this regard, specifically medially collapsed posterior alveolar segments and a protruded and inferiorly positioned premaxillary segment. To optimize the surgical result, fixed orthopedic appliances can be used to expand the posterior segments and/or retract the premaxillary seg-

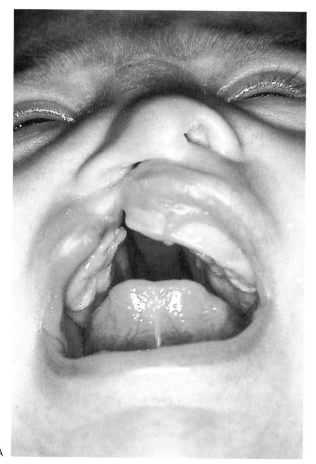

A

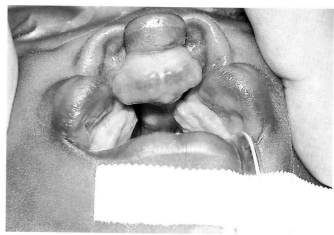

B

Fig. 69.1 Unrepaired complete clefts of the lip and palate. **(A)** Unilateral. **(B)** Bilateral; note the posterior arch collapse, the protrusive premaxilla and the separation of the lip segments.

ment, thereby more closely approximating the cleft segments. Posterior expansion can be achieved by a pin- or screw-retained 'jackscrew' type or spring-loaded appliance (Fig. 69.2). These can also retract the premaxilla with the addition of another screw component, or elastic bands between the premaxillary segment and the posterior portion (Fig. 69.3). Retraction of the premaxillary segment can also be achieved by extraoral elastic traction across the premaxilla (Fig. 69.4), either alone, or in conjunction with an active posterior expansion appliance or passive posterior 'molding' appliance (maintains posterior alveolar width as the anterior

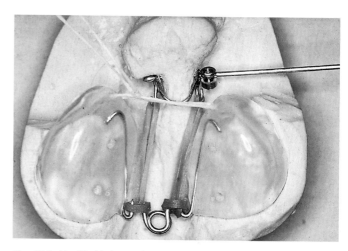

Fig. 69.3 Modified infant orthopedic expansion appliance to retract the premaxilla. Appliance shown on the plaster cast of the patient; note the anterior stainless steel portion which pierces the premaxilla and the elastic bands extending between the two portions of the appliance to retract the premaxilla.

Fig. 69.2 An example of an infant orthopedic expansion appliance utilizing a midpalatal screw (jackscrew) for posterior expansion.

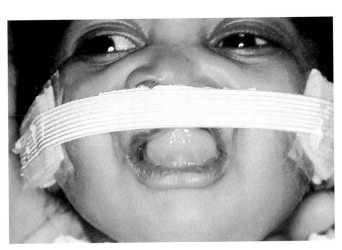

Fig. 69.4 An extraoral elastic traction band across the premaxilla to provide retraction.

portion is being 'molded'). Alternatively, a preliminary surgical procedure, such as lip adhesion, can be carried out following the expansion. The elastic force of the healing lip serves to retract the premaxilla for the later definitive lip repair. Some craniofacial centers routinely use fixed presurgical orthopedic treatment, whereas at other centers simple elastic traction is considered sufficient. Different assessments of the potential iatrogenic risks of presurgical expansion (damage to the tooth buds, aspiration of materials, additional anesthetic and surgical procedures etc.) versus the positive benefits in treatment needs or outcomes[5-7] influence the treatment choice. At some centers advocating early orthopedic treatment, primary alveolar bone grafting or periosteoplasty is accomplished at the same time as the lip closure. Purportedly these additional procedures provide a better arch form, fewer fistulae and a decreased need for future secondary bone grafting. To date, the long-term benefits of these procedures are still controversial.[5,7]

PRIMARY DENTITION STAGE

Depending on the development of speech and other factors, surgical closure of the palate generally occurs between 9 and 18 months of age. Following this, the typical cleft-affected patient will still have a cleft of the maxillary alveolus and may have one or more fistulae on the buccal and/or lingual side of the alveolus. Generally, the patient at this age also has all the primary incisors, with the complete primary dentition appearing by $3\frac{1}{2}$ years of age. Orthodontic treatment from this age until the beginning of the mixed dentition phase is relatively rare. Treatment indications at this stage are identical to those in non-cleft individuals,

i.e. to control or eliminate deleterious habits, functional shifts or space loss after premature loss of primary teeth. Digit habits can be successfully overcome in cleft-affected patients if they are willing to comply with treatment, consisting of fixed or removable habit appliances, which can also serve to correct crossbite where present. However, in the presence of a maxilla without bony continuity across the palate or alveolus, the corrected crossbite will need to be retained until some form of bony continuity (usually accomplished by secondary bone grafting) is provided. If this will not be established in the near future, and in the absence of a functional shift of the mandible due to the crossbite, it is often in the patient's best interest to postpone crossbite correction until immediately prior to the bone graft.

Independent of a habit, crossbite interference should be eliminated when practicable in cases where the patient must actively shift their mandible to achieve maximum intercuspation. This is most easily done by selective reduction of the interfering teeth, but may require orthodontic expansion. The rationale for elimination of these functional shifts is to prevent consequent unfavorable jaw growth. Orthodontic expansion at this stage, which may involve anterior and/or posterior expansion (Fig. 69.5), is possible but may require long-term retention.

In the absence of treatment between the primary and mixed dentition stages, patients should at least be monitored for eruption and dental development. Any significant delay in dental age, particularly in short-statured patients, should raise suspicion of growth hormone deficiency (as clefting, a midline defect, is often associated with other midline defects, such as pituitary or cardiovascular anomalies).

MIXED DENTITION

Once the permanent teeth begin to erupt and the patient enters the mixed dentition stage, it is important to assess future orthodontic treatment needs. Relatively rapid changes in the dentition, as well as the developing social and self-awareness of the patient at this age, makes orthodontic evaluation and the development of long-term treatment objectives mandatory.[8] Standard orthodontic records (nominally consisting of panoramic and cephalometric radiographs, facial and intraoral photographs, clinical examination notes and dental models) are therefore indicated at this stage in most cases. In addition, selected periapical and/or occlusal radiographs to assess missing/supernumerary teeth and/or bone quantity and anatomy in the cleft site may be indicated. These records are necessary to develop an orthodontic diagnosis and tentative treatment options, as well as

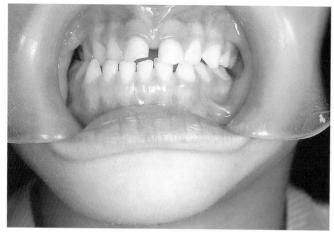

A

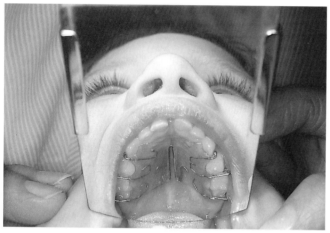

B

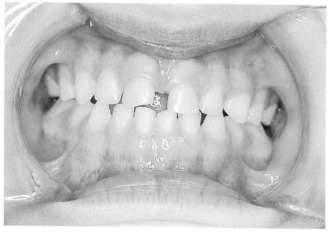

C

Fig. 69.5 An example of a functional shift in the primary dentition. **(A)** Full intercuspation; note the shift of the dentition and midlines. **(B)** Removable maxillary expansion appliance; note the hemisection of the acrylic and the stainless steel wire spring to provide for expansion. **(C)** Expansion after 5 months of appliance wear.

to provide an initial benchmark for subsequent development and growth. Future treatment needs and options should be presented to the patient and parents at this time. It is important to prepare them for the compliance, co-operation, expense, and patience required in orthodontic treatment.

Many cleft-affected patients will be missing teeth in the cleft area and others will have supernumerary primary and/or permanent teeth. A tentative decision should be made at this time as to which teeth will be maintained and which will be removed. For teeth to be removed, the timing of the extractions should be determined based on the location and prognosis of the teeth. If the teeth are erupted in the area of the cleft they can serve to maintain bone in the region until the graft is accomplished. However, if the teeth are removed at the same time as the graft is placed, the residual soft-tissue defect may compromise wound closure. One acceptable compromise is to maintain the teeth until a very short time prior to the graft and then extract them, so that the bone will still be maintained but the soft tissue will be healed by the time of the graft.

Most patients with cleft alveoli present in the mixed dentition stage with a posterior crossbite and malaligned maxillary incisors. These patients will typically benefit from expansion of the collapsed maxillary segment(s) and elimination of traumatic occlusion in preparation for alveolar bone grafting. Radiographs (panoramic, maxillary occlusal or periapical) of the cleft area are necessary to assess the development of the adjacent unerupted teeth, as the bone graft is ideally placed when the root of the erupting adjacent lateral incisor or canine is half to two-thirds completed.[9,10] The grafted bone is then most likely to be present in sufficient amounts to allow eruption of the adjacent tooth, which brings its periodontal attachment with it, inhibiting further bone resorption.[9,11] The majority of these teeth erupt spontaneously, but it may occasionally be necessary to surgically uncover and place orthodontic traction on the adjacent tooth to achieve eruption.[9]

For maximum stability of the maxilla during bone healing, consistent with sound orthopedic principles, traumatic occlusion of teeth in the cleft region should be eliminated prior to alveolar bone grafting. This may be done through alignment of the offending (usually maxillary incisor) teeth. However, as it is fairly common to have only a thin layer of bone along the cleft side of the roots of adjacent teeth, it is often best to delay their orthodontic alignment until after the graft. If the teeth are aligned prior to the bone graft, great care must be used to prevent moving the roots into the cleft site. In addition, a period of retention prior to the bone graft allows reformation of the cortical bone along the root prior to surgical exposure. Denudation of the roots

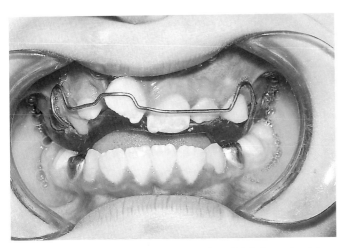

Fig. 69.6 Removable appliance in a right unilateral cleft lip- and palate-affected patient. The appliance was made prior to the bone graft, with posterior occlusal coverage to prevent traumatic occlusion of the incisors postoperatively. Note the bends in the labial bow to maintain passivity of the bow prior to the bone graft. Following the bone graft the labial bow can be adjusted to align the central incisor.

during the grafting procedure may result in periodontal defects, ankylosis, root resorption and/or decreased alveolar bone mass upon healing. Alternatively, orthodontic alignment can be postponed until after graft placement, and a full-time bite splint (Fig. 69.6) can be used to prevent any traumatic occlusion during graft healing.

Besides the elimination of traumatic occlusion, expansion may also be indicated prior to the bone graft to realign the maxillary segments and improve surgical access to the graft site. The maxillary segments must not be expanded beyond the limits of surgical closure, therefore the amount and timing of pre-graft expansion should be planned in consultation with the surgeon on each case. The ideal expansion from an orthodontic perspective would provide coordinated maxillary and mandibular arch forms. If achievement of these orthodontic objectives will result in a poor prognosis for the graft, a choice must be made between delaying the graft until adolescence and uniting the segments with an orthognathic surgical procedure, or performing the graft without expansion and attempting expansion later, or accepting the crossbite. Delaying the graft until adolescence, however, may have deleterious effects on erupting adjacent teeth or on the orthodontic movement of adjacent teeth, resulting in significant periodontal defects and even loss of these teeth. Expansion in unilateral cleft lip- and palate-affected patients is fairly predictable after alveolar bone grafting, although ideal arch form may be compromised. This is less predictable in the bilateral cleft lip and palate situation, probably because of increased scarring and lack of a functional maxillary midline suture to expand.

In the typical unilateral or bilateral complete cleft case

expansion is limited by the resistance of the zygomatic buttresses and the scar tissue present. This scar tissue can be quite resistant to expansion, especially in patients who exhibit impressive amounts of maxillary collapse owing to the scarring. Adequate expansion can be achieved with a number of different appliances: removable appliances incorporating jackscrew devices or wire springs (see Fig. 69.5); fixed spring appliances (such as a quad-helix, W-arch or various combinations of these; Fig. 69.7); or fixed jackscrew devices such as the Hyrax appliance (Fig. 69.8). Appliance selection in any given case should be based on the direction and extent of expansion desired, the teeth present, the expected resistance of the tissue, access to the cleft area by

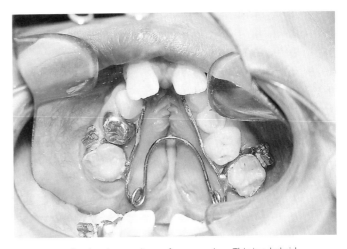

Fig. 69.7 A fixed-spring appliance for expansion. This is a hybrid appliance, being essentially a W-arch expander but incorporating the two posterior helices of the quad-helix.

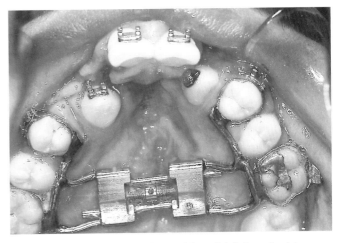

Fig. 69.8 A fixed 'Hyrax' expander in a bilateral cleft lip and palate patient. Note the posterior placement of the expander, which allowed surgical access for the bone graft. Also note the canines, which have erupted through the grafted bone and are now ready for orthodontic alignment. The expander has been maintained passively for the bone graft healing and will be retained to augment the orthodontic anchorage while moving the canines to the facial.

the surgeon, and the anticipated compliance of the patient. Removable appliances are preferred for hygiene but lend themselves to problems of compliance, lack of retention and loss. Fixed appliances require less patient compliance and generally have fewer retention problems, but are a greater hygiene problem and can lead to decalcification and caries if not properly maintained. The spring appliances apply lighter forces and are under the control of the orthodontist, with the quad-helix generally providing lighter forces over a greater range of activation than the W-arch. They can be activated to expand the segments differentially, which is quite useful as the lesser segment (or posterior segments in a bilateral cleft patient) is often more collapsed anteriorly than posteriorly. The jackscrew type of appliance is very rigid, can generate very high forces and result in rapid movement, but requires periodic activation by the patient or a parent. They are designed and constructed to provide a certain amount and direction of expansion. Reactivation of spring-loaded appliances may be necessary several times before the desired expansion is achieved, generally requiring 4–6 months with good compliance. It must be recognized that any fistulae the patient may have (including those that may be 'unknown' to the patient and/or clinician) will tend to be enlarged during the expansion, and this should be pointed out to the patient. Such fistulae are generally closed at the time of the alveolar bone graft. Appliance design should ensure unimpeded surgical access at the time of the bone graft (see Figs 69.7, 69.8), particularly in bilateral cleft patients. If, following expansion, the appliance components are in a position to interfere with the surgery, then the appliance should be modified beforehand. The appliance should be conducive to good oral hygiene, as poor oral hygiene has been implicated in bone graft failure.[12] For proper healing of the graft the expansion must be maintained for 4–6 months afterwards, either by retention of the passive expansion appliance or by replacement with a removable acrylic retainer or fixed lingual arch (Fig. 69.9). Where the cleft is complete and bilateral it is important to stabilize a mobile premaxilla at the time of the graft and until the graft has been incorporated into the host bone.[12] This will require from 6 weeks to 6 months, depending on such variables as graft size, tissue stretch and/or scarring, occlusal stability, and individual variations in bone and soft-tissue healing capacity. A full-time maxillary splint or heavy labial or lingual fixed appliance can be used to provide this stability.

An alternative approach advocates alveolar bone grafting at a younger age (5–7 years), orthodontically 'stimulating' the graft shortly afterwards by rapid expansion with a fixed expansion (usually a jackscrew type) appliance.[13] The proponents of this protocol claim shorter orthodontic treat-

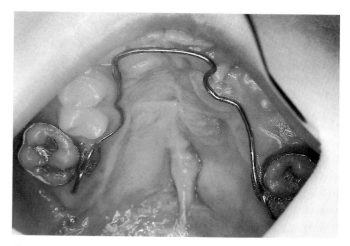

Fig. 69.9 Fixed lingual arch to maintain expansion after placing an alveolar bone graft.

ment times and the prevention of maxillary horizontal hypoplasia by earlier anterior crossbite correction. In theory, this rapid expansion could have an effect similar to distraction osteogenesis at the cleft site, but objective long-term comparative studies are lacking. Initial maxillary incisor alignment can often be effected with fixed orthodontic appliances immediately following the bone graft. Generally, at this point the patient is given a 'vacation' from active treatment and placed in retention. A removable acrylic retainer with plastic pontics can be used to mask missing or unerupted teeth until comprehensive orthodontic treatment is begun. A temporary bonded lingual retainer (0.0175″ multitwist archwire) can also be used to retain spaced incisors (Fig. 69.10).

Following stabilization of the bone graft and initial incisor alignment an orthodontic assessment is indicated to develop treatment objectives and future treatment needs. Clinical and cephalometric evaluation is necessary at this point to

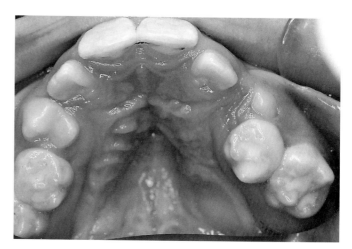

Fig. 69.10 Lingually bonded 0.0175″ twist wire to retain the central incisor alignment.

consider the general pattern of maxillary and mandibular growth that has been expressed and can be expected in these patients. Discordant monozygotic twin studies have revealed differences based on the type and severity of the cleft.[14] Maxillary and mandibular growth is essentially unaffected in patients with clefts of only the lip and alveolus, with the cleft twins exhibiting thinner upper lips and more upright maxillary incisors. Clefting of only the palate can result in a shorter posterior face height, a steeper mandibular plane angle, and maxillary and mandibular retrognathia. Complete unilateral clefting of the lip and palate (Fig. 69.11) can result in a failure of the maxilla to grow anteriorly, resulting in a posterior and inferior displacement. The mandible tends to be of a normal size but deflected inferiorly, resulting in an increased mandibular plane angle and anterior face height. Consequently, patients with very flat profiles, increased face heights and/or class III skeletal relationships will generally exhibit a worsening of their condition with further growth. Significant skeletal deformities are best treated with a combination of orthodontics and surgery in one stage at a later age, or in multiple stages in very severe cases. Sufficiently young (generally 8 years of age or less[15-18]) mild maxillary deficient cleft-affected patients may benefit from orthopedic forces for maxillary protraction. In order to effect orthopedic changes the patient must apply the forces (350–500 g per side) over 10–24 hours a day for an

average of 12–15 months' total treatment time.[15-18] This treatment is provided by bonded full occlusal coverage acrylic splints[18] or fixed banded (including bands on the primary canines and primary second molars or first permanent molars)[15-17] intraoral appliances, generally incorporating some provision for concomitant maxillary expansion and with hooks at the canine area for engagement of elastics.

The extraoral protraction force is applied via elastic force to a facial mask, of which many different styles are commercially available. These differ in their incorporation of various pads, bands and frame styles, and can even include an American football style helmet. Several different styles can be kept on hand to include the patient in the selection process, which seems to help with compliance. Regardless of the mask type, the elastic force is applied in a forward and slightly downward (generally 15–25 degrees down relative to the occlusal plane) direction, taking care not to impinge on the lips.[15-17]

Verdon[15] has also advocated the use of elastics and independent posterior intraoral appliances to apply the expansive, as well as the protractive, forces.

During the treatment period the correction of anterior crossbites and improvement of the prognathic profile is fairly predictable, although variable.[17,18] Studies of this treatment indicate that the immediate therapeutic effect is one of limited maxillary skeletal advancement (1–3 mm), maxillary dental advancement, and counterclockwise or posterior rotation of the mandible.[15-18] Tindlund and Rygh[17] have reported that significant anterior skeletal advancement with this therapy occurs only in unilateral cleft cases, with bilateral cleft patients exhibiting almost exclusively (90%) dentoalveolar advancement.

Although the immediate benefits of this therapy have been well studied, the long-term effects have not been determined in large clinical trials. Young and compliant patients with mild maxillary deficiencies who can benefit from, or at least tolerate, the effects of maxillary dental protrusion and downward and backward displacement of the mandible, are the best candidates for this treatment option.

Orthognathic surgery or distraction osteogenesis, rather than orthopedic protraction, should be planned in patients with true mandibular prognathism, severe mandibular retrognathism, skeletal open bite, moderate to severe maxillary deficiency, or who have limited or no craniofacial growth remaining. Even in seemingly ideal candidates it should be stressed that further growth may compromise the orthopedic effects, necessitating camouflage orthodontic treatment or orthognathic surgery for an acceptable result.

The most challenging patients, as a group, to the orthodontist are those with complete bilateral cleft lip and palate. Because of the lack of an intact circumoral musculature

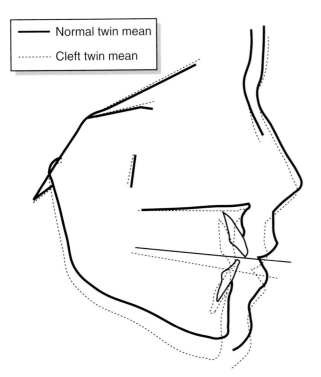

Fig. 69.11 Stylized mean cephalometric superimpositions of monozygotic twins discordant for complete unilateral cleft of the lip and palate. The non-cleft twin means are depicted as solid lines and the cleft-affected twin means are depicted as dotted lines.[14]

Normal twin mean
Cleft twin mean

and bony continuity in the maxilla, the premaxilla is typically mobile and connected to the rest of the skull by a vomerine 'stalk' with an attendant vomerine–premaxillary suture. In addition, these individuals suffer from more severe tissue deficiencies, which can be accentuated by surgical repairs, scar contracture, and oral and nasal dysfunction. In terms of orthodontic treatment, these deficiencies often pose a number of problems: minimal coverage of the maxillary incisors by the upper lip, a shallow maxillary labial vestibule, a short and tight upper lip with protrusive lower lip, large fistulae, palatal webs over the maxillary molar area, missing maxillary lateral incisors, ectopically erupting teeth, and hypoplastic or missing central incisors. The timing of the surgical correction of these problems, if indicated, must be coordinated between the surgeon and the orthodontist. At the mixed dentition stage many of these patients will exhibit a protrusive and mobile premaxilla which may contain anywhere from four to no incisors (usually two central incisors). Anterior crossbites are frequently observed owing to posterior rotation of the premaxilla and retroclination of the maxillary incisors (sometimes to the extreme of having the facial surfaces of these teeth occluding with the mandibular incisors). Even when there is no crossbite there is often a severe discrepancy between the three maxillary segments, with the premaxillary segment protrusive and inferiorly displaced relative to the posterior segments. The ideal vertical position of the premaxilla can be difficult to assess because of the common hypoplasia of the nose and/or upper lips, leading to the illusion of a premaxilla overdeveloped vertically (Fig. 69.12). If the premaxilla is truly malpositioned, this can usually be corrected by pre-graft orthopedic movement. However other than fairly simple tipping movements of the premaxilla around the vomerine stalk, this can be difficult,

depending on the amount and type of movement required, the compliance of the patient, and the teeth available for appliance anchorage. The premaxillary segment can be surgically repositioned at the time of alveolar bone grafting, although this is rarely necessary and requires great care to prevent the loss of perfusion of the premaxilla.[19] The relative protrusion of the premaxilla at an early age is not an indication of excessive maxillary growth potential in these patients. In fact, from age 4 to maturity the forward growth rate of the premaxilla has been shown to be half that of non-cleft patients, whereas mandibular growth is essentially the same.[20] This amounts to a functional 'headgear' effect, generally resulting in an acceptable maxillary/mandibular relationship by adolescence.[20,21] This must be taken into account in young candidates for premaxillary repositioning procedures, who should, in fact, be treated to increased overjet at the time of surgery.

PERMANENT DENTITION

When the typical patient is approximately 12–14 years old, in the very late mixed or early permanent dentition stage, it is appropriate to obtain complete new diagnostic records (lateral and panoramic radiographs, supplementary periapical and/or occlusal radiographs, photographs, models and a clinical examination) and reassess their comprehensive treatment plan, in collaboration with the other members of the team. The most common problems seen at this point include missing, supernumerary and/or malformed teeth adjacent to the cleft area, some residual maxillary constriction, a displaced maxillary dental midline, and frenal or periodontal

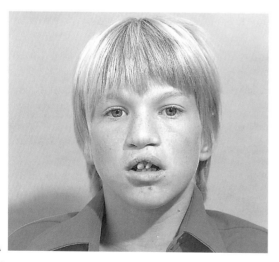
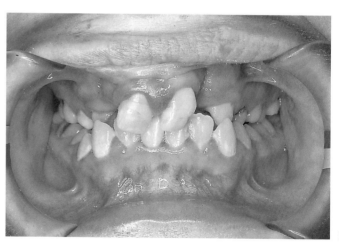

Fig. 69.12 A young patient with a repaired bilateral cleft lip and palate. **(A)** Facial view, note the excessive amount of incisors displayed at rest. **(B)** Dental view, note the vertical position of the maxillary incisors in this view appear to be within normal limits compared to the maxillary posterior segments and mandibular teeth.

abnormalities in the cleft. In addition, these patients not uncommonly exhibit delayed dental development, altered eruption patterns, missing permanent teeth outside the immediate cleft area, and/or supernumerary teeth. Most of those with an underlying mild to moderate class II or 'weak' class I pattern can be treated with orthodontics alone, whereas those with a class III pattern or a severe class II pattern (such as some patients with Pierre–Robin syndrome or craniofacial microsomia (Fig. 69.13) will require orthognathic surgery or distraction osteogenesis for an acceptable result.[22]

An important treatment planning consideration for many of these patients involves missing teeth, usually the lateral incisor(s). Sometimes a tooth may be physically present but compromised (reduced periodontial attachment, impacted, hypoplastic, poor root form or size etc.). A decision must be made whether or not to treat the patient with canine substitution or prosthetic replacement. This decision should be based on several factors: the alignment of the crown and root of the canine, the morphology and color of the canine, the presence of residual fistulae, the presence or absence of a good bony fill from the alveolar graft, the maxillary midline, the occlusal relationships of the posterior segments, spacing, crowding, the presence and prognosis of the maxillary premolars, and the general maxillary to mandibular skeletal and facial relationships. In cases where the maxillary dental midline is on or off to the non-cleft side, the canine has erupted mesially with reasonable root position adjacent to the maxillary central incisor, the canine is fairly small and white in color, both premolars are present

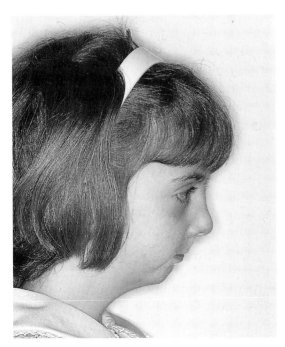

Fig. 69.13 A patient with Pierre-Robin syndrome, note the significant mandibular retrognathia.

on the affected side, and the molar and canine relationships on that side are class II, canine substitution can be an excellent choice. Conversely, prosthetic replacement of the missing lateral incisor is best in cases where the maxillary canine is in either a class I relationship or has its crown displaced mesially but the root still positioned distally, the maxillary midline is off to the cleft side, the incisors are retroclined, there are other teeth missing or with a poor prognosis on the affected side, and where the molars are in a good class I relationship bilaterally. In skeletal class III patients the choice of substitution or replacement will also depend on whether orthognathic surgical procedures are planned, in which case the space may be required to decompensate the maxillary central incisors. If interdental osteotomies are planned to expand the posterior portion, or insufficient bone exists preoperatively to support the teeth, some space should be left which the surgeon will close at the time of surgery.

Prosthetic replacement of lateral incisors, if indicated, can be accomplished through removable prostheses, fixed partial dentures or osseointegrated dental implants. The latter should not be placed prior to the completion of active vertical facial growth (best assessed by serial cephalometric films), and a minimum of 7 mm space should be obtained for their future placement.

As previously mentioned, children with skeletal problems (true mandibular prognathism, severe mandibular retrognathism, skeletal open bite, moderate to severe maxillary deficiency or poor facial profiles), who will require orthognathic surgery in the long term, ideally would not begin their comprehensive orthodontic treatment until approximately 1–1.5 years prior to the proposed surgery date. Generally, a more predictable final result is achieved if the orthognathic surgery is done at the completion of active craniofacial growth. This usually occurs at 14–16 years of age for females and 16–18 years of age for males, but is quite variable individually. Serial lateral cephalometric radiographs, demonstrating no significant change over at least a 6-month interval, are the preferred technique for assessing craniofacial growth completion. Preoperative orthodontic treatment is usually begun in our clinic based on these age estimates, adjusted for the individual patient based on that patient's general development (i.e. early, average or late pubertal development). It is stressed to the patient and parents that this is an estimate and that growth will be followed with serial radiographs during the orthodontic phase to assure completion of growth. If the patient is orthodontically ready for the surgical procedure prior to growth completion, he or she can be maintained in that condition with fixed appliances until surgery; however, if the surgery date is anticipated to be 6 months or more away, we commonly remove the fixed appliances and place the patient in removable retainers until growth is completed. This is indicated for dental hygiene as well as convenience and compliance. The patients and parents appreciate this 'vacation' from active treatment, and understand that the orthodontic treatment following the orthognathic surgery is very important and will require frequent visits and good compliance.

Prior to the comprehensive preoperative orthodontic treatment, limited treatment can be provided to address crowding, functional issues, psychological issues, and/or to eliminate or prevent traumatic occlusion. The benefits of such treatment must be realistically weighed against the risks of patient/parent 'burnout', as well as the increased risk of decalcification, root resorption and periodontal problems associated with increased treatment time. The goals and end-points of such limited treatment should be clearly defined initially, so that orthodontic treatment does not become a lifelong affair for these patients.

The most common orthognathic surgical need in cleft-affected patients is maxillary skeletal augmentation. This may involve all three planes of space, necessitating skeletal advancement, expansion and vertical displacement. In cases of open bite, mandibular asymmetry, mandibular protrusion or mandibular retrusion, the surgical procedure may include the mandible. It is the orthodontist's responsibility to develop a comprehensive treatment plan for the final occlusion and skeletal relationships in concert with the surgeon and/or prosthetic dentist. In addition, the effect of these procedures on the patient's facial esthetics and functional abilities to breathe and speak must be considered, with appropriate input from the respective specialists.

Preoperative orthodontic treatment almost always involves full fixed appliances, and often results in an apparent 'worsening' of the malocclusion as the previous natural dental compensations are removed in order to align the teeth properly with respect to their skeletal components. This effect should be explained to patients and parents in advance. Errors on the side of excessive decompensation are preferred over inadequate decompensation, as errors of this type allow a more aggressive surgical correction. This in turn will allow any minor skeletal relapses that might occur postoperatively to be managed orthodontically and still result in a satisfactory outcome. Preoperatively, orthodontic establishment of the mandibular arch form should occur early in the treatment. This will often involve the reversal of existing dental compensations by expansion of upright, lingually tipped molar crowns, and flaring and leveling of mandibular incisors. Because of the typical dental compensations and the need to expand the lower arch, extractions for crowding should be carefully assessed in these cases. The orthodontist

should not attempt to actively close or deepen the bite preoperatively in any patient who originally presented with an open bite or minimal overbite. Instead, in the preoperative phase the orthodontist should allow the open bite to persist or even open further, as the surgeon is expected to close the bite skeletally. Any extrusive posterior tooth movements should be performed preoperatively on these patients to minimize the prospect of the open bite recurring later.

Impressions and models are necessary during the preoperative orthodontic treatment in order to assess arch and occlusal compatibility in all open bite, asymmetric, maxillary constriction and class III patients, and are recommended in other surgery patients as well. Common problem areas are the canines (the mandibular and maxillary canine dimensions are often not compatible, creating a problem at surgery) and molars (especially second molars, which may have significant interferences and so should generally be banded/bonded fairly early in treatment). All patients should be prepared for surgery by having large, rectangular, stainless steel archwires placed, which should have been in place for a sufficient time (generally 6–8 weeks minimum) to be essentially passive. Ideally, a few days before surgery these archwires should be removed and impressions made for the final model surgery and surgical splint construction. This is the ideal time to place lugs at appropriate positions on the archwires for intra- and postoperative ligatures and elastics. The wires should be marked for lug positions prior to removal in this case. A high-speed dental handpiece and fine finishing burr to lightly 'score' the archwire is preferred for marking in our clinic. Some means of identifying the right and left sides of the wires, the arch, and/or the occlusal/gingival side of the wires is also necessary, as it is important that the wires are returned to the patient in the same orientation as when they were removed. Soldered lugs are preferred to the crimp-on lugs or tied-on ligature 'hooks', owing to their robustness, and it is better to have too many than too few. If the patient is scheduled for a segmental osteotomy, the archwire can be segmented at this time, or left intact to be sectioned in the operating room. The risk of debonding brackets is less if they are segmented while out of the mouth, and the ends of the wire, where sectioned, can be rolled for patient comfort. However, if the surgery is postponed for any reason, the segments are now unfortunately free to move independently. The archwires should be tied in with all-steel ligatures: no elastic ligatures or elastic 'chain' or thread should be used. The model surgery should be done with, or at least approved by, the patient's orthodontist. It is generally agreed that cleft-affected orthognathic surgery patients are at greater risk for maxillary relapse, because of the extra soft-tissue stretch from previous lip and palate repair scars and tissue deficiencies. In order to minimize this risk, the following measures should be explored: rigid fixation, overadvancement to a weak class I relationship, overexpansion of the maxilla, maintenance of a large (0.040 in) expanded buccal wire postoperatively, bone grafting, postoperative extraoral traction (such as a reverse-pull headgear), and maxillary strut fixation. Posteroanterior relapse should be monitored by carefully observing the molar, canine and incisor relationships, particularly during the first 3 months postoperatively. If suspected, a lateral cephalometric radiograph should be obtained and, if relapse is present, it should be addressed by class III elastics or reverse-pull headgear (reverse-pull headgear is preferable in cases requiring control of the vertical component of force, as in patients who had an open bite preoperatively). The use of class III elastics can open the bite by extruding the posterior maxillary teeth. To compensate for this, a vertical-pull chin cup, straight vertical-pull headgear and/or thick posterior bite blocks can be used in conjunction with the elastics. Final lip and/or nose revisions are often best accomplished after orthodontic and orthognathic surgical procedures have been completed. This is an important consideration to allow the surgeon to tailor the final lip balance, nasal form etc. to the final position of the maxilla and anterior teeth.

To review, cleft patients will typically require intermittent surgical and orthodontic care from the time of birth to early adulthood. Multiple phases of active orthodontic treatment at various times, followed by periods of retention or observation, are indicated over continuous long-term treatment. Prior to instituting treatment at any particular stage, the clinician should consider whether there is, in fact, a problem for the patient; if it is likely to worsen with time; whether treatment will prevent or minimize further problems; and whether the degree of improvement warrants treatment at this time. Very few patients require orthopedic intervention prior to lip closure, and this would be accomplished at the specific request of the surgeon involved. Also rare is treatment in the primary dentition stage, which should be confined to the elimination of parafunctional habits or functional shifts. Treatment generally begins in the early mixed dentition stage, usually involving maxillary expansion and incisor alignment to eliminate traumatic occlusions or crossbites, often in preparation for an alveolar bone graft. Most patients will require comprehensive orthodontic treatment, instituted in the late mixed or early permanent dentition stage. The more severely affected patients will require orthodontic treatment in conjunction with orthognathic surgical procedures, which should be delayed for facial growth completion.

REFERENCES

1. Latham RA 1980 Orthopedic advancement of the cleft maxillary segment: a preliminary report. Cleft Palate Journal 17:227–233
2. Graber TM 1949 Craniofacial morphology in cleft palate and cleft lip deformities. Surgery Gynecology and Obstetrics 88:359–369
3. Berkowitz S. 1985 Timing of cleft palate closure – age should not be the sole determinant. Journal of Craniofacial Genetics and Developmental Biology (Suppl 1):69–83
4. Mestre JC, DeJesus J, Subtelny JD 1960 Unoperated oral clefts at maturation. Angle Orthodontics 30:78–85
5. Millard DR, Berkowitz S, Latham RA, Wolfe SA 1988 A discussion of presurgical orthodontics in patients with clefts. Cleft Palate Journal 25:403–412
6. Huddart AG 1973 An evaluation of pre-surgical treatment. British Journal of Orthodontics 1:21–25
7. Subtelny JD 1990 Orthodontic principles in treatment of cleft lip and palate. In: Bardach J, Morris HL, (eds) Multidisciplinary management of cleft lip and palate. pp 615–636 WB Saunders, Philadelphia.
8. Moore RN 1986 Orthodontic management of the patient with cleft lip and palate. Ear Nose Throat Journal 65:46–58
9. El Deeb M, Messer LB, Lehnert MW, Hebda TW, Waite DE 1982 Canine eruption into grafted bone in maxillary alveolar cleft defects. Cleft Palate Journal 19:9–16
10. Hall HD, Werther JR 1991 Conventional alveolar cleft bone grafting. Oral and Maxillofacial Surgery Clinics of North America 3:609–616
11. Bergland O, Semb G, Abyholm FE 1986 Elimination of residual alveolar cleft by secondary bone grafting and subsequent orthodontic treatment. Cleft Palate Journal 23:175–205
12. Vig KWL, Turvey TA 1985 Orthodontic – surgical interaction in the management of cleft lip and palate. Clinics in Plastic Surgery 12:735–748
13. Boyne PJ 1991 Bone grafting in the osseous reconstruction of alveolar and palatal clefts. Oral and Maxillofacial Surgery Clinics of North America 3:589–597
14. Simmons KE, Johnston MC. Craniofacial morphology of monozygotic twins discordant for clefts of the lip and/or palate. In preparation.
15. Verdon P 1989 Utilisation raisonnée du masque orthopédique facial. Orthodontie, Tours
16. Tindlund RS, Per Rygh, Boe OE 1993 Orthopedic protraction of the upper jaw in cleft lip and palate patients during the deciduous and mixed dentition periods in comparison with normal growth and development. Cleft Palate and Craniofacial Journal 30:182–194
17. Tindlund RS, Per Rygh 1993 Maxillary protraction: different effects on facial morphology in unilateral and bilateral cleft lip and palate patients. Cleft Palate and Craniofacial Journal 30:208–221
18. Buschang PH, Porter C, Genecov E, Genecov D, Sayler KE 1994 Face mask therapy of preadolescents with unilateral cleft lip and palate. Angle Orthodontics 64:145–150
19. Vig KWL, Turvey TA, Fonseca RJ 1996 Orthodontic and surgical considerations in bone grafting in the cleft maxilla and palate. In: Turvey TA, Vig KWL, Fonseca RJ (eds) Facial clefts and craniosynostosis. Principles and management. pp 396–440 WB Saunders, Philadelphia
20. Vargervik K 1983 Growth characteristics of the premaxilla and orthodontic treatment principles in bilateral cleft lip and palate. Cleft Palate Journal 20:289–302
21. Friede H, Pruzansky S 1972 Longitudinal study of growth in bilateral cleft lip and palate from infancy to adolescence. Plastic and Reconstructive Surgery 49:392–403
22. Ross RB 1987 Treatment variables affecting facial growth in complete unilateral cleft lip and palate. Cleft Palate Journal 24:3–77

Controversies in clefts

70

A. MARK BOUSTRED/STEPHEN B. COHEN

INTRODUCTION

The field of cleft lip and palate surgery abounds with controversy, for which there are several reasons. First, the final assessment of treatment results must wait until the child is fully grown, as surgical maneuvers in children may have an important influence on facial growth. This long endpoint of treatment makes trials of different therapeutic maneuvers a very lengthy process. Another important factor is the difficulty of distinguishing whether a deformity is due to an inherent defect in the tissues themselves, or is a secondary effect of surgery. For example, is the deficiency in midfacial growth due to the tissues being hypoplastic and lacking in normal growth potential, or is it an unwanted side effect of surgery on the palate at an early age? A lack of uniformity in the choice of treatment modalities in a particular center, as well as changes of treatment protocol or random selection of treatment type with changing vogues in surgery, further hampers critical assessment and comparison of results. This chapter will attempt to address common controversies in cleft surgery. These are discussed in chronological order, as they present themselves in the growing child with a cleft.

FEEDING

The child with an open cleft palate is compromised in its ability to generate sufficient negative intraoral pressure to enable normal feeding. Consequently such children work themselves into a state of exhaustion during feeding and fall asleep, only to wake up hungry after a short period. Feeding can be assisted either by modifications to the bottle and method of feeding, or by the use of a palatal obturator, which closes the defect and allows the infant to generate

sufficient negative pressure for feeding (Fig. 70.1). Palatal obturators are generally effective, but may involve further costs and visits for making the apparatus and enlarging it as the child grows. A simpler approach that is successful in many infants is to deliver the food into the mouth without the infant having to suck it out of the breast or bottle. The bottle nipple should be long enough to deliver milk well into the oral cavity. Either the nipple can be modified by increasing the size of its opening so milk drips out spontaneously, or a 'squeeze' bottle can be used. So-called 'cleft palate nipples', which attempt to obturate the cleft with a rubber flange, are rarely satisfactory. The child is best fed at a 45-degree angle to help prevent feed from entering the nose. Angled bottles can be helpful, but are not essential. More air is generally swallowed, and the infant requires a longer 'burping' session after feeding. Breast milk is best and, for the mother who is willing to expend the extra effort, can be obtained with a breast pump. This is fed to the child from a bottle, and at the end of the feed, the infant can be placed on the breast for 'nurture nursing'. At the author's institution (SRC) all newborns with cleft lip and palate are seen by a nutritionist and an occupational therapist. Those who do not gain weight with nipple and bottle modification

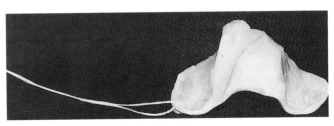

Fig. 70.1 Selectively ground away acrylic obturator, contoured to permit the symmetrical orthopedic repositioning of the premaxilla. Note: Dental floss safety line for removal of device (Rutrick RE, Cohen SR, Black PW, et al. Presurgical orthopedic management of the unilateral cleft lip and palate newborn patient. *Operative Techniques in Plastic and Reconstructive Surgery*. 1995;2:3:159–163).

receive obturators. We have shown significant benefits with the use of obturators in both rate of feeding and weight gain.[1]

PREOPERATIVE ORTHODONTICS

The goal of preoperative orthodontics is to move the abnormally positioned maxillary arches and premaxilla in the case of the bilateral cleft palate into a normal relationship prior to surgery. The soft tissues follow their bony foundation, and the cleft lip elements move closer together under the influence of the orthodontic forces, narrowing the cleft. This provides a more normal bony foundation and a more symmetrical face, upon which a tension-free lip repair can be performed. Some surgeons almost always use preoperative orthodontics, some use it occasionally, particularly in wide clefts, and some do not use it at all.

Several different appliance designs have been used (Fig. 70.2). These can be applied extraorally to the soft tissues of the lip, thus indirectly acting upon the maxillary arch, or intraorally, acting directly on the bony arches. The simplest extraoral device is a surgical tape applied across the upper lip from cheek to cheek. A more sophisticated version includes a head bonnet, to which an elasticized strap is attached and applied to the upper lip. These devices are most valuable in the patient with a protruding premaxillary segment in the bilateral cleft palate. They are economical and simple to apply, but do require some understanding and cooperation from the parents, who need to apply new tape or adjust

straps at regular intervals. These devices can be effective and have few negative points apart from their visibility, possible trauma to skin, and the parental involvement.

More controversial is the use of intraoral devices. These can be passive or active, as well as self or pin (bone) retained. Passive devices are simple palatal obturators molded for self-retention. They span the palatal cleft, facilitating feeding and helping prevent maxillary arch collapse. The major problem with such devices is that they may need adjustment or replacement in a rapidly growing child, thus imposing financial and time burdens upon the family. Pin-retained devices exert an active molding force upon the maxillary segments. The best example is the Latham coaxial screw device, used in the bilateral cleft to expand collapsed lateral arches and to reposition the projecting premaxilla.[2,3] Other forms of active devices can be used. The sequence for the Latham device in unilateral and bilateral clefts is dental impressions and device fabrication, with placement at around 6 weeks of age, removal with gingivoperiosteoplasty and lip adhesion at 2–3 months, followed by definitive lip repair at approximately 6 months of age (Fig. 70.3). The indications in the author's experience are severe premaxillary protrusion in bilateral clefts and, possibly, very wide complete unilateral clefts with extremely discordant lesser and greater maxillary arches. We prefer to use either a bonnet with elastic traction and/or taping with a palatal

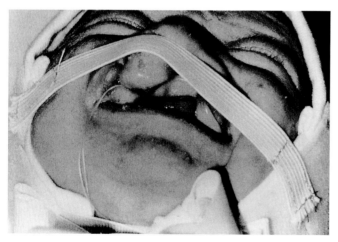

Fig. 70.2 Elastic traction placed across the cleft lip and attached to Velcro (Velcro USA Inc., Manchester, NH) side panels as needed to control the direction of segmental remodeling. The obturator is in place, and a safety line is taped to the face (Rutrick RE, Cohen SR, Black PW, et al. Presurgical orthopedic management of the unilateral cleft lip and palate newborn patient. *Operative Techniques in Plastic and Reconstructive Surgery.* 1995;2:3:159–163).

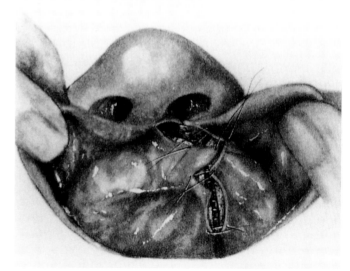

Fig. 70.3 Following reposition of the maxillary segments with the pinned Latham device, lip adhesion is achieved by extending the excision along the mucocutaneous edges of the lip cleft short of the planned marks for the future rotation–advancement. The mucosae of the lip edge are turned back and sutured along the edges of the periosteoplasty and to each other across the cleft for nasal closure. The muscles and skin are approximated, which achieves a gentle lip adhesion (Millard DR, Latham RA. Improved primary surgical and dental treatment of clefts. *Plast Reconstr Surg.* 1990;86:856–871).

obturator in bilateral and complete unilateral cleft lip and palate. In the patient with bilateral cleft lip and palate, when the maxillary arches are collapsed the premaxilla cannot be retracted posteriorly. In these cases a small jackscrew can be placed in the palatal obturator, and maxillary expansion can be performed while the premaxilla is retrodisplaced. If necessary, a passive palatal obturator can be used to prevent maxillary collapse during remodeling. The benefits of maxillary arch alignment preoperatively are twofold. First, the hard tissues (and therefore the soft tissues) of the cleft are optimally aligned for lip repair, permitting as tension-free a repair as possible, and a gingivoperiosteoplasty can be accomplished with the possibility of avoiding alveolar bone grafting in up to 50% of cases[4] (see following section). Some surgeons still advocate preliminary lip adhesion for wide clefts, although most would proceed with formal lip repair, warning parents that a revision is likely to be needed. Antagonists of presurgical orthodontics maintain that once an effective muscular lip repair has been achieved, the underlying arch will be effectively molded and that presurgical orthodontics has virtually no effect on the eventual occlusion in the permanent dentition.[5,6]

The major disadvantages of intraoral pin-retained orthodontic molding appliances is their expense, the need for anesthesia for insertion, and the need for adjustment. However, given available resources and cooperative and competent parents, an appropriate device in a properly selected patient will yield great dividends.

Stenting of the cleft nasal deformity has been combined with presurgical maxillary arch alignment.[7] Using acrylic stents attached to the palatal orthopedic device, the deformed nostril is progressively molded to help correct the deformity, lengthen the columella and expand the vestibular skin deficiency. Results have been encouraging; however, like other operative techniques it is time-consuming, requiring weekly visits and careful monitoring.

LIP REPAIR, TIMING AND TYPE OF REPAIR

TIMING

The lip is usually repaired at 2–3 months of age in an infant who is thriving and in the absence of other more pressing medical problems. The 'rule of 10s' is still appropriate: a weight of at least 10 lb, hemoglobin of 10 gm, and an age of at least 10 weeks. By 3 months of age the anesthetic risks are reduced, as fetal physiology has been replaced by that of a normal infant. It should be mention-

ed that these principles were established at a time when pediatric anesthesia was riskier. Improved anesthetic techniques permit earlier lip and palate repair, if indicated. Neonatal repair of the cleft lip and, in some centers, lip and palate as a single stage, is performed by a few surgeons.[8] However, the majority operate on these children at 2–3 months of age. The anesthetic risks of operating in the neonate for a non-emergent condition outweigh the possible advantages of healing with less scarring and avoidance of social embarrassment for the parents. Until clear advantages have been demonstrated with neonatal repair (such as improved maternal bonding or reduced scarring) we prefer to wait until the baby is 2–3 months old.

Deferring lip repair beyond 3 months of age is unnecessary unless the infant's medical condition precludes operation at this stage or presurgical orthodontics are incomplete. This latter exception ought not to delay lip repair significantly.

TYPE OF REPAIR: UNILATERAL CLEFTS
(Fig. 70.4)

Need for lip adhesion

The need for preliminary lip adhesion was partly discussed earlier. Nowadays, most surgeons reserve this procedure for difficult cases with particularly wide clefts. However, many routinely prefer a full repair, which is amenable to revision if needed. Revision can be carried out at the time of palate repair or later, depending on the severity of the residual deformity. Proceeding with a formal lip repair at the first operation allows maximal use of the available tissue, and repair methods can be used which place the scar such that revision can be readily performed.

Type of lip repair: unilateral clefts

In former times this was a much more hotly debated subject. There are three groups of lip repair in common use today (see Davies[a] for a classification):

- *Rotation–advancement*[10,11] This is probably the most widely used method, of which multiple modifications have been made.[12]
- *Triangular flap* The flap involves the upper lip (Davies Z-plasty) or the lower lip (Tennison–Randall) or, historically, both upper and lower lips (Skoog, Trauner). Triangular flap techniques at the upper or lower lip are still used today; however, many surgeons believe they are rarely appropriate in view of the disadvantages, listed in Table 70.1. Others reserve the

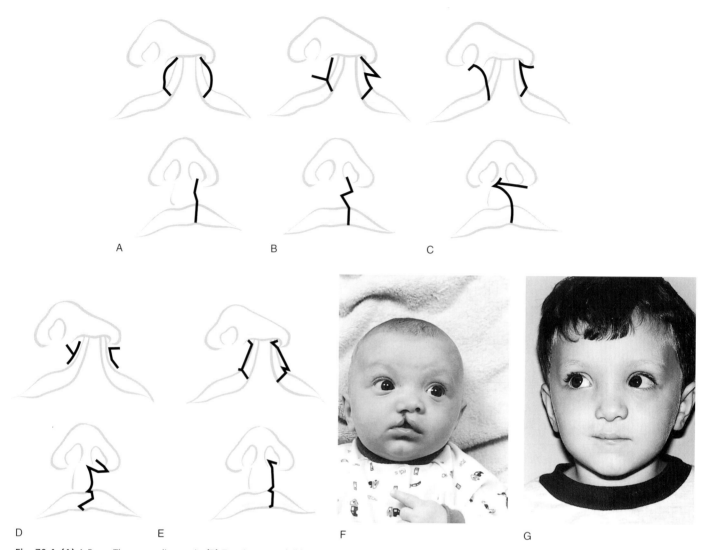

Fig. 70.4 (A) A Rose–Thompson lip repair. **(B)** Tennison–Randall lip repair. **(C)** Millard rotational advancement. **(D)** Modified Z-plasty. **(E)** Nakajima repair. **(F)** Preoperative photograph of a 3-month-old boy with right narrow, but complete, unilateral cleft lip and palate. **(G)** Postoperative photograph of the same child at age 3 following Millard rotational advancement repair.

technique for very wide clefts and cases with marked lip height discrepancy. The modified Davies Z-plasty[13] and Nakajima[14] repairs place the triangular flap high on the lip, along the nostril sill. The height deficiency of the medial lip element is lengthened by placing a triangular flap at the nostril sill and a small white roll flap. These techniques avoid the major disadvantages of triangular flap repairs by positioning the flap where it is not readily visible, and the vertical scar along the philtral line.

- *Straight-line* Rose–Thompson. The advantages and disadvantages of each type of repair are listed in Table 70.1.
- *Delaire technique* The Delaire technique,[14a,14b] which is popular in Europe, is based on functional closure of the lip and nasal aperture, careful dissection of all muscles involved, anatomic repositioning of all structures of the lip and the nasal entrance, and wide subperiosteal dissection and release of the circumoral musculature. Wide subperiosteal dissection is necessary from the nasal ridge to the infraorbital rim, and the body of the zygoma down to the zygomatic crest, as well as from the vomer and nasal septum up to the anterior aspect of the nasal bones and the upper rim of the septum. In addition, the various muscles of the lip and nostrils must be dissected, separated, correctly repositioned and reinserted (especially the transverse part of the nasal muscle, the levator, the depressor septi, and the peripheral part of the obicularis oris muscle). Functional musculoskeletal correction of secondary unilateral cleft lip deformities is also possible with the Delaire approach.

Table 70.1 Unilateral cleft lip repairs – pros and cons

Repair	Advantages	Disadvantages
Millard rotation–advancement	Allows adjustments as operation proceeds Minimal amount of tissue is discarded Scars placed in anatomically correct position, in the line of the philtral column (except in its uppermost part) Nostril sill reinforced and built up Ease of revision, with rerotation if necessary (short lip)	A more difficult technique for the beginner to master The approximation of two convex curves leaves the majority of bulk in the center of the lip and not on the lower free border. This may cause a pouting appearance in wide clefts Tendency to early contracture of the long vertical lip scar Technically difficult in wide clefts, with necessity for wide soft tissue undermining Difficulty in obtaining adequate lip length in a cleft with a marked lip height discrepancy. In such cases the repaired lip will end up shorter than the normal side. A small Z-plasty can be added just above the white roll to ameliorate this problem at the time of the initial repair (or at a secondary procedure), or the lip can be revised at a later stage with rerotation. Many surgeons prefer this later approach as it avoids scars which cross the philtral column Tendency towards a constricted nostril on the cleft side Scar across the base of the columella
Triangular flap repairs Tennyson–Randall	Relatively inexperienced surgeons can obtain reasonable results Achieves excellent lengthening of the shortened cleft side Cupid's bow preserved and well aligned Of particular value in the wide cleft Only a small amount of tissue is discarded	Horizontal scars at triangle site transgress normal anatomic features of lip, i.e. pass across philtral column, flattening and obscuring it. (This is much less of a problem with the modified Davies Z-plasty and the Nakajima repairs, where the triangular flap is placed in the upper lip or nostril sill) Cleft side may end up too long. To avoid this the cleft side repair should be designed 1 mm shorter than the non-cleft side Difficult to revise
Nakajima	Minimal tissue discarded Straight line scar is easy to revise Scar placed in line of philtral column (except for upper portion) Triangular flap hidden at nostril sill	May form vertical contracture
Straight line repair (Rose–Thompson)	Scar orientation good Uncomplicated by small flaps Easy method of repair for minor clefts	May form vertical contracture Poor procedure for wide cleft: too much tissue is discarded, difficulty achieving adequate length laterally, difficulty preserving natural cupid's bow

TYPE OF REPAIR: BILATERAL CLEFTS
(Fig. 70.5)

Repair of bilateral cleft lip has so far been less successful in accomplishing a normal-looking lip than has unilateral repair. Several types of bilateral lip repair are in common use today:

- Straight line closure (Veau III);
- Manchester, Broadbent and Wolf;[15]
- Millard;[16]
- Mulliken;[17]
- Black;[18]
- Noordhoff.[19]

Space does not permit detailed discussion of each of these operations. Early repairs discarded the prolabium; however, its potential for growth was later realized to be important and modern repairs use it to form the midportion of the lip. The ideal width of the prolabial segment to be used for the midlip is controversial. Narrowing it down to 3–4 mm at its base results in a more natural philtrum but runs the risk of compromising the blood supply. However, the prolabium often widens and lengthens considerably with growth, and many patients with initial 6–7 mm philtral repairs end up with an unnaturally wide philtrum.

The Veau III method is the simplest giving good results except when the prolabium is very small. For these cases a Millard repair is preferable. The essential difference between the Manchester and Millard methods is that the former keeps the prolabial white roll, whereas the latter introduces a new white roll from the lateral lip elements. A dis-

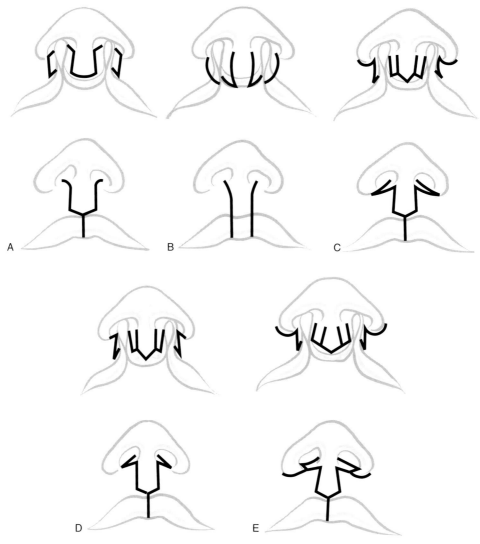

Fig. 70.5 (A) Veau III. **(B)** Broadbent and Woolf (modified Manchester). **(C)** Millard. **(D)** Noordhoff. **(E)** Mullikan.

advantage of using the prolabium for the white roll and adjacent vermilion is the color differences that may exist with the lateral lip elements.

All the above, with the exception of the Manchester and the Veau III, involve a complete orbicularis repair. Manchester felt that this would in most instances produce a lip that is too tight. Many surgeons using other methods will simply bring the orbicularis to the margins of the pro-labium if full repair in the midline is going to be too tight.

Forked flaps are used in several of the methods. Most surgeons have now abandoned techniques where the forked flaps are stored as excess tissue for later use (Millard, Mulliken). However, the techniques of Black and Noordhoff use small forked flaps for reconstructing the nasal floor, if necessary.

The author finds Black's method useful and would like to highlight it (Figs 70.6, 70.7). This repair uses the prolabial white roll and vermilion for the cupid's bow. The lateral prolabial elements are preserved, undermined, and brought together to form a well-lined labial sulcus, which allows freedom of movement of the lip and a more natural (non-tethered) smile. Procedures which fail to create an adequate labial sulcus, leaving the lip bound to the bone as a unit, may place abnormal stresses on the central maxilla and restrict growth, or place abnormal vertical stress on the premaxilla, potentiating a downward movement. The vertical suture lines simulate the philtral columns with the C-flaps, breaking these lines into a Z and bringing the nasal floors and anterior nasal sills to the proper height and width. Full muscle reconstruction is performed. Patients with very wide bilateral clefts or a prominent premaxilla present as difficult problems. The roles of preoperative orthodontics and lip

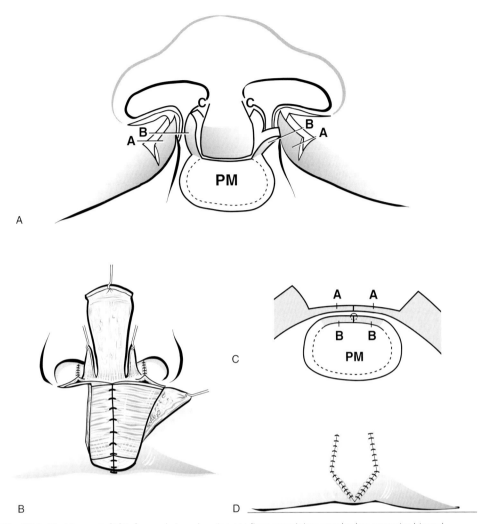

Fig. 70.6 Black's repair **(A)** Infranasal view showing 'A' flaps remaining attached as posterior hinged turndown flaps, and 'B' flaps remaining attached to the premaxilla. Incisions continue directly posteriorly from tip of lateral advancement flaps and from lateral base of triangular 'C' flaps into face along cleft margins in preparation of repair of nasal floor. **(B)** Nasal floor is closed first, then lip lining ('A' flap) closed. Muscles repaired. At this stage the prolabial flap may be dropped ('C' flap) may be rotated into place and skin may be repaired. **(C)** Infranasal representation of lining of labial sulcus. **(D)** Finish skin repair. (From Black PW. Bilateral cleft lip. *Clinics in Plastic Surgery*. 1985;12:627–641).

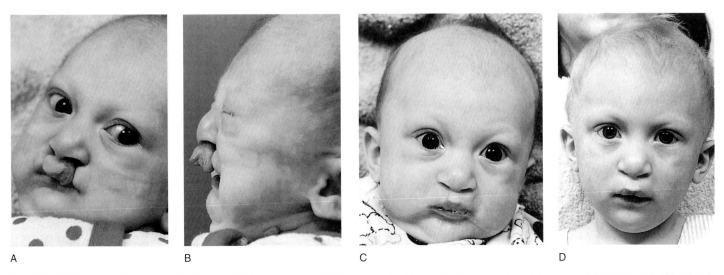

Fig. 70.7 **(A)** Three-month-old girl with bilateral cleft lip, frontal view. **(B)** Three-month-old girl with bilateral cleft lip, lateral view. **(C)** Three-month-old girl with bilateral cleft lip at age 6 months. **(D)** Three-month-old girl with bilateral cleft lip at age 2 years. Nasal reconstruction will be performed at 3–5 years of age.

adhesion have been discussed. Some advocate sequential closure of each lip side in the patient with a very wide bilateral cleft; however, closure of the second side (2–3 months after the first) must usually be performed under extreme tension, and accurate marking at this time may be difficult owing to distortion of the prolabium by the previous operation. The author has never had to stage lip closure for wide bilateral clefts. Surgical setback of the prominent premaxilla should be limited to those patients in whom the above methods have failed, owing to the negative impact on growth from interference with the vomer/nasal septum.

SINGLE-STAGE LIP AND PALATE REPAIR

There have been several advocates of a single-stage repair of the lip and palate.[20,21] The advantages, in terms of reducing the number of operations and accomplishing velopharyngeal competence at an early stage, are significant. Initially surgeons were reluctant to perform a single-stage procedure, owing to the magnitude of the operation and the anesthetic considerations. With improvements in anesthesia, however, the operation can be safely performed without increased risk. This approach has particular advantages in underdeveloped populations, where return visits are logistically difficult. The major concerns are whether single-stage surgery affects facial growth more negatively than does staged surgery, and whether fistula rates and speech results are acceptable. These questions remain unanswered. For this reason, most surgeons have preferred to do staged repairs of the lip and palate.

TIMING AND TYPE OF PALATE REPAIR

TIMING

The most important considerations influencing the time of closure of the palatal cleft are the onset of speech development and the influence of early surgery on facial growth. Ideally, the palatal cleft should be closed prior to the onset of speech development. However, many believe that the earlier the repair, the greater the negative impact on facial growth (and the greater the degree of technical difficulty). Infants start to babble from 6 to 9 months of age and most have spoken their first word by 13 months. Competent velopharyngeal function is critical for normal speech development. In patients with a hypoplastic maxilla following cleft lip and palate repair it is difficult to know how much of this hypoplasia is attributable to an intrinsic growth deficiency of the facial tissues and how much is a secondary negative effect of surgery. In most centers about 20% of patients

with repaired cleft lip and palate will require orthognathic surgery to correct deficient maxillary growth, yet studies of adolescents and adults with unrepaired clefts have shown normal maxillary growth.[22,23] Palatal surgery is generally held to be the most important negative influence, although posterior pharyngeal flaps also contribute to the deficiency in maxillary growth. Clinical and laboratory studies have demonstrated that lip repair alone can retard facial growth.[24,25] Palatal surgery in childhood does impair facial growth, but no differences have been shown in the degree of underdevelopment of the maxilla among children operated on at different ages according to the different protocols: early repair at 3–9 months, delayed repair at 12–24 months, late repair at 2–5 years, or early soft palate repair at 3–9 months with delayed hard palate repair up to 15 years.[26–30] Significantly better speech results have been obtained when the palatal repair has been completed before the age of 1 year.[31–33] A lower fistula rate and more normal lip and nose anatomy have also been reported following early surgery, and these benefits offset the disadvantages of increased technical difficulty and a longer operation time.[34,35] An additional advantage of early surgery is the preservation of hearing, afforded by earlier protection of the Eustachian tube, and a reduced incidence of middle ear disease.[26,31,36]

Because there is no evidence that earlier surgery in childhood interferes to a greater degree with facial growth than later surgery in childhood, and as normal speech development takes precedence over facial growth, the trend has been towards early surgery. Maxillary hypoplasia can be corrected in adolescence with orthognathic surgery, whereas late speech problems are not easily corrected. Exactly what constitutes 'early' is debatable, but a cut-off at the age of 1 year seems appropriate.

ONE STAGE OR TWO?

Closure of the palate can be accomplished in one or two stages. The rationale behind a two-stage operation is that closure of the soft palate would narrow the hard palate defect and facilitate closure, while reducing the negative impact upon facial growth. The reduced surgical dissection required for a narrower hard palate defect, operating at an age when the maxilla was considered less sensitive to surgically induced growth impairment and following facial growth, was hoped to be beneficial. Late two-stage closure, as popularized by Schweckendiek, delayed the second stage to late childhood. Unfortunately this approach has been unsuccessful, with uniformly poor speech results, even with the use of palatal obturators.[30,37] Other surgeons have performed the second stage during the second year of life; however, assessment of these patients also failed to show any difference in facial growth.[30] This approach was based upon a questionable understanding of facial growth, as maxillary growth is centered on the tuberosity area and not the palatal shelves. There is still a role for a two-stage procedure in the patient with a very wide palatal cleft, which would be difficult to close satisfactorily without the development of a fistula or excessive palatal scarring. Closing the soft palate first can reduce the hard palate defect to manageable proportions.

TYPE OF PALATAL REPAIR

Techniques used for closing the cleft palate fall into several categories:

- Hard palate
  von Langenbeck/bipedicled flaps;
  Pushback – Veau – Wardill–Kilner, with unipedicled flaps;
  Vomer flaps;
- Soft palate
  Layered closure;
  Intravelar veloplasty;
  Furlow.

The lack of prospective trials comparing different methods makes it difficult to establish which is the best. Most reports have been retrospective.[38] There are different degrees of clefting, which greatly affect the ease of obtaining successful palatal closure, and it is probable that there are differences between patients in the neuromuscular functional ability of the velopharynx and, therefore, in the potential for achieving satisfactory velar function following cleft palate closure. The patient with a hypoplastic muscle with deficient innervation and abnormal physiology cannot be compared to one with more favorable muscle development. Likes must be compared to accurately determine the results of different procedures. The surgeon's skill and technique are very important, further confounding comparison of different reports. Simple closure by the von Langenbeck method (bipedicled mucoperiosteal flaps) and its modifications remains popular because of its simplicity. Bardach and Salyer's modification, with division of the anterior part of the bipedicled flap, turning it into an unipedicled flap – the 'two-flap palatoplasty' – has been useful, simplifying the dissection and preservation of the greater palatine artery pedicle. This is essentially a throwback to the Veau–Wardill–Kilner type of repair. The disadvantages of this technique include denuded areas of palatal bone at the lateral releasing incisions and the midline longitudinal scar, with the risk of contracture, a tendency toward anterior fistula formation, and little palatal lengthening. However, modifications have enabled the extent of denuded palatal bone to be minimized,

and in narrow and moderate clefts the lateral releasing incisions can be avoided altogether, or partially or completely closed. Pushback techniques, introduced by Dorrance in 1925 and refined by Veau in 1931 and later Wardill and Kilner, both in 1937, have generally fallen into disrepute as they leave relatively large areas of denuded hard palate anterolaterally, and the concern is that spontaneous healing of these areas results in increased scarring and growth restriction. Furthermore, it is not certain whether the palatal lengthening gained by these procedures is maintained. The fistula rate is possibly higher, and it seems that the presence of a functioning muscular sling in the velum is more important than the length of the palate. Many modifications have been described to line the denuded areas and hopefully prevent contracture, but these have not gained wide popularity. A prospective study comparing von Langenbeck's repair with V–Y pushback and von Langenbeck's repair combined with a primary pharyngeal flap, found no differences in speech results but greater blood loss with the V–Y pushback and more respiratory obstruction with the pharyngeal flap.[39]

The use of vomerine flaps remains controversial. Although some have reported interference with midfacial growth[40] they are widely used, particularly in more severe clefts, and many surgeons feel that the negative impact upon growth has been overemphasized and that the benefits of obtaining a good nasal closure, reducing the incidence of palatal fistula and improving nasal physiology, outweigh the disadvantages.

Role of intravelar veloplasty (IVV)

The role of intravelar veloplasty (IVV)[41,42] remains controversial. The hypothesis that dissection of the levator muscle off its abnormal insertion on the hard palate, with suture across the midline recreating the anatomy of the levator sling, would be beneficial for velar function is certainly attractive. The addition of IVV to the von Langenbeck repair has been reported to markedly improve speech results.[43] However, Marsh's[44] prospective study found no significant improvement in velopharyngeal function with the addition of IVV. This study has come under criticism that the procedure as performed was inadequate and not extensive enough. Favorable results have been reported by others in both primary and secondary operations.[45,46] It is probable that there is a population of cleft palate patients in whom the levator muscle or its innervation or neural control is defective, and an IVV in this subset of patients might not make a significant difference. We do not currently have the ability to routinely determine in which patients levator neuromuscular function is deficient. If this were possible, it might allow the surgeon to select candidates for primary IVV in whom the procedure would have a greater chance of success.

Palate repair with primary pharyngoplasty

Because the majority of patients with cleft palate (80%) will achieve satisfactory speech without the use of a pharyngoplasty, it cannot be recommended for routine use in primary palate repair, particularly as it can be associated with significant airway obstruction in the infant (see discussion on VPI and pharyngoplasty). There may be a small subset of patients with gross 'velopharyngeal disproportion' in whom the experienced surgeon feels that velopharyngeal competence will not be achieved with standard palatal repair, and here there may be a role for primary pharyngoplasty. The author has no experience with infant pharyngoplasty or flap.

Furlow Z-plasty

Furlow reported on his novel technique of cleft palate repair by double opposing Z-plasty in 1978, publishing it in 1986.[47] This ingenious technique has the advantages of reorientating and retropositioning the levator muscles in a more anatomic position with minimal dissection of the muscles, thus reconstructing the levator sling with minimal scarring around the muscles, lengthening the soft palate, elevating the palate superiorly, narrowing the nasopharyngeal orifice and minimally dissecting the hard palate without leaving bare areas. It is hoped that this procedure will have a minimal effect on the growth of the midface; however, it has not been performed often enough to be able to assess its effects on facial growth. Several studies have shown that the procedure provides for good speech in the majority of cases.[48-51] It has been criticized as having a high incidence of oronasal fistulae, but most of these have occurred early on in various authors' series, underlining the fact that there is a learning curve with this procedure, which takes longer to perform and is technically more difficult than others. Seagle found no difference in the incidence of VPI in patients undergoing Furlow repair compared to intravelar veloplasty in a prospective study[52] (Seagle 1997, personal communication).

VELOPHARYNGEAL INCOMPETENCE (VPI) IN CLEFT PATIENTS

Normal speech cannot be produced without a competent velopharyngeal mechanism. Children learning to talk who have velopharyngeal incompetence (VPI) will develop compensatory mechanisms in an attempt to deal with the loss of oral pressure (or dental arch collapse). Once velopharyngeal competence has been achieved, these compensatory mechanisms must be unlearned and this can prove problematic, particularly in the older child, who can continue talking abnormally. The sooner VPI is effectively treated, the fewer and less established the compensatory mechanisms will be, hence the better the prognosis for speech. The earlier a diagnosis of VPI can be made, the sooner remedial surgery can be performed and the better the final speech result. However, making this diagnosis in small children can be difficult owing to their limited ability to cooperate with standard investigations. The assessment of velopharyngeal function is performed on several levels, as indicated below. Children of 3–4 years will vary in their ability to cooperate with the more invasive of these tests (nasendoscopy, fluoroscopy). However, a skilled investigator with good rapport may succeed in gaining this vital information, allowing the surgeon to proceed with remedial surgery at a relatively early stage (2.5 years).

1. A perceptual evaluation of resonance, nasal air escape, and articulation is performed.
2. Velopharyngeal closure is screened. Patients who fail steps 1 and 2 proceed on to:
3. Objective assessment with computerized instruments for acoustic and non-acoustic velopharyngeal function;
4. Imaging with some combination of dynamic flexible fiberoptic nasendoscopy, radiography or fluoroscopy (during speech).

Articulation is evaluated separately, bearing in mind the age-appropriateness of articulation and the presence of compensatory misarticulations.

Minimal standards for the evaluation and treatment of patients with cleft lip/palate or other craniofacial anomalies have been developed, including assessment of velopharyngeal function [ACPCA, March 1993 # 52].

CHOICE OF SECONDARY OPERATION FOR VPI

Which secondary procedure is best for achieving velopharyngeal competence in the previously repaired cleft palate is controversial. Pharyngeal flaps were the mainstay of treatment for many years and remain a standard and acceptable approach. However, dissatisfaction with the significant side effects of these procedures, and their flagrantly antiphysiologic basis, has led surgeons to seek alternatives. Pharyngeal flaps are associated with snoring, obstructive sleep apnea, airway compromise, difficulty in clearing nasal secretions, and hyponasality in a significant number of patients.

The following procedures are commonly performed for secondary VPI:

- Pharyngeal flap, superiorly or inferiorly based;
- Sphincter pharyngoplasty;
- Intravelar veloplasty, Furlow palatoplasty;
- Posterior pharyngeal wall augmentation with a variety of materials, autogenous and alloplastic;
- Palatal lift obturators.

Which procedure should be used in which patient? This choice still depends largely upon the experience and bias of the surgeon, rather than upon data. However, certain trends are developing which seem to have a rational basis. Rather than simply performing a pharyngeal flap on all patients with VPI, each patient should be analyzed carefully as to their particular problems.

In patients with 'small' VPI and a gap between the posterior pharynx and the soft palate of less than 5 mm there is evidence that a Furlow palatoplasty may be beneficial.[48,52,53] Other factors that may help in the accurate selection of patients for a Furlow procedure include a circular or sagittal pattern closure and a good response to biofeedback speech therapy. The same type of patient who is suitable for a Furlow may also be suitable for a radical muscle correction or IVV.[46] Both these procedures are more anatomically correct and may have physiologic bases for correcting VPI. Posterior pharyngeal wall augmentation with a variety of materials is another operation which may benefit patients with mild VPI. However, the exact site of placement is critical and the material used for augmentation may not last, or may shift position or become infected (particularly if prosthetic), and other options are generally favored. If the VPI is small then any method should have a good result.

Patients with more severe VPI and wider gaps will generally need some sort of pharyngoplasty. The pharyngeal flap requires medial movement of the lateral pharyngeal walls against the obturating flap, so that the lateral gaps (ports) are adequately closed during speech. It should be wide enough and be placed at the point of maximum lateral wall movement. Pharyngeal flaps have been modified (made shorter) in an attempt to lessen airway obstruction, and nasopharyngeal tubes placed for nasal breathing postoperatively until the patient can breathe orally, apparently with improved results.[54] The various sphincter pharyngoplasties require velar elevation to be successful, and should be positioned on the pharynx at the height of maximum velar elevation, which should be identified relative to the anterior

tubercle of the first cervical vertebra.[55–57] Sphincter pharyngoplasty is associated with a lower incidence of obstructive sleep apnea.

TIMING AND TYPE OF NASAL REPAIR

The enormous number and variety of operative procedures described for correction of the cleft lip nasal deformity is testament both to the inadequacy of many techniques and to the difficulty of the deformity. Some believe that the nasal tissues are hypoplastic, but others feel they are simply deformed but present. Anatomic dissections of infants with clefts lend support to the hypoplastic concept, as the alar cartilage on the cleft side is frequently not only deformed, but also smaller.

TIMING

There are several schools of thought concerning the timing of cleft rhinoplasty:

- Primary nasal repair – at the time of the lip repair;
- Early repair – before puberty;
- Late repair – after puberty

The advantages of primary repair include the attractiveness of a single-stage operation; correction completed at an early age, helping reduce psychosocial problems; the ability to correct abnormal muscle insertions and vectors of pull, which distort the cleft nose while it is accessible and exposed during the lip repair; and the possibility that early correction will allow more normal growth and development of the nose. It is hoped that early repair, usually performed in the preschool years, will avoid the difficulties of operating on the small infant nose but provide the benefit of correction before the child enters school, thereby avoiding psychosocial problems that generally do not become important until the age of 6 years. Antagonists of primary repair believe the risk of causing surgical injury to an infant's nose, with the possible attendant growth problems, is too high and that easier and more effective surgery can be performed on older children or adolescents. They maintain that the scarring secondary to the operation will interfere with nasal development and may cause distortion; that most patients will require corrective nasal surgery at a later stage anyway, even if they have undergone primary or early correction; and that many cleft patients require multiple other operative procedures, giving the surgeon ample opportunity to perform a rhinoplasty at another time. Advocates of primary and early repair[58–62] have shown excellent results on long-term follow up, without evidence of interference with nasal growth. However, poorly performed early surgery would certainly be detrimental. Cartilage has a limited wound healing capacity, and fractured or transected cartilage retains weak areas that can give rise to deformity. Animal experiments have demonstrated facial underdevelopment following resection of the anterior and basal part of the nasal septum, but repositioning of the alar cartilages is a different issue. Primary or early nasal septal surgery is best avoided unless absolutely necessary for functional reasons, and should then be performed conservatively. However, careful repositioning of the alar cartilages can be safely performed in the infant or preschool child. On balance, the best time for cleft rhinoplasty is still debatable. Good results can be obtained with a variety of approaches, and a superiority of one over the other has yet to be demonstrated. When deformity is mild, nasal surgery can be delayed until puberty, but if it is severe interventions corrective surgery should be performed in the preschool years.

TYPE OF REPAIR

Cleft rhinoplasty can address several areas of deformity: the bony foundation (maxilla), dorsum, septum and tip. The extent and number of maneuvers performed will depend on the degree of 'perfection' desired by the patient, balanced against their willingness to undergo repeated operations, the availability of resources, and a realistic appraisal by the surgeon of the law of diminishing returns. A more radical correction can be safely performed in the older patient, whereas in the infant and preschool child the extent of correction must be balanced against the possibility of injury and growth disturbance to the delicate nasal structures.

Operations to improve the bony foundation are generally reserved until skeletal maturity has been reached. Occasionally this may be performed at a younger age, when maxillary hypoplasia is so extreme that psychosocial issues force the surgeon's hand. In this case the prime indication is not so much the nose, but rather the entire midfacial recession. The choice of operation is not controversial, with the Le Fort I osteotomy and its modifications being the mainstay.

Most surgeons prefer to delay septal surgery until skeletal maturity, unless the deformity is severe, with functional airway problems. There are degrees of airway compromise, and possible gains from surgery must be weighed against the possible negative effect on growth.

The number and variety of surgical procedures described for addressing deformities of the nasal tip preclude the discussion of individual operations; however, they can be classified into several types.

- Repositioning of the alar cartilages can be performed with sutures alone or with mobilization/dissection of the cartilages, followed by suture suspension/modification.
- Alar subunit rotations.
- Procedures addressing nasal and lip muscle abnormalities.[63]
- Alar reconstruction by cartilage grafting/augmentation.
- Stenting techniques.[64]
- Columella reconstruction.
- Ancillary procedures addressing nostril stenosis, vestibular webs, alar rim webs, vestibular skin deficiency etc.

The approach to the nasal tip structures can be 'open' or 'closed'. Most surgeons performing primary cleft rhinoplasty have used 'closed' or limited approaches, via the existing lip incisions or limited incisions in the nasal vestibule (rim, infracartilaginous etc.). Some have used an open approach for primary repair;[65] however, long-term follow up is not yet available. There is one long-term review of possible untoward effects from early correction using an open approach.[66] Data is becoming available on the safety of the open approach in the infant or preschool child. Most surgeons have used an open approach in the adolescent with apparent safety when properly performed.

The facial degloving approach (Figs 70.8, 70.9) has been used by the author for early secondary rhinoplasty in bilateral cleft nasal deformity. The midface degloving procedure as advocated by Black is conducted through circumvestibular incisions with a dart on the nostril floor. A second incision is carried out in the upper buccal sulcus, and the upper lip is elevated over the cartilages. The cartilages are mobilized, trimmed and sutured in the midline. Conchal cartilage can be added for dorsal tip projection. When the lip and nasal incisions are closed, the columella lengthens by conforming to the underlying rebuilt cartilaginous skeleton. This avoids external incisions, as employed in the Cronin approach, and forked flaps (Millard), which give an unnatural appearance to the columella. The unilateral cleft nasal deformity is approached via a standard open rhinoplasty. Cartilage grafting is used whenever necessary. Recently, we have carried out primary rhinoplasty employing extensive undermining of the cartilages and placement of nasal stents as described by Nakajima.[64] With this approach, one must be cautious of producing nasal stenosis.

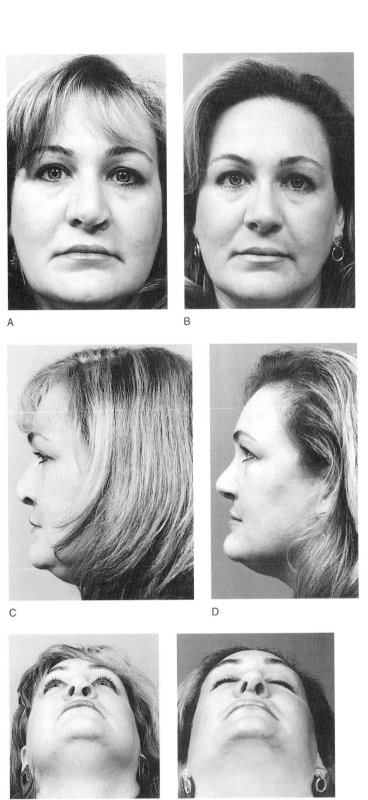

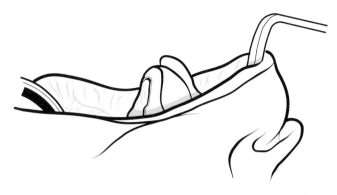

Fig. 70.9 Artist's depiction of midface degloving technique. Note that the upper lip and nasal skin envelope have been drawn up to expose the lower lateral and upper lateral cartilages.

Fig. 70.8 **(A)** Preoperative frontal photograph of 39-year-old woman with unilateral cleft lip and nasal deformity. **(B)** Postoperative frontal photograph following an open structure rhinoplasty with cartilage rearrangement and tip rhinoplasty. **(C)** Preoperative lateral photograph. **(D)** Postoperative lateral photograph. **(E)** Preoperative submental view. **(F)** Postoperative submental view.

ALVEOLAR BONE GRAFT AND GINGIVOPERIOSTEOPLASTY

The bony cleft of the hard palate generally is not problematic to the patient as long as an adequate soft-tissue repair has been performed. However, the bony defect of the alveolus is problematic, because of the resultant instability of the maxillary arches. Furthermore, teeth that erupt into the cleft are inadequately supported and most will be lost. For these reasons the surgeon must help the patient to attain a complete and stable maxillary arch. Attempts to accomplish this can be divided into those performed in infancy (primary) or at a later date (secondary).

PRIMARY BONE GRAFTING

Primary bone grafting of alveolar and palatal defects was popularized in the 1960s and 1970s from several centers in Europe by Schmid, Johanson and Schrudde, each with some variation in the particular technique used. However, Friede and Johansen's[67] long-term report on adolescents who had undergone primary bone grafting in infancy showed pronounced midfacial and alveolar growth impairment, and most surgeons no longer perform this technique, although there are still many advocates who maintain it can be performed without adversely affecting maxillary growth when accompanied by appropriate maxillofacial orthodontics.[68–73]

SECONDARY BONE GRAFTING

Secondary bone grafting is a well established procedure, the most favorable timing being just before the canine teeth erupt. Some controversy still exists as to the best source of the graft. Most surgeons utilize buccal and gingival flaps to bring attached gingiva over the cleft site. Rarely, buccal mucosal flaps are used, and reasonably good tooth eruption has been reported with this technique.

TYPE AND SOURCE OF BONE GRAFT

Cancellous bone is a much richer source of osteoprogenitor cells than is cortical bone. The diffusion and revascularization vital for graft survival takes place much more readily in cancellous bone grafts, and they heal and become fully incorporated earlier and more completely than do cortical bone grafts.[74]

The better survival of grafts taken from bones of membranous origin, particularly when used in craniofacial reconstruction, has been much debated.[75] Most problems relating to graft resorption and loss probably pertain more to cortical than to cancellous bone grafts. It is probable that much of the improved survival reported with calvarial grafts is related to the bony architecture and thickness of the diploe, rather than to an intrinsic superiority of the bone itself.[76] When a cancellous bone graft is required, whether the site of origin is membranous or endochondral is probably less important than when a cortical graft is needed, and other factors become relatively more important in selecting a source of graft. The quantity and quality of cancellous bone available at a particular donor site are important. Donor site morbidity, ease of harvesting, time taken for harvesting, and the possibility of simultaneous harvesting by a second operator are important considerations. When the calvaria is used as a donor site the scar can be hidden in the hair and postoperative pain is not a problem. However, potentially serious complications such as dural tear or cerebral injury can occur, although their incidence is minimal when the operator is well versed in this technique. The donor site can conveniently be included within the operative field in craniofacial procedures. However, simultaneous graft harvesting is not possible, and the operative time is increased.

The ilium is an abundant source of cancellous bone graft and permits simultaneous harvesting by a second operator, but donor site morbidity is a major consideration. This can be great in relation to the amount of bone removed, with problems of postoperative bleeding and hematoma, pain, limping, hyperesthetic and anesthetic patches and, more rarely, ileus and abdominal hernia. These problems have been reduced with the use of less extensive techniques. Most surgeons now favor the ilium as the source for alveolar bone graft, and are supported by recent studies.[77,78]

There have been several reports of minimally invasive techniques for harvesting iliac bone. Bone biopsy techniques have been modified for alveolar graft harvest (the Craig bone biopsy set, the CORB biopsy needle). However, both of these require special instrumentation, have a higher risk of perforation of the cortex with its attendant problems and, as they use power tools, may cause heat injury to the graft. It has been shown that cranial graft harvested by a cranio-

tome has a less well preserved haversian system and osteocyte population than that harvested by Hudson brace, translating into less successful results in alveolar cleft bone grafting.[79] A minimally invasive technique has been described by the author whereby a Volkman's spoon (curette) is used to access the iliac medullary cavity via a short stab incision.[80] With this technique, sufficient quantities of cancellous bone can be harvested with minimal donor site morbidity and early pain-free ambulation.

PERIOSTEOPLASTY

Periosteoplasty, or 'boneless bone grafting', was championed by Skoog in the 1960s and 1970s and performed at the time of the lip closure. He used a flap of maxillary periosteum taken from the external surface of the maxilla laterally, and based medially at the edge of the pyriform aperture. This flap was transposed medially to establish periosteal continuity across the alveolar defect. The basis of this procedure was the premise that new bone would form from the periosteum and fill in the alveolar defect. In their early experience, bridging bone was noted in 81% of patients.[81] However, on long-term followup Skoog's method showed no distinct advantage relative to stability of the maxillary segments. Regarding midfacial growth, these patients were found to have bimaxillary retrognathia; however, the degree was within limits for unilateral clefts.[82] Rintala, formerly a protagonist of periosteoplasty, abandoned the procedure because new bone formation was inadequate in most patients to prevent lateral maxillary arch collapse, and 70% of his patients eventually required later bone grafting.[83] Furthermore, concerns of a deleterious effect on maxillary growth caused most surgeons to abandon the procedure. Ross noted that any soft-tissue procedure on the alveolus before the age of 10 years resulted in a vertical growth deficiency in the anterior maxilla.[84]

Several centers have persisted with periosteoplasty, modifying the technique so that the mucoperiosteum adjacent to the cleft is used to accomplish closure.[85-87] The Scandinavian group did not use preoperative orthopedics, and the bony gaps generally were large. The above protagonists of gingivoperiosteoplasty maintain it is essential that the maxillary segments be well aligned with a minimal gap for the procedure to be successful. Lip adhesion alone cannot be relied upon to accomplish this (however, if a palatal obturator is used after adhesion and gradually reduced in size to help guide alignment, a decent arch configuration can be obtained). The mucoperiosteum adjacent to the cleft is raised to develop flaps anteriorly and posteriorly, and these are closed across the bony cleft, creating a tunnel in which

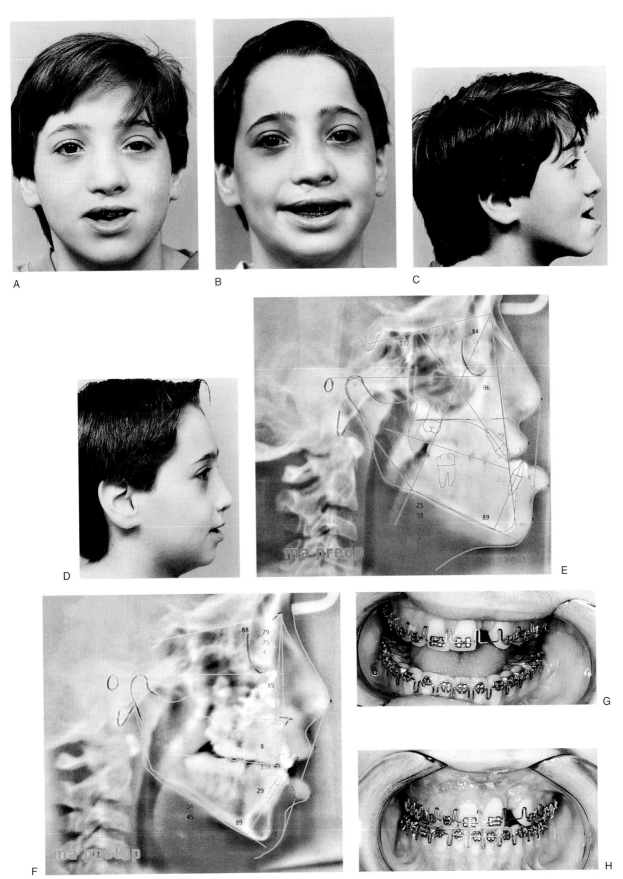

Fig. 70.10 (A) Preoperative frontal photographs of a 12-year-old boy with unilateral cleft lip and palate, with severe midface retrusion and class III malocclusion. **(B)** Postoperative frontal view following maxillary advancement and mandibular setback. **(C)** Preoperative lateral view. **(D)** Postoperative lateral view following orthognathic surgery. **(E)** Preoperative cephalogram. **(F)** Postoperative cephalogram. **(G)** Preoperative occlusion. **(H)** Postoperative occlusion.

bone can form, closing the alveolar cleft. If successful, the advantages are closure of the cleft, stabilization of the maxillary segments, avoidance of oronasal fistula and raw areas, no need for later bone grafting, and successful eruption of the canine tooth. Even if insufficient bone is formed in the cleft, later bone grafting is facilitated by the presence of a mucoperiosteal bridge. Millard did not indicate in how many patients this approach was successful, but did comment that bone bridging was visible in 'most' patients who had been X-rayed. Brusati and Mannuci reported the formation of bridging bone in 100% of their patients.[87] The real question is whether this bridging bone is adequate to obviate the need for secondary bone grafting. Cutting[4] states that if the maxillary gap is less than 2 mm, adequate bone will form following gingivoperiosteoplasty in approximately 50% of patients.

The major concern with this new generation of periosteoplasty procedures is the question of its influence on facial growth. In a preliminary study comparing children with unilateral clefts, no impairment of maxillary growth following gingivoperiosteoplasty was found; however, the numbers were small and followup short.[88] Supporting data from long-term followup are required before primary gingivoperiosteoplasty can be recommended as a routine treatment. The senior author prefers a pragmatic approach to setting up the maxillary segments for gingivoperiosteoplasty. If premaxillary traction with a palatal obturator aligns the maxillary segments, the gingivoperiosteoplasty can be done at the lip repair. More commonly, lip closure aligns the palatal shelves and gingivoperiosteoplasty is done at the time of palate repair which is carried out at 6 months of age.

EARLY TREATMENT OF SEVERE SKELETAL DEFORMITIES

With increased safety in performing orthognathic surgery, some surgeons believe maxillary advancement should be performed in a select group of patients with persistent severe class III malocclusion in childhood, rather than waiting

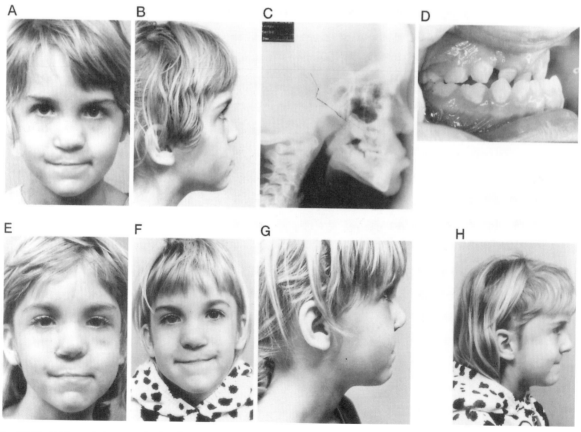

Fig. 70.11 (A) Frontal photograph of a 4½-year-old girl with right unilateral cleft lip and palate. **(B)** Lateral photograph. Note midfacial retrusion in upper/lower lip relations. **(C)** Preoperative cephalogram demonstrating severe maxillary midfacial hypoplasia. **(D)** Preoperative occlusal photograph showing class III malocclusion. **(E)** Postoperative frontal photograph taken 4 weeks after maxillary midface distraction device is removed. **(F)** Postoperative frontal photograph taken 8.5 months after distraction of a maxillary midface. **(G)** Postoperative lateral photograph taken 4 weeks after the devices were removed. Note the improvement in malar midface position in upper/lower lip relations. **(H)** Postoperative lateral photograph taken 8.5 months after surgery. (Cohen SR et al 1997: Maxillary – midface distraction in children with cleft lip and palate: a preliminary report. Plast. Reconstructive Surgery 99: 1421–1428).

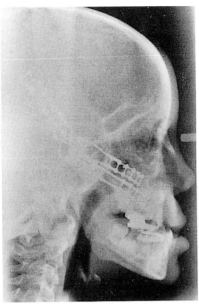

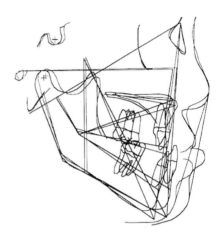

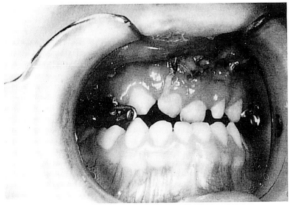

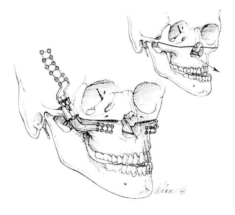

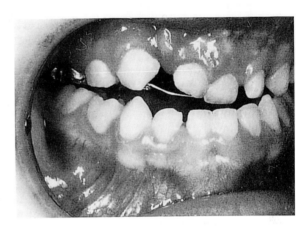

Fig. 70.12 (Above, left) Postoperative cephalogram 5 weeks following placement of bilateral maxillary distractors and just prior to removal. Note the improvement in skeletal and soft-tissue profile. (Above, right) Cephalometric analysis. Note: the movement in the vertical direction, with more sagittal movement at molars. Maxillary and dental movement did not correlate with the clinical results of dentition, which are much better than cephalometric analysis would suggest. One problem is the difficulty in determining the global superimposition because of the slightly different magnifications in the preoperative and postoperative cephalograms. The other problem is that because of vertical maxillary lengthening, the mandible has autorotated open with the chin moving retrograde, removing some of the pseudoprognathism present preoperatively. (Center, left) Postoperative occlusion showing substantial correction of class III malocclusion at the canine, which is now slightly class II. (Center, right) Postoperative occlusion 8.5 months after surgery. (Below) Artist's depiction of modified high Le Fort osteotomies with placement of internal distraction devices. (Cohen SR et al 1997: Maxillary – midface distraction in children with cleft lip and palate: a preliminary report. Plast. Reconstructive Surgery 99: 1421–1428).

for adolescence. The psychologic benefits of correcting a severe deformity are felt to outweigh the disadvantages of relapse requiring reoperation. Indeed, these patients are operated on with the realization that a readvancement will probably be required in many at late adolescence, but the magnitude of later surgery may be reduced (Fig. 70.10).

Craniofacial distraction techniques offer the hope of being able to accomplish the above in a less invasive fashion at a younger age, possibly with less interference with growth and easier later revisional surgery. Distraction is performed in the 6-year-old with unilateral or bilateral cleft lip and palate and severe class III malocclusion. High Le Fort I or modified Le Fort III may be used (Figs 70.11, 70.12). Distraction is combined with transverse maxillary expansion. When the distraction devices are removed or headgear discontinued, an alveolar bone graft can be placed. The use of these techniques in cleft patients is still developing.

REFERENCES

1. Burstein F, Cohen S, Oddo J, Simms C et al 1996 The feeding obturator: indications and results. Fifty-third Annual Meeting, American Cleft Palate–Craniofacial Association. San Diego, California
2. Georgiade N, Latham R 1975 Maxillary arch alignment in the bilateral cleft lip and palate infant, using the pinned coaxial screw appliance. Plastic and Reconstructive Surgery 56:52–60
3. Latham R, Kusy R, Georgiade N 1976 An extraorally activated expansion appliance for cleft palate infants. Cleft Palate Journal 13:252–261
4. Cutting C 1997 Advances in cleft lip and palate. Perspectives and Advances in Plastic Surgery Symposium. Snowbird
5. Huddart A 1979 Presurgical changes in unilateral cleft palate subjects. Cleft Palate Journal 16:147–157
6. Huddart A 1984 Late findings in dental occlusion in unilateral clefts with presurgical treatment. Third International Symposium on the Early Treatments of Cleft Lip and Palate, Zurich, Switzerland
7. Maull D, Cutting C, Brecht L, Grayson B 1997 Long-term effect of presurgical nasoalveolar molding on three-dimensional nasal shape in unilateral clefts. American Cleft Palate–Craniofacial Association, 54th Annual Meeting, New Orleans
8. Desai S 1990 Cleft lip repair in newborn babies. Annals of the Royal College of Surgeons of England 2:101–103
9. Davies D 1971 Cleft lip repair. Fifth World Congress of Plastic and Reconstructive Surgery. Butterworths, London
10. Millard DRJ 1976 Cleft craft – the evolution of its surgery. 1. The Unilateral deformity. Little Brown, Boston
11. Trier WC 1985 Repair of the unilateral cleft lip: the rotation–advancement operation. Clinics in Plastic Surgery 12:573–594
12. Noordhoff M, Chen Y, Chen K, Hong K, Lo L 1995 The surgical technique for the complete unilateral cleft lip–nasal deformity. Operative Techniques in Plastic and Reconstructive Surgery 2:167–174
13. Fernandes D, Hudson D 1993 The modified Z-plasty for unilateral cleft lip repair. British Journal of Plastic Surgery 46:676–680
14. Nakajima T, Yoshimura Y 1993 Early repair of unilateral cleft lip employing a small triangular flap method and primary nasal correction. British Journal of Plastic Surgery 46:616–618
14a. Delaire J 1978 Theoretical principles and technique of functional closure of the lip and nasal aperture. Journal of Maxillofacial Surgery 6:109–116
14b. Schendel SA Delaire J 1981 Functional musculoskeletal correction of secondary unilateral cleft lip deformities: combined lip/nose correction and LeFort I osteotomy. Journal of Maxillofacial Surgery 9:108–116
15. Broadbent T, Woolf R 1974 Bilateral cleft lip: one-stage primary repair. CV Mosby, St Louis
16. Millard DRJ 1977 Cleft craft – the evolution of its surgery. II. The bilateral and rare deformities. Little Brown, Boston
17. Mulliken J 1995 Bilateral complete cleft lip and nasal deformity: an anthropometric analysis of staged to synchronous repair. Plastic and Reconstructive Surgery 96:9–26
18. Black P 1985 Bilateral cleft lip. Clinics in Plastic Surgery 12:627–641
19. Noordhoff M 1986 Bilateral cleft lip reconstruction. Plastic and Reconstructive Surgery 78:45–54
20. Farina R 1958 Bec-de-lièvre unilateral total. Annalesde Chirurgie plastique 111:199–205
21. Davies D 1970 The radical repair of cleft palate deformities. Cleft Palate Journal 7:550–561
22. Ortiz-Monasterio F, Serrano A, Barrera G, Rodriguez-Hoffman H, Vinageras E 1966 A study of untreated adult cleft patients. Plastic and Reconstructive Surgery 38:36–41
23. Boo-Chai K 1971 The unoperated adult cleft of the lip and palate. British Journal of Plastic Surgery 24:250–257
24. Bardach J, Klausner E, Eisbach K 1979 The relationship between lip pressure and facial growth after cleft lip repair: an experimental study. Cleft Palate Journal 16:137–146
25. Onizuka T, Isshiki Y 1975 Development of the palatal arch in relation to unilateral cleft lip and palate surgery: a comparison of the effects of different surgical approaches. Cleft Palate Journal 12:444–451
26. Desai S 1983 Early cleft palate repair completed before the age of 16 weeks: observations on a personal series of 100 children. British Journal of Plastic Surgery 36:300–304
27. Bishara S 1973 The influence of palatoplasty and cleft length on facial development. Cleft Palate Journal 10:390–398
28. Blijdorp P, Egyedi P 1984 The influence of age at operation for clefts on the development of the jaws. Journal of Maxillofacial Surgery 12:193–200
29. Nystrom M, Ranta R 1990 Effect of timing and method of cleft palate repair on dental arches at the age of three years. Cleft Palate Journal 27:349–352
30. Witzel M, Salyer K, Ross R 1984 Delayed hard palate closure: The philosophy revisited. Cleft Palate Journal 21:263–269
31. Randall P, LaRossa D, Fakhraee S, Cohen M 1983 Cleft palate closure at 3 to 7 months of age: a preliminary report. Plastic and Reconstructive Surgery 71:624–628
32. Dorf D, Curtain J 1982 Early cleft palate repair and speech outcome. Plastic Reconstructive Surgery 70:74–81
33. Barimo Jea 1987 Postnatal palatoplasty, implications for normal speech articulation – a preliminary report. Scandinavian Journal of Plastic Reconstructive Surgery 21:139–143
34. McComb H 1989 Cleft lip and palate: new directions for research. Cleft Palate Journal 26:145–147
35. Lehman Jjea 1990 One-stage closure of the entire primary palate. Plastic and Reconstructive Surgery 86:675–681
36. Blijdorp P, Muller H 1984 The influence of the age at which the palate is closed on the rhinological and otological condition in the adult cleft patient. Journal of Maxillofacial Surgery 12:247–254
37. Bardach J, Morris H, Olin W 1984 Late results of primary veloplasty: the Marburg project. Plastic and Reconstructive Surgery 73:207–218
38. Roberts C, Semb G, Shaw W 1991 Strategies for the advancement of surgical methods in cleft lip and palate. Cleft Palate–Craniofacial Journal 28:141–149
39. Wray C, Dann J, Holtmann B 1979 A comparison of three

techniques of palatorrhaphy: in-hospital morbidity. Cleft Palate Journal 16:42–45

40. Delaire J, Precious D 1985 Avoidance of the use of vomerine mucosa in primary surgical management of velopalatine clefts. Oral Surgery 60:589–597

41. Kriens O 1971 Fundamental anatomic findings for an intravelar veloplasty. Cleft Palate Journal 7:27–37

42. Edgerton M, Dellon A 1971 Surgical retrodisplacement of the levator veli palatini muscle. Plastic and Reconstructive Surgery 47:154–167

43. Trier W, Dreyer T 1984 Primary von Langenbeck palatoplasty with levator reconstruction: rationale and technique. Cleft Palate Journal 21:254–262

44. Marsh JL, Grames L, Holtmann B 1989 Intravelar veloplasty: a prospective study. Cleft Palate Journal 26:46–50

45. Cutting C, Rosenbaum J et al 1995 The technique of muscle repair in the cleft soft palate. Operative Techniques in Plastic and Reconstructive Surgery

46. Sommerlad B, Henley M, Birch M, Harland K, Moiemen N, Boorman J 1994 Cleft palate re-repair – a clinical and radiographic study of 32 consecutive cases. British Journal of Plastic Surgery 47:406–410

47. Furlow LJ 1986 Cleft palate repair by double opposing Z-plasty. Plastic and Reconstructive Surgery 78:724–738

48. Randall P, La Rossa D, Solomon M, Cohen M 1986 Experience with the Furlow double-reversing Z-plasty for cleft palate repair. Plastic and Reconstructive Surgery 77:569–576

49. Hoffman W 1992 Current techniques in palate repair. Perspectives in Plastic Surgery 6:32–45

50. Grobbelaar A, Hudson D, Fernandes D, Lentin R 1995 Speech results after repair of the cleft soft palate. Plastic and Reconstructive Surgery 95:1150–1154

51. Chen K, Noordhoff S 1994 Experience with Furlow palatoplasty. Chang Keng I Hsueh – Chang Gung Medical Journal 17:211–219

52. Chen P, Wu J, Chen Y, Noordhoff M 1994 Correction of secondary velopharyngeal insufficiency in cleft palate patients with the Furlow palatoplasty. Plastic and Reconstructive Surgery 94:933–941

53. Hudson D, Grobbelaar A, Fernandes D, Lentin R 1995 Treatment of velopharyngeal incompetance by the Furlow Z-plasty. Annals of Plastic Surgery 34:23–26

54. Shprintzen R, Singer L, Sidoti E et al 1992 Pharyngeal flap surgery: operative complications. International Anesthesia Clinics 30:115–124

55. Orticochea M 1983 A review of 236 cleft patients treated with dynamic muscle sphincter. Plastic and Reconstructive Surgery 71:180–188

56. Jackson I, Silverton J 1977 The sphincter pharyngoplasty as a secondary procedure in cleft palates. Plastic and Reconstructive Surgery 59:518–524

57. Riski J, Serafin D, Riefkohl R et al 1984 A rationale for modifying the site of insertion of the Orticochea pharyngoplasty. Plastic and Reconstructive Surgery 73:882–894

58. Anderl H 1990 Primary unilateral cleft lip and nose reconstruction. In: Bardach J, Morris H (eds) Multidisciplinary management of cleft lip and palate. WB Saunders, Philadelphia

59. Ortiz-Monasterio F, Olmedo A 1981 Corrective rhinoplasty before puberty: a long-term follow-up. Plastic and Reconstructive Surgery 68:381–391

60. McComb H 1986 Primary repair of the bilateral cleft lip nose: a 10-year review. Plastic and Reconstructive Surgery 77:701–716

61. Salyer K 1986 Primary correction of the unilateral cleft lip nose: a 15-year experience. Plastic Reconstructive Surgery 77:558–568

62. Tan K, Piggot R 1993 A morbidity review of children with complete unilateral cleft lip nose at 10+/−1 years of age. British Journal of Plastic Surgery 46:1–6

63. Talmant J-C 1993 Nasal malformations associated with unilateral cleft lip – accurate diagnosis and management. Scandinavian Journal of Plastic Reconstructive Surgery and Hand Surgery 27:183–191

64. Nakajima T, Yoshimura Y, Sakakibara A 1990 Augmentation of the nostril splint for retaining the corrected contour of the cleft lip nose. Plastic and Reconstructive Surgery 85:182–186

65. Trott J, Mohan N 1993 A preliminary report on open tip rhinoplasty at the time of lip repair in unilateral cleft lip and palate: the Alor Setar experience. British Journal of Plastic Surgery 46:363–370

66. Takato T, Yonehara Y, Susami T 1995 Early correction of the nose in unilateral cleft lip patients using an open method: a 10-year review. Journal of Oral and Maxillofacial Surgery 53:28–33

67. Friede H, Johanson B 1982 Adolescent facial morphology of early bone grafted cleft lip and palate patients. Scandinavian Journal of Plastic and Reconstructive Surgery 16:41

68. Nylen B et al 1974 Primary early bone grafting in complete clefts of the lip and palate. A follow-up study of 35 cases. Scandinavian Journal of Plastic and Reconstructive Surgery 8:79

69. Nordin KE et al 1983 Early bone grafting in complete cleft lip and palate cases following maxillofacial orthopedics. 1. The method and the skeletal development from seven to 13 years of age. Scandinavian Journal of Plastic and Reconstructive Surgery 17:33–50

70. Larson O et al 1983 Early bone grafting in complete cleft lip and palate cases following maxillofacial orthopedics. II. The soft-tissue development from seven to 13 years of age. Scandinavian Journal of Plastic and Reconstructive Surgery 17:51–80

71. Larson O, Ideberg M, Nordin K-E 1983 Early bone grafting in complete cleft lip and palate cases following maxillofacial orthopedics. III. A study of the dental occlusion. Scandinavian Journal of Plastic and Reconstructive Surgery 17:81–92

72. Larson O, Ideberg M, Nordin K-E 1983 Early bone grafting in complete cleft lip and palate cases following maxillofacial orthopedics. IV. A radiographic study of the incorporation of the bone grafts. Scandinavian Journal of Plastic and Reconstructive Surgery 17:93–98

73. Rosenstein S et al 1991 The case for early bone grafting in cleft lip and palate: a second report. Plastic and Reconstructive Surgery 87:644–654

74. Burchardt H 1987 Biology of bone transplantation. Orthopedic Clinics of North America 18:187–196

75. Kusiak J, Zins J, Whitaker L 1985 The early revascularisation of membranous bone. Plastic and Reconstructive Surgery 76:510–516

76. Hardesty R, Marsh J 1990 Craniofacial onlay bone grafting: a prospective evaluation of graft morphology, orientation, and embryonic origin. Plastic and Reconstructive Surgery 95:5–14

77. Cohen M, Figueroa A, Haviv Y et al 1991 Iliac versus cranial bone for secondary grafting of residual alveolar clefts. Plastic and Reconstructive Surgery 87:423

78. La Rossa D, Buchman S, Rothkopf D, Mayro R, Randall P 1995 A comparison of iliac and cranial bone in secondary grafting of alveolar clefts. Plastic and Reconstructive Surgery 96:789–797

79. Sadove A, Nelson C, Eppley B, Nguyen B 1990 An evaluation of calvarial and iliac donor sites in alveolar cleft grafting. Cleft Palate Journal 27:225–228

80. Boustred A 1997 Minimally invasive iliac cancellous bone graft harvesting. Plastic and Reconstructive Surgery 99:1760–1764

81. Hellquist R, Skoog T 1976 The influence of primary periosteoplasty on maxillary growth and deciduous occlusion in cases of complete unilateral cleft lip and palate. Scandinavian Journal of Plastic and Reconstructive Surgery 10:197–208

82. Hellquist R, Ponten B 1979 The influence of infant periosteoplasty on facial growth and dental occlusion from five to eight years of age in cases of complete unilateral cleft lip and palate. Scandinavian Journal of Plastic and Reconstructive Surgery 13:305–312

83. Rintala A, Ranta R 1989 Periosteal flaps and grafts in primary cleft repair: a follow-up study. Plastic and Reconstructive Surgery 83:17–22

84. Ross R 1987 Treatment variables affecting facial growth in complete unilateral cleft lip and palate. Part 3: Alveolus repair and bone grafting. Cleft Plastic Journal 24:33–44

85. Smahel Z, Mullerova Z 1994 Facial growth and development in unilateral cleft lip and palate during the period of puberty: comparison of the development after periosteoplasty and after

primary bone grafting. Cleft Palate–Craniofacial Journal 31:106–115

86. Millard D, Latham R 1990 Improved primary surgical and dental treatment of clefts. Plastic and Reconstructive Surgery 86:856–871

87. Brusati R, Mannucci N 1992 The early gingivoalveoloplasty – preliminary results. Scandinavian Journal of Plastic and Reconstructive Surgery and Hand Surgery 26:65–70

88. Wood RJ, Grayson BJ, Cutting CB 1997 Gingivoperiosteoplasty and midfacial growth. Cleft Palate–Craniofacial Journal 34:17–20

71

Cleft rhinoplasty

JEAN-CLAUDE TALMANT

INTRODUCTION

Over the past two decades the simultaneous correction of unilateral complete cleft lip and nasal deformity has confirmed that the outcome of primary alar cartilage repositioning is more successful when done in a synchronous repair, and that early cartilage repositioning does not interfere with growth of the nasal tip. It is today a certain and well accepted practice, with more than 25 years of follow-up.

Thanks to this experience, the challenge is now to achieve in a single-stage procedure the same kind of results in primary repair of the bilateral complete cleft lip and nasal deformity, including primary lengthening of the columella. To be safe this surgery should be very precise, the concept simple and the technique reproducible even when preoperative orthopedics are not available.

As primary correction of the nasal deformity, based on a sound anatomic knowledge, is today the ideal treatment, secondary revision or correction for esthetic or functional reasons is always possible from 6 years of age.

The same principles must guide the surgeon in both primary and secondary surgery: in cleft lip–nasal repair. Everything must be done to restore all functions, the major one being nasal ventilation. This functional approach, emphasized by Delaire, must be a constant concern and is more demanding than the simple layered closure with orbicularis muscle realignment, termed functional repair of the lip.

Among the numerous functional concerns of the surgeon, two points are essential. First, if the repaired baby sleeps with his mouth closed, we really can expect normal facial growth. Labial competency and a patent airway should be preserved or restored early.[1–8] Secondly, surgery is the main cause of dysfunction and facial growth disturbance, owing to scarring of the lip, the nostril and the palate. Procedures that create secondary scars, especially at the level of the palate, are the worst and must be avoided.[9–17]

ANATOMY

PATHOGENESIS OF NASAL DEFORMITY: THE ROLE OF THE FACIAL ENVELOPE

The functional approach is an accurate and careful attempt to create the best esthetic and functional result. It should be based on a good knowledge and understanding of the normal and pathologic anatomy of the cleft lip and nose.

However, this pathologic anatomy remains controversial. Usually hypoplasia and displacement of the maxillary segments are regarded as the main causes of the deformity.[18–23] The logical conclusion of this concept is to restore a normal maxillary arch by early preoperative orthopedics.

In our opinion the basic defect is one of muscle, and the most effective orthopedic treatment is an anatomic and balanced muscular reconstruction. A few authors have cited muscle imbalance on both sides of the unilateral cleft as being an important factor, yet the influence of muscle imbalance remains poorly understood.

Mechanical features of the facial envelope

When the author was studying with Tessier, he saw him dissecting the platysma and working with the conviction that each muscle of facial expression is an element of a network covering the whole face. He coined the term 'the facial SMAS', which is made of two layers: superficial and deep.

The superficial musculoaponeurotic system (SMAS) is a continuous fibromuscular layer which interconnects the musculature through an aponeurosis, thus distributing their forces. It is the *continuity* which gives it its morpho-functional and surgical importance.

The global concept of the facial envelope,[3] which involves the elastic soft tissue covering the face and neck (skin, muscles and mucosa), permits a better grasp of their morphofunctional influences than studies limited to individual muscles or even to the SMAS. The mechanics of the facial envelope introduce a new essential feature that alters the distribution of the forces.

Bleschmidt has published the fascinating face of a 7.5-week-old fetus that looks very sad, with deep paranasal folds, but at this age, there are no functional muscles at all. The two paranasal folds are a mechanical phenomenon, closely connected with the existence of the oral split. It is well explained by the theory of elasticity. The facial covering, made of ectomesenchyma, is stretched by the growing brain and the growing facial processes. As soon as the oral split appears and breaks the continuity of the facial envelope it concentrates the vertical stress laterally, just behind each commissure, in the shape of two commissural folds; each one goes up from the mental tubercle of the mandibular body to a place just above and behind the nostril.

At the mesenchymal stage of the embryo this mechanical phenomenon seems able to organize the fascicular arrangement of the facial muscles, which looks like a diagram of the local stresses. Once the individual muscular cells mature and become contractile they orientate themselves toward the axis of local stress, just like iron filings in a magnetic field.

This mechanical phenomenon is also probably able to individualize or even to capture the alar cartilage from the nasal capsule in order to allow the control of the facial envelope on this part of the external nose, which works like a nozzle with an adaptable neck usually called the nasal valve.

The disposition of the muscles in two layers in the area of the oral commissure (the buccinator is the deep layer) is not a matter of chance. According to the theory of the resistance of materials, the principle of stratification is the best way to improve the resistance of the commissure of a split when submitted to strong vertical stretch.

At any time, the facial muscles have to compromise with these mechanical phenomena as they work in an ensemble where the commissural folds divide the facial envelope into three anatomic sectors, one central and two lateral. The central or labial one corresponds to the premaxilla and the incisor arches. From a mechanical point of view the lips have much greater freedom of action than the cheeks. In the infant, when labial activity dominates, the commissural folds are smooth. Laterally there are two retrocommissural or bucconasal sectors, gathering on each side, the cheek and the lateral wall of the external nose above the nostril.

With advancing age the labionasal folds become much deeper and sharper as the buccal activity becomes the dominating one and pulls them back. Each lateral sector corresponds to the lateral aspect of the maxilla and the lateral border of the piriform aperture. The canine takes its place in the front of the lateral segment of the maxillary dental arch, under its commissural fold control.

The nasal valve is under the control of the facial envelope

When there is nasal airway obstruction the functional adaptation of the facial covering will be a distal pull on the commissural folds to prevent the collapse of the neck of each nasal valve. Such a facial posture stresses the underlying frame and is unfavorable to the eruption and positioning of the maxillary canine or lateral incisor. The adenoid nose is another kind of adaptation, with increased activity of the incisor bands of the orbicularis oris muscle. These two muscles shorten the lip to orientate the nostril forward, but at the same time compress the maxillary arch at the lateral incisor level; as well as bringing the commissural folds nearer, they hinder the transverse development of the piriform aperture and increase the work of breathing. The functional unlocking of the adenoid nose would be an anterior expansion of the intermaxillary suture to give more width to the piriform aperture. Indeed, this clinical case is closely related to the problem of cleft lip and palate patients.

Facial envelope, hypoplasia and growth mechanisms

Any interruption of the facial envelope in its anterior region will disturb the whole facial balance and will automatically change the arrangement of the muscles inside the SMAS itself, resulting in skeletal deformity and problems of subsequent facial growth. Hypoplasia, displacement of the maxillary segments and deformity of the lower lateral cartilage are all direct consequences of the rupture of the facial balance. A knowledge of these musculoaponeurotic structures in the region of the lower lateral cartilage, the anterior nasal spine and the nasal septum is therefore essential in both normal and cleft subjects, as correction of the nasal deformity can be achieved only when the surgeon is fully aware of the modified arrangement of the muscles and of their relationships.

A cleft lip and palate is above all a muscular cleft. Irrespective of the mechanism of the cleft there is always a primary hypoplasia, at least on the cleft side of the philtrum, where there is no muscle at all, and in the premaxilla, where frequently one tooth and its surrounding bone are missing. We can do nothing about this primary hypoplasia.

Because the cleft is muscular, imbalance and dysfunction are immediate and cause secondary hypoplasia. This has been confirmed by Mooney, who has shown that the hypoplasia of the premaxilla is noticeable only after the 14th week of embryologic life, more than 8 weeks after the day when the cleft appeared.[30] Thus it is highly probable that the lack of development of the anterior nasal spine, the premaxilla and the maxilla is the result of the growth mechanism operating under abnormal anatomic relationships.[23–30]

We can correct the secondary hypoplasia by reconstructing a normal forward growth unit, which associates septum, vomer, premaxilla, septopremaxillary ligament and labionasal muscles in front of the midline. Without being dogmatic, it is difficult to deny the interest of the early septal traction model of midfacial growth during embryological life and the first 2.5 years of postnatal life.[23] This is particularly striking, with the protuding premaxilla of the bilateral cleft being thrust forward by a septum free of the restraint of the facial envelope and of the continuity of the maxilla. After the first 2.5 years of postnatal life the forward sliding of the vomer on its maxillary surface is still necessary to the balance and harmonious reconciliation of maxillary forward growth, nasal septum growth and forward and downward growth of the vomer.

To be successful, the repair should:

- Reconstruct a normal muscular anatomy in front of the midline;
- Preserve the potential growth of each component of the forward growth unit, specially of the vomer, by avoiding the use of vomerine mucosa in primary management of the velopalatine cleft.[12]

This latter point is controversial, but a number of studies have stressed the risk associated with interference with facial growth. There are now new timings which allow the closure of the bony palate without the use of vomerine mucosa and without secondary epithelialization of denuded bone. It might be wise to take advantage of this opportunity.

PATHOGENESIS OF THE CLEFT LIP NOSE DEFORMITY: THE MUSCULAR DEFECT AND ITS CONSEQUENCES

In a complete unilateral cleft asymmetry makes the deformity more evident and easier to understand. Chronology is also an important point to consider when studying the cleft lip nose deformity.

On the cleft side, from the first day of the defect – that is, from the 36th day of gestation – the interruption of the facial envelope in the region of the anterior nasal spine occurs when the only frame is the cartilaginous nasal capsule. The earliest point of ossification in the maxilla appear about 2 weeks later, at a time when the muscle precursors are already present. This means that the abnormal musculature is present during the formation of the bones, virtually all of which takes place at the direction and under the influence of asymmetric and distorted muscular forces. Normally the muscles of the face, which migrate from the second branchial arch, reach the midline the week after the fusion of the facial processes. In cases of total cleft, the muscles of the lip and of the sill of the nostril remain on the external edge and do not insert on their corresponding part of the midline. As early as the 8th week of embryologic life, important anomalies of the nasal septum are already present.[23] The nasal septum is curved or bent toward the non-cleft side, and forms a convex curvature relative to the cleft side. This is probably proof of the septal ability to push forward, as in the absence of noticeable muscle it deforms as soon as it encounters asymmetric resistance from the facial envelope as a result of its rupture.

It is easy to understand that the distribution of the stresses inside the ruptured facial envelope is altered, and that the consequences for the organization of the SMAS will not be limited to the margin of the cleft.

From the studies of surgeons such as Fara we are familiar with the description of the lateral muscle fibers which bend cranially, parallel to the cleft in a more or less jumbled pattern, insert in the skin and the vermilion, and are more or less mature. But now we must extend our field of vision beyond the margin of the cleft, and think globally. The facial imbalance involves the network of the SMAS itself. Once the individual muscular cells become contractile, they orientate themselves toward the modified axis of the local stress. The meshes of the net will be more or less enlarged and deformed.

As stated by Randall,[31] in a review of the history of cleft lip nasal repair, if we except the excellent publications of McCoomb[21] and of Veau,[32] little has been published on the study of gross anatomy by dissection of stillborn infants, and of microscopic anatomy by examination of serial cuts of faces of cleft fetuses. The conclusions of these studies, and of a few theses or publications and of personal observations, are now presented.

The normal anatomy

The normal anatomy of the muscles of the lip and the nostril is probably well known to every reader, but it seems important to ensure that the terminology used will be understood.

The septopremaxillary ligament, initially described by

Latham, is the aponeurotic structure which links the septum to the premaxilla. The ligament and its median sagittal expansion receives the terminal insertions of the nasolabial muscle, distributing and transmitting their forces to the periosteum of the premaxilla and the maxilla, thus directly soliciting the interincisive suture.

In the premaxilla area there are two planes of muscle insertions:

- A deep vertical one which comes from the nose: the nasalis muscle;
- A superficial horizontal one: the orbicularis oris muscle. This plane is better known but its complexity is often not appreciated.

The deep plane is essentially constituted by the constrictor nasi muscle complex or nasalis muscle. Its superior part is the transverse muscle, which lies on top of but remains separated from the upper lateral cartilage, after which it sweeps down around the lower cartilage, joining laterally with the myrtiform head to insert on to the maxilla, and terminates medially in the floor of the nostril. The myrtiform head arises from the maxilla between the apex of the lateral incisor and the canine, and then ascends toward the nostril sill. It joins the fibers of the transverse muscle laterally and terminates medially in a fan shape in the anterior mucosa of the floor of the nose.

Either of the two heads of the constrictor muscle complex is capable of being a constrictor and of having an independent action, but in fact they work in concert with the whole facial envelope.

The superficial plane is the orbicularis oris muscle, which is composed of three strata:

- The oblique bands originate from the depressor anguli oris in the labial commissure. The more internal fibers run vertically, adjacent to the philtral column, and are part of the bulk of the philtral crests. Superficially these fibers insert into the cutaneous part of the upper lip. The strongest part of the oblique bands inserts into the septopremaxillary ligament in front and above the ANS. Some fibers interweave with the terminal insertion of the depressor nasi septi into the foot plate.
- The horizontal fibers are continuous medially just beneath the philtral dimple and extend from one commissure to the other. At the commissure they intermingle with numerous other muscles of facial expression.
- The incisal bands are formed deep to the oblique bands within the incisive fossa, below the myrtiform, and run superficially to insert into the free end of the upper lip.

The structure of the philtrum is mainly the consequence of decussation of muscle fibers in the midline, with oblique and vertical extensions into the dermis of the lateral aspect of the philtral ridges, whereas there is a relative absence of muscle fiber insertion into the dermis of the dimple, as shown by St Lee.

Anatomy of the cleft lip nose

When a cleft occurs the facial envelope loses its anterior support on the nasal septum and the muscles cannot reach the midline. This will disorganize the whole SMAS.[6-8] On the cleft side the facial envelope falls and is retracted and displaced posteroinferiorly, as can be seen on the alar base and the commissure of the lips.

The vestibular lining of the lateral wall and of the sill of the nostril is stretched and vertically elongated. This stretch can only be made worse by the opposing action of the levator muscles and the orbicularis oris. The lower lateral cartilage, normally overlying the upper lateral cartilage, is pulled inferiorly from the upper cartilage with a considerable distension of the nasal fold. The vestibular lining is much more lengthened than the external skin, as if it were turning inside out, like taking off a surgical glove.

The transverse part of the constrictor nasi muscle slips down into the space thus created between the upper and lower lateral cartilages, as illustrated by Chateau.[24] A well known print of McComb's[21] shows accurately the abnormal situation of the transverse muscle on the cleft side in a unilaterally cleft stillborn infant.

The constrictor nasi muscle is unique in the SMAS (Fig. 71.1) in that it has two fixed insertions: its transverse part lies on top of, but remains separated from, the upper lateral cartilage, after which it sweeps down around the lower lateral cartilage, joining with the myrtiform head to insert onto the premaxilla and into the floor of the nose. In the complete unilateral cleft, because of its two fixed insertions, the nasal muscle resists the posterior displacement of the SMAS. However, it can move anteriorly during contraction, so that it covers the inferior part of the lower lateral cartilage and forces the lateral crus to torque inferomedially. The upper part of the nostril web is tipped up by the rotated lower edge of the lateral crus, and the lower part of the web is deformed by the strong myrtiform head of the nasal muscle and an excess of connective tissue.

In 1995 we published[8] the picture of a frontal section through the nostrils of a 14-week-old human fetus with a complete cleft on the left side, where we can see an evident concentration of muscle cells corresponding to the transverse part of the nasalis muscle, close to the deformity of the lower lateral cartilage on the cleft side. Higher-power views confirm this, which is seen on each of the serial cuts.

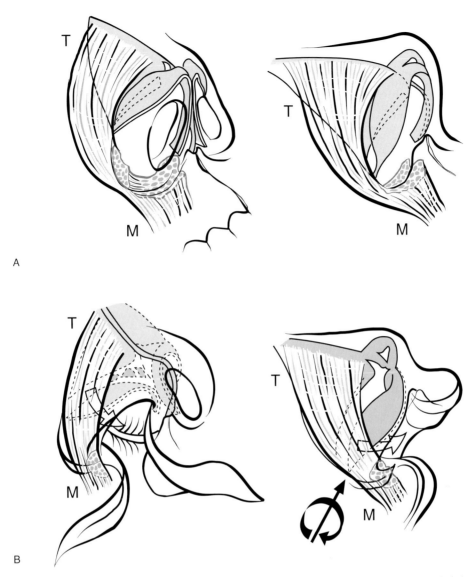

Fig. 71.1 The nasalis muscle with its two heads: the transverse muscle (T) and the myrtiform muscle (M), in a normal subject **(A)** and in a complete unilateral cleft subject **(B)**. In a unilateral cleft the nasalis muscle, with its two fixed insertions, resists the posterior displacement of the facial envelope. Its anterior sliding in relation to the other structures induces caudal rotation of the lateral crus. The myrtiform becomes the strongest anchorage point of the facial envelope, and is located in the base of the nasal web.

On a frontal section through the nostrils of a 21-week-old human fetus[8] with a complete cleft on the left side, we have seen the same asymmetry. In this case the serial cuts showed that the nasalis muscle is slightly globular, with staining indicating delayed maturation. Probably this relates to the new role of the nasal muscle, which is now the strongest anterior anchorage point of the facial envelope on the cleft side, as Veau stressed 68 years ago. The nasalis muscle is close to the deformed cartilage but separated by abundant connective tissue, which we have all seen, especially in the most everted nostrils. Below the myrtiform, which is the inferior part of the nasalis muscle, we have seen the insertions of the incisive head of the orbicularis oris muscle.

Contrary to what has been said by certain authors, it is not its absence that explains the muscle-free area laterally to the wing of the nose, but rather the vertical distension of the region.

Between the 10th and 15th weeks of embryologic life the deformity of the cleft lip nose is complete, and is the same as in a newborn. This knowledge is of prime importance before surgical research on cleft fetuses can be carried out. There is strictly no parallel between a surgically created cleft in a normal fetus immediately repaired, and the surgical repair in utero of a spontaneous cleft, where the associated cleft lip nose deformities will persist. In the best case the nasal outcome would be the same as in a lip adhesion. The

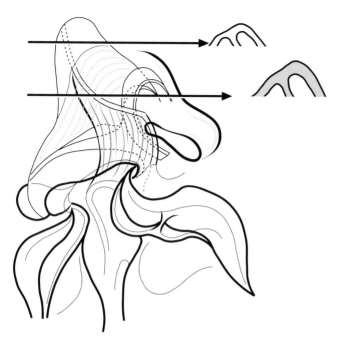

Fig. 71.2 Deformity of the bony and cartilaginous structures of the nose in a unilateral complete cleft, with a double curvature of the septum. Note the depression and retraction of the nasal bone and of the upper lateral cartilage on the cleft side.

in utero repair should not have to be redone to be of value.

The rest of the nose is also deformed (Fig. 71.2). The dorsum is deviated toward the non-cleft side. The septum forms a strong convexity in the cleft, that is, a convexity from behind forward by a curvature of the septum, and a convexity from above to below by luxation of the septovomerian junction and lateral inclination of the vomer. This deformation, which appears very early, even though the musculature because of its delay in evolution is almost absent, can only be made worse by the asymmetric forces exerted on it from the midline, carrying the nasal bone, the septum, the anterior nasal spine and the columella toward the non-cleft side. On this side the concavity of the septum is filled by the hypertrophic inferior turbinate. Irrespective of its deviation, the nasal bone is very asymmetric. The loss of support of the facial envelope in the midline causes a depression and retraction of the whole SMAS on the cleft side, which will deform in the same way all the hemiface and particularly the nasal structures. This is obvious at the level of the upper lateral cartilage.

The columella is shorter on the cleft side and may look almost absent when the cleft is very wide and the premaxilla very protruded. This feature is particularly striking in total bilateral clefts. The shortness of the columella is explained by three different mechanisms.

The columella itself is not elongated by the normal dif-ferential of forward growth between the nasal septum and the premaxilla. In Latham's hypothesis[33] the columella is wanted tissue and this analysis of the defect induces to bring tissue into the columella. The result of such a procedure, especially in bilateral clefts, is frequently a nose with too large nostrils, which is paradoxical when the columella itself remains imperfect.

The infra tip part of the columella disappears in the broad and flat nasal tip as the domes and the alar cartilages are pulled apart from each side of the septum. In fact, the circumference of the nostril is normal and the columella is hidden in the tip of the nose, from whence it can be extracted by proper repositioning of the splayed genua. In our opinion this mechanism is the most important, as we have seen a severe complete bilateral cleft where the columella was of a normal length, because in this particular case, which was a bilateral number 3 facial cleft, the alar bases had lost their continuity with the facial envelope and were no longer subject to the posteroinferior pull of the facial envelope. In this case, the explanation of Latham does not work properly. We are more and more convinced that the columella is inside the nose, and this concept is very promising in primary repair of the bilateral cleft lip with simultaneous lengthening of the columella.[34–40]

The inferior part of the columella is in fact the superior part of the center of the upper lip in front of the anterior nasal spine, which participates in the projection of the nose. The correct response is a good muscular repair in front of the anterior nasal spine.

Indeed, in a complete bilateral cleft the septum is usually sagittal and the nasal deformity is symmetrical and looks like the addition of two unilateral clefts. Usually, however, the degree of the deformity is parallel to the width of the bony cleft, and to the protrusion of the premaxilla.

PRIMARY CORRECTION OF COMPLETE UNILATERAL CLEFT LIP AND NASAL DEFORMITY

The muscular structures of the cleft side do not play their normal part because they do not have their terminal insertions in the midline. The primary repair of the unilateral cleft lip nasal deformity must include an anatomic muscular reconstruction of the lip and the nostril sill, and the correction of the deformity of the lower lateral cartilage.

Many surgeons still consider the skin the more important tissue. New designs and new flaps are the answer to all the problems, especially to increase the height of the lip and to lengthen the columella. Ingenious modifications and refinements have been brought to Millard's technique to improve the efficiency of the C flap[41] or to give more skin to the lateral lip. In our opinion, the main quality of Millard's technique is the principle of rotation of the philtrum and the advancement of the lateral lip element, with its perfect final scar. But the height of the lip depends overall on the muscular repair. We cannot understand why so many surgeons still use a triangular flap repair derived from the Tenisson technique when the lip does not need a Z-plasty to be lengthened but rather a good muscle repair. In cases of bilateral cleft, a Z-plasty on both sides may look like a caricature that will be very difficult to improve.

The accuracy of the muscular repair also deeply influences the repositioning of the alar base, and of the lower lateral cartilage, the shape and the patency of the nostril, with correction of the curtain-like obstruction of the nostril web, and the achievement of a proper level and width of the nostril sill. For all these reasons, the lip repair is part of the correction of nasal the deformity and cannot be dissociated from it.

Timing

Our timing of the primary repair has evolved towards a synchronous repair of the soft palate, the lip and the nostril at 6 months of age. This is a reasonable compromise to achieve in one step such a long and careful procedure. For 24 years I have closed the lip and nostril at 6 months of age, without early preoperative orthopedic treatment, as I consider an anatomic muscular reconstruction is the best approach.

To avoid the use of vomerine mucosa and the bad scarring of the raw area along the alveolar bone that results from the V-Y push-back procedures of palatal closure, I changed the timing 14 years ago.[13–17] Now I close the soft palate during the first operation, at the same time as the lip, that is, at 6 months of age.

After the first operation the remaining palatal cleft narrows to such an extent that by 18 months of age the residual fissure can be closed in two planes with only the fibromucosa of the palatal shelves, without undermining the vomerine mucosa or incising laterally.

PRIMARY SURGICAL PROCEDURE

On the lip, the primary surgical procedure is designed to systematically correct the abnormal anatomy.

The cutaneous incisions (Fig. 71.3)

These are rather similar to those used in Millard's procedure,[22] with only a few modifications:

- The perialar incision is not useful if the muscular repair is well understood. The adjustment of the level of the alar base and of the width of the nostril sill is the result of the muscular suture.

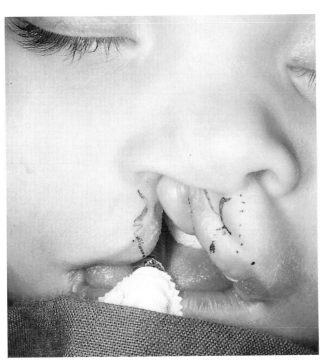
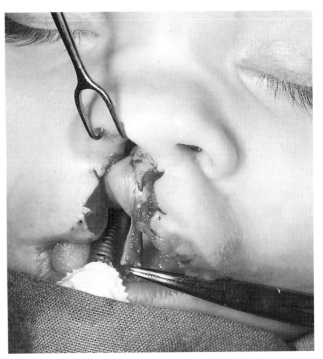

A   B

Fig. 71.3 Markings for the primary repair of a unilateral complete cleft. The principle of Millard's technique – rotation of the philtrum and advancement of the lateral lip element – are respected. The design is simplified, and none of the incisions recommended to increase the height of the lip are used.

- The nasal skin of the nostril sill is never included in the lateral lip element, as it is unnecessary to obtain a normal height.
- The indication for the back cut is exceptional, and it is used more for lengthening the columella than the lip.

As mentioned above, the key points of Millard's design are the concept of rotation of the philtrum and lateral advancement, but above all the incorporation of the C flap in the base of the columella and the perfect placement of the final scars are considerable advantages. The height of the lip depends directly on the muscular reconstruction. It is very rare to reconstruct a lip that is too short with this technique, but the beginning surgeon can achieve an excess of height, which is the risk of full muscle repair without correcting the original vertical distension by crossing of the two muscular planes. Last but not least, the feeling of this 'cut as you go' method is perfectly adapted to this kind of muscle repair where the eye is the only guide.

Freeing the displaced structures

Repositioning of the displaced muscular and cartilaginous structures must be prepared for laterally by wide subperiosteal undermining, to allow repositioning of the facial envelope in relation to the midline, and suturing without tension. On the medial side the periosteum is respected in front of the interincisive suture. The septal mucoperichondrium is widely elevated on the cleft side, and the alar cartilage is freed by a blind but accurate dissection from its connections with the skin, the upper lateral cartilage, the septum, the periosteum of the piriform aperture, and the contralateral lower lateral cartilage. The advancement of the alar base frequently needs an incision in the mucoperiosteum of the nasal vestibule along the piriform aperture, which will be closed by a labial mucosal flap. More details about the nasal dissection are given below.

The muscular suture

The muscular suture is prepared by short subcutaneous undermining of the edges. On the lateral side the orbicularis oris muscle is separated from the superficial nasolabial muscle (essentially the levator muscles), and on the opposite side a space is opened between the periosteum and the orbicularis oris beyond the midline.

Muscle suturing takes place essentially in two planes, deep and superficial. The crossing direction of these two planes corrects the vertical distension of the lip.[6,8]

The reconstruction of the constrictor nasi muscle complex represents the deep plane (Fig. 71.4). Its simple suture medially on to the nasal septum would result in the muscle lying horizontally, which would not only raise the nasal floor but also pull the web of the nostril toward the midline, thus obstructing the nasal airway. This obstruction is compounded by the concomitant lowering of the junction of the upper lateral cartilage and the nasal septum in the upper part of the web (Fig. 71.5). The myrtiform, which is the inferior maxillary head of the constrictor nasi muscle complex, is identified as the deeper muscle just below the web of the nostril, where it is not dissected. In order to obtain the correct level of the future nasal sill, its reinsertion must be accomplished inferomedially so that it is sutured to the periosteum and connective tissue overlying the facial aspect of the premaxilla, in the region of the developing lateral incisor. In primary surgery it may be useful to reinforce its reinsertion on to the premaxilla by passing through the mucosa of the labial sulcus. With experience the surgeon learns the correct placement of this suture, which stabilizes the level of the nostril sill.

A more superficial plane is now created by passing a suture from the deep superior part of the lateral orbicularis oris muscle to the periosteum and the fibrous tissue at the base of the septum, just in front of the anterior nasal spine. By their crossing directions, these first two surgically created muscle insertions have a correcting effect on the vertical distension of the nasolabial region, a distension which is usually not written about but one which can almost always be observed by an excess in height between the point of implantation of the alar base and the mucocutaneous line of the upper lip. On some occasions a suture between the nostril sill and the orbicularis muscle contracts the residual excess of height in this area, with or without a skin excision just below the alar base.

Specifically, functional continuity of the orbicularis oris muscle is achieved in two planes after its separation from the nasolabial levator muscles. The deep part of the muscle from the cleft side is sutured to the deep muscular fibers of its counterpart across the midline. The superficial part, however, is sutured so that the resultant muscular junction is just lateral to the midline, thus mimicking a philtral ridge.

The nasolabial levator muscles will be sutured to their counterparts and to the opposite orbicularis oris muscle at the end of the operation. Final vertical adjustment of the height of the lip and of the width of the nasal sill can be made by crossing sutures between the nasal and labial parts of the superficial plane on both sides (for example, between the opposite foot plate and the orbicularis oris muscle).

Correction of the nasal deformity

The principle of correction is to lift the alar cartilage and at the same time to push the transverse muscle out of the

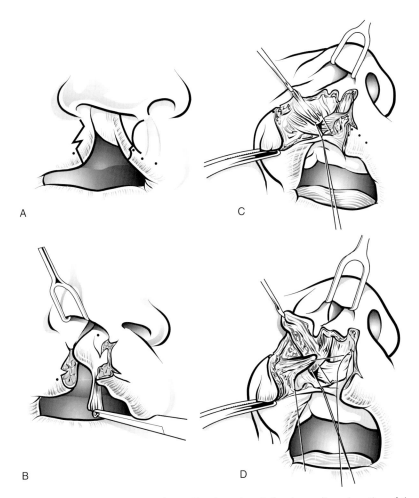

Fig. 71.4 The muscular suture in two planes. The deep plane is the descending reinsertion of the myrtiform head of the nasalis muscle on the lateral aspect of the premaxilla. The superficial plane is the ascending reinsertion of the orbicularis oris muscle on the anterior nasal spine. **(A)** marking; **(B)** Incision; **(C)** Muscular suture, deep plane; **(D)** Muscular suture, superficial plane.

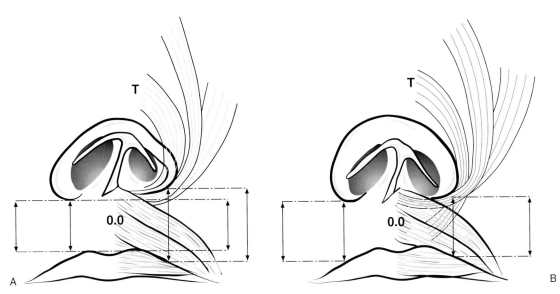

Fig. 71.5 (A) The incorrect suture of the myrtiform head of the nasalis muscle on the anterior nasal spine raises the nasal floor and pulls the nasal web toward the midline, thus obstructing the nasal airway. **(B)** The crossing direction of the two planes stabilizes the nostril sill at a good level and corrects the lateral vertical distension of the lip.

web, and prevent relapse by recreating a stable concave nasal fold and redraping the vestibular lining. It must be understood that in order to reposition the lower lateral cartilage accurately it is more important to meticulously free around the cartilage and carefully reconstruct the muscle of the nasal sill, than it is to perform complex fixation procedures. The normal overlying relationship between the dome of the alar cartilage and the upper lateral cartilage at the top of the nasal valve should be meticulously re-established. To achieve this, the dissection of the muco-perichondrium from the septum and from the two sides of the upper lateral cartilage must be very extensive, with elongation of the mucosa in front of the inferior border of the upper lateral cartilage to allow complete projection of the dome with respect to the upper lateral cartilage. A good instrument for this work is a Freer's double curved elevator, which is very efficient for lengthening the mucosa between the upper and lower cartilages, and pushing up the inferior aspect of the alar cartilage in order to round and spread out the folded dome. This lengthening is carried on along the web, which is the most retracted area of the nostril. Freeing the dome and the splayed genua is not enough. This cartilaginous area is folded into a concave curvature and, since the 3 months of embryologic life, has been embedded in a fibrous perichondrium, rupture of which is necessary to invert the curvature into a convex one.

Now it is time to reshape the nostril and to maintain the correction. Personally I have abandoned direct sutures between the nasal cartilages, and use mattress sutures to recreate the concavity of the base of the nasal fold during the first week, with nasal splinting, made of a thin sheet of silastic. To achieve good splinting of the nostril it is better to adopt the sandwich principle, with one sheet of silastic inside the nostril and one externally. Thus dead spaces are avoided and the new relationship between the apparently redundant vestibular lining, which slips inside the nose with respect to the external skin, is maintained. With this method it is easier to smooth out the ridge of the nostril web, to adjust the lift of the nostril rim, and to support the dome. The recent evolution of this method is the consequence of its application in the primary synchronous repair of nasal deformity in complete bilateral cleft, as discussed later.

Modeling the nasal splint (Fig. 71.6)

Custom-made appliances have been used by a few surgeons for primary alar cartilage repositioning. Mulliken,[38,39] one of those most involved in the difficult task of primary lengthening of the columella in complete bilateral clefts, has abandoned splinting, which failed to prevent post-

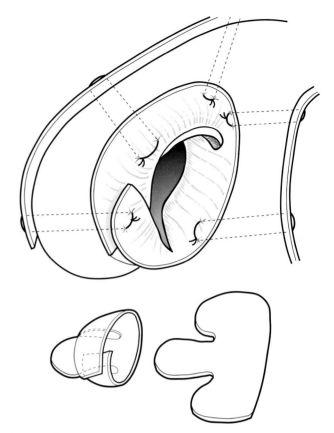

Fig. 71.6 The custom-made appliance used to reposition the freed lower lateral cartilage and the vestibular lining. The posterior half of a square piece of silastic is tailored into a shamrock shape. The superior notch is placed astride the free border of the upper lateral cartilage and the superior leaf supports the dome and recreates its concavity. The internal splint is secured to a contralateral piece of silastic through the septum, and to an external piece, to close the dead space and control the sliding displacement of the external skin with regard to the vestibular lining.

operative collapse of the dome, and prefers a semi-open approach, with direct suture between the alar dome and the ipsilateral upper lateral cartilage at the level of its junction with the septum.

In contrast, the results I have achieved in secondary lengthening of the columella and reshaping of the nasal tip by simple alar cartilage repositioning and splinting have convinced me that it is an interesting to explore and to improve primary cleft surgery.

For a 6-month-old baby the nasal splint (Fig. 71.6) is made from a non-reinforced sheet of silastic® (ref 500–5) cut into a 3 × 3 cm square. The posterior half is divided into three equal leaves like a shamrock. The middle one of these is left intact and will be placed along the septum. The superior and inferior leaves are reduced in length and trimmed to avoid any sharp continuity with the middle one. The superior notch will be placed astride the junction of the upper lateral cartilage with the septum, and the superior leaf will be modeled to round and support the dome and deepen the concavity of the nasal fold, in order to settle the normal position of the lower lateral cartilage overlying the upper lateral cartilage. The inferior leaf pushes down the nasal sill and conforms the concavity of the base of the nasal fold.

The splint is secured by monofilament nylon sutures to a contralateral piece of silastic through the septum. The remodeling of the nostril is then resumed using through-and-through sutures between the inner splint and an external piece of silastic. While the sutures are being placed the redundant vestibular lining which is not actually in excess is pushed inside the nose, with a sliding redraping with respect to the external skin. Indeed, only a complete freeing of the different cartilages, and of the vestibular lining with respect to the external skin, allows the achievement of a stable result after remodeling, with the custom-made appliance left in place for 6–7 days. When the nursing conditions are good a prolonged inner splinting assures both a good esthetic result and a patent airway.

During the first few days the splint is filled with petroleum gauze to prevent any maceration of the lip sutures from the nasal secretions.

The advantages of the method are:

- To limit the extent of the skin incisions that jeopardize its viability (especially in bilateral clefts), and to leave less scarring, with subsequent retraction of the nostril and relapse.
- To close any dead space and thus prevent bad scarring

and retraction of the thick skin of the nasal tip.

- To create new relationships between the vestibular lining and the external skin, and, thanks to this redraping inside the nose, to lift the alar rim and to correct without excision the redundant skin in the soft triangle, which is useful to restore the internal concavity of the dome.
- To elevate the dome and return the lower lateral cartilage to its normal position overlying the upper lateral cartilage, without abnormal fixation by sutures linking the alar dome with the upper lateral cartilage. The external skin and the vestibular lining slide in opposite directions, and this is the only method except the open approach of Trott[40] that can lift the alar dome and the alar rim without shortening the nose. Such a feature is particularly interesting when dealing with a complete bilateral cleft lip nasal deformity.
- To smooth out the curtain-like obstruction of the nasal web by redraping the apparently redundant skin of the everted nostril inside the nose. The success of this correction depends on a wide undermining of the inner skin of the nostril up to the nostril rim.
- The transparency of the silastic allows visual control when the sutures are tied, so it is easy to prevent any risk of skin necrosis.

The results of primary repair of the cleft lip nasal deformity in unilateral complete cleft with or without minor secondary revisions are illustrated in Figures 71.7, 71.8 and 71.9. If

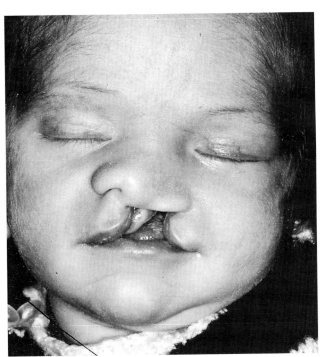
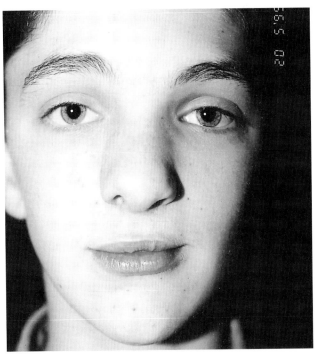

Fig. 71.7 Result at 16 years of age of the primary closure of a wide unilateral complete cleft lip and palate, after minor revision of the nostril and the septum at 8 years of age.

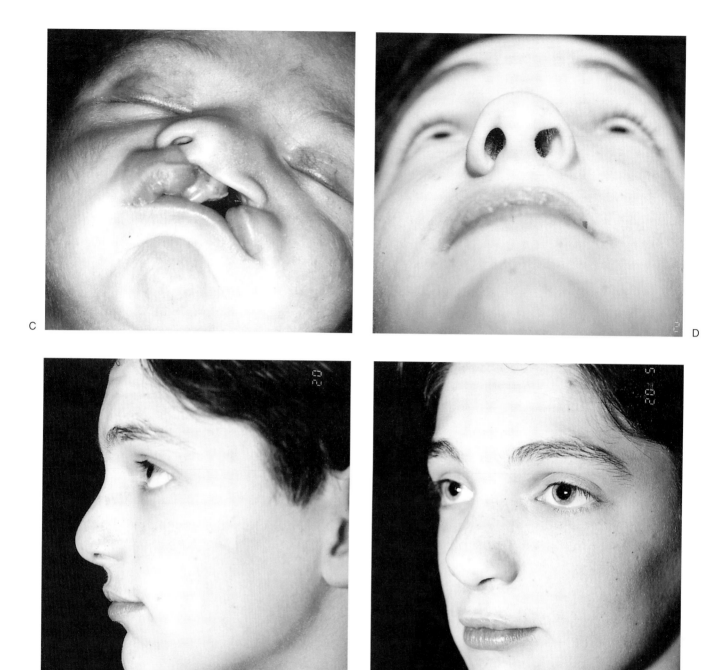

C

D

E

F

experience improves the predictability of the results, the anatomic principles of muscular reconstruction and of repositioning of the lower lateral cartilage are precious guides to achieve corrections close to the normal anatomy. Recent refinements developed to lengthen the columella at the time of the primary bilateral cleft lip repair have already benefited the unilateral cleft lip nose deformity. Now we can expect a more perfect primary repositioning of the dome with less scarring. Secondary revision will be both rarer and easier.

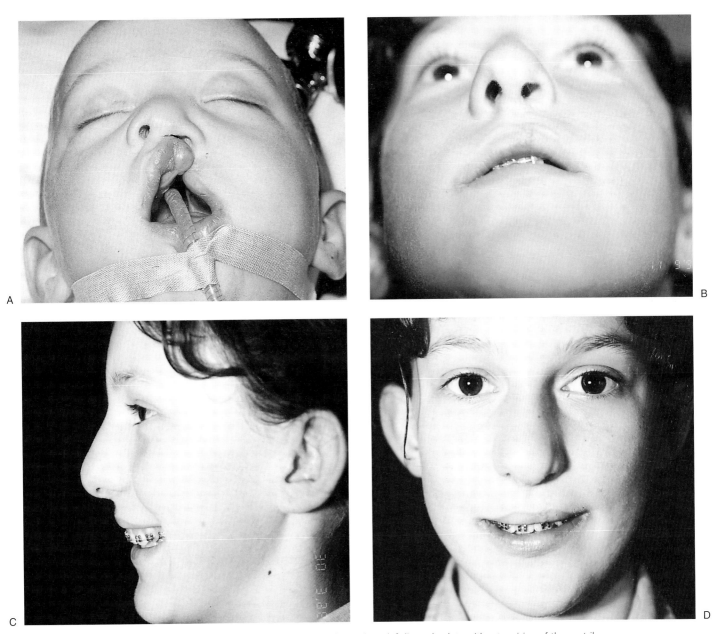

Fig. 71.8 Result at 13 years of age of the primary repair of a unilateral complete cleft lip and palate without revision of the nostril.

BILATERAL COMPLETE CLEFT LIP AND NASAL DEFORMITY

The correction of bilateral complete cleft lip and nasal deformity remains the most difficult challenge in the field of this surgery. Whereas the progress of the outcome of primary correction of unilateral complete cleft lip and nasal deformity is striking, and the practice is considered as not threatening for nasal cartilage growth nor facial growth, the bilateral complete cleft has not taken advantage of this experience of synchronous repair to the same degree.

The main problem is the very short columella, which is the pedicle of the prolabial flap during primary surgery: when the lip was repaired on both sides in a single step, the nasal correction was postponed for a second stage to preserve the blood supply to the prolabial flap. When an attempt was made to correct the nasal deformity during the first operation, it was only a partial release and elevation of the lateral crura of the lower lateral cartilage. The dissection was incomplete in the area of the dome, the medial crura and the septum to avoid jeopardizing the viability of the prolabial flap. The result was less than satisfying, with a tiny columella, a broad tip and flared alae. At the level of the lip an excess of height, with too-high implanted alar

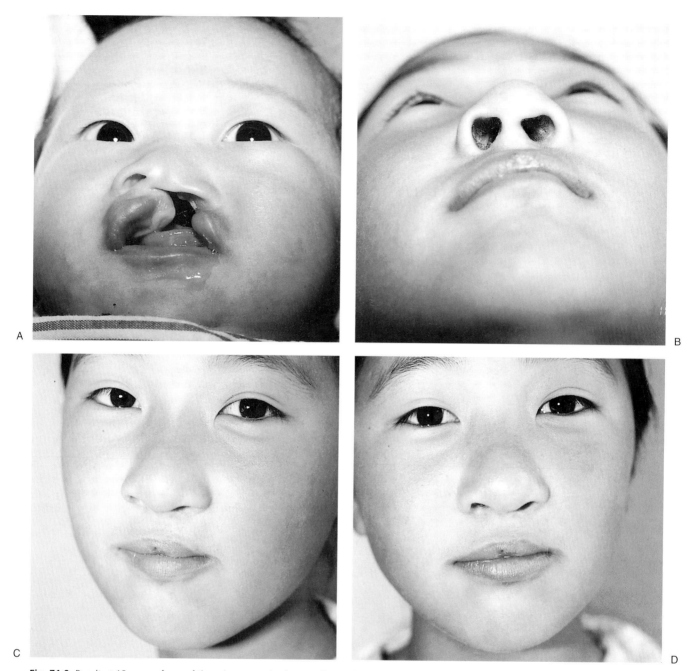

Fig. 71.9 Result at 12 years of age of the primary repair of a complete unilateral cleft lip and palate (minor revision of the alar rim and reposition of the septum at 9 years of age).

bases, was usual. In the worst cases the medial crura were pulled inferoposteriorly and a strong web inside either nostril pulled the alar domes apart from the septum. The complete bilateral cleft is a remarkable testing ground for different techniques of primary repair of the complete unilateral cleft. Among them, only the most anatomic and logical techniques can be associated in a bilateral synchronous lip and nasal repair, without increasing in a caricaturist way their own typical deformities. For example, in unilateral clefts the Z-plasty technique, closely related to Tennison's method,

may look quite good when the scars are inconspicuous. However, a Z-plasty is not necessary to achieve an adequate lip height and the scar goes through the philtrum without justification. In primary bilateral complete cleft lip and nose repair it is simply impossible to close the two clefts in the same step using Z-plasty, and after repair in two successive procedures the natural tendency to an excessive lip height in bilateral cleft is especially striking with Z-plasty.

Evolution of ideas about the pathogenesis of the short columella

The usual teaching was that there is a skin defect in the columella and that the solution was to bring tissue into it. The most popular technique was the forked flap procedure described by Millard,[42] taking the tissue from the lateral prolabium to bring it into the columella. In primary surgery the forked flaps are 'banked' either in or below the nasal sill, from where they are secondarily redeemed to be incorporated into the columella.

In secondary surgery the forked flaps are taken from the typically wide prolabium and transposed directly.

Another way is to take secondary tissue from the nose. The most common technique, described by Cronin,[43] is a medial rotation of bilateral bipedicled flaps from the nasal floor and alae.

These primary or secondary procedures have in common their own scars and distortions. Most techniques create a transverse scar in the columellar labial junction. With the two lateral vertical scars, and the inferior horizontal scar of the cupid's bow reconstructed by two lateral cutaneovermilion mucosal flaps, the philtrum is circumscribed by a square scar. Even if the result looks quite good at rest, these scars frequently become obvious with smiling, especially the transverse scars. It is difficult to achieve a natural nasolabial angle: it may be too sharp and retracted when smiling, or obtuse at rest, with a drift of the columellar base into the upper lip, contributing to an elongated lip.

The columella itself may be unnatural, too thin or too wide. An excess of length with growth is possible when the forked flap is performed in early childhood, as stressed by Pigott.

The new concept: the columella is inside the nose

In bilateral clefts there is frequently a need for a reduction of enlarged nostrils by excision of the alar bases, which improves the flared and everted look. This indication is unknown in unilateral cases, where the repaired nostril is rather smaller than the contralateral one, and induces one to think about the cause of such enlarged nostrils. The most logical explanation is that skin has been brought into the columella from the lip after an incorrect analysis of the defect. In fact, the circumference of the nostril is normal and the columella is inside the nose, but has more or less completely disappeared into its broad tip.

From an anatomic point of view the bilateral complete cleft nasal deformity is a reproduction of the unilateral complete cleft nasal deformity but on both sides. The very protruding premaxilla increases the effect of separation on the midline. On either side the alar cartilages are pulled apart from the septum, with the same degree of deformity as can be seen in the most severe complete unilateral cleft. For this reason, the features of a complete unilateral cleft lip nose deformity are at their maximum in bilateral clefts, especially in those with a short columella and the splayed medial crura and genua.

The posterior retraction and fall of the facial envelope explains the ptosis and eversion of the vestibular lining and the lowering of the lower lateral cartilage from its normal position overlying the upper lateral cartilage. On either side, the forward sliding displacement of the transverse muscle forces the lateral crura to torque inferomedially.

During recent years a few attempts have been made to primarily correct the nasal deformity at the same time as the repair of the lip on both sides.

McCoomb tried a primary forked flap procedure to lengthen the columella before closing the bilateral cleft lip in a second step.[34] However, 15 years later he became dissatisfied with this and published a primary open approach to the alar cartilages, with a V-Y lengthening of the columella, that is an interesting demonstration in favor of the concept that the columella is inside the nose. To prevent skin necrosis the synchronous repair of the lip is limited to a long lip adhesion.[35]

Cutting[44] is in favor of bringing tissue from the lip into the columella with an ingenious unwinding prolabial flap. It is a very inventive technique that does not completely eliminate the risk of a secondary scar in the nasolabial angle to correct asymmetry. However, today there are too many arguments in favor of the concept of 'the columella being inside the nose to follow Cutting.

Since Morel Fatio,[37] Broadbent & Woolf,[36] the way is definitely open with the work of Mulliken,[38,39] who has evolved toward a synchronous primary repair of the complete bilateral cleft lip and nasal deformity with a semi-open approach to the alar cartilages and some trimming of the redundant vestibular lining.

Like McCoomb and Cutting, Mulliken needs a good correction of the maxillary arch prior to surgery, and uses the pin-retained Georgiade Latham appliance. The Alo Setar experience of Trott[40] has convinced me that the primary synchronous repair of the complete bilateral cleft lip and nasal deformity is feasible in every circumstance and in countries without preoperative orthopedics. Now, reassured as to the quality of the blood supply to the prolabial flap during a synchronous repair, with a semi-open approach to the nose and an unprepared maxillary arch, I have been doing synchronous repairs for more than 2 years.

Nevertheless, I have made substantial modifications from my own experience of the anatomy and the surgical correction of the complete unilateral cleft lip nasal deformity.

The following principles should be emphasized:

- The primary synchronous repair of bilateral complete cleft lip and nasal deformity should be feasible in every socioeconomic circumstance and country, and as a correct concept should be available everywhere.
- No preoperative orthopedics, the best orthopedic treatment being a balanced muscular repair with a patent airway and as little scarring as possible. Indeed, for cleft palate teams where preoperative orthopedics are available the primary surgical treatment is the same, but with the risk of closing and locking too early the bony cleft in the only area where there is always a primary hypoplasia in relation to the lateral incisor.
- Synchronous repair of the bilateral complete cleft lip and nasal deformity without an open approach, to avoid jeopardizing the viability of the prolabium and to limit unnecessary scars, with their own complications, retractions and distortions.
- Dissection of the nasal cartilages under the perichondrium, beginning medially on the septum and laterally on the caudal end of the lateral crura. The dissection is precise, without exposure of the lower lateral cartilage, especially the dome and medial crura, and does not threaten the blood supply to the prolabial flap. The nasal mucosa is elongated, particularly between the upper and lower lateral cartilages. The retraction of the perichondrium which hinders the rounding of the dome should be ruptured subcutaneously to allow complete unfolding of this embedded area in front of the top of the nasal web.
- Reposition secured by custom-made appliances, without dead space. The inner and external splinting, adjusted with precision, can secure the projection of the dome and drape the redundant vestibular lining in the proper position without trimming. In the absence of direct sutures between the ipsilateral upper and lower cartilages, redraping the vestibular lining inside the nose may preserve the length of the nose.
- Complete repositioning of the alar bases of the nostrils, on both horizontal and vertical axes. This last point, stressed by Mulliken in his previous papers, is very important, not only to correct the flared nostrils, but to push up the domes by the elasticity of cartilaginous arches whose bases are gathered in the proper position. It is also important to prevent a too high position of the alar bases, with excessive lip height. Nevertheless, an ideal and stable transverse position of the alar bases is difficult to achieve as there is a strong tendency to relapse.

PRIMARY CORRECTION OF BILATERAL CLEFT LIP AND NASAL DEFORMITY IN A SYNCHRONOUS REPAIR

Twenty-five years ago I adopted Millard's design, with a cutaneovermilion mucosal flap on both sides to reconstruct the cupid's bow. With 20 years' experience I have come back to techniques that preserve the cutaneovermilion junction of the prolabium, for two reasons:

- To achieve the ideal white roll of the cupid's bow, we need to incorporate this particular structure from the lateral lip elements. It is a sacrifice that reduces the final length of the lip from one commissure to the other when it is already too tight.
- The transverse scar along the cupid's bow gives a good appearance at rest, but is frequently obvious with smiling, and this defect increases with age. In practice, only an unscarred cupid's bow is perfect.

INCISIONS (Fig. 7.10)

The medial prolabial flap is 6–8 mm wide. On either side the lateral prolabial flaps are no longer 'banked' but are trimmed at the end of the operation and sutured to the alar bases to build the nasal sill.

Just behind the lateral prolabial flap is designed an additional mucosal flap, taken from the lateral aspect of the premaxilla with a superior pedicle based on the columella, which is itself separated from the septum for a few millimeters. This second flap is included in a back-cut of the septal mucosa, just below the junction of the upper lateral cartilages with the septum. It provides a lining to the area of the dome and assists in lengthening of the columella by protecting the foot plates from the posteroinferior pulling usually observed when the lip is closed on both sides. This flap is easy to handle as the rotation is less than 90 degrees, and is very useful. This flap has another important advantage: it allows control of the position of the nasolabial angle and hinders the drift of the columella into the upper part of the lip.

On both sides the cutaneous incisions are the most simple, and preserve as much as possible the dry mucosa that will reinforce the central vermilion.

DISSECTION

This step of the operation is the key to a complete and stable repair where muscles and nasal cartilages find their normal relationships.

On both sides, after a back-cut in the labial sulcus, a wide

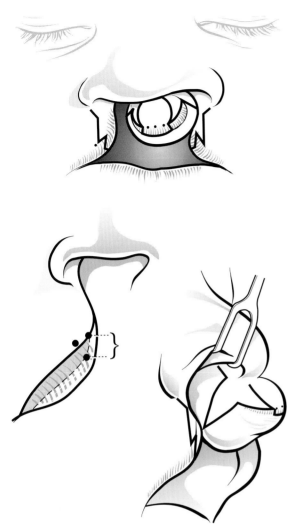

Fig. 71.10 Primary repair of bilateral complete cleft lip and palate. **(A)** Incisions on the prolabium and on the lateral lip elements. **(B)** Detail of the lateral incision to preserve the dry mucosa. **(C)** Marking of the additional mucosal flap undermined from the lateral aspect of the premaxilla, and of the back-cut in the septal mucosa just below the upper lateral cartilage.

subperiosteal undermining on the lateral segment of the maxilla from the malar area to the nasal bone and from the orbital rim to the piriform aperture allows the advancement of the cheek and the lateral part of the lip to the midline. Along the piriform aperture the nasal mucosa is widely undermined from the medial wall of the maxilla.

On the midline (Fig. 71.11), the prolabial flaps and the posterior mucosal flaps are undermined without touching the periosteum on the anterior aspect of the premaxilla. A short cut is made between the septum and the columella, and the perichondrium of the inferior border of the septum is incised to open the way for the Freer's dissector, for a wide subperichondrial undermining of the septum and its junction with the two upper lateral cartilages. A precise dissection exposes their two sides and joins the piriform aperture

laterally. The mucosa between the upper and lower cartilages is elongated. The dissection is resumed from the piriform aperture and begins on the caudal end of the lower lateral cartilage. The superficial face of the lateral crura is widely separated from the skin without exposure, and its inner face is slightly undermined along the cephalic border. A last undermining is made along the ridge of the nasal web, where the vestibular lining is separated from the caudal border of the lateral crura up to the dome. The dome itself is not dissected, but the blunt end of any instrument – a skin hook, for example, – can be pushed up its inferior face to round it by rupture of the perichondrium, which locks the retracted shape. The skin between the nasal web and the nostril rim is also undermined to allow a complete redraping of the vestibular lining.

To preserve the blood supply to the prolabial flap, no dissection is made on the midline between the medial crura and the dome.

Laterally, a back-cut is made in the vestibular lining close to the piriform aperture to allow elevation of the alar base and of the lower lateral cartilage. A mucosal flap from the lateral lip element will provide the lining needed.

MUCOSAL SUTURES

The mucosal flap from the lateral part of the premaxilla is included in the back-cut of the septal mucosa, just below the upper lateral cartilage. Then the nasal floor is repaired and the labial mucosa of the sulcus sutured laterally, and approximated to the mucosa of the premaxilla.

MUSCULAR REPAIR (See Fig. 71.11b)

The myrtiform head of the nasalis muscle, which is the deeper muscle in front of the nasal fold, is sutured to the lateral aspect of the premaxilla. To secure this suture it is wise to tighten it on the mucosa of the labial sulcus, but only after the more superficial suture of the two orbicularis muscles in front of the midline is completed. At the same time, the suture of the nasalis muscle will deepen the nasal floor and the labial sulcus.

The superior suture of the orbicularis muscle is suspended to the fibrous tissue of the septal area just in front of the anterior nasal spine. A strong suture takes the dermis of both alar bases, and is passed through the fibrous tissue in front of the anterior nasal spine. Care must be taken when tightening this suture, to correct as best as possible the interalar width close to 24 mm, as stressed by Mulliken, who also emphasizes the vertical positioning of the nostril.

The vertical distension between the alar base and the lateral white roll should be corrected by vertical compression of

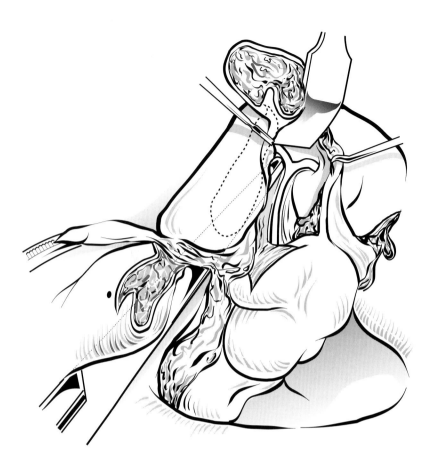

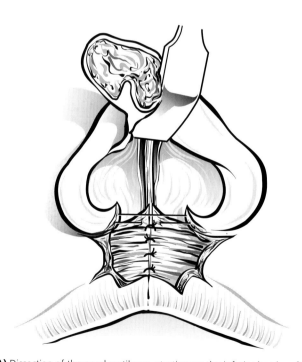

Fig. 71.11 (A) Dissection of the nasal cartilages, starting on the inferior border of the septum. The septum and the two upper lateral cartilages are denuded on both sides. The perichondrium is undermined far laterally and the undermining is resumed from the piriform aperture and extended along the superficial side of the lower lateral cartilage and its cephalic and caudal border. **(B)** Muscular suture of the orbicularis oris suspended to the anterior nasal spine, and suture between the alar bases and the anterior nasal spine.

the different planes. Usually the previous crossing suture of the two muscular planes is not enough in bilateral cases. To lower the alar base and control the excessive height of the lip just below the nostril, a skin excision is made on the superior edge of the lateral lip element (in a cyma shape, as described by Mulliken) and the dermis of the nostril sill is sutured to the orbicularis oris muscle, deepening the nostril sill and controlling the height of the lateral lip element.

BUILDING THE PHILTRUM

The prolabial flap is inserted between the two lateral lip elements and the central vermilion is made from three pieces of dry mucosa, with meticulous suturing.

SECURING THE CORRECTION OF THE NASAL DEFORMITY (Fig. 75.12)

After completion of the suturing of either nasal sill, the lower lateral cartilages and the vestibular lining are ready to configure the nasal tip. As in unilateral complete cleft, a custom-made appliance is placed in each nostril and the first step is to lengthen the columella from the base to the tip, using two or three through-and-through sutures from

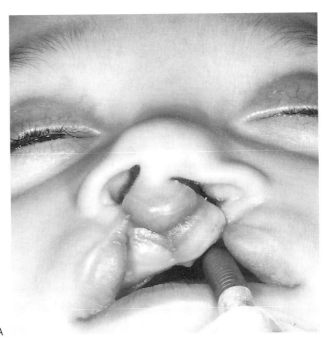

A

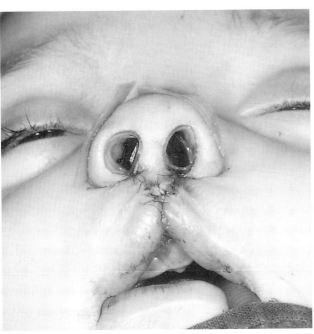

B

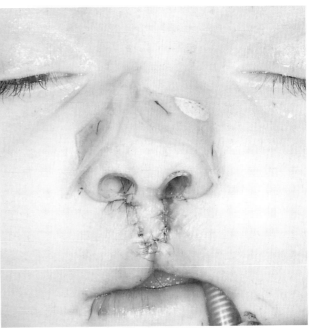

C

Fig. 71.12 The custom-made appliances are placed to secure the repositioning of the lower lateral cartilages and lengthen the columella.

one side to the other, along the posterior edge of the medial crura and the genua. The principle is then to push the vestibular lining inside the nose to deepen the concavity of the nasal fold in front of the alar base, and to elevate the lateral crura and re-establish its normal overlaping position with regard to the upper lateral cartilage.

The additional use of an external piece of silastic allows closure of the dead space and ensures good contact between the alar cartilages with the skin and the vestibular lining, a condition which minimizes the scar and is a promise of stability. Any trimming of skin and vestibular lining is unnecessary, as it is easy to observe after removal of the

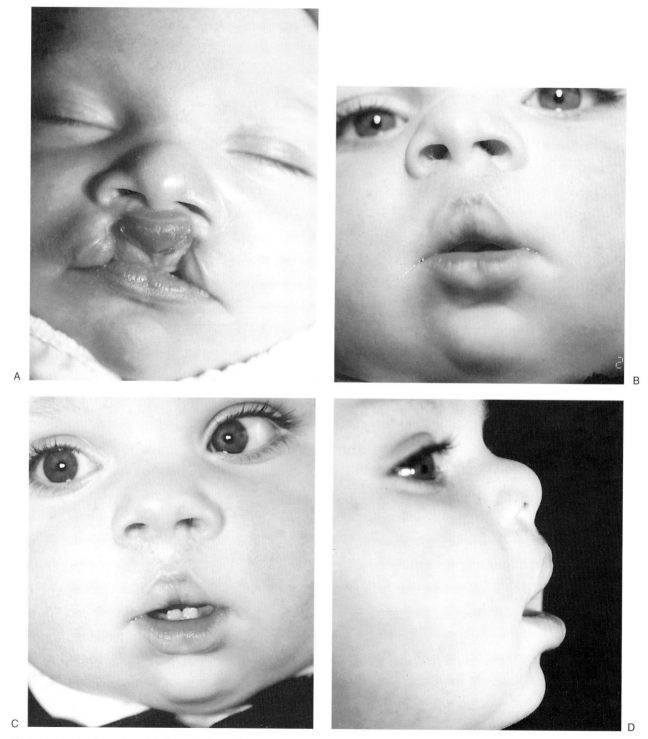

Fig. 71.13 Bilateral complete cleft lip and palate with Simonard's bands. Results 6 month after synchronous repair of the lip, the columella and the soft palate.

appliances 6 or 7 days later that there is no excess of tissue. It is probably important to respect the vestibular lining and redrape it to stabilize the shape of the nasal tip, and to preserve the best nasal valve mechanism possible, with independence between the upper and lower lateral cartilages. Another point to consider is that with this technique the vestibular lining is rolled inside the nose, but the external skin can be lengthened. So we do not have the shortening of the nose that usually accompanies other techniques of correction (except for Trott's technique). The use of sutures

tied on a bolster is not new, but the transparency of the silastic gives good visual control during the whole procedure of remodeling, and makes it precise and reproducible as well as safe for the viability of the skin. With experience of more than 2 years this primary lengthening of the columella has been found uneventful, and its principle being similar to the correction of the deformity of the lower lateral cartilage in unilateral clefts, we believe that the outcome will be the same in bilateral clefts (Figs 71.13, 71.14).

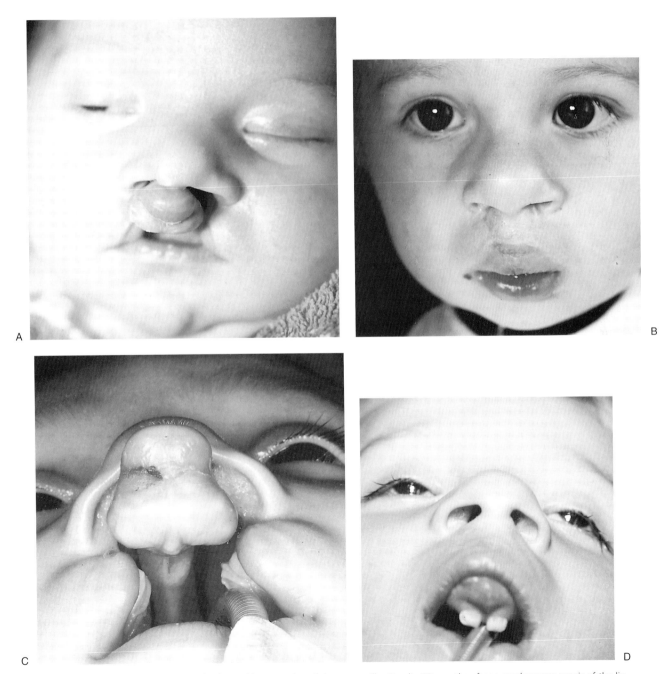

A

B

C

D

Fig. 71.14 Bilateral complete cleft lip and palate with protrusion of the premaxilla. Results 12 months after a synchronous repair of the lip, the columella and the soft palate.

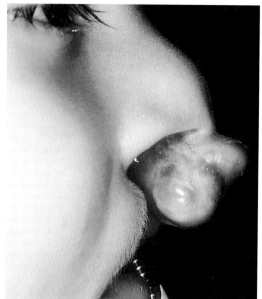

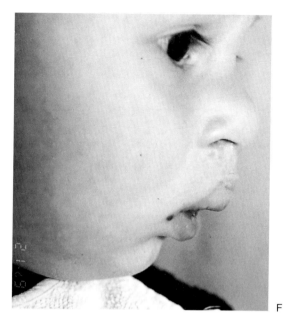

COMPLICATIONS AND SECONDARY SURGERY FOR RELAPSES AND DEFORMITIES

Nasal breathing and labial competency are prerequisites for good subsequent facial growth. Our experience is that we can expect normal development when the young patient repaired with a cleft lip and palate sleeps with his mouth closed. If this condition is not initially fulfilled, a patent airway should be reestablished as early as 6 years of age if necessary.[4–8]

NASAL BREATHING IMPAIRMENT

After more than 24 years primary surgery associated wide subperichondrial undermining of the septum and a repositioning of the lower lateral cartilage after a subcutaneous dissection, allows us to conclude that this early nasal surgery does not hinder nasal cartilage growth, nor facial growth.

SCAR CONTRACTION OF THE NOSTRIL

All small nostrils are surgical complications, but we have never seen stenosis of the nostril when prolonged primary internal splinting (4 months) was feasible. Slightly retracted nostrils are very uncommon with conventional primary splinting during the first week. The new technique of simultaneous external and internal splinting without dead space seems safer than conventional splinting. When retraction occurs it is usually limited to the nostril sill which can be corrected by a simple Z-plasty. However, in three of our oldest patients before the use of custom-made appliances, we had to repair a stenosis of the nasal valve. These patients had in common bad scarring of the lip and the use of primary forked flaps or primary Z-plasty inside the nostril.

The correction of the nostril stenosis can be effected by a simple procedure: deep incisions open the retracted scar in the nasal sill and the area of the junction of the upper lateral cartilage with the septum. These areas are grafted with cheek mucosa, and the shape of the nasal valve is modeled by a custom-made appliance as described above. If good nursing preserves the patency of the splint, it is easy to maintain it for 4 months and so prevent retraction.

RESIDUAL NASAL DEFORMITIES

Nasal breathing impairment is caused not only by retraction, but is frequently the consequence of combined deformities on the cleft side. The curtain-like obstruction of the nostril web is in contact with a convex curvature of the septum. The nasal sill is slightly retracted and too elevated, and the junction of the upper lateral cartilages is too low. On the contralateral side the inferior border of the septum is deviated toward the nostril, and the large concave curvature of the septum is filled with a very hypertrophic inferior turbinate.

On the cleft side, the constriction of the maxilla narrows the piriform aperture and the nasal floor.

INDICATIONS

After proper evaluation of the different causes, each deformity is corrected accurately and in a very conservative way. Thus in the case of a constriction of the maxilla, orthopedic expansion is carried out as early as 4 years of age. If the vertical deformity of the lateral segment of the maxilla is large, a periosteogingivoplasty before 6 years of age is followed by a spontaneous bony fusion and correction of the vertical deformity. In more conventional cases (unilateral complete cleft) the periosteogingivoplasty is performed between 8 and 12 years of age combined with a bone graft.

The deviated and deformed septum should be repositioned with as little resectioning as possible. To prevent relapse of the cleft lip septal deformity, it is frequently necessary to do a simultaneously partial resection of the hypertrophic inferior turbinate in the concavity of the septum, otherwise it would push the septum back into its previous position. The hypertrophied of the inferior turbinate, at least on the contralateral side, is an established feature of cleft patients. A bilateral hypertrophy of the inferior turbinate is also not exceptional.

The curtain-like nasal obstruction is in close relation with the deformity of the lower lateral cartilage. A marginal incision along the caudal border of the lower lateral cartilage allows good exposure of the lateral crura, the dome and the medial crura.[6] The dissection involves also the upper lateral cartilage and the septum. With a contralateral marginal incision it is possible to achieve perfect exposure of all the cartilaginous structures of the tip of the nose without any other incision, specially without an open approach. Such a bilateral dissection is sometimes useful to correct significant unilateral cleft lip nose deformity, but is always the first step in lengthening of the columella in the bilateral cleft lip nose deformity. Custom-made stents as described above are always useful to model and maintain the shape of the columella, and of the tip of the nose.

LATE NASAL CORRECTIONS

When primary surgery is performed in accordance with the anatomic and functional principles developed above, and any residual defects are corrected in early childhood, development even through the growth spurt of adolescence is usually uneventful.

By adolescence the indications for and technique of rhinoplasty are very similar to those in non-cleft patients. Deviated or unharmonious noses can be improved with the same techniques, but with caution, as there are always previous scars and some bony hypotrophy on the cleft side. These already scarred patients do not need the additional stigma of unjustified rhinoplasty.

In our opinion the recent promotion of the open approach to cleft rhinoplasty may induce surgeons to believe that the most difficult rhinoplasty is now easy, and that to pile up cartilaginous or bony grafts is enough to create a balanced nose, whereas the simple repositioning of the deformed cartilages is the best solution. To add a lot of material to reshape the nose does not give the assurance of a long-term esthetic result, and may be detrimental to the airway. Obviously well trained surgeons may have good results with the open approach, but they could surely achieve the same results without external scarring. My criticism is that inexperienced surgeons could think that this new approach changes a difficult operation into an easy one. More scars in the tip of the nose will cause additional difficulty in case of secondary revision for residual defects. It is an evident drawback of the open approach, the solution to which will often be a rhinoplasty without skin incision.

SEVERE CLEFT LIP NOSE SEQUELAE

After a correct primary muscular reconstruction of the lip and repositioning of the lower lateral cartilage, the functional approach philosophy will guide the management of the residual deformities during early childhood.

Breathing through the nose, even during sleep, is a prerequisite for normal facial growth. This assumption is far from the usual teaching. In fact, secondary alar revision, septal surgery and turbinate resection are often postponed until the late teens, when facial growth is almost complete and can no longer be influenced.

It is in this context that we encounter severe cleft lip nasal sequelae after poor primary surgery, especially at the level of the palate, with bad scarring, retraction and subsequent dysfunction.

This section on the treatment of residual cleft lip nose deformity will not be a 'cookbook' with a collection of tricks to achieve good and stable results under any circumstances. More pragmatically, it will be a logical guide towards an anatomic repair of the remaining deformity.

Despite the numerous and inventive techniques of secondary correction, with new designs, new flaps, piling up of cartilage grafts with or without an open approach, few are the adequate responses to this technique. As with post-trauma reconstructive surgery, most are used only for morphologic purposes, without a clear concept of the specific deformity and of the imperative necessity for nasal ventilation. If we except the rare cases of agressive previous surgery verging on mutilation, hypoplasia is too often a poor excuse for our bad results. In fact, there is no substantial lack of skin, muscle or cartilage. In the worst case only the lateral incisor, with its surrounding bone, is absent.

EVALUATION OF SECONDARY DEFORMITIES

As discussed earlier, in the section on primary surgery, we have to replace each structure in its correct position to restore normal anatomy. It is the way to re-establish simultaneously both morphology and function. What has not been done at the first attempt should be thus done secondarily (Figs 71.15, 71.16, 71.17).

A clear view of the deformity is essential. Both partial relapse of the original deformity and scarring and drawbacks from the previous surgery are the causes of cleft lip nasal sequelae. The first step in the treatment is a complete and precise clinical evaluation of the deformity at each level. Of course an understanding of the true nature of the defect is part of the diagnosis and will give the key to treatment.

The quality of facial growth, of the relationship between the maxilla and the mandible, and the condition of the alveolar cleft are not the subject of this chapter. However, the bony platform is such an important point, which greatly influences nasal and labial morphology, that its assessment is an important part of the diagnosis. The chronology of the different steps for correction of the maxillary deformity depends on the age of the patient and many other conditions, such as socioeconomic circumstances. In the most common cases, the secondary revision will be the opportunity to bone graft the alveolar cleft while improving esthetics and function. In the older patient, after the adolescence growth spurt, a Le Fort I osteotomy may be indicated,[45] but the simultaneous correction of the cleft lip nose deformity is a difficult challenge, especially the nose. I prefer a two-stage correction.

The clinical evaluation of the labial and nasal deformities is made difficult because the landmarks are misleading. If the vertical axis is clearly deviated toward the non-cleft side, the horizontal plane is difficult to determine. To improve judgment changing the angle of vision is very useful, as it is surprising to see how different and more acute is the perception of the asymmetry when the examining physician, placed behind and above the patient, inverts the image. The same effect can be obtained with a mirror.

The horizontal reference we have to re-establish is the line of the alar bases. This will be the datum line to appreciate the asymmetry of the nostril rims or of the domes above, and of the height of the lip below. The cupid's bow should be horizontal, but also the height of the lip must be measured laterally between the alar bases and the white roll along the vermilion, as it is almost always higher on the cleft side. At each level symmetry of the landmarks with respect to the midline is assessed. This concerns the alar domes, the shape of the columella, the interalar width, the nostril sills, the circumference of the nostrils, and the volume of the alar lobules. Deviation of the dorsum and of the tip of the nose, the retraction of the nasal bone and the upper lateral cartilage on the cleft side, can be appreciated.

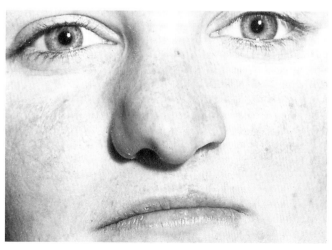
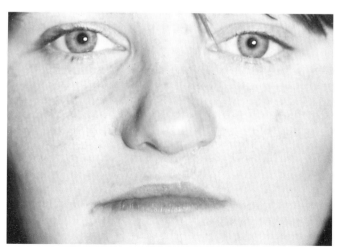

A

B

Fig. 71.15 Sequelae of a complete unilateral cleft lip and palate. Correction by complete reopening of the cleft and simultaneous muscular repair and repositioning of the nasal cartilages. Pre-A,C,E and Post-B, D, F

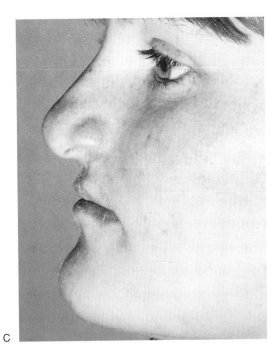

C

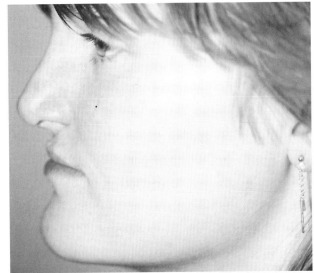

D

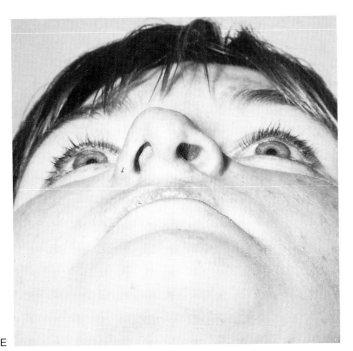

E

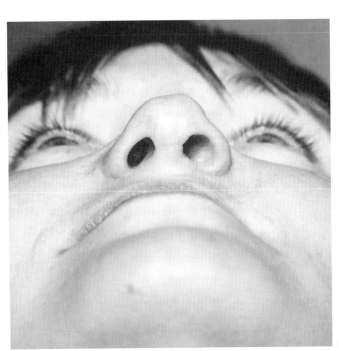

F

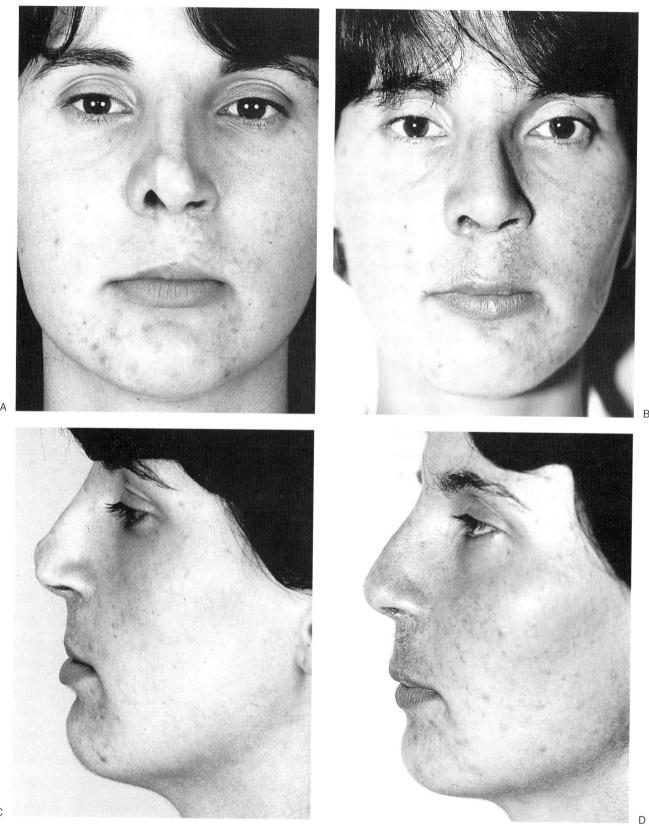

Fig. 71.16 Sequelae of a complete unilateral cleft lip and palate. Correction in two steps: after a complete reopening of the cleft the muscular repair was associated with cartilage repositioning. In a second step an Abbe flap was achieved to balance the two lips. Pre-A, C and Post B, D.

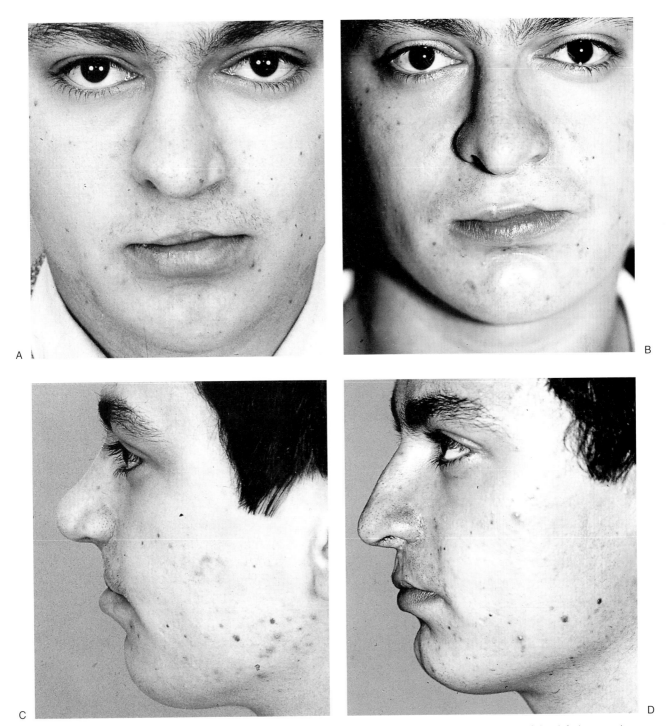

A
B
C
D

Fig. 71.17 Sequelae of a complete unilateral cleft lip and palate. Correction in three steps: after a complete reopening of the cleft the muscular repair was associated with cartilage repositioning. In a second step a rhinoplasty was necessary to achieve a more balanced nose. The third step was an Abbe flap.

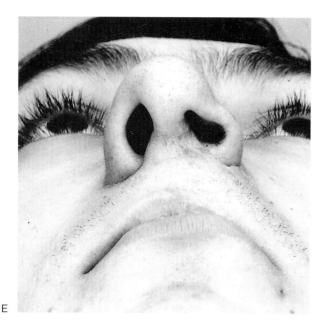

E

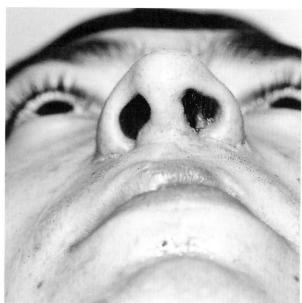

F

An important point to consider when making the decision regarding secondary revision is the quality of the lip repair, as a combined lip/nose may be the best way of correcting the greatest number of defects.[46] When the defects are recognized and the surgeon is involved in the whole treatment of the cleft lip and palate, from the first operation to the end result, a secondary revision with a complete reopening of the cleft is the opportunity to correct the asymmetry at each level.[6] Too often the surgeon, like the patient, focuses on the nose, ignoring the lip with a poor muscular repair, a flat look, a depressed scar and asymmetrical positioning of the alar bases, on the pretext of not re-entering the lip for fear of worsening the scar. An excellent scar with a poor morphologic result is proof that the patient has a good aptitude for unnoticeable scars even if the repair has been technically less than ideal. Why should the scar be worse if the surgery is more skilfully carried out, especially with a better muscular repositioning and less skin tension?

The suppleness of the lip and its aptitude for smiling, whistling, pouting and grimacing will be a crucial step in the evaluation. During motion, the deformities and the scars are usually more noticeable. This will encourage the surgeon to improve the repair through a complete reopening and with precise management, to reduce as much as possible the number and extent of the final scars.

The functional assessment also considers nasal ventilation.[2-8] Its clinical evaluation, especially during sleep, is of a greater value than any measure of airflow and nasal resistance. The main goal of treatment should be to restore the nasal airway to break the patient of the habit of mouth breathing by correcting the retracted scars of the nostril sill and the nasal floor; the deformity of the septal cartilage and the vomer; the hypertrophy of the inferior turbinate, particularly in the septal concavity of the non-cleft side (and sometimes on the cleft one); the vertical shortening of the nasal valve, with lowering of the upper lateral cartilage and elevation of the nostril floor; and the curtain-like obstruction of the nasal valve raised by the oblique ridge of the caudal border of the rotated lower lateral cartilage.

HOW TO DECIDE ON A COMPLETE REOPENING OF THE CLEFT

If both alar bases are in good symmetry with regard to the midline transversally and vertically, and the lip needs only minor revision, it will be enough to perform a secondary rhinoplasty without re-entering the lip. In this particular case we are in the situation discussed earlier, regarding immediate follow-up of the primary surgery. To restore nasal ventilation by septal surgery, turbinectomy or additional repositioning of the lower lateral cartilage through a marginal incision is an adequate response to the most common problem. When correcting the deviation of the dorsum in the same step, the surgeon should be aware of the frequent hypotrophy of the ascending process of the maxilla on the cleft side, where a lateral osteotomy is not always necessary.

On the contrary, asymmetrical implantation of the alar

bases (usually too high and retracted on the cleft side), depressed and enlarged or scarred and narrowed nostril sills, associated with a noticeable labial defect as regards height, flat look, poor adjustment of the white line or of the thickness of a lateral vermilion, and bad scarring, are the indications to completely reopen the cleft, especially if there is an anterior fistula of the bony alveolar cleft with insufficient underlying bone support and remaining cleft gingiva.

COMPLETE REVISION OF THE UNILATERAL CLEFT LIP NOSE DEFORMITY

Reopening the cleft is the best way to restore the proper condition before any other treatment and to start again on a good anatomic basis.[6]

Incision (Fig. 71.18)

If the labial scar is vertical, a simple excision will be the solution to reopen the cleft. In our opinion, rotation of the philtrum and advancement of the lateral lip are the basic principles of unilateral repair. When the scar is a Z-plasty it may be good to turn it into a Millard design if the cutaneous sacrifice to eliminate the horizontal scar remains reasonable. However, a compromise to shorten the horizontal scar and simultaneously preserve a good suppleness of the lip is often necessary.

Dissection (Fig. 71.19)

This is probably the most important step, which justifies the whole procedure, as only completely freed structures can be moved and fixed in their proper anatomic relationships.

As in primary surgery the bony cleft, the nasal cartilages and the muscles are exposed by a wide subperiosteal and

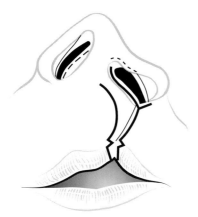

Fig. 71.18 Incision in a complete reopening of the unilateral cleft. The most usual design is vertical, even if the previous scar is a Z-plasty.

subperichondrial undermining then mobilized and repositioned.

On the lateral side the lip and the cheek are elevated from the underlying lateral maxillary segment. The lateral nasal mucosa and the vestibular lining of the nostril are separated from the maxilla. A back-cut in the vestibular lining along the piriform aperture allows advancement of the cheek and of the alar base toward the midline. On the premaxilla, the dissection preserves enough fibrous tissue on the lateral part of its anterior aspect and in the area of the anterior nasal spine to allow a strong reinsertion of the lateral muscles.

The septum and the vomer are exposed on both sides. As in primary surgery, the lower and upper lateral cartilages are separated from the overlying skin through a double approach from the piriform aperture and from the midline. The caudal end of the lateral crura is separated from its fibrous connections with the periosteum of the piriform aperture. A marginal, or more precisely an infracartilaginous, incision extended inferiorly along the caudal border of the lower lateral cartilage is often useful to complete the dissection of the whole lower lateral cartilage. It is thus possible to free the folded dome embedded in a fibrous perichondrium. When the perichondrium of the superficial side and of the cephalic border of the lower lateral cartilage is excised, the dome rounds up like a flower opening. At the end of the dissection, the vestibular lining and its attached lower lateral cartilage is completely separated from the superficial skin. The only differences between the primary surgery and the complete secondary revision are, in the latter case, the retraction of the previous scars and the direct approach, which allows a better freeing of the dome. When the surgeon is struggling against a Tennison Z-plasty, scars along the white roll, or any of the numerous nasal scars of an open approach or primary 'trimming' along the nostril rim, he will understand that unjustified incisions during primary surgery have serious drawbacks and will reject such procedures.

The repair from the bone to the skin

The bony cleft
The repair starts with the bony cleft being closed on its nasal, palatal and gingivovestibular sides and bone grafted if necessary. We consider the iliac crest to be the best donor site.

Sometimes the mucosal incisions of the lip and in the area of the bony cleft have to be adapted to the local conditions.

When the alveolar cleft is in good approximation the best solution is to perform a gingivoperiosteoplasty. Indeed,

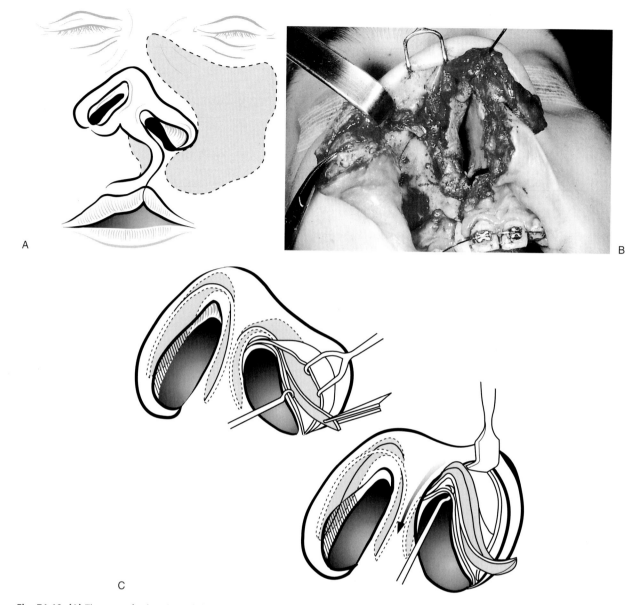

Fig. 71.19 (A) The area of subperiosteal dissection in a complete revision of a unilateral cleft. **(B)** Laterally, wide subperiosteal undermining and a back-cut along the piriform aperture allow the advancement of the cheek and of the lateral lip toward the septum. In the midline the dissection preserves enough fibrous tissue on the lateral part of the premaxilla, and in the area of the anterior nasal spine, to allow a strong reinsertion of the lateral muscles. Through the dissection of the bony cleft and a unilateral interseptocolumellar incision, the septum and the vomer are undermined on either side, as is the cleft side upper lateral cartilage. **(C)** The lower lateral cartilage is widely undermined from the skin and separated from the other cartilages through an infracartilaginous incision.

such a procedure necessitates another kind of dissection, preserving the continuity of the gingiva with the mucosa of the sulcus, and should be planned before starting the incision.

It is also important to preserve and enlarge the excision of the labial scar and turn it into a mucosal island flap[6] (Fig. 71.20) to provide more lining for the nostril sill and nasal floor when needed. The mucosal flap is left attached to the deep submucous plane of the lateral lip. In this last case, a 4-month nostril splinting will prevent the scar from retracting.

The septum

Through complete reopening of the cleft it will be easier to expose and correct the deviated and twisted nasal septum and vomer. Repositioning, partial resection and reinforcement with cartilage grafts combine to preserve a good and symmetrical nasal support[47] but at the same time smooth out the sharp angulation of the septovomerian junction in the cleft side and the cartilaginous curves with luxation of the caudal border on the non-cleft nostril. In a few cases the resection of the vomer must involve the posterior nasal spine to open the cleft nasal fossa.

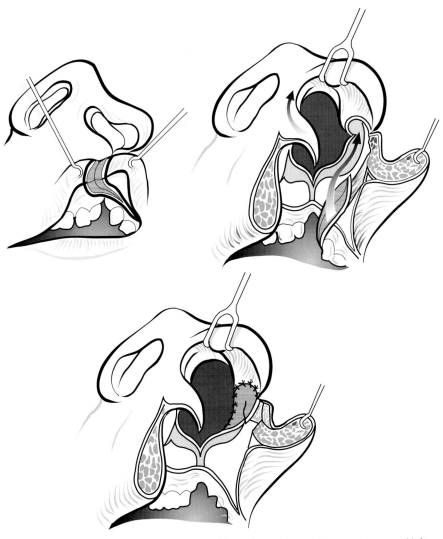

Fig. 71.20 A lateral mucosal island flap is saved from the excision of the scarred tissue and left attached to the deep submucous plane of the lateral lip. This flap provides extra lining to the nostril floor.

Sometimes on the cleft side, the vertical hypertrophy of the inferior turbinate needs to be reduced. Much more frequently the non-cleft side inferior turbinate is huge and fills the concavity of the septum. Its partial resection is necessary to prevent the septum from complete relapse and to clear the airway. The resected septal cartilage and bone are preserved for grafting if necessary.

The muscles

Thanks to the wide subperiosteal dissection and the back-cut of the vestibular lining along the piriform aperture, it is easy to advance the cheek, the alar base and the lip toward the midline, in order to repair as anatomically as possible the different muscular planes of the lip, and to replace the lower lateral cartilage in its normal position overlying the

upper lateral cartilage. The best way to know how to correct each defect is to be involved in the primary surgery, with a clear vision of the pathologic anatomy of the muscles and of the subsequent nasal cartilages deformities, so that at each level the surgeon understands where the muscle repair has been incorrect and how to free and reposition the structures concerned. Experience and expertise in this field are indispensable. Details of the muscular repair technique are to be found in the section on primary repair.

The majority of surgeons exaggerate the role of the skin this is the most common fault of the plastic surgeon. They should know that the height of the lip, the vertical and transverse position of the alar base, the level of the nostril sill, the shape of the philtrum, and the depth of the labial sulcus are all direct consequences of the muscular repair.

Indeed, to influence morphology by muscle repair in an area where the muscles have close connections with the dermis, we should respect these connections and limit the dissection between the muscle and the skin or the mucosa to the immediate proximity of the cleft.

A wide subcutaneous dissection of the muscles is inadequate, as it hinders a sharp repositioning of the landmarks. Mobilization of the muscles, allowing their repositioning, must be by wide subperiosteal undermining.

Subperiosteal undermining, after experimental studies, especially in beagles and rabbits[9–11] has been considered harmful to subsequent growth. Mainly for this reason many surgeons have missed the best means to advance the retracted facial envelope toward the midline and so to reposition anatomically, without tension, the muscles in the area of the cleft.

A recent study in the rabbit[48] has shown that wide subperiosteal undermining on the anterior aspect of the maxilla without other work, especially without creating a cleft by removing bone, does not interfere with facial growth, whereas the same extensive undermining between the periosteum and the muscles in the same circumstances hinders facial growth. As the blood supply to the periosteum is provided from the muscles, this conclusion is not surprising, and confirms my clinical experience of over 25 years with cleft patients. The periosteum is the interface between the bone and the facial envelope, but the periosteum is part of the facial envelope. The only way to restore the normal relationship of the retracted facial envelope with the structures of the midline is to advance the whole facial envelope, widely undermined subperiosteally from the lateral maxillary segment. Another confirmation of the favorable influence of mobilization of the whole facial envelope, with its periosteum, is the early periosteogingivoplasty. Before 6 years of age, in the bilateral cleft with an important vertical deformity between the premaxilla and the lateral maxillary segment. There is a spontaneous horizontalization and fusion of the maxillary arch. It seems that the bone, after a short delay, follows the displacement of the facial envelope.

The nasal repair

A final important point is that the usual teaching, especially for ENT surgeons, is that the septal and in general the nasal surgery must be postponed until the age of 15 so as not to interfere with nasal cartilage growth and facial growth. Other specialists, such as orthodontists, know that nasal breathing is necessary for good facial growth. At the beginning of this chapter we discussed the importance of the facial envelope, which controls the nasal valve and regulates nasal ventilation. We must remember that the functional adaptation of the facial envelope when there is a nasal obstruction is always unfavorable to the transverse development of the maxillary arch at the lateral incisor level. This knowledge is important in cleft patients, who are often predisposed by the primary surgery to nasal airway obstruction for anatomic reasons, and as a consequence of scarring in the area of the nasal valve. Nasal ventilation even during sleep is necessary for normal facial growth, secondary to good positioning of the tongue and perfect labial competency. To turn the habit of oral ventilation in a young patient into nasal ventilation requires efficient restoration of the nasal airway early enough in childhood to permit re-education before the labial incompetency worsens, as this will worsens by the increasing anterior facial height. Effective improvement of the nasal airway, confirmed by measurement of airflow and nasal resistance, will be possible only if the habit of nasal ventilation is associated with good tongue positioning and labial competency. In our opinion, the nasal obstruction should be assessed by clinical examination and treated by adequate and conservative repositioning and resectioning as early as 6 years of age.

Fixation of the nasal cartilages

With increasing experience, I am convinced that the quality of the nasal correction depends more on the extent of cartilage freeing and on the muscular repair of the nostril sill than on complex fixation procedures. When both bases of the alar cartilage are in their proper position, the elasticity of the freed alar dome rounds up and projects the tip of the nose. I no longer use direct sutures,[6] preferring to combine internal and external splinting, exactly as in primary surgery. This technique is more precise especially to lengthen the columella, to give to the dome its normal position overlying the upper lateral cartilage, and to deepen the nasal fold. At the same time it is possible to maintain the septum and to control the length of the nose, as with this technique the skin may be lengthened while the vestibular lining is rolled inside. All the details of double splinting are to be found in the section on primary surgery.

The residual deformities after complete unilateral reopening

Even after long experience, the immediate result of a complete reopening of the cleft lip nose deformity is rarely perfect. If most defects have disappeared the less inconspicuous ones become more acute, and must be reevaluated on the lip and on the nose. Each can be improved in a tertiary revision.

Residual alar drooping is one of the most common defects. As a result of incomplete freeing of the lower lateral cartilage, the alar dome is pushed down by the caudal rim of the upper lateral cartilage, or sometimes by the deviated caudal end of the septum. In some cases, the alar drooping is associated with a residual oblique ridge inside the nostril, caused by the rotated caudal border of the lateral crura. The best solution is to treat the real cause of the defect by a new dissection of the lower lateral cartilage using a marginal incision approach. A tiny resection, or repositioning of the caudal septum or of the caudal end of the upper lateral cartilage, followed by nostril splinting, is often enough to lift the alar dome into the proper position. In some cases, especially in everted nostrils, there is an excess of skin and subcutaneous tissue along the caudal border of the lateral crura. In this particular case, it might be wise to place the lateral part of the infra-cartilaginous incision inside the nostril a few millimeters more anteriorly along the cartilage, so that this excess can be trimmed just before closure. The advantage of such an anatomic correction is to respect the normal vestibular concavity of the dome and the delicate curvature of the alar rim at its junction with the columella. The nostril rim is a landmark and should not be violated. An unscarred alar rim is more precise, mobile and natural. The temptation of most surgeons is to lift the alar rim by trimming the skin in this area.[22] In our opinion it is better to respect the normal anatomy, and any adjustment in this area must be very conservative. Other surgeons, inspired by Tajima,[22,49–52] rather than trimming the skin of the alar margin have incorporated this ellipse of skin in a 'reverse U' flap, which is lifted into the nose by suspension to the opposite alar cartilage and to the upper lateral cartilages. Actually, Tajima's procedure is very similar to the anatomic repositioning of the lower lateral cartilage I perform through an infracartilaginous incision, but I need no extra skin from the alar margin, nor permanent cartilaginous suspension. The extent of my dissection is more important, the alar base is repositioned anatomically, and the double splinting allows simultaneous lengthening of the external skin while the vestibular lining and its lower lateral cartilage is pushed inside the nose to recreate the nasal fold and the concavity of the dome. I believe that the alar rim is a landmark to be respected, and I cannot approve the transposition of an alar rim flap into the nostril to lengthen the columella on the same side and simultaneously lift the alar rim. When this procedure is done on both sides in bilateral clefts,[53] or is associated with an onlay conchal cartilage graft on the lower lateral cartilage in unilateral cleft,[54] my feeling is the same: I think that such procedures are disconnected from the normal anatomy and are as inadequate as the creation of a dimple in the philtrum by including a conchal cartilage graft subcutaneously.

Correction of the bridge of the nose

When the dorsum of the nose is deviated with a convex curvature on the opposite side and the hump has excessive proportions, it may be necessary to perform a rhinoplasty. The surgeon should plan this procedure with the greatest care and forethought, and take a few important details into account.

The ascending process of the maxilla and the nasal bone on the cleft side are usually hypotrophic or retracted. For this reason lateral osteotomy is not always indicated on the cleft side, or must be done with the greatest care. Narrowing the nose may worsen nasal ventilation, and this risk is increased when the nasal valve is deformed by a distorted septum and by retraction from scars, as in cleft noses.

When the hump is excessive it must be adjusted only after complete stabilization of the projection of the tip of the nose. After 25 years' experience in secondary surgery of cleft lip nose, with complete reopening, wide undermining and muscular reconstruction, I am convinced that it is impossible to predict the proportion of projections of the tip of the nose and of the nasolabial angle that will persist for 6 months or a year later. For this simple reason, rhinoplasty to harmonize the nasal proportions should be done as a tertiary procedure, except for minor adjustments. In this kind of rhinoplasty, the reduction must be especially prudent. It is better to preserve a mild convexity of the dorsum to balance the nasal tip than to increase the surgical stigma of these already scarred patients by making a small nose. When removing the hump, a crushed septal cartilage graft is very useful to straighten the bridge and to hide the asymmetry of the bony nose and of the twisted septum. This grafting on bridge gives a natural look without excessive narrowing, facilitates a good balance with the tip of the nose, and preserves nasal ventilation.

The length of the nose in this kind of patient should be spared if possible, as it is better for the lip to be in the shadow of the nasal tip.[46]

At a time when the open approach is frequently advocated for difficult rhinoplasties, especially secondary and the cleft rhinoplasty,[55,56] it is necessary to explain my own choice of internal rhinoplasty with submucosal dissection by intercartilaginous or infracartilaginous incisions.

During the complete revision of the lip and the nostril, the reopening of the cleft and the unilateral interseptocolumellar incision give a good view of the septum and the upper lateral cartilages. At the same time, to gain good access to the lower lateral cartilage, an infracartilaginous or marginal incision is perfect.

In a tertiary rhinoplasty an intercartilaginous and interseptocolumellar incision on the non-cleft side, and an infracartilaginous or marginal incision on the cleft side, are enough to carry out a complete submucosal dissection and any remodeling of the bony and cartilaginous structures to correct the deviation and adjust the nasal proportions. When securing the correction with internal and external splinting, an appreciation of the morphologic result obtained by progressive repositioning of the structures is easy and clear. At each step this procedure allows good control, especially to reshape the nasal fold, to lengthen the columella, to replace the vault of the dome in its normal position overlying the upper lateral cartilage, and to balance the level of the alar rim in relation to the opposite side. The precision of remodeling by double splinting is a real advantage when the adjustment of the length of the nose and the projection of the tip is made difficult by thick skin in the supratip area.

In unilateral cleft rhinoplasty, the design of the open approach has frequently been adapted to lengthen the columella. Numerous variations have been published since the original Rethis' incision, modified by Erich, Potter, Bardach, Spira, Cronin and many others.[55,56] The essential aim of the external approach is to suture the alar cartilages under direct vision, and often to add grafts of cartilage. However, it is more difficult to appreciate the immediate effect of these procedures, as the elevated skin must be replaced and sutured before judging. When examining the published results, some scars remain noticeable, and the symmetry of the nostrils and the tip of the nose is incomplete, with partial relapse, which is a reflection of the insufficient freeing of the nasal cartilages. Frequently, suture of the domes creates a notch on the cleft alar rim and worsens the narrowing of the nasal valve by pulling the lateral crura toward the septum. It always shortens the nose, in contrast to internal dissection, where the double splinting allows achievement of two apparently incompatible objectives at the same time: lengthening the nose and projecting the tip. Piling up cartilage grafts to improve the look is often detrimental to the airway. The surgeon must also be a sculptor, to reshape the external nose and also to restore a normal airway. The best solution is not to build a strong and thick nose but to respect the normal anatomy, where one layer of cartilage is enough to meet both objectives. Of course it is possible to do through an open approach what we can do by a conventional internal approach, but why add an external scar if there is no evidence that this is superior, and this scar will be one more difficulty in correcting a relapse?

The last refinements (Fig. 71.21)

Careful analysis of the final result of unilateral cleft rhinoplasty often finds an asymmetry between the two alar lobules. Usually, the cleft side is smaller, especially in the front view, where its vertical height is less than on the opposite side. The best solution in this case is to reduce the non-cleft alar lobule just 1 mm above the alar facial junction.[22] The excision usually preserves the vestibular skin of the nostril, but is adapted to adjust the width of the nostril sill. The alar lobule skin excision can be used as a graft when indicated along the alar rim. I frequently use it as a dermal graft inserted in a very superficial tunnel just inside the vertical labial scar, to fill it and create the shape and volume of the philtrum.

When the height of the lip is excessive between the alar labial junction and the white roll, and the nostril sill is positioned too high, a skin island flap taken from the highest part of the lip just below the alar labial junction is transposed on a deep muscular pedicle inside the nostril sill, through a parallel incision. After closure, the effect of this is to correct the height of the lip and simultaneously to lower the nostril sill.

The particularities of secondary rhinoplasty in bilateral clefts

As in unilateral clefts, the usual defects are an association of relapse of the original deformity with scarring and drawbacks from the previous surgery. The scars of the bilateral Tennisson repair are frequently very noticeable and are a serious handicap for this method at a time when repair with vertical scars has given proof of better results with a good follow-up.

With the recent concept that the columella is inside the nose, we should achieve a new generation of results where the columella will be of normal length without scarring between the lip and the nose. Any surgeon interested in the field of secondary surgery of bilateral cleft lip nose should read the section devoted to primary surgery. In the light of the simultaneous primary repair of the lip and of the columella, it will be understood that the secondary bilateral cleft lip nose can be more often corrected by anatomic repositioning of the lower lateral cartilages through marginal incisions, both for lengthening the columella and for a better definition of the tip of the nose.

In most secondary cases the columella has already been lengthened by Millard's technique using forked flaps, or by advancement flaps from the nostril sill and alae according to Cronin. One of the usual drawbacks of these procedures is an excessive nostril circumference, with enlarged sills and

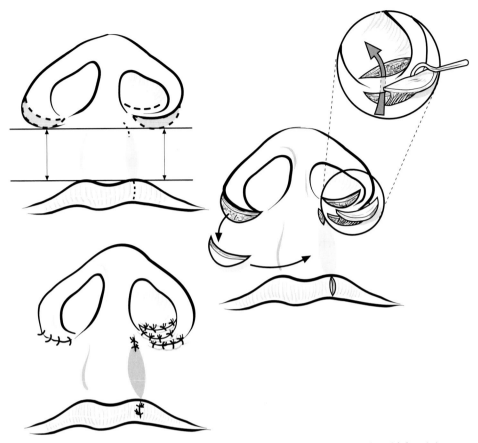

Fig. 71.21 The last refinements. On the cleft side, the excessive alar lobule is reduced **(A)** and the excised skin is prepared as a dermal graft **(B)** to be placed under the vertical scar of the lip to simulate a philtral column **(C)**. On the cleft side, the excess of height of the lateral lip **(A)** is turned into an island skin flap **(B)** to lower the nostril sill **(C)** and correct the lip at the same time.

various degrees of lengthening of the columella, from short to overlong. These enlarged nostrils must at some time be reduced. Such a phenomenon is almost unknown in unilateral cleft lip noses, and induce one to think that the columella has been lengthened after an incorrect analysis of the defect. In fact, the columella is in the broad tip of the nose, from where it can be extracted by proper repositioning of the lower lateral cartilages without any skin flap supplied from the lip.

How can a bilateral cleft lip nose previously repaired by Millard's forked flap procedure or Cronin's technique be corrected (Fig. 71.22)?

The associated defects in most cases are an excess of height of the lateral lip, between the alar lobule and the vermilion, and a poor muscular repair in the midline, with a scarred philtrum. The width of the nostril sills and the length of the columella are inadequate.

As in secondary repair of unilateral clefts, the basic aim is to restore the horizontal datum line of both alar bases, with a good muscular repair of the orbicularis oris muscle in front of the anterior nasal spine, and of the nostril sills.

It is possible to revise both sides in the same step,[6] with a complete reopening of one side, where a periosteogingivoplasty and a bone graft can be associated if necessary, and a partial repair of the soft tissue on the other side, where the vermilion is left intact to preserve the blood supply to the philtrum (Fig. 71.22). With this procedure it is easy, after wide bilateral subperiosteal undermining, to adjust the length of the columella, the width of the nostril sills and the height of the lip on either side at the same time. Both lower lateral cartilages can be freed and repositioned at the same time. The correction of the nose is done with exactly the same technique as in primary repair of the bilateral cleft, discussed in the first section of the chapter. The dissection through the midline, starting along the septum and continued on both sides of the upper lateral cartilages, is completed by an infracartilaginous approach on either nostril. The correction is maintained by double splinting.

The quality of the lip repair depends on the amount of tissue the surgeon has at his disposal, especially at the level of the white roll and the vermilion. If the lip is too tight, an Abbe flap will be indicated. The need to perform an

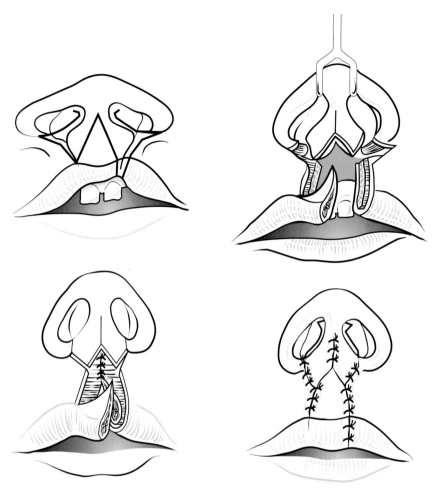

Fig. 71.22 Complete bilateral revision in a single-stage procedure. The prolabial part of the lip is left attached to the vermilion of the lateral lip on one side. A wide subperiosteal dissection on both sides allows a symetrical reconstruction of the lip, of the columella and of the nostril sills.

Abbe flap for the unilateral cleft lip nose sequelae is rare, and in this case the technique must be adapted by proper excision to place the flap in the midline to simulate the philtrum but eliminate the lateral scar as much as possible.

In bilateral sequelae a great number of patients have a tight lip, which is more frequent when the white line of the cupid's bow is reconstructed from the lateral white roll, as in Millard's technique. It is a sacrifice of at least 10 mm in a lip that is already too tight. For these reasons the Abbe flap has a good future, but we can hope it will become infrequent with the new primary surgery.

If the Abbe flap is performed to reconstruct the middle part of the lip and the columella during a complete secondary revision (Fig. 71.23), I usually prefer to do it in a tertiary step, under local anesthesia and neurolept analgesia, to avoid any lip kinking from the endotracheal tube. The best esthetic result is obtained when the Abbe flap reconstructs only the philtrum and its vermilion, in a

lip prepared to be symmetrical and where both vertical scars are excised reconstructed by a triangular flap 12 mm wide. The natural curvature of the lower lip simulates a philtral dimple, and its white roll the cupid's bow. The tip of the flap should not be placed exactly in the nasolabial angle, to avoid any depression at this level. The scar of the donor area in the center of the inferior lip is short and vertical, which is far less noticeable than a Y scar in the mentolabial fold.

Many papers have been published where the Abbe flap is used in a secondary revision without anatomic muscular repositioning, to restore at the same time the philtrum, the nostril sills and the columella, with more or less complex scars in the recipient lip and in the donor site. This is not the correct way. As little scarring as possible should be a permanent concern, especially in bilateral clefts. Cleft surgery is not like reconstructive surgery for cancer or gunshot injuries. If we except very unusual cases, the level of our

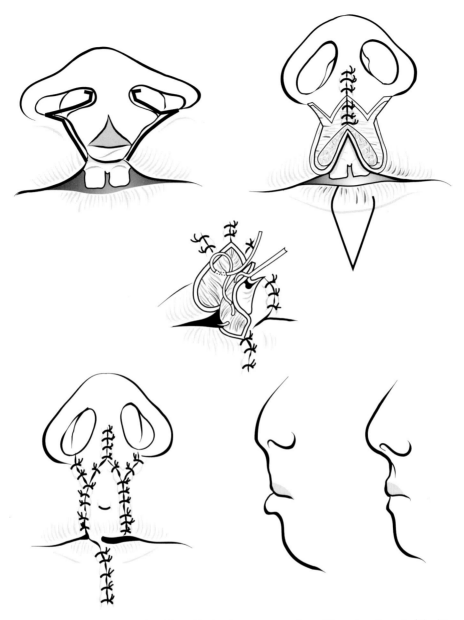

Fig. 71.23 Complete bilateral revision with simultaneous correction of the columella and of the lip by an Abbe flap.

current knowledge should make us very exigent as to the final result in cleft patients: the only acceptable scars are the vertical ones in the lip.

CONCLUSION

This chapter finishes as it began, with comment about the pathologic anatomy of cleft lip and nose. We believe that this reflects the philosophy of the functional approach.

Every surgeon involved in cleft surgery who would like to improve their results should turn their attention to the permanent role of the muscles. From their influence on the cleft lip nose deformity during fetal life, to the facial consequences of their functional adaptation to nasal obstruction in the growing patient, they are the key to many of our questions. The surgeon must learn to create muscular balance and avoid hindering the muscular work by scarring, and also to avoid functional adaptation by incorrect repositioning of the cartilaginous structures which are the support of a major function, nasal ventilation.

REFERENCES

1. Levignac J, Chalaye JC, Mahe E, Riu R 1986 Morphologie du nez. Importance du mécanisme orificiel. Annales de Chirurgie Plastique 31:309–318
2. Talmant J, Rouvre M, Thibult JL, Turpin P 1982 Contribution à l'étude des rapports de la ventilation avec la morphogénèse cranio-faciale. Déductions thérapeutiques concernant l' ODF. In: Rapport du 55è Congrès de la SFODF. Paris, Prelat
3. Talmant J 1995 Nose breathing and facial covering mechanics: a relationship orthodontists have to control. In: Bollender CJ, Bounoure G, Barat Y (eds) Extraction versus non extraction, SID, Paris, pp 74–86
4. Talmant JC 1982 La narine du bec-de-lièvre unilatéral. Peut-on concilier esthétique et ventilation normale? L'orthodontie Française 53:451–456
5. Talmant JC 1984 Correction de la narine du bec de lièvre unilatéral: ses grands principes. Annales de Chirurgie Plastique 29:123–132
6. Talmant JC 1990 Sequelles labio-narinaires des fentes labio-maxillo-palatines. In: Levignac J, Chirurgie des lèvres. Masson, Paris, pp 81–97
7. Talmant JC 1993 Nasal malformations associated with unilateral cleft lip. Scandinavian Journal of Plastic and Reconstructive Surgery and Hand Surgery 27:183–191
8. Talmant JC 1995 Reflexions sur l'étiopathogénie des fentes maxillo-palatines et l'évolution de leurs traitements. Annales de Chirurgie Plastique et Esthetique 40:639–656
9. Bardach J, Mooney M, Giedrojc-Juraha ZL 1982 A comparative study of facial growth following cleft lip repair with or without soft tissue undermining: an experimental study in rabbits. Plastic and Reconstructive Surgery 69:745–754
10. Bardach J, Bakowska J, McDermott-Murray J, Mooney M, Dusdieker L 1984 Lip pressure changes following lip repair in infant with unilateral cleft of the lip and palate. Plastic and Reconstructive Surgery 74:476–481
11. Bardach J, Kelly KM, Jakobsen MA 1988 Simultaneous cleft lip and palate repair. An experimental study in beagles. Plastic and Reconstructive Surgery 82:31–41
12. Delaire J, Precious D 1985 Avoidance of the use of vomerine mucosa in primary surgical management of velopalatine clefts. Oral Medicine, Oral Pathology 60:589–597
13. Malek R, Psaume J 1983 Nouvelle conception de la chronologie et de la technique chirurgicale du traitement des fentes labio-palatines. Résultats sur 220 cas. Annales de Chirurgie Plastique et Esthétique 28:237–247
14. Poupart B, Coornaert H, Debaere PA, Treanton AM 1983 Fentes labio-palatines: est-il loisible de laisser ouvert le palais osseux. (Etude de 62 cas avec un recul de 6 ans et plus.) Annales de Chirurgie Plastique et Esthetique 28:325–336
15. Ross RB 1987 Treatment variables affecting facial growth in complete unilateral cleft lip and palate. Cleft Palate Journal 24:3–77
16. Schweckendiek W 1979 Primary veloplasty: long term result without maxillary deformity. Cleft Palate Journal 15:268–274
17. Schweckendiek W, Kruse E 1986 Two stages palatal repair. The Marburg approach. In: Early treatment of cleft lip and palate, Hotz M (ed) Hans Huber, Berne, pp 114–118
18. Anderl H 1990 Primary unilateral cleft lip and nose reconstruction. In: Bardach J, Morris HL (eds) Multidisciplinary management of cleft lip and palate. WB Saunders, Philadelphia, pp 184–196
19. Bardach J, Cutting C 1990 Anatomy of the unilateral and bilateral cleft lip and nose. In: Bardach J, Morris HL (eds) Multidisciplinary management of cleft lip and palate. WB Saunders, Philadelphia, pp 150–159
20. McComb H 1985 Primary correction of unilateral cleft lip nasal deformity: a 10 year review. Plastic and Reconstructive Surgery 75:791–799

21. McComb H 1990 Anatomy of the unilateral and bilateral cleft lip nose. In: Bardach J, Morris HL (eds) Multidisciplinary management of cleft lip and palate. WB Saunders, Philadelphia, pp 144–149
22. Millard DR 1976 Cleft craft: the evolution of its surgery. Vol I, The unilateral deformity. Little, Brown, Boston.
23. Siegel MI, Mooney MP, Kimes KR, Gest TR 1985 Traction, prenatal development, and the labioseptopremaxillary region. Plastic and Reconstructive Surgery 76:25–28
24. Chateau JP 1976 Etudes anatomiques du complexe musculaire naso-labial. Incidences sur la chirurgie reconstructive des fentes labiales. Thèse Médicale, Nantes
25. Delaire J 1975 La cheilo-rhinoplastie primaire pour fente labio-maxillaire congénitale unilatérale. Essai de schématisation d'une technique. Revue de Stomatologie 76:193–216
26. Delaire J 1979 La cheilo-rhinoplastie fonctionnelle secondaire. Revue de Stomatologie 80:218–224
27. Kernahan DA, Dado DV, Bauer BS 1984 The anatomy of the orbicularis muscle in unilateral cleft lip based on a three-dimensional histologic reconstruction. Plastic and Reconstructive Surgery 73:875–881
28. Kimes KR, Mooney MP, Siegel MI, Todhunter J 1992 Growth rate of the vomer in normal and cleft lip and palate human fetal specimens. Cleft Palate–Craniofacial Journal 29:38–43
29. Mooney MP, Siegel MI, Kimes KR, Todhunter J 1988 Development of the orbicularis oris muscle in normal and cleft lip and palate human fetuses using three-dimensional computer reconstruction. Plastic and Reconstructive Surgery 81:336–344
30. Mooney MP, Siegel MI, Kimes KR, Todhunter J 1991 Premaxillary development in normal and cleft lip and palate human fetuses using three-dimensional computer reconstruction. Cleft Palate–Craniofacial Journal 28:49–54
31. Randall P 1992 History of cleft lip nasal repair. Cleft Palate–Craniofacial Journal 29:527–530
32. Veau V 1928 Etude anatomique du bec-de-lièvre unilatéral total. Annales d'Anatonie Pathologique et d'Anatomie Normale 5:601–632
32a. Lee ST 1988 A histological study of the piltrum. Annals Academy of Medicine 17:328–334
33. Latham RA 1973 Development and structure of the premaxillary deformity in bllateral cleft lip and palate. British Journal of Plastic Surgery 26:1–11
34. McCoomb H 1990 Primary repair of the bilateral cleft lip nose: a 15-year review and a new treatment plan. Plastic and Reconstructive Surgery 86:882
35. McCoomb H 1994 Primary repair of the bilateral cleft lip nose: a 4 year review. Plastic and Reconstructive Surgery 94:37–47
36. Broadbent TR, Woolf RM 1984 Cleft lip nasal deformity. Annals of Plastic Surgery 12:216
37. Morel-Fatio D, Lalardrie JP 1966 External nasal approach in the correction of major morphological sequellae of the cleft lip nose. Plastic and Reconstructive Surgery 38:116
38. Mulliken JB 1992 Correction of the bilateral cleft lip nasal deformity: evolution of a surgical concept. Cleft Palate–Craniofacial Journal 29:540–545
39. Mulliken JB 1995 Bilateral complete cleft lip and nasal deformity: an anthropometric analysis of staged to synchronous repair. Plastic and Reconstructive Surgery 96:9–26
40. Trott JA, Mohan NA 1993 A preliminary report on one-stage open tip rhinoplasty at the time of lip repair in bilateral cleft lip and palate. The Alo Setar experience. British Journal of Plastic Surgery 46:215–222
41. Salomonson J 1996 Preserving aesthetic units in cleft lip repair. Scandinavian Journal of Plastic and Reconstructive Surgery and Hand Surgery 30:111–120
42. Millard DR Jr 1958 Columella lengthening by a forked flap. Plastic and Reconstructive Surgery 22:454

43. Cronin TD 1958 Lengthening the columella by use of skin from nasal floor and alae. Plastic and Reconstructive Surgery 21:417

44. Cutting C, Grayson B 1993 The prolabial unwinding flap method for one-stage repair of bilateral cleft lip, nose and alveolus. Plastic and Reconstructive Surgery 91:37–47

45. Schendel SA, Delaire J 1981 Functional musculo-skeletal correction of secondary unilateral cleft lip deformities: combined lip–nose correction and Le Fort I osteotomy. Journal of Maxillofacial Surgery 9:108–116

46. Tessier P, Delbet JP, Pastoriza J, Aiaich R 1969 Sequelles labiales et nasales du bec-de-lièvre complet, chez l'adolescent. Relation avec les malformations et deformations du maxillaire. Annales de Chirurgie Plastique XIV:312–327

47. Jonsson C-E 1993 Secondary correction of the unilateral cleft nose deformity with an endonasal technique. European Journal of Plastic Surgery 16:143–148

48. Mannucci N, D'Orto O, Di Francesco A, Brusati R 1997 A comparison of the effect of supraperiosteal versus subperiosteal dissection of the growing maxilla in rabbit: an experimental study. In: Lee ST, Huang M (eds) Transactions 8th International Congress on Cleft Palate and Related Craniofacial Anomalies, Singapore, Stamford Press, pp. 125–130

49. Tajima S, Maruyama M 1977 Reverse-U incision for secondary repair of cleft lip nose. Plastic and Reconstructive Surgery 60:256–261

50. Nakajima T, Yoshimura Y, Kami T 1986 Refinement of the 'reverse-U' incision for the repair of cleft lip nose deformity. British Journal of Plastic Surgery 39:345–351

51. Tolhurst DE 1983 Secondary correction of the cleft lip nose deformity. British Journal of Plastic Surgery 36:449–454

52. Dibbel DG 1982 Cleft lip nasal reconstruction: correcting the classic unilateral defect. Plastic and Reconstructive Surgery 69:264–270

53. Van der Meulen JC 1992 Columellar elongation in bilateral cleft lip repair: Early results. Plastic and Reconstructive Surgery 89:1060–1067

54. Thomson HG 1985 The residual unilateral cleft lip nasal deformity: a three-phase correction technique. Plastic and Reconstructive Surgery 76:36–43

55. Cronin TD, Denkler KA 1988 Correction of the unilateral cleft lip nose. Plastic and Reconstructive Surgery 82:419–431

56. Tschopp HM 1988 The open sky rhinoplasty for correction of secondary cleft lip nose deformity. Scandinavian Journal of Plastic and Reconstructive Surgery 22:153–158

Evaluating outcomes – a statistician's perspective

72

COLIN CRYER

INTRODUCTION

The focus of this chapter will be the issues that need to be addressed in answering the research question: What combination of treatment and care results in the best outcomes for complete unilateral cleft lip and palate? This could be in terms of:

- What surgical interventions are the best;
- What timing;
- What sequencing;
- Effective use of ancillary services;
- The experience of the surgeon etc.
- A combination of these.

Cleft lip and palate (CLP) is a relatively rare occurrence, unusual in that the defects are major for the child and disturbing for the family, and yet are amenable to treatment with potentially good outcomes.[1] The above question is important, because deciding on the success or failure of a particular combination of treatment and care is not a simple matter. It also raises a number of supplementary questions, which will be outlined below and discussed further.

- *What are the appropriate outcomes to measure?* There are many potential outcomes that can be considered relating to growth, cosmetic appearance, physical functioning, speech and language development, and psychosocial state. Some procedures may have an excellent outcome as measured by one or more of these variables, but have a poor outcome on others.
- *When should the outcome be assessed?* There is an interest in measuring the outcomes at – in some sense – the optimal time. Who decides what this optimal time is? From a professional surgical perspective, a good facial appearance in adulthood with normal skeletal relationships might be a

goal. Hence, from this perspective the optimal time of measurement would be in adulthood. However, it may be that what matters to a particular patient is their facial appearance in childhood, so that normal relationships are least affected, and so from that perspective the optimal time of measurement is in childhood.

- *What combination of factors can lead to the best outcome?* This begs the question: What are the factors that could potentially affect the outcome(s)? This could include the surgical procedure used, surgical timing, the skill and experience of the surgeon, the timing and procedures of orthodontic treatment, the timing and techniques of speech therapy, and the composition, activities and dynamics of the team involved in treatment and care.
- *From whose perspective should this question be answered?* Should the identification of the combination of treatment and care that results in the best outcomes be considered from the professionals' or from the patient's/parent's perspective? There are a number of professionals involved in the treatment of cleft lip and palate, and they are likely to view the importance of different outcomes differently, i.e. the surgeon, the orthodontist, the speech therapist etc. However, it is the patient's and his or her family's perspective that is of paramount importance. Different patients and their families may put different levels of importance on the outcomes. Consequently, there will be no one answer to the headline question for all families.
- *How can this question be answered?* From the author's perspective some part of the answer to this question will be obtained using methods of statistical inference, that is, methods that allow one to make statements about the true underlying position from sample (or incomplete) data. The domain of the methods of statistical inference includes both the research and the analysis methods used.

Assume, for example, that a research study has been carried out to compare two different approaches to the treatment and/or care of the patient, and that a difference between the two interventions has been found. The question is, is it real or a statistical artefact caused by chance or bias? The main source of bias is confounding; however, other sources include selection and information bias. The choice of research methods, and the choices made in the detail of the methods, is important in determining whether one can dismiss an observed difference as a possible chance finding or one due to bias, and thus whether one can conclude that a real difference in effect has been found.

• *What is confounding bias and what can be done about it?* In studies used to answer the headline question there is the likelihood of a mixing of the effects of a number of factors associated with treatment, care, prognosis etc., e.g. between volume of surgery, surgical procedures and timing, and level of organization of the team. This is called *confounding*. It is a common reason for bias in these types of study, and is a reason why many previous studies have resulted in misleading conclusions. Statistical devices do exist to control confounding. They untangle the differences, and can be used when certain conditions hold.

• *What other sources of bias are there, and what can be done about them?* If it were possible to control or eliminate all confounding, there are still many other sources of bias that could mislead the scientist into making unjustified conclusions when a difference is observed. One reason is errors in the measurement of the outcome(s), or in the measurement of those variables that can affect the outcome(s) considered. This has been called *information bias*. Another reason is systematic differences in the characteristics between those who were selected for the study and those who were not, i.e. *selection bias*.

• *Could the apparent effects observed be due to chance?* Typically, chance is measured by a p-value in the context of a hypothesis test, that is, a null hypothesis of no difference is set up, the data are collected, a significance test is carried out, and a p-value is obtained. The sorts of tests appropriate for research in this area are discussed later. The p-value measures the probability of obtaining the difference observed, or something more extreme, if the null hypothesis is true. If the p-value is small, we usually conclude that the difference is statistically significant and the null hypothesis is rejected.

Chance is influenced by a number of things, including the number of patients included in the study, the scale of measurement of the outcome variable(s), and the distribution of the measurements in the groups being compared. The study size required to detect modest differences in effect is quite large, and so this tends to present a major

problem for the CLP researcher owing to the relatively rare occurrence of clefts.

• *What research methods are appropriate?* Among the research methods, the paradigm of clinical research is the randomized controlled trial (RCT). Can this method be used to answer the headline question? In this chapter I will describe the characteristics of the RCT, and also discuss some of its limitations in this research environment. Some alternative methods that have been used are observational studies: the cohort study, intercenter studies, studies using historical controls (before–after), case series, and single case studies. Each of these has its problems. Nevertheless, they can and have contributed information to the overall picture, and so although the information produced thus far is incomplete, it can and should be used to address the key question posed.

• *Can traditional methods be used to find a statistically significant answer?* Some classical methods of analysis (described later) may help to answer the headline question, but all of them have limitations for this purpose.

• *Where do we go from here?* Both the methods of design and those of analysis are limited in their ability to answer the headline question. So, where do we go from here? There are a number of ideas that should be considered, and these are described later. However, more radical thinking is required.

• *What alternative methods of analysis are there?* At least one radical thinker has proposed a non-classical statistical approach to answering this sort of question: a decision theoretic approach.[1] In my view, the most cogent statistical decision analysis is carried out within a framework of Bayesian statistical theory. This will be described through illustration.

This approach makes it explicit who is deciding what outcomes are most important. In fact, it allows one to analyse the data from different people's perspectives (the different professionals', the patient's and the family's) to come up with perhaps conflicting answers. The advantage of this is that it makes clear what the priorities are from the different perspectives and so allows debate to proceed, both rationally and with sensitivity to other people's views.

The approach provides a means of breaking into the difficult problem of determining how the outcomes can be maximized when aggregated across all the important dimensions.

• *Aims of the chapter* This chapter aims to provide further explanation and insight into each of the above topics, and will highlight a potential way forward to answering the headline question: What combination of treatment and care results in the best outcomes for complete unilateral cleft lip and palate?

WHAT ARE THE APPROPRIATE OUTCOMES TO MEASURE?

A program of treatment and care can be evaluated using process measures, outputs or outcomes.

- Process is the measurement of those procedures that are aimed at the efficient treatment of the patient, e.g. the frequency with which the surgical team meets to discuss its activities.
- Output is the activity of the team, e.g. the number of new patients treated in one year.
- The outcomes are the consequences for the patient of the actions of the team, and are the physical and psychological effects of the treatment and care program (e.g. facial appearance, speech, depression).

Although the process and output measures are often useful intermediary measures, the outcomes are of primary importance and I will concentrate on these here.

In Table 72.1 examples of outcomes associated with facial appearance, growth, function, psychosocial state and patient satisfaction, used by investigators in the field of CLP research, have been listed. A recent guide to practice, monitoring and evaluation, produced by the American Association of Oral and Maxillofacial Surgeons,[3] has divided outcomes into: 'Favorable therapeutic outcomes' and 'Known risks and complications associated with therapy'. The goal is to achieve the first and avoid the second, and the outcomes can reflect either of these. Their list of outcomes is too extensive to reproduce here, and so the reader is referred to the source.

The goal of treatment and care of the cleft lip and palate patient is to achieve 'normalcy.[4] This is likely to be impossible to define or to achieve. Nevertheless, keeping this overall goal in mind may help us to place the myriad of outcomes that have been proposed in their proper context. In attempting to achieve 'normalcy', the primary outcomes are those that affect the way in which the patient interacts with the external world, i.e. cosmetic appearance, functional and psychosocial outcomes. Some procedures may have an excellent outcome as measured by one or more of these variables, but have a poor outcome on others. Whatever the outcome, there is a desire for it to be both *reliable* (i.e. reproducible) and *valid*.

The term *validity* means that the variable should be a true measure. For example, if one wished to measure facial appearance a valid variable might be one which was a direct measure by subjective assessment, and was such that the variable scored highly for good facial appearance and low for poor facial appearance. On the other hand, much effort

Table 72.1 Outcomes used in cleft lip and palate research

Dimension	Examples
Facial appearance	*Nasolabial appearance*: Nasal form. Nasal deviation. Vermilion border. Nasal profile. Nasal asymmetry. Width of nose. Length width and angulation of nostrils. Lip length. Lip deviation. Lip height. General esthetic appearance.
Growth	*Craniofacial form and soft-tissue profile*: Length of the maxilla. Prominence of the alveolar process. Maxillary prominence (s-n-ss). Mandibular prominence (s-n-pg). Maxillary length (ss'-pm.) Maxillomandibular relationship (ss-n-sm). Anterior facial angle (nsl-ml). Cranial base angulation (n-s-ba). Lower face angulation (NL-ML). Anterior face height. Lower face height (ss'-gn). Facial contour. Left–right dominance. Lip protrusion. Lip pressure. Width of nasal cavity. Mandibular width. *Nasopharyngeal characteristics*: Nasopharyngeal depth. Minimum of posterior pharyngeal wall and soft palate. *Dental*: Goslon Yardstick. Subjective assessment of plaster mouth casts. Occlusion (Crossbite. Overjet). Radiographic appearance. Vertical development (incisors and cuspids). Anterior–posterior development (incisor and buccal segments). Transverse development (cuspids and first molars). Position of upper central incisor. Relative teeth height. Arch width and depth.
Function	*Speech*: Articulation. Intelligibility. Nasal resonance (hypernasality, hyponasality). Nasal emission. Phonology. Language. Voice. Velopharyngeal insufficiency. Oral motor skills. *Hearing*: Audiometry. (Otitis media)
Psychosocial	Educational level achieved. Type of occupation. Monthly income. Marital status.
Patient satisfaction*	Technical. Bureaucratic. Medical behaviour. Nursing care.

*Not identified for cleft lip and palate specifically, but from a general review of audit and quality of care.[2]

has gone into obtaining cephalometric measurement of the cleft patient. However, as a measure of appearance the cephalometric measurements (e.g. maxillary prominence) need to have good correlation with facial appearance to be described as having high validity for the measurement of this concept. Fortunately, a number of these cephalometric measures do have good correlations. As they are not direct measures, they can be termed *indicators*.

Reliability, on the other hand, is a measure of the reproducibility of the measure if carried out repeatedly. Of particular interest is the intra- and the inter-rater reliability, which measures the reproducibility of measures within the same rater, and between two or more raters, respectively.

FACIAL APPEARANCE

Table 72.1 indicates that the direct assessment of facial appearance (more specifically nasolabial appearance) has been achieved almost exclusively using subjective assessments of aspects of the form of the nose and the lips. Although direct subjective assessments are a valid measure for some aspects of facial appearance they may suffer from problems of reliability, which have been found to be poor for this type of measurement.[4]

Indirect measures such as cephalometric measurements, on the other hand, were found to have good reliability, but can only be regarded as indicators of facial appearance owing to the indirect nature of the correspondence between them and facial appearance.

Subjective impressions of appearance using photographs and cephalometric measures may both have their validity compromised by the fact that two-dimensional views are being used to assess a three-dimensional phenomenon.[4] With care, however, this can be less of a problem. Furthermore, some aspects of facial appearance are dynamic, and so static assessments through photographs and cephalograms may pose a problem. For example, these media do not allow lip function to be assessed.[4] These limitations are discussed further below.

GROWTH

The measurement of growth is problematic because of the many changes that take place in the face during development. However, this is an area where a substantial amount of work has been done in both developing and using outcomes that measure aspects of the skeleton, the soft-tissue profile, the form of the mouth and palate, and the relative positioning and height of the teeth.

The main outcome measurements that have been used by many investigators are aspects of the craniofacial form obtained from cephalometric measurements. Landmark points on the skeleton have been identified that are now standardly used to derive the angles between certain points and planes of the facial skeleton, or distances between the landmarks which can be related to normative values. In a similar way, aspects of the soft-tissue profile can be measured geometrically to complement these skeletal form measures. A number of these are listed in Table 72.1.

For measurements in the mouth, investigators have used both objective and subjective measures. A well used measure is the Goslon Yardstick, which was developed in a collaborative study between Great Ormond Street, London, and a center in Oslo. It is measured from the subjective impressions of dental casts, and has been found to be a 'reliable, robust and rapid means of discriminating between the quality of dental arch relationships in crosscenter studies.'[5] It is nevertheless based on subjective impressions, albeit with relatively good reliability. On the other hand, distances between teeth using reference points have been measured to give more objective measurements.

FUNCTION

Speech and language

Speech as an outcome has been considered by a number of investigators. Assessments have been made on the basis of tape recordings of standard phrases subjected to speech analysis to detect particular variables of speech, as indicated in Table 72.1.[6] Although the variables measured tend to be subjective assessments, they have been found to have acceptable reliability. Objective measures, for example nasal pressure, have been used to measure some dimensions of speech.[7]

Hearing

Relatively little has been published in CLP research related to hearing. Given that the AAOMS[3] identifies improved middle ear health and/or function as one of the favorable outcomes, and chronic otitis media with effusion as a known risk and complication associated with the repair of cleft palate deformities, more attention should be given to this area.

PSYCHOSOCIAL

The psychological impact of the facial appearance, speech and other functions associated with cleft lip and palate can be extremely large, and can affect cognitive development, behavior, self-concept, educational progress and social development.[8] It can result in significant social and psychological handicap as a result of responses from peers, teachers and others, as well as self-perceived limitations.[9,10] In addition, the psychosocial impact includes pain, suffering, disruption of family life, and the sense of loss of control.[4] This results in significant effects on, for example, educational attainment, employment and marital status.[11] Despite all the above, little attention has been given to this area in the CLP literature.

SATISFACTION

'Achieving and producing health and satisfaction, as defined for its individual members by a particular society or subculture, is the ultimate validator of the quality of care.'[12]

The general focus of the literature dealing with patient satisfaction is on the process aspects of medical care, and these include the institutional characteristics of healthcare, medical behavior (including interpersonal behavior and technical competence), nursing care, and the values and attitudes of non-medical staff,[2] as opposed to the other outcomes of care. Devlin's[2] overview of audit and quality in clinical care makes the observation that, in general, the views of the medical professional in terms of what is the major influence on patient satisfaction is the technical competence of the medical staff, whereas the patients themselves have a much more rounded view, being also concerned with interpersonal relationships and the behavior of the staff.

It is known that certain groups assess their satisfaction higher than others: older people and males, for example, and some lower, such as people with poor psychological health. A further complication in measuring patient satisfaction is that satisfaction with nursing care is a large determinant of satisfaction with care in general.

Again, the assessment of patient satisfaction has been neglected in CLP research.

DISCUSSION

Although much work has been done on the development of a number of outcome measures in CLP research, particularly cephalometric measurements, they still have their problems. One particular problem is that they are two-dimensional measures for phenomena in three dimensions.

Three-dimensional measures

Three-dimensional methods are available through, for example, laser scanning, which is non-invasive, rapidly obtainable, can be viewed from varying directions, and is claimed to permit analysis away from the midline to an accuracy of 1 mm.[13] Other three-dimensional methods include stereophotogrammetry.[14]

Although promising, three-dimensional measures may not be the answer to some of the problems highlighted for two-dimensional cephalometric measures, i.e.

- Individual analysis may be dependent on profile orientation.
- The landmarks used to assess growth provide no information on shape or changes in the segments joining them.
- The determination of landmarks relies on expert opinion to create homologous points.[13,15]

There are a number of reasons, some similar to those for two dimensions, why it is difficult to make measurements in three dimensions. In order to make measurements landmark points are set, and so the limitations of using and the problems of identification of landmarks are similar to those described above. Other difficulties include:

- Landmark points are difficult to identify, leading to the introduction of measurement error.
- There are currently no normative data available.
- They are currently relatively subjective measurements and lack reliability.[16]

These types of approach looks promising; however, as with all measurement methods the goal is a standardized measure with good reliability and validity, which at this early stage of development is yet to be achieved.

Dynamic measures

Both two- and three-dimensional measurements are based on a snapshot in time, and so cannot measure movement. For example, a major goal of the treatment and care of cleft lip and palate patients is the achievement of good appearance and function in the nasolabial area. Consequently there is an interest in assessing the symmetry of lip movement, and this is not captured by more traditional methods of measurement. This problem has been addressed in a number of ways, including the use of video recording.[17] As in the discussion above, the measurement goal is a standard measurement instrument with good reliability and validity, which is still to be achieved.

Multiattribute health index

Some have endeavored to produce a multiattribute health index to summarize outcomes on a number of dimensions.[18] In such an index, the outcomes would be combined together in a weighted combination. A limitation of this may be that the same weights are applied for each patient, whereas the importance attributed by each patient to each outcome is likely to be different (see below). Consequently, in this area of research such an instrument seems inappropriate.

WHEN SHOULD THE OUTCOME BE ASSESSED?

Some authors have classified outcomes into two types, proximate and ultimate.[19] Proximate outcomes are those that are observable shortly after the intervention and may, for example, include the skeletal relationships of the face, or the physical appearance of the face a short time after surgery. On the other hand, the ultimate outcome may be viewed as the long-term effects of the intervention. For example, because the relationships of the facial skeleton change throughout the growth period, those measured in childhood can be regarded as *proximate*, and those measured in adulthood can be regarded as *ultimate* outcomes.

However, investigators are interested in measuring the outcomes at what could be considered the optimal time. Who decides what this optimal time is? From a professional perspective a good facial appearance in adulthood with normal skeletal relationships might be a goal, and so from this perspective the optimal time of measurement would be in adulthood. However, it may be that what matters to a particular patient is their facial appearance in childhood, so that normal relationships are least affected. From this perspective the optimal time of measurement is in childhood.

This question is considered further later in the chapter.

WHAT COMBINATION OF FACTORS CAN LEAD TO THE BEST OUTCOME?

To help answer this question it would be useful to know what are the factors that could potentially affect the outcome(s). These could include the composition, activities and dynamics of the team involved in treatment and care; the procedures used; the timing; the skill, and the experience of the surgeon, the orthodontist, the speech therapist etc.

Little is known about the effectiveness of most forms of treatment and care for cleft lip and palate patients. The promotion of particular techniques by enthusiastic practitioners has done much to shape current practice.[4] Particular controversy exists about the relative contributions to the outcome of the surgical procedure used, surgical timing, surgical skill, and the experience of the surgeon as measured by the volume of cleft lip and palate surgery.

A consensus conference of professionals experienced in the diagnosis and treatment of craniofacial anomalies in the USA in 1991 agreed a number of resolutions, of which an abridged list is presented:

- Management is best provided by a multidisciplinary team of specialists.
- The best care is provided by teams who see sufficient numbers of patients each year to maintain expertise.
- The best time for first evaluation is in the first few weeks of life.
- From the first contact, the family needs to be provided with psychological help.
- Parents should be given information to assist them in making decisions, helping to prepare them and the child for the procedures that are to follow.
- Care should be coordinated by the team and should be

sensitive to the particular needs (including social and cultural) of the family.
- Appropriate documentation is essential during the lengthy follow-up.
- Evaluation of treatment effects should include satisfaction, psychological outcomes and social effects, as well as growth function and appearance.[8]

These factors, summarized in Table 72.2, reflect professional consensus but are not at present supported by research evidence.

Many different surgical procedures are used by cleft lip and palate teams. Shaw and colleagues[20] reported that 34 teams presenting their treatment programs to a conference described 34 different ones. The literature, however, generally fails to resolve the uncertainty of what is/are the best treatment program(s). Some of the reasons for teams adopting different treatment regimens are:

- The differing types of skills available in each of the surgical teams;
- The operator's proficiency with a particular technique;
- Lack of documentation on the relative merits of the techniques, leading to ignorance of what is the best;
- Different perspectives on what are the most important outcomes.[1]

The American Association of Oral and Maxillofacial Surgeons[3] identified a number of factors that can affect both beneficial and adverse outcomes, based on 'best available knowledge'. These include:

- The age of the patient;
- Patient and family understanding of the condition and therapeutic goals;
- Patient's and family's compliance with treatment;
- Severity of the cleft deformity and velopharyngeal incompetence;
- Language and hearing problems;
- Presence of other major disease, and abnormalities;
- Hospital and professional staff's familiarity and experience;
- Potential for scarring;
- Inadequate nutrition, growth and development;
- Access to care.

Some examples of treatment and care factors discussed in the literature are highlighted below.

SURGICAL PROCEDURE AND TECHNIQUE

Iatrogenic effects

How much contemporary surgery interferes with growth, and which of lip or palatal surgery is more harmful, is a

Table 72.2 Selected treatment factors affecting cleft lip and palate outcomes

	Factors	Outcomes
Team	Multidisciplinary composition. No. of patients seen per year. Time patient first seen. Evaluations at regular intervals. Degree of team working. Qualification of members. Experience of members. Degree of CPD. Centralized and comprehensive records. Audit and external peer review. Liaison with PHC.	
Facility	Size. Appropriateness.	
Audiologic care	Pattern of assessment before age 1 year. Provision of hearing aids where necessary. Liaison with educational services.	
Cleft lip and palate surgery	Time and type of surgical repair. Timing of bone grafting of alveolar clefts in relation to dental development. Use of presurgical maxillary orthopedics. Use of primary nasoplasty. Muscle reconstruction in repair of palate. Assessment of nasal patency and velopharyngeal mechanism. Type of intervention used for each of these.	Appearance
Craniofacial and maxillofacial surgery	Use and timing of orthognathic surgery when orthodontic treatment fails. Use of pre- and post-treatment speech evaluations. Use of model surgery and prediction tracings if surgical procedure may alter dental occlusion.	Growth Function
Dental care	Degree of monitoring of dental growth, facial growth and development, and dental disease. Appropriateness or lack of referral for caries control, preventive measures and space management. Management of malocclusion. Use of orthodontic appliances. Use of surgical correction and orthodontic treatment for facial deformity.	Psychosocial wellbeing
Nursing care	Assistance with feeding. Offer basic information. Weekly assessments of nutritional intake during 1st month of life. Preparation of family on what to expect. Demonstration of acceptance of facial anomaly. Use of hospital nurses in postoperative care.	Satisfaction
Otolaryngeal care	Assessment and treatment (as necessary) of ear disease or malformation. Assessment and treatment of airways problems.	
Psychosocial services	Frequency of screening interviews parental competence, child management skills, and parent–child relationship, with referral where necessary. Guidance provided to parents on behavior management, teasing, rejection etc. Screening for cognitive development, behavior, self-concept, educational progress, psychosocial development, and referral where necessary. Use of support groups. Availability of social skills training.	
Speech/language services	Frequency of evaluation before age 5, and after 5. Type of evaluations: laryngeal function. Use of speech–language services, or surgery, when problems identified. Velopharyngeal function, and interventions used.	

Based on information produced by a consensus conference of professionals involved in the treatment and care of cleft lip and palate.[8]

matter of dispute. Various authors have suggested iatrogenic effects of surgery. In complete clefts of the lip and palate, surgery appears to affect facial growth, which becomes more apparent as the child reaches maturity.

It has been postulated that those most at risk of maxillary distortion after surgery are those with a significant deficiency of tissue. However, the specific cause, be it lip surgery or palatal surgery, remains uncertain. Nevertheless, it has been reported that the potential for good maxillary growth can be safeguarded if the surgery is performed atraumatically.[21]

Below are some examples of surgery that have been shown to affect one or more of the outcomes of interest. However, there have been a number of contradictory findings reported, and this leads to a degree of uncertainty regarding the true effects.

Example 1: Lip repair

A number of studies found that the growth of the basal maxilla and the alveolar process was impaired following lip surgery, both in patients with accompanying palate repair and in those with lip repair only. Lip pressure after surgery may influence the growth of the maxilla, as it was found to be much higher than in a non-cleft control group.[21]

Example 2: Palate repair

It has been postulated that scar tissue in the region of the maxillary/palatine and palatine/pterygoid sutures acts to prevent the maxilla's normal forward and downward translation. Scars on the dental arch could cause an inward deflection of the dentoalveolar processes, resulting in anterior and transverse crossbite.[21]

Particular procedures

The literature reflects the uncertainties with regard to the benefits and problems associated with particular procedures. Two examples are given below.

Example 1: Single-layer vomer flap

There are different opinions regarding the benefits and drawbacks of a single-layer vomer flap to close the hard palate. The six-center Eurocleft study showed that the two best centers (as measured by the Goslon yardstick) both used this procedure at the time of lip closure.[21] However, this result was confounded by the volume of surgery carried out by the members of the surgical teams, and the consistency of protocols.

Example 2: Push-back procedures

Some work has indicated that push-back procedures are more harmful than alternatives in that they result in maxillary growth restraint and a higher incidence of crossbite; others, however, have not found this problem. One group found no evidence that push-back procedures results in better speech.[21]

SURGICAL TIMING

There is a consensus that the timing of surgery is important in achieving good outcomes. Although this might be agreed, there is less agreement as to what is the best timing for different types of surgery. Two examples are given below.

Example 1: Time of lip closure

Surgical repair of the cleft lip is usually carried out in the first 6 months of life.[8] The time of lip closure is thought to influence maxillary growth restraint, the most popular time being 3 months. Some operate on newborns, but it is speculated that this leads to greater growth disturbance.[21]

Example 2: Time of hard palate repair

Early hard palate repair is thought to impair maxillary growth, whereas late repair is thought to impair speech.[22] On the other hand, a review of a number of studies indicated that maxillary prominence did not differ between those centers practicing early closure of the hard palate using the vomer flap, compared with other one-stage palatoplasty, including push-back, and those where hard palate closure is carried out at 4–8 years of age.[21] Witzel et al[23] indicated that the beneficial effect of delaying hard palate repair on growth is unproven, and may not be effective unless delayed to beyond 12 years of age. A consensus conference in the USA agreed that the cleft palate should be closed by the age of 18 months.[8]

CLEFT TEAM

The cleft lip and palate team may include individuals from a large number of areas of professional practice, including surgical (plastic and maxillofacial), speech and language therapy, psychological and dental professionals. The American Cleft Palate–Craniofacial Association[8] states that it is essential for team members to be trained and experienced in craniofacial anomalies. Each team must be responsible for ensuring that its members have the required qualifications and experience, and should assist then in keeping up with current practice.

The effective functioning of this team, and the health outcomes associated with craniofacial team management, has received little research attention. However, the effectiveness of that team has been postulated by both clinicians and administrators to be an important factor associated with beneficial outcomes. Effective team working is thought to have many advantages over fragmented community-based care, where the patient is treated by a number of independent specialists.[24]

VOLUME OF SURGERY

An analysis of the available evidence leads to the conclusion that the existence of a causal link between the experience of the surgeon (in terms of volume of surgery) and the quality of outcome is 'unproven'. However, there seems to be more evidence in support of such a link than against.

The evidence from other health areas points to the fact that surgery of any kind should be carried out by high-volume operators.[21] This fits with our own intuition that the quality of outcome would be improved if the surgeon has carried out high volumes of relevant surgery. However, there is only weak evidence[25] from cleft lip and palate research to support this. This comes from a study in which the significant differences between centers could have been due to a number of reasons, only one of which was the volume of surgery.

If such a relationship does hold, there is little or no evidence to help in deciding the volume threshold below which one could expect an unacceptable proportion of poorer outcomes. It has been stated that a cleft palate team that takes on at least 50 new or recall patients with cleft lip and palate per year generates experience and maintains professional skills and team function.[24] In a survey of 224 cleft and craniofacial teams, predominantly from the USA, Strauss and Ellis[24] found that teams performed a mean of 21 cleft lip repairs per year, and a mean of 25 cleft palate repairs. However, 17% and 14%, respectively, of teams performed five or fewer procedures per year.

The six-center Eurocleft study showed that the two best centers as measured by the Goslon Yardstick had high-volume surgical operators, and the worst had low-volume operators.[20,26] However, the limitations of this study meant that the effects of particular surgical procedures, the consistent use of protocols and the volume of surgery could not be separated because of confounding, and so the observed differences could be due to any one or a combination of these factors.

SURGICAL PROTOCOLS

The use of consistent surgical protocols within a team may increase the likelihood of a beneficial outcome. The six-center Eurocleft study showed that the two best centers as measured by the Goslon Yardstick had consistent surgical protocols and the worst had inconsistent protocols.[20,26] As mentioned earlier, however, the surgical procedure, consistent surgical protocols and volume of surgery of the operators were confounded.

DENTAL CARE

Patients with cleft lip and palate will require dental care as a result of their condition, and the type and quality of treatment and care will influence some aspects of the outcome of the program. The necessary procedures should monitor craniofacial growth and correct dental problems and abnormal jaw relationships in order to achieve the best function and cosmetic appearance.[8]

SPEECH AND LANGUAGE

Patients with cleft lip and palate will have some degree of speech disorder. The nature and quality of therapy will influence language development and speech quality. There should be regular assessment, with systematic measurement of progress. This may include surgical or prosthetic intervention to improve speech.[8]

PSYCHOLOGICAL SERVICES

The psychological impact of this condition can be great, and screening for cognitive development, behavior, self-concept, educational progress and social development, with referral for guidance and counseling for both the parent and child, are necessary to try and minimize this impact.[8]

AUDIOLOGICAL CARE

Some patients with clefts have abnormalities which make them susceptible to ear disease. Surveillance and intervention are required to reduce hearing disorders, and also to reduce the detrimental effect on speech and language which can be caused by hearing loss. The nature and quality of

the surveillance and treatment may influence the outcomes of hearing and speech.[8]

CONCLUSIONS

Many factors can affect the outcome of treatment and care in cleft lip and palate patients. In addition, with such a large number of possible outcome measures, the estimation of the independent effects of each of the factors is doubly difficult.

FROM WHOSE PERSPECTIVE SHOULD THIS QUESTION BE ANSWERED?

Should the identification of the package of treatment and care that results in the best outcomes be considered from the professionals' or from the patient's/parent's perspective? There are a number of professionals involved in the treatment of cleft lip and palate and they are likely to view the importance of different outcomes differently. However, it is the patient's and the family's perspective that is of paramount importance.

PATIENT'S PERSPECTIVE

Different patients and their families may put different levels of importance on the outcomes. Some families may regard cosmetic appearance as of paramount importance and be willing to compromise on other outcomes. Others might put the greatest weight on the psychosocial factors, and thus endeavor to minimize the psychological effect of the condition, with less emphasis on the other dimensions. Others might consider that physical functioning (speech, breathing, eating, hearing) take the greatest priority and be willing to compromise on other outcomes. There is therefore no one answer to the key question for all families. On the other hand, a favorable outcome in one dimension is often accompanied by favorable outcomes in the others, in which case the answer to the question would be less dependent on particular patient preferences.

RELATIVE IMPORTANCE OF APPEARANCE, SPEECH AND HEARING

Some work[1] has indicated that for the attributes of cosmetic appearance, speech and hearing, almost everyone gave the lowest weight to hearing. Specialists were split in their view of the relative importance of cosmetic appearance and speech: just less than half favored cosmetics, and just more than half favored speech. The mothers of the patients were also split, with the balance going slightly the opposite way, whereas fathers favored good speech over appearance in almost all cases. Krischer[1] speculated that the mother's value systems were similar to the surgical team's than the father's, as the mother tends to have a closer relationship with the team than does the father. It should be noted that assessments on which these findings were based were self-completed questionnaires, whereas they are most rigorously assessed by interview. Consequently, these findings can only be regarded as indicative.

HOW CAN THE RESEARCH QUESTION BE ANSWERED?

I am endeavoring to find an answer to the research question: What combination of treatment and care results in the best outcomes for complete unilateral cleft lip and palate? From my perspective, some part of the answer to this question will be obtained using methods of *statistical inference*, that is, methods that allow one to make statements about the true underlying position from either sample or incomplete data. The domain of statistical inference includes both the research and the analysis methods.

INFERENCE

A schema giving the general structure of statistical inference is shown in Figure 72.1. To illustrate the general framework within which statisticians operate, consider the Eurocleft study. This arose out of an International Conference on Cleft Lip and Palate and Related Craniofacial Anomalies. Orthodontists from six centers formed a research group in which one of the principal pieces of work was a comparative study of treatment outcomes in UCLP between the centers. The subjects included in the study were aged

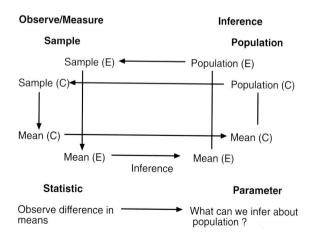

Fig. 72.1 The structure of statistical inference.

8–10 at the time of record collection, and the outcomes considered were based on craniofacial form (as measured by cephalometry), dental arch relationships (from casts of the dentition), and facial appearance (based on photographs of the face). The nature of the surgery provided, the case load of individual surgeons and the organization of cleft teams differed from center to center.[20] For illustration, a simplified version of this study will be used in which only centers C and E are compared, using as an outcome facial appearance assessed using subjective impressions of masked photographs.[27]

Statisticians refer everything back to a population. The population to which this work refers is for both centers, the catchment population aged 8–10 who are or will undergo surgery for UCLP. This definition assumes a steady state, i.e. that what we observe today can be used to make inferences about what will happen tomorrow.

Having defined the population, the next step is to take a sample. In this case, the sample includes those who were treated and who were born in the years 1976–1979, for whom there were usable color photographs for assessment. Of the 151 UCLP patients treated at the centers satisfying the entry criteria, 36 did not have usable photographs. In addition, not all the patients seen at the centers during this period were included. For some centers, where there were more than 30 patients seen during the period, patients were selected at random.

This process produced the sample for whom subjective assessments were carried out on the four dimensions of nasal form (frontal view), deviation of the nose (relative to an imaginary vertical midline), shape of the vermilion border, and nasal profile, including the upper lip. For illustration, only the nasal deviation will be considered. The mean nasal deviation for Center C was larger than that for Center E, where a high score means poor appearance and a low score good appearance (Fig. 72.2).

Even though there was a difference between the means for recent patients treated in Centers C and E, this could be for a number of reasons. What we wish to do is to make a statement about the whole population from which these patients were drawn – in this case the means for the catchment populations of Centers C and E. That is, we want to know whether the difference we have observed is real or an artifact due to bias or chance (Fig. 72.3).

REASONS FOR AN OBSERVED DIFFERENCE

There are two reasons why an observed difference could be a statistical artifact: *bias* and *chance*. Significance tests are usually used to assess chance, which is measured by the *p*-value (i.e. the probability of obtaining the difference observed

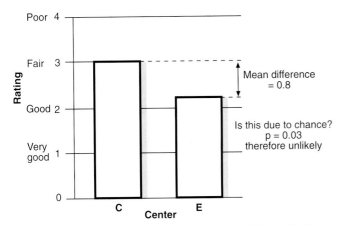

Asher-McDade et al. Cleft-Palate Craniofacial Journal 1992; 29: 409-412

Fig. 72.2 Mean nasal deviation score for two Eurocleft study centers.

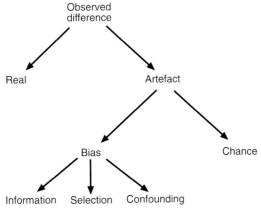

Fig. 72.3 Statistical reasons for obtaining an observed difference between groups.

or something more extreme if there is no true difference in the means). 'Chance' deals with random deviations from the truth. If the only reason why the results observed differ from reality is chance, when more and more data are collected, the result observed will get closer and closer to the true answer. On the other hand, 'bias' describes systematic deviations from the truth. If the results are subject to bias, larger and larger samples will not help – just give a more and more precise estimate of the wrong answer.

Almost 20 years ago, Sackett[28] published a paper listing a large number of potential biases that can occur in analytical studies. The main ones are confounding bias, information bias and selection bias (see below).

INTERPRETATION OF RESULTS

In the Eurocleft study it was observed that for nasal deviation 'there was a significant difference in the ratings between centres.'[27] The principal difference was between Center C and Center E, which had the following treatment regimens:

For center C:

- The lip was closed within the first 6 months.
- The palate was closed at approximately 1 year of age.
- Surgical management varied and many different surgeons were involved in the primary procedures.

For center E:

- Lip closure was at 3 months using a Millard procedure.
- The anterior part of the hard palate was closed at 3 months by a vomer plasty.
- The remainder of the palate was closed at 18–20 months using a modified von Langenbeck procedure.
- Three surgeons were involved who had completed 33, 14 and 3 lip repairs, respectively, for complete UCLP, and six who had completed 17, 11, 10, 6, 3 and 3 palate repairs, respectively.

In all studies, the way in which the results are interpreted and reported is crucial. It is important that no claims are made that are not supported by the data. Shaw and Williams[29] have implied that a possible cause of the difference observed between centers is the volume of surgery carried out by the surgeons, and that a solution to this would be to have specialist high-volume centers. Although this is appealing, such a conclusion would not be justified on this evidence alone, as there are many different reasons why Center E appears more effective than Center C, and the volume of surgery may not be one of these. This type of study must be seen as hypothesis generating. In order to make that statement with confidence, further evidence would be required based on analytical studies or trials (see below).

WHAT IS CONFOUNDING BIAS AND WHAT CAN BE DONE ABOUT IT?

The original purpose of the Eurocleft work was to assist the clinician in selecting precise programs of care that have the best overall chance of success. However, because of the confounding between center, treatment package, organization within the centers, surgeons' experience and caseload, and with other factors, it is only speculation that the problems of outcome may be ascribed to low-volume operators and non-standardization of procedures within a center.[25]

Consider the specific question: Do low-volume operators produce less desirable outcomes as measured by subjective assessment of nasal deviation? We have observed that patients from Center C were assessed as having on average significantly worse nasal deviation than those from Center E. During the period 1976–1979 (the years of birth of the subjects) there were 10 surgeons operating in Center C, among whom the maximum number of lip repairs carried out on patients with unilateral cleft lip and palate was five, and the maximum number of palate repairs was seven. In contrast, in Center E only three surgeons carried out lip repair on patients with unilateral cleft lip and palate, and the number of patients treated by each surgeon was 33, 14 and 7, respectively. Six surgeons carried out palate repair in Center E; the numbers of patients treated were 17, 11, 10, 6, 3 and 3.[20] Consequently, these results for Centers C and E are consistent with high-volume operators producing better outcomes.

However, the range of treatments in the two centers differ quite markedly. If lip closure at 3 months of age using the Millard procedure, closure of the anterior part of the hard palate using vomer plasty at the same time, and closure of the remainder of the palate at 18–20 months of age using a modified von Langenbeck procedure is more effective and has better outcomes than the range of procedures used in Center C, then this might be the reason for the difference between the results for the two centers, rather than the volume of surgery carried out by each of the operators.

In addition, the organization of the teams at each center was different, ranging from highly centralized to very decentralized.[25] Again, if as speculated by these authors, centralized organization of the treatment and care team results in a greater likelihood of a favorable outcome, this would be consistent with the observed results.

Consequently, at least three possible reasons for patients at Center E having a greater likelihood of a favorable outcome are: volume of surgery carried out by the surgeons, the surgical procedures used and their timing, and the level of organization of the treatment and care teams. We know that there is a statistically significant difference between the mean nasal deviations for Center E compared to those for Center C, but we do not know which, if any, of the above is the true reason, or what combination of these factors has resulted in this superior outcome. There is a mixing of the effects of volume of surgery, surgical procedures and timing, and level of organization, and from the information presented these effects cannot be untangled. This mixing of effects is called *confounding*, and is a common reason for bias in these types of study, and why many previous studies of this nature have resulted in misleading conclusions. This is illustrated in Figure 72.4.

Observational studies (of which the Eurocleft study is an example) always carry the risk of confounding. So, even if the study were not subject to other forms of bias, observed differences could be due either to the factors given above, or to a number of other factors that affect the outcome, e.g.:

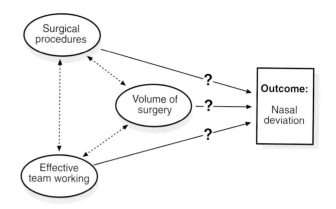

Fig. 72.4 An illustration of confounding.

- Age
- Sex
- Social class
- Ethnic group (ethnic differences in craniofacial form implies that ethnic group will be related to many outcomes)
- Severity of the cleft deformity.

Statistical devices do exist to control confounding, i.e. to untangle the differences, and these can be used when certain conditions hold. One that was used in this study was restriction: i.e. a limited age range was used, and minority ethnic groups were excluded to eliminate any chance of confounding with these variables.

Matching has also been used in some cleft studies to control confounding. For example, in a study investigating the effect of pharyngeal flap surgery on facial growth, as measured from cephalometric radiographs, patients to be compared were matched on cleft type, sex, mandibular growth direction and absolute cranial base size.[30] Matching ensures that the groups to be compared have almost identical distributions for each of the variables for which matching has been arranged: the likelihood is removed that an observed difference can be attributed to differences between the groups in these variables. It should be noted that it is very difficult to organize successful matching on more than one or two variables, unless the study size is very large.

Some fairly sophisticated multivariable statistical techniques exist to reduce the effect of confounding. These attempt to untangle the contribution of each variable on the outcome(s) and are described later. Unfortunately, very few reported studies have used these methods. Those that do not will be subject to quite substantial confounding bias, and hence are likely to produce misleading results.

WHAT OTHER SOURCES OF BIAS ARE THERE AND WHAT CAN BE DONE ABOUT THEM?

Continuing with the same example of Eurocleft Centers E and C, the difference in nasal deviation observed could be an artifact due to the confounding with other factors that might affect the likelihood of a favorable outcome. If it were possible to control or eliminate all confounding, there are still many other sources of bias that could mislead the scientist into making unjustified conclusions. There could be bias caused by errors in the measurement of the outcome(s), or in the measurement of those variables that can affect the outcome(s) considered. This has been called *information bias*. There could also be systematic differences in the characteristics between those who were selected for the study and those who were not, i.e. *selection bias*.

INFORMATION BIAS

Information bias results from flaws in measuring the outcome or other data. The ideal is to collect data by objective measurement, which gives little opportunity for error and hence far less chance of information bias. Examples of this would be the measurement of height, weight etc. On the other hand, concepts such as pain, beauty etc. are measured by subjective impression. They are less precise and so are more prone to information bias. This is the situation that we have in the Eurocleft study dealing with facial appearance.[27]

One essential methodological step when dealing with the sort of assessment which is subject to information bias is the training and calibration of raters on a 'training set' of patients. However, even with this there will still be information bias.

In historical studies, where records are used to obtain information on factors affecting the outcome, the quality of data from the records is of major importance. Records will not contain complete information on some factors, and may not include any on some other important risk factors for the outcome. The use of poor-quality data will lead to information bias.

Information bias can be split into two types, differential and non-differential. If there is a choice (research methods can be chosen to influence the type of bias that is introduced), then non-differential information bias is to be preferred.

Non-differential information bias

What is non-differential information bias? An example would be where the raters' assessment of nasal form, nasal deviation, vermilion border or nasal profile is not completely accurate; however, the likelihood and the degree to which raters get their assessment wrong is independent of center. In other words, on average the rate and extent of misclassification for patients from Center C is the same as for Center E.

In order to illustrate this, let us further simplify the outcomes used in the Eurocleft paper dealing with nasolabial appearance.[27] Consider an outcome that is assessed as either 'Good' (i.e. equivalent to a rating of 'very good' or 'good' on the original scale) or 'Bad' (i.e. equivalent to a rating of 'fair', 'poor' or 'very poor' on the original scale). Assume that if one could find an objective and error-free means of measuring the appearance, the results would be as shown in Table 72.3a. These hypothetical error-free results show a rate ratio between centers of 2.43 (= 87%/36%) and a rate difference of 51% (= 87%−36%).

Further assume that all the raters tend to incorrectly rate as 'Good' more frequently than they incorrectly rate as 'Bad', as follows:

- They rate 20% of those that are in reality 'Good' as 'Bad'.
- They rate 10% of those that are in reality 'Bad' as 'Good'.

This gives the results shown in Table 72.3b. The rate ratio is now 1.94, and the rate difference is 34%.

Table 72.3 A hypothetical example of non-differential information bias

(a)	*Hypothetical error-free results*			
		Good	Bad	Total
	Center C	5 (36%)	9	14
	Center E	26 (87%)	4	30
	Rate ratio:		2.43	
	Rate difference:		51%	
(b)	*Actual observations*			
		Good	Bad	Total
	Center C	5 (36%)[a]	9[b]	14
	Center E	21 (70%)[c]	9[d]	30
	Rate ratio:		1.94	
	Rate difference:		34%	

[a]5−1+1=5
[b]9−1+1=9
[c]26−5+0=21
[d]4−0+5=9

Whichever way it is measured, the difference between the two centers appears less, when subject to non-differential information bias, than the true difference. Generally this type of bias 'waters down' any difference that exists (in technical jargon, non-differential information bias results in the observed difference that is biased towards the null value). The reason why this bias is preferable to some others is that its direction can be predicted. In the presence of this sort of bias, the investigator knows that if a significant difference is found between groups or centers, then in the presence of no other bias the true difference is even greater than that observed.

Differential information bias

The worst type of information bias is that which affects the groups differentially, e.g. when the probability of misclassification differs between centers. For example, in the Eurocleft study six raters were used, one from each of the six centers. Assume that the rater from Center E was not blind to the center, and that he or she tends to rate Center E patients more favorably than patients from the other centers. In other words, his or her probability of classifying the patient's appearance as 'Good' when it should have been 'Bad' is higher when dealing with the patients from his or her own center than for patients from other centers. If the other raters were blind, they would not favor any particular center in their assessment. Overall, this situation would tend to favor one center over the others, in this case Center E.

The problem with this type of bias is that it is unpredictable: the investigator usually cannot predict which way it will affect the results. Some ways to deal with this are to have:

- Blinding of the raters;
- Random order of assessment;
- Independent and qualified raters.

Note that these do not prevent misclassification: what they do is to try and ensure that the information bias is the same for each center, and that its effect is therefore predictable.

The Eurocleft study can be commended for having implemented the first two, but the degree to which the first is achieved may be open to question. Even though an attempt was made to mask the identity of the patients, it is unlikely to have been successful in all cases. Raters may be familiar with some of the cases and thus be able to identify the pictures, consequently undermining the attempt to have blind assessment. Although they have not used inde-pendent raters, they have done the next best thing and taken a rater from each of the six centers in the study.

SELECTION BIAS

Selection bias is the error caused by the systematic differences in characteristics between those who are selected for study and those who are not. The usual way to avoid selection bias is to use:

- An objective method of assessing the eligibility of the patient for the study;
- Blind assessment of eligibility for the study;
- Random selection of those eligible.

For the same example, within the Eurocleft study dealing with nasolabial appearance[27] the potential sources of selection bias are:

- The choice of patients for treatment in the hospital;
- Among those patients, the choice of which to include in the study.

Difficulties could arise if the severity of cases treated in the centers differed, as it would seem reasonable to suppose that for the more severe cases the likelihood of a favorable outcome in terms of appearance would be less. So, if Center C is treating more severe cases than Center E, this would be one reason why the scores for Center C are on average worse than for Center E.

It was also reported that photographs, from which the assessment of appearance was to be made, were not available for 36 of the 151 patients considered in the study, i.e. almost a quarter of the study population. It is highly unlikely that the patients with the missing photographs were similar in every way to the patients included in the study, and so this would result in selection bias. If the level of bias was different in each of the centers, and for example the missing photographs were for the least severe cases, and each center had different proportions of missing photographs, this would bias each center's results to different degrees. We are told that Center E had no missing photographs. If Center C had a high proportion of missing photographs and these were for the least severe patients, then the patients included in the study from Center C would be more severe overall than for Center E. In this case a difference in the facial appearance between the two centers would be observed, even though there was no difference in the effects of the surgery, the effects of the teams, the experience of the surgeons etc. It would be simply due to the selection bias.

COULD THE APPARENT EFFECT BE DUE TO CHANCE?

CHANCE

It was indicated earlier that there are three reasons why a difference between groups of patients exposed to different interventions can be observed. It could be a real difference in the effect of the intervention, it could be due to bias, or it could be due to chance. Typically, chance is measured by a p-value in the context of a hypothesis test. That is, a null hypothesis of no difference is set up, the data are collected, a significance test is carried out and a p-value obtained. The sorts of tests appropriate for research in this area are discussed later.

The p-value measures the probability of obtaining the difference observed, or something more extreme, if the null hypothesis is true. In the comparison between Centers C and E in the Eurocleft study, we are told that for the outcome 'nasal deviation' $p < 0.05$.[27] What this says is that if the null hypothesis is true, there was a less than 5 in 100 chance of observing a difference of the magnitude obtained or larger. So, the difference obtained was unlikely to be due to chance alone. Another way of saying this, is that if there is no real difference between two centers, then in 100 studies comparing the two you would expect to find a difference at least as large as the one obtained less than five times out of 100. If the p-value is small, we usually conclude that the difference is statistically significant and the null hypothesis is rejected. Chance is influenced by:

* The number of patients included in the study;
* The scale of measurement of the outcome variable(s);
* The distribution of the measurements in the groups being compared.

STUDY SIZE REQUIREMENTS

Implications for study size

In carrying out a statistical test there are two types of error that can be made:

* False claim of a difference between groups – type I error;
* Failure to detect a real difference between groups – type II error.

If the convention of rejecting the null hypothesis when $p < 0.05$ is followed, this is effectively setting the proportion of times that a type I error is made at 0.05, i.e. 5% of the time.

The study size is one of the things that controls the type II error rate. The probability of not making a type II error is called the power of the test. The desire is to choose a study size such that the power of the test is large, i.e. such that the probability is large of rejecting the null hypothesis of no difference if a real difference in the effect of exposure to the interventions exists.

Scales of measurement

The study size requirements depend on the type (measurement scale) of outcome data to be used in a comparison. Typically, in discussing such issues, measurement scales are divided into three types:

* Interval or ratio scale data, for which an assumption of normally distributed residuals apply;[31]
* Ordinal data (or interval/ratio scale data, for which the assumption of normally distributed data does not apply);
* Nominal or categorical data.

The first of these can otherwise be described as measurement data; some of the cephalometric measures fall into this category.

Ordinal data are outcomes measured on a semiquantitative scale. That is, if a higher score is assigned to one individual (A) than to another (B), this indicates that the outcome for A is in some sense better than that for B, but the difference between the score does *not* represent the magnitude of the difference in the outcomes. For example, educational level achieved by the cleft lip and palate patient could be a psychosocial outcome of interest. The study by Ramstad et al[11] in Norway considered educational attainment classified as:

1. Second level, second stage I
2. Second level, second stage II
3. Third level, first stage I
4. Third level, first stage II
5. Third level, second stage I and II.

This represents an ordinal scale, with the worst outcome at the top with the lowest score, and the best at the bottom with the highest.

Finally, nominal or categorical data are those for which the outcome is a set of categories, rather than a score in which ordering of outcomes or magnitude of differences in outcomes are implied. Type of crossbite is an example of this type of variable, classified as 'no crossbite', 'buccal', 'anterior', and 'anterior and buccal'.[32]

Estimating study size

When estimating the number of patients required for a study, the investigator needs to be able to identify the size of the difference between the groups that should be detected, i.e. usually this would be the minimum clinically significant difference. Table 72.4 shows a number of scenarios for nominal/categorical data and for interval/ratio scale data, and the study size requirements for the simplest situation of detecting a difference between two groups. For each part of the Table it is assumed that the null hypothesis of no difference between the two groups will be rejected if $p < 0.05$, i.e. the significance test is operating at a 5% level of significance (the probability of a type I error is 0.05). Also, for both parts of the Table the study sizes have been provided to ensure a power of 95%, i.e. a 95% chance of finding the stated difference statistically significant.

The methods of treatment and care for CLP have reached a stage of development such that differences in effect of two different treatments will be relatively small. Therefore, study sizes need to be arranged to detect treatments that result in relatively small improvements.[33]

Nominal/categorical data

For nominal/categorical data with two categories (binary data), the study size requirement depends solely on the magnitude of the difference in population proportions that the investigator wishes to detect. If the two categories being measured are 'success' or 'failure', Table 72.4 shows the study size requirements for different examples of popu-

lation success rates for the two groups: labeled treatment and control. To be able to detect huge differences in the treatment effect compared to the control (ie. 75% versus 25%) only very modest numbers of patients per group (22) are required. However, only in exceptional cases would this level of difference be expected. More realistic scenarios are shown in the bottom three rows of the table. For example, to detect a difference between a real treatment effect of 60% success, compared to a control success of 50%, would require 638 patients per group. Unfortunately, this number of patients would be beyond the ability of most investigators to recruit.

Interval/ratio scale

For interval/ratio scale data the study size requirements depend on the magnitude of difference between population means that the investigator wishes to detect, and the magnitudes of the standard deviations of the data for each of the two populations being compared. To use the statistical tests such as the T-test and the F-test (in an analysis of variance), the assumption is made that the standard deviations (or variances) of the groups being compared are equal, and that the data observed follow a normal distribution. This is the situation presented in Table 72.4.

The second row of Table 72.4, under the heading Interval/Ratio Scale, shows that there is a study size requirement of 26 patients per group if the population difference in group means is 1 standard deviation. This is almost large enough for such a difference to be obvious to the eye without carrying out statistical tests. The requirement to detect smaller differences is more realistic and is shown below this (0.5 and 0.25 of a standard deviation differences). It can be seen that as the difference that one wishes to detect halves, the study size requirement quadruples.

Ordinal data

The study size requirements for ordinal data lie in between those for interval/ratio scale data and for nominal/categorical data. Consider outcomes measured on an ordinal scale with many points, which tend towards a quantitative scale, e.g. depression and anxiety scales derived from a battery of questions, each of which is an ordinal scale with multiple categories. The study size requirements for these scales are similar to those for outcomes measured on an interval/ratio scale. For ordered categorical data with only a small number of categories, however, the study size requirements are more similar to those for nominal/categorical data. Examples of this type of scale would be the nasolabial appearance measures used in the Eurocleft study.[27]

Table 72.4 Example of estimated study size requirements

Nominal/categorical data Sig level = 5%; Power = 95%			Interval/ratio scale data Sig level = 5%; Power = 95%	
Control (% success)	Treatment (% success)	No. of Patients per group[a]	Difference in means (no. of SDs)	No. of Patients per Group[b]
25	75	22	2	7
30	60	66	1	26
50	70	150	0.5	104
50	60	638	0.25	416
50	55	2587		

[a]Rothman KJ, Boice JD 1982 Epidemiologic analysis with a programmable calculator. Epidemiology Resources Inc., Boston. Schlesselman JJ 1974 Sample size requirements in cohort and case-control studies of disease. American Journal of Epidemiology 99: 381–384. Walter SD 1977 Determination of significant relative risks and optimal sampling procedures in prospective and retrospective comparative studies of various sizes. American Journal Epidemiology 105: 387–397
[b]Armitage P 1971 Statistical methods in medical research. Blackwell, London, pp 184–188

Loss to follow-up

The study sizes quoted are those required to be entered into the analysis. If it is expected that there will be 20% loss to follow-up of patients in the study, then the number of patients entered into the study = target study size divided by 0.8. So, if the target study size in each group is 80, with 20% loss to follow-up, the number of patients entered into the study would be 80/0.8, i.e. 100 patients per group.

How large should the power be?

It should be noted that when calculating study size, 95% power should be aimed for. To plan for lower power will not result in great savings in study size, but may compromise the study's ability to detect a real difference.

Investigators should think long and hard about the value of a study which has inadequate power. For example, I have been presented with study designs for which the power of the study is as low as 20%. This means that in four out of five such studies the work will not detect a clinically significant difference. This could only be justified if the study was being carried out with the specific intention of contributing to some form of subsequent meta-analysis (see below). If study size, and hence power, is small then the interpretation of a non-significant result becomes problematic. In this case, the investigator would not know whether the non-significant result was because there were no clinically significant differences between the groups, or was due to lack of power to detect a difference.

Choice of scale

The study size requirements are far lower for data measured on an interval/ratio scale than for nominal/categorical data. Consequently, if there are a limited number of patients available for a study there may be sufficient to detect a clinically meaningful difference if the outcome is measured on an interval/ratio scale, whereas for the same study size a real difference in the effects of treatment is unlikely to be detected if the outcome is measured using a categorical outcome.

Examples

Semb and Shaw[21] have commented that in their opinion the Eurocleft study size was too small. They have provided examples of study size requirements for two outcomes, and these are given below.

Cephalometry

Cephalometric measures are usually treated as an interval/ratio scale, with normally distributed observations. For the maxillary prominence the study size requirement per group to detect a 1.5 degree difference at 9 years of age between two centers is 117; 1.5 degrees was the maximum difference observed between two of the six Eurocleft centers. Furthermore, study sizes need to be increased by around 80% if all mutual pairwise comparisons are of interest for the six-center study, and by almost 50% if one center acts as a reference and the other five are compared against it.[25] Sample size requirements would decrease substantially with age, owing to the increasing divergence of the cleft population growth curve from the normal growth curve with age.[34] Nevertheless, the study size requirement is still likely to exceed the number of patients of similar ages treated by most centers.

Goslon Yardstick

For a comparison of occlusion in study models using the Goslon Yardstick, Shaw and colleagues[25] have indicated that to pick up a mean difference of 0.75 between two centers requires a study size of 19 per group, and for an all-pairs comparison between six groups would require 34 per group. They also noted that the maximum difference between two centers in the Eurocleft study was 0.87, implying that the study size requirements would be even less.

Their presentation is somewhat contentious, however, as the calculations assume that it is appropriate to use methods suitable for data measured on an interval/ratio scale, which have normally distributed errors, for the analysis of the Goslon score. The Goslon Yardstick[35] is an effective but somewhat crude 5-point scale used to assess dental arch relationships. It is by nature an ordinal scale. The sample size calculations for an ordinal scale are complex; however, for this level of measurement the study size requirements would be more similar to those of a categorical scale than those for interval/ratio data. To analyse the data using methods appropriate for ordinal data (see below) would give substantially greater study size requirements than those presented.

Other scenarios are presented by a number of authors associated with the Eurocleft study.[25,34,36]

Implications

The study size required to detect small differences is large, and thus tends to present a major problem for the CLP researcher owing to the relatively rare occurrence of the condition. Most centers would have difficulty recruiting enough patients for a single-center study or trial. This, then, is one of the methodological difficulties that needs to be overcome when endeavoring to address the headline question that introduced this section.

The number of cleft lip and palate patients may decrease in future. It is now possible to detect fetuses with cleft lip by the 14th week of gestation, and even earlier in some cases, using transvaginal sonography.[37] In two-thirds of cases, cleft lip is associated with cleft palate.[38] In a small study in Israel, 15 cases of cleft lip were detected by routine screening with sonography, and 14 of these were terminated.[39] This decision was reached after the parents had consulted with other parents of children who had cleft lip and/or palate. Also, the parents of the child who was born indicated that should a subsequent fetus be detected with cleft lip, then they would have the pregnancy terminated. Furthermore, the authors reported that eight plastic and 15 maxillofacial surgeons indicated that they would prefer terminating fetuses with detected clefts; the paper does not report how many surgeons were questioned.[39] It seems that the only people not asked were the affected patients themselves.

This problem of large sample size requirements and small numbers of patients per center will be considered alongside other problems associated with researching this problem, in later sections.

WHAT RESEARCH METHODS ARE APPROPRIATE?

Among the available research methods, the paradigm of clinical research is the randomized controlled trial (RCT). Can this method be used to answer the headline question? In the early 1990s, a cleft lip and palate research methods paper stated that, 'The main thrust of clinical research should undoubtedly be the planning and initiation of well-designed, ethical, and efficient randomised controlled trials.[34] However, many would disagree with this statement because of the methodological difficulties that exist with the use of RCTs for clinical research relating to cleft lip and palate.

In this section I will describe the characteristics of the RCT, and also discuss some of its limitations in this research environment. Some alternative methods that have been used are observational studies, prospective and retrospective cohort studies, intercenter studies, studies using historical controls (before and after), case series, and single case studies. Each of these has its problems. Nevertheless, they can all contribute to the overall picture, and so although the information produced to date is far from complete, it should be used to address the headline question. One problem is that the accuracy of information provided by research diminishes as the validity of the study diminishes.

In general the RCT has the highest validity, and case series and single case studies have the lowest.

Case reports are used to provide the initial anecdotal evidence of the success or otherwise of a particular procedure. Case series have then been used to provide information on the procedure for a wider cross-section of patients. However, they cannot be used to provide evidence of the superiority of one procedure over another, particularly for cleft lip and palate research at this time, where only small average improvements in outcome resulting from one technique rather than another might be expected. Consequently, this section will only consider comparative studies, as these are the only type that can hope to answer the headline question at this current stage of knowledge.

I would like to acknowledge the helpful discussions provided by Roberts et al[34] and by Shaw et al[4] in giving insight into some of the problems associated with the application of these methods to answer cleft lip and palate research questions. However, the following discussion reflects my own opinions, and I suspect that Shaw, Roberts and their colleagues would not agree with a number of the statements made.

RANDOMIZED CONTROLLED DESIGN

The ideal design for quantitative evaluation is the true experimental design, which should include the following five elements:

- A representative sample of the target population or program recipients;
- One or more baseline measurements (i.e. preceding the intervention);
- An unexposed group, or a group exposed to a control treatment, for comparison;
- Random assignment of the sample to experimental and control groups;
- One or more postintervention assessments.[40]

In a clinical context the randomized controlled trial is regarded as the epitome of scientific validity. This design is particularly necessary for evaluation when the differences in expected outcomes are small compared to the variation between patients.[19]

A schema of RCT design is shown in Figure 72.5. As regards the characteristics just mentioned:

- The RCT usually focuses on a particular subgroup that is more homogeneous than the total patient population, e.g. unilateral complete cleft lip and palate cases are often used to the exclusion of other cleft cases. From such trials, generalization can therefore only be made to this specific group of patients.

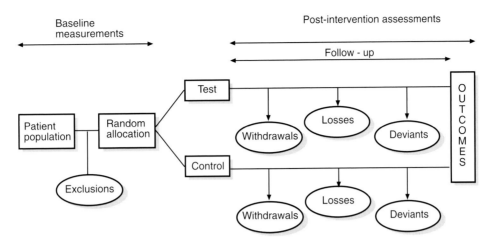

Fig. 72.5 The structure of a randomized controlled trial.

- Within cleft lip and palate research, baseline measurements of prognostic variables are essential.
- Within an RCT treatment is determined at random, which avoids conscious and unconscious bias in treatment allocation, and thus removes significant confounding bias. It ensures balance between treatment groups for all variables causally related to the outcome, known or unknown. If the research question relates to the comparison of two surgical interventions, then to be a true RCT each surgeon involved should use both surgical techniques, and the one used on a particular patient should be determined at random. This can result in a number of problems, both ethical and practical (see later).
- Patients are followed up over time. A number of problems can occur during the long period of follow-up that should occur in CLP research, relating to withdrawal of patients from the study, loss to follow-up (which is likely to be less of a problem than in some other settings), and patients being treated in a way that deviates from the trial protocol.
- At the appropriate times the outcomes are measured.

It is interesting to note that few RCTs have been carried out in this area, and very few, if any, have incorporated long follow-up times.[4,34] There are a number of practical problems associated with the use of RCTs that have tended to make these very difficult to carry out in this setting:

1. The problem of accruing sufficient patients to obtain a meaningful result, and ethical problems, have been barriers to their use (see discussion at the end of the section).
2. A particular surgeon would be required to use each of the procedures being tested. However, a surgeon is likely to be more familiar with one procedure and hence to obtain better results with it than with a less familiar procedure. This could result in bias against innovation.
3. Working to a standard protocol may not permit the necessary latitude for the surgeon to adapt the procedure to the unique nature of the cleft being presented: a procedure may be successful when used on some clefts but not others.[41]

With regard to (2) above, it has been suggested that a standardization phase be used to compensate,[42] but the effectiveness of this has been questioned.[41] Shaw has suggested that the need for effective training and standardization of surgeons tends to mean that only the simpler techniques can be successfully included in RCTs, as they are easier to learn. He argues that this does not pose a problem, since it is more likely that simpler procedures will be more readily adopted anyway.

THE COHORT STUDY

The cohort study attempts to simulate a randomized controlled trial, but without the randomization. This should be regarded as a second-choice method to be used where RCTs are not ethically, practically or economically possible.

As in an RCT, a population of patients is defined and followed up over time, and the outcome assessed. The aim is to collect data on all factors that could influence the outcome, including the interventions used.

The investigator does not influence which patient receives which intervention, and so this type of study is termed 'observational'. This category also includes intercenter studies.

Data can be collected prospectively or retrospectively (Fig. 72.6) Retrospective cohort studies appear to have been carried out in much greater numbers than prospective cohort studies in CLP research. Unfortunately, the descriptions authors provide make it impossible in some cases to

Prospective cohort

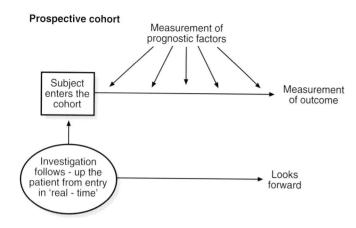

Retrospective cohort

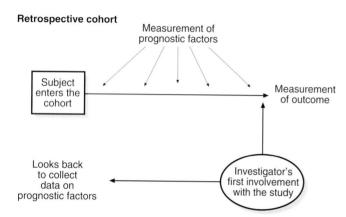

Fig. 72.6 The structure of a prospective and retrospective cohort study.

determine whether a study they are presenting is prospective or retrospective. (Journal editors could rectify this problem by insisting on a structured abstract for study reports, in which this information is made explicit.)

Prospective cohort study

In a prospective study the patients are followed prospectively from diagnosis to assessment. As with RCTs, information is collected prospectively on the treatment and care program, on other factors affecting the outcomes, and on the outcomes themselves, and consequently information bias can be minimized. The availability of this information also means that the groups to be compared can be chosen with the confidence of knowing what the similarities and differences are between them and between the interventions used. However, also like RCTs, they exhibit the same problems in terms of the length of time needed to accrue the necessary number of patients, and the length of follow-up required.

The major problem of a prospective cohort study is that the treatment groups being compared will not be equiva-

lent in the characteristics that influence the outcome. For example, treatment choices for the patient may be made on information unavailable to the researcher. Also, the success of the surgical technique is likely to be highly influenced by the surgeon carrying it out, and in this kind of design the investigator will rarely be able to separate out the effects of the surgical procedure used from the timing and the skill and experience of the surgeon.

Retrospective cohort study

The retrospective cohort study attempts to simulate an RCT retrospectively. A group of patients whose outcomes can be assessed close to the start of the study are considered. Other data are collected retrospectively. The patients are identified from their records and followed up retrospectively, using either their records and/or interviews to collect information on factors that could influence the outcome, including interventions. The advantage of these types of study are that they can be carried out relatively rapidly, and they do not run the risk of subject dropout. They have been used to provide useful information that has influenced the management of cleft cases and improved care.[41]

For this type of study, however, there are even more potential problems than for the prospective cohort study:

- The difficulty of tracing all the patients, or their details, retrospectively;
- The difficulty of obtaining clearly described treatment protocols from 10–20 years ago;
- The relevance of those treatment protocols to today;
- The information available on treatment, the severity of the cleft and other prognostic factors, may be missing or difficult to interpret;
- Treatment choices may have been made on the basis of information unavailable to the investigator.

There may be a great deal of variation in the prognostic factors which could result in a lack of comparability between the groups being compared. This matters if these variables have a great affect on the outcomes being measured.

Intercenter comparisons

An intercenter comparison is an example of a cohort study, either prospective or retrospective. They have been used by a number of research groups because of the small number of cases of cleft subtype generated in a single center.

The main problem with intercenter comparisons in this field is the confounding between surgical technique, surgical skill, volume of surgery, use of ancillary services, and the organization of the cleft team. It is unlikely that the independent effects of these factors could be estimated using this type of study. Consequently, it makes the interpretation of the results extremely difficult. As indicated by Shaw and his colleagues on a number of occasions,[4,34] intercenter studies should therefore be regarded as hypothesis-generating studies, and not confirmatory areas. Consequently, no firm conclusions can be drawn from these studies: they should just be a stepping stone to further analytical research.

HISTORICAL CONTROL STUDIES

These studies compare the treatments used in one period of time with those used in a subsequent period. They can arise naturally from changes of therapy in a single center, and are particularly valuable when there are durable records obtained in standard ways (radiographs, study casts, speech recordings etc.). However, there are a number of problems associated with historical control studies:

- They often arise from changes of personnel, and so there will be confounding between surgeon and the treatments being compared.
- New techniques are likely to be introduced by a more experienced surgeon, and if previous procedures were carried out by an average surgeon better results might be expected just on competence alone.
- Other changes of treatment and care, including changes in ability and the techniques used, will have occurred during the extensive follow-up period that is required.

The methodological problems with, and hence the bias introduced by, historical control studies are such that the results from this type of work are potentially highly misleading. Examples have been cited where the results of historical control studies have been contradicted by subsequent RCTs.[4,34]

PROBLEMS

There are a number of problems associated with each type of research method, some of which have been highlighted by others in the application of research methods to CLP research.[34]

Ethical problems

Ethical problems are peculiar to experimental designs, i.e. the RCT. There can be no second chance for a surgeon if the chosen procedure results in a poor outcome for a patient, so there is a strong imperative to use the best option. This is compounded by the fact that many surgeons have strong opinions about what is the best option, and so they would see it as personally unethical to use techniques that they think are less effective. Also, participation in randomization may jeopardize the surgeon's credibility with his or her patients. On the other hand, Shaw argues that participation in a trial may be beneficial to the patient. Trials tend to introduce a level of rigor that raises the level of care provided, which has been demonstrated in some cancer trials.[42]

Study size

Study size is a potential problem owing to the rarity of the condition (<2 births per 1 000), the subtypes that exist, and the potential study size requirements for most of the outcomes considered. Because only a relatively small number of patients of a particular cleft subtype are treated at a particular center, this presents a problem for the research investigator, which could become worse in the light of the potential for screening for cleft lip and palate, leading to the abortion of affected fetuses.[39]

Most of the studies and trials that have been carried out in cleft research are characterized by the small number of patients included. Small study sizes will pose a problem whatever the type of study, as in most instances differences in treatment effects will be small. We have seen that large study sizes are required to detect small differences, and that the number of patients required for a study in which the outcome is qualitative (categorical data) or semiquantitative (ordinal data) is larger still. Also, larger study sizes are advisable should there be a problem with confounding, as there is more opportunity to control confounding caused by several variables when analyzing studies involving a large number of patients.

Some of the other problems are as follows.

- *Information bias* is a large potential problem in retrospective studies in particular, principally because of the dependence on records for details of the treatments used, on other prognostic variables and, in some instances, for the measurement of the outcomes themselves.
- *Selection bias*, i.e. the representativeness of cases selected for research, can be a problem in all types of research design. However, it can be a particular problem for RCTs because of the strict entry criteria used in trials, often leading to the exclusion of large numbers of patients. This limits the inferences that can be made.
- *Confounding bias* is a problem, especially in observational studies, because it is very difficult to separate out the effects of each of the prognostic factors

(e.g. the treatment package, the skill and experience of the surgeon, the effect of ancillary staff, preoperative anatomy etc.). The use of randomization in large RCTs removes this problem.

- The *long follow-up time* can cause particular problems. The time between initial treatment and the measurement of some outcomes should ideally be in the order of 10 or maybe 20 years (facial appearance, facial growth).

- There are many outcomes of interest: facial appearance, function, social and psychological impairment. This increases the complexity of investigating the relative effectiveness of interventions, particularly when some outcomes show benefit and at the same time others show disbenefit from a particular intervention.

- The fact that some outcomes are still in development means that there will be a further lack of standardization in the way they are assessed. This is particularly problematic for rare conditions such as CLP, where investigators depend on combining information from several centers, often retrospectively, in their attempt to obtain a definitive answer.

- Some outcomes are particularly subjective, and so controlling the size of information bias, whatever the research design, presents particular difficulties.

The discussion has indicated problems with all of the potential research methods available. It can be concluded that no method is entirely satisfactory, and so whichever is chosen some bias will be introduced. The goal of study design is to minimize that bias.

There are a number of areas where improvements in the methods used in CLP research could be made, and these are discussed below.

CAN TRADITIONAL ANALYSIS METHODS BE USED TO FIND A STATISTICALLY SIGNIFICANT ANSWER?

Classical methods of analysis have been used when attempting to answer the headline question. I will list some that have been used, as well as some alternative classical approaches. However, all these methods are, in my view, too limited to be able to answer the headline question.

Table 72.5 shows some appropriate analytical methods that should be, and have been, used to compare independent samples in cleft lip and palate research. This includes the situation where two treatment methods are compared using patients who can be regarded as independent of one another. This is in contrast to studies or trials where there is a close matching between, for example, pairs of patients. Classically, this occurs in studies that use twins.[51] Some authors, however, have treated pairs of patients, defined by loose matching criteria, as dependent cases or matched pairs. For example, Jonsson et al[32] matched 11 subjects who had received one program of treatment with 11 others who received another program, and these were matched 'with respect to the morphology and the size of the alveolar processes and the size of the cleft'. It may be just acceptable to use paired methods of analysis (e.g. the paired *t*-test, or the Wilcoxon matched pairs signed rank analysis[31])

Table 72.5 Appropriate analytical methods for independent samples in cleft lip and palate research

	2 Groups, no confounders	>2 Groups, no confounders	2 or more groups, confounders
Interval/ratio data (Normally distributed residuals) e.g. I1. Maxillary prominence[43] I2. Intercanine width[44]	2 sample *t*-test[31]	One-way analysis of variance (ANOVA) and multiple comparison test (e.g. Duncan's multiple range test)[31]	Unbalanced multiway ANOVA, analysis of covariance (ANCOVA) or general linear modeling[47]
Ordinal data (Or non-normally distributed residuals) e.g. O1. Nasolabial appearance[27] O2. Goslon scores[35] O3. Speech scores[45] O4. Level of education achieved[11]	Wilcoxon rank sum test or Mann–Whitney U test[31]	Kruskal–Wallis test[31]	Proportional odds regression[48]
Nominal/categorical data e.g. C1. Type of crossbite[32] C2. Hypernasality[46] C3. Marital status[11]	χ^2-test or Fisher's exact probability test[31]	χ^2-test[31]	Multiple linear logistic regression (binary outcome) or loglinear modeling[49,50]

for data matched in this way. However, for study sizes more appropriate for this type of work a preferable approach would be to treat the observations as independent and control for the matching variables in the analysis, using regression techniques (see below).

Table 72.5 illustrates three scenarios. First, the situation where two groups are compared and there are no confounders, shown in the first column. These methods would be appropriate for an analysis of an RCT in which, for example, two treatments were being compared. Alternatively, it could be used to provide a preliminary analysis of observational study data (e.g. from a cohort study); however, such an analysis would need to be followed up with something more sophisticated to control for potential confounding. The second column shows a comparison with more than two groups, with no control of confounding, and would be used in a similar situation to that described for the first column, but where three or more interventions were being compared.

The third column shows the methods to be used when there are either two or more groups to be compared, but the data originate from an observational study where there is confounding by other variables (e.g. by age, sex, surgeon's experience, preoperative morphology), and thus need to be controlled. An appropriate set of methods used in this situation fall into the class of generalized linear models,[52] and specific types of modeling method are highlighted in the table. These methods tend to be more complex than the ones listed in the first two columns; however, they are readily available to users of standard statistical software such as SAS[47] and SPSS.[53] These methods should be used in the majority of analytical studies in the field of cleft lip and palate research. Unfortunately, relatively few CLP studies have been analyzed using these more sophisticated methods, with a number of exceptions.[43,54,55]

The Table divides the methods into those that are appropriate for:

- Interval or ratio scale data, for which an assumption of normally distributed residuals applies;
- Ordinal data (or interval/ratio scale data for which the assumption of normally distributed data does not apply);
- Nominal or categorical data.

For a description of scales of measurement, see earlier.

Examples of each of these outcomes are shown in Table 72.5, which highlights that care must be taken when deciding how the data from a study or trial should be analyzed. However, there are many other situations that could be considered, and in each case the appropriate analytical method needs to be chosen. Some further examples are as follows.

Table 72.5 deals with the comparison of groups: i.e.

one treatment program against another. However, the study variable of interest might instead be a continuous measure. For example, Long et al[56] were interested in whether the width of the cleft affected the success of secondary alveolar bone grafts. They used as outcomes aspects of the bone architecture, e.g. ratios of alveolar bone heights. These were treated as interval/ratio measures with normally distributed errors. In this case simple regression analysis can be used to assess the association between a continuous independent and dependent variables. If control of confounding is required, then multiple linear regression or general linear modeling can be used.[47]

To answer the headline question a follow-up study is the ideal design. Particularly when following subjects prospectively, repeat measures are generated, i.e. measures of the same outcomes which are collected at different ages e.g. maxillary recession. For example, Semb and Shaw[57] addressed the question: Does the facial development change following a pharyngeal flap? Repeat cephalograms were used, at different ages for the child, to assess whether outcomes such as maxillary protrusion, maxillary length etc. were the same in the pharyngeal flap group as in controls. A repeat measures analysis of variance[58] was the appropriate method to choose (provided that the assumptions of the method were satisfied).

Finally, some have addressed the question of simultaneous assessment of multiple outcomes. An empirical approach to this is that exemplified by the analysis used by Brothers et al[7] who compared the speech results of 21 patients who underwent the Furlow double-opposing Z-palatoplasty with those of 10 patients who underwent the Wardill–Kilner procedure. Multiple outcomes were of interest, which included hypernasality, nasal emission and overall velopharyngeal adequacy for speech. These were considered simultaneously using a multivariate analysis of variance. This tests an overall hypothesis of no differences, on any of the dimensions, between the two groups. If the sample size was large enough it was a reasonable hypothesis to test, and, provided the assumptions of the technique hold (e.g. normally distributed data – which is questionable in this instance), it is an appropriate technique to apply. If a statistically significant difference is found then one would wish to do more work to identify what those differences are.

With the exception of the above technique, the ones described are suitable for assessing outcomes on one dimension only. However, if contradictory results were obtained for different outcomes (e.g. facial appearance and speech), then a way of resolving these contradictions would need to be found. This is discussed later. First, however, a number of more traditional approaches to improving research in this area will be considered.

WHERE DO WE GO FROM HERE?

A number of problems need to be overcome if the headline question is to be answered satisfactorily. These include ethical problems associated with RCTs, the large study sizes necessary, confounding bias (particularly for observational studies), information bias (particularly in retrospective studies), selection bias, long follow-up times, and the many outcomes that are of interest, some of which are still in development and a number of which are highly subjective in nature.

The methods of both design and analysis are limited in their ability to answer the headline question. So, where do we go from here? There are a number of ideas that should be considered:

- Plan for meta-analyses of future studies and trials;
- Improved record systems;
- Identification of valid and reliable indicators of the outcomes;
- Develop widely accepted, valid and reliable measuring instruments.

META-ANALYSIS

A meta-analysis takes the results from a number of small trials/studies, which alone are not big enough to provide useful information in their own right, and combines them to obtain a more definitive answer. The information in a meta-analysis is an estimate of the magnitude of the relative effect of the intervention compared with a control. Also taken into account in this process is the precision of these estimates, expressed either as standard errors or as confidence intervals.

For example, if for the control intervention the rate of success is 50% as measured by some valid outcome, and for the test intervention it is 60%, then the measure of relative effect – the rate ratio (RR) – is 1.2. If there were 100 patients being compared in each group, the confidence limit around this rate ratio estimate would be 0.93 to 1.54. In this case, the result of the χ^2-test to compare the two proportion gives $p = 0.16$. From the p-value it can be concluded that there is no significant difference between test and control. Consistent with this, from the 95% confidence interval, one can conclude that the data are consistent with a real difference of between 0.93 and 1.54, and hence with a rate ratio of 1, i.e. with the true rate of success for the control group being the same as the rate of success for the test group. However, it says more than that: it says that the results are also consistent with a true relative difference between the two groups, ranging from the control group having a true success rate 7% better than the test group, to the test group having a true success rate 54% better than the control group.

If there was a second study with 100 patients in each of the test and control groups, and an observed 52% success in the control group and a 64% success in the test group, then this would give an estimated rate ratio of 1.23, with 95% confidence interval: 0.97 to 1.56 ($p=0.086$). This again is not statistically significant.

If these results are combined using a meta-analysis, it gives a combined estimate of RR = 1.22, with a 95% confidence interval of 1.02 to 1.45 ($p=0.027$) (Fig. 72.7). These results are consistent with the test result being at

Hypothetical meta-analysis of treatment for CLP

Study	Success/patients		Rate ratio	95% Confidence interval		P-Value
	Test	Control				
1	60/100	50/100	1.20	0.93	1.54	P=0.16
2	64/100	52/100	1.23	0.97	1.56	P=0.09
Combined	124/200	102/200	1.22	1.02	1.45	P=0.03

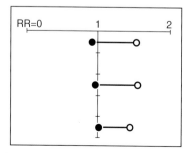

Fig. 72.7 Hypothetical meta-analysis of treatment for CLP.

least 2% better than the control, but it could be as much as 45% better. Meta-analysis has therefore turned two non-significant results into a combined statistically significant result. This can be extended to combining as many studies or trials as are available dealing with like interventions and outcomes.

Meta-analysis can either be used retrospectively on studies already completed and published, or planned prospectively. It has been used (retrospectively) to combine the results of a number of small trials, which individually showed no significant effect, to produce a significant result (e.g. the effect of cytotoxic chemotherapy in the treatment of breast cancer[59]). The analysis of a multicenter clinical trial, in which the number of patients from any particular center is insufficient to compare the interventions within that center, can be regarded as a design for which the analysis is a form of meta-analysis. However, a meta-analysis is more flexible than multicenter trials insofar as the trials from which the results are combined do not have to conform to exactly the same protocols.

Meta-analysis techniques may be one way of solving the problems of small numbers of patients. However, the current situation with CLP research is much more variable and uncertain than described above. The validity and practicability of combining the results from the trials and studies in existence is uncertain, particular when carried out in different countries, with slightly different outcomes, and different interventions in each. This is not a technique that can be applied in an uninformed manner, and often calls for a number of caveats as part of the conclusions.

I suspect that a retrospective meta-analysis of previously published work may not be possible. However, exploration of the feasibility of planning for a meta-analysis which includes the next generation of CLP patients is likely to be more fruitful.

IMPROVED RECORD SYSTEMS

The next suggestion is similar to the last in that it proposes an infrastructure to facilitate future research, in this case retrospective studies.

One of the major weaknesses of retrospective studies is missing information, or information that has not been collected in a valid or reliable form. If those who treat CLP patients could agree a set of data that is required for the evaluation or audit of treatment, this would be the first step to establishing a data infrastructure to form the basis of future research. This would include information on treatments, prognostic factors and outcomes.

There is a need for recognition among all professionals involved in the treatment and care of CLP patients that all

such patients are future research subjects; all data should be collected with this in mind. Before this can be implemented, however, an agreed set of measures needs to be developed for outcome, treatment and other prognostic variables. As a starting point, the following should be routinely collected in clinical files:

- Diagnoses
- A complete medical history
- Treatment plans and goals
- Social and psychological history
- Dental and orthodontic findings and history
- Intraoral dental casts
- Facial photographs
- Lateral cephalometric radiographs.[24]

These data relate to the principal outcomes perceived to be of concern, and the likely prognostic factors for these outcomes. The collection of this information should conform to particular standards in order to ensure that it can be included retrospectively in research studies. This is not a new idea. Preliminary work to set up a regional cleft lip and palate database was reported in 1994,[60] and has been discussed by various authors.[25,61]

IDENTIFICATION OF VALID AND RELIABLE OUTCOME INDICATORS

One of the problems of CLP research is the long time period between intervention and measurement of the outcome. This results in either prospective studies and trials not being carried out, or major compromises being made in their design.

If it were possible to identify/develop indicators that are measured a relatively short time after treatment, which are highly correlated with the outcomes, this would be a major step forward. As with any other measurement instrument, the requirements for these indicators would be their validity and reliability. For these 'early predictor' indicators, validity would need to be assessed against long-term outcome.

This has been proposed previously,[34] when it was noted that existing longitudinal data would be a starting point for this type of investigation.

Some work has already been carried out to investigate this possibility. A number of authors have suggested that the measurement of dental arch relationships using the Goslon Yardstick at age 10, and perhaps as young as age 5, is a good indicator of longer-term outcomes.[5,25,33,62] If the same could be achieved for a wide range of other outcomes, the problem of long follow-up times could be reduced.

WHAT ALTERNATIVE METHODS OF ANALYSIS ARE THERE?

The previous discussion has indicated that traditional methods of research design and analysis have limitations when endeavoring to answer the headline question, and so more radical thinking is required. One such radical thinker has proposed a non-classical statistical approach to answering this sort of question: a decision theoretic approach.[1] Petitti[59] has stated that 'Decision analysis is useful when the clinical or policy decision is complex and information is uncertain. The method is particularly useful in examining issues when at least some of the consequences of the decision are distant in time from the decision.' This describes the situation of cleft lip and palate research perfectly.

In my view, the most cogent statistical decision analysis is carried out within a framework of Bayesian statistical theory.[63,64] Individual trial and study results cannot be expected to provide an answer to the headline question on their own, but they can be viewed as changing our level of uncertainty regarding the relative effectiveness of a particular (aspects of an) intervention. The Bayesian statistical approach makes it explicit who is deciding what outcomes are most important. In fact, it allows one to analyze the data from different people's perspectives (the different professionals, the patient's and their family's) to produce perhaps conflicting answers. The advantage of this is that debate can proceed rationally, sensitive to the views of others. The approach provides a means of breaking into the difficult problem of determining how the outcomes can be maximized when aggregated across all the important dimensions.

There are five steps in a decision analysis:[65]

1. The problem is identified and bounded.
2. The problem is structured through the construction of a decision tree.
3. Information necessary to fill the decision tree is obtained.
4. The decision tree is analyzed.
5. A sensitivity analysis is carried out.

These will be described in turn, but first a simple example is presented.

A HYPOTHETICAL EXAMPLE

A simplified hypothetical example of the application of this approach, taken from Krischer,[1] is shown in Figure 72.8. This deals with an outcome on just one dimension – speech – measured by the percentage of words that are intelligible to a listener.[66] In this example there are three alternative

Example of Bayesian decision theory - Speech

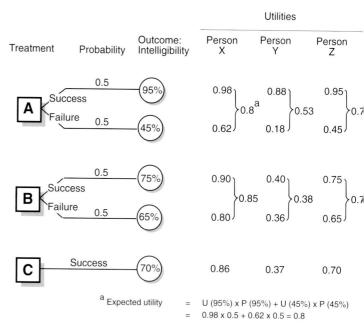

$$^a \text{Expected utility} = U(95\%) \times P(95\%) + U(45\%) \times P(45\%)$$
$$= 0.98 \times 0.5 + 0.62 \times 0.5 = 0.8$$

Fig. 72.8 Example of Bayesian decision theory – speech

treatments, A, B and C. If treatment A is successful, the outcome is that the patient will be 95% intelligible; however, if it is unsuccessful they will be 45% intelligible. The probability of success is 0.5 or 50%, and the probability of failure is 50%. For treatment B there is 50% chance of success, and in this case the patient's intelligibility is 75%; the chance of failure is 50%, in which case their intelligibility will be 65%. For treatment C there is only one outcome: 70% intelligibility with certainty.

In this example, three people have had their utilities assessed for a range of outcomes for speech. That is, the value that these three people place on each of the outcomes was assessed. Person X was risk averse. Such people tend to avoid options that could result in the worst outcome, i.e. treatment A (if treatment A fails the result will be the worst level of intelligibility out of all possible treatment options). For this person there was very little difference between treatments B and C; however, their risk averseness led them to favor treatment C. Person Y was a risk taker, tending to put much greater utility on the best outcomes and attributing little utility to mediocre outcomes. For this person the correct decision was treatment A, as they had a chance of obtaining an excellent outcome of 95% intelligibility. Person Z was risk neutral. Their change in utility from one outcome to another directly reflected the improvement from one outcome to another. In this case, person Z would be equally happy with all three treatments, as the expected level of intelligibility for each was 70%.

In all three cases, the correct decision for the particular person was obtained by maximizing their expected utility. For each person this resulted in a different decision, reflecting the type of personality for whom the utility assessment was based.

The general message from this hypothetical example is that the personality types and the preferences of each patient were different and, as a consequence, led to different optimal treatment decisions. Ideally, therefore, treatment packages should be individualized to reflect these differences.

THE STEPS IN A DECISION ANALYSIS

Identifying and bounding the problem

This consists of stating the problem concisely and breaking it down into its component parts, the first of which is to identify the initial alternative courses of action. This is usually followed by identification of the second and subsequent courses of action. The final part is the identification of the outcome(s).

A requirement of decision analysis is the identification of all possible outcomes considered relevant. This operation would obviously need to be simplified because of the large number of outcomes that exist. Only the most important outcome variables would be considered, and identification of these would require consensus between the professionals involved as well as the patients and families.

Structuring the problem

For this part a decision tree is constructed which shows graphically each component of the decision problem and its potential consequences.

Obtaining information to fill the decision tree

This step includes finding the probabilities of the proximate and long-term outcomes from sources such as literature reviews, primary data collection, and consultation with experts. This step also includes estimating the utilities associated with each of the outcomes. Each of these is discussed below.

Analysing the decision tree

The final result of this step is an estimate of the probability of occurrence of each of the possible outcomes, and from this an estimate of the expected utility associated with each of the decisions.

To obtain the probability of occurrence of each of the outcomes requires the application of Bayesian methods. It also requires the combining of probabilities for the occurrence of outcomes on several dimensions. Both of these are described below.

Sensitivity analysis

The goal of a sensitivity analysis is to examine the sensitivity of the conclusions to the assumption made, including the prior beliefs on which the analysis was based. This is also discussed below.

UTILITY THEORY

The decision-making in the example above was dependent on the probability of occurrence of each outcome and the benefits that each patient placed on each of the outcomes. The benefits associated with each of the outcomes are measured using utility, a concept which is at the center of work surrounding quality adjusted life years (QALYs) as an outcome.[67]

Utility theory is based on a set of axioms first presented by von Neumann and Morgenstern in 1947,[68] and this mathematical theory covers the properties of utility measures. Further developments led to multiattribute utility theory, which provided a way of exploring the utility associated with multidimensional outcomes and the utilities of outcomes on the constituent dimensions.[69] Methods of utility assessment usually comprise a series of value judgments related to the range of permissible outcomes (standard gambles[67]). Typically, this is achieved by asking the person to express preferences from among a series of scenarios. As utility scales need to be defined over all possible outcomes for each of the dimensions considered – appearance, growth, function, psychosocial and satisfaction – this process can be long and involved.

Under certain assumptions, utility measures can be made for each of the variables separately and then combined with weights to reflect the relative importance attached to a particular type of disablement. The weights are derived from the person making an assessment of how much of an attribute on one dimension (e.g. appearance) they would be willing to sacrifice for a given increase in another attribute (e.g. speech). An illustration of the outcome of this process was given earlier.

There are potential ethical problems associated with the assessment of utilities for a patient and their family. The assessment involves making choices between sets of hypothetical outcomes for treatment and care. Although hypothetical, the patient and their family are likely to personalize these, and this could cause significant distress. Those who believe that the benefits do not outweigh the cost of distress will deem the work unethical.

BAYESIAN METHODS

The example above showed the application of Bayesian decision theory, which is based on combining the probability of the occurrence of each of the possible outcomes with its associated utility. The decision is made that maximizes the expected utility. The framework for the estimation and combination of probabilities, which is necessary for the derivation of the probabilities associated with each of the outcomes, is based on Bayesian theory, a branch of statistical theory.

The application of Bayesian methods has been far more limited than the classical methods (e.g. hypothesis testing), but there have been a number of applications in the medical arena, notably clinical decision analysis/computer-assisted diagnosis, as well as non-medical applications, such as artificial intelligence and guidance systems, which have shown remarkable success in some cases.

Bayesian methods take their name from the Reverend Thomas Bayes, who developed and proved a very elegant theorem which, in its simplest form, gives a way to update our beliefs about a situation, using measurements and observations to produce a new set of beliefs.

$$\text{Prior beliefs} \rightarrow \text{Data} \rightarrow \text{Posterior probabilities}$$

For example, we might be completely ignorant about whether on average a test intervention is better or worse than a control before we collect any data assessing the effects of the two interventions. We could therefore write our prior beliefs as:

$$P(C > T) = P(T > C) = 0.5$$

When we collect some data and find that the control intervention has been successful 50% of the time, and the test intervention 60% of the time, our beliefs are modified. Using Bayes' theory it is possible to derive new values for $P(C > T)$ and $P(T > C)$. For example, if the above data resulted in an estimate of the $P(T > C = 0.85)$, this means that we are 85% certain that the test intervention is better than the control intervention (Fig. 72.9).

The theory has a great deal of flexibility in a number of ways:

1. The prior beliefs can be modified to describe the beliefs of each individual or groups of individuals (e.g. surgeons have different beliefs regarding the effectiveness of each of the plethora of surgical interventions available). The result of the analysis depends on the prior belief, and if each individual has a different prior belief their individual analyses will give different posterior probabilities for the outcome. However, these differences only reflect the diversity of experience and opinion within any group.

2. The examination of the effect of using different prior beliefs can be used to carry out a sensitivity analysis to judge how critical those prior beliefs are in estimating the probability of each outcome.

3. The beliefs can be updated any number of times through the collection of new data, or the incorporation of data from trials and studies in a sequential fashion, e.g.

$$\text{Prior} \rightarrow \text{Data}(1) \rightarrow \text{Posterior}(1) \rightarrow \text{Data}(2) \rightarrow \text{Posterior}(2) \rightarrow \text{etc.}$$

Consequently, it can be used in a manner similar to meta-analysis.

4. The technique allows one to incorporate subjective assessments of the strength of evidence associated with the different experimental designs that generated the information used for updating the beliefs. The known or suspected biases in those studies can be built into the analysis as uncertainties.

5. It can be used to estimate the size of the difference between the interventions, as well as just the probability

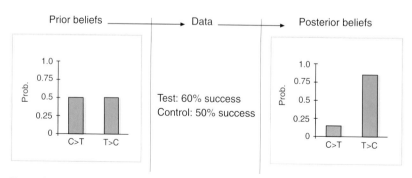

Key: C>T = Control better than test intervention
T>C = Test better than control intervention

Fig. 72.9 An illustration of Bayesian theory.

of one being better than another. This is essential for judging clinical significance.

6. As has been described, it can facilitate decision-making in the presence of incomplete information, i.e. even when the result is not statistically significant. It could also be used to highlight those areas where the greatest uncertainties exist due to lack of evidence, which should be a stimulus to future research.

The theory can be viewed as a coherent framework within which existing information about the likelihood of outcomes occurring, given the various interventions, can be marshalled.

COMBINING PROBABILITIES

The application of Bayesian decision theory involves combining probabilities in order to derive the probabilities of each combination of possible outcomes, across all the dimensions considered. Figure 72.10 gives a hypothetical and simplified example of this. What it shows are the probabilities of good appearance (and, conversely, poor appearance) following a particular intervention, as well as the probabilities of good and poor speech following the same intervention.

Figure 72.10 shows that the probability of the person having good appearance is 0.75, and of poor appearance 0.25. If the person has good appearance, the probability of their having good speech is 0.7, and of poor speech 0.3. On the other hand, if the outcome is poor appearance the probability for good speech is shown to be 0.95, and for poor speech 0.05. Consequently, the probability of having an outcome of good speech depends on whether the person has good appearance (0.70) or poor appearance (0.95) as

an outcome. By combining probabilities, the probability of each of the four outcomes shown can be produced, as shown in the right-hand column of Figure 72.10.

In a decision analysis, probability trees similar to this would need to be produced for each of the treatments to be compared. By combining information on the probabilities of each of the outcomes, with their utilities, the treatment with the largest expected utility could be identified, and this is the treatment most suitable for the patient.

ESTIMATING PROBABILITIES

In order to estimate the probabilities for each of the main treatment outcomes, there is a need for a comprehensive and highly structured review of the literature. Some literature reviews already exist, and so it may be possible to use these as a starting point for the estimation of the probability of each of the outcomes. However, the difficulties of obtaining information on, or of deriving, these probabilities should not be underestimated. Many involved in the treatment of CLP would agree that the outcomes that have been measured most routinely using standard methods are aspects of craniofacial form. However, Ross[61] found that the literature presenting cephalometric measurements could not be summarized because of variability between studies in the following: age and sex of the patient, cleft type, choice of cephalometric measurement, and operators' interpretation of landmarks from which the measurements were derived.

The general concern is that the literature is incomplete for estimating the probability of a range of different outcomes following the various interventions. This may force us to rely heavily on expert opinion (transformed into prior beliefs) of the effect of interventions, until the appropriate

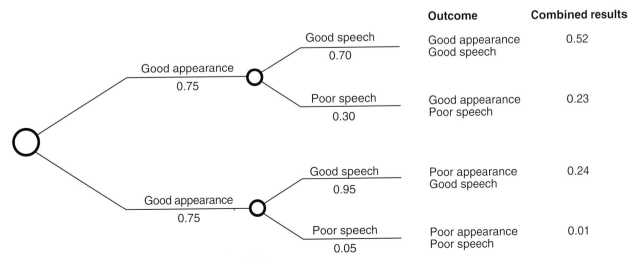

Fig. 72.10 Hypothetical example of combining probabilities.

research evidence is available. One goal of any analysis should be to clearly identify our ignorance and uncertainty, where it exists. Virtually no elements of treatment have been evaluated using rigorous experimental design.[34] Nevertheless, it is only by pursuing this approach that the gaps in our knowledge will be identified, and research carried out to fill them.

AN APPLICATION OF DECISION THEORY

Through the application of the sorts of approaches described above, Krischer[1] suggested that the differences in decision-making observed in CLP treatment and care are due, at least in part, to the way in which the different levels and types of disablement are viewed by the different specialists, e.g. their views on the relative values to be placed on cosmetic, dental, speech, hearing and psychological outcomes. For example, he examined the situation where preoperative orthopedics are used by some teams but not by others. He discovered that the team using preoperative orthopedics gave greater weight to cosmetic outcomes than did those that used purely surgical interventions. Each of these teams were making decisions consistent with their values. For the team using preoperative orthopedics, the decision that maximized their expected utility was to do so. For the other teams the decision that maximized their expected utility was not to use preoperative orthopedics. Neither decision was wrong. Although different decisions were reached, both were consistent with the value systems of the respective teams.

CONCLUSIONS

I believe that Bayesian decision theory offers the potential to make significant progress. It provides the means to marshal existing information into a coherent framework, and then to use it to make coherent choices. Nevertheless, to apply Bayesian decision theory is a major research project, but one worth investigating.

Having said this, there is still a need to carry out good research concurrently to provide more information on the efficacy of treatments, to use more sophisticated methods of analysis of those studies and trials to untangle the effects of confounding and reduce the effects of other sources of bias, to improve record systems, to identify valid and reliable indicators of the outcomes, and to develop widely accepted, valid and reliable measuring instruments. Some practitioners and researchers are already engaged in work that aims to address some of these needs, but what is missing is a coherent framework to which all this work can contribute.

REFERENCES

1. Krischer JP 1976 The mathematics of cleft lip and palate treatment evaluation: measuring the desirability of treatment outcomes. Cleft Palate Journal 14:165–180
2. Devlin HD 1990 Audit and the quality of care. Annals of the Royal College of Surgeons 73 (Special Suppl): 3–11
3. American Association of Oral and Maxillofacial Surgeons 1995 Parameters of care for oral and maxillofacial surgery. A guide for practice, monitoring, and evaluation. Journal of Oral and Maxillofacial Surgery 53 (Suppl 5):105–136
4. Shaw WC, Roberts CT, Semb G 1996 Evaluating treatment alternatives: measurement and design. In: Turvey TA, Vig KWL, Fonseca RJ (eds) Facial clefts and craniosynostosis. Principles and management. WB Saunders, London pp 756–766
5. Mars M, Asher-McDade C, Brattstrom V et al 1992 The RPS. A six-centre international study of treatment outcome in patients with clefts of the lip and palate: Part 3. Dental arch relationships. Cleft Palate–Craniofacial Journal 29:393–397
6. Lohmander-Agerskov A, Friede H, Lilja J, Soderpalm E 1996 Delayed closure of the hard palate: a comparison of speech in children with open and functionally closed residual clefts. Scandinavian Journal of Plastic and Reconstuctive Surgery and Hand Surgery 30:121–127
7. Brothers DB, Dalston RW, Peterson HD, Lawrence WT 1995 Comparison of the Furlow double opposing Z-palatoplasty with the Wardill–Kilner procedure for isolated clefts of the soft palate. Plastic and Reconstructive Surgery 95:969–977
8. American Cleft Palate–Craniofacial Association 1993 Parameters for the evaluation and treatment of patients with cleft lip/palate or other craniofacial anomalies. Cleft Palate–Craniofacial Journal 30 (Suppl 1): S1–S12
9. Clifford E 1987 The cleft experience: new perspectives on management. Charles C Thomas, Springfield
10. MacGregor FC 1990 Facial disfigurement: problems and management of social interaction and implications for mental health. Aesthetic Plastic Surgery 14:249–257
11. Ramstad T, Ottem E, Shaw WC 1995 Psychosocial adjustment in Norwegian adults who had undergone standardised treatment of complete cleft lip and palate. I Education, employment and marriage. Scandinavian Journal of Plastic and Reconstructive Surgery and Hand Surgery 29:251–257
12. Donabedian A 1966 Evaluating the quality of medical care. Milbank Memorial Fund Quarterly: Health and Society 44:166
13. McCance AM, Moss JP, Fright WR, Linney AD, James DR 1997 Three-dimensional analysis techniques – Part 2: Laser scanning: a qualitative three-dimensional soft-tissue analysis using a color-coding system. Cleft Palate–Craniofacial Journal 34:46–51
14. Berkowitz S, Pruzansky S 1968 Stereophotogrammetry of serial casts of cleft palate. Angle Orthodontics 38:136–149
15. Mardia KV 1989 Comment: some contributions to shape analysis. Statistical Science 4:108–111
16. Mishima K, Sugahara T, Mori Y, Sakuda M 1996 Three-dimensional comparison between palatal forms in infants with complete unilateral cleft lip, alveolus, and palate (UCLP) with and without Hotz's Plate. Cleft Palate–Craniofacial Journal 33:245–251
17. Morrant DG, Shaw WC 1996 Use of standardised video recordings to assess cleft surgery outcome. Cleft Palate–Craniofacial Journal 33:134–142
18. Boyle MH, Torrane GW 1984 Developing multi-attribute health indexes. Medical Care 22:1045–1057
19. Tulloch JFC, Antczak-Bouckoms AA 1996 A methodological approach to outcome assessment. In: Turvey TA, Vig KWL, Fonseca RJ (eds), Facial clefts and craniosynostosis. Principles and management. WB Saunders, London pp 745–755
20. Shaw WC, Asher-McDade C, Brattstrom V et al 1992 The RPS. A

six centre international study of treatment outcome in patients with clefts of the lip and palate: Part 1. Principles and study design. Cleft Palate–Craniofacial Journal 29:393–397

21. Semb G, Shaw WC 1996 Facial growth in orofacial clefting disorders. In: Turvey TA, Vig KWL, Fonseca RJ (eds) Facial clefts and craniosynostosis. Principles and management. WB Saunders, London pp 28–56

22. Bardach J, Morris HL, Olin WH 1984 Late results of primary veloplasty: the Marburg project. Plastic and Reconstructive Surgery 73:207–215

23. Witzel MA, Sayer KE, Ross BR. 1984 Delayed hard palate closure. The philosophy revisited. Cleft Palate Journal 21:263–269

24. Strauss RP, Ellis JHP 1996 Comprehensive team management. In: Turvey TA, Vig KWL, Fonseca RJ (eds) Facial clefts and craniosynostosis. Principles and management. WB Saunders, London pp 130–142

25. Shaw WC, Dahl E, Asher-McDade C et al 1992 The RPS. A six centre international study of treatment outcome in patients with clefts of the lip and palate: Part 5: General discussion and conclusions. Cleft Palate–Craniofacial Journal 29:393–397

26. Molsted K, Asher-McDade C, Brattstrom V et al 1992 The RPS. A six centre international study of treatment outcome in patients with clefts of the lip and palate: Part 2. Craniofacial form and soft tissue profile. Cleft Palate–Craniofacial Journal 29:393–397

27. Asher-McDade C, Brattstrom V, Dahl E et al 1992 The RPS. A six centre international study of treatment outcome in patients with clefts of the lip and palate: Part 4. Assessment of nasolabial appearance. Cleft Palate–Craniofacial Journal 29:393–397

28. Sackett DL 1979 Bias in analytical research. Journal of Chronic Diseases 32:51–63

29. Shaw WC, Williams AC, Sandy JR, Devlin HB 1996 Minimum standards for the management of cleft lip and palate: efforts to close the audit loop. Annals of the Royal College of Surgeons of England 78:110–114

30. Long RE, McNamara JA 1985 Facial growth following pharyngeal flap surgery: skeletal assessment on serial lateral cephalometric radiographs. American Journal of Orthodontics 87:187–196

31. Altman DG 1991 Practical statistics for medical research. Chapman & Hall, London

32. Jonsson G, Stenstrom S, Thilander B 1980 The use of a vomer flap covered with autogenous skin graft as a part of the palatal repair in children with unilateral cleft lip and palate. Arch dimension and occlusion up to the age of five. Scandinavian Journal of Plastic and Reconstructive Surgery 14:13–21

33. Atack NE, Hathorn IS, Semb G, Dowell T, Sandy JR 1997 A new index for assessing surgical outcome in unilateral cleft lip and palate subjects aged five: reproducibility and validity. Cleft Palate–Craniofacial Journal 34: (in press).

34. Roberts CT, Semb G, Shaw WC 1991 Strategies for the advancement of surgical methods in cleft lip and palate. Cleft Palate–Craniofacial Journal 28:141–149

35. Mars M, Plint DA, Houston WJB, Bergland O, Semb G 1987 The Goslon Yardstick: a new system of assessing dental arch relationships in children with unilateral clefts of lip and palate. Cleft Palate Journal 24:314–322

36. Shaw WC, Asher-McDade C, Brattstrom V et al 1992 The RPS. International clinical audit for cleft lip and palate – a preliminary European investigation. In: Jackson IT, Somerlad BC (eds) Recent advances in plastic surgery, No. 4. Churchill Livingstone, Edinburgh, pp 1–15

37. Bronshtein M, Blumenfeld I, Kohn J, Blumenfeld Z 1994 Detection of cleft lip by early second trimester transvaginal sonography. Obstetrics and Gynecology 84:73–76

38. Melnick M 1989 Cleft lip and cleft palate: etiology and pathogenesis. In: Kernahan DA, Rosenstein SW, Dado DV (eds) Cleft lip and palate. Williams and Wilkins, Baltimore pp 3–7

39. Bronshtein M, Blumenfeld I, Blumenfeld Z 1996 Early prenatal diagnosis of cleft lip and its potential impact on the number of babies with cleft lip. British Journal of Oral and Maxillofacial Surgery 34:486–487

40. Green LW, Lewis FM 1986 Measurement and evaluation in health education and health promotion. Mayfield Publishing Co., Palo Alto

41. Berkowitz S 1995 Ethical issues in the case of surgical repair of cleft palate. Cleft Palate–Craniofacial Journal 32:271–276

42. Shaw WC 1995 Ethical issues in the case of surgical repair of cleft palate – commentary. Cleft Palate–Craniofacial Journal 32:277–280

43. Semb G 1988 Effect of alveolar bone grafting on maxillary growth in unilateral cleft lip and palate patients. Cleft Palate Journal 25:288–295

44. Huang C-S, Cheng H-C, Chen Y-R, Noordhoff MS 1994 Maxillary dental arch affected by different sleep position in unilateral complete cleft lip and palate infants. Cleft Palate–Craniofacial Journal 31:179–184

45. McWilliams BJ, Randall P, LaRossa D, et al 1996 Speech characteristics associated with the Furlow palatoplasty as compared with other surgical techniques. Plastic and Reconstructive Surgery 98:610–619

46. Haapanen M-L 1995 Effect of method of cleft palate repair on the quality of speech at the age of 6 years. Scandinavian Journal of Plastic and Reconstructive Surgery and Hand Surgery 29:245–250

47. SAS Institute 1989 SAS/STAT user's guide, version 6, 4th edition, volumes 1 and 2. SAS Institute, Cary, NC

48. McCullagh P 1980 Regression models for ordinal data. Journal of the Royal Statistical Society B 43:109–142

49. Kleinbaum DG 1992 Logistic regression. A self-learning text. Springer-Verlag, New York

50. Fienberg SE 1980 The analysis of cross-classified categorical data The MIT Press, Cambridge MA

51. Laatikainen T, Ranta R, Nordstrom R 1996 Craniofacial morphology in twins with cleft lip and palate. Cleft Palate–Craniofacial Journal 33:96–103

52. McCullagh P, Nelder JA 1989 Generalised linear models, (2nd edn). Chapman & Hall, London

53. Norusis MJ 1993 SPSS for Windows. Base system user's guide, release 6.0. SPSS, Chicago

54. Heliovaara A, Ranta R 1993 One-stage closure of isolated cleft palate with the Veau–Wardill–Kilner V to Y pushback procedure or the Cronin modification. III. Comparison of lateral craniofacial morphology. Acta Odontologica Scandinavica 51:313–321

55. Molsted K, Dahl E, Skovgard LT, et al 1993 The RPS. A multicentre comparison of treatment regimens for unilateral cleft lip and palate using a multiple regression model. Scandinavian Journal of Reconstructive Surgery and Hand Surgery 27:277–284

56. Long RE, Spangler BE, Yow M 1995 Cleft width and secondary alveolar bone graft success. Cleft Palate–Craniofacial Journal 32:420–427

57. Semb G, Shaw WC 1990 Pharyngeal flap and facial growth. Cleft Palate Journal 27:217–224

58. Winer BJ 1971 Statistical principles in experimental design, 2nd edn. McGraw-Hill, New York

59. Petitti DB 1994 Meta-analysis, decision analysis, and cost effectiveness analysis. Methods of quantitative synthesis in medicine. OUP, Oxford

60. Luther F, Cook PA 1994 The development of a regional cleft lip and palate database – a preliminary report. British Journal of Orthodontics 21:291–295

61. Ross RB 1987 Treatment variables affecting facial growth in complete unilateral cleft lip and palate. Part 1: Treatment affecting growth. Cleft Palate Journal 24:5–23

62. Atack N, Hathorn I, Mars M, Sandy J 1997 Study models of 5 year old children as predictors of surgical outcome in unilateral cleft lip and palate. European Journal of Orthodontics 19: (in press)

63. Lilford RJ, Thornton JG, Braunholtz D 1995 Clinical trials and rare diseases: a way out of the conundrum British Medical Journal 311:1621–1625

64. Lilford RJ, Braunholtz D 1996 The statistical basis of public policy: a paradigm shift is overdue. British Medical Journal 313:603–607

65. Weinstein MC, Fineberg HV 1980 Clinical decision analysis. Saunders, Philadelphia

66. Subtelny JD, Van Hattum RJ, Myers BB 1972 Ratings and measures of cleft palate speech. Cleft Palate Journal 9:18–27

67. Torrance GW, Feeny D 1989 Utilities and quality-adjusted life years. International Journal of Technology Assessment in Health Care 5:559–575

68. von Neumann J, Morgenstern O 1947 Theory of games and economic behaviour. Princeton University Press, Princeton

69. Keeney RL, Raiffa H 1976 Decisions with multiple objectives: preferences and value tradeoffs. Wiley, New York

Surgical planning

73

LARRY M. WOLFORD/R. THEODORE FIELDS

INTRODUCTION

Dentofacial deformities affect approximately 20% of the population. Patients with dentofacial deformities may demonstrate various degrees of functional and esthetic compromise. Such malformations may be isolated to one jaw, or they may extend to multiple craniofacial structures. They may occur unilaterally or bilaterally and may be expressed to varying degrees in the vertical, horizontal and transverse facial planes. Many patients with dentofacial deformities can benefit from corrective orthognathic treatment. This chapter will focus primarily on diagnosing and treatment planning for the correction of dentofacial deformities.

Orthognathic surgery is the art and science of diagnosis, treatment planning and execution of treatment, by combining orthodontics and oral and maxillofacial surgery to correct musculoskeletal, dento-osseous and soft-tissue deformities of the jaws and associated structures.

Successful orthognathic surgery demands the understanding and cooperation of the oral and maxillofacial surgeon, orthodontist and general dentist. Each must provide a proper diagnosis and treatment plan, perform the necessary treatment, and refer for necessary treatment outside their respective areas of expertise. Support from other dental and medical professionals may be necessary to provide the optimal functional and esthetic outcome that results in patient satisfaction. These specialists may include periodontists, prosthodontists, endodontists, neurosurgeons, ophthalmologists, otolaryngologists, plastic surgeons and speech pathologists.

Moderate to severe occlusal discrepancies usually require combined orthodontic treatment and orthognathic surgery to obtain the most stable result with optimal function and esthetics. The orthodontist is largely limited to the movement of teeth and alveolar bone with little appreciable effect on basal bone. The orthodontist's role is thus to align and decompensate the teeth in relation to the upper and lower jaws. The oral and maxillofacial surgeon can move the facial skeleton, but cannot provide detailed alignment and precise interdigitation of the teeth. The oral and maxillofacial surgeon, therefore, repositions the jaws and facial structures as dictated by the existing deformities and therapeutic goals. In order for patients to receive 'state-of-the-art' care in correcting their deformities, the orthognathic team must be able to:

1. Correctly diagnose existing deformities.
2. Establish an appropriate treatment plan.
3. Execute the recommended treatment.

The basic therapeutic goals, and examples, for orthognathic surgery are provided in Table 73.1.

Specific therapeutic goals for orthognathic surgery vary from patient to patient. These goals are directed towards the correction of specific musculoskeletal, dento-osseous, and soft-tissue deformities. The specific therapeutic goals may include one or more of the following:

- Correct masticatory and/or swallowing abnormalities.
- Establish a functional occlusion through normalization of the occlusal relationship, overbite, overjet, occlusal plane angulation and transverse dimension.
- Correct the inability to open or close the jaws.

Table 73.1

Basic therapeutic goals	Examples
Function	Normal mastication, speech, ocular function, respiratory function
Esthetics	Establish facial harmony and balance
Stability	Avoid short- and long-term relapse
Minimize treatment time	Provide efficient and effective treatment

- Correct associated TMJ dysfunction, pathosis or pain.
- Correct structural abnormalities resulting from over- or underdevelopment.
- Decrease or eliminate myofascial pain and/or headaches.
- Correct abnormalities relating to respiratory compromise, i.e. sleep apnea, airway obstruction, nasal septal deviation, snoring, choanal atresia, hypertrophied turbinates, nasal polyps, etc.
- Correct speech problems, i.e. hyper- or hyponasal speech, velopharyngeal incompetence, articulatory speech dysfunction, etc.
- Improve stability of orthodontic results.
- Improve dental and periodontal health.
- Improve psychosocial impairments.

Diagnostic factors and risk factors are conditions that may modify the treatment planning and affect the outcome of the surgical procedures. Awareness of potential risk factors is mandatory for proper treatment planning and for proper preoperative patient counseling. Common diagnostic and risk factors are:

- Type of congenital or development deformity.
- Type of acquired deformity.
- Type of musculoskeletal/dento-osseous deformity.
- Type of malocclusion.
- Respiratory problems.
- Sinus or nasal airway disease and/or pathosis.
- Speech problems.
- TMJ dysfunction or pathosis.
- Masticatory and/or swallowing difficulties.
- Psychosocial impairment.
- Bone and/or soft-tissue pathoses.
- Infection.
- Bleeding dyscrasias.
- Allergies or hypersensitivity to surgical materials.
- Abnormal osseous and/or soft-tissue anatomy.
- Compromised vascularity at the surgical site.
- Systemic or localized diseases that may interfere with normal healing.
- Myofascial pain dysfunction.
- Ocular or orbital deformity and/or impairment.
- Severity of esthetic facial deformity.
- Poor patient compliance.
- Previous orthodontic and/or orthognathic surgery.
- Neuromuscular abnormalities.

PATIENT EVALUATION

Thorough evaluation and diagnosis is one of the most important aspects of overall patient management. Failure to recognize major functional and esthetic problems may lead to compromise, complications and unfavorable outcomes. Patient evaluation for orthognathic surgery may be divided into four main areas:

1. Patient concerns, or chief complaints.
2. Clinical examination.
3. Radiographic and imaging analysis.
4. Dental model analysis.

This diagnostic sequence may identify patients who are candidates for orthognathic surgery and determine whether ancillary medical or surgical procedures may be beneficial. Such patients may require further specialist evaluation for speech, audiometry, periodontics, general dental, psychologic, neurologic, ophthalmologic, medical or other concerns.

PATIENT CONCERNS

A patient's ultimate satisfaction with treatment outcome often depends upon attention to the patient's chief concerns.[1,2] While a change in appearance may be an improvement in the eye of the surgeon and may normalize a patient's profile according to cephalometric standards, such a change may be undesirable to the patient. Understanding the patient's concerns, motivations and expectations will help define treatment parameters and provide insight to the psychologic health of the patient. Specific questions that may help identify the patient's chief concerns include:

1. What are your concerns or problems?
2. Have you had previous treatment for this condition and what has been the outcome?
3. Why do you want treatment?
4. What do you expect from treatment?

This assessment of patient concerns will help develop a preliminary problem list and will help identify patients with unrealistic expectations. Patients with unrealistic expectations must be counseled so that they understand the treatment limitations and the likely outcomes before initiating orthodontic or surgical therapy. Patients who maintain unrealistic expectations are best not treated. It is important that patients thoroughly understand all the treatment options, the anticipated outcomes and the potential risks and complications. Situations involving an uninformed patient or a patient with unrealistic expectations often result in dissatisfaction and may create medicolegal difficulties. Accordingly, the surgeon and orthodontist must be careful not to mislead the patient into perceiving greater expectations than can be provided.[3–5]

SYSTEM-ORIENTED PHYSICAL EXAMINATION

Usually orthognathic surgery is performed on healthy patients. This does not, however, diminish the significance of presurgical evaluation, including medical and dental histories, physical examination and appropriate laboratory studies.[6] Obtaining an appropriate and current medical history may affect treatment planning and may help the surgeon to avoid potentially life-threatening complications. Patient examination should rule out or identify patients with difficult airways, connective tissue or autoimmune diseases, bleeding disorders, or other pathologic conditions that may preclude or modify surgery. An appropriate systemic assessment should be performed for every patient.

PATIENT PREPARATION FOR DENTOFACIAL EXAMINATION

The patient is best evaluated while sitting upright in a straight-backed chair with the examiner seated directly opposite at eye level. The patient should generally be examined with his/her pupillary plane parallel to the floor. Compensatory positioning may be appropriate for patients exhibiting orbital dystopia. The ears also may be used to establish a plane parallel to the floor. The patient's head should be oriented so that the clinical Frankfort horizontal plane (ClFH), defined as a line from the tragus of the ear to the bony infraorbital rim, is parallel to the floor (Fig. 73.1B). This is a reproducible position that mimics the 'natural' standing head posture of most individuals with normal jaw structures. This position may be used to obtain standardized measurements throughout the treatment sequence.[7] Patients with dentofacial deformities often develop alternative head postures for functional reasons or to make the deformity less obvious. It is important to adjust such compensatory head postures during clinical, radiographic and photographic evaluation by orienting the ClFH parallel to the floor.[8] Following surgical-orthodontic correction, the 'natural' head posture often reverts to a more normal position because functional and esthetic compensation is usually no longer necessary. Selecting a standardized and reproducible head position aids in proper diagnosis, as well as evaluation of post-treatment results.

Once the head is oriented properly, the mandibular condyles should be seated in the glenoid fossae with the teeth lightly touching together. Although it is important to evaluate centric occlusion, the definitive clinical examination relative to surgical-orthodontic diagnosis and treatment planning should be performed with the patient in centric relation. Failure to evaluate in centric relation may result in a misdiagnosis or incomplete diagnosis, inappropriate or compromised treatment plan, and unacceptable or compromised treatment outcome. To obtain centric relation, have the tip of the patient's tongue positioned at the most posterior aspect of the palate while gently closing together. An alternate method of obtaining centric relation is to have the patient relax the mandible and, while keeping the condyles seated, manipulate the mandible upward until the first teeth touch, and ask the patient to hold that position.

For proper evaluation, the patient's lips should be relaxed and not forced together. This relaxed lip posture will allow evaluation of vertical facial height and the morphology and drape of the soft tissues. Relaxation of the lips allows evaluation of tooth-to-lip measurements, possible lip incompetence, and coincidence of the dental midlines. Combined with mentalis muscle relaxation, lip relaxation also allows evaluation of the chin position and the presence or absence of skeletal abnormalities such as vertical maxillary excess or vertical maxillary deficiency. The lip posture is frequently overclosed with vertical maxillary deficiency patients.

FACIAL EVALUATION

For vertical facial analysis, the face is most easily divided into equal thirds (Fig. 73.1A). The upper facial third extends from the hairline to the glabella. The middle third extends from the glabella to the subnasale. The lower third extends from the subnasale to the soft-tissue mentum. Orthognathic surgery most commonly alters the lower third of the face, with some influence on the middle third.

In addition to this vertical analysis, pretreatment facial evaluation should also address the frontal and lateral facial

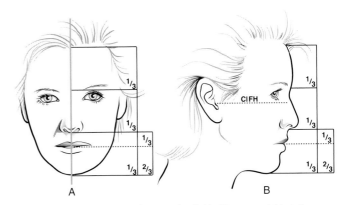

Fig. 73.1 (A) Vertically, the face can be divided into equal thirds for assessment. The lower third of the face can be divided into thirds with the distance from subnasale to upper lip stomion equaling one-third, and lower lip stomion to soft-tissue mentum equaling two-thirds. This ratio provides optimal vertical facial balance in the lower third of the face. **(B)** In profile, the face is divided in the same manner. Head orientation is important, with the clinical Frankfort horizontal (ClFH) oriented parallel to the floor. Clinical Frankfort horizontal is a line from the tragus of the ear to the bony infraorbitale.

planes. Evaluation from the frontal view should include the following 14 anatomic relationships:

1. The forehead, eyes, orbits and nose are evaluated for symmetry, size and deformity.
2. The normal intercanthal distance is 32 ± 3 mm for Caucasians, and 35 ± 3 mm for black-skinned people and orientals (Fig. 73.2)
3. The normal interpupillary distance is 65 ± 3 mm (Fig. 73.2).
4. The intercanthal distance, alar base width and palpebral fissure width should all be equal (Fig. 73.2).
5. The width of the nasal dorsum should be one-half the intercanthal distance, and the width of the nasal lobule should be two-thirds the intercanthal distance.
6. A vertical line through the medial canthus and perpendicular to the pupillary plane should fall on the alar bases ± 2 mm (Fig. 73.2).
7. The upper lip length is measured from subnasale to upper lip stomion. The normal upper lip length is 22 ± 2 mm for males and 20 ± 2 mm for females (Fig. 73.3).
8. A normal tooth to upper lip relationship exposes 2.5 ± 1.5 mm of incisal edge with the lips in repose (Fig. 73.4).
9. The facial midline, nasal midline, lip midlines, dental midlines and chin midline all should be congruent, and the face should be reasonably symmetrical, vertically and transversely (Figs 73.5, 73.6).

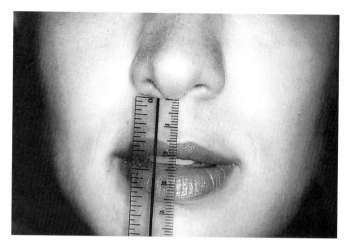

Fig. 73.3 Upper lip length is measured from subnasale to upper lip stomion. For males the normal value is 22 ± 2 mm, and for females 20 ± 2 mm.

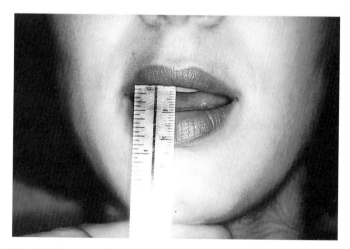

Fig. 73.4 The normal upper tooth-to-lip relationship is 2.5 ± 1.5 mm.

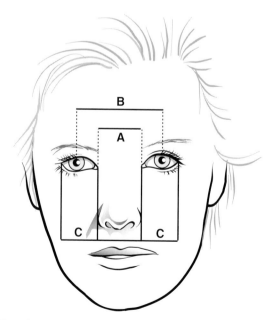

Fig. 73.2 The transverse facial balance includes a normal intercanthal distance of 32 ± 3 mm for Caucasians, and 35 ± 3 mm for blacks and orientals. The normal interpupillary distance is 65 ± 3 mm. The width of the palpebral fissures should equal the intercanthal distance.

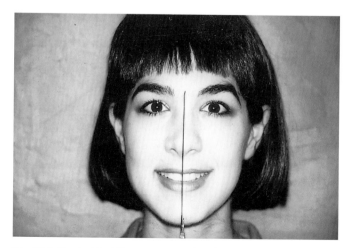

Fig. 73.5 The facial midlines are assessed, including the nasal, maxillary and mandibular dental midlines, and the chin midline, relative to the facial midline. Left to right facial symmetry is also evaluated.

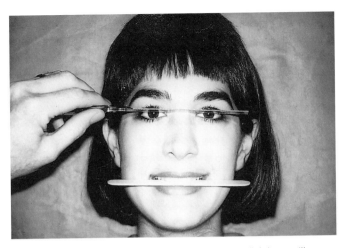

Fig. 73.6 Transversely, the occlusal plane should parallel the pupillary plane, providing there is no orbital dystopia.

10. If the patient's lips are overclosed, the jaws should be rotated open until the lips just begin to separate. The condyles should remain seated in centric relation. The true lip length and the tooth-to-lip relationship may then be evaluated.

11. The smile is frequently one of the patient's chief concerns. When smiling, the vermilion of the upper lip should fall at the cervicogingival margin with no more than 1–2 mm of exposed gingiva. In addition to this relationship, surgical decisions also must consider the tooth-to-lip relationship with the lips in repose, because many factors may influence lip posture during animation. The amount of upper lip elevation during smiling may be affected by:

    (a) anteroposterior position of the maxilla and mandible in relation to the cranial base as well as to each other;

    (b) amount of overjet and overbite;

    (c) angulation of the anterior dentoalveolus;

    (d) occlusal plane angulation;

    (e) clinical crown length;

    (f) neuromuscular function.

    Each of these factors may contribute to inaccuracies in the determination of the proper maxillary vertical position if this position is determined only by evaluation of the tooth-to-lip position during smiling.

12. The lower eyelid should be level with or slightly above the most inferior aspect of the iris. The sclera between the inferior aspect of the iris and the lower lid ('scleral show') may indicate infraorbital hypoplasia or exophthalmos.

13. The distance from glabella to subnasale and subnasale to mentum should be approximately in a 1 : 1 ratio

providing that the upper lip length is normal (Fig. 73.1A).

14. The length of the upper lip should be one-third the length of the lower facial third; i.e., lower lip stomion to soft-tissue mentum should be twice the vertical dimension of the upper lip, providing that the upper lip is normal in length (Fig. 73.1A).

LATERAL VIEW

Evaluation of the lateral plane is usually the most valuable assessment in determining vertical and anteroposterior problems of the jaws.

1. The distance from glabella to subnasale and from subnasale to soft-tissue menton should be in a 1 : 1 ratio if the upper lip length is normal (Fig. 73.1B).

2. With the maxilla in the normal anteroposterior position and the upper lip of normal thickness, the ideal chin projection is 3 ± 3 mm posterior to a line through subnasale that is perpendicular to the clinical Frankfort horizontal plane (Fig. 73.7).

3. The morphology and relationships of the nose, lips, cheeks and chin are evaluated.

4. The cervicomandibular angle is evaluated in reference to the chin position.

5. The length of the upper lip should be one-third the length of the lower facial third; i.e., lower lip stomion to soft-tissue mentum should be twice the vertical

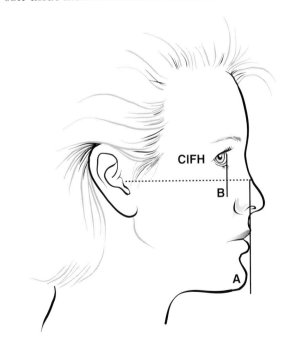

Fig. 73.7 A line perpendicular to the clinical Frankfort horizontal through the subnasale should be 3 ± 3 mm anterior to the chin. **(A)** A line tangent to the globe, perpendicular to clinical Frankfort horizontal, should fall on the infraorbital soft tissues ± 2 mm **(B)**.

dimension of the upper lip if the upper lip is normal in length (Fig. 73.1B).

6. The upper lip supralabrale should be 1–3 mm anterior to the subnasale.
7. A line perpendicular to Frankfort horizontal and tangent to the globe, should fall on the infraorbital soft tissues ± 2 mm (Fig. 73.7).

ORAL EXAMINATION

Oral examination helps identify functional and esthetic deformities of the dento-osseous and soft-tissue structures. Thorough oral examination should address the following issues:

- Occlusal relationship (Class I, Class II, Class III).
- Anterior overbite or open bite.
- Anterior overjet and any crossbites.
- Health of the dentition.
- Tooth size discrepancies.
- Curve of Wilson.
- Curve of Spee.
- Dental crowding or spacing.
- Missing, decayed, retained primary, non-salvageable teeth.
- Discrepancies between centric occlusion and centric relation.
- Periodontal evaluation.
- Transverse, A-P, or vertical asymmetries.
- Anatomic or functional tongue abnormalities.
- Record any masticatory difficulties.
- Any other pathologic processes.

Occlusal factors to be evaluated in the oral examination are discussed under 'Dental model analysis'.

PERIODONTAL EVALUATION

Several periodontal factors must be evaluated prior to orthognathic and orthodontic treatment. Patients with pre-existing periodontal disease or gingivitis have an increased risk of disease exacerbation during orthodontic treatment and post treatment, particularly in areas where interdental osteotomies may be required.[9] Factors that can adversely affect periodontal health in relation to orthognathic surgery include smoking, excessive alcohol or caffeine consumption, bruxism and clenching, connective tissue/autoimmune diseases, diabetes and malnutrition.[10] All periodontal disease should be addressed prior to orthodontics and surgery.

Inadequate attached gingiva, most frequently associated with the mandibular anterior teeth, may contribute to the development of periodontal problems such as gingival retraction, tooth sensitivity and bone loss. In areas of inadequate attached gingiva, gingival grafting should be considered. When indicated, free gingival grafts or free connective tissue grafts should be performed before the initiation of orthodontics. Gingival grafting should occur before orthodontic treatment because orthodontic tipping and surgical incisions for genioplasty, subapical osteotomies and vertical interdental osteotomies may all dramatically worsen periodontal problems and further deplete attached gingiva. Providing adequate attached gingival tissue before orthodontic and surgical intervention will protect this tissue and minimize tissue retraction.

Orthognathic surgical techniques must protect the periodontal tissues and minimize vascular compromise to the bone, teeth and soft tissues. Care should be made to maintain bone around the necks of each of the teeth at the interdental osteotomy sites. Orthodontics can facilitate interdental osteotomies by tipping the roots of the teeth away from the osteotomy site. Several studies demonstrate that with such orthodontic assistance and careful surgical technique, interdental osteotomies have a minimal effect on the periodontium.[11–14] The failure to identify risk factors, poor surgical technique and lack of attention to detail can result in devastating periodontal complications.

TEMPOROMANDIBULAR JOINT

The temporomandibular joints (TMJ) provide the foundation for orthognathic surgery. Presurgical TMJ dysfunction or undiagnosed TMJ pathosis can result in unfavorable outcomes such as postoperative pain, condylar resorption, malocclusion, jaw dysfunction and facial deformity.[15]

The TMJs should be assessed prior to treatment and periodically throughout treatment. Basic TMJ factors to consider include:

1. The patient history may reveal headaches, ear problems, myofascial pain, TMJ dysfunction, clicking and popping, crepitation, limited opening, pain, difficulty chewing, progressive development of an open bite, shifting of the mandible, or neck and shoulder problems. Etiologic factors, time of onset, signs and symptoms, previous treatments and outcomes, symptom frequency and duration, parafunctional habits, and other modifying factors should be recorded.
2. Polyarthridities or other systemic conditions should be identified or ruled out. These conditions may include connective tissue or autoimmune diseases such as: rheumatoid arthritis, systemic lupus erythematosis, scleroderma, sarcoidosis, reactive arthritis, psoriasis,

psoriatic arthritis, Sjögren's disease, ankylosing spondylitis and Reiter's syndrome.[15]

3. Clinical examination should assess pain, function and joint noise. Deviation of the mandible during opening may, for example, indicate a unilateral closed lock or fibrous ankylosis. Joint noises such as clicking and popping may suggest articular disc displacement. Crepitation within the joint may indicate osteoarthritis or perforation of the retrodiscal tissues.

4. Panoramic radiographs, transcranial radiographs, transpharyngeal radiographs, tomograms, CT scans, MRI and other imaging modalities should be obtained and evaluated as indicated.

5. Existing TMJ conditions should be properly diagnosed and discussed with the patient. Conditions requiring correction should be properly sequenced and treatment planned. The patient should be informed of any abnormal TMJ findings and how such conditions may influence their orthodontic and orthognathic outcome, even if these conditions do not require intervention.

THE NOSE

A history should be taken relative to previous nasal trauma, nasal airway obstruction, allergies, sinus problems, predominate mouth breathing versus nasal breathing, esthetic concerns and previous surgery.

A functional and esthetic nasal evaluation should include thorough examination of internal and external nasal structures. Esthetic evaluation of the external nasal anatomy should be performed from frontal and profile views. Scars, lesions, soft-tissue thickness, asymmetries and evidence of previous surgeries should be noted. From the frontal view, the normal intercanthal distance is 32 ± 3 mm (Fig. 73.2). The normal dorsal width is one-half this measurement and the normal lobule width is two-third this distance. The nasal dorsal length should fill most of the middle third of the face. No more than one-third of the vertical dimension of the nares should be visible from the frontal view.

From the clinical and radiographic profile view, the nasion should be at the same vertical level as the upper palpebral crease. The nasal dorsum should be straight to slightly concave. The normal nasolabial angle ranges from 90 to 105 degrees (Fig. 73.8). The normal nasal projection angle, measured by a line tangential to the nasal dorsum relative to a line perpendicular to the Frankfort horizontal, is 34 degrees for females and 36 degrees for males. The columella should extend 3 to 4 mm below the lateral alar rims. There should be a 2:1 ratio from the base of the nose to the anterior extent of the nares, and from the anterior aspect of the nares to the tip of the nose. The nares should

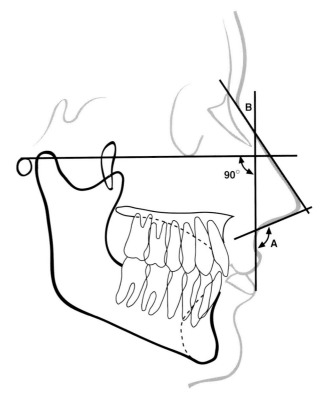

Fig. 73.8 The normal nasolabial angle is 90–105 degrees **(A)**. The normal nasal projection angle with a line tangent to the dorsum of the nose and the angle created by a line perpendicular to Frankfort horizontal should be 36 degrees for males and 34 degrees for females **(B)**.

be symmetric. Radiographic films most helpful in identifying nasal and paranasal sinus pathoses include the lateral cephalometric radiograph, Water's view, posteroanterior cephalometric radiograph, soft-tissue nasal radiographs and CT scan.

A thorough intranasal examination should be performed to identify any existing airway obstruction or pathosis, including nasal septal deviation, hypertrophied turbinates, nasal polyps or nasopharyngeal adenoids.

RADIOGRAPHIC EVALUATION

TYPES OF IMAGING TECHNIQUES

The three most routine radiographs used in the diagnosis of dentofacial deformities are: (i) the lateral cephalometric radiograph; (ii) the panoramic radiograph; and, when indicated, (iii) the periapical radiograph. Panoramic and periapical radiographs can be helpful to determine tooth alignment, root angulation and existing pathoses. Other imaging modalities such as posteroanterior cephalograms, TMJ tomograms, transcranial radiographs, Water's view images, MRI and CT scans may be required as determined by individualized patient needs.

LATERAL CEPHALOMETRIC RADIOGRAPH

The lateral cephalometric radiograph is one of the most important tools in the diagnosis of jaw deformities. It is used to analyze skeletal, dentoalveolar and soft-tissue relationships in the anteroposterior and vertical dimensions. For proper positioning, the patient's head should be postured so that the jaws are in centric relation with the teeth lightly touching and the lips relaxed. The head should be positioned so that the clinical Frankfort horizontal plane is parallel to the floor. Appropriate intensifying screens should be used so that both hard- and soft-tissue structures are properly exposed and visible on the radiograph. If the patient's bite is overclosed (such as in vertical maxillary deficiency), then a second lateral cephalometric radiograph should be taken with the condyles still seated in centric relation but the mouth opened until the lips just begin to separate. This posture will allow assessment of soft-tissue as well as bony structures without distortion of the lips. Anteroposterior cephalometric radiographs may be helpful, particularly in diagnosing and treatment planning patients with significant transverse asymmetries.

CEPHALOMETRIC ANALYSIS VERSUS CLINICAL DIAGNOSIS

There are numerous cephalometric analyses available to evaluate lateral cephalometric radiographs. Regardless of the specific analysis the clinician uses, it is important to understand that there may be significant differences between the clinical evaluation and the values obtained from cephalometric analysis. When a significant difference occurs, the clinical evaluation is far more important for treatment planning.[16] Cephalometric analysis is only an aid to clinical assessment and should not be used as the sole diagnostic tool.

CORRECTED FRANKFORT HORIZONTAL

In cases where the cephalometric values do not correlate with the clinical impression, adjustments should be made in the reference cranial base structures (i.e., corrected Frankfort horizontal line). Values should be adjusted to correlate with the clinical impression for use in diagnosis and treatment planning. The Frankfort horizontal plane may be aberrantly positioned due to vertical malposition of porion or orbitale, and/or anteroposterior malposition of nasion. A proper Frankfort horizontal plane also may be

difficult to locate due to difficulty in the radiographic identification of porion or orbitale. A corrected Frankfort horizontal plane to correlate the cephalometric values for maxillary and mandibular positions with the clinical impression provides a cephalometric analysis that will assist in diagnosis and treatment planning (Fig. 73.9). Cephalometric analysis tempered with good clinical judgment can be a valuable tool in establishing the most appropriate orthodontic and surgical treatment plan.

CEPHALOMETRIC ANALYSIS

There are many reasonable cephalometric analyses available for clinical decision-making. The authors use an analysis which evaluates 14 cephalometric relationships. This analysis permits a rapid diagnostic assessment as follows:

1. *Maxillary depth* is an angular measurement formed by the Frankfort horizontal and a line from nasion through point A (NA line). The normal value is 90 ± 3 degrees (Fig. 73.10A).
2. *Mandibular depth* is the angle formed by the Frankfort horizontal and a line from nasion through point B of

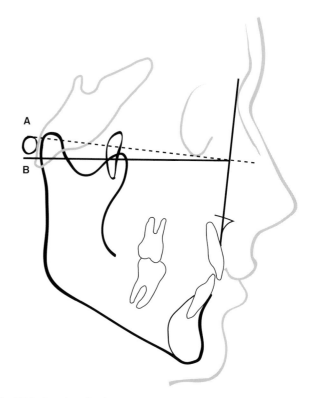

Fig. 73.9 Occasionally, the anatomic Frankfort horizontal plane **(A)** may not correlate to the clinical impression or the patient's deformity. In such instances, a corrected Frankfort horizontal plane (CFH) can be constructed **(B)** so that the numerical cephalometric values will correlate to the clinical diagnosis of the patient.

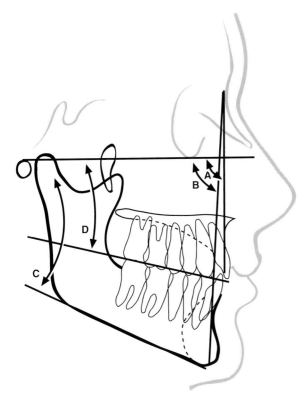

Fig. 73.10 A normal maxillary depth is 90 ± 3 degrees (**A**). The normal mandibular depth is 88 ± 3 degrees (**B**). The normal mandibular plane angle to Frankfort horizontal is 25 ± 5 degrees (**C**). The normal occlusal plane angle is 8 ± 4 degrees (**D**).

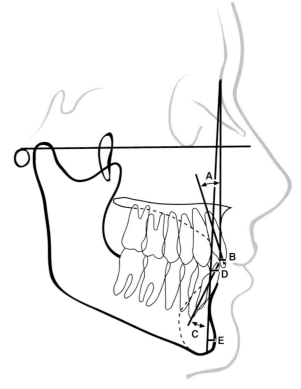

Fig. 73.11 The long axis from the upper incisor to the NA line has a normal value of 22 ± 2 degrees (**A**). The labial surface of the upper incisor should be 4 ± 2 mm anterior to the NA line (**B**). The long axis of the lower incisor to the NB line has a normal value of 20 ± 2 degrees (**C**). The labial surface of the mandibular central incisors should be 4 ± 2 mm anterior to the NB line (**D**). Hard-tissue pogonion should be 4 ± 2 mm anterior to the NB line with a 1 : 1 ratio, with the position of the labial surface of the mandibular central incisors anterior to the NB line (**E**).

the mandible (NB line). The normal value is 88 ± 3 degrees (Fig. 73.10B).

3. *The Frankfort mandibular plane angle* (FMA) is the angle created by a line from the mentum through the gonion relative to the Frankfort horizontal. The normal value is 25 ± 5 degrees (Fig. 73.10C).

4. *Occlusal plane angulation* is determined from a line drawn tangent to the buccal groove of the mandibular second molar through the cusp tips of the premolars and the angle of this line relative to the Frankfort horizontal. The normal value is 8 ± 4 degrees. The occlusal plane has significant influence on function and esthetics, particularly when double jaw surgery is performed (Fig. 73.10D).

5. *Upper incisor angulation* relates the long axis of the maxillary incisor to the NA line and is normally 22 ± 2 degrees. The labial surface of the incisor tip should be 4 ± 2 mm anterior to the NA line. Upper incisor angulation is very important in establishing the presurgical orthodontic goals (Fig. 73.11A,B).

6. *The lower incisor angulation* relates the long axis of the mandibular incisor to the NB line and is normally 20 ± 2 degrees. The labial surface of the incisor tip should be 4 ± 2 mm anterior to the NB line. It is also

important to assess the lower incisor angulation in determining the presurgical orthodontic goals (Fig. 73.11C,D).

7. *The pogonion projection* is measured from the most protrusive point of bony pogonion to the NB line with a normal relationship of 4 ± 2 mm. Optimal mandibular balance is achieved when the labial surface of the lower incisors and pogonion are in a 1 : 1 ratio anterior to the NB line (Fig. 73.11E).

8. *The upper lip length* is measured from the base of the nose (subnasale) to the inferior part of the upper lip (upper lip stomion). The normal length of an adult male lip is 22 ± 2 mm. For a female, it is 20 ± 2 mm. Upper lip length is the basis for establishing vertical facial dimensions in the lower third of the face, because the upper lip length usually is not easily altered. This measurement is the basis for establishing the vertical length of the lower two-thirds of the lower third of the face (Fig. 73.12A).

9. *The upper tooth-to-lip relationship* is measured from the relaxed upper lip stomion to the incisal edge of the

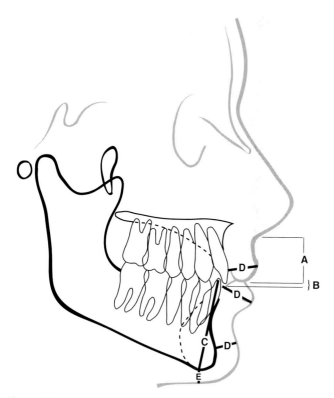

Fig. 73.12 Normal upper lip length for a male is 22 ± 2 mm, and for females 20 ± 2 mm **(A)**. Normal tooth-to-lip relationship is 2.5 ± 1.5 mm **(B)**. The lower anterior dental height is measured from the mandibular central incisor tips to hard-tissue mentum **(C)**. It has a normal value of 44 ± 2 mm in males, and 40 ± 2 mm in females. An important interrelationship is two times the upper lip length should equal the lower anterior dental height. The soft-tissue thickness of the upper lip, lower lip and chin area usually ranges from 11 to 14 mm, but more importantly should be a 1 : 1 : 1 ratio **(D)**. The soft-tissue thickness in the mentum is normally 7 ± 2 mm **(E)**.

upper incisor. The normal value is 2.5 ± 1.5 mm. This evaluation is important in establishing the vertical dimensions of the face, particularly when there are vertical dysplasias present in the maxilla (Fig. 73.12B).

10. *The lower anterior dental height* is measured perpendicular to Frankfort horizontal from the lower incisor tip to a line tangential to the hard tissue mentum. The average lower anterior dental height for a male is 44 ± 2 mm, and for females, it is 40 ± 2 mm. For optimal balance in the lower third of the face, the lower anterior dental height should be approximately twice the upper lip length. If the upper lip is longer than normal, then the lower anterior dental height should be longer than normal so that the facial dimensions will be balanced in the lower facial third (Fig. 73.12C).

11. *The soft-tissue thicknesses of the upper lip, lower lip and chin area* is normally between 11 to 14 mm. More

importantly, there should be a 1:1:1 ratio. Variations in this ratio may influence treatment planning decisions with regards to the lips and chin (Fig 73.12D).

12. *The soft-tissue thickness of the mentum* is measured perpendicular to Frankfort horizontal from hard tissue mentum to soft tissue menton. The normal dimension is 7 ± 2 mm. Excessive thickness or thinness of this area may influence alterations in the height of the anterior mandible (Fig. 73.12E).

13. *The nasal projection angle* is a line tangent to the soft tissue of the nasal dorsum and a line perpendicular to Frankfort horizontal through soft-tissue nasion. Normal is 34 degrees for females and 36 degrees for males (Fig. 73.8B).

14. *The nasolabial angle* is a line tangent to the columella through the subnasale, and a line tangent to the upper lip. The normal range is 90–105 degrees (Fig. 73.8A).

DENTAL MODEL ANALYSIS

Dental model analysis is important in establishing proper diagnoses and treatment goals, particularly in reference to orthodontics. Proper dental model analysis improves the understanding and development of the presurgical orthodontic goals. Nine basic dental model evaluations that should be made include:

1. Arch length measurements.
2. Tooth size analysis.
3. Tooth position.
4. Arch width analysis.
5. Curve of occlusion (curve of Spee).
6. Cuspid-molar position.
7. Tooth arch symmetry.
8. Buccal tooth tipping (curve of Wilson).
9. Missing, broken down or crowned teeth.

ARCH LENGTH MEASUREMENTS

These measurements should correlate the widths of the teeth relative to the amount of alveolar bone available. The evaluation of arch length and cumulative dental width helps to identify the presence or absence of crowding or spacing. This evaluation helps to determine if teeth need to be extracted, spaces need to be created or spaces need to be closed (Fig. 73.13).

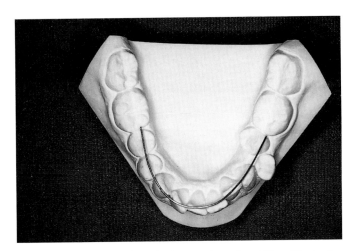

Fig. 73.13 The arch length evaluation correlates the widths of the teeth in relation to the amount of alveolar bone available. It also helps in determining if extractions are indicated and what specific orthodontic mechanics may be necessary to properly align the teeth.

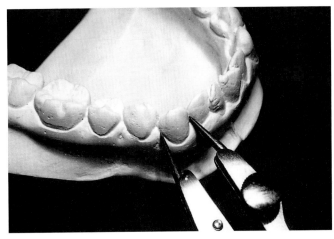

Fig. 73.14 A tooth size analysis evaluates the combined widths of the six mandibular anterior teeth in relation to the six maxillary anterior teeth. Measurements are made at the widest mesial-distal dimension. Evaluation of the tooth size compatibility is necessary so that appropriate orthodontic treatment can be utilized to correct the problem before surgery.

TOOTH SIZE ANALYSIS

This relates the relationship of the mesiodistal width of the upper teeth compared to the lower teeth. Although tooth size discrepancies can occur in the premolar and molar areas, this analysis is used primarily in relation to the anterior six maxillary and mandibular teeth. Many patients with dentofacial deformities will have anterior tooth size discrepancies, often with a decreased maxillary tooth width (most commonly attributable to small lateral incisors) in relation to the mandibular teeth. In such cases, even proper tooth alignment with all spaces closed often precludes the establishment of a good Class I cuspid relationship. Instead, an end-on or slight Class II cuspid–molar occlusal relationship often results.

Bolton's analysis is a method of correlating the widths of the upper and lower anterior six teeth. The summation of mesiodistal widths of the upper anterior six teeth measured at the contact level, divided into the combined width of the lower anterior six teeth, yields a value called the intermaxillary Bolton's index (Fig. 73.14). The average index is 77.5 ± 3.5 mm. A simple conversion of this method would be to measure the width of the lower anterior six teeth and multiply that sum by 1.3. This results in a calculated ideal upper arch width. The difference between the calculated and the actual values determines the tooth size discrepancy. Usually the lower teeth are relatively larger than the upper teeth. Tooth size discrepancies can also occur in the premolar and molar areas, where the maxillary and mandibular teeth should be approximately the same mesiodistal width. The management of tooth size discrepancies will be discussed later.

TOOTH POSITION

Tooth position in the context of orthognathic analysis refers primarily to the angulation of the maxillary and mandibular incisors in relation to the basal bone. The dental models are correlated with the cephalometric evaluation and the ideal axial inclination of the incisors is determined. The tooth position analysis determines whether extractions are necessary, spaces need to be created or eliminated, and what mechanics are needed to align and level the arches or segments of the arches.

ARCH WIDTH ANALYSIS

This refers to the evaluation of the intra-arch widths between the maxilla and the mandible. This is best analyzed by holding the models in the occlusal position that is to be achieved with the orthodontic and surgical correction, and then assessing the transverse relationship. For example, if a patient has a true skeletal Class III occlusion with a Class III cuspid–molar relationship, then the models are positioned in a Class I cuspid–molar relation and the transverse relationship evaluated. Likewise, a skeletal Class II patient in a Class II cuspid–molar relationship should be evaluated by positioning the models into a Class I cuspid–molar relationship. The transverse relationship can also be evaluated by placing the models into a Class II molar position to determine if a Class I cuspid and a Class II molar relationship would be best for that particular patient. Arch width analysis is helpful in determining presurgical orthodontic mechanics, as well as contributing to the selection of the appropriate surgical procedures.

CURVE OF OCCLUSION (CURVE OF SPEE)

The curve of occlusion has significant influence on whether the curve of occlusion in the arches will be corrected orthodontically, if extractions will be necessary, or if surgical intervention is indicated to level the occlusal plane. If an accentuated curve of occlusion in the lower arch is leveled orthodontically, the lower incisors will move anteriorly approximately 0.6–1 mm for every vertical millimeter of leveling required (Fig. 73.15). Also, it is important to understand that after about 2 mm of leveling the lower arch by intrusion of the lower incisors, the orthodontics become less stable. Correcting a reverse curve of occlusion, particularly in the lower arch, by extruding the incisors may not provide a stable result. To correct a reverse curve, surgical leveling of the arches is preferred. Surgical leveling may be achieved by subapical osteotomies or bilateral body osteotomies in the mandible or a segmental procedure in the maxilla.

CUSPID–MOLAR POSITION

The cuspid–molar position dictates the occlusal functions. It is usually preferable to have a Class I cuspid–molar relationship; however, a Class II molar relationship is very acceptable. A Class III molar relationship is less desirable, but it may be indicated in some cases.

TOOTH ARCH SYMMETRY

Tooth arch symmetry compares the left to right symmetry within each arch. There may be a significant asymmetry within the arch, such as a cuspid on one side being more anteriorly positioned than the cuspid on the opposite side. This problem often occurs when one side of the arch is missing a tooth. Correction may require special orthodontic mechanics, unilateral extraction or additional surgical procedures.

BUCCAL TOOTH TIPPING (CURVE OF WILSON)

This evaluates the position of the occlusal surfaces of the maxillary posterior teeth, in a medial-lateral direction (Fig. 73.16). If the occlusal surfaces of the maxillary posterior teeth are tipped buccally, it may be difficult to achieve a proper occlusal relationship. It is even more difficult, in the presence of a transverse maxillary deficiency with pre-existing buccal tipping, to correct the problem orthodontically, orthopedically, or even with surgically assisted orthopedic expansion. The buccal tipping will usually worsen with these mechanics. Even with surgically assisted rapid palatal expansion, the palate only expands approximately one-third the amount of the expansion that occurs at the occlusal level thus, increasing the curve of Wilson. Surgical expansion is usually advantageous because the palate can be expanded by a greater amount than the occlusal level if indicated, thus, decreasing the curve of Wilson, and segments of the maxilla can be repositioned in all three planes of space.

MISSING, BROKEN DOWN OR CROWNED TEETH

Missing, broken down or crowned teeth may influence treatment design. If a tooth is non-restorable and requires extraction in a potential osteotomy location, the extraction

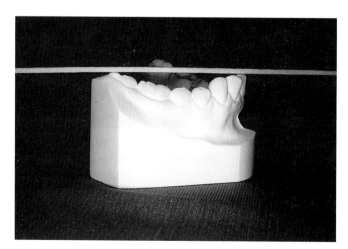

Fig. 73.15 An accentuated curve of occlusion is seen, with mid buccal teeth being several millimeters below a line tangent to the incisors and second molars. For every millimeter of vertical leveling, the lower anterior teeth will come forward 0.6–1 mm.

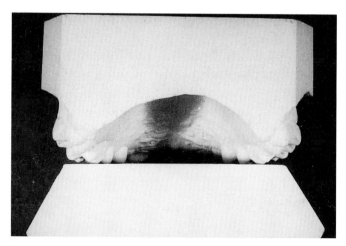

Fig. 73.16 The upper dental model is being evaluated from a posterior direction, showing significant buccal tipping (increased curve of Wilson), with the palatal cusp tips being significantly lower than the buccal cusps.

space may need to be closed orthodontically or the space maintained. In some cases, it may be helpful to maintain the tooth to improve stability during surgical alignment of the jaws or segments thereof, with removal postsurgery.

DENTAL MODEL SURGERY

Many techniques for model surgery have been proposed. In two-jaw surgery, most techniques advocate positioning the maxilla first, and fabricating an intermediate splint with the intact mandible and the repositioned maxilla. An alternative technique, however, may provide improved surgical accuracy by avoiding intraoperative maxillary shifting during the placement of intermaxillary fixation due to excessively thin maxillary walls or due to intermaxillary instability during large mandibular advancements.[17]

This alternative technique involves repositioning the mandible first, rigidly stabilizing it, and then repositioning and stabilizing the maxilla. After mounting the dental models on a semiadjustable articulator using a facebow transfer and centric bite registration, the models are carefully trimmed. The mandibular model and its base are trimmed flat on the anterior aspect. The base of the mandibular model is then trimmed to form a rectangular column of plaster beneath the model, using the initial anterior surface as the starting reference plane (Fig. 73.17). Next, the maxillary model and the base are trimmed flat from the canine to molar region bilaterally, with these cuts parallel to the dentition. The anterior and posterior aspects of the maxillary model and base are then trimmed flat, parallel to each other and perpendicular to both the base and the

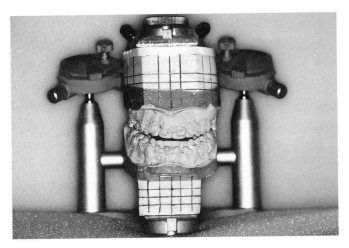

Fig. 73.17 The base of the mandibular model is trimmed to form a rectangular column of plaster beneath the model. Placement of the reference lines allows better control of mandibular orientation when moving it anteroposteriorly or transversely.

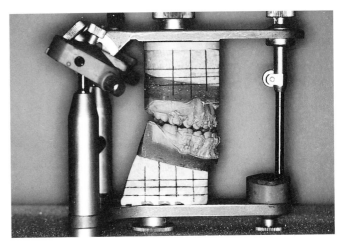

Fig. 73.18 The maxillary model is trimmed so that the plaster walls are trimmed parallel in relation to the buccal aspects of the posterior teeth.

anteroposterior midline (Fig. 73.18). Three horizontal reference lines are then drawn 5 mm apart around each of the models. Three to five vertical lines are then placed on each side of the models. The reference lines quantify anteroposterior, vertical and transverse movements of the mandible relative to the maxillary teeth and articulator base.

Measurements are taken from the surgical treatment objective (STO) (prediction tracing) to determine the position of the mandible for model surgery. The STO is superimposed over the original cephalometric analysis. A pencil point held at the condylar area allows rotation of the STO, in relation to the underlying cephalometric tracing, until the first dental contact occurs between the mandible on the STO and the maxilla on the original cephalometric tracing (Fig. 73.19). This spacially orients the anteroposterior vertical and occlusal plane orientation of the repositioned mandible relative to the uncut maxilla. The mandibular plaster model is then cut free of its base and repositioned into its new position as predetermined by the STO and prediction tracings (Fig. 73.20). The incisal pin is not altered vertically at all. Any interferences on the plaster base are removed from either the inferior base attached to the mounting ring or the undersurface of the resected mandibular model. The mandible is then secured in its new position with sticky wax or glue. An intermediate splint is fabricated to aid in positioning the mandible at the time of surgery.

The maxillary model is then cut off its base at the approximate level of the anticipated Le Fort osteotomy. The maxilla should be sectioned to obtain the best functional and occlusal relationship. Interferences are trimmed, and the maxillary occlusion is interdigitated to the best possible dental relationship and fixed to the maxillary base

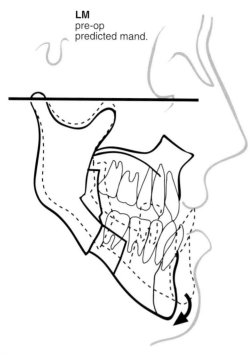

Fig. 73.19 To determine the anteroposterior position of the mandible in relation to the unoperated maxilla, a pencil point is held in the midpoint of the condylar head. The prediction tracing is rotated so that the mandible on an STO articulates with the maxilla on the cephalometric tracing where initial tooth contact is projected to occur. This relates the anteroposterior position of the mandible in relation to the unoperated maxilla. This relationship should then be reproduced in to the model surgery.

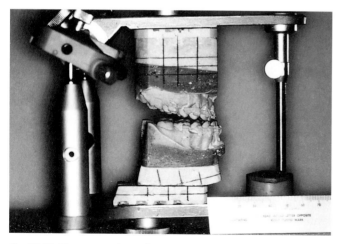

Fig. 73.20 The mounted mandibular model is repositioned on the articulator to correlate to the anteroposterior movements achieved on the STO. The resultant interdental relationship can be duplicated in surgery with the use of an intermediate splint made on the models in this position.

(Fig. 73.21). To maximize accuracy, the plaster is removed or wax is added between the mobilized segments and the stable base to simulate vertical changes. In cases where the maxilla has been expanded or where spaces have been created in the interdental cut area, we generally prefer to use a

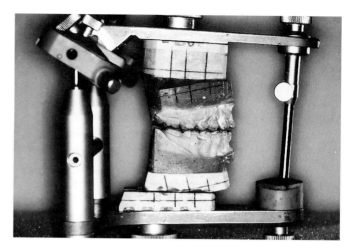

Fig. 73.21 The maxilla is then mobilized and sectioned, if indicated, and placed into occlusion to maximize the dental intercuspation.

modified palatal splint to provide transverse stabilization (Fig. 73.22). This splint creates transverse stability by interdigitating along the palatal surfaces of the dentition. The palatal soft tissues must be protected and waxed out, providing approximately 2 mm of clearance so that the splint will not restrict blood flow.

It is preferable to use a palatal splint without occlusal coverage. Most commonly we section the maxilla into three pieces between the lateral incisors and canines. Once the segments are properly positioned and stabilized, the palate is waxed out with a 2 mm thickness of wax so that the palatal mucosa is not impinged, as this could cause vascular compromise to the maxillary segments (Fig. 73.22). This splint design provides transverse stability of the maxillary

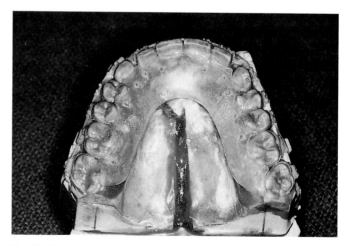

Fig. 73.22 Transverse stability of the segmentalized maxilla can be achieved using a palatal splint. The soft tissues on the palate must be waxed out, providing approximately 2 mm of wax relief. This splint does not cover the occlusal surface of the teeth. The transverse palatal stability is achieved by contact of the splint against the palatal aspects of the maxillary teeth.

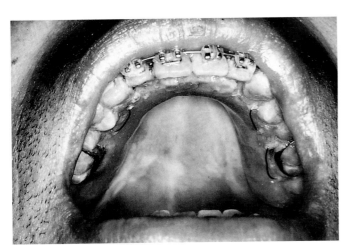

Fig. 73.23 The maxillary splint is seated and secured. Light gauge wires engage the teeth from first molar to first premolar bilaterally. The anterior teeth are usually not ligated into the splint.

arch, yet allows a maximal occlusal interrelationship. These splints can be wired in place for 1–2 months, and then continued for an additional 2–3 months as a removable appliance to maximize the transverse stability.

Interdental holes are placed in the splint so that it can be ligated to the teeth. We usually ligate individual teeth from the first molars to the first premolars. The anterior teeth are not ligated into the splint as a rule, but the interdigitation of the splint to those teeth can help maintain the anteroposterior position (Fig. 73.23). We prefer this splint to an occlusal covering splint, because we feel that it significantly decreases occlusal discrepancies and allows maximal interdigitation of the maxillary and mandibular teeth, thus decreasing potential postsurgical occlusal problems. Shifting between the reference lines on the mobilized portion of the models and the stable bases will be very useful at the time of surgery to help correlate the movements. With accurate prediction tracings, model surgery and splint fabrication, the surgery is greatly simplified. When the mandible is positioned first, the only measurement required during surgery is the vertical position of the maxillary central incisors. Proper use of the mandibular inferior border reciprocating saw blade[18] reduces the risk of a bad splint and facilitates predictable mandibular first surgical sequencing.

Maxillary surgery can be performed first, but segmental surgery requires the construction of both intermediate and final splints. With a final splint that covers the occlusal surfaces of the maxillary teeth, the intermediate splint must join the mandibular teeth and the undersurface of the final splint. Surgical stability may be compromised if the maxilla is repositioned first and mandibular advancement is required, particularly when large mandibular advancements are required. Mandibular advancement may stress the maxillary bone plates to the degree that the maxillomandibular complex can rotate backward before rigid fixation is applied to the mandible. This may result in a functional and esthetic compromise.

ORTHODONTICS WITHOUT PRIOR SURGICAL CONSIDERATION

Occasionally, orthodontic treatment is initiated before the need for surgery is recognized. When this situation arises, the orthodontist and surgeon should compare the pretreatment records with records that show the patient's present condition. The stability of the orthodontic mechanics must be assessed. If there are concerns about instability of the dental alignment within the arches, then the arch wires can be sectioned to allow vertical and transverse relapse while maintaining the correction of any rotations. The teeth should be allowed to settle for 4–6 months if significant unstable movements have been performed such as rapid palatal expansion, orthodontic expansion, orthodontic closing of open bites, or dental extrusion or intrusion. The patient should be re-evaluated with new records after stabilization to establish the proper diagnosis and treatment goals.

DIAGNOSTIC LIST

Before developing a treatment plan, establish a list of all existing problems evident from clinical, radiographic, dental model and other indicated evaluations. This problem list should include: skeletal imbalances, occlusal problems, esthetic concerns, temporomandibular disfunction (TMD) and/or myofascial pain, missing teeth, crowns, bridges, endodontically treated teeth, dental implants, periodontal problems or other functional disorders. The diagnostic list includes all functional, esthetic and dental problems, as well as any other medical factors that may affect treatment outcomes. The treatment plan is formulated from the problem list.

INITIAL SURGICAL TREATMENT OBJECTIVE

The surgical treatment objective (STO), or prediction tracing, is a two-dimensional projection of the osseous, dental and soft-tissue changes resulting from surgical orthodontic correction of orthodontic and orthopedic deformities.[19]

The purposes of the STO are threefold: (i) establish orthodontic goals; (ii) to develop surgical objectives; and (iii) to create the predicted facial profile which can be used as a visual aid in patient consultation.

The STO has significant importance in two phases of treatment planning. The initial STO is prepared before treatment to determine orthodontic and surgical goals. The final STO is prepared after active orthodontic treatment and before surgery to determine the exact vertical and anteroposterior changes to be achieved. The STO is important in establishing treatment objectives and projected results, as both a diagnostic aid and a treatment planning blueprint.

PRESURGICAL ORTHODONTIC GOALS

Before performing an initial STO, presurgical orthodontic treatment goals must be established by clinical examination, dental model evaluation and cephalometric analysis. The basic orthodontic goal is to upright the teeth over basal bone while also satisfying spatial requirements. Specifically, the ideal initial presurgical orthodontic goals are:

1. Position the long axis of the maxillary central incisors so that their final position will be approximately 22 degrees to the NA line, with the labial face of the incisors 4 mm anterior to that line.
2. Position the long axis of the mandibular central incisors so that their final position will be approximately 20 degrees to the NB line, with the labial face of the incisors 4 mm anterior to that line.
3. Satisfy arch length requirements in regards to crowding or spacing.

These ideal incisor positions to the NA and NB lines provide the most practical method for establishing the presurgical orthodontic goals.

A complete orthodontic treatment plan should be developed prior to the initiation of compensations, and identifying proper anchorage. By overlying a second acetate sheet on the original cephalometric tracing, the presurgical orthodontic goals can be simulated by tracing the teeth into the desired presurgical orthodontic position. The orthodontist can then determine the required orthodontic mechanics to meet the presurgical goal.

When developing the initial STO for mandibular but not maxillary surgery, the surgical reference lines are drawn on the original cephalometric radiograph to mimic actual surgical cuts (Fig. 73.24). All landmarks that remain unchanged with the mandibular movement are traced onto the STO acetate sheet, including the cranial base struc-

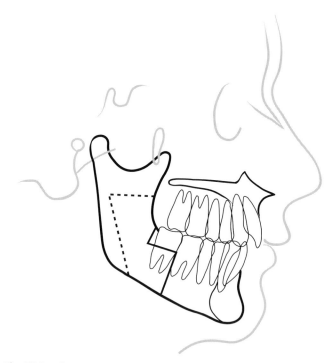

Fig. 73.24 The surgical reference lines in the mandible are drawn on to the radiograph in the areas where they will actually be performed at the time of surgery.

tures, the maxilla, the soft tissue of the nose and the upper lip. The STO acetate sheet is then repositioned so that the mandibular dentition is in the best fit with the maxillary dentition and the distal portion of the mandible is traced into its new position. The proximal segment is then traced in its original position, or rotated around the condyle until the distal and proximal segments have the best fit. Shifts between the surgical reference lines will indicate bone to be removed or spaces that will be created (Fig. 73.25). The chin is then evaluated, and any indicated chin procedure is drawn on the STO. The soft tissues are then drawn in to complete the STO.

With only maxillary surgery, the most important surgical decision is determining the vertical position of the maxilla. The anteroposterior position of the maxilla on the prediction tracing will be determined by the position of the mandible. The surgical reference line for the maxillary osteotomy is drawn on the original cephalometric tracing to simulate the level of surgery (Fig. 73.26). The basic landmarks that will remain unchanged should be traced on the acetate sheet of the STO. These landmarks include the cranial base, frontal bone and nasal bones. A horizontal line at the proper vertical position of the maxillary incisal edges is drawn parallel to the Frankfort horizontal (Fig. 73.27). The acetate sheet is then rotated around the midpoint of

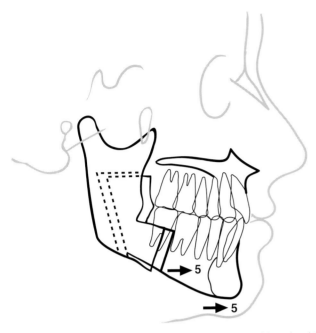

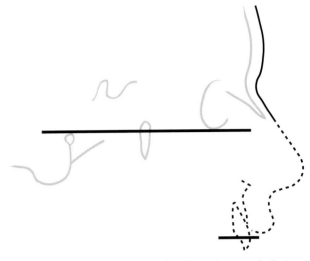

Fig. 73.27 On the STO, the stable landmarks are drawn and a horizontal line is used to determine the vertical position of the maxillary central incisors. This line is drawn parallel to the Frankfort horizontal.

Fig. 73.25 The mandible has been advanced to its new position, the chin assessed, and the soft tissues traced to complete the prediction tracing. The shift between the surgical reference lines indicates the amount of advancement to occur.

the mandibular condyle until the mandibular incisors are 1–2 mm above the incisor tip reference line to correlate to the amount of vertical maxillary change to be achieved with the treatment. The mandible is then traced onto the STO (Fig. 73.28). The maxilla, whether segmented or one piece, is then placed into the best fit of the dental segments. The teeth, bony structures and soft tissues are then traced in accordingly (Fig. 73.29).

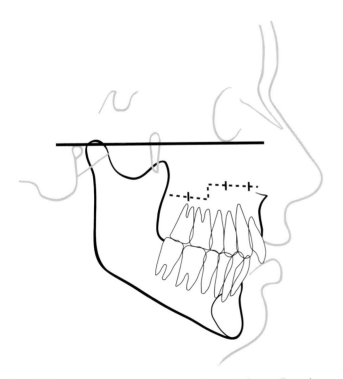

Fig. 73.26 The surgical reference lines are drawn on the maxilla at the actual location where these cuts will be performed. It is preferable to use the maxillary step osteotomy with the step in the zygomatic buttress area.

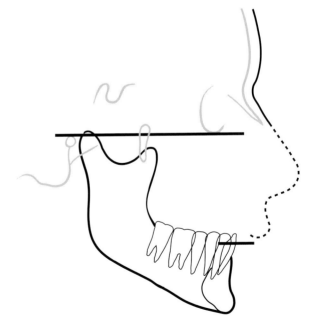

Fig. 73.28 From the original cephalometric radiograph, the mandible is rotated upwards in relation to the horizontal reference line on the STO tracing until the lower central incisors are approximately 2 mm above that line. The mandible is then traced in its new position, indicating the final position of the mandible in relation to the stable cranial-based structures.

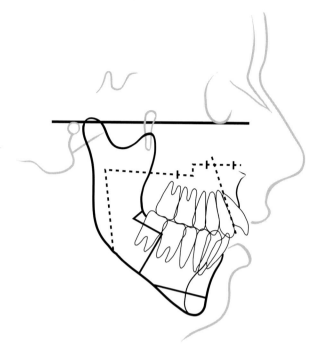

Fig. 73.29 The segments of the maxilla are then positioned into occlusion with the mandible and the new relationships are traced onto the prediction tracing, including the surgical reference lines and soft tissues.

DOUBLE JAW SURGERY

After the cephalometric tracing is complete, the surgical reference lines are drawn on it to mimic the actual position of the surgical sites (Fig. 73.30). There are three critical decisions when planning double jaw surgery:

1. The vertical position of the maxillary incisor.
2. The anteroposterior position of the maxillary incisor.
3. The occlusal plane angulation.

These lines are drawn on the STO after tracing all stable landmarks (Fig. 73.31A). The anterior maxillary segment on the cephalometric tracing is positioned on the STO by placing point A on the NA line and the incisor tip is placed on the vertical and anteroposterior reference lines and tracing it onto the STO (Fig. 73.31B). With the mandible positioned onto the STO in relation to the maxillary incisors and the occlusal plane angulation (Fig. 73.32), the distal mandibular segment is traced onto the STO. The

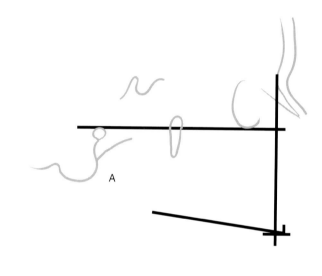

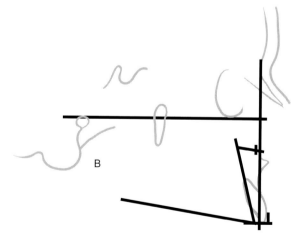

Fig. 73.31 (A) The vertical position of the maxillary central incisors is selected and a horizontal line is drawn to mark that position. The anteroposterior position of the labial surfaces of the maxillary central incisors is determined by placing a short vertical line 4 mm anterior to the normal maxillary depth. The occlusal plane angle (normal 8 ± 4 degrees) is selected based on functional and esthetic goals. **(B)** The anterior maxillary segment is aligned and positioned by placing the incisal tips of the maxillary central incisors on the horizontal reference line. The vertical surface should be placed against the anterior reference line and point A on the normal maxillary depth line. The anterior maxilla and the surgical reference lines are then traced.

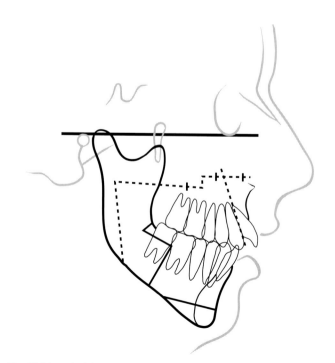

Fig. 73.30 In double jaw surgery, the surgical reference lines are drawn on the cephalometric tracing to mimic the actual position of the surgical cuts.

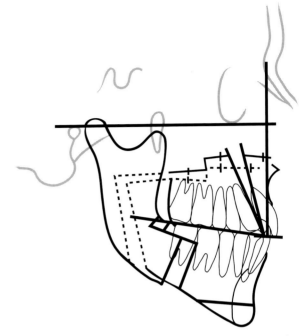

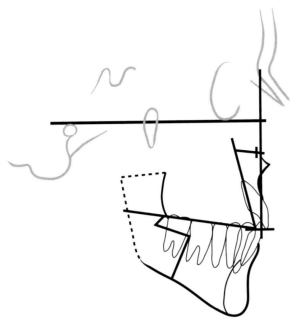

Fig. 73.32 The mandible is positioned into the best fit in reference to the maxillary incisors and the occlusal plane angle reference line. The distal mandibular dental segment and surgical reference lines are then traced.

Fig. 73.34 The posterior segment of the maxilla is then positioned and integrated with the best fit into the mandible. The surgical reference lines are appropriately traced.

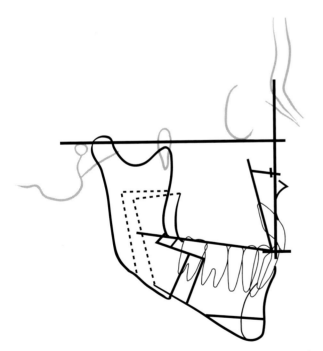

Fig. 73.33 The proximal segment is rotated until the *buccal* horizontal surgical reference lines contact each other. The proximal segment and surgical reference lines are then traced.

ed onto the STO, the chin position then should be determined. The NB line provides a convenient reference for determination of the anteroposterior position of bony pogonion. There should be a 1:1 ratio between the distances from the labial surface of the mandibular central incisors to the NB line and from the pogonion to the NB line (Fig. 73.35). The vertical dimension of the anterior mandible is measured from the tip of the mandibular central incisors to hard-tissue mentum. For optimal esthetics, this dimension should equal twice the upper lip length. Appropriate alteration of the bony chin is traced onto the STO. The soft tissues are then added to complete the STO. Skeletal, dental and soft-tissue changes on the STO are compared to the original cephalometric tracing. These changes should be recorded on the STO. The STO now provides the blueprint for dental model surgery and the actual surgical procedures.

SOFT-TISSUE CHANGES

Soft-tissue changes discussed here assume an alar base cinch suture and an intraoral V–Y closure are used to close the maxillary incision. Upper lip supralabrale advances approximately 80% the amount of maxillary advancement (Fig. 73.36A). In maxillary setbacks, the upper lip will move posteriorly about 50% the amount of anteroposterior movement of the maxilla (Fig. 73.36B). Superior repositioning of the maxilla will lengthen the upper lip about

proximal mandibular segment is then aligned onto the STO with the distal segment and traced (Fig. 73.33). The posterior segment of the maxilla is positioned onto the STO to interdigitate best with the mandibular dentition (Fig. 73.34). The surgical reference lines are traced onto the STO with each segment. Once the maxilla and mandible are position-

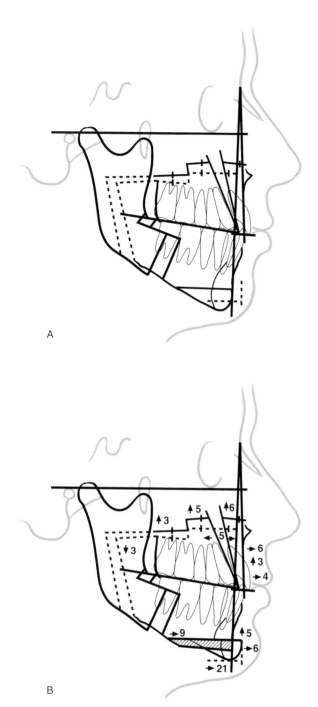

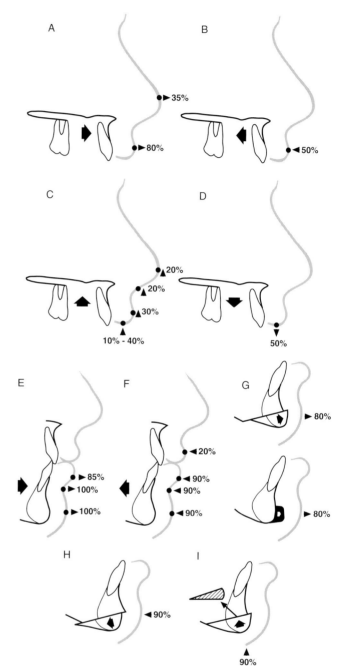

Fig. 73.35 (A) The NB line is drawn to determine the anteroposterior position of the chin. An ideal relationship is when the labial surfaces of the mandibular central incisors and the chin are both 4 ± 2 mm anterior to the NB line. The vertical height of the mandible, as measured from the mandibular central incisor tips to hard-tissue menton, should equal twice the upper lip length for optimal facial balance. **(B)** Indicated chin alterations are made and the soft tissues drawn.

50% the amount of downward movement of the maxilla (Fig. 73.36D). Mandibular advancement will advance soft-tissue pogonion approximately 100% at pogonion. With mandibular advancement, lower lip infralabrale will advance approximately 85% (Fig. 73.36E). As the mandible is moved posteriorly, soft-tissue pogonion will move backward, approximately 90% the amount of bony movement (Fig.

Fig. 73.36 (A) The upper lip moves forward approximately 80% the amount of maxillary advancement and the nasal tip will elevate approximately 35%. **(B)** When the maxilla is moved posteriorly, the upper lip will retract about 50% of the maxillary movement. **(C)** With superior repositioning of the maxilla, the upper lip will shorten vertically 10–40% the amount of vertical movement, depending on soft-tissue management. **(D)** The upper lip will lengthen approximately 50% the amount of downward movement of the maxilla. **(E)** With mandibular advancement, the soft tissues at the menton will advance approximately the same distance as the anteroposterior movement of the pogonion. The lower lip will advance about 85%. **(F)** As the mandible is moved posteriorly, the soft tissue at pogonion will move posteriorly approximately 90% the amount of bony movement. The upper lip will move posteriorly approximately 20% the amount of mandibular movement. **(G)** Either osseous or alloplastic chin augmentation will produce approximately an 80–85% soft-tissue advancement. **(H)** As the chin is set posteriorly, the soft tissues will change about 90% the amount of anteroposterior movement. **(I)** As the osseous chin is moved superiorly, the soft tissues change about 90% of the vertical bony movement.

73.36F). For chin augmentations, either osseous or allo-plastic, soft tissues will advance approximately 80–85% the amount of anteroposterior hard-tissue augmentation (Fig. 73.36G). The vertical lengthening of the chin will cause about 100% of soft-tissue vertical change at the menton. Posterior movement of the chin will result in about 90% posterior movement of the soft tissues (Fig.73.36H). Vertical reduction of the chin with a wedge ostectomy, and moving the inferior border of the mandible superiorly, will result in about 90% vertical soft-tissue change (Fig. 73.36I).

THE FINAL SURGICAL TREATMENT OBJECTIVE

The final STO is performed on a lateral cephalometric tracing after active presurgical orthodontic treatment has been completed and immediately before surgery. The same basic approach to STO construction is used as described for the initial STO. Correlation of the model surgery to the final STO prediction tracing should provide an accurate surgical guide.

DEFINITIVE TREATMENT PLAN

The definitive treatment plan is formulated based on the patient's concerns, clinical evaluation, radiographic analysis, dental model evaluation, initial STO and other relevant studies. The general sequencing of treatment is described below.

DENTAL AND PERIODONTAL TREATMENT

Any indicated periodontal or general dental maintenance, prevention or restoration should be performed prior to orthodontic and surgical intervention. The dental objective is to maintain as many teeth as possible and stabilize the periodontium. Temporary crowns and bridges should be placed where necessary for the orthodontic and surgical phases of treatment. Definitive restorations should be fabricated and delivered after surgery and orthodontics are completed. Periodontal management may include scaling and curettage, as well as gingival grafting, to provide adequate attached gingiva. Gingival grafting is most commonly needed in the anterior mandible. Providing adequate attached gingiva and good periodontal health are most important when orthodontic mechanics will tip the mandibular anterior teeth forward and when anterior vestibular incisions are necessary to perform genioplasty, subapical osteotomies or anterior body osteotomies. Inadequate attached gingiva will likely result in periodontal stripping and loss of supportive bone.

EXTRACTIONS

Extractions are sometimes necessary to correct for arch length and dental width discrepancies. Premolars are the most common teeth extracted, usually related to excessive crowding or overangulated incisors. Ideally, third molars should be removed at least 9–12 months prior to mandibular osteotomies, particularly when traditional sagittal split surgical techniques are planned. Early removal allows the extraction sites to heal properly and provide stable bony interfaces for the osteotomized bony margins. The presence of the third molars significantly weakens both proximal and distal segments and may increase the risk of unfavorable splits or mandibular fractures.

Use of the inferior border osteotomy technique[18] usually allows safe removal of the mandibular third molars at the time of sagittal split osteotomy, but the safest technique is still early removal of the mandibular third molars. Maxillary third molars also may be removed at the same time as the maxillary osteotomies. If removing maxillary third molars during orthognathic procedures, it is preferable to remove them after mobilization of the maxilla to minimize the risk of unfavorable fracture in the tuberosity region. Removing maxillary third molars during orthognathic surgery may provide poor bony interfaces in the tuberosity region, cause fracture of tuberosity bone, and restrict placement of rigid fixation plates. If the maxillary third molars are removed prior to orthognathic surgery, they should be removed 9–12 months before, to allow adequate healing and to optimize the vertical bony support in this region.

PRESURGICAL ORTHODONTICS

The orthodontist is responsible for moving the teeth to a more desirable position over basal bone in preparation for surgical repositioning. Primary presurgical orthodontic goals include:

1. *Position the teeth over the basal bone* and eliminate dental compensations. The desired dental positions are established according to clinical evaluation, initial STO and dental model analysis. Surgically assisted rapid palatal expansion, orthopedic expansion, orthodontic expansion or distraction osteogenesis may be used to help position teeth over basal bone without extraction in the crowded arch. These types of expansions must be performed carefully because of the potential for transverse orthodontic relapse. Long-term retention is required to maintain a stable occlusal result.

2. *Align and level the teeth* within their respective arches as determined by the cephalometric, dental model and clinical analyses. When there are excessive curves or reverse curves in the occlusion (curve of Spee), it must be determined whether to level orthodontically or to

use surgery such as mandibular body osteotomies, subapical osteotomies and/or segmentalization of the maxilla. Surgical procedures are typically more stable in the leveling of significant occlusal curves.

3. *Adjustment for tooth size discrepancy.* Tooth size discrepancies usually occur because of small maxillary lateral incisors. This situation decreases the combined mesiodistal width of the six maxillary anterior teeth, such that proper arrangement with the six lower anterior teeth is difficult. An end-on Class II cuspid relationship often results. If the Bolton analysis indicates a significant tooth size discrepancy, it may be impossible to achieve a Class I canine relationship at the time of surgery without appropriate presurgical orthodontic adjustments. For some patients, tooth size discrepancy may be treated best by closing spaces and recontouring the interproximal contact areas to reduce the width of the lower teeth. For other patients, it may be more appropriate to open spaces between the maxillary anterior teeth, usually adjacent to the lateral incisors. These spaces can be eliminated postsurgically by placing crowns or veneers. Occasionally, osteotomies may be indicated to create space to correct for tooth size discrepancies. Vertical osteotomies between the lateral incisors and canines can allow adjustment for up to 2–3 mm of tooth size discrepancy. Extraction of a lower incisor may be considered when the tooth size discrepancy is greater than 5 mm and significant crowding or overangulation of the lower incisors is present.

4. *Correction of rotated teeth.* Dental rotations may be evaluated from the dental models and direct clinical assessment. If the rotations do not interfere with the establishment of the desired dentoskeletal relationship, they may be corrected postsurgically. Most rotations, however, are corrected during the presurgical orthodontic phase.

5. *Divergence of roots adjacent to surgical sites.* If interdental osteotomies are planned, it may be necessary for the orthodontist to tip the adjacent tooth roots away from the area of the planned osteotomy to prevent damage to the teeth. Periapical radiographs are helpful in assisting with this determination. If the roots are too close together, postsurgical periodontal problems may develop with loss of interdental bone and teeth.[10,11]

6. *Coordination of upper and lower arch widths.* Certain transverse arch width discrepancies can be corrected with stable and predictable orthodontic movements.Others may require dentofacial orthopedics, surgically assisted rapid palatal expansion or surgical expansion. The stability of maxillary arch expansion after orthodontic, orthopedic or surgically assisted rapid palatal expansion may be predicted as follows:

(a) The bite is more likely to open anteriorly if the incisors have significant initial vertical inclination. These techniques should not be used when there is a significant pre-existing open bite. If the maxillary incisors are overangulated, then the bite will deepen anteriorly as the spacing is closed.

(b) Buccal tipping of the maxillary posterior teeth will increase the curve of Wilson. These techniques are not recommended when significant pretreatment buccal tipping exists.

(c) Long-term or permanent retention will be necessary to counterbalance the orthodontic relapse seen in many of these patients.

(d) In late adolescent and adult patients, surgical assistance is likely to be necessary to expand the maxilla orthodontically or orthopedically, because the midpalatal suture is no longer amenable to orthodontic expansion.

Surgical expansion of the maxilla at the time of the Le Fort I procedure using multiple segmentation of the maxilla, stabilization with bone plates and hard-tissue grafting of the palate and lateral maxillary walls allows stable expansion when appropriate final splints are used.

SURGERY

The surgical procedures used to correct existing musculoskeletal deformities must provide optimal functional and esthetic results with good stability. New records should be taken before surgery, and the patient should be re-evaluated to determine the progress and readiness for surgery. A new STO should be performed to determine the final position of the jaws and to predict the resultant profile. For double jaw surgery, a simulated surgery is then performed on the facebow-mounted dental models to determine how the dento-osseous structures will be repositioned. The preferred surgical sequencing is listed below:

1. TMJ management.
2. Mandibular ramus sagittal split osteotomies.
3. Removal of mandibular third molars.
4. Subapical and/or body osteotomies.
5. Application of rigid fixation to mandible.
6. Maxillary osteotomies and mobilization.
7. Removal of maxillary third molars.
8. Turbinectomies/nasoseptoplasties.
9. Maxillary segmentation, application of rigid fixation and appropriate grafting.
10. Genioplasty.

11. Facial augmentation.
12. Rhinoplasty.
13. Submental/submandibular suction lipectomy.

This sequencing will help achieve optimal outcomes, whether performed at one or more operations.

POSTSURGICAL ORTHODONTICS

When rigid skeletal fixation is used, postsurgical orthodontics can usually begin 4–8 weeks after surgery. The teeth and osseous segments can be moved rapidly during the first few months following surgery. The orthodontist should see the patient every 1–2 weeks for adjustments during the first 2–3 months of postsurgical orthodontics so that changes may be monitored closely. Once the initial healing phase is complete and the occlusion is stable, the appointment intervals can be extended to a more traditional time frame. The final positioning of the teeth usually takes from 3 to 12 months of postsurgical orthodontic treatment, but sometimes longer, depending on the orthodontic requirements. Although reasonable stability from surgical healing occurs in approximately 3–4 months, the final postsurgical healing phase may take 9–12 months.

DEFINITIVE PERIODONTAL AND GENERAL DENTAL MANAGEMENT

Definitive periodontal treatment, such as esthetic periodontal surgery and mucoperiosteal flap procedures, may be performed at this time. Lastly, definitive restorations and prosthetic tooth replacement complete the treatment. Ancillary treatment such as rhinoplasty or speech therapy may be sequenced as indicated for each specific patient.

SURGICAL PROCEDURES

There are many surgical procedures available to correct dentofacial deformities. Orthognathic surgeons should have experience with these procedures and a thorough understanding of reasonable treatment goals in order to develop a plan that provides optimal functional and esthetic results. The surgeon must be aware of the potential risks and complications that can occur with each of these procedures. This knowledge will enable the surgeon to develop an optimal treatment plan and alternative treatments according to his or her level of skill. The surgeon must be able to communicate to the patient the existing problems, the magnitude of these problems, the recommended treatment, alternative treatment options, and the potential risks and complications.

GENIOPLASTY PROCEDURES

Genioplasty procedures can alter the position of the chin in all three planes of space. Chin position is most commonly changed by use of a sliding osteotomy or by the addition of an alloplastic implant.

OSSEOUS PROCEDURES

When the bony chin is to be repositioned, a soft-tissue pedicle must be maintained to ensure viability to the osteotomized segment. The traditional horizontal osteotomy (Fig. 73.37A) or the tenon and mortise technique can be used. Stabilization can be achieved by wiring, bone screws and/or bone plates.

Anteroposterior augmentation

The usual limiting factor for chin advancement is the anteroposterior dimension of the symphysis, unless the osteotomized segment is surgically tiered. If the chin is narrow transversely, advancement will tend to make the face appear even more tapered. Soft-tissue change is approximately 80–85% of the amount of bony augmentation (Fig. 73.36G). Over time, anterior bone resorption can occur with an osseous result of 80% compared to the original amount of advancement. Soft tissue may also regress posteriorly.

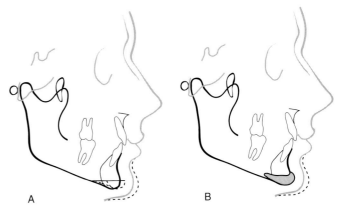

Fig. 73.37 (A) An osseous genioplasty can be used to augment the chin, move it posteriorly, alter its vertical position or change the transverse postion of the chin. **(B)** Alloplastic implants can be used to augment the chin anteriorly. They are less effective for vertical augmentation.

Anteroposterior reduction

Optimal soft-tissue change is achieved by performing a horizontal sliding osteotomy and moving the chin and attached soft tissues posteriorly. The chin usually appears wider after this procedure and the labiomental fold decreases. Soft-tissue change, if soft tissue remains attached to the anterior and inferior aspect of the chin, is usually 90% of the anteroposterior bony reduction. Shaving of the anterior aspect of the bony chin may result in only 20–30% posterior movement of the soft tissue in relation to the amount of bone removed. Care should be taken to ensure the soft tissues 'follow' the hard tissue. Not infrequently failure to do so will leave a mobile soft-tissue mass which may be pulled inferiorly by mentalis, to produce an unattractive ptosis of the chin.

Vertical augmentation (down-graft)

Vertical augmentation is best accomplished with a horizontal osteotomy and inferior repositioning of the chin segment. This technique usually requires bone or synthetic hard-tissue grafting. Soft-tissue change is approximately 100% of the osseous change.

Vertical reduction

The most predictable vertical reduction is with a wedge resection and rotation of the inferior chin segment superiorly. When soft tissue remains attached to the inferior border, the soft-tissue change will be approximately 90% of the vertical osseous change. If the inferior border is resected and removed, then the vertical soft-tissue change will be only 25–30% of the amount of bone removed.

Transverse repositioning

Transverse repositioning is used to correct asymmetric chins. A horizontal osteotomy is performed, and the chin is shifted, and sometimes rotated, transversely and stabilized.

Lateral augmentation

By splitting the chin segment in the midline, the segments can be expanded and stabilized. If a large expansion is planned, the midline defect may require bone or synthetic bone grafting. Narrowing of the chin can be accomplished by rotating the segments medially, but the effectiveness of this technique is limited.

AGE FOR OSSEOUS GENIOPLASTY

Perform after 12 years of age to allow for eruption of the permanent mandibular canines and premolars.

ALLOPLASTIC AUGMENTATIONS

Various synthetic materials can be used to augment the chin (Fig. 73.37B). Rigid stabilizaton of implants is critical because mobility may result in malposition and infection. Most infections of chin implants occur when there is improper fixation or inadequate soft-tissue closure. The following recommended technique is safe and provides good long-term stability:

1. Perform the chin implant as the last step, after all other orthognathic procedures are completed and the associated incisions are closed.
2. After exposure and preparation of the implant area, thoroughly irrigate with sterile saline or an antibiotic solution.
3. Change gloves and wash off glove powder before handling implant.
4. Stabilize the implant to the mandible to eliminate mobility and migration by using bone screws, plates or intraosseous wiring.
5. Close the incision in two layers with reapproximation of the mentalis muscle layer and tight mucosal closure.

Some of the alloplastic materials commonly used for chin augmentation are described below.

Porous block hydroxyapatite (Interpore 200)

This is preshaped in two segments (left and right) to facilitate adaptation to the bony chin. Usually the bony chin and the inner surface of the implant will require contouring. The better the bone–implant interface, the greater the bony growth into the implant.[20–22] Stabilization of the implant is best achieved with bone screws. Although a high degree of predictability can be achieved with this implant material, it is somewhat brittle and difficult to handle. No bone resorption is clinically evident beneath this implant. There is approximately 80–85% soft-tissue change relative to the anteroposterior implant dimension.

Silastic

Silastic often causes significant bone resorption. Silastic implants are also difficult to stabilize. There is approximately 80–85% soft-tissue change. This is not a recommended technique.

Hard-tissue replacement

Hard tissue replacement (HTR; Walter Lorenz Co., Jacksonville, Florida, USA) is a porous material composed of polymethylmethacralate beads, bonded together and coated with calcium hydroxide. The standard performed chin implant is constructed in three segments with titanium hinges to facilitate mandibular adaptation. Custom-made implants are also available. The chin implant is stabilized to the mandible with a bone screw in the middle segment of the implant. Bone resorption is not clinically evident beneath the implant, but no osseous ingrowth occurs. Soft-tissue change is approximately 80–85% of the implant thickness.[23]

Age for alloplastic augmentation genioplasty

This may be performed after eruption of the mandibular anterior teeth.

Complications

There are several potential complications associated with osseous and alloplastic augmentation:

- Loss of osteotomized bone segment.
- Bone resorption.
- Infection.
- Displacement/malalignment.
- Paresthesia of lower lip and chin.
- Lower lip ptosis.
- Mentalis muscle dysfunction.
- Unsatisfactory esthetic outcome.

Loss of the osteotomized bone segment may occur secondary to avascular necrosis. Avascular necrosis usually occurs due to loss of tissue attachment or secondary to infection. Loss of the segment may require further alloplastic or bone graft reconstruction. A large amount of bone resorption can be expected if a free bone graft is used to augment the chin or if the soft-tissue pedicle to the mobilized chin segment is stripped excessively. Pedicled osseous genioplasties usually undergo anterior bone resorption of about 10–20%. Infection is most commonly caused by avascular necrosis, contamination and wound breakdown. Special situations may require removal of wires, screws, alloplasts or bone with later reconstruction. Displacement of the alloplast may occur secondary to trauma or inadequate stabilization. This may require additional surgery to restabilize the implant. Lower lip ptosis may be caused by inadequate positioning, resuspension or stabilization of the mentalis muscle and associated soft tissues. Normally, when relaxed, the lower lip should be level with the lower incisor edges. Correction of lower lip ptosis requires repositioning and resuspension of the mentalis muscles. Anesthesia or paresthesia of the lower lip and chin may result from trauma to the inferior alveolar and/or mental nerve branches from incision design, dissection, retraction or direct injury when performing osteotomies. Nerve injury may be avoided by careful incision placement, careful dis-

section, minimal nerve retraction and carefully planned bone cuts. If nerve transection is directly visualized, immediate repair is indicated.

MANDIBULAR SUBAPICAL PROCEDURES

These procedures are designed to alter portions of the mandibular dental alveolus and can be divided into three types: anterior, posterior and total subapical osteotomies.

ANTERIOR MANDIBULAR SUBAPICAL OSTEOTOMY

Osteotomy design involves vertical interdental osteotomies joined by a horizontal osteotomy at least 5 mm below the apices of the associated teeth (Fig. 73.38). A horizontal vestibular incision is used for access. The vascularity to the mobilized segment is maintained by the lingual soft-tissue

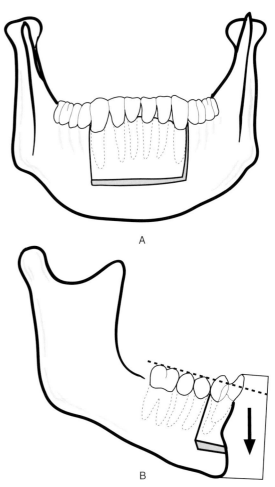

Fig. 73.38 (A, B) Vertical interdental osteotomies are performed with a connecting horizontal osteotomy. The horizontal osteotomy should be positioned at least 5 mm below the apices of the teeth to minimize the risk of dental devitalization.

pedicle. Indications for anterior mandibular subapical osteotomy include: leveling the occlusal plane, changing the anteroposterior position of the mandibular anterior teeth, correcting asymmetries and changing the axial angulation of the mandibular anterior teeth.

Contraindications to these procedures should be identified prior to presurgical orthodontic treatment. Tooth roots too close together at the interdental osteotomy site may cause root amputation, ankylosis, periodontal defects or loss of teeth and bone. Severe periodontal problems may also result from excessive removal of interdental bone. Major changes in vertical position may worsen pre-existing periodontal problems in area of vertical osteotomy. A relative contraindication is the necessity for multiple single- or two-tooth segments, because of a high incidence of tooth and bone loss.

If a tenon and mortise technique[24] is used and the segment is to be moved posteriorly, the tenon should be based on the mobilized segment. When the segment is being moved forward, the tenon should then be based on the inferior segment. Bone screws, interosseous wiring or bone plates can be used to stabilize the bone segments. Soft-tissue closure is achieved by suturing the muscle layer first to resuspend the lower lip and then tight mucosal closure.

POSTERIOR MANDIBULAR SUBAPICAL OSTEOTOMY

Posterior mandibular subapical osteotomy is a difficult procedure that may result in a tenuous blood supply to the mobilized segment. Usually the inferior alveolar neurovascular bundle is detached from the segment so that the vascular supply is primarily from lingual periosteum and muscle. Morbidity to the inferior alveolar nerve is high. The procedure is technically more difficult in patients with high mandibular plane angles and decreased posterior vertical mandibular height.

TOTAL MANDIBULAR SUBAPICAL OSTEOTOMY

Total mandibular subapical osteotomy is also a technically difficult procedure, but if performed below the inferior alveolar bundle, the mobilized segment maintains a good blood supply. This procedure is complicated by the fact that it is most often indicated in patients with a low mandibular plane angle. The neurovascular bundle sometimes must be dissected free of the mandible prior to performing the osteotomy. The risk of inferior alveolar nerve injury is high. Indications include a retruded dentoalveolus with a strong chin, and transverse discrepancies with an accentuated

curve of occlusion. While there are few absolute contraindications, there are several relative contraindications and precautions for this difficult procedure. Decreased anterior and posterior mandibular height, for example, increases the technical difficulty of performing the osteotomy. When the dentoalveolus needs to be advanced considerably beyond the stable chin point, there may be better treatment alternatives.

AGE FOR SURGERY

Although there are no studies refering to the vertical growth effects of interdental osteotomies, it is recommended that surgery should be performed in females after the age of 14 and males after the age of 16.

POSSIBLE COMPLICATIONS

These include the loss of teeth and bone, periodontal defects, lower lip paresthesia/anesthesia and pathologic fracture. Anesthesia or paresthesia of the lip, teeth and gingiva may occur secondary to trauma of the inferior alveolar or mental neurovascular bundle. This usually resolves in a few weeks to several months. If the neurologic deficit lasts

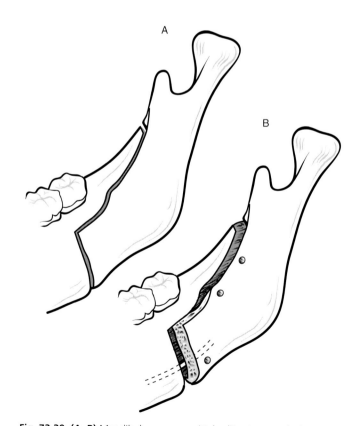

Fig. 73.39 (A, B) Mandibular ramus sagittal split osteotomy is the most common technique used for mandibular advancement. Rigid fixation significantly improves the stability and predictability of this technique.

longer than 1 year, the prognosis for recovery is poor. If the nerve is severed, primary repair will give the best result. Teeth and gingiva in subapical segments will commonly exhibit an extended period of anesthesia or paresthesia.

MANDIBULAR RAMUS SURGERY

Mandibular sagittal split ramus osteotomy is the most common mandibular orthognathic procedure. This osteotomy technique was originally described by Trauner and Obweigeser in 1957. The bilateral sagittal split ramus osteotomy can be used for mandibular advancement or setback, control of the occlusion, and position of the condyle. The technique has undergone numerous modifications. The most recent modification maximizes bony interface by splitting the mandible at the inferior border, providing controlled positioning of the proximal segment (Fig. 73.39).[18] Even with large advancements, bone grafting is rarely required. Indications for sagittal split ramus osteotomies include mandibular advancement, setback (Figs 73.40, 73.41) and correction of mandibular asymmetries. Contraindications include severe decreased posterior mandibular body height, extremely thin medial–lateral width of ramus, severe ramus hypoplasia and severe asymmetries.

The advantages of sagittal split surgery include:

- Healing is quick because of a good bony interface.
- It can advance or set back the mandible, correct most asymmetries and alter the occlusal plane.
- Rigid fixation can be used, eliminating the need for maxillomandibular fixation (MMF). Rigid fixation, when properly applied, significantly improves the stability and predictability of results.
- Modifications can maintain the angle of the mandible in the original spatial position, even in large advancements.
- Major muscles of mastication remain in the original spatial position.

The disadvantages of sagittal split surgery include:

- There is an increased incidence of nerve damage, although this is usually temporary.
- Unfavorable splits may occur.
- It must create a fracture on the lingual aspect of the ramus.
- It is difficult to correct significant asymmetries.

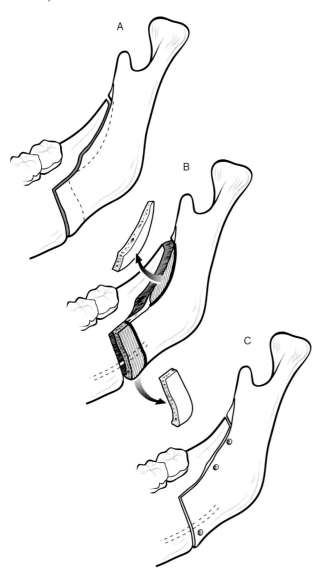

Fig. 73.40 (A) For mandibular prognathism, the sagittal split is completed in a similar fashion as for mandibular advancements. **(B)** Bone from the proximal segment must be removed from the anterior and superior aspects. **(C)** The segments can be interdigitated and rigid fixation used to stabilize the segments.

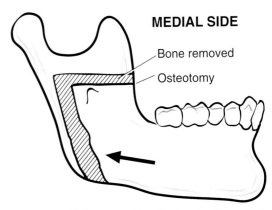

MEDIAL SIDE

Bone removed

Osteotomy

Fig. 73.41 For mandibular prognathic patients, using the sagittal split ramus technique, where it moves posteriorly along the occlusal plane angle, the posterosuperior aspect of the distal segment is moved superiorly and posteriorly creating bony interference. This will require removal of bone above the medial cut, and along the posterior aspect of the proximal segment posterior where the vertical fracture occurs.

VERTICAL OBLIQUE OSTEOTOMY (subcondylar osteotomy) (Fig. 73.42)

Either extraoral or intraoral approaches can be used.

Indications:

- Mandibular setback.
- Small movements (unless temporalis, medial pterygoid and masseter muscles are detached from the distal segment).
- Asymmetries of mandible requiring setback.
- Large movements may require coronoidectomies.

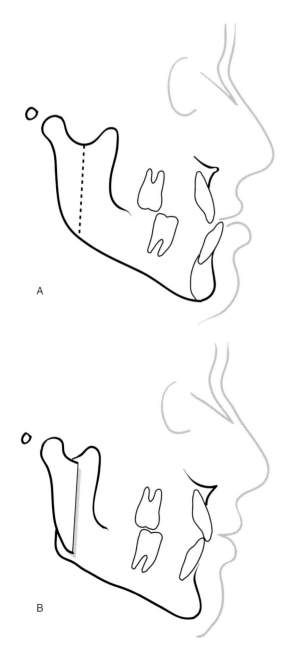

A

B

Fig. 73.42 (A, B) The vertical oblique osteotomy of the mandibular ramus can be used to set the mandible posteriorly.

Stabilize segments with intraosseous wiring or rigid fixation for the most predictable results. This procedure is designed to allow the condyle and posterior border of the mandible to remain essentially in their original positions, while the mandibular ramus and body are moved posteriorly. This procedure involves making a vertical cut from the sigmoid notch to the angle of the mandible.

Contraindications:

- Large setbacks (unless temporalis, medial pterygoid and masseter muscles are detached from the distal segment).
- Large advancements.
- Lengthening the ramus (unless temporalis, medial pterygoid and masseter muscles are detached from the distal segment).

Advantages:

- Technically easy.
- Can correct mandibular prognathism or asymmetries.

Disadvantages:

- Unless segments are wired, it may be difficult to control the position of the condyle. Condylar sag may result in open-bite postoperatively.
- Healing time may be increased because of poor bony interface between segments.
- Difficult to use rigid skeletal fixation (i.e., bone screws) through an intraoral approach, so usually requires 4–8 weeks of MMF.
- May require relatively long-term interarch elastics to control occlusion following removal of MMF, because of increased healing time and lack of condyle positional control.

MANDIBULAR RAMUS INVERTED 'L' OSTEOTOMY (Fig. 73.43)

Both extraoral and intraoral approaches are acceptable procedures for mandibular setbacks. Indications include small or large setbacks, asymmetries, mandibular advancements, ramus lengthening, presence of a thin ramus mediolaterally and severe decrease in posterior mandibular body height. Contraindications include abnormal posterior location of the mandibular foramena and mandibular advancements without grafting.

Advantages:

- Can correct mandibular prognathism or asymmetries.
- Coronoid process and temporalis muscle remain basically in original position.

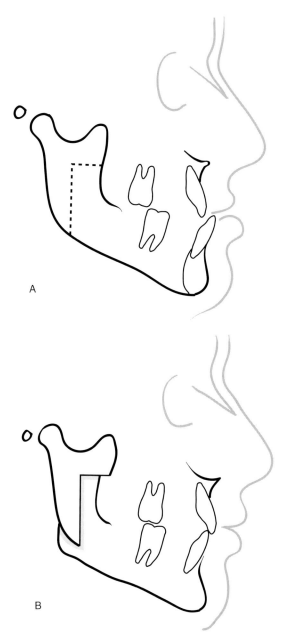

Fig. 73.43 (A, B) The inverted L osteotomy can be used to set the mandible posteriorly. A greater distance can be achieved than by the vertical oblique osteotomy. It also allows vertical lengthening or shortening of the ramus without affecting the major muscles of mastication.

- Can set back mandible a great distance.
- Can lengthen ramus or advance the mandible when used with bone or synthetic bone for grafting.
- May be able to use rigid skeletal fixation.

Disadvantages:

- Usually requires bone or synthetic bone grafting for significant ramus lengthening or mandibular advancement.

- Healing time may be increased compared to other techniques because of poor approximation of the segments when grafts are not used.

Affects on growth

Ramus procedures have no significant affect on rate of growth, but alteration of the position and orientation of the proximal segment can alter the vector of subsequent mandibular growth.

Age of surgery

Surgery can be performed predictably from the age of 12 years and older. With the sagittal split osteotomy, it is best to use it after the second molars are erupted so they are not injured prior to eruption.

COMPLICATIONS OF MANDIBULAR RAMUS SURGERY

Early relapse

Early relapse is usually related to improper condylar positioning or slippage between segments during the healing phase. Relapse is usually significantly less with rigid fixation when compared to non-rigid methods.

Condylar sag

Condylar sag, the most common complication of mandibular ramus surgery, is usually caused by intraoperative improper positioning of the condyle by the surgeon, joint edema or hemarthrosis such that the condyle is not fully seated. If not corrected, the mandible will shift posteriorly following the release of MMF, creating a Class II open-bite. The preferred method of correction for condylar sag is to immediately reposition the mandibular segments (particularly if rigid fixation is used). Alternatively, correction may be achieved by the release MMF with removal of stabilization wires, screws and/or plates, to position jaws in slight Class III relationship for a short period of time. Condylar sag can be avoided by careful surgery, proper seating of the condyle and stabilizing segments with screws, plates and/or wires. If interosseous wires are used to stabilize the segments, include skeletal stabilization such as circummandibular wires, infraorbital suspension wires or piriform suspension wires to adequately stabilize the segments.

TMJ hemarthrosis or edema

Other possible complication of mandibular ramus surgery

are TMJ hemarthrosis and edema. This may displace the condyle downward and forward. Hemarthrosis and joint edema are caused by traumatic surgery or fluid effusion into the bilaminar tissues or joint spaces. This can occur with wire or bone screw stabilization. Treatment for hemarthrosis includes aspiration of the joint spaces prior to stabilization of the segments, or intraoperative occlusal adjustment to compensate for condylar displacement. For edema, several minutes of firm upward pressure on the proximal segment will help to express the majority of the fluid from the bilaminar tissue, allowing the condyle to seat more appropriately. The application of rigid fixation and careful surgical techniques will prevent these complications.

Unfavorable splits or fractures

Other complications of mandibular ramus surgery include unfavorable splits or fractures. These fractures most commonly occur at the buccal cortex of the proximal segment or vertically through the third molar area of the distal segment. Management requires careful completion of split and stabilizing segments with interosseous wires, screws and/or bone plates.

Extrusion of teeth

Extrusion of teeth may also complicate ramus surgery. This is fairly common when interosseous wiring and MMF are used for stabilization of the mandibular segments. Extrusion also may occur with postsurgical elastics, particularly when there is an associated postsurgical malocclusion. Causes of tooth extrusion include: improper skeletal stabilization, advancement greater than 5 mm, short tooth roots, mobile teeth, condylar sag and periodontal disease. If extrusion occurs, there is a potential for orthodontic relapse. Treat by extensive orthodontics or reoperate later. Prevent extrusion by careful orthodontics and surgery, and adequate skeletal stabilization.

Periodontal defects

Periodontal defects are most commonly caused by extrusion or protrusion of teeth, particularly in the lower arch. Poor hygiene may also contribute to the development of postsurgical periodontal defects. Pre-existing periodontal problems can worsen with orthodontics and surgery. Improperly performed interdental osteotomies may result in vascular and periodontal compromise. The difficulty of postsurgical dental hygiene in the presence of numb teeth and gums may predispose a patient to periodontal disease.[25,26] Treatment should include frequent professional dental hygiene visits with special attention to home care regimens. The prevention of periodontal disease should include appropriate presurgical periodontal management, good presurgical orthodontics, careful surgery, adequate skeletal stabilization and proper oral hygiene techniques.

Temporomandibular joint dysfunction

TMJ dysfunction is one of the more common complications that may occur with orthognathic surgery. Any spacial alterations in condylar position, in relation to the fossa, can affect the health and wellbeing of the TMJ, occlusion and masticatory muscles. Postsurgical TMJ dysfunction may result from several situations:

1. Pre-existing TMJ conditions, recognized or unrecognized, often worsen by surgical alteration of the jaw relationships.[15]
2. Intraoperative or postsurgical joint trauma may precipitate TMJ problems.
3. Overloading of a joint may create a TMJ dysfunction problem. Common causes for overloading include large mandibular advancement, opening the bite posteriorly with splints and then using posterior vertical elastic mechanics after splint removal, and Class III elastics.
4. Long-term MMF, while required with interosseous wiring, will interfere with normal nutritional factors and function of the disc and articular cartilage. This may result in an increased potential for degenerative changes.
5. Abnormal postsurgical muscle function such as bruxing and clenching may create a TMJ problem.
6. Pre-existing connective tissue/autoimmune diseases affecting joints, bacterial contamination of the joints, malnutrition, diabetes and other medical conditions can interfere with subsequent healing, creating continued pathologic changes within the TMJs.

The types of TMJ dysfunction that may arise after orthognathic surgery include:

1. Internal derangements with subluxation or dislocation of the articular disc. The treatment will depend on severity and may include non-surgical approaches, anthroscopy, or open joint procedures to reposition the discs or replace the discs.
2. Perforation of the articular disc or bilaminar zone, usually due to disc dislocation as a result of trauma or overloading of the joint (i.e., orthodontic mechanics, bruxism or clenching, and large surgical advancement). The perforation usually occurs posterior to the disc in the bilaminar tissues. Depending on the severity, it may

be treated by non-surgical methods, arthroscopy or open joint procedures to facilitate repair.

3. Degenerative joint disease may be as minor as sclerotic changes of the condylar head or may be as severe as progressive resorption of the condyle. These conditions may require no treatment, non-surgical treatment, arthroscopy, or open joint procedures to reposition the disc, replace the discs, replace the condyles, or replace the condyles and the articular surfaces of the glenoid fossae.

4. Muscle dysfunction such as trismus, clenching, bruxism and myofascial pain may require no treatment, non-surgical treatment, physical therapy or medical therapy. Anthroscopy and open joint procedures may be considered if the TMJ is the cause of the muscle dysfunction.

5. Hypomobility may be due to disc dislocation, intracapsular adhesions, pain, a steep articular eminence, osteoarthritic changes, fibrous or bony ankylosis. Treatment depends on the severity of the condition and may include no treatment, non-surgical treatment, arthroscopy or open joint procedures.

6. Hypermobility is uncommon as a postsurgical complication and is rarely encountered, unless the condition was pre-existing. If it does occur, however, it may be related to chewing or stretching of the capsule and associated ligaments during the surgery.

7. Pain can be a result of TMJ pathosis, malalignment of the jaws with occlusal interferences, development of muscle imbalances or dysfunction, a neurologic or vascular disorder, or referred pain of dental origin. The treatment depends on the causative factor.

Prevention of postsurgical TMJ dysfunction is based on proper evaluation, diagnosis and management of patients both before and after orthognathic surgery.[16] Pretreatment and presurgical evaluation of the TMJs should include appropriate clinical and imaging examination. Pre-existing TMJ disease should be identified and managed appropriately. The joints should not be overloaded by using excessive forces such as Class III elastics. Patients with a history of nocturnal clenching and bruxing may require medications postsurgically to decrease the overloading effects of these habitual patterns.

Mandibular advancements will increase the resting pressures within the joints until the soft tissues have a chance to re-equilibrate with the mandibular alignment. It is especially important to maintain a closed bite posteriorly with surgery unless the surgeon is expecting a significant vertical relapse in the area. Surgically creating a posterior open-bite may require vertical elastics to close the open-bite, which may overload the joint. Careful surgery minimizing the loading forces on the joint and appropriate management of the TMJ presurgically, intraoperatively and postsurgically will minimize TMJ complications.

Nerve injury

Several nerve complications are also commonly encountered with mandibular ramus surgery. The inferior alveolar nerve or its branches may be injured during ramus, body, subapical and chin procedures.[17–19] With these procedures it is not uncommon to have a temporary neuropraxia (Type I) nerve injury. The etiology may be edema, manipulation, stretching or mild pinching of the neurovascular bundle. If this problem occurs, recovery may take from 2 weeks to several months.

Axonotomesis (Type II) injury is caused by a crushing or significant stretching of the nerve. This can cause degenerative changes within the distal portion of the nerve and may take from 3 months to 2 years to recover, depending on the severity and location of the injury.

Neurotomesis (Type III) nerve injury is a result of severance or resection of the nerve. Recovery is unpredictable. The best chance for successful recovery is an immediate direct anastomosis. Delays in surgical management may result in atrophy of the distal portion of the nerve that will significantly decrease the quality of recovery with delayed repairs.

If the inferior alveolar nerve is severed in a prognathic correction, generally the nerve can be directly repaired without any significant tension on the nerve. However, if the nerve is cut during a mandibular advancement, the appropriate method for management when performing a primary or secondary repair may require decortication of the lateral aspect of the mandible overlying the neurovascular bundle up to and including the mental nerve area. The anterior portion of the inferior alveolar nerve can be cut to allow posterior repositioning of the distal portion of the inferior alveolar nerve and mental nerve. The repair must be completed with minimal tension. Primary repairs will yield the best results. Secondary repair will yield poorer results, especially with long delays (over 6 months). The result of the repair will depend on the type and extent of nerve injury, the length of time since the injury, the quality and type of repair, the amount of tension on the repaired nerve, and the vascularity of the area where the repair is being performed. If a nerve graft is required, the size, length and fascicular pattern will affect the results. With a nerve injury requiring a delayed surgical repair, the return of total and completely normal sensation is unlikely.

Infections

Infections usually occur due to breakdown of an incision with contamination or avascular necrosis. Indicated treatment includes culture and sensitivity, appropriate antibiotics, conservative debridement, and copious and frequent irrigation with saline. The most common surgical area to become infected is the mandibular sagittal split incision area. If properly managed, there is little to no consequence. *Candida albicans* infections are also very common intraorally in some patients. Systemic antibiotics may increase the incidence of candida infection.

Nonunion

Nonunions are usually caused by poor segment alignment and inadequate bony contact, or mobility. Nonunions are best treated early by providing stability and adequate bony contact between segments. A long-term nonunion may require reoperation with possible bone or synthetic bone grafting. Nonunions may be prevented by careful surgery, appropriate immobilization of segments, proper stabilization and adequate bone contact between segments.

Growth disturbance and considerations

Growth disturbances may occur as a result of ramus surgery. Continued growth of the mandible can occur presurgically or postsurgically in young patients with mandibular prognathism, or in adolescents or adults as a result of condylar hyperplasia, osteochondroma, or other pathologic conditions. Condylar hyperplasia is a common condition in growing skeletal Class III patients. Treatment options for growing condylar hyperplasia patients include: (i) operating after growth is complete; (ii) operating prior to the cessation of growth with possible additional surgery at a later time; and (iii) performing a high condylectomy to stop the growth, performing orthognathic surgery at the same time or at a second operation.

Adolescent patients demonstrating unilateral or bilateral condylar hyperplasia can continue to have mandibular growth into their mid-twenties. The deformity will continue to worsen beyond the normal growing years. A high condylectomy removing the lateral and medial component of the top of the condyle has been shown by Wolford & Le Banc to cease growth.[27] The articular disc is repositioned over the condylar stump and any additional orthognathic procedures performed. The growth of the mandible will stop except for appositional growth of the chin. It is generally recommended that this surgery should not be performed before the age of 13–14 years in females and 15–16 years in males.

Trauma or other injury to the TMJ in growing children may cause severe mandibular deficiency. Also in certain TMJ pathoses, deficient growth may occur (i.e., juvenile rheumatoid arthritis, idiopathic condylar resorption, ankylosis, etc.) If a TMJ is involved, surgery may be required to correct the TMJ pathosis, with orthognathic procedures to correct the jaw deformity. Most likely, no further significant growth of the mandible will occur in these conditions unless a growth center transplant, such as a sternoclavicular or costochondral graft, is used. These growing grafts may yield unpredictable results, but the sternoclavicular graft seems to have a greater normal growth potential than the costochondral graft.

Ramus, body or subapical surgery should not cause a significant growth disturbance, unless the body or subapical procedures damage adjacent roots resulting in ankylosis. Ankylosis may result in vertical deficient growth of the alveolar process.

Bleeding problems

In ramus osteotomies, the most common major vessels involved in bleeding problems include: inferior alveolar, facial, retromandibular, masseteric and maxillary vessels. In mandibular body osteotomies, bleeding involvement may include the inferior alveolar, lingual and facial vessels. Hemorrhage control is initially performed with pressure packing, identification of causative vessel(s) and hemostasis by cauterization, avitene, other hemostatic agents or ligation. Secondary bleeding is rare, but can be controlled by local tamponade or re-exploration of the wound.

MANDIBULAR BODY SURGERY
(Fig. 73.44)

Mandibular body surgery can be divided into anterior body and posterior body surgery. Anterior body surgery refers to osteotomies anterior to the mental foramen, including the symphysis area. Posterior body surgery involves osteotomies around and adjacent to the mental foramen area or further posterior in the body. Posterior body surgery requires specific management of the inferior alveolar neurovascular bundle for its preservation. The basic indications for mandibular body osteotomies include: (i) occlusal plane leveling; (ii) mandibular setback; (iii) removal of edentulous space or teeth and associated bone; (iv) narrowing or widening of the mandible; (v) lengthening of the mandible; and (vi) distraction osteogenesis. Contraindications include adjacent roots that are too close together and vascular compromise to adjacent soft tissue and bone.

The osteotomies should be performed so that there will be maximum bony interface following the repositioning of

interface, inaccurate position of the bony segments or inadequate stabilization of the segments. Nonunion or malunion may necessitate additional surgery to reposition and stabilize the segments.

Loss of teeth and bone

The loss of teeth and bone may occur secondary to vascular compromise, resulting in infection, osteomyelitis or avascular necrosis. Vascular insufficiency can be devastating and may require hyperbaric oxygen treatment, as well as secondary procedures that restabilize the bone segments.

Infections

Infection or osteomyelitis may require antibiotics and debridement. Infection is rare unless there is major damage done to the bone, teeth and soft tissues during surgery.

Periodontal defects

Periodontal defects may occur as a result of vascular compromise or inadvertent removal of the cervical interdental bone. Defects also may occur by creating tears or vertical incisions in the osteotomy area.

Nerve damage

Anesthesia or paresthesia of the lower lip, chin and gums are the most common complications of mandibular body surgery. Generally, neurosensory deficit is temporary. It is usually caused by edema and manipulation of the neurovascular bundle. In an anterior body osteotomy, where the anterior branch of the inferior alveolar nerve is sacrificed, the anterior teeth and gingiva may be numb for many months or permanently. If an inferior alveolar or mental nerve injury is encountered during the surgery, immediate repair is indicated.

SIMULTANEOUS MANDIBULAR BODY AND RAMUS PROCEDURES

Simultaneous ipsilateral mandibular body and ramus procedures can be accomplished providing that the soft tissues are appropriately managed. Maintaining the integrity of the inferior alveolar neurovascular bundle, particularly in posterior segments, is important. Careful management and protection of the lingual tissues is also vital. When mandibular sagittal split ramus osteotomies are performed in conjunction with mandibular body procedures, it is generally recommended to complete the sagittal split procedure prior to the body osteotomies. If the body osteotomies are

POTENTIAL COMPLICATIONS FOR MANDIBULAR BODY SURGERY

Nonunion or malunion

Nonunion or malunion usually result from a poor bony

Age for surgery

This surgery is recommended after the age of 14 in females and 16 in males.

Effects on growth

Interdental osteotomies should not affect vertical alveolar growth, unless a tooth root is injured, resulting in ankylosis, which could result in deficient vertical growth.

the segments. Rigid fixation is preferred for stabilization of the segments. Significant bony gaps may interfere with healing. Precise treatment planning, in the model surgery, and the prediction tracing is paramount for success in body osteotomies. Rigid fixation improves the stability and facilitates healing.

Combining body osteotomies and sagittal splits of the ramus allows flexibility and movement of the posterior and anterior segments independent of each other.

Fig. 73.44 (A, B) Mandibular body osteotomies can be performed in any area of the mandible to move the anterior segment of the mandible posteriorly, or alter the vertical and transverse position.

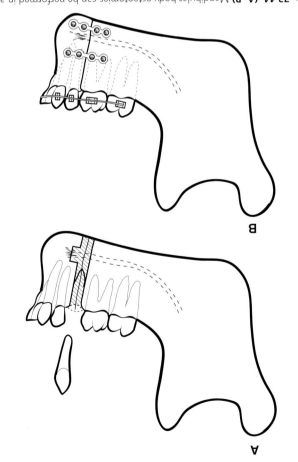

performed first, even with rigid fixation, the prying forces necessary to complete the sagittal split may displace the body segments. If vertical oblique, or inverted 'L' osteotomies are performed along with body osteotomies, either procedure may be completed first. Once both the ramus and body osteotomies are completed, the occlusal split can be used to align the segments appropriately for stabilization, preferably rigid fixation.

MAXILLARY PROCEDURES

Maxillary deformities can occur in all three planes of space (anteroposterior, vertical and transverse). Surgical procedures must be custom designed for each patient. The maxilla can be repositioned superiorly, inferiorly, anteriorly, posteriorly, or transversely, and in one or more segments, depending on the nature of the deformity. Segmentalization of the maxilla will permit the arch to be widened, narrowed, leveled or improve the arch symmetry.

There are four basic maxillary Le Fort I surgical designs. The osteotomies can be completed with a tapered fissure bur or a reciprocating saw. Preservation of the descending palatine vessels is important, because approximately 80% of blood flow to the maxilla normally comes from these vessels.[28,29] Some surgeons, however, routinely coagulate these vessels and some studies have shown that pulpal blood flow is not altered when compared with preservation of the vessels. Circumvestibular incision is usually adequate, even with segmentalization. However, pedicle flaps may be necessary in patients with compromised vascularity to the maxilla (i.e. reoperated maxillas, cleft deformities, very small segments). The basic maxillary osteotomy procedures are detailed below.

Traditional Le Fort I osteotomy (Fig. 73.45)

This is made with a straight line cut from the piriform rim area (4–5 mm above apices of teeth) to the pterygoid plate area. Surgical separation is also recommended at the pterygoid plate–tuberosity area, lateral nasal walls and septum/vomer area. Be aware of the 'ramping' effect of this osteotomy design, particularly with maxillary advancement or setback. The ramping effect occurs due to the horizontal osteotomy not being parallel to the Frankfort horizontal plane.

Maxillary step osteotomy (Fig. 73.46)

Horizontal cuts are made parallel to the Frankfort horizontal plane (4–5 mm above the canine apex) from piriform rim to zygomatic buttress. In the buttress region, a vertical step is made (usually 5–8 mm in length) and the horizontal osteotomy is continued posteriorly at a lower level to the pterygoid plates, usually parallel to the Frankfort horizontal plane.[30] This design permits straight forward or backward movement of the maxilla and eliminates ramping. The maxillary step provides an additional area for grafting with bone or synthetic bone if indicated. The maxillary step provides an anteroposterior reference point to help facilitate repositioning of the maxilla.

High Le Fort I osteotomy

Anterior maxillary osteotomies are made close to the infra-orbital rim, carefully preserving the infraorbital nerve. This osteotomy is directed posteriorly at the buttress area at a lower level. Completion of the osteotomies are as described for the traditional Le Fort I osteotomy.

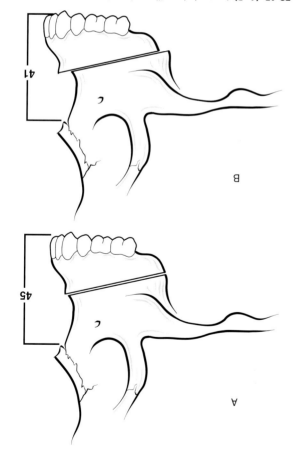

Fig. 73.45 (A, B) A retruded maxilla undergoing a Le Fort I osteotomy for advancement. The traditional Le Fort I generally angles the osteotomy from a higher position anteriorly to a lower point posteriorly in the zygomatic buttress area. This creates a slope along the lateral maxillary wall. As the maxilla is advanced forward, it also moves superiorly along the bony ramp.

SEGMENTALIZATION OF THE MAXILLA

Segmentalization of the maxilla has several advantages over one-piece Le Fort I osteotomies. The authors use segmentalization in approximately 95% of maxillary surgeries. Segmentalization of the maxilla has several benefits:

• Correction of transverse excesses or deficiencies.
• Correction of asymmetry (i.e., one cuspid is more anterior than the opposite cuspid as corrected by advancing one side more than the other side).
• Correction of transverse vertical deformities.
• Correction of accentuated or reverse curves of occlusion.
• Elimination or creation of spacing within the arch.

Segmentalization of the maxilla includes one or more interdental osteotomies coupled with midline or parasagittal osteotomies of the palate to permit repositioning of the maxilla in two or more segments. Orthodontic preparation should diverge the roots adjacent to the predetermined interdental osteotomy sites. Careful interdental vertical cuts should correlate to the model surgery and STO. Palatal cuts can be made with a bur, saw or osteotome, being careful to protect the integrity of the palatal mucosa. With a circumvestibular incision, the blood flow to the anterior maxillary segment is primarily from the palatal mucosa. Tears or injuries to the palatal mucoperiosteum may lead to periodontal defects or avascular necrosis of the anterior segments. Interdental bone should be preserved around the necks of teeth and over roots. For three-piece maxillary surgery, it is frequently advantageous to make interdental cuts between the lateral incisor and canine rather than the canine and first premolar, because this allows for:

• Control of incisor angulation.
• Ability to level the occlusion.
• Expansion or constriction of the posterior maxilla from the canines through the molars.
• Adjustment for tooth size discrepancies in the anterior arch by creating space between the lateral incisors and canines.

Elimination of this spacing may require dental restorations.

Maxillary horseshoe osteotomy

This is designed to keep the horizontal palatal shelf attached to the nasal septum and lateral nasal walls, while mobilized the maxillary dentoalveolus.[31] For superior movements, the dentoalveolus is telescoped over the stable palatal bone, maintaining the nasal airway dimensions. This technique may be used in select cases of vertical maxillary excess.

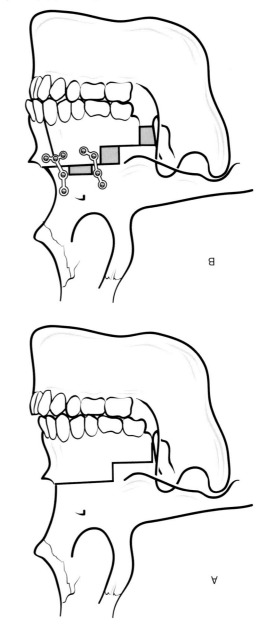

Fig. 73.46 **(A)** The maxillary step osteotomy allows straightforward or posterior movement of the maxilla. The horizontal cuts are made parallel to the Frankfort horizontal plane. **(B)** If the maxilla is advanced significantly, then it is necessary to graft with bone or synthetic bone along the horizontal osteotomy, at the maxillary step, and in larger advancements between the tuberosity and the pterygoid plates.

STABILIZATION

There are several acceptable methods for fixation of the maxilla to aid in stabilization and healing. Rigid fixation with bone plates and screws is a far superior technique to interosseous wiring and suspension wiring techniques.

Rigid fixation

Rigid fixation for maxillary surgery implies the use of bone plates. Ideally, a minimum of four bone plates should be used. Each side should have a plate in the piriform rim area and one plate in the zygomatic buttress area. For each plate, a minimum of two bone screws should be placed above the osteotomy and two screws below. The bone plates must be adapted so they are passively positioned against the bone, so that when the bone screws are inserted and tightened, the maxilla will not be displaced. Surgery must be more precise and exacting when using rigid fixation than with other fixation techniques. Rigid fixation offers more stability than interosseous wiring or suspension wiring techniques.[32]

Intraosseous wiring

Wire fixation is not the recommended technique for securing the maxilla because of the inherent instability. However, circumstances may exist for its use. Four wires should be used, bilaterally, in the piriform rim areas and in the zygomatic buttress areas. Suspension wires for the maxilla and circummandibular wires for the mandible will improve stability. Vertical and anteroposterior relapse is significantly greater than with rigid fixation. Bony interfaces are necessary with this technique to provide vertical stability.

Suspension wires

Several types of suspension wires may be used. Infraorbital suspension wires are placed through the inferior orbital rim. Zygomatic buttress suspension wires are placed through the buttress. Piriform rim suspension wires pass through the piriform rim area. Relapse or positional change of the maxilla is significant compared to rigid fixation with bone plates.

Suspension wiring can be used in conjunction with intraosseous wires. However, the types of skeletal movements with predictable results is very limited, particularly in double jaw surgery. The use of these techniques is discouraged because of their inherent instability and the high predictability with rigid fixation.

Threaded Steinmann pins

Threaded Steinmann pins can be placed horizontally through the zygomatic buttress (above the osteotomy) and directed laterally out into the arch.[30] The pin is then bent downward at almost 90 degrees and attached to the first molar headgear tube or other orthodontic appliance. This technique is indicated when stability is required but bone plating is inadequate, or secondary to thin bone or large advancements or expansions where there is extreme difficulty adapting bone plates.

Surgical stabilizing appliance (splint)

These appliances may assist in repositioning and stabilizing the jaws and/or segments thereof. An intermediate splint is used to reposition and rigidly stabilize one of the jaws, so that the jaw can then be used as a reference to reposition the other jaw (Fig. 73.47). A final splint assures proper repositioning of the jaws or segments, in relation to each other. The final splint may also prevent transverse maxillary relapse.

An occlusal splint is constructed on properly positioned dental models to fit in between the occlusal surfaces of the upper and lower teeth. It may be secured to either jaw by wire fixation. A palatal splint (Fig. 73.22) is designed to help stabilize maxillary segments and fits along the palatal aspects of the crowns, but it does not cover the occlusal surfaces. The palatal soft tissues must be relieved in the construction so no impingement occurs that could compromise the blood flow to the maxillary segments. A lingual splint is designed similarly to stabilize a segmented mandible.

BONE OR SYNTHETIC BONE GRAFTING

Bone or synthetic bone grafting is frequently required to fill bony defects, improve surgical stability and enhance healing, especially with large movement (above 7 mm).

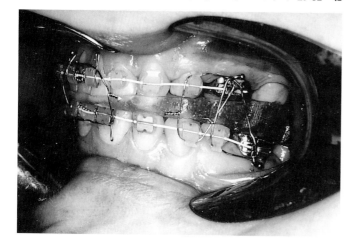

Fig. 73.47 An intermediate splint is made on dental models, and is used to reposition one jaw into a predetermined position in relation to the stable jaw. Demonstrated here is the intermediate splint used to reposition the mandible, which will be rigidly stabilized then followed by maxillary repositioning.

Autogenous bone

Iliac crest, tibia or cranial bone may provide the best quality bone for grafting. These grafts obviously require a second surgery site. The healing process may be longer for autogenous bone grafts than for porous block hydroxyapatite (PBHA). Autogenous grafts also are more difficult to contour than PBHA.

Porous block hydroxyapatite

Porous block hydroxyapatite (PBHA) is a bone graft substitute (Fig. 73.48) used in orthognathic surgery.[20–22,33,34] With this material, bone and soft-tissue growth occur through the pores and is complete by 3–4 months, with bone maturation occurring after that (Fig. 73.49). PBHA is easier to work with and stabilize than bone, but it is brittle and must be stress shielded (requires four bone

plates for stabilization) during its initial healing phase. This material causes no adjacent bone resorption and rarely becomes infected, even when exposed to the maxillary sinus. It does not significantly resorb with time. If exposed to the oral or nasal cavity, it will most likely become infected and require removal. However, with careful management of the soft tissues, this risk is minimal.

AFFECTS ON GROWTH

Le Fort I osteotomies for the normal growing maxilla or the deficient growing maxilla effectively eliminates further anteroposterior growth, although vertical alveolar growth remains essentially unchanged.[35] With a normal growing mandible, a Class III occlusion may develop. Although vertical maxillary excess patients also have the anteroposterior component of growth affected, the vertical alveolar growth continues at the same excessive growth rate as presurgery, thus usually maintaining a stable occlusal relationship, but with a downward and backward growth vector. Patients with cleft palates including alveolar clefts, have deficient growth effects in all three planes of space.

The maxillary horseshoe technique (Fig. 73.50), or maxillary dentoalveolar osteotomy, keeps the palatal bone attached to the septum and lateral nasal walls. This technique demonstrates good maxillary growth postsurgically in patients with vertical maxillary excess.[36] Anteroposterior growth as well as horizontal and vertical may be maintained.

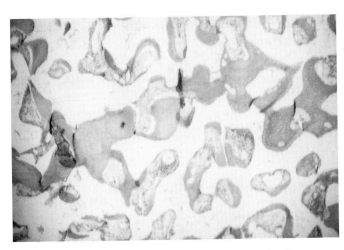

Fig. 73.48 Porous block hydroxyapatite (PBHA) is a bone graft substitute with pores ranging from 190 to 230 μm. It is composed of pure hydroxyapatite.

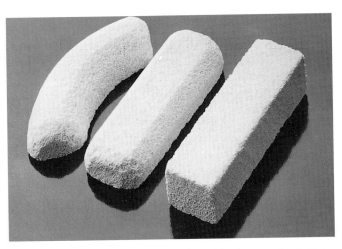

Fig. 73.49 Histologic assessment of a PBHA graft 8 months after surgery demonstrates good bony ingrowth without evidence of inflammation (×23).

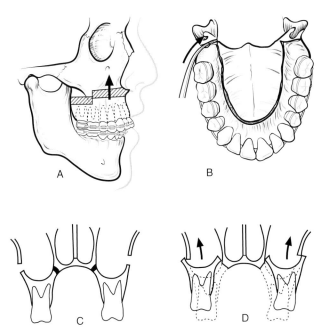

Fig. 73.50 (A–D) The maxillary horseshoe technique maintains the attachment of the palatal bone to the septum, but mobilizes the remaining maxillary dentoalveolus.

AGE FOR SURGERY

Patients with normal or deficient growth of the maxilla should be deferred for surgery until maxillary growth is essentially complete, which is generally 15 years of age for females, and 17–18 years for males. Operating prior to completion of growth may result in the development of a Class III occlusal tendency. Vertical maxillary excess patients can be operated earlier, around 13 years for females and 14–15 years for males, with the understanding that subsequent growth will be downward and backward because the vertical alveolar bone growth will continue at the presurgical rate.

ANCILLARY PROCEDURES IN MAXILLARY SURGERY

There are a number of additional procedures that can be carried out to enhance the quality of results with maxillary surgery. These procedures can have both esthetic and functional effects.

The alar base cinch suture (Fig. 73.51)

With maxillary surgery, the intra-alar base width will almost always increase when maxillary surgery is performed. The reasons for this are:

- The soft tissues, particularly the periosteum and musculature, are detached from the lateral walls of the maxilla in the perinasal area.
- Superior or anterior movements of the osseous structures in the piriform area will cause widening of the alar base because of the increased prominence of the supportive skeletal structures.
- The tissue edema that normally occurs with maxillary surgery will cause the alar base width to increase.

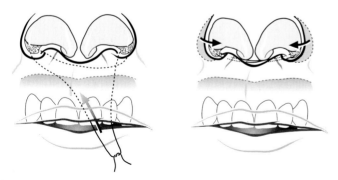

Fig. 73.51 The alar base cinch suture is placed intraorally through the fibroadipose tissue of the alar base on one side, and in a figure-of-eight fashion through the opposite side and secured. This controls the transverse width of the alar bases.

Therefore, an alar base cinch suture is usually indicated in maxillary surgery to help assure a more refined and esthetic result. The use of the alar base cinch suture significantly improves the controllability of the width of the alar bases.[37] The alar base cinch suture should be performed following maxillary stabilization and prior to closure of the incision. The suture is placed intraorally with a large curved needle. The needle is passed through adjacent soft tissue of the alar base and directed upwards to catch the fibroadipose tissue at the alar base. The needle is passed from the lateral to the medial direction. The procedure is performed on the opposite alar base are again approaching from a lateral to medial direction, resulting in a figure-of-eight pattern. The suture is then tightened until the desired width of the alar base is achieved. The suture material of choice is 2–0 PDS. The alar base cinch suture: controls the alar base width; improves nasal tip projection; decreases nasolabial angle prominence; decreases lip shortening; and helps maintain the anteroposterior thickness of the upper lip, particularly at the superior portion of the upper lip.

V–Y closure (Fig. 73.52)

A V–Y closure of the circumvestibular incision can also assist in the esthetic improvement of the upper lip. A predetermined amount of vertical closure is performed before the horizontal aspect of the incision is closed. A 4–0 chromic suture is usually preferred for this closure. The alar base cinch suture and V–Y closure help to minimize lip shortening, maintain lip thickness, improve the amount of vermillion exposed and support the upper lip tubercle.

Septoplasty

Once the maxilla has been mobilized and downfractured, direct access to the nasal septum is easily obtained. The entire septum, including the cartilaginous portion, vomer and perpendicular plate of the ethmoid bone, can be approached. The perichondrium and periosteum are carefully dissected off the septum to expose the underlying septal bone and cartilage (Fig. 73.53). The septum is treated by removing, cutting or repositioning the involved bone and cartilage. Low tension transeptal suturing may reapproximate the septal mucosa and help avoid the development of a septal hematoma. Indications for septoplasty include: (i) correction of nasal airway obstruction created by a deviated nasal septum; (ii) correction of a deviated septum that is causing an esthetic concern; (iii) removal of bone spurs; or (iv) prevention of postsurgical deviation of the septum when the maxilla is being advanced or moved superiorly.

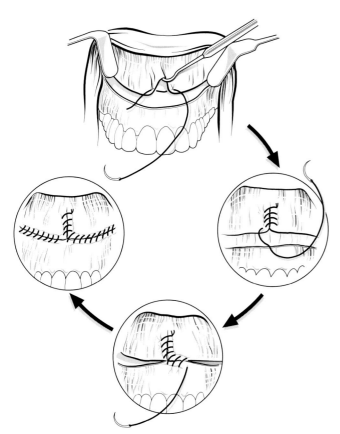

Fig. 73.52 V–Y closure of the maxillary vestibular incision helps to maintain the thickness and length of the upper lip and the amount of vermillion exposed.

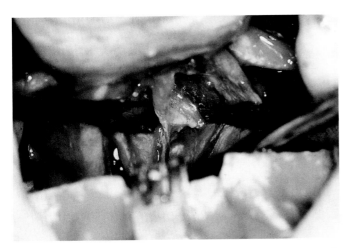

Fig. 73.53 The mucoperiosteum and perichondrium have been reflected from the nasal septum, revealing a large septal spur on the left side. This structure can be removed, and any septal deviations corrected, by incising, excising, and/or removing portions of the septal bone and cartilage.

Inferior turbinoplasty or turbinectomy

Nasal airway obstruction is common in patients with maxillary deformities, particularly those with vertical maxillary excess. The nasal airway obstruction may be due to large inferior turbinates. Approximately 80% of functional nasal airway occurs from the top of the inferior turbinate to the nasal floor. Enlargement of the turbinates can be absolute or relative. Absolute enlargement means that the bone or soft tissue of the turbinates is larger than normal, causing an obstruction. Relative enlargement is when normal sized turbinates cause obstruction because of the decreased transverse width of the nasal cavity. This is more evident in patients with vertical maxillary excess deformities where the transverse width of the functional nasal cavity is frequently less than normal. In addition, patients requiring maxillary superior repositioning procedures will have a further decreased functional airway available as the nasal floor is moved upward, thus increasing the need for turbinectomies, in order to maintain a functional nasal airway. Indications for removing a portion or all of the inferior turbinates include: nasal airway obstruction created by the turbinates; hypertrophy of the bone or soft-tissue components of the turbinates; and superior repositioning of the maxilla such that additional space is required to move the maxilla upward and/or maintain a good functional nasal airway.

The turbinates are approached following downfracture of the maxilla. An incision is made through the mucoperiosteum of the nasal floor, exposing the turbinate from its anterior aspect to its posterior extent (Fig. 73.54). A partial turbinectomy is performed by direct excision of bone and mucosa (Fig. 73.55). Hemostasis is achieved by electrocautery. The nasal floor mucoperiosteum is then closed with 4–0 chromic suture. The same procedure is performed bilaterally.

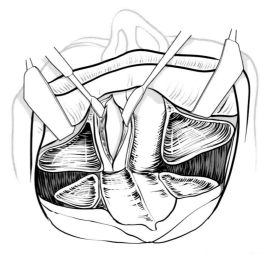

Fig. 73.54 An incision is made through the mucoperiosteum of the nasal floor to expose the turbinate from the anterior aspect to its posterior extent. This approach is performed unilaterally or bilaterally, depending on where the nasal airway obstruction is occurring in reference to the turbinates.

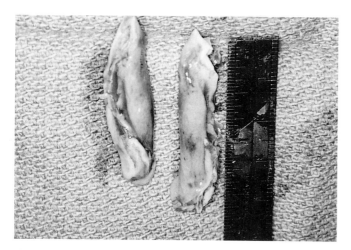

Fig. 73.55 Partial turbinectomies are performed, removing the inferior portion.

Third molar removal

Third molars may be indicated for removal in orthognathic cases for any of the following reasons: (i) impacted tooth; (ii) inadequate space within the arch for the tooth to erupt and be a functional tooth; (iii) malalignment of the third molar creating lack of function; (iv) associated pathology with the tooth; (v) recurrent pericoronitis; and (vi) location within the osteotomy site that may render structural weakness within the jaw component. The timing for removal of third molars in relation to orthognathic surgery may be important. Maxillary third molars, whether they are impacted or erupted, can be taken out at the same time as the orthognathic surgery, or should be taken out a minimum of 9 months to 1 year prior to the surgery. If removed prior to surgery, it will take 9–12 months for the socket area to adequately heal. Orthognathic surgery within 6 months of extraction may result in an unfavorable fracture through the tuberosity, resulting in mobilization of the anterior aspect of the maxilla but with the posterior tuberosity area remaining attached to the pterygoid plates and to the palatine bone. This may cause extreme difficulty in mobilizing and repositioning the maxilla. When removed at the time of surgery, the third molars are most easily extracted following the downfracture of the maxilla. This helps prevent aberrant fracturing through the tuberosity area.

Impacted or erupted mandibular third molars may cause extreme thinning of the lingual cortex. If the surgeon performs the 'traditional' sagittal split procedure, usually the inferior border and portion of the lingual cortex may fracture off with the proximal segment. With an impacted third molar, particularly in high-angle cases, it is quite possible to get a vertical fracture in the third molar area through the lingual cortical plane. This results in a separate posterior segment of the distal portion of the mandible that may create difficulty in stabilization. If mandibular third molars are to be removed prior to orthognathic surgery, they should be removed 9–12 months before. Performing the surgery sooner can result in a weakened lingual plate which may increase the potential for a vertical fracture through the third molar area when the traditional sagittal split technique is used. Mandibular third molars can be removed safely at the same time as the sagittal split osteotomy surgery, when the inferior border modification is used.[18] Even in cases with a high mandibular plane angle, retaining a portion of the lingual cortex at the inferior border of the mandible on the distal segment will help to prevent aberrant fractures through the third molar socket area. Another option is to leave the third molar alone and remove it at a later time. Removal during the sagittal split osteotomy procedure enables good visualization of the inferior alveolar nerve and should help decrease trauma to the nerve during the removal of the impacted tooth. Erupted mandibular third molars are usually best extracted following completion of the sagittal split procedure.

COMPLICATIONS OF MAXILLARY SURGERY

Relapse

Relapse occurs by postoperative settling of the maxilla back towards its original position. Advancements and downgrafts are the most difficult movements to stabilize. With maxillary advancements, there is a tendency for the maxilla to settle posteriorly, often with counterclockwise rotation. Improperly stabilized maxillary downgrafts tend to experience upward relapse.

Relapse occurs most commonly in patients who have thin maxillary bone or in patients where inadequate stabilization is present. Relapse can also occur in patients with parafunctional habits such as bruxing or clenching. Even with rigid fixation, bruxing and clenching can cause bone plates and screws to migrate through bone, allowing maxillary settling. This untoward movement is minimized by applying bone plates at the lateral borders of the piriform rim and zygomatic buttresses. Optimal stabilization can be achieved with bone plates at each of these vertical facial buttresses and at least two bone screws above the osteotomy in each plate, and two bone screws below the osteotomy in each plate, appropriate grafting and medications if indicated to control parafunctional problems. Controlling bruxism and clenching may be achieved with muscle relaxers (i.e., Flexeril, Robaxin), tranquilizers (i.e., Valium), antidepressants (i.e., Elavil) and antiseizure medication (i.e., Klonopin). For significant maxillary advancements, downgrafts or any movement where there is minimal or no bony interface, bone grafting will be necessary in the areas of bony voids to maximize stability and provide bony continuity, by promoting healing and minimizing the likelihood of relapse. These movements may require synthetic or autogenous bone grafts.

Postoperative patient evaluation should include the assessment of surgical stability. Early detection of relapse allows conservative countermeasures and corrections. Orthodontic or orthopedic therapy may provide positional control. Orthodontic compensations may mask small positional changes or functional shifts. With more significant relapse either in the early postoperative period or at longer follow-up, reoperation may be necessary.

Maxillary settling

Maxillary settling differs from relapse in that relapse involves movement of the maxilla back towards its preoperative position. Settling involves posterior or vertical maxillary movement as a result of inadequate stabilization regardless of the original maxillary position. Both situations may occur when there is inadequate bony interface or inadequate vertical stabilization. Settling occurs much more commonly with interosseous wiring than with rigid fixation. Settling may also occur by fracture or displacement of interpositional hydroxyapatite or bone grafts. With instability, the maxilla tends to move upward with counterclockwise rotation of the mandible, often leading to a Class III occlusal tendency. Parafunctional habits such as clenching or bruxing may predispose patients to this condition. Discontinuance of such habits may assist with obtaining a stable result. Identification and treatment of maxillary settling are similar to those procedures described for maxillary relapse.

Transverse relapse

Transverse relapse most commonly occurs in segmental maxillary osteotomies with expansion transversely. The transversely expanded maxilla may collapse medially, creating posterior crossbites. Reasons for such collapse include: (i) lack of soft-tissue mobilization at the time of expansion; (ii) inadequate grafting and stabilization along the palatal midline; (iii) poorly adapted bone plates; (iv) unstable presurgical orthodontic movements; and (v) hyperfunctional buccinator muscle activity. The avoidance of transverse collapse requires careful surgical technique, including: adequate stabilization with midpalatal grafts, freeing up the soft tissues for a tension-free closure and using parasagittal incisions so that the midline graft will remain covered by soft tissue. Various techniques can be used to provide transverse stability to the expanded maxilla, including placement

of: (i) a bone plate placed across the nasal floor; (ii) a heavy-gauge circumferential arch wire in the molar head-gear bracket tubes; (iii) a transpalatal arch bar to help maintain the palatal width; (iv) an occlusal coverage splint; and (v) a palatal splint without occlusal coverage.

Condylar distraction

This occurs most often when there are interferences in the tuberosity or pterygoid plate area. Although the teeth may be in occlusion, the condyles can be distracted or protracted out of the fossae as the maxillomandibular complex is rotated to its new position. Sometimes the interferences are very subtle and can fool even the most experienced surgeon.[38,39] This problem is most common when the posterior aspect of the maxilla is moved upward or the maxilla is moved posteriorly. Prevention is achieved by assuring that there are no bony interferences. If the problem is not identified until after surgery, then the patient will most likely require reoperation. Minor problems may be corrected by orthopedic forces such as headgear. However, usually the most predictable results can be achieved by addressing the situation surgically.

Bleeding

Bleeding can be a very significant problem in orthognathic surgery.[40,41] With maxillary surgery, the most common bleeding areas are: (i) descending palatine vessels and the anterior or posterior palatine vessels; (ii) posterior superior alveolar vessels; (iii) pterygoid plexus; (iv) incisive canal vessels; (v) internal maxillary artery; and (vi) vessels associated with the nasal septum and turbinates.

When hemorrhage does occur, it is usually best to identify which vessel is involved and approach it systematically. Initially, compression with gauze packing will usually control and stop excessive hemorrhage. For small to medium sized vessels, electrocautery can be used. Avitene or Surgicel can also be placed in areas of bleeding or oozing to help with hemostasis. Ligation of vessels with suture or vascular clips is usually recommended for moderate to large vessels or if other more conservative means are unable to control the bleeding.

Delayed bleeding is most often related to damage to the descending palatine vessels. The bleeding occurs generally 5 days to 3 weeks post surgery and is usually the result of a damaged or torn vessel that ruptures. This problem can be life threatening if control of the bleeding is not achieved. The management of delayed bleeding generally involves the placement of anterior and posterior nasal packs. An Epistat, inflatable nasal pack or Foley urinary catheter can be used by positioning and inflating the balloons for tamponade. Once the packs are placed, they should not be removed for at least 48 hours. Then the balloon can be released. If bleeding recurs, then the packing must be placed once again for another 48 hours. If bleeding continues to be a problem, selective embolization can be applied or ligation of the offending vessel can be accomplished, which may require remobilization of the maxilla for access to the descending palatine vessels.

Avascular necrosis

This condition develops when the vascular supply to the segments is severely compromised. Initially, the gingiva becomes dusky in appearance. When blanching pressure is placed upon the tissues and removed, the tissue does not refill with blood. The tissue will begin to slough, usually within 12–24 hours. Bone and tooth roots may become exposed with or without infection. Eventually, bone and teeth may be lost. If this problem is identified or suspected, early treatment includes hyperbaric oxygen therapy. This should be initiated immediately with 20–30 dives. Conservative debridement (i.e., minimal removal of tissue) and good oral hygiene are important to maximize regain of viability of some of the involved bone. Reconstructive procedures, as necessary, are determined by the extent of the deformity. Avoidance of this problem is best achieved by a careful flap design and careful surgery.

Periodontal defects

Periodontal problems are usually caused by one of the following factors: (i) trauma to adjacent soft tissue and bone; (ii) avascular necrosis; (iii) tearing of the interdental soft tissue through the papilla; (iv) removal of the bony collar around the neck of the teeth; (v) vertical incisions at interdental areas; and (vi) damage to palatal tissues resulting in vascular compromise with subsequent loss of teeth and bone.[9,10,42]

Recommended treatments for periodontal defects include: (i) Local periodontal procedures as necessary; (ii) gingival grafting of soft tissue or bone; and (iii) debridement and reconstruction. The avoidance of periodontal problems is achieved by careful surgery to preserve vascular supply to the area, with careful management to the soft tissue in the area.

Nerve injury

The infraorbital nerve frequently receives trauma primarily from retraction. Under normal situations, a temporary neurosensory deficit may persist from a few days to several months.

Permanent injuries to this nerve are rare, but direct trauma to the nerve can occur.[43,44] One of the more damaging type of injuries is the severe stretch injury. If the anterior, middle and posterior branches of the superior alveolar nerves are cut, numbness to the teeth and buccal gingiva may remain for a considerable period of time. It may take from 1 to 1.5 years to regain sensibility.[45]

Infection

Infections can occur in the maxilla around bone plates, interosseous wires, hydroxyapatite grafting, bone grafting and debris. Infection may also arise as a sinusitis or in response to avascular necrosis. Osteomyelitis of the maxilla occurs rarely in orthognathic surgery. Periapical abscesses can also cause infection in the area. Treatment considerations include debridement, antibiotics and irrigation.

Nonunion

Nonunion usually occurs because of the lack of a bony interface, excessive mobility or infection. Excessive muscle activity, parafunctional habits, occlusal interferences or aberrant jaw function also can contribute to the mobility of the maxilla.

Treatment may include the following techniques:

1. Eliminate infection using antibiotics, irrigation, debridement or other treatment as necessary.
2. Eliminate parafunctional habits, interarch elastics or occlusal interferences.
3. Wait for approximately 6 months to see if tightening occurs.
4. If no improvement, reoperate to remove fibrous tissue from the osteotomy area, restabilize with rigid fixation and graft with either porous block hydroxyapatite or autogenous bone.

SPECIAL CONSIDERATIONS

In order to obtain the optimal functional and esthetic results, it is frequently necessary to perform double jaw surgery. Appropriate treatment planning and sequencing of the various procedures are necessary to achieve optimal outcomes. There are options in the sequencing of double jaw surgery of either repositioning the maxilla first, or the mandible first. These two basic approaches will be discussed.

Repositioning of the maxilla first

When the maxilla is repositioned first, considerations must

be evaluated relative to forces that may be placed on the repositioned maxilla by whatever indicated procedures are necessary in the mandible. The recommended treatment sequence would be:

1. Perform sagittal split osteotomies, but do not complete the splits.
2. Perform maxillary osteotomies, segment and mobilize.
3. Complete intranasal procedures if indicated (turbinectomies, nasoseptoplasty, etc.).
4. The application of maxillary splints, rigid fixation, and grafting as necessary with porous block hydroxyapatite or bone.
5. Completion of mandibular sagittal split osteotomies, place into final splint, apply intermaxillary fixation and rigid fixation.
6. Other procedures (i.e., genioplasties, facial augmentation, rhinoplasty, etc.).

In performing the sagittal split osteotomies on the mandible, a bite block is generally necessary in order to perform the medial osteotomy cuts and a lot of prying and forces may have to be placed on the mandible to separate the segments. During instrumentation, forces can inadvertently be placed on the maxilla, displacing it from its original position. It is usually best to perform all of the surgical cuts for the mandibular ramus sagittal split osteotomy except for the final splitting of the mandible. This way, most of the force that may displace the maxilla is completed and the mandible can be used as a reference to reposition the maxilla.

If appropriate and accurate model surgery is performed, the maxilla can be repositioned anteroposteriorly, transversely and vertically using the mandible as the base reference. Bone plates should be employed in double jaw surgery because of increased stability requirements. If a one-piece maxilla is planned, then a monoblock type splint can be constructed from the model surgery to position the maxilla at surgery. If segmentalization of the maxilla is planned, a final splint will need to be made along with an intermediate splint to articulate with the lower teeth and undersurface of the final splint. The mandible will need to be repositioned into its final position to construct the final splint. Then utilizing a second mounted mandibular model, a common intermediate splint can be made to interdigitate between the lower teeth and the lower occlusal imprint of the final splint. Following repositioning of the maxilla, the sagittal splits are then completed and the mandible is set into its final position and appropriate stabilization is applied. Mandibular segmental body osteotomies are generally performed after the sagittal splits are complete. Once all of the soft tissues are closed, then the chin and other procedures can be performed.

Repositioning the mandible first

It has been these authors' experience that repositioning the mandible first, in most cases, provides overall improved predictability of the final esthetic outcome.[17] The sequencing when the mandible is repositioned first is:

1. Completion of mandibular sagittal split osteotomies, repositioning with intermediate splint, application of intermaxillary fixation and application of rigid fixation.
2. Completion and mobilization of maxillary osteotomies.
3. Intranasal procedures such as turbinectomies, nasoseptoplasties, etc.
4. Application of final splint, intermaxillary fixation, rigid fixation to the mandible and grafting, if indicated, with porous block hydroxyapatite or bone.
5. Other procedures (i.e., genioplasty, other facial augmentation, rhinoplasty).

This sequencing technique works particularly well when the occlusal plane angle is to be decreased and the mandible is to be rotated in a counter-clockwise direction. An intermediate splint is necessary and is made from the models where the mandible has been accurately repositioned with the maxilla remaining in its original place. The anteroposterior and vertical position of the mandible being repositioned in the model surgery is determined from the prediction tracing and clinical assessment. The mandibular surgery is completed using an intermediate splint for repositioning and then application of rigid fixation. The maxillary model is then repositioned to occlude and function with the mandible. The final splint is applied if warranted. Frequently, however, we prefer to use no final splint, but place the maxillary segments into the best functional relationship and apply intermaxillary fixation, rigid fixation and grafting if necessary. A palatal splint is our preferred method of stabilizing an expanded maxilla.

OCCLUSAL PLANE ALTERATION

The correction of dentofacial deformities often requires double jaw surgery to achieve a quality functional and esthetic result. An often ignored, but important, cephalometric and clinical interrelationship in the diagnosis and treatment planning for the correction of dentofacial deformities is the occlusal plane angulation. The occlusal plane angle is formed by the Frankfort horizontal and a line tangent to the cusp tips of the lower premolars and the buccal groove of the second molar. The normal value for adults is 8 ± 4 degrees. An increased occlusal plane angle is usually reflected in an increased mandibular plane angle, and a decreased occlusal plane angle usually correlates with a decreased mandibular plane angle.

Traditional management in double jaw surgery, regardless of the steepness of the presurgical occlusal plane, either maintains the presurgical occlusal plane angulation, establishes the occlusal plane angle by autorotation of the mandible (usually in an upward and forward direction) or selectively increases the occlusal plane relative to FH to 'improve' stability. Although these methods may achieve an acceptable relationship of the teeth in centric relation, they may not provide the optimal functional and esthetic relationship of the musculoskeletal structures and the dentition. As the occlusal plane increases in steepness and begins to approach the slope of the TMJ articular eminence, certain functional problems may develop, including:

- Loss of canine rise occlusion.
- Loss of incisal guidance.
- Development of working and non-working posterior dental functional interferences.

If the clinician believes in the 'protected occlusion philosophy', there may be concern over the application of the traditional treatment modalities of increasing the angulation of the occlusal plane in certain types of cases.

Morphologic facial types

There are two facial types that may benefit for occlusal plane alteration: the low occlusal plane (LOP) brachycephalic type and the high occlusal plane (HOP) dolichocephalic type.

Low occlusal plane facial type

The LOP facial type patient may be indicated for an increase in occlusal lane (IOP) angulation. Some of the basic clinical and radiographic characteristics of the LOP facial type include:

- Decrease occlusal plane angulation (OP <4 degrees).
- Low mandibular plane angulation.
- Prominent mandibular gonial angles.
- Strong chin in relation to the mandibular alveolus (anteroposterior macrogenia).
- Most often Class II malocclusion although Class I or Class III also occur.
- Often an accentuated curve of Spee in the mandibular arch and sometimes a reversed curve in the maxillary arch.
- Anterior deep bite.
- Decreased angulation of the maxillary incisors as in the Class II, Division 2 malocclusion, but may also have overangulated incisors.
- Decreased angulation of the mandibular incisors.

Surgical increase of the occlusal plane

Patients demonstrating the LOP facial type may benefit functionally and esthetically by increasing the occlusal plane angle with a clockwise rotation of the maxillomandibular complex to fall within the normal range (8 ± 4 degrees). To illustrate the specific changes associated with a clockwise rotation of the jaws, a case with a Class I occlusion is used and the maxillary central incisor edge functions as the center of rotation (Fig. 73.56). The following changes occur:

- Occlusal plane angle increases.
- Mandibular plane angle increases.
- Chin rotates posteriorly.
- Posterior facial height decreases.
- Perinasal bone structures advance.
- Maxillary incisor angulation decreases.
- Mandibular incisor angulation increases.

Clockwise rotations have become one of the most acceptable methods for treating patients and should provide adequate stability, because all of the muscles of mastication will remain basically the same length or will shorten. The center of rotation of the maxillomandibular complex will effect the esthetic change. If the point of rotation is at the incisor tips, then the perinasal area will advance and the chin will rotate posteriorly. If the point of rotation is at point A, then the perinasal area will not be affected as significantly, but the upper incisor edge and the inferior aspect of the upper lip will rotate posteriorly and the chin will rotate even further posteriorly. Pure vertical or antero-

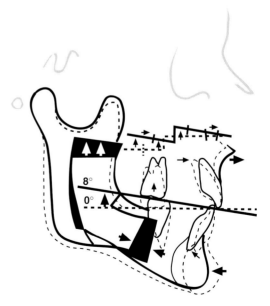

Fig. 73.56 In surgical increase of the occlusal plane (IOP) the chin rotates posteriorly in relation to the incisor tips, the perinasal areas advance. The posterior facial height decreases, the maxillary incisor angulation decreases, and the mandibular incisor angulation increases.

posterior movements (without rotation) will not affect the occlusal plane angulation or incisor angulation. These movements will, however, have an influence on lip function and esthetics.

The surgical approach to increase the occlusal plane as compared with decreasing the occlusal plane may vary in sequencing of maxillary and mandibular osteotomies during surgery. Accurate presurgical prediction tracings and accurate model surgery simplify the surgery and enhance the accuracy and stability of the treatment outcome.

With the LOP facial type, most surgeons may find it easier to reposition the maxilla first with rigid fixation, creating a posterior open-bite that can be set up with an intermediate splint (made from accurate model surgery). The mandible is then moved into proper alignment with the maxilla by using ramus osteotomies (preferably sagittal split osteotomies). Usually, bone must be removed from the medial aspect of the proximal segment, directly above the level of the medial horizontal cut. This bone is consistently an area of interference if it is not removed. The use of rigid fixation eliminates the need for intermaxillary fixation (IMF) after surgery and is most helpful in achieving a predictable outcome when properly applied. Care must be taken not to overload the joints.

High occlusal plane facial type

The characteristics of the (HOP) facial type generally include:

- Increased occlusal plane angulation (OP >12 degrees).
- Increased mandibular plane angulation.
- Anterior vertical maxillary excess and/or posterior vertical maxillary deficiency.
- Increased vertical height of the anterior mandible and/or decreased vertical height of the posterior mandible.
- Decreased projection of the chin (anteroposterior microgenia).
- Anteroposterior mandibular deficiency.
- Decreased angulation of maxillary incisors, although overangulation can occur.
- Increased angulation of mandibular incisors.
- Class II malocclusion is most common, although Class I and Class III malocclusions can also occur.
- An anterior open-bite may be accompanied by an accentuated curve of Spee in the upper arch.
- In more pronounced cases where the occlusal plane approaches the slope of the articular eminence, the following may occur: loss of incisal guidance; loss of canine rise occlusion; and the presence of working and non-working dental interferences in the molar areas.

- The more severe cases may demonstrate moderate to severe sleep apnea symptoms as a result of the tongue base being displaced posteriorly and constricting the oropharyngeal airway (normal oropharyngeal airway space is 11 ± 2 mm).

Surgical decrease of the occlusal plane

In the HOP facial type, the indicated surgical correction may include a counter-clockwise rotation of the maxillomandibular complex. For illustrative purposes, a Class I case is used with the maxillary incisor edge as the center of rotation (Fig. 73.57). The anatomic changes that occur include:

- Occlusal plane angle decreases.
- Mandibular plane angle decreases.
- Maxillary incisor angulation increases.
- Mandibular incisor angulation decreases.
- Projection of the chin increases relative to the lower incisor edges.
- Posterior facial height may increase.
- Prominence of the mandibular angles may increase.
- Perinasal area moves posteriorly in relation to the maxillary incisor edges.
- Incisal guidance and canine rise occlusion improves and posterior working and non-working interferences are eliminated.
- Oropharyngeal airway increases.

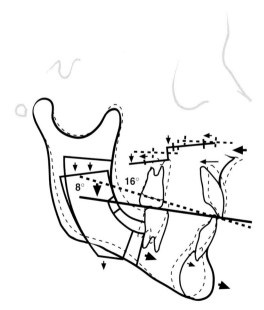

Fig. 73.57 The surgical decrease of the occlusal plane (DOP) results in increased projection of the chin, decreased prominence of the perinasal areas, maxillary incisor angulation increases, mandibular incisor angulation decreases, and there is an increase in the oropharyngeal airway.

The center of rotation will affect the esthetic relationship of the jaws with the other facial structures. If the center of rotation is at the maxillary incisor edge, as in Figure 73.57, the perinasal area, subnasale area and the nasal tip will move posteriorly and the chin will come forward. If rotation is around point A or higher, then the perinasal area and the nose will be less affected, but the maxillary incisor edges will come forward, increasing the antero-posterior support to the upper lip. The chin will also come further forward. When decreasing the occlusal plane angle and advancing the mandible, the oropharyngeal airway will increase approximately 50% of the advancement measured at the genial tubercles. Figure 73.58 demonstrates the significant esthetic difference that the alteration of the occlusal plane can make.

It is important to evaluate the status of the TMJ before surgery, particularly when decreasing the occlusal plane angulation. The movement association with decrease of the occlusal plane (DOP) will increase pressure in the joints until the muscles, soft tissues, and dento-osseous structures have a chance to readapt. If the joints are healthy and stable, they should be able to withstand the increased loading through the adaptation phase. Conversely, patients with pre-existing TMJ disorder must be carefully assessed and appropriately managed, so that the joints will be stable when the surgery is performed.

When the occlusal plane angle is decreased, it is usually easier to first set the mandible into its new position, creating a posterior open-bite. An intermediate splint will help align the mandible in its new position and then rigid fixation is applied to the mandible. Usually four or five 2-mm-diameter bicortical screws inserted perpendicular to the bone will provide more than adequate stability. We prefer to place three screws along the ascending ramus and two screws at the inferior border. Using the inferior border osteotomy technique makes the sagittal split much more predictable and provides bone interface at the inferior border between the proximal and distal segments. This makes the maxillary surgery much easier to perform with better positional accuracy. Stabilization of the maxilla is achieved with four bone plates and porous block hydroxyapatite or bone grafting to fill any osseous defects. In some cases, the vertical height of the ramus may be increased. However, because most of the cases requiring this type of movement are skeletal and occlusal Class II malocclusions, the distal segment moves inferiorly, but anteriorly to the pterygoid-masseteric sling. In Class III skeletal and occlusal relations, as the ramus portion of the distal segment must move down through the sling (which can occur in Class III facial types with high occlusal and mandibular angles), the pterygoid-masseteric sling can be split to allow the postero-inferior aspect of the distal segment to rotate down through the sling. The bone will eventually remodel back up to the height of the sling. Rigid fixation eliminates IMF and usually light guiding elastics are all that are necessary to control the occlusion post surgery.

PRESURGICAL ORTHODONTIC GOALS FOR LOW OCCLUSAL PLANE AND HIGH OCCLUSAL PLANE FACIAL TYPES

Since alteration of the occlusal plane will significantly affect the inclination of the teeth, it is imperative, when establishing presurgical orthodontic goals, to know the specific intended alteration of the occlusal plane. For instance, in the LOP facial type, it may be desirable to increase the maxillary incisor angulation above normal, anticipating a decrease in incisor angulation as the occlusal plane angle is surgically increased. Conjointly, it may also be desirable to decrease the mandibular incisor angulation below normal, knowing that as the occlusal plane is increased, the mandibular incisor angulation will also increase. The change in degrees of the respective occlusal planes will reflect the same change of degrees in the decrease of the maxillary incisor angulation and increase of mandibular incisor angulation.

In the HOP facial type, decreasing the angulation of the maxillary incisors below normal during the presurgical orthodontic phase may be indicated, so that when the occlusal plane is surgically decreased, the same angulation change will occur with an increase in the maxillary incisor angulation and a decrease in the mandibular incisor angulation.

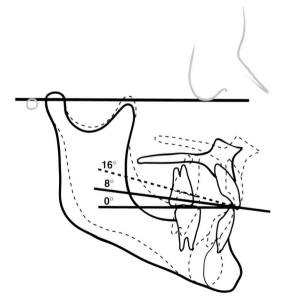

Fig. 73.58 With the fulcrum located at the incisor tips, the changes created by increasing the occlusal plane or decreasing the occlusal plane can be appreciated.

If the maxilla is segmentalized in either the LOP or HOP facial type, then the presurgical orthodontic goals, relative to the maxillary incisor angulation, will not be as critical as they are for a one-piece maxilla. If sectioned bilaterally, between the lateral incisors and canines, the following movements can be accomplished:

- Optimal maxillary incisor angulation.
- Adjustments for tooth size discrepancies between the maxillary and mandibular anterior teeth.
- Corrections of transverse and anteroposterior arch discrepancies.
- Leveling the curves of Spee and Wilson.

TONGUE ASSESSMENT

An enlarged tongue can cause dentoskeletal deformities, instability of orthodontic and orthognathic surgical treatment, and create masticatory, speech and airway management problems. Understanding the signs and symptoms of macroglossia will help identify those patients who can benefit from reduction glossectomy (surgical reduction of the tongue size) to improve function, esthetics and treatment stability. There are a number of congenital and acquired causes of true macroglossia. Examples include:

- Muscular hypertrophy.
- Glandular hyperplasia.
- Hemangioma.
- Lymphangioma.

Macroglossia occurs commonly in conditions such as Down syndrome and Beckwith–Wiedemann syndrome. Acquired factors may include acromeglia, myxedema, amyloidosis, tertiary syphilis, cysts or tumors, and neurologic injury.[46] There are specific clinical and cephalometric features that may help the clinician identify the presence or absence of macroglossia. Not all these features are always present, and their existence is not necessarily pathognomonic for the diagnosis of macroglossia. The clinical features and the radiographic features are listed at the end of the section. Most open-bites are not related to macroglossia. In fact, it has been established that closing open-bites with orthognathic surgery will allow a normal tongue, which is a very adaptable organ, to readjust to the altered volume of the oral cavity, with little tendency towards relapse.[47,48] If true macroglossia is present with the open-bite, then instability of the orthodontics and orthognathic surgery are likely to occur, with a tendency for the open-bite to return. Pseudomacroglossia is a condition in which the tongue may be normal in size, but it appears large in relation to its anatomic interrelationships. This can be created by:

- Habitual posturing of the tongue.
- Hypertrophied tonsils and adenoid tissue displacing the tongue forward.
- Low palatal vault, decreasing the oral cavity volume.
- Transverse, vertical, or anteroposterior deficiency of the maxillary or mandibular arches that decreases the oral cavity volume.
- Mandibular deficiency.
- Tumors that displace the tongue.

Pseudomacroglossia must be distinguished from true macroglossia because the methods of management may be different.

The clinical features of true macroglossia are:

- Grossly enlarged and/or wide, broad and flat tongue.
- Open-bite (anterior or posterior).
- Mandibular prognathism.
- Class III malocclusion with or without anterior and posterior crossbite.
- Chronic posturing of the tongue between the teeth at rest (rule out habitual posturing of a normal sized tongue).
- Buccal tipping of maxillary posterior teeth (increased curve of Wilson).
- Buccal tipping of mandibular posterior teeth (reverse curve of Wilson).
- Accentuated curve of Spee in the maxillary arch.
- Reverse curve of Spee in the mandibular arch.
- Increased transverse width of mandibular and maxillary arches.
- Diastemata in the mandibular or maxillary dentition.
- Crenations on the tongue (scalloping).
- Glossitis (due to excessive mouth breathing).
- Speech articulation disorders.
- Asymmetry in the maxillary or mandibular arches associated with an asymmetric tongue.
- Difficulty eating and swallowing (severe cases).
- Instability in orthodontic mechanics or orthognathic surgical procedures that in normal circumstances would be stable.
- Airway difficulties, such as sleep apnea, secondary to oral or oropharyngeal obstruction.
- Drooling.

The cephalometric radiographic features of macroglossia are:

- Tongue fills the oral cavity and extrudes through an anterior open-bite.
- Mandibular dentoalveolar protrusion or bimaxillary dentoalveolar protrusion.
- Overangulation of the maxillary anterior teeth.
- Overangulation of the mandibular anterior teeth.

- Disproportionately excessive mandibular growth with dentoalveolar protrusion.
- Decreased oropharyngeal airway.
- Increased gonial angle.
- Increased mandibular plane angle.
- Increased mandibular occlusal plane angle.

Tongue surgery

Reduction glossectomy (surgical reduction of the tongue)

Patients with true macroglossia may be candidates for reduction glossectomy. The most common technique used is the keyhole or midline elliptical excision and anterior wedge resection. The tongue flaps are then sutured back together in a straight line (Fig. 73.59). In the presence of musculoskeletal deformity with a malocclusion and true macroglossia, there are basically three choices on surgical sequencing:

1. Stage I: reduction glossectomy; Stage II: orthognathic surgery.
2. Stage I: orthognathic surgery; Stage II: reduction glossectomy.
3. Perform the orthognathic surgery and reduction glossectomy in one surgical stage.

The option of performing the reduction glossectomy first as an isolated procedure and the orthognathic surgery second, has the following advantages as compared with the

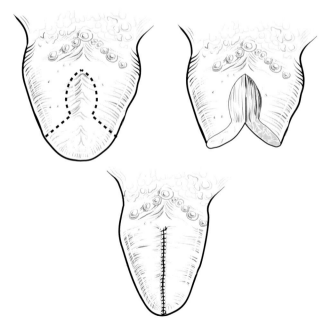

Fig. 73.59 The keyhole procedure (midline elliptical incision and anterior wedge resection) is the most common technique used for reduction glossectomy.

combined procedure: (i) less airway concern; (ii) no inter-maxillary fixation required; and (iii) presurgical orthodontics when performed after the reduction glossectomy will be more stable and predictable. Performing the reduction glossectomy as the primary stage is indicated when extensive orthodontics are necessary before the orthognathic surgery, and the size of the tongue impedes the required orthodontic movements. Reducing the size of the tongue in these cases is indicated to facilitate the stability of the presurgical orthodontics. The second sequencing option would be indicated if occlusal instability developed after orthodontics and orthognathic surgery as a result of an enlarged tongue. The development of dentoskeletal changes directly related with tongue size, such as an anterior open-bite or a Class III occlusal tendency, would indicate that reduction glossectomy may be beneficial. In performing the treatment simultaneously with rigid fixation, it is usually helpful to complete the orthognathic surgery first. Once the orthognathic surgery is rigidly stabilized, a reduction glossectomy can be performed. Because a reduction glossectomy generally causes a transient but significant increase in the size of the tongue, secondary to edema, performing the tongue procedure last may allow the occlusion to be better established before the onset of edema. However, if the tongue is extremely large, the reduction glossectomy may need to be sequenced first to allow the proper occlusion to be established when the orthognathic surgery is performed. With the surgical procedures, care must be used so that the lingual, hypoglossal and glosso-pharyngeal nerves are not injured. Although the indications for reduction glossectomy are few, when the procedures are indicated, the following conclusions can be appropriately drawn:

1. Reduction glossectomy can significantly improve functional and esthetic outcomes.
2. The anterior resection combined with the midline keyhole type procedure is the best technique.
3. Improved function relative to airway, speech and mastication can be anticipated.
4. If the excessively large tongue is causing significantly unfavourable mandibular growth, reduction of the tongue may help control the problem.[46]

TEMPOROMANDIBULAR JOINT MANAGEMENT

Dentofacial deformities and TMJ problems often coexist. Appropriate treatment should be provided for both conditions. When coexisting conditions do exist, separate or simultaneous management may be indicated. In most cases TMJ problems should be corrected first. If surgery is required, it must be decided whether at a single operation where both the TMJ and orthognathic surgeries are performed, or at separate operations. Arthroscopy is not recommended, particularly where the mandible requires advancement. Arthroscopy usually displaces the disc further forward. Continued condylar function on the bilaminar tissues may result in continuing and often increasing pain, joint dysfunction and sometimes results in condylar resorption. The senior author recommends open joint surgery for TMJ reconstruction in orthognathic surgery patients.

Surgical TMJ treatment modalities are determined from patient history, clinical assessment, etiology, time since onset, TMJ anatomy, duration of symptoms, type of previous treatment, number of previous surgeries and presence of systemic or other local conditions.

A brief description of the types of TMJ problems and treatment recommendations follow. Surgery is of course the treatment of last resort, after conservative measures have failed.

Articular disc displacement

In patients with TMJ articular disc displacement with reduction or without reduction, the health of the disc and surrounding joint structures should be carefully evaluated. With a salvageable disc and healthy condylar and fossa elements, treatment should be targeted at stable disc repositioning and ligament repair. Articular disc repositioning and ligament repair with a Mitek suture anchor and artificial ligaments may provide improved stability over other traditional techniques.[49,50] There is a high success rate if this is performed within the first 4 years of the onset of symptoms. After 4 years, the success rate decreases.[51]

Articular disc dislocated/condyle and fossa in good condition

When the articular disc is dislocated, and non-salvageable without perforation, but the condyle and fossa are in good condition, there are two basic surgical approaches for TMJ management.

1. Arthroscopy is a consideration, particularly if no orthognathic surgery is required. Arthroscopy is not recommended for the Class II patient requiring mandibular advancement or any procedure where increased TMJ loading will occur as a result of the orthognathic surgery.
2. If the disc requires replacement, one of the following techniques, in order of author preference, can be

considered: (i) sternoclavicular disc graft; (ii) temporal fascia graft; (iii) dermal graft; and (iv) auricular cartilage graft.

The sternoclavicular joint is the most similar joint in the body to the TMJ functionally, structurally and histologically. The articular disc is very similar to the TMJ articular disc. A split thickness or full thickness disc graft can be harvested and stabilized to the condyle with a Mitek anchor and also to the medial capsule, lateral pterygoid muscle, bilaminar tissue and lateral capsule. Although a relatively new technique, initial results are most favorable.

Temporal fascia, dermal and auricular cartilage grafts will thin with loading, may perforate, and may result in further degenerative changes of the disc replacement tissue, fossa, and condyle in a significant percentage of patients, and require further surgery.[52]

Articular disc salvageable/condyle non-salvageable

When the disc is salvageable, but the condyle is non-salvageable (i.e., trauma with degeneration of the condyle), reconstruction of the condyle can be accomplished with one of the following techniques: (i) sternoclavicular graft; (ii) costochondral graft; and (iii) total joint prosthesis. The authors prefer a split thickness sternoclavicular graft, without the sternoclavicular disc, for autogenous condylar replacement. A split thickness graft usually fits nicely into the glenoid fossa. Rib grafts can be used, but they are not as strong and they may warp if loaded, resulting in difficulty in managing the occlusion. Total joint prostheses (FDA approved prostheses) are a very predictable procedure but long-term outcomes are not known because the prosthesis has only been available for 9 years. Total joint prostheses would be indicated if previous open TMJ surgery has been performed.

Articular disc and condyle non-salvageable/fossa salvageable

When the articular disc and condyle are not salvageable, but the fossa is in good condition, the following treatment options are available: (i) sternoclavicular graft including the articular disc; (ii) costochondral graft; and (iii) total joint prostheses. The autogenous tissue we prefer is the sternoclavicular graft because of its strength, available length, good medullary bone, articular disc and similarity to the TMJ. The costochondral graft lacks strength and can warp under loading, resulting in difficulty in controlling the occlusion postsurgery. The total joint prosthesis works well in this situation.

Idiopathic condylar resorption

Idiopathic condylar resorption is a poorly understood but well-documented condition that can affect the TMJs. This condition is most commonly seen in teenage females as they progress through their pubertal growth spurt, and then it can proceed to either self-arrest or result in complete loss of the condylar head and neck. It may be hormonally mediated and is seen predominantly in high occlusal plane/high mandibular plane angle facial types. In this progressive disease process, the articular discs are always dislocated. If the disc is salvageable, repositioning it, removing the hypertrophied synovial and bilaminar tissues, and stabilizing the disc with a Mitek anchor, has been proved by Wolford et al[49,50] to be a very stable approach to treating this condition. Orthognathic surgery can be done at the same operation or performed at a second operation. If the TMJs are not addressed, orthognathic procedures will generally cause further resorption of the condyles, resulting in a Class II anterior open-bite skeletal and dental relationship.

Other degenerative joint conditions

There are a number of conditions in which degenerative joint conditions preclude the use of autogenous tissues for a predictable outcome. These conditions include:

- Degenerative changes resulting in a non-salvageable disc and condyle, with degenerative changes also in the fossa.
- Two or more previous surgical procedures to the TMJ.
- The presence of connective tissue/autoimmune disease, affecting the joint, such as psoriatic arthritis, psoriasis, lupus, scleroderma, Sjögren's syndrome, ankylosis spondylitis, reactive arthritis and rheumatoid arthritis.

These conditions are best treated by condylectomy, discectomy, joint debridement and reconstruction with an FDA-approved total joint prostheses (preferably custom-made) and fat grafts to the TMJ area generally harvested from the abdomen or buttock. Wolford & Karras[53] have demonstrated that fat grafts packed around the prosthesis significantly reduce fibrosis and heterotopic bone formation around joints, improving treatment outcomes, and significantly decreasing the risk of further surgery being required for removal of these unfavorable tissues. With the use of custom-made total joint prostheses, significant mandibular deformities can be corrected by repositioning the mandible on a reproduced three-dimensional model of the patient's TMJ and jaw anatomy. A custom-made joint prosthesis can then be designed to fit the TMJ an the new position of the

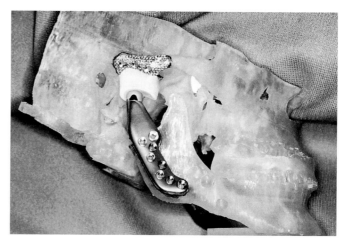

Fig. 73.60 The custom-made total joint prosthesis is constructed from a 3D plastic model of the patient's jaws and joints (TMJ Concepts system).

mandible (Fig. 73.60). With total joint prostheses, the TMJ can be reconstructed, and the mandible can be repositioned into its most ideal position. Simultaneous maxillary surgery and other procedures can also be performed.

Active condylar hyperplasia

Active condylar hyperplasia is a condition in which the condyles and, thus, the mandible continue to grow and develop into the mid twenties. There are two basic vectors of growth: (i) vertical growth, usually unilateral causing vertical facial elongation on the involved side; (ii) horizontal growth, causing horizontal elongation of the mandible. Active condylar hyperplasia can be treated predictably in the mid teen years with high condylectomies, removing both the medial and lateral condylar poles, and recontouring the remaining condylar head to conform to the fossa. The articular disc is repositioned over the remaining head of the condyle, usually with a Mitek anchor. This predictably eliminates any further growth of the mandible, and simultaneous orthognathic surgery can be carried out at the same time, to correct the associated jaw deformities. With this technique, postsurgical jaw function is typically very good.

Osteochondroma of the condyle

Osteochondroma of the condyle is a relatively rare condition, but is the most common neoplastic conditiion that can occur in the TMJ. Growth is usually similar to vertical condylar hyperplastic growth. This condition can occur at any age, but is most commonly seen from the teenage years up through the forties. The abnormal condylar growth may be very slow or rapid, and the presenting symptoms may include facial asymmetry, malocclusion, lateral open-bite on the involved side, or the development of TMJ symptoms. Frequently, outgrowth from the condylar head can occur medially, anteriorly, laterally, posteriorly and vertically, and can usually be identified by radiographic, CT or MRI imaging. This outgrowth of the tumor usually creates an uneven articular surface on the condylar head. There are two basic approaches to correcting this pathology. First, a low condylectomy can be performed with recontouring of the lower portion of the condylar neck. The articular disc then is repositioned over the 'new' head, and stabilized. Other orthognathic procedures are then performed at the same operation. Second, a low condylectomy can be performed with reconstruction of the condyle using a sternoclavicular graft, costochondral graft or a total joint prosthesis. Other required orthognathic procedures can be performed at the same operation or at a later operation.

Autogenous tissues are most successful when no more than one previous surgery has been performed, no connective tissue, autoimmune or inflammatory diseases are present, and when the fossa is still in good condition. Once there have been two or more previous surgeries, any of the above diseases or there is significant degenerative change in the fossa, an FDA-approved total joint prostheses may be the treatment of choice. With any of the above TMJ joint techniques, orthognathic surgery can be performed simultaneously, or at a secondary stage. It is important to understand that TMJ pathology should be corrected first, and then the orthognathic procedures performed whether it is all done simultaneously, or in two separate operations.

SIMULTANEOUS ORTHOGNATHIC SURGERY AND RHINOPLASTY

Nasal airway difficulties can usually be corrected at the time of the orthognathic surgery, while the maxilla is mobilized and rotated inferiorly. This gives good access to perform nasoseptoplasty, partial turbinectomy, removal of nasal polyps or other indicated procedures. External nasal deformities can be corrected at the same time as the orthognathic surgery, or at a secondary procedure. For some patients, it may be more convenient and practical to carry out the rhinoplasty procedures at the same time as the orthognathic surgery.[54,55] The use of rigid fixation for the orthognathic surgery is paramount because of the necessity to maintain a good oral airway, as the nasal airway is often obstructed with mucous, packing, edema and blood clots, rendering it ineffective as an airway immediately after surgery and for the following first week or two. Surgical sequencing would include performing all of the orthognathic surgery with application of rigid fixation first through a nasal endotracheal tube. There are two basic approaches to airway management when performing the required change from the nasoendotracheal tube to the oral endotracheal tube. Following completion of the orthognathic portion and release of intermaxillary fixation, one option is to remove the nasal endotracheal tube and insert an oral endotracheal tube. The second technique involves stabilizing the tube intraorally with a clamp and then pulling the nasal portion of the tube out through the mouth, thus eliminating the need to change out the tube and eliminating the use of the laryngoscope. Each of these techniques provides complete and unobstructed access to the nasal structures. Extreme care must be taken by the anesthetist during oral intubation to ensure that excessive pressure is not placed on the maxilla or mandible that could displace the dento-osseous segments. The alternative to simultaneous surgery is to perform the orthognathic surgery first, then secondarily perform the rhinoplasty.[56] The rhinoplasty should not be carried out as the first surgical stage.

Performing rhinoplasty at the same time as orthognathic surgery is very challenging. Because of the edema that is present from just performing the orthognathic aspect, as well as any spatial changes of the underlying dento-osseous structures, significant alteration and distortion of the soft tissues in and around the nose, cheeks and upper lip will occur. Careful planning must be done before the surgery to incorporate the expected final soft-tissue changes from just the orthognathic surgery and then very carefully plan and execute the rhinoplasty procedures at the same time as the orthognathic surgery. The nasal dorsum will appear more retruded than it actually will be after the facial edema has resolved.

REFERENCES

1. Wilmot JJ, Barber HD, Chou DG, Vig KW 1993 Associations between severity of dentofacial deformity and motivation for orthodontic-orthognathic surgery treatment. Angle Orthodontist 63:283–288
2. Kiyak HA, Vitaliano PP, Crinean J 1988 Patients' expectations as predictors of orthognathic surgery outcomes. Health Psychology 7:251–268
3. Finlay PM, Atkinson JM, Moos KF 1995 Orthognathic surgery: patients expectations; psychological profile and satisfaction with outcome. British Journal of Oral and Maxillofacial Surgery 33:9–14
4. Ouellette PL 1978 Psychological ramifications of facial change in relation to orthodontic treatment and orthognathic surgery. Journal of Oral Surgery 36:787–790
5. Kiyak HA, McNeill RW, West RA et al 1982 Predicting psychologic responses to orthognathic surgery. Journal of Oral and Maxillofacial Surgery 40:150–155
6. Holtzman LS, Burns ER, Kraut RA 1992 Preoperative laboratory assessment of hemostasis for orthognathic surgery. Oral Surgery Oral Medicine Oral Pathology 73:403–406

7. Houston WJ 1991 Bases for the analysis of cephalometric radiographs: intracranial reference structures or natural head position. Proceedings of the Finnish Dental Society 87:43–49

8. Claman L, Patton D, Rashid R 1990 Standardized portrait photography for dental patients. American Journal of Orthodontics and Dentofacial Orthopedics 98:197–205

9. Schultes G, Gaggl A, Karcher H 1998 Periodontal disease associated with interdental osteotomies after orthognathic surgery. Journal of Oral and Maxillofacial Surgery 56:414–417

10. Wolford LM 1998 Periodontal disease associated with interdental osteotomies after orthognathic surgery. Journal of oral and Maxillofacial Surgery 56:417–419

11. Dorfman HS, Turvey TA 1979 Alterations in osseous crestal height following interdental osteotomies. Journal of Oral Surgery 48:120–125

12. Shepard JP 1979 Long-term effects of segmental alveolar osteotomy. International Journal of Oral Surgery 8:327–332

13. Kwon H, Philstrom B, Waite DE 1985 Effects on the periodontium of vertical bone cutting for segmental osteotomy. Journal of Oral and Maxillofacial Surgery 43:953–955

14. Fox ME, Stephens WF, Wolford LM et al 1991 Effects of interdental osteotomies on the periodontal and osseous supporting tissues. International Journal of Adult Orthodontics and Orthognathics 6:39–46

15. Reiche-Fischel O, Wolford LM 1996 Changes in temporomandibular joint dysfunction after orthognathic surgery. Journal of Oral and Maxillofacial Surgery (Suppl 3):84–85

16. Chaconas SJ, Fragiskos FD 1991 Orthognathic diagnosis and treatment planning: a cephalometric aproach. Journal of Oral Rehabilitation 18:531–545

17. Cottrell DA, Wolford LM 1994 Altered orthognathic surgical sequencing and a modified approach to model surgery. Journal of Oral and Maxillofacial Surgery 52:1010–1020

18. Wolford LM, Davis WMcL 1990 The mandibular inferior border split: a modification in the sagittal split osteotomy. Journal of Oral and Maxillofacial Surgery 48:92–94

19. Wolford LM, Hilliard FW, Dugan DJ 1985 Surgical treatment objective: a systematic approach to the prediction tracing. St Louis, Mosby pp 1–74

20. Wolford LM, Wardrop RW, Hartog JM 1987 Coralline porous hydroxylapatite as a bone graft substitute in orthognathic surgery. Journal of Oral and Maxillofacial Surgery 45:1034–1042

21. Holmes RE, Wardrop RW, Wolford LM 1988 Hydroxylapatite as a bone graft substitute in orthognathic surgery: histologic and histometric findings. Journal of Oral and Maxillofacial Surgery 46:661–671

22. Moenning JE, Wolford LM 1989 Coralline porous hydroxylapatite as a bone graft substitute in orthognathic surgery: 24-month follow-up results. International Journal of Adult Orthodontics and Orthognathic Surgery 4:105–117

23. Karras SC, Wolford LM 1998 Augmentation genioplasty with hard tissue replacement implants. Journal of Oral and Maxillofacial Surgery 56:549–552

24. Wolford LM, Moenning JE 1989 Diagnosis and treatment planning for mandibular subapical osteotomies with new surgical modifications. Oral Surgery Oral Medicine Oral Pathology 68:541–550

25. Omnell ML, Tong DC, Thomas T 1994 Periodontal complications following orthognathic surgery and genioplasty in a 19-year-old: a case report. International Journal of Adult Orthodontics and Orthognathic Surgery 9:133–139

26. Fox ME, Stephens WF, Wolford LM, El Deeb M 1991 Effects of interdental osteotomies on the periodontal and osseous supporting tissues. International Journal of Adult Orthodontics and Orthognathic Surgery 6:39–46

27. Wolford LM, Le Banc J 1986 Condylectomy to arrest disproportionate mandibular growth. Abstract presentation. In: American Cleft Palate Association Annual Meeting, New York, NY

28. Bell WH, Fonseca RJ, Kennedy JW et al 1975 Bone healing and revascularization after total maxillary osteotomy. Journal of Oral Surgery 33:253–267

29. Bell WH, You ZH, Finn RA, Fields RT 1995 Wound healing after multisegmental LeFort I osteotomy and transection of the descending palatine vessels. Journal of Oral and Maxillofacial Surgery 53:1425–1433

30. Bennett MA, Wolford LM 1985 The maxillary step osteotomy modification and Steinmann pin stabilization. Journal of Oral and Maxillofacial Surgery 43:307–311

31. Epker BN, Wolford LM 1980 Dentofacial deformities: surgical–orthodontic correction. St Louis: Mosby, pp 242–245

32. Satrom KD, Sinclair PM, Wolford LM 1991 The stability of double jaw surgery: a comparison of rigid versus wire fixation. American Journal of Orthodontics 6:550–563

33. Wolford LM, Moenning JE 1988 Interpore 200 porous hydroxyapatite as a bone graft substitute in orthognathic surgery: two-year follow-up in 49 patients. Interpore International, 1–3

34. Wardrop JE, Wolford LM 1989 Maxillary stability following downgraft and/or advancement procedures with stabilization using rigid fixation and porous block hydroxyapatite implants. Journal of Oral and Maxillofacial Surgery 47:336–342

35. Mogavero FJ, Buschang PH, Wolford LM 1997 Orthognathic surgery effects on maxillary growth in patients with vertical maxillary excess. American Journal of Orthodontics and Dentofacial Orthopedics 111:288–296

36. Epker BN, Schendel SA, Washburn M 1982 Effects of early surgical superior repositioning of the maxilla on subsequent growth: III. Biomechanical considerations. In: McNamara JA, Carlson DS, Ribbens (eds), The effects of surgical intervention on cranial growth. Monograph No 12, Craniofacial Growth Series Ann Arbor, Michigan: Center for Human Growth and Development, University of Michigan, pp 231–250

37. Guymon M, Crosby DR, Wolford LM 1988 The alar base cinch suture to control nasal width in maxillary osteotomies. International Journal of Adult Orthodontics and Orthognathic Surgery 2:89–95

38. Kaplan PA, Tu HK, Koment MA et al 1988 Radiography after orthognathic surgery. Part II. Surgical complications. Radiology 167:195–198

39. Mavreas D, Athanasiou AE 1992 Tomographic assessment of alterations of the temporomandibular joint after orthognathic surgery. European Journal of Orthodontics 14:3–15

40. Lanigan DT, Hey JH, West RA 1990 Major vascular complications of orthognathic surgery: hemorrhage associated with LeFort I osteotomies. Journal of Oral and Maxillofacial Surgery 48:561–573

41. Lanigan DT, Hey JH, West RA 1990 Aseptic necrosis following maxillary osteotomies: report of 36 cases. Journal of Oral and Maxillofacial Surgery 48:142–156

42. Carroll WJ, Haug RH, Bissada NF: The effects of the LeFort I osteotomy on the periodontium. Journal of Oral and Maxillofacial Surgery 50:128–132

43. Jones DL, Wolford LM, Hartog JM 1990 Comparison of methods to assess neurosensory alterations following orthognathic surgery. International Journal of Orthodontic and Orthognathic Surgery 5:35–42

44. Jones JK, Van Sickels JE 1991 Facial nerve injuries associated with orthognathic surgery: a review of incidence and management. Journal of Oral and Maxillofacial Surgery 49:740–744

45. Kohn MW, White RP Jr 1974 Evaluation of sensation after segmental alveolar osteotomy in 22 patients. Journal of the American Dental Association 89:154–156

46. Wolford LM, Cottrell DA 1996 Diagnosis of macroglossia and indications for reduction glossectomy. American Journal of Orthodontics and Dentofacial Orthopedics 110:170–177

47. Turvey TA, Journot V, Epker BN 1976 Correction of anterior open bite deformity: a study of tongue function, speech changes, and stability. Journal of Maxillofacial Surgery 4:93–101

48. Wickwire NA, White RP Jr, Proffit WR 1972 The effect of mandibular osteotomy on tongue position. Journal of Oral Surgery 30:184–190

49. Wolford LM, Cottrell DA, Karras SC 1995 Mitek mini anchor in maxillofacial surgery. In: Proceedings of SMST-94, The First International Conference on Shape Memory and Superelastic Technologies. MIAS, Monterey, CA, 477–482

50. Fields RT Jr, Cardenas LE, Wolford LM 1997 The pullout force for mini and micro suture anchor systems in human mandibular condyles. Journal of Oral and Maxillofacial Surgery 55(Suppl):483–487

51. Wolford LM, Karras SC 1994 Simultaneous TMJ and orthognathic surgery. Journal of Oral and Maxillofacial Surgery 52:98–99

52. Henry CH, Wolford LM 1995 Reconstruction of the temporomandibular joint using a temporalis graft with or without simultaneous orthognathic surgery. Journal of Oral and Maxillofacial Surgery 53:1250–1256

53. Wolford LM, Karras SC 1997 Autologous fat transplantation around temporomandibular joint total joint prostheses: preliminary treatment outcomes. Journal of Oral and Maxillofacial Surgery 55:245–251

54. Cottrell DA, Wolford LM 1993 Factors influencing combined orthognathic and rhinoplastic surgery. International Journal of Adult Orthodontics and Orthognathic Surgery 8:265–276

55. Waite DD, Matukas VJ, Sarver DM 1988 Simultaneous rhinoplasty procedures in orthognathic surgery. International Journal of Oral and Maxillofacial Surgery 17:298–302

56. Schendel SA, Carlotti AE 1991 Nasal considerations in orthognathic surgery. American Journal of Orthodontics and Dentofacial Orthopedics 100:197–208

Orthodontic role in planning – clinical aspects

74

LINDSAY J. WINCHESTER/DAVID R. YOUNG

A combined approach involving orthodontics and surgery will be required for those patients who present with severe skeletal and dentofacial discrepancy which cannot be treated by orthodontics alone. Proffitt & Ackerman (1985)[1] describe the 'envelope of discrepancy' which illustrates the limits of orthodontic treatment alone; orthodontics combined with growth modification and surgical correction (Fig. 74.1). Clearly, therefore, in a growing child a case will require surgery if it is too severe to be corrected by orthodontics and growth modification. In an adult surgery will be required in those cases where the jaw discrepancy is too severe to camouflage with orthodontic tooth movement, or where an increase in long-term stability is desired, including the following:

- Gross class II or class III.
- Long face syndrome/anterior open-bite cases.
- Very deep overbite cases in non-growing individuals.
- Severe asymmetries.
- Syndromes.

TREATMENT PLANNING

Diagnosis and planning for orthognathic cases involves a systematic team approach by both orthodontist and maxillofacial surgeon. Additional specialists may also be involved, including a restorative dentist, a periodontist, a pedodontist and a psychologist. The aims of treatment are a functional stable occlusion with good facial and dental esthetics. Orthognathic surgery is not without its risks and should not be undertaken without thorough planning and careful assessment of the patient's ability to cope with all aspects of treatment.

REASON FOR ATTENDANCE

The first stage in treatment planning is to ascertain the

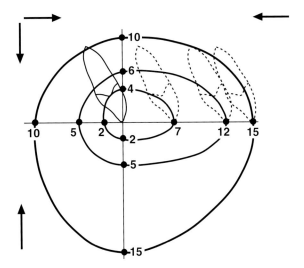

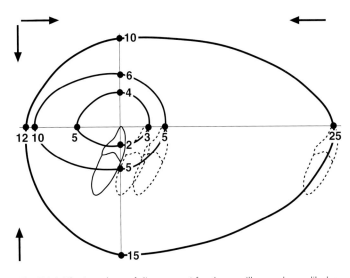

Fig. 74.1 The 'envelope of discrepancy' for the maxillary and mandibular arches. The inner circle indicates the limits of orthodontic treatment (camouflage); the middle circle, tooth movement combined with growth modification; the outer circle, combined orthodontic and surgical treatment. (Reproduced from Proffitt & Ackerman.[1])

reason for presentation. The patient may be concerned with his/her facial and/or dental appearance, the psycho-social impact of which can be very significant.[2] Patients may also present for reasons of function, such as difficulty in eating certain foods associated with an anterior open-bite, or with a traumatic occlusion associated with a deep overbite. Less common presenting complaints include speech problems and poor oral hygiene associated with severe dentofacial abnormality. Patients who dislike the arrangement of their teeth are often poorly motivated to maintain good dental health, which in turn can lead to periodontal problems and further unfavorable tooth movement. There is evidence to suggest that some severe malocclusions may be associated with temperomandibular joint dysfunction,[3] and this too can be a presenting symptom.

As well as identifying the patient's complaints, their expectations should also be elicited. Patients require careful assessment of their psychologic status to ensure that their expectations are realistic and that the patient's problem list is compatible with that of the clinician. It is particularly important to identify the dysmorphophobic type of patient who may present with a relatively mild deformity, which he or she perceives as being responsible for entirely inappropriate problems. There are also some patients who have un-realistic expectations of being able to change their inherent racial appearance to that of another race by embarking on orthognathic treatment. A psychologic referral may be required to confirm a diagnosis of dysmorphophobia. These patients are clearly unsuitable for orthognathic treatment, as they will inevitably be disappointed with the outcome.

HISTORY

It is important to take a thorough medical and dental history. Extremes of facial discrepancy can be associated with general medical conditions such as acromegaly (class III cases) or chronic juvenile arthritis and muscular dystrophy (class II cases with open-bites). Such medical conditions will complicate orthognathic treatment and may make treatment inherently unstable if not adequately controlled. Most pre-existing medical conditions, with careful management, will not preclude orthodontic-surgical correction, but it is essential to discuss all the risk factors and potential complications with the patient. It is also important to establish the patient's social history so that treatment timings can be coordinated with work, school, exam and domestic responsibilities.

Caries, periodontal disease and temperomandibular dysfunction need to be controlled prior to commencing orthognathic surgery. Cases requiring restorative/periodontal therapy should be diagnosed in conjunction with the relevant specialists at the initial treatment planning stage. In patients with caries, periodontal disease or periapical pathology, the choice of extractions may be dictated by the prognosis of the teeth. If there is a lack of attached gingivae, which is mainly seen in the anterior mandibular area, this should be treated by free gingival grafting prior to any orthodontic tooth movement. It is important to record any problems related to the masticatory muscles and temporomandibular joints prior to commencing treatment, to avoid any conflict as to whether symptoms were pre-existing or arose during treatment. If any significant abnormalities are detected these require investigation and treatment before orthognathic treatment can commence. It is important for patients to realize that orthognathic treatment to correct dentofacial deformity is unpredictable in its affect on pre-existing temporomandibular dysfunction, which may even worsen after such treatment.[4]

The patient's growth status needs to be carefully established. In most cases it is desirable to delay surgical treatment until growth has declined to that of adult levels. This is particularly important in the timing of surgery for class III cases, and in anterior open-bite cases exhibiting severe backward rotation of the mandible, where late mandibular growth would affect the stability of the end result. In class II cases surgery to advance the mandible can be carried out at a younger age as late growth is unlikely to be detrimental, although it is usual to defer treatment until after the adolescent growth spurt. Growth rate can be assessed by serial height recordings, lateral cephalograms and study models while monitoring a patient through the adolescent years. Height measurements taken at 4-monthly intervals can be plotted on growth charts to see when growth is tailing off.

In asymmetry cases it is important to establish if the condition is progressive. In the case of hemifacial microsomia and post-traumatic ankylosis of the condyle, the asymmetry is progressive and early intervention to prevent the abnormal from affecting the normal is indicated. Other asymmetries are most likely to become evident after the adolescent growth spurt and it is important to differentiate between condylar hyperplasia, hemimandibular elongation and hemimandibular hypertrophy.[5] If the condylar head is actively proliferating then the condition is less likely to burn itself out. A ^{99m}Tc-labeled bone scan may be a useful diagnostic aid in determining whether or not there is increased activity in the condyle, although clinical findings will often be sufficient to demonstrate the need for surgical intervention. The orthodontist is experienced in monitoring growth and has an important role in diagnosing these complex cases.

CLINICAL EXTRAORAL EXAMINATION

The patient should be sitting upright (or standing) with

the Frankfort–mandibular plane parallel to the floor for correct assessment of facial esthetics, balance and symmetry. The aim is to identify whether the maxilla, the mandible or both are abnormal.

Frontal analysis

Frontal face esthetics are particularly important, as this is how the patient most often views him- or herself and is viewed by others. Several facial parameters should be evaluated and measured. The facial thirds, trichion (hairline) to glabella (eyebrows), glabella to subnasale and subnasale to gnathion should be approximately equal in dimension (Fig. 74.2A). Particular attention is placed on examination of the middle and lower thirds. Orbital rims are checked for equal height and symmetry. The intercanthal width (34 ± 4 mm) should equal the alar base width; the width of the mouth should approximate the distance between the inner margins of the iris of the eyes; and the width of the mandible at the gonial angles should approximate the distance between the orbits (Fig. 74.2B). Sclera exposure is normal when the lower eyelid just touches the lower border of the iris. If more sclera is visible, the alar base is wider than normal, or if there is perinasal hollowing then this may indicate maxillary hypoplasia.

It is essential to assess the lips at rest and during function, as they play an important role in facial esthetics. The amount of tooth visible beneath the upper lip is extremely significant in deciding whether the maxilla requires impaction or inferior repositioning. At rest 2–3 mm of tooth should be visible, with the whole central incisor being exposed to the gingival margin on smiling. If an excess of gingivae is exposed on smiling or at rest this must be measured. Care must be taken when recording these measurements if the upper lip is of abnormal morphology. Normally the upper lip tubercle hangs slightly inferior to the vermillion on either side of it, but it can be particularly pendulous or very superior in some patients, where a compromise from the ideal tooth exposure may produce the best esthetics. The upper lip length should be recorded (average 20 mm in females, 22 mm in males). The lower lip vermillion should be exposed approximately 25% more than the upper lip at rest, with an average interlabial separation of up to 3 mm, and the lip line should be a third of the way between the base of the nose and the chin. A deep labiomental fold may be associated with a reduced lower anterior face height and a reduced fold the converse. Lower anterior mandibular height should be in the range 49 ± 3 mm (for males) and 42 ± 3 mm (for females),[6] and deviation from this may require a genioplasty to

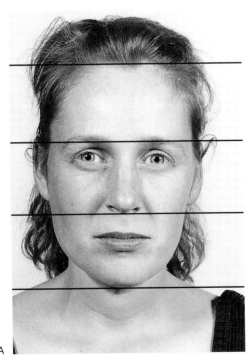 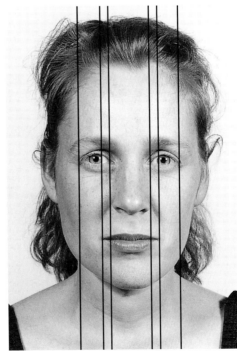

Fig. 74.2 Frontal face analysis. (**A**) Facial thirds – trichion to glabella, glabella to subnasale, and subnasale to menton – should be equal. (**B**) Intercanthal width should approximate alar base width, commissure width should approximate the distance between the outer margins of the iris, and the width of the mandible at the gonial angles should approximate the orbital width.

correct. In a well-proportioned face the ratio of bizygomatic width to face height is 0.88 for males and 0.86 for females, with a ratio of bigonial to bizygomatic width of around 0.70.[7] The shape and symmetry of the chin in relation to the whole face is also important. Looking from above the patient, down the centre of the face, the skeletal and dental centrelines are recorded. Any major skeletal asymmetry may necessitate a posteroanterior cephalogram, or ideally laser scanning, 3D computerized tomography (CT) together with stereolithograph models for further investigation.

Profile analysis

From the lateral view it is important to further assess the vertical as well as the anteroposterior relationship. The face is again examined in facial thirds, to check the anterior soft-tissue facial heights (Fig. 74.3).[8] The shape of the forehead and the presence of any frontal bossing should be noted. The nasal dorsum and tip are examined, recording any dorsal hump or nasal tip rotation, either upwards or downwards. This has particular relevance when considering maxillary advancements and impactions, as the nose tip will tend to be rotated upwards. The nasolabial angle should be 100 ± 10 degrees and gives an indication of whether the upper incisors should be proclined, retroclined or maintained, if surgery to the maxilla is not planned. An obtuse nasolabial angle may be associated with maxillary hypoplasia and therefore be improved by maxillary advancement.

In the lower third of the face the lips, chin and chin–neck contour are assessed. The overall balance of this part of the face is a good indicator of facial deformity. The relative prominence or retrusion of either jaw is assessed in relation to the true vertical line dropped from the most prominent part of the forehead, perpendicular to the Frankfort plane. Any obvious deviation of the upper or lower lips from this line will indicate a discrepancy (Fig. 74.4). Other helpful analyses include the zero meridian, a true vertical dropped from soft-tissue nasion, from which the soft-tissue chin should be within 0 ± 2 mm,[8] (Fig. 74.5), and the Holdaway line, whereby a line extended from the soft-tissue chin through the upper lip should bisect the nose (Fig. 74.6).[9] Chin projection should be considered in relation to the whole profile, notably the forehead and nose, to determine overall balance. The

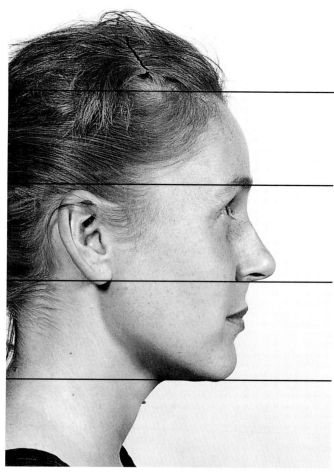

Fig. 74.3 Profile analysis: the face is examined in facial thirds to check anterior soft-tissue heights. The facial thirds should be approximately equal.

submental region is examined for lax skin or excess fatty tissue, which is often associated with a short throat length (mean 57 ± 6 mm). This may be a contraindication for a mandibular setback or may necessitate additional procedures such as liposuction.

Facial analysis must be considered alongside the general stature of the patient, as a well-built person may suit a slightly prognathic mandible, whereas a patient with a small physique may not. The clinical extraoral examination therefore results in an identified problem list which is subsequently confirmed by cephalometric analysis. By far the most important aspect of diagnosis is the clinical examination and it is erroneous to try and dictate surgical procedures on the basis of cephalometric values alone.

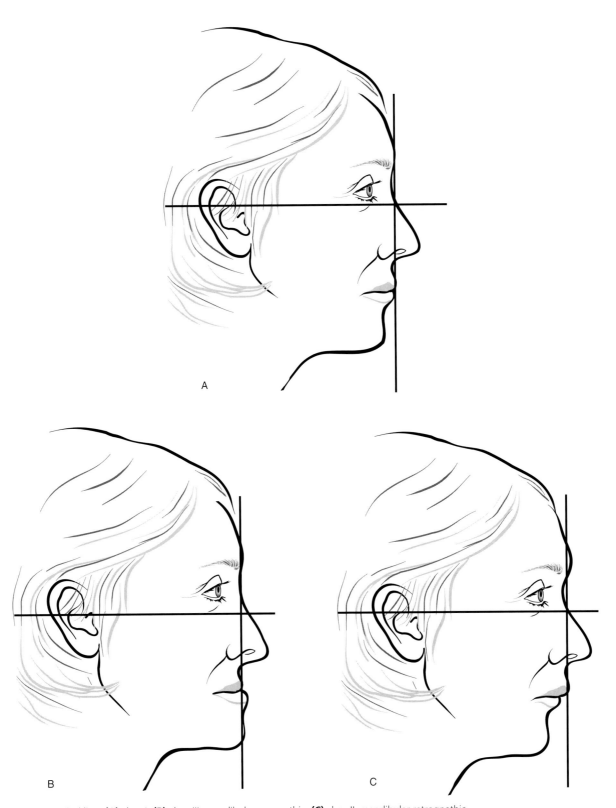

Fig. 74.4 The true vertical line: **(A)** class I; **(B)** class III, mandibular prognathic; **(C)** class II, mandibular retrognathic.

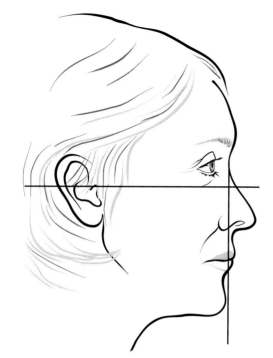

Fig. 74.5 The Zero meridian.

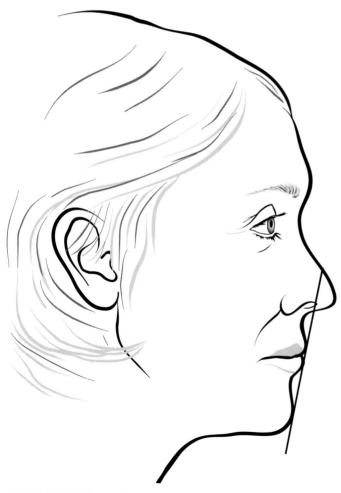

Fig. 74.6 The Holdaway line.

CLINICAL INTRAORAL EXAMINATION

A routine orthodontic diagnosis is carried out to assess the dental relationship, crowding, spacing and general condition of the dentition. The amount of dental compensation for the skeletal discrepancy is assessed in all three planes of space: anteroposteriorly, laterally and vertically. Particular attention is paid to any abnormality of the occlusal plane, such as a cant of the maxilla in asymmetry cases or a step in the occlusal plane in anterior open-bite cases.

As well as carrying out an evaluation of the static occlusion, it is also important to assess the functional occlusion, noting any discrepancy between centric occlusion and centric relation, and checking for parafunctional activity and associated wear of the teeth. Any displacements on closing may either increase or decrease the apparent skeletal discrepancy observed clinically in all three planes of space.

DIAGNOSTIC RECORDS

Diagnostic records are used as an adjunct to the clinical examination, not as a substitute. The minimum requirements for planning a surgical-orthodontic case will include photographs, a panoramic radiograph, an anterior occlusal radiograph, a lateral cephalograph and two sets of study models (one may be articulated on a semiadjustable articulator).

Extraoral photographs should include frontal face with lips relaxed, frontal face smiling, three-quarters face and profile. Intraoral photographs should include the teeth in occlusion (front, left and right) and occlusal mirror shots.

Radiographs are examined for pathology, caries, periodontal disease, root morphology/length, amount of bone available for tooth movement and the presence of any unerupted teeth, notably wisdom teeth. Any abnormal findings may require further diagnostic radiographs. A thorough cephalometric analysis should be carried out as described later.

Study models enable a more detailed analysis of the static occlusion as well as allowing model surgery and a trial diagnostic setup if required. Some cases may present with tooth size discrepancies or with teeth of poor prognoses which necessitate a diagnostic setup to evaluate the result of a certain extraction program. The need for articulation of study models at the initial planning stage is controversial, but it may be necessary if maxillary superior repositioning is planned, to determine the effect of mandibular autorotation. In cases with large displacements it may also be useful to mount models in centric relation to aid treatment planning. In most cases, however, it is sufficient to determine arch compatibility by articulating the pre-treatment study models by hand, reserving the need for a facebow recording and articulated models to immediately before surgery.

Recently the techniques of videoimaging and facial laser scanning have been used to aid diagnosis and treatment planning, providing enhanced patient communication. As these techniques improve they may become more prominent in the planning of such cases.

FORMULATING A TREATMENT PLAN

Having collated all the information from the clinical examination and the diagnostic records, a problem list is formulated and prioritized. Possible solutions to the problem list are then considered and discussed with the patient to allow a definitive treatment plan to be formulated. Prediction tracings and feasibility model surgery are used to aid decision making as well as to provide a means of conveying information to the patient. The surgical procedures are decided first, followed by the orthodontic plan.

PRESURGICAL ORTHODONTICS

A modern understanding of facial growth and dental/skeletal relapse post-osteotomy has allowed the development of orthodontic mechanics which have transformed the quality of combined orthodontic/surgical outcome. The key to definitive results is the correct diagnosis of the skeletal/dental discrepancy and subsequent prescription of appropriate orthodontic mechanics. Presurgical orthodontics should enable the ultimate skeletal and soft-tissue changes to be achieved by the planned surgical procedures, and should also enhance postsurgical stability. The principles of presurgical orthodontics are:

- Arch alignment.
- Arch leveling.
- Decompensation.
- Arch coordination.

ARCH ALIGNMENT

Good arch alignment is achieved by using the preadjusted edgewise system of fixed appliances to provide bodily control of teeth in all three planes of space. The choice of slot size of the appliance is a matter of personal preference. It is important to ensure that rigid archwires are used at the time of surgery to enhance surgical stabilization, and it will be necessary to work up to 17×25 wires in a 0.018-inch system

and 19×25 wires in a 0.022-inch system. If segmental mechanics are planned, then the use of a 0.022-inch slot size, which allows the use of a 21×25 wire, is recommended for adequate control. If segmental surgery is planned it is advantageous to place either 0.022-inch standard edgewise brackets on the canines or 0.022-inch preadjusted edgewise brackets of the contralateral side to allow the canines to be positioned upright, rather than mesially inclined, to ensure that the canine roots are away from the osteotomy cuts. Similarly if segmental osteotomies are planned through extraction sites, adequate space (2–3 mm) must be left between the roots of the teeth as well as the crowns, therefore extraction series preadjusted brackets, which tend to approximate the roots, should not be used.

The relief of crowding, leveling, correction of rotations and occlusal interferences is as much a part of presurgical orthodontics as routine treatment, because if left it can prevent arch compatibility and limit surgical outcome. Teeth should be aligned by arch expansion if it is desirable to keep the incisors proclined; for example, in a class II case where the upper arch is narrow, there is minimal/moderate crowding and the upper incisors are providing good lip support. If arch length reduction is desirable and the incisors require retraction, then extractions should be carried out; for example, in a class II case where the lower incisors need to be retracted to decompensate.

ARCH LEVELING

Arch leveling frequently accompanies arch alignment in conventional orthodontic treatment, but it may not be desirable in all surgical cases. As the mandible is moved surgically either backwards or forwards it is the lower incisor position which controls the vertical lower anterior face height. In patients with reduced lower anterior face height, where an increase in face height is required to improve facial balance, the curve of Spee should not be leveled presurgically. The curve of Spee can be maintained with full arch mechanics by wiping a curve into sequential lower stainless steel archwires. The mandible is surgically advanced to produce a 'three-point landing', occluding only posteriorly and on the incisors (Fig. 74.7). The canines and premolars are then extruded, as described under postsurgical orthodontics. This is a common scenario in the class II division 2 patient with reduced face height and deep overbite. Controversy exists as to the size of lateral open-bite which can be reduced postsurgically. There is no research evidence, and a range exists from 4 to 10 mm that clinicians will accept as possible to close with elastics. If the proposed lateral open-bite is thought to be too large, then the curve of Spee will need to be partially reduced presurgically, with

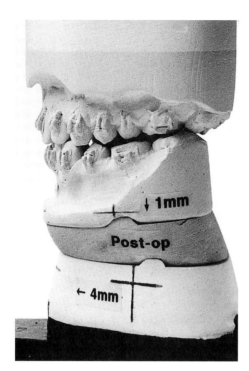

Fig. 74.7 Model surgery for a patient with reduced lower anterior face height, where the lower arch has not been leveled presurgically, producing a 'three-point landing'.

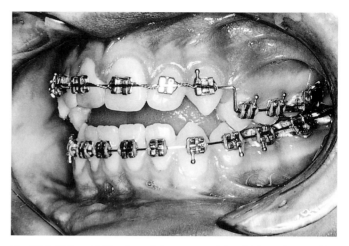

Fig. 74.8 Differential leveling of the upper arch in a high-angle open-bite case allows segmental surgery to impact the posterior maxilla, together with auto-rotation of the mandible to close the anterior open-bite. The upper canine brackets are placed on the opposite side to normal to ensure that the roots of the canines are mesially inclined, away from the osteotomy cuts.

an inevitable limitation of increase in the anterior lower face height postsurgically. If the latter produces an undesirable esthetic result and it is desirable to increase the face height further, then surgical techniques such as an augmentation genioplasty may be considered. Alternatively if there is a marked step in the lower occlusal plane, this can be maintained with sectional orthodontic mechanics prior to an anterior mandibulotomy set-down.

Patients with a normal or increased lower anterior face height should generally have their arches leveled by intruding the incisors to prevent further increase in face height which would be esthetically and functionally undesirable. The ability to intrude incisors orthodontically depends on the root and bone morphology. Teeth with short spindly roots may be very prone to resorption if intruded.[10] Successful intrusion requires light forces in the range of 10–20 g per tooth,[6] which are best provided by Burstone, Ricketts, Bioprogressive or Tip-edge type mechanics. Full arch mechanics will invariably achieve leveling by some proclination of the incisors which may or may not be desirable. If such incisor proclination is undesirable then extractions may be necessary to retract the incisors.

The long-face patient with an anterior open-bite also requires careful management in relation to arch leveling. In the upper arch it will be necessary to maintain a step in the occlusal plane presurgically if segmental surgery is planned (Fig. 74.8). Differential surgical leveling to intrude the

posterior buccal segments will level the arch and reduce the open-bite by allowing autorotation of the mandible. If a LeFort I maxillary impaction is planned in such a case, the maxilla will be impacted more posteriorly. The upper arch in this instance will have full arch mechanics, which should aim to extrude the molars and premolars and intrude the upper labial segment, to worsen the open-bite presurgically. Research has shown that these cases often relapse due to either surgical relapse[11] or unfavorable growth rotations.[12] The importance of these orthodontic tooth movements, which are inherently unstable, is to try and minimize postsurgical relapse. Following removal of the fixed orthodontic appliances the intruded incisors will tend to extrude, and the extruded molars and premolars will tend to intrude again, so counteracting any tendency for the open-bite to recur as a result of vertical skeletal relapse. Orthodontic mechanics to achieve these aims include increased curves of Spee in the upper archwires, reversed curves of Spee in the lower archwires, box/check interarch elastics to extrude the buccal segments and reciprocally intrude the upper labial segment, J-pull headgear to the upper labial segment and cervical-pull headgear to the upper molars.

DECOMPENSATION

Dental compensation in all three planes of space can occur in patients with skeletal discrepancy. Although this compensation reduces the skeletal/dental and soft-tissue discrepancy, it limits optimal surgical correction. Orthodontic decompensation aims to eliminate this camouflage, resulting in treatment objectives which are frequently the total opposite to those of conventional treatment. Patients invariably will look worse before surgery, as the full extent of their skeletal discrepancy becomes apparent with orthodontic decompensation (Fig. 74.9). It is important to warn patients of this fact before commencing the presurgical orthodontic phase of treatment.

Anteroposteriorly the incisors are generally placed at a normal angulation to their skeletal bases if feasible, irrespective of the maxillo-mandibular angle. In class II division 1 malocclusions the upper incisors are usually left in their original position or proclined, while the lower incisors are usually retroclined, so increasing the overjet, and allowing maximal mandibular advancement. An extraction pattern in such cases may involve the loss of upper second premolars and lower first premolars or lower first premolars only. Class III interarch elastics may be used to facilitate the anteroposterior decompensation (Fig. 74.10). If there is excessive spacing in the upper arch, protraction headgear can be used to close the space from behind, while maintaining incisor proclination. In a class II division 2 malocclusion the upper incisors will invariably require considerable proclination, and the upper arch may often be managed by non-extraction.

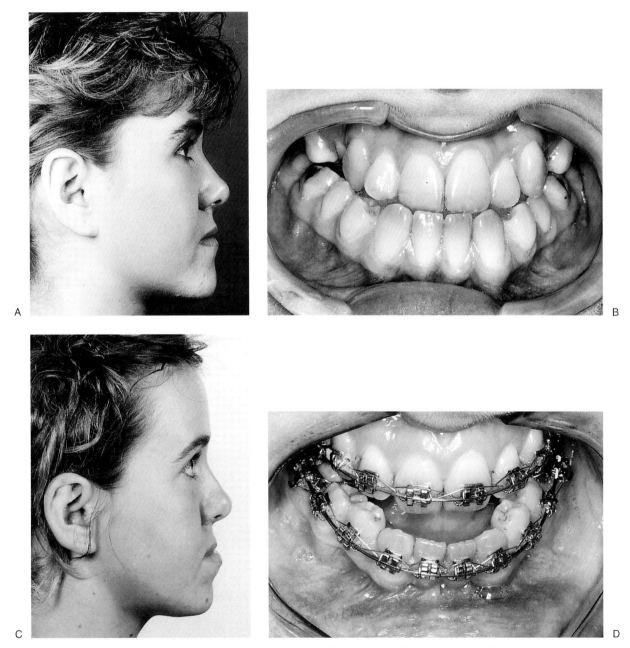

Fig. 74.9 The full extent of the skeletal discrepancy becomes evident with orthodontic decompensation in class III patient: **(A,B)** before decompensation, **(C,D)** after presurgical orthodontics.

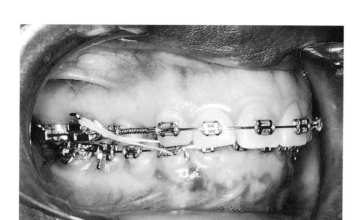

Fig. 74.10 Class III elastics are frequently used to facilitate decompensation of a class II case. Lower incisors are retroclined and upper incisors proclined.

The use of Roth incisor brackets, with increased crown torque, can be advantageous in class II cases. In a class III case the upper incisors are usually retracted and the lower incisors are generally proclined. Such cases often have small, crowded maxillas and may require extraction of upper first premolars, together with expansion in some cases, to facilitate decompensation. Treatment is often complicated by previous premolar extractions and no residual spacing, necessitating the use of headgear, nickel–titanium distalizers or magnets to distalize the upper buccal segments and create space for incisor retraction. It may also be necessary to consider extraction of the upper second molars in such cases. Roth incisor brackets generally have too much torque for class III surgical cases. The lower arch in a class III case is often managed by non-extraction, with class II elastics aiding decompensation (Fig. 74.11). If crowding is severe enough to warrant extractions, lower second premolars are the preferred choice.

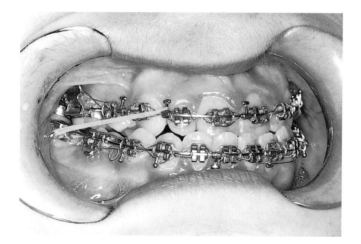

Fig. 74.11 Class II elastics facilitate decompensation in a class III case. Lower incisors are proclined and upper incisors are retroclined.

The amount of incisor decompensation which is either desirable or feasible may vary from the ideal. On stability grounds complete decompensation to a standardized norm is not always required for a definitive surgical result. In some cases full decompensation can produce an excessive skeletal/dental discrepancy that requires surgical movements in excess of 10 mm, with increasing potential for surgical relapse. An example of this would be a class III case with a well-aligned, proclined upper labial segment, with good lip support and acceptable incisor show, where decompensation of the lower incisors alone will allow adequate esthetic correction with mandibular surgery. In such a case decompensation of the maxillary incisors may make the discrepancy so large as to require bimaxillary surgery to correct. Full decompensation may also be limited on anatomic grounds, for instance when there is insufficient alveolar bone, unfavorable root morphology (blunted, pipette shaped or resorbed) or teeth of poor prognosis (a history of trauma, transplanted teeth or periodontally involved teeth). Inadequate attached gingivae may also limit decompensation and is particularly a problem in the lower incisor region. A free gingival graft may need to be placed to facilitate decompensation under these circumstances. Additional dental factors may limit decompensation. Where the lower labial segment is crowded and proclination is required, then alignment can occur simultaneously with decompensation. If however the lower labial segment is upright and spaced, but proclination of the lower incisors is still required, then there will be a tendency to open up further spaces and full decompensation may not be desirable. In the case of differential impaction of the maxilla full decompensation of the upper incisors is not required. The upper incisors should be left slightly more proclined in this case, so that when the maxilla is impacted more posteriorly the upper incisors will not be overly uprighted in the face, or their vertical incisor show increased.

Decompensation should also be considered in the transverse dimension. It is important to determine whether a crossbite tendency is skeletal or dental in origin. Small discrepancies up to 4–6 mm in upper and lower arch widths can usually be corrected orthodontically, however orthodontic expansion is inherently unstable and the addition of surgery to the treatment plan does not decrease the potential for orthodontic relapse. If there is considerable tipping of the molars and premolars in an attempt to compensate for transverse skeletal discrepancy, the teeth should be decompensated and surgical expansion of the maxilla carried out instead. Some transverse arch discrepancies are extremely difficult to correct presurgically due to interocclusal locking and in these circumstances it may be advisable to carry out the surgery first, eliminating the interference and allowing more efficient orthodontic tooth movement. If a transverse discrepancy exists at the time of surgery then a final acrylic wafer is essential to prevent the patient developing a lateral displacement postsurgically. The guideline is that not more than a half-cusp crossbite should be left for postsurgical correction.[5] Decompensation in the vertical dimension is achieved in the leveling phase of treatment as discussed above.

ARCH COORDINATION/COMPATIBILITY

Presurgical orthodontics should produce arches which are compatible both vertically and laterally. In the vertical dimension the second or third molars often present a problem presurgically, especially in high angle cases, where the planned postsurgical occlusion may be propped open on the terminal molars. It is important not to elongate the upper terminal molars, which can be avoided by positioning the bands as occlusally as possible.

Laterally the intermolar and intercanine widths need to be coordinated. Expansion of the upper arch can be carried out using sequentially rigid archwires or a quadhelix, which is useful for differential expansion. Rapid maxillary expansion is not recommended in adults due to the potential risk to the roots and periodontium,[13] although it can be used if surgically assisted, by splitting the palate before expanding. It is important to also correct any dental centreline discrepancies before surgery and this may necessitate removal of teeth, even when well aligned, to prevent unwanted rotational surgical movements, especially in the maxilla. In the case of mandibular asymmetry, if there is compensatory tilting of the lower incisors, they will need to be uprighted thereby worsening the discrepancy, to allow correct positioning of the chin in the midline at the same time as achieving coincident dental centrelines. Coordination of the arches should be checked with 'snap models' prior to surgery so that orthodontic adjustments can be made. In class III cases with narrow upper arches the upper canines frequently require extensive expansion to avoid occlusal interference in the planned postsurgical occlusion. In cases with narrow maxillary arches the palatal cusps of the molars will often interfere in the planned postsurgical position, due to inadequate torque control. The use of Roth molar bands, with increased buccal root torque, can help to avoid this problem. Full size rigid archwires are essential to provide torque control and maintain expansion, but must be in place for a sufficient period of time to achieve such tooth movements. If this does not allow transverse arch coordination, surgical expansion will be required.

Efficient presurgical orthodontics should be completed within 12–18 months, with the intention of setting up the case for finishing within 6 months of surgery. Orthodontic movements which must be carried out before surgery include anteroposterior positioning of the incisors, and intrusion, whereas extrusion (leveling), root paralleling and correction of minor crossbites can be completed in the postsurgical phase.

DEFINITIVE SURGICAL PLANNING

The details of surgical planning are discussed in Chapter 79. The orthodontist should work closely with the surgeon during this final planning phase of treatment. From the orthodontic aspect it is important for the final archwires to have been passive for at least 8 weeks prior to surgery to avoid any unwanted tooth movements after the intermediate and final wafers have been constructed. Repeat lateral cephalometric radiographs, panoramic radiographs, photographs and study models are taken at this stage. The final archwires should ideally be removed for the final planning models to prevent distortion of the impressions, but must be replaced exactly to avoid unwanted tooth movements. It is often easier to place ribbon wax over the brackets, ensuring that the occlusal surfaces of the teeth are not obscured, prior to taking impressions. A facebow recording allows the models to be articulated on a semiadjustable articulator, which is mandatory if a maxillary procedure only (involving autorotation of the mandible) or bimaxillary procedure is planned. Having planned the extent of surgical movement clinically, the cephalometric radiograph can be used to confirm the feasibility of surgery and probable resulting soft-tissue profile, followed by the model surgery and construction of intermediate and final wafers. Wafers should have the facility to be made removable in the postsurgical phase of treatment, by placing circle hooks in the molar, canine and incisor regions. The patient can then use elastics to place the wafer around the upper brackets (Fig. 74.12). When segmental surgery is planned it may be necessary for the orthodontist to bend up a heavy auxiliary wire to stabilize the segments, in addition to the final wafer, during the initial postoperative phase. This wire can be placed in the headgear tube and ligated to the base archwire at the time of surgery. Attachments need to be placed by the orthodontist, if the orthodontic brackets do not carry integral hooks, to aid surgical stabilization. It is important to avoid distorting the final wires when these attachments are placed. Brass hooks can be soldered onto the archwires or crimpable hooks can be placed, but light Kobayashi ligatures should be avoided as they are insufficiently rigid.

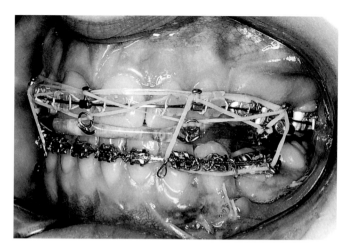

Fig. 74.12 The final wafer is made removable with elastics between the circle hooks of the wafer and the surgical hooks on the upper archwire. Trimming of the posterior lower occlusal surfaces of the wafer, together with box elastics and a light 'memoflex' lower archwire, allows rapid extrusion of the lower molars and premolars in the postsurgical phase of treatment.

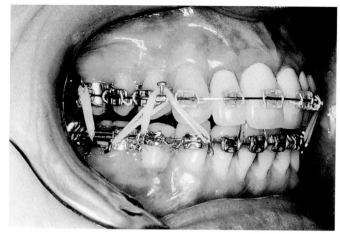

Fig. 74.13 The use of light lower archwires and settling elastics settles the occlusion in the vertical dimension.

POSTSURGICAL ORTHODONTICS

The postsurgical phase of treatment should be completed within 4–6 months of surgery, as patients' motivation and cooperation will be limited at this stage.[14] The routine use of rigid internal fixation has enabled the postsurgical orthodontic phase of treatment to start sooner after surgery than was possible with interosseous wire fixation or intermaxillary fixation (MMF), due to enhanced stability. In all but the most well interdigitating postoperative occlusions an interocclusal wafer is recommended to guide the patient into the new occlusal position, utilizing light interarch elastics. The wafer can usually be removed to allow orthodontic settling after about 2–4 weeks, once there is good bony union and the patient has reasonable opening. The archwires are either sectioned or changed to lighter wires to allow settling in the vertical dimension, together with the use of interarch elastics (Fig. 74.13). Braided rectangular archwires may be used to produce specific tooth movements while maintaining torque. In mandibular advancements the elastics should have a class II element, and in mandibular setbacks they should have a class III element. The patient should be seen at 2- to 3-weekly intervals by the orthodontist at this stage to continue to guide the final occlusal position by judicious elastics and to avoid any displacements or deviations of the mandible while the final intercuspal position is being established. In high angle cases, with open-bite tendencies, the amount of postoperative vertical elastics in the buccal segments should be kept as minimal as possible to avoid opening the bite. Leveling of the lower arch in patients with reduced face heights, where there is a marked curve of Spee, may take slightly longer than the ideal. The interocclusal wafer is made removable, so that the patient can take it out for cleaning. The lower canines and premolars are then extruded utilizing box elastics and a flexible archwire in the lower arch, together with sequential occlusal trimming of the wafer (Fig. 74.12). Ideally there should be some residual lower arch spacing to allow leveling without proclination of the lower incisors.

Where segmental surgery has been carried out finishing procedures involve the removal of standard edgewise brackets, or brackets of the opposite side on canines, replacing them with the appropriate preadjusted bracket to produce correct inclination of the teeth adjacent to the osteotomy cuts.

Retention will be no different than that required for routine orthodontic cases, but it must be remembered that expansion, either surgical or orthodontic, will need to be retained for at least a year, as it is inherently unstable.[15] Definitive restorative treatment is best carried out at the end of retention when any tooth movement has stabilized.

REFERENCES

1. Proffitt WR, Ackerman JL 1985 A systematic approach to orthodontic diagnosis and treatment planning. In: Graber TM, Swain BF (eds) Current orthodontic concepts and techniques, 3rd edn. St Louis: CV Mosby, 1985
2. Macgregor FC 1990 Facial disfigurement: problems and management of social interaction and implications for mental health. Aesthetic Plastic Surgery 4:249–257
3. Ingervall B, Mohlin B, Thilander B 1980 Prevalence of symptoms of functional disturbances of the masticatory system in Swedish men. Journal of Oral Rehabilitation 7:185–197
4. Onizawa K, Schmelzeisen R, Vogt S 1995 Alteration of temporomandibular joint symptoms after orthognathic surgery: a comparison with healthy volunteers. Journal of Oral and Maxillofacial Surgery 53:117–121

5. Obwegeser HL, Makek MS 1986 Hemimandibular hyperplasia – hemimandibular elongation. Journal of Maxillofacial Surgery 14:183–208

6. Riolo ML, Moyers RE, McNamara JA, Hunter WS 1974 An atlas of craniofacial growth. Monograph number 2, Craniofacial growth series. University of Michigan

7. Proffitt WR, White RP 1991 Surgical–orthodontic treatment. Missouri: Mosby-Year Book

8. Ricketts RM, Bench RW, Gugino CF, Hilgers JJ, Schulof RJ 1979 Bioprogressive therapy – book 1. Rocky Mountain Orthodontics

9. Holdaway RA 1983 A soft tissue cephalometric analysis and its use in orthodontic treatment planning. American Journal of Orthodontics 84:1–28

10. Levander E, Malmgren O 1988 Evaluation of the risk of root resorption during orthodontic treatment: a study of upper incisors. European Journal of Orthodontics 10:30–38

11. Lake SL, McNeil RW, Little RM, West RA 1981 Surgical mandibular advancement: a cephalometric analysis of treatment response. American Journal of Orthodontics 80:376–394

12. Houston WJB 1988 Mandibular growth rotations – their mechanisms and importance. European Journal of Orthodontics 10:369–373

13. Barber AF, Sims MR 1981 Rapid maxillary expansion and external root resorption in man: an SEM study. American Journal of Orthodontics 79:630–652

14. Kiyak HA, Hohl T, West RA, McNeil RW 1984 Psychological changes in orthognathic surgery patients: a 24 month follow-up. Journal of Oral and Maxillofacial Surgery 42:506–512

15. Phillips C, Medland WH, Fields HW, Profitt WR, White RP Jr 1992 Stability of surgical maxillary expansion. International Journal of Adult Orthodontics and Orthognathic Surgery 7:139–146

Orthognathic surgical techniques 75

DAVID E. FROST

INTRODUCTION

The artistic aspect of orthognathic surgery has been developing and improving for decades. The scientific aspect of these procedures has been investigated by clinical and academic surgeons in multiple arenas around the world. Volumes of textbooks have been published to detail the variations in orthognathic techniques to achieve stable predictable surgical results.[1–6] This chapter is a small compendium and synopsis of surgical techniques to treat skeletal deformities of the maxilla and mandible. It is not intended to encompass the multitude of surgical procedures which have historically been used to treat variations in skeletal deformities. I do not intend to cover diagnosis, treatment planning, advantages or disadvantages of the different surgical procedures, rather it is my goal to discuss the surgical procedure itself, some of the pitfalls which one encounters in the surgical procedure, and techniques which can be used to avoid problematic results.

The rapid advance in the ability to perform some of these surgical procedures can be partially attributed to the development of instrumentation. There is wide individual variation among surgeons – I have chosen to include a section on instruments and will reference those instruments as they are used in the appropriate procedures. While these instruments are available from a number of manufacturers and suppliers, I have used one individual manufacturer/supplier to standardize my instrument selection (KLS Martin LP, Jacksonville, Florida).

INSTRUMENTS

The significant advances in orthognathic surgical technique have been brought about by intensive research by basic scientists, clinicians and academicians as well as by innovative development of surgical instrumentation. In this section of the text I want to familiarize the reader with various instruments and their use. To this end I have selected one supply company for the instrumentation. It should be noted that numerous supply companies have a plethora of selection of similar instruments. My goal here is not to promote one particular company, but rather to make the reader aware of the unique uses of some of the instruments.

General instruments useful in all types of orthognathic surgery would include periosteal elevators (Fig. 75.1), which

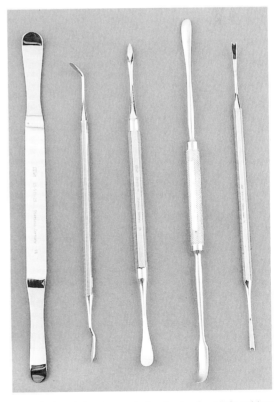

Fig. 75.1 Periodontal elevators and wire director from left: Seldon; Woodson; #9 periosteal; Freeier; wire director (gauze packer).

come in a variety of sizes and shapes. The Woodson periosteal elevator is useful for elevating and retracting flaps of tissue between teeth, on the palatal aspect of a downfractured segmentalized Le Fort osteotomy, and in removing bony fragments over a neurovascular bundle. The Freeier periosteal elevator is useful in developing soft-tissue flaps between teeth, in the pyriform aperture area, and as a retractor for mucosa in the ramus region. A #9 Molt periosteal elevator is most widely used for elevation of subperiosteal flaps and completing the dissection in all subperiosteal planes explored in orthognathic surgical procedures. The Seldon periosteal elevator is rarely used to elevate periosteum but acts as a wide retractor useful in the sagittal split osteotomy, the total subapical osteotomy, and for retraction around the perpendicular plates of the palatine bone and the descending palatine vessels in a Le Fort I osteotomy.

The toe-in and toe-out (tip down and tip up) Obwegeser type retractors (Fig. 75.2) are useful in all aspects of orthognathic surgery. The toe-in (tip down or curve down) retractor is most useful to retract subperiosteal flaps. The toe-in tip should be placed on bone. This allows for atraumatic retraction of the flaps. The toe-out retractor (tip up or curve up) is best utilized to retract soft tissue in any plane other than subperiosteally. The toe-out retractor is also used to retract the tunneled tissue in the pterygomaxillary

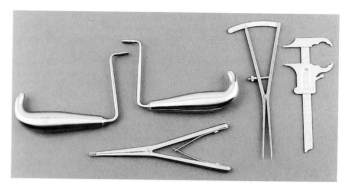

Fig. 75.3 Tessier mobilizers, Turvey palatal expander, Boley gauge and Castroviejo calipers.

fissure region during the Le Fort I osteotomy procedure. The toe-out retractor can be used to position the proximal segment of a sagittal split osteotomy. These retractors come in various widths. Some are available with serrations on the end which allow for better gripping of the bone but are more prone to cause trauma to soft-tissue flaps.

A number of instruments and modifications of instruments have been designed for use in the Le Fort I osteotomy (Fig. 75.3). Some of these can be adapted for use in other procedures as well. Specific instruments utilized for the Le Fort I would include the Tessier mobilizers which are placed in the disjunction between the tuberosity of the maxilla and the pterygoid plates. These mobilizers are paired and are utilized either individually or together to mobilize and retract the downfractured maxilla. The Turvey palatal expander is a modification of a craniofacial instrument designed by Tessier. It is used to place passive pressure in the palatal osteotomy sites of segmentalized Le Fort I osteotomies. It is useful in achieving passive expansion and mobilization of the segments. The Castroviejo calipers and Boley gauge are used to reference intraoperative measurements. The Boley gauge is commonly used to measure the distance between the dorsal nasal pin and a maxillary tooth, while the Castroviejos are used to measure distances between reference holes placed around an osteotomy cut.

Numerous osteotomes are used both in the maxillary and the mandibular orthognathic surgical procedures (Fig. 75.4). The small 'spatula' osteotomes are useful in the interdental osteotomies of the maxilla and in beginning the sagittal split osteotomy at the superior border. A sequential size selection of small thin osteotomes is helpful. The pterygomaxillary junction region can be separated with a variety of pterygomaxillary chisels which have been modified by a number of clinicians. The main goal of these chisels is to deliver the force in a near perpendicular direction. As it is impossible to enter the fissure from a perpendicular direction the modifications all deal with the angulation of

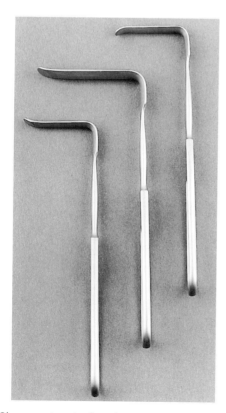

Fig. 75.2 Obwegeser type toe-in and toe-out retractors. Various sizes. From right (top) medium toe-in; large toe-out; medium toe-out.

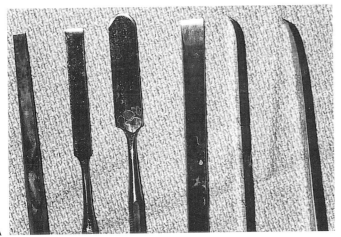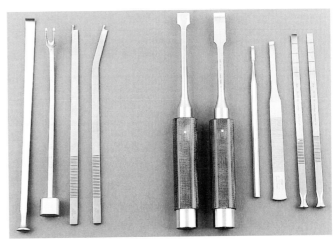

Fig. 75.4 Osteotomes and chisels. **(A)** Small spatula osteotomes and slightly curved chisels – close up. **(B)** From left: selection of pterygomaxillary chisels; nasal double- and single-guarded osteotomes; fiber-handle Obwegeser type splitting osteotomes and a variety of specialty osteotomes.

the cutting edge, its width and handle design. Presented here are a number of selections of pterygomaxillary chisels.

A selection of fiber-handle osteotomes is useful for completing the mandibular ramus procedures (Fig. 75.4B), specifically the sagittal split. They can also be adapted to some difficult downfractures of the Le Fort I osteotomy (see text below). A selection of guarded osteotomes is useful for completing posterior maxillary wall osteotomies as well as lateral nasal wall osteotomies and separation of the nasal septum from the floor of the nose. These come in differing lengths with various degrees of curvature. The guarded aspect is to keep the dissecting end of the osteotome in the subperiosteal plane.

Mandibular surgical procedures require some specialized instrumentation (Fig. 75.5). In the sagittal split osteotomy the Obwegeser channel retractor, the Terry modified channel retractor, the ramus pusher for stripping of the temporalis attachment and the 'notched ramus retractor' are all useful for dissection and exposure of the medial and lateral aspect of the ascending ramus. The Hargis J stripper can be used as a retractor for the maxilla or as a stripping instrument to remove medial pterygoid and lateral aspects of the masseter attachment from various segments of a sagittal split and a transoral vertical ramus osteotomy.

For the transoral vertical ramus osteotomy the dissection remains totally lateral. The vertical nature of the osteotomy requires special instrumentation for visualization and adequate, safe placement of the oscillating saw (Fig. 75.6). Brauer right and left retractors for the sigmoid notch allow for superior protection of the masseteric artery as it traverses the sigmoid notch. The Merrill–LeVasier is placed on the posterior border of the ramus to develop adequate retraction for placement of the oscillating saw.

As mentioned above, many different sizes and shapes of

osteotomes are used to complete the splitting of the ramus for a sagittal osteotomy. The small osteotomes, larger fiber-handle osteotomes, and intermediate-sized chisels and osteotomes are all useful. Two specially designed instruments have gained great popularity in the past few years (Fig. 75.7). The Smith inferior border splitters are used to begin the split at the inferior aspect of the vertical leg of a sagittal osteotomy. These splitters allow for levering against a dense portion of the distal mandible. The upper border spreader, also designed by Smith, allows for wide disbursement of pressure on the lateral and medial cortexes as the sagittal osteotomy begins to separate. This instrument also allows for some retraction of the segments for visuali-

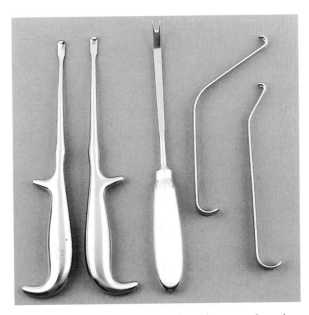

Fig. 75.5 From left: J strippers; ramus pusher; Obwegeser channel retractor and Terry modified channel retractor.

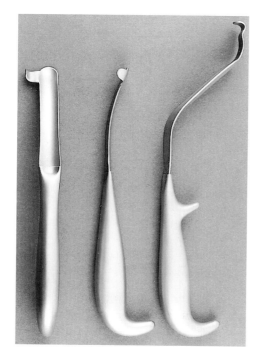

Fig. 75.6 Transoral vertical ramus osteotomy – specialized retractors. From left: Brauer left and right sigmoid notch retractors; Merrill–LeVasier ramus retractor.

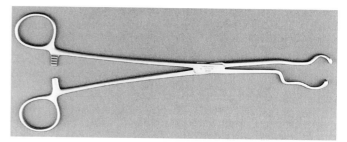

Fig. 75.8 Wolford modified upper border clamp.

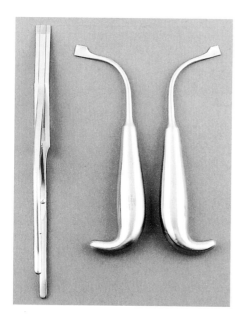

Fig. 75.7 Specialized sagittal split instruments. From left: Smith upper border spreader and lower border right and left splitters.

zation of the neurovascular bundle if it needs to be removed from the proximal segment.

Figure 75.8 shows the Wolford modified upper border clamp. This instrument is introduced transorally to aid in the stabilization of the proximal distal segment relationship while rigid fixation is applied. There are multiple modifica-

tions of this clamp. In essence, the clamp is an Alyce type clamp which has been modified to allow for gripping of the bone of a ramus area without undue pressure being applied. The clamp should be placed at the area of maximum bony contact (Fig. 75.8).

There are numerous other instruments which have unique applications in orthognathic surgery. Unless they were specifically referenced in this text I have elected to not include them in the instrumentation section. Individual surgeon preference and idiosyncrasies will dictate certain individual choices for instrumentation. The KLS Martin Company of Jacksonville, Florida, supplied the instruments and illustrations for this section of the text.

MAXILLARY OSTEOTOMIES – LE FORT I LEVEL SURGERY

The most popular and useful approach to skeletal correction of maxillary deformities is via the total maxillary osteotomy or Le Fort I osteotomy.[7-9] The surgical procedure has been developed to allow for multiple modifications to correct three-dimensional deformities of the maxillary complex. Downfracturing of the maxilla allows for segmentalization and three-dimensional repositioning of the dentoalveolar complex. This versatile operation allows for elongation, shortening, forward advancement or retrusion and differential leveling of the entire complex.[9-12]

Adequate anesthesia is achieved with nasotracheal intubation and low-profile draping of the tubes. Adequate stabilization of the nasotracheal tube is easily established with a pillow case type head drape and secure taping of the tube to the head. This allows for rotation of the head in any direction as the need occurs during surgery. It also prevents the potential dislodgment of the nasal endotracheal tube.

Once adequate anesthesia has been achieved, local anesthetic is infiltrated into the buccal vestibule and the palate. 0.5% Lidocaine with 1:200 000 epinephrine is adequate. Approximately 10 ml infiltrated in the buccal vestibule and palate on each side will give adequate hemostasis during the early soft-tissue dissection. In the average patient we have found it unnecessary to go to extremes for hypotensive anesthesia for the completion of these osteotomies. Anesthetic management of these patients is beyond the scope of this chapter and will not be dealt with further.

The soft-tissue incision is a full-thickness periosteal incision from the buttress of the zygoma to the buttress of the zygoma with attention in the midline to a V-ing of the incision to allow for esthetic closure.[13,14] The incision can be made with a scalpel or electrocautery. Electrocautery seems to control some hemorrhage at the time of the incision, however no long-term studies have justified its use over the more traditional scalpel. Layered incisions are possible, but serve no advantage for the dissection. Once the periosteum has been incised, blunt instruments are used to elevate a mucoperiosteal flap superiorly. Adequate visualization is most important, so the flaps should be elevated superiorly to identify the pyriform aperture, the infraorbital foramen and its exiting neurovascular bundles, and the buttress of the zygoma. Tunneling subperiosteally posteriorly under the buttress of the zygoma is done with periosteal elevators to allow for exposure of the pterygomaxillary junction. The periosteal elevator should be maintained on the bone and in a subperiosteal plane with angulation as it proceeds posteriorly to incline inferiorly or towards the hamular process of the sphenoid bone. This will alleviate the potential problem of entering the pterygomaxillary fissure and concomitant increased hemorrhage.[15,16] A cheek retractor with the tip pointing out (toe-out) is placed in the pterygomaxillary junction region to allow for adequate soft-tissue retraction and exposure of the posterior aspect of the maxilla.

The inferior soft tissue is not stripped from the bone except in areas where interdental osteotomies are planned. The anterior nasal spine soft tissue is elevated and the pyriform is visualized completely. The dissection on one side and the bony cuts are completed prior to starting the dissection on the opposite side. The rationale for this approach is to minimize the oozing blood loss and edema in an area which will not be approached surgically for some time.

The soft tissue of the nasal pyriform aperture is reflected and the nasal mucoperiosteum is elevated with appropriately shaped periosteal elevators (#9 periosteal or Freeier elevator). The anatomy of the pyriform aperture and the floor of the nose should be familiar to all experienced surgeons. It should be noted that the pyriform opening actually extends inferiorly into the floor of the nose. The Freeier elevator with the strong curve allows for easy elevation of the soft tissue while maintaining bone contact. Frequently there are nasal/septal deviations and cartilaginous and osseous spurs on the septum which make the dissection of the mucoperiosteum difficult. It is important to maintain an intact nasal layer where possible. Care in this portion of the dissection will decrease bothersome hemorrhage both interoperatively and postoperatively.

Once the nasal layer has been dissected, it is prudent to place a periosteal elevator or a ribbon retractor to protect the mucoperiosteum of the nasal floor during the osteotomy cuts. This also can be used to protect the endotracheal tube or nasoesophageal stethoscope which will be in the nares for the operation.

As may be preferred by some surgeons, reference marks can be placed in a vertical fashion in the lateral wall of the maxilla, or bone reference holes a standardized distance apart (15 mm seems to be a reasonable distance) can be placed in a vertical fashion in the buttress and in the pyriform rim region (Fig. 75.9).[17–19] Alternatively, a non-threaded K wire or Steinmann pin can be placed in the nasal dorsum and a reference distance taken from that K wire to the anterior dentition to allow for determination of the amount of superior repositioning of the anterior maxilla (Fig. 75.10).[20,21] I find it preferable to place the K wire in the nasal dorsum for the anterior measurement as well as placing reference holes posteriorly in the buttress region to allow for accurate posterior/superior repositioning.

Once the reference measurements have been taken and recorded, the lateral osteotomy may be completed using either a reciprocating saw or a rotary instrument (Fig. 75.11). In the maxilla with very thin lateral walls, often encountered with vertical maxillary excess and long-face syndrome patients, a rotary instrument such as a small fissure bur or a round bur may be preferable to a reciprocating saw. The reciprocating saw is generally much quicker and gives a

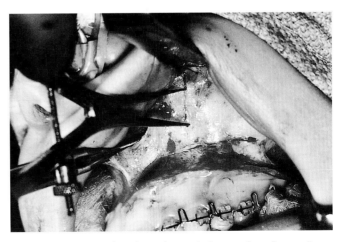

Fig. 75.9 Calipers used to place reference holes or scribe reference line for maxillary repositioning.

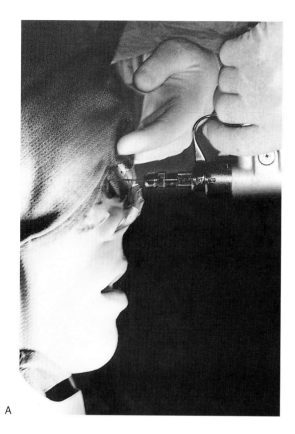

A

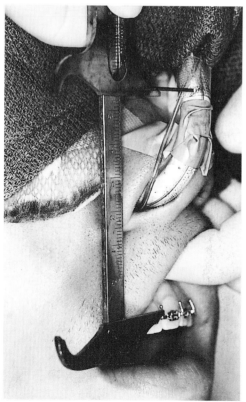

B

Fig. 75.10 (A) K wire being placed in nasal dorsum. **(B)** Boley gauge to measure vertical maxillary relationship pre-osteotomy.

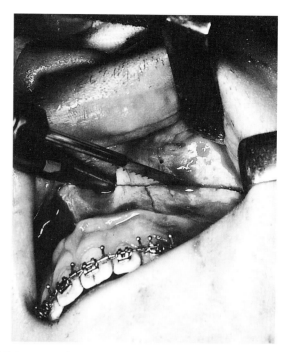

Fig. 75.11 Le Fort I level horizontal osteotomy with reciprocating saw. *Note*: nasal soft–tissue protection with osteotome.

smooth cut, however the vibration of the saw can fracture the maxillary wall. The experienced surgeon will note that the osteotomy is only through the lateral wall of the maxilla until the anterior aspect of the nose is reached. This area has a triangular-shaped wedge of bone which is the junction of the lateral wall of the nose and the lateral wall of the maxillary sinus. This thickened area of bone can be cut with either the reciprocating saw or the rotary instrument. The retracting osteotome or ribbon retractor in the nasal cavity prevents laceration of the soft tissues or of the endotracheal tube.

A saw also has the disadvantage of not being able to be adequately angled to allow for customization of the bone cuts. This customization is often beneficial in the posterior region when trying to do a step osteotomy to allow for position of graft material or planned high cuts to allow for esthetic augmentation of the paranasal region.

Once the bony cut has been made from the lateral aspect at the pterygomaxillary fissure region to the pyriform aperture region the reciprocating saw can be turned and placed into the maxillary sinus and a cut from inside to outside can be done to allow for the posterior lateral wall of the antrum to be adequately osteotomized (Fig. 75.12). This cut should be done from inside out with the toe-out cheek retractor protecting the soft tissues in the pterygoid fissure area.

A curved single-guarded osteotome can be used to complete the osteotomy of the posterior lateral aspect of

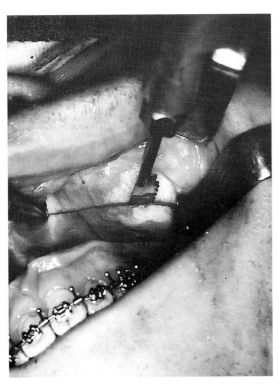

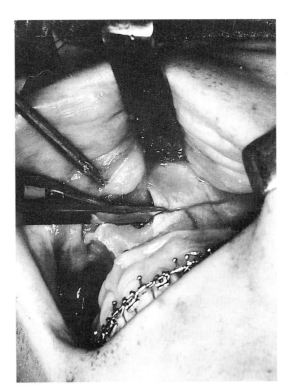

Fig. 75.12 Reciprocating saw cutting from inside out to allow for the posterior wall to be sectioned.

Fig. 75.13 Single-guarded nasal osteotome completing the lateral nasal osteotomy.

the maxilla to the pterygoid plates. Care and attention should be used in the direction of this osteotome and the depth achieved. It is not intended to cleave off the pterygoid plates at this time, nor is it desirable to traverse through the descending palatine vasculature. The osteotome is generally used to start a cleavage point. The prudent surgeon would also keep this osteotomy as low as possible in the pterygomaxillary plate region to avoid the superior vascular structures, both venous and arterial, which reside in and traverse the pterygomaxillary fissure region. The area is then packed, usually with an absorbent gauze, and attention is directed to the contralateral side.

The soft-tissue dissection is done on the opposite side at this time. I delay the soft-tissue dissection until after the entire osteotomy has been completed on one side. This gives less opportunity for ooze and hemorrhage to occur. The length of exposure also leads to increased edema. The surgical procedure is similar on the contralateral side.

Attention is then directed to the lateral nasal walls. The soft tissue is retracted medially bilaterally with periosteal elevators and a straight single-guarded nasal osteotome is introduced down the lateral nasal wall to allow for separation of the superior bone from the soon-to-be downfractured maxilla (Fig. 75.13). The osteotome is malleted posteriorly until the perpendicular plates of the palatine bone are reached. Do not mallet into the perpendicular plates of the

palatine bone as the descending palatine vessels can easily be transected or perforated and cause significant hemorrhaging. The nasal septum is removed from the superior aspect of the palate by using a double-guarded nasal septal osteotome (Fig. 75.14). Prior to the introduction of the osteotome, the nasal mucoperiosteum and perichondrium is stripped as far as possible posteriorly and superiorly to allow for the osteotome to be passed and not cause any tears in the nasal mucosa. This is often difficult because of

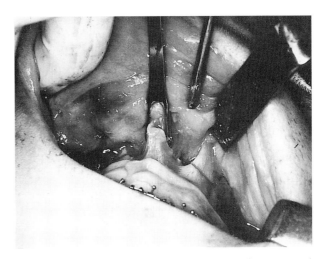

Fig. 75.14 Double-guarded nasal septal osteotome used to separate the palate from the nasal septum; guards should be subperiosteal.

the frequency of bony spurs which occur in this area. A few extra moments of soft-tissue dissection and retraction will prevent a lengthy period of time spent suturing rents in the nasal mucosa.

The packs placed at the posterior aspect of the pterygomaxillary fissure region and the junction of the horizontal osteotomy are then removed, a toe-out cheek retractor is placed to retract the mucosa, and a heavily curved pterygomaxillary chisel is introduced. The chisel is directed inferiorly at the junction of the pterygoid plates with the posterior maxilla. The index finger of the nondominant hand is generally introduced into the oral cavity at the hamular notch region in the area of the junction of the pterygoid plates with the posterior maxilla. This finger can easily palpate the properly placed osteotome as it is moved to the ideal position. Once this osteotome is firmly seated in position, it should be levered laterally as far as possible to allow for the vector of force to be delivered in as close to a perpendicular direction to the junction of the pterygomaxillary plates and the posterior maxilla as is feasible. A sharp rap on the osteotome is delivered by the surgical assistant. Generally one or two raps will allow the osteotome to wedge between the junction of the pterygoid plates and the maxilla. This bone cut does not have to be completed – merely starting it will allow for the direction of the fracture to proceed in an appropriate fashion. The area is packed and a similar procedure is completed on the contralateral side.

Retraction (toe-in retractors placed on bone) is placed under the flaps to allow for adequate visualization and then digital downward pressure is applied to the anterior maxilla. This will generally allow for passive inferior repositioning of the maxilla. This 'downfracture' maneuver should not require a great degree of pressure. If excessive force is required, the head must be stabilized by another assistant. Again, if excessive force is required, the bone cuts should be examined to be sure they are complete, the osteotome should be reintroduced in the lateral nasal wall and in the horizontal cut as it moves posteriorly towards the junction of the pterygoid plates. The pterygomaxillary osteotome can also be reintroduced and malleted again to assure the complete break of the plates from the maxilla. If downfracturing does not proceed easily at this time I find it helpful to place a thin wide osteotome (fiber-handle osteotome – see instrument section) in the lateral nasal wall area, posteriorly to the perpendicular plate of the palatine bone region, and then with a rotational movement aid in completing the fracture through the perpendicular plate of the palatine bone. I find that this is usually the area where the osteotomy holds up and prevents easy downfracturing. This can be done bilaterally with two thin wide

osteotomes, one placed on each side. The maxilla is then easily downfractured with digital pressure in the anterior region.

Once the maxilla is downfractured, the pterygomaxillary retractors (Tessier mobilizers) are placed in the inferior and posterior aspect of the downfractured maxilla. Pressure and manipulation with these allows for free mobilization of the maxilla. The bony impingements can be fractured and the maxilla mobilized with these instruments. One of the retractors can be removed and that side packed. A toe-out cheek retractor or Tessier is placed in the contralateral side to allow for adequate retraction of the soft tissues. The bony interferences and impingements in the posterior aspect of the maxilla can now be removed with a rongeur or rotary instrument as necessary. The descending palatine vessels are identified and either retracted or clipped as necessary.[22] I generally prefer to place vascular clips on the vessel, one superiorly and one inferiorly, and to incise the vessel between them. The area of most bony interference to passive superior repositioning is generally the area that this vessel traverses, so consequent to adequate superior repositioning of the maxilla this vessel generally needs to be clipped and bone removed in the posterior medial aspect of the sinus wall and at the area of the perpendicular plates of the palatine bone (Fig. 75.15). If the maxilla is to be inferiorly repositioned to any significant degree this vessel

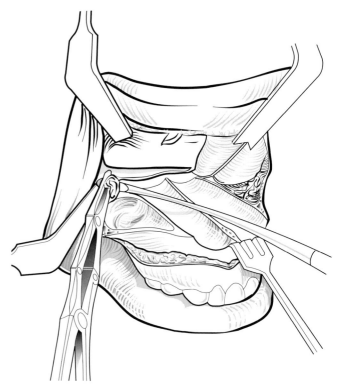

Fig. 75.15 Removal of bone around the perpendicular plate of the palatine bone. The descending palatine vessels may be ligated.

must be clipped to avoid a possible laceration in the stretching process of inferior repositioning. Similarly, the vessel will be placed under a significant amount of tension if the maxilla is to be advanced to any degree. While a number of reports[23–25] of avascular problems have occurred secondary to inappropriate manipulation of this vessel and soft-tissue pedicles, this author believes that the majority of these are secondary to inappropriate flap design and improper management of the soft-tissue pedicles rather than the sacrifice of this single vessel either unilaterally or bilaterally. In a number of institutions with various surgeons and various degrees of expertise in junior faculty, we have noted no vascular problems related to sacrifice of this vessel. Once the area has been debrided, antral mucoceles and polyps removed and the bone smoothed for the planned repositioning of the maxilla, the area can be packed and the procedure completed on the opposite side.

SEGMENTALIZATION

The maxilla can be segmentalized for repositioning of dento-osseous segments. This is easily done with the maxilla in the downfractured position. The interdental osteotomy cuts for segmentalization can be started with the maxilla still in the intact position. This allows for the lateral cortical cuts to be completed while the maxilla is stable and not moving around. A small fissure bur, an oscillating saw or a sagittal saw can be used to complete these interdental cuts. While the saws are somewhat quicker, the loss of fine touch in using the saws can be detrimental. For this reason it is preferred to use a small fissure bur to make the lateral cortical scoring cuts and then use a small thin spatula osteotome to complete the cuts through to the palate.

In general, segmentalization is done: (a) between the central incisors for a two-piece maxillary osteotomy for expansion; (b) between the canine and the premolar for a three-piece maxillary osteotomy for posterior expansion and differential superior repositioning; or (c) between the canine and the lateral incisor, for differential superior repositioning and for expansion including the canines. It has become more frequent in recent years to segmentalize between the canine and the lateral incisor. This is due in part to a number of reasons, one of which is the fact that the canines are routinely angled posteriorly by the orthodontist to allow for proper axial inclination. It seems to be problematic with some orthodontists when creating the space for an interdental osteotomy between the canine and the bicuspid region. There has been a tendency in recent years for the orthodontist to prefer nonextraction management of cases and this results in a minimal amount of space for an interdental osteotomy between the canine and the

first premolar. It is generally necessary to expand the inter-canine distance as well. To avoid the necessity of a four-piece maxillary osteotomy and to allow for proper posterior and canine expansion the osteotomy between the lateral incisor and the canine is used.

The interdental osteotomies can be started with adequate retraction of the soft tissue (Woodson elevator) and the use of a small fissure bur to score the lateral cortex (Fig. 75.16). The handpiece should be angled in such a fashion anterior to posteriorly as to prevent inadvertent damage to one of the adjacent teeth. It should be remembered that the premolar palatal root is generally anterior to the buccal root and will be damaged if the handpiece is not angled more posteriorly, bringing the cutting edge anteriorly. I find it easier and potentially less hazardous to use a rotary instrument such as a fissure bur rather than the reciprocating or sagittal saw. The reciprocating saw or sagittal saw may be quicker to complete the osteotomies between the teeth, but there is much less touch or feel as the bone is sectioned. This could lead to inadvertent damage to a tooth. Scoring the lateral cortex to the marrow and then using a small spatula osteotome to complete the cut to the palate places the adjacent teeth at less risk (Fig. 75.17). This allows for the osteotome to possibly touch against the tooth but not damage the tooth as readily as the powered instruments will. A finger is inserted on the palate to palpate the osteotome as it 'greensticks' or cuts the palatal cortex.

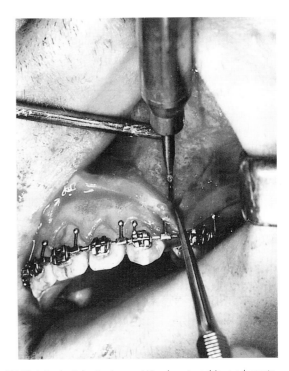

Fig. 75.16 Interdental osteotomes: Woodson to achieve adequate retraction, small fissure bur to begin osteotomy.

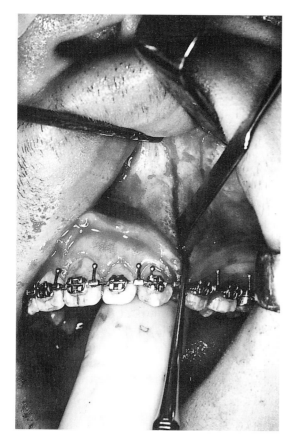

Fig. 75.17 Spatula osteotome to complete interdental osteotomy. Note finger on palate to palpate the completion of the osteotomy without damage to the palatal soft tissue.

A channel retractor can be placed at the posterior aspect of the hard palate over the posterior nasal spine with the maxilla in the downfractured position. This retractor is then gently elevated to tip up the posterior aspect of the downfractured maxilla. Concomitant retraction on the anterior maxilla will aid in visualization of the downfractured maxilla from the palatal side (Fig. 75.18). This allows for easy completion of the palatal segmentalization. These osteotomy cuts are done with rotary instruments. The segmentalization for expansion is easily done in a parasagittal fashion along the nasal side of the lateral nasal wall. This avoids roots, vascular structures and thin palatal mucosa. If excessive expansion is necessary (greater than 7 mm) parasagittal cuts should be done bilaterally. This permits more relaxation of the soft tissue over the palate. A resultant free piece of bone is developed in the midpalatal area. This should not have all the periosteum stripped off and should not result in a free graft. Turvey palatal expanders can be introduced to aid in expansion. I have found it most useful to strip some of the underlying mucoperiosteum from the dento-osseous segments to allow for passive expansion. The anterior transpalatal osteotomy between the inter-

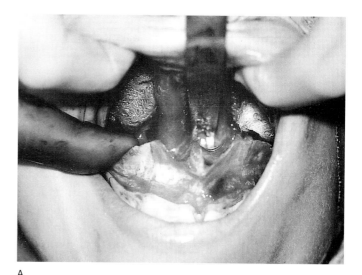

A

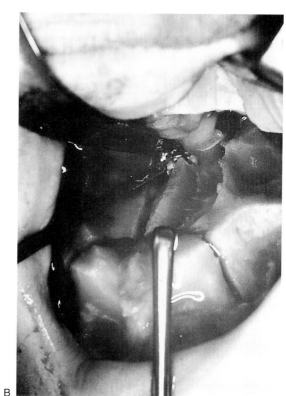

B

Fig. 75.18 (A) Channel retractor placed over posterior nasal spine with maxilla downfractured. Aids in retraction and visualization.
(B) Segmentalized, expanded maxilla in downfractured position with channel retractor over posterior nasal spine. J stripper over pyriform for retraction.

dental osteotomies of the canine premolar interspace is also easily completed with the maxilla tilted down and forward. Periodic relaxation on the channel retractor will allow for vascular perfusion to continue during this short but critical phase of the surgery.

Once the osteotomies are completed, the segments are mobilized. A Woodson instrument can be used to strip periosteum from the inferior aspect of a segment to allow for its adequate expansion and mobilization. When the segments have been adequately mobilized a pre-bent orthodontic archwire replaces the existing archwire. This is secured with ligature ties. The pre-bent archwire has been fabricated from the model surgery. It can be bent with lugs or it can have clamp-on lugs placed at appropriate sites for use in intermaxillary fixation. An auxiliary heavy archwire which is placed in the headgear tubes can be used to add stability for maxillary expansion cases. The archwire gives dental stabilization to the segments. A prefabricated interocclusal acrylic splint is routinely used to tie the segments together at the occlusal surface. The benefit of the splint is that it gives a reproducible position to the dentition, allows the mandible to be wired to this finalized occlusion, and allows for the maxillomandibular complex to be referenced to the stable condyles as the maxilla is rotated superiorly. With the splint wired to the maxillary dentition the patient is placed in intermaxillary fixation with a heavy stainless steel wire placed bilaterally. For open-bite cases, an intermaxillary fixation wire in the anterior area is also used. While applying posterior and superior pressure on the angle of the mandible to seat the condyles appropriately, the maxillomandibular complex is passively rotated superiorly. Any impingements are identified and relieved until the vertical position of the maxilla is achieved as dictated by the preoperative planning. In the area of the perpendicular plates of the palatine bone liberal removal is indicated, especially with superior repositioning. Small impingements in this area can cause distraction of the condyles when rotating the maxillomandibular complex superiorly. This can lead to a postoperative anterior open-bite discrepancy. The critical reference point is the distance from the K wire to the upper incisor bracket. The amount of predicted superior repositioning or inferior repositioning is measured and the maxilla is held in place at this position. As a second check, the posterior measurement of the planned superior repositioning or inferior repositioning is verified using the previously placed reference holes. Some parallax occurs when a large amount of expansion, or anteroposterior repositioning occurs, and this should be taken into consideration when making this measurement. In general, with an intact mandible, the anterior measurement from K wire to incisor bracket will allow for adequate determination of the final maxillary position. The anterior–posterior position is dictated by the intact mandible being used for a rotational reference.

Once the appropriate position has been determined, the maxilla can be stabilized with small bone plates. The monocortical fixation devices after the Champy technique are most widely adaptable to this procedure.[26–29] Heavier

plates are utilized if the maxilla is being inferiorly repositioned. Bone grafting is appropriate for inferior repositioning as well as for any substantial gaps between the mobilized inferiorly repositioned maxilla and the stable superior bony base. Plate selection, position and number are determined based on the requirements for stabilization, the anatomy of the patient, and the number of segments. In general, a single X-shaped bone plate on the lateral maxillary wall bilaterally is sufficient for single-piece maxillary osteotomies (Fig. 75.19). For segmentalized osteotomies an X-shaped or an L-shaped plate in the posterior segment and a single vertical plate on either side of the pyriform aperture for the anterior segment is adequate. Some surgeons prefer to place an anterior plate and posterior transosseous wires or no posterior plates at all to allow for passive positioning of the posterior complex. This is theoretically to aid in prevention of the postoperative complication of residual anterior open-bite. Personally I have not had this problem and believe that the attention to prevention of anterior open-bite is best achieved when the maxillomandibular complex is passively positioned superiorly. The surgeon's

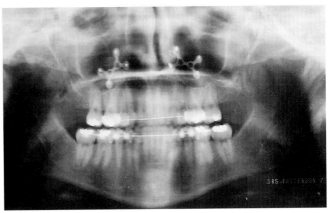

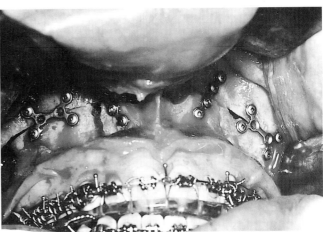

Fig. 75.19 (A) Panoramic radiograph showing X-shaped bone plate for stabilization to Le Fort I osteotomy. **(B)** Operative view of X-shaped bone plates posteriorly in segmentalized osteotomy.

manipulation of the condylar complex must not allow for any distraction of the condyle down in the glenoid fossa. This will prevent the sequela of postoperative anterior open-bite.

Once stabilization has been completed, the intermaxillary fixation is released and the bite is again verified, with the condyle and the mandibular complex being passively rotated into the splint. The splint can be removed and the bite verified with the dentition as well. If there is any segmentalization or expansion, the splint should be ligated to the maxillary dentition after the verification of occlusion has been completed.

The incision is generally closed in layers with a permanent OO Prolene type stitch being used to cinch the alar base musculature together (Fig. 75.20) and then a slowly resorbable stitch such as 4.0 Vicryl being used in a con-

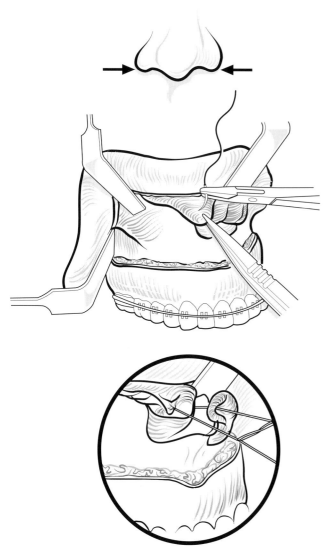

Fig. 75.20 Alar base cinch suture. Both sides are sutured together across the midline.

tinuous over and over fashion to close the mucosa. V–Y advancement of the midline or multiple modifications of V–Y advancement are advocated to maintain vermilion bulk.[13,14]

MANDIBULAR SURGERY – SAGITTAL SPLIT OSTEOTOMY

The sagittal split osteotomy was introduced to the American oral and maxillofacial surgery arena by Drs Trauner and Obwgeser some forty years ago.[30,31] Since that introduction, numerous modifications and permutations of the osteotomy have been suggested, utilized, perfected or abandoned. I present for you in this discussion a basic osteotomy technique which has been utilized for many years as an acceptable procedure for advancement or reduction of the mandible. The use of rigid fixation is readily adaptable to this osteotomy technique.[32] The bilateral sagittal split osteotomy for advancement procedures is the most commonly used and popular orthognathic corrective procedure today. The use of the osteotomy for posterior repositioning is widely used but frequently overshadowed by the vertical subsigmoid osteotomy which will be described in another section of this chapter.

TECHNIQUE

The sagittal split is accomplished via an intraoral approach with an incision starting on the anterior aspect of the vertical ramus. The incision is carried inferiorly through the lateral aspect of the retromolar fossa to the buccal of the second or terminal molar. The incision angles laterally and anteriorly, continuing forward a distance necessary to allow for adequate retraction and visualization. This varies with the amount of advancement or setback of the mandible. It is important to keep the incision lateral to allow for easy closure of the wound with the teeth in fixation. In this period of rigid internal fixation, it may not be necessary to suture the incision with the patient in intermaxillary fixation, however the possibility always exists that this may be required due to inadequate, improper or troublesome splits. The incision is started superiorly enough to allow for exposure of the ascending ramus. I prefer to carry this incision through the periosteum on the initial cut. The periosteum and mucosa are reflected to expose the lateral cortex of the mandible. As the ascending ramus is approached a notched ramus retractor is introduced to allow for stripping of the insertion of the temporalis muscle. The attachment of the temporalis can be very tenacious, but it must be removed to at least the level of the sigmoid notch and preferably higher.

This assures easy access to the medial aspect of the mandible and better visualization for the medial bone cut. Once the notched ramus retractor has been placed and the dissection carried superiorly a periosteal elevator is introduced along the bone in a subperiosteal fashion and directed horizontally on the medial aspect of the mandible. Starting at about the level of the sigmoid notch, the periosteal elevator is passed horizontally to an area posterior or proximal to the lingula. This periosteal elevator is then replaced with a Seldon periosteal elevator or retractor. The Seldon is angled to allow the inferior edge of the retractor to engage the bone and the superior edge of the retractor to develop a pocket or area for the suction tip and saw or drill to be placed. This pocket allows for the Seldon to protect the inferior neurovascular bundle as it enters the lingual foramen. A double-ended dental curette can then be introduced to identify the sigmoid notch. It is important to identify the sigmoid notch superiorly and the entrance of the neurovascular bundle to the lingual foramen inferiorly. Splitting the distance between these two structures will allow for an appropriate medial osteotomy. I personally prefer to err on the side of being slightly low or closer to the lingula than to the sigmoid notch. As the mandible goes superiorly in this area, the amount of medullary bone decreases and there is a significant chance of fused cortices – this makes for a potential horizontal osteotomy of the ramus which is a difficult complication to manage.

Using adequate retraction and irrigation, a rotary instrument or reciprocating saw of choice can be utilized to make the initial cut. It is my preference to use a Lindemann bur in a handpiece to make this cut. Terminate the posterior aspect of the cut just behind the entrance of the neurovascular bundle into the lingual foramen. The medial cut is only through the inner cortex or down to bleeding bone. It is feathered or tapered as it approaches the posterior aspect of the bony cut (the depth of the Seldon retractor helps determine this) so that when splitting occurs the split is directed medially through the lingual cortex rather than through the posterior aspect of the mandible. The original descriptions through the posterior aspect allowed for more bone contact but required greater stripping of soft tissue and entailed increased risk of bleeding intraoperatively and postoperative loss of blood supply to the proximal segment.

When the osteotomy has been completed on the medial aspect, an absorbent gauze is packed in the area and the Seldon retractor removed. Relaxation on the notched ramus retractor can allow for the easy exposure of the lateral aspect of the mandible. Subperiosteal dissection is carried forward and inferior to an area opposite the first and second molar interspace. The lateral exposure is completed to the inferior

border. A lateral channel retractor is placed at this time to assist in retraction. If difficulty is encountered in placing this retractor, a special periosteal stripper can be used to assist in removing the attachments to allow for passive placement of the retractor. Usually this is not necessary. Attention should be paid to the minimal stretching and pulling of the periosteum in this area. Posteriorly, the lateral-inferior dissection should end before the antegonial notch. The lateral subperiosteal dissection on the soon-to-be proximal segment of the ramus should be minimal. At this point, I prefer to use a number eight (#8) round bur or a small fissure bur in a rotary handpiece to place a cut vertically from the channel retractor to the external oblique ridge. This cut is through the lateral cortex and is generally made anterior to the second molar, extending from the inferior border superiorly to the external oblique ridge. It extends through cortex to marrow. Observation for the neurovascular bundle is important when completing the lateral bony cut. Frequently the neurovascular bundle lies close to the lateral cortex, and the rotary instruments have the potential to damage the neurovascular bundle when making the cortical cut. I round the angle at the external oblique ridge to begin the connection of the medial horizontal cut with the lateral vertical cut. At this time, switch to a small fissure bur (701) to connect the two osteotomies if not already done. The fissure bur may also be used at the depth of the channel retractor, cutting posteriorly to initiate the inferior border split.

All of these bone cuts can be done equally as well with a reciprocating saw. It should be noted when using the reciprocating saw that the cut begins at the superior horizontal osteotomy going through the cortex only, then changing to a sagittal osteotomy immediately and decreasing the depth of the saw as it approaches the distal aspect of the second molar. The osteotomy is carried forward through the lateral cortex to the area of the external oblique ridge which would normally join with the vertical cut.

The reciprocating saw is removed and is placed in a vertical fashion on the lateral aspect of the mandible in the channel retractor. With the channel retractor angled anteriorly and the handpiece turned slightly anteriorly, the reciprocating saw can be used to complete the vertical cut as well. It is slightly quicker to use the reciprocating saw, but also slightly more traumatic to the adjacent soft tissues. Visibility for the assistants is compromised with the saw. Whichever is preferred by the individual operator, the cuts should be only through the cortex to allow for protection of the vascular and neural structures that traverse the mandible in this area.

Once the vertical and horizontal cortical cuts have been connected, the split can be accomplished. The limits of the split are defined by the horizontal and vertical bony cuts. A small spatula osteotome which has been specially thinned for this technique is driven along the vertical cut to ensure that the inferior cortex has been adequately split. This thin osteotome is then stepped along the connection between the vertical cut and the horizontal cut, with the handle of the osteotome being leaned medially to allow the cutting edge of the osteotome to stay as close to the lateral cortex as possible. It is lightly malleted to a depth of a few millimeters, and is repositioned along the distance between the vertical and the horizontal osteotomy. Once the initial split has occurred, the osteotome is introduced again at the anterior/superior extent of the osteotomy and a second slightly wider osteotome is introduced lateral to the initial osteotome. This again is malleted, a millimeter or two deeper than the original osteotome. This allows for continuation of the cut or splitting along the same cleavage plane and helps ensure that the split remains close to the lateral cortex. If the nerve is encountered, it can be separated from the proximal segment as it is visualized. In general, it is not seen at this point of the dissection. This two-osteotome technique is then continued from the vertical osteotomy to the horizontal osteotomy. It is restarted in the anterior extent, this time with the initial osteotome being malleted to the depth of the cut, the second osteotome being placed buccal to that and malleted slightly deeper, and then a third, broader osteotome (thicker) being placed between the two and gently rapped. This will begin a separation of the superior aspect of the osteotomy. This is done from anterior to posterior along the sagittal aspect of the split (Fig. 75.21). Once adequate superior splitting has begun to occur, a specially developed inferior splitting

osteotome can be introduced at the depth of the channel retractor (Fig. 75.21). These osteotomes are pared for individual use on the right and left ramus. The cutting edge of the osteotome is introduced at the depth of the vertical cut and, as the pressure is applied to the distal inferior bony aspect of the mandible, the proximal segment begins to split away from the distal segment. This begins the splitting of the inferior border. If done in concert with placement of a splitting osteotome (wide fiber-handle osteotome) at the superior border, the sagittal split is frequently completed. If not, the superior border splitting osteotomes are introduced and rotated in such a fashion as to allow the levering blade of the osteotome to engage the cortical bone and apply pressure to split the mandible (Fig. 75.22). If the nerve is encountered, it is carefully separated from the proximal segment, usually with a curette or a Woodson instrument. If the split along the inferior border is incomplete, the thin osteotome can be used to assist in its completion. Once the bone is completely separated, toe-in cheek retractors are placed in the osteotomy to retract the proximal segment. The distal segment is manipulated and brought forward. The neurovascular bundle is visualized or oftentimes is still covered by a layer of medullary bone. A special J-shaped stripping periosteal elevator is introduced into the split of the osteotomy with the stripping element being placed along the inferior border of the distal segment (Fig. 75.23). This stripper is then carefully but firmly moved along the inferior aspect of the distal segment anteriorly to the extent of the dissection and posteriorly to the neurovascular bundle's entrance into the distal segment. This allows for removal of any muscular attachments of the medial pterygoid and helps with a passive

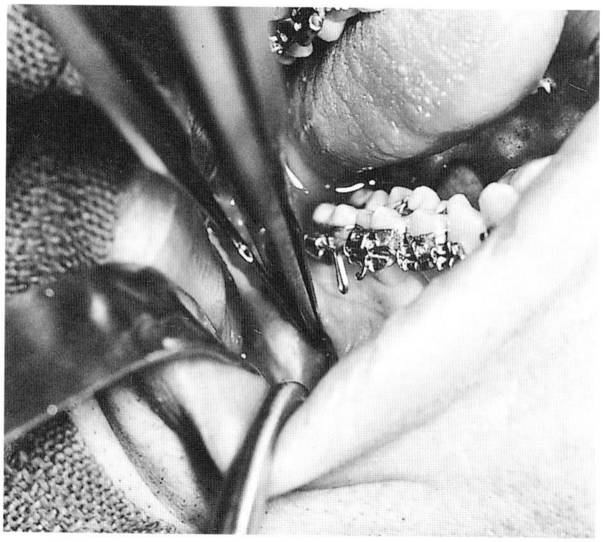

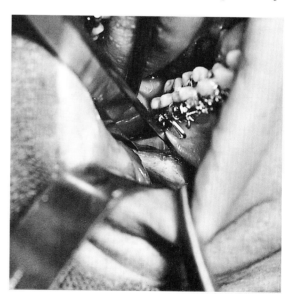

Fig. 75.21 Three osteotomes in place – beginning the separation. Smith inferior border spreader at inferior aspect.

Fig. 75.22 Fiber-handle osteotome being used in conjunction with inferior border spreader.

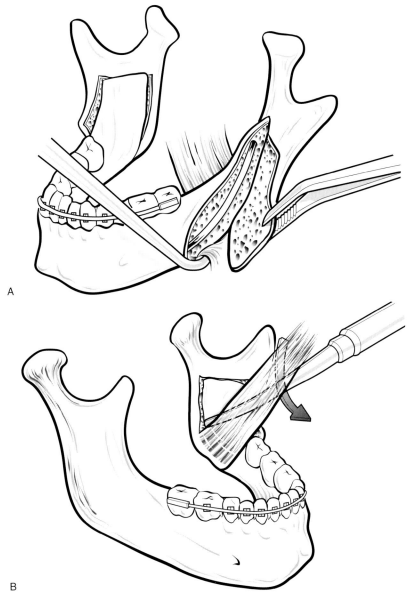

Fig. 75.23 (A,B) J stripper used to remove muscle attachments from medial aspect of distal segment. Used through the osteotomy split.

advancement of the mandible. If the osteotomy is being used for posterior repositioning, the J stripper can be turned around and placed in the osteotomy cut but with the 'J' portion engaging the proximal segment. The proximal segment is most at risk for loss of blood supply, so judicious retraction and stripping is advised. In general, the only area that needs to be stripped is that which might impinge on or prevent the passive posterior repositioning of the proximal segment. This is generally at the angle of the mandible and the posterior aspect of the ramus. The shape of the mandible means that frequently the split will occur high on the medial aspect. This gives a 'short' split inferiorly. The neurovascular bundle often forms the inferior margin of

the split when it is completed in this fashion. This makes inferior placement of bone screws difficult but the advantage is that it leaves more medial muscular attachment to the proximal segment and prevents some of the loss of the gonial angle secondary to ischemia.[33] If changes in the mandibular occlusal plane are anticipated with counter-clockwise rotation of the anterior aspect of the occlusal plane, then this modification or anatomic variation of this split has some theoretical advantages in maintaining good angular morphology.

The area is then irrigated with copious amounts of saline and examined for any bony irregularities that might interfere with the passive repositioning of the distal segment or with the proper adaptation of the proximal segment to the distal segment. These bony irregularities could compress or injure the neurovascular bundle.[34] They are easily removed with a rasp, file or rotary instruments.

The procedure is completed bilaterally and then the patient is passively advanced into the planned occlusion. A splint is applied between the maxillary and mandibular dentition and the patient is placed in intermaxillary fixation with interdental wires. I prefer to use one 25 gauge wire in the second molar/first molar region, another 25 gauge wire in the first molar/second bicuspid region, and for selected cases a third wire in the canine/central incisor region. Once the intermaxillary fixation has been secured, the proximal segment is positioned into the glenoid fossa with appropriate care to the seating of the condyle. The passivity with which the proximal segment aligns with the distal segment is important. The magnitude of advancement at the vertical bone cut is examined and verified with the presurgical estimate. The proximal segment is manipulated or positioned with a Coker clamp placed on the superior aspect of the proximal segment and a gauze packer placed at the inferior aspect. The force on the proximal segment is then directed posteriorly and superiorly with light pressure being placed at the angle of the mandible to vertically and anteriorly seat the condyle. The condyle should be positioned passively with no undue pressure either posteriorly or superiorly. The bone gap between the proximal and distal segment, the bony interface, the amount of advancement and the condyle position are all assessed by the surgeon at this time. If the segment position is appropriate, then a clamp can be placed in the superior aspect to stabilize it or alternatively a toe-out cheek retractor pressed against the lateral aspect of the proximal segment will hold the position while a transosseous hole is drilled for placement of the initial screw.

Transcutaneous or transoral screw placement is acceptable.[35–37] It is also possible to stabilize the osteotomy with transoral or percutaneous placement of monocortical plates to stabilize the proximal–distal segment relationship.[38] Specially designed plates which are L-shaped allow for easy transoral placement and stabilization and also allow for adjustment should the condyles not be properly seated. Adjustment can be performed by removing the anterior screws, repositioning the proximal segment, and replacing the screws. If this technique is used, it must be remembered that the screws are placed monocortically. Bicortical screw placement in the proximal aspect of the bone plate would eliminate the ability to adjust the plate distal segment position. Although this technique is acceptable and gives good stabilization it should not be misconstrued as rigid fixation. When using this technique I generally place

the patient in intermaxillary fixation for one to two weeks.

If transoral screw placement is to be used, it can be done quite readily as soon as the condyle is positioned. If using the transoral screw technique, lag screwing is not beneficial. The first screw should be placed at the point of maximum contact between the proximal and distal segments.[35] In general, the screws placed transorally are at an oblique angle and will be slightly longer than those which are placed transcutaneously.[39] Once the initial screw has been placed and tightened into position, two other screws can be placed in a linear fashion at the superior border, or an L pattern with two screws at the superior border and one at the inferior aspect can be placed.

If the surgeon prefers the transcutaneous approach or if there is a significant amount of splaying of the segments with the advancement, then a transcutaneous approach is ideal.[40] If using the transcutaneous approach it is beneficial to place the screw insertion apparatus through the cheek with the cheek retractor in place for this apparatus prior to the final positioning of the condyle. Once the screw placing apparatus is applied, the condyle is again passively repositioned as described above.

A clamp is advisable for stabilization of the proximal and distal segment relationship. This clamp should not be so tight as to cause a torqueing of the segments and should be placed at the superior border at the point of maximum bony contact.

If placing percutaneous screws, one can use either the three screws in a linear fashion at the upper border or some L-shaped arrangement of screws. Lag screwing is possible in the transcutaneous approach as long as there is not a significant gap between the segments which would be closed by the use of a lag screw. The use of a lag screw in a gap position without a shim to prevent torqueing would cause the condyles to deviate laterally.[32]

Condylar positioning devices have been advocated by some surgeons to ensure proper repositioning of the condylar head in the glenoid fossa. These devices potentially stabilize the condyle in the presurgical relationship either to the maxilla, the zygomatic buttress or some other stable reference point. Although this concept is interesting, the devices are extremely time consuming, cumbersome, and have not consistently demonstrated acceptable results.[41] It has been our practice not to use the condylar repositioning devices; in over two hundred sagittal splits with rigid internal fixation no reoperation or temporomandibular joint surgery because of the relationship of the condyle has been necessary.

Once the proximal–distal segment relationship has been stabilized with the screw fixation bilaterally, the intermaxillary fixation is released. As the fixation is released the patient is held in maximum occlusion by the surgeon. When the fixation wires have been removed the mandible is gently rotated open and closed in a hinging fashion by the surgeon. Prematurities or irregularities or tendency towards a retropositioning of the mandible should all be noted. If the prematurities or discrepancies are felt to be secondary to the splint, modifications in the splint can be performed. The splint can be removed and the occlusion verified, with midline position being critical. If there is a marked class II retropositioning of the mandible, then the intermaxillary fixation should be reapplied, the screws removed and the condylar position repeated. The procedure needs to be repeated until the condyles are seated in such fashion that the occlusion can be reproducibly verified. The surgeon should also move the jaw into right and left lateral excursive positions to verify that there are no changes in temporomandibular joint function.

There is a variable amount of torqueing of the condyles which occurs during surgery. This torqueing, along with general surgical retraction and manipulation, causes edema in and around the temporomandibular joint. This may account for some immediate occlusal discrepancies and marginal reproduction of the occlusion. This intercapsular edema as well as pericapsular edema can also cause the 'condylar sag' or inferior repositioning of the condyle which is commonly seen after ramus surgery. For this reason, place the patient in light to medium class II training elastics immediately following the final verification of condylar position. The splint is generally left in place until the patient returns to active orthodontic care – approximately four weeks. The elastics are maintained for the first two to three weeks following surgery. The splint can now be fixated to the maxillary dentition with a simple 28 gauge wire through the occlusal surface of the splint and around the maxillary orthodontic appliances. Generally, one wire in each quadrant is acceptable.

The incision is closed with a simple over and over resorbable suture after copious irrigation of the medial and lateral dissections. Pressure dressings and drains are not necessary.

An alternative to rigid fixation is the use of wire osteosynthesis. Since the early popularization of rigid fixation by multiple authors[39,40] the alternative forms of fixation have been rarely used. The use of wire osteosynthesis to stabilize the proximal–distal segment relationship in a sagittal osteotomy is a time-honored technique which still is a useful alternative. It does require the placement of maxillomandibular fixation for a period of at least eight weeks.[42] The best results for stabilization of the proximal segment relationship with wire osteosynthesis were achieved utilizing the inferior border wire as described by Booth.[43] This technique should still be considered for patients who have potential large torqueing movements with rigid fixation, patients who reject rigid fixation, and when inadvertent or improper splitting occurs and causes a complication which cannot be managed with some other form of rigid fixation.[44] It has been my experience that this is a rare situation.

THE VERTICAL SUBSIGMOID OSTEOTOMY

This osteotomy is used for correction of mandibular sagittal excess and mandibular sagittal excess with slight amounts of apertognathia (open-bite). It has commonly been referred to in the literature as a transoral vertical ramus osteotomy (TOVRO) or an intraoral vertical ramus osteotomy (IVRO).[45–47]

IVRO: SURGICAL TECHNIQUE

A mucoperiosteal incision is made over the external oblique ridge and extends from the level of the occlusal plane of the maxilla interiorly. The length is approximately 3 cm. The periosteum is incised at the anterior border of the mandible, and subperiosteal dissection is carried out on the lateral surface of the mandible only. This dissection is completed with periosteal elevators and extends from the sigmoid notch to the antegonial notch region.

The notched ramus retractor is used for stripping the temporalis tendon insertion off the coronoid process. This aids in better identification of the sigmoid notch. A Brauer retractor is positioned in the sigmoid notch and a J-shaped stripper is introduced to the posterior border of the mandible. This stripper is run vertically at the subperiosteal level along the posterior aspect of the ramus to the angle. This allows for adequate stripping and ease in placement of the LeVasier–Merrill retractor. This retractor is quite bulky and requires a significant amount of stretching of the periosteum for easy insertion (Fig. 75.6). The oscillating saw is then introduced into the cup of the LeVasier–Merrill retractor and an osteotomy is completed from the sigmoid notch inferiorly with intent to complete the inferior extent of the osteotomy at the inferior aspect of the angle of the mandible. The antilingular prominence on the lateral aspect of the mandible is thought to mirror the position of the lingula.[48] The saw should be kept posterior to that position. The bone cut is made with a 120 degree beveled oscillating saw blade (Fig. 75.24). This beveled blade is utilized so that the angle of the bone cut will minimize medial displacement of the proximal segment caused by

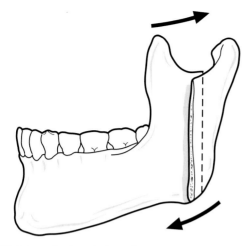

Fig. 75.24 Schematic of surgical cuts for IVRO.

pull of the medial pterygoid musculature. If a 90 degree blade is used the proximal segment may tend to retract medially, making its lateral positioning difficult.

When the osteotomy cut is completed a periosteal elevator can be introduced in the osteotomy site to aid in lateral mobilization of the proximal segment. As this segment is mobilized laterally it can be grasped with a Coker or manipulated and held laterally with the periosteal elevator. Residual muscle attachments on the proximal segment can be removed using the periosteal elevator. Inferior muscle attachments on the distal segment of the mandible can be removed in a similar fashion with a periosteal elevator or with the reintroduction of the J stripper. It is important to release this muscle attachment as it can prevent passive posterior repositioning and lead to some relapse. A gauze pack is placed to assure that the segment is adequately retracted laterally and then attention is directed to the opposite side. After completion of the osteotomy bilaterally, the mandible is placed into the occlusal splint and the patient is placed in intermaxillary fixation. The position of the proximal segments is checked bilaterally. They should passively rest lateral to the distal segment on the ascending ramus. Some inferior bony prominences on the proximal segment may need to be removed. The sharp prominences will resorb passively over time, but in general this can be improved upon by judicious removal of this inferior extension. Areas of bony interference which might cause torqueing of the condyle usually occur at the depth of the sigmoid notch on the distal segment. With the Brauer retractor placed, a triangular-shaped piece of bone from the sigmoid notch on the distal segment interiorly into the osteotomy site can be removed. This will also minimize the rotation and distraction of the condyle laterally and inferiorly in the glenoid fossa. The segment may be wired in place with a transosseous wire

placed through a bur hole in the distal segment and around the proximal segment or with no wire fixation and just passive manipulation of the condyle into the fossa. It is possible with some degree of manipulation even to place a screw to stabilize this segment.[49,50] I prefer not to place screws in this procedure because the predictability and reliability of the condylar position is minimal. The potential for torqueing with the screw or stabilizing the condyle in an inappropriate position is fairly significant. Rather, when the patient is placed in intermaxillary fixation, the condyle is manipulated into the appropriate position and seated into the fossa; the area is then irrigated copiously with saline and the incision closed with a continuous over and over resorbable suture.

The intermaxillary fixation is maintained for two weeks and then the patient is treated similar to a condylar fracture. The intermaxillary fixation is released, 'strong' or 'heavy pull' elastics are placed in the anterior, and the patient is functioned into the splint.

This operation is significantly less difficult and time consuming than the sagittal osteotomy for posterior setback. It also has less potential for neurosensory alterations than the sagittal ramus osteotomy. It still has not maintained high degrees of popularity, mainly because of the potential for relapse and the lack of easy adaptability to rigid internal fixation. It should be maintained as a viable option in orthognathic surgery for management of patients with concomitant temporomandibular joint problems and mandibular sagittal excess. It can also be done unilaterally and combined with a unilateral sagittal split for some asymmetry problems.

COMBINED MAXILLARY AND MANDIBULAR OSTEOTOMIES (STAGING/SEQUENCING)

Skeletal deformities which require surgical correction in both the maxilla and the mandible are treated in one operation. The sequencing is generally determined by the preference of the surgeon. Some thoughts and rationale for sequencing will be given.

It is my preference to complete the surgical bony cuts without splitting the mandible prior to proceeding to the maxillary osteotomy. The maxillary surgical procedure is then completed and stabilized, followed by completion of the mandibular surgery.

The rationale which supports the completion of the bony cuts in the mandible prior to the splitting evolved from the original techniques of maxillary surgery when the maxilla was somewhat unstable and was placed in its position with intraosseous wires. With the common use of rigid internal fixation it is my preference to complete the bony cuts for any genioplasties or chin procedures prior to starting the other aspects of the osteotomy. This prevents the vibration on the rigid fixation of the mandible which is a necessary part of the genioplasty. I still prefer to complete the bony cuts of the ramus sagittal split prior to completing the maxillary procedure. This eliminates the potential for some of the manipulation after the maxilla has been stabilized. Once the mandibular cuts have been completed the areas are packed and the maxillary osteotomy is completed. With the intact stable mandible used to relate the maxillary position, the maxilla is then stabilized and attention is directed to the mandible for its final splitting and repositioning. The genioplasty is stabilized as the final procedure. This is an important consideration when doing model surgery and preparing intermediate and final splints.

As an alternative it is possible to split the mandible first, use an intermediate splint to fixate the mandible to the unoperated maxilla, and then stabilize the maxilla to the operated and repositioned mandible. The only danger in so doing is that the stabilization and fixation of the mandible is generally more challenging than for the maxilla. If an improper or misdirected split of the mandible occurs, rigid fixation may be even more problematic. This could mean having to abort the procedure. However, if the maxilla was done first, the mandible could still be stabilized to the appropriately positioned maxilla. Therefore it has been my preference to complete the maxillary surgery prior to the completion of the mandibular surgery.

TOTAL SUBAPICAL OSTEOTOMY

The total subapical osteotomy is used to treat patients with class II dentoalveolar retrusion and balanced facial skeletal morphology. These patients have the opportunity to be treated by sagittal split advancement osteotomy of the ramus, but this results in a prognathic appearance of the lower face. The combination of a reduction genioplasty with the mandibular advancement treats the bony deformity but can produce an unesthetic soft-tissue result.[51,52] The total subapical osteotomy allows for satisfactory correction of the occlusal disharmony and excellent esthetics.

MacIntosh first described the indications and technique for total subapical osteotomy, listing the indications as infantile apertognathia, relapse from prior ramus osteotomies, and condylar agenesis and hypoplasia.[53] The most frequent indication I have seen includes mandibular dentoalveolar hypoplasia with good chin projection, lateral open-bite

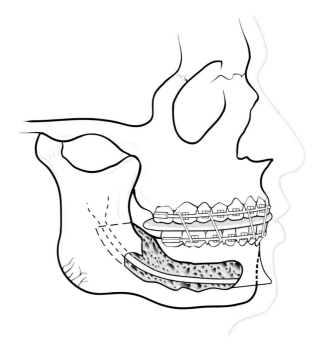

Fig. 75.25 Schematic of correction with lingual split modification of total subapical osteotomy.[57]

deformities, or mandibular vertical alveolar deficiency. True skeletal anterior apertognathia should not be treated in the mandible.[11] There have been a number of modifications of the original description of MacIntosh's technique.[54–57] The technique which will be described here is a further modification which has been used successfully for a number of years (Fig. 75.25).[58]

TECHNIQUE

A curvilinear incision is made in the buccal sulcus from one ascending ramus area to the other. The incision is at least one centimeter and preferably two centimeters from the mucogingival junction, allowing for the largest possible labial tissue pedicle. The incision is carried to bone with blunt dissection to identify the mental foramina and neurovascular bundle (NVB) (Fig. 75.26). Once exposed, the NVB is removed from the mandible. This is done essentially following the technique originally described by Fitzpatrick.[59] First, a circumferential osteotomy of the mental canal is completed with a surgical bur and the circular bony fragment is mobilized and removed. Decortication over the inferior alveolar canal is then performed with horizontal parallel bone cuts following the course of the neurovascular bundle. The cortical bone is removed with an osteotome and the medullary bone with a curette (Fig. 75.27). The mental nerve is retracted slightly so the incisal branch of the inferior alveolar nerve can be severed with a

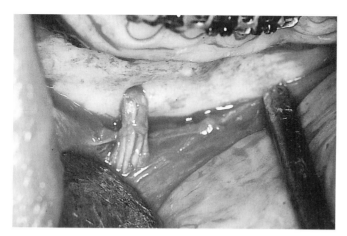

Fig. 75.26 Neurovascular bundle identified prior to decortication.

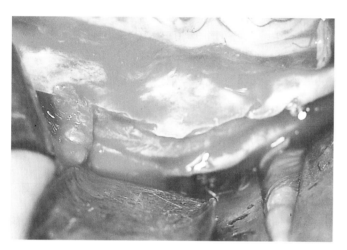

Fig. 75.27 Neurovascular bundle decorticated to ascending ramus, ready for retraction.

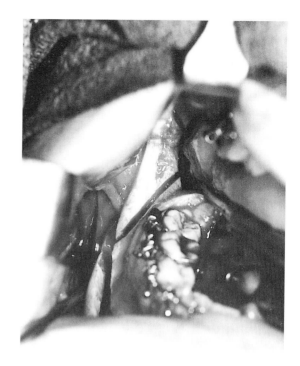

Fig. 75.28 Lingual split (inferior to lingular) bone cut converted to horizontal osteotomy through decorticated canal. Note neurovascular bundle below retractor exiting the ramus laterally.

number 11 surgical blade. The neurovascular bundle can then be removed easily from the canal until it reaches the area of the ramus where the nerve crosses to the medial aspect and courses toward the lingula. Usually at this position the neurovascular bundle is 1.0–1.5 cm proximal to the second molar. At this point the nerve is retracted and protected while the osseous surgery is completed. One surgical modification which frequently makes the neural management easier is the introduction of the surgical operating microscope and the use of a diamond bur to aid in the decortication and removal of the neurovascular bundle from the canal. The neurosensory deficits noted in our series of patients have not exceeded those expected in the combined sagittal split and reduction genioplasty group of patients.

The medial subperiosteal dissection is performed inferior to the lingula. This allows a ribbon retractor or other instrument to be placed subperiosteally and angled toward the bone *superiorly* to protect the neurovascular bundle as

it enters the mandibular foramen (Fig. 75.28). The horizontal to vertical osteotomy is then completed similar to a sagittal split in the ramus but below the lingula. The vertical osteotomy can then be converted to a horizontal osteotomy as the alveolar portion of the mandible joins the ramus. The osteotomy is continued through the mandibular canal to join a similar osteotomy from the contralateral side.

Once the osteotomies are connected, there should be easy mobility of the dentoalveolar segment. Care should be taken to ensure that each bony cut is completed prior to any 'prying' or a fracture of the inferior border of the mandible may occur. The area most prone to this fracture is at the junction of the ramus and body osteotomy.

The dentoalveolus may be segmentalized to allow for three-dimensional changes.[59,60] Care is taken to strip a minimal amount of soft tissue from the interdental bone when segmentalization is completed. The blood supply to this area has already been compromised somewhat.[33] After the segment or segments have been repositioned, stabilization is completed by placing an occlusal acrylic splint to index the bite to the maxilla. The patient is placed in intermaxillary fixation and the vertical references verified. The dentoalveolar osseous segment can then be stabilized to the basal bone of the mandible with individual bone screws, with bone plates, or with circum-mandibular wires (Fig. 75.29). The innate stability of this osteotomy eliminates the need for any long-term intermaxillary fixation.

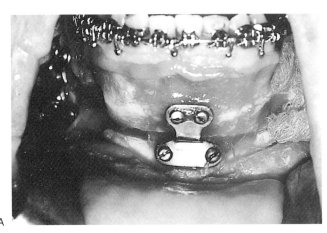

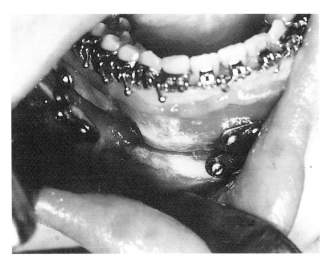

Fig. 75.29 (A) Frontal view of stabilization with inverted chin plate. **(B)** Lateral view; neurovascular bundle repositioned in 'canal'.

Once the segments are stabilized in their new positions, the neurovascular bundle is replaced in the bony canal. The previously removed lateral cortical bone can be particulated and placed as a graft; alternatively a resorbable bone substitute may be used. The incision is closed in a continuous over and over fashion using a resorbable suture. No special suturing techniques are necessary, however a pressure dressing to the chin and labial mental fold area will help prevent hematoma formation.

The class II occlusion with deficiency of the mandible is most effectively treated with orthodontic preparation and ramus surgery. When combined with reduction genioplasty to treat class II dentoalveolar deficiency alone, an acceptable occlusal result follows but an unacceptable appearance of the chin and labial mental fold region will often occur (Fig. 75.30). The total alveolar osteotomy with a retro-molar osteotomy or a sagittal split osteotomy effectively corrects the deformity, however it is difficult to manage the sagittal split and there is a lack of bone contact if the retromolar osteotomy is used. The approach described above involves a lingual split in the sagittal plane below and medial to the neurovascular bundle in the ramus and has the advantage of maximum bone contact with less difficulty completing the split.

Although there are limits to the amount of dento-alveolar advancement that is possible while maintaining bone contact, the limit has not been encountered in my series of cases. The procedure provides predictable excellent stability and is easily adapted to the correction of lateral open-bites, vertical deficiencies, and anterior/posterior dentoalveolar deficiencies. The procedure allows for the muscular position of the mandible to remain unchanged.

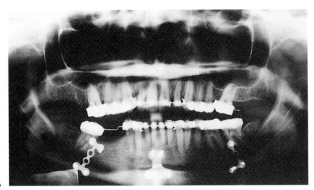

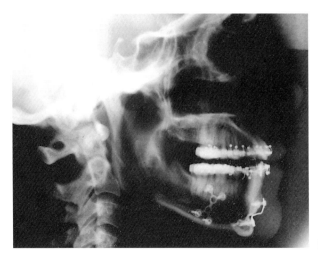

Fig. 75.30 (A) Panoramic radiograph of completed total subapical osteotomy with bone plate stabilization. **(B)** Lateral cephalometric radiograph of different patient showing profile and use of inverted chin plate for stabilization.

REFERENCES

1. Bell WH (ed) 1992 Modern practice in orthognathic and reconstructive surgery. Vols I, II and III. WB Saunders, Philadelphia

2. Bell WH, Proffit W, White RP (eds) 1980 Surgical correction of dentofacial deformities. Vols I and II. WB Saunders, Philadelphia

3. Bell WH (ed) 1986 Surgical correction of dentofacial deformities: new concepts. WB Saunders, Philadelphia

4. Peterson LJ, Indresano AT, Marciani, RD, Roser SM (eds) 1992 Principle of orthognathic surgery. In: Peterson LJ, Indresano AT, Marciani RD, Roser SM (eds) Principles of oral and maxillofacial surgery. Vol III. JB Lippincott, Philadelphia, Part IX, chs 47–56

5. Proffit WR, White RP 1990 Surgical-orthodontic treatment. CV Mosby-Yearbook, St Louis

6. Epker BN, Fish LC 1986 Dentofacial deformities: integrated orthodontic and surgical correction. CV Mosby, St Louis

7. Willmar K 1974 On LeFort I osteotomy. Scandinavian Journal of Plastic and Reconstructive Surgery (suppl 12)

8. Proffit WR, Phillips C, Turvey TA 1987 Stability following superior repositioning of the maxilla by LeFort I osteotomy. American Journal of Orthodontics and Dentofacial Orthopedics 92:151

9. Wolford LM, Hilliard FW 1981 The surgical-orthodontic correction of vertical dentofacial deformities. Journal of Oral Surgery 39:883

10. Wardrop RW, Wolford LM 1989 Maxillary stability following downgraft and/or advancement procedures with stabilization using rigid fixation and porous hydroxyapatite implants. Journal of Oral and Maxillofacial Surgery 47:326

11. Frost DE, Fonseca RJ, Turvey TA, Hall DJ 1980 Cephalometric diagnosis and surgical-orthodontic correction of apertognathia. American Journal of Orthodontics 78:657–669

12. Bell WH, Turvey TA 1974 Surgical correction of posterior cross-bite. Journal of Oral Surgery 32:811

13. Hackney FL, Nishioka GJ, VanSickels JE 1988 Frontal soft-tissue morphology with double V-Y closure following LeFort I osteotomy. Journal of Oral and Maxillofacial Surgery 46:850–855

14. Schendel SA, Williamson LW 1983 Muscle reorientation following superior repositioning of the maxilla. Journal of Oral and Maxillofacial Surgery 41:235

15. Turvey TA, Fonseca JR 1980 The anatomy of the internal maxillary artery in the pterygopalatine fossa: its relationship to maxillary surgery. Journal of Oral Surgery 38:92

16. Newhouse RF, Schow SR, Kraut RA, Price JC 1982 Life-threatening hemorrhage from a LeFort I osteotomy. Journal of Oral and Maxillofacial Surgery 40:117

17. Epker BN, Fish LC 1986 Dentofacial deformities, integrated orthodontic and surgical correction, Vol I. CV Mosby, St Louis

18. Epker BN 1981 Superior surgical repositioning of the maxilla; long-term results. Journal of Maxillofacial Surgery 9:199

19. Maloney F, West RA, McNeill W 1982 Surgical correction of vertical maxillary excess: a reevaluation. Journal of Maxillofacial Surgery 10:84

20. Johnson DG 1985 Intraoperative measurement of maxillary repositioning: an ancillary technique. Oral Surgery, Oral Medicine, and Oral Pathology 61:266

21. Nishioka GJ, Van Sickels JE 1989 Modified external reference measurement technique for vertical repositioning of the maxilla. Oral Surgery, Oral Medicine, and Oral Pathology 64:22

22. Bell WH, Fonseca RJ, Kennedy JW, Levy BM 1977 Bone healing and revascularization after total maxillary osteotomy. Journal of Oral Surgery 33:253

23. Westwood RM, Tilson HB 1975 Complications associated with maxillary osteotomies. Journal of Oral Surgery 33:104

24. Lanigan DT 1988 Injuries to the internal carotid artery following orthognathic surgery. International Journal of Adult Orthodontic and Orthognathic Surgery 4:215

25. Lanigan DT, Tubman DE 1987 Carotid-cavernous sinus fistula following LeFort I osteotomy. Journal of Oral and Maxillofacial Surgery 45:969

26. Champy M 1980 Surgical treatment of mid-face deformities. Head and Neck Surgery 2:451

27. Harle F 1980 LeFort I osteotomy using miniplates for correction of the long face. International Journal of Oral Surgery 9:427

28. Van Sickels JE, Jeter TS, Aragon SB 1985 Rigid fixation of maxillary osteotomies. A preliminary report and technique article. Oral Surgery, Oral Medicine, and Oral Pathology 60:262

29. Tucker MR, White RP 1991 Maxillary orthognathic surgery. In: Tucker MR, Terry BC, White RP, Van Sickels JE (eds) Rigid fixation for maxillofacial surgery. JB Lippincott, Philadelphia

30. Trauner R, Obwegeser H 1957 Surgical correction of mandibular prognathism and retrognathia with considerations of genioplasty. Oral Surgery 10:677–681

31. Obwegeser H 1964 Indications for surgical correction of mandibular deformity by sagittal splitting technique. British Journal of Oral Surgery 1:157–168

32. Tucker MR, Frost DE, Terry BC 1991 Mandibular surgery. In: Tucker MR, Terry BC, White RP, Van Sickels JE (eds) Rigid fixation for maxillofacial surgery. JB Lippincott, Philadelphia

33. Epker BN 1984 Vascular considerations in orthognathic surgery. I. Mandibular osteotomies. Oral Surgery, Oral Medicine, and Oral Pathology 57:472

34. Nishioka GJ, Zysset MK, Van Sickels JE 1987 Neurosensory disturbances with rigid fixation of the bilateral sagittal split osteotomy. Journal of Oral and Maxillofacial Surgery 45:20

35. Foley WL, Frost DE, Paulin WB, Tucker MR 1989 Internal screw fixation: comparison of placement pattern and rigidity. Journal of Oral and Maxillofacial Surgery 47:720

36. Foley WL, Frost DE, Paulin WB, Tucker MR 1989 Uniaxial pull-out evaluation of internal screw fixation. Journal of Oral and Maxillofacial Surgery 47:277

37. Carter TB, Frost DE, Tucker MR 1989 Cortical thickness in human mandibles: clinical relevance to the sagittal split ramus osteotomy. Journal of Oral and MaxilloFacial Surgery 47 (suppl 1):86

38. McDonald WR, Stoelinga PJ, Blijdorp PA, Shoenaers JA 1987 Champy bone plate fixation in sagittal split osteotomies for mandibular advancement. International Journal of Adult Orthodontic and Orthognathic Surgery 2:89

39. Turvey TA, Hall JD 1986 Intraoral self-threading screw fixation for sagittal osteotomies: early experiences. International Journal of Adult Orthodontic and Orthognathic Surgery 4:243

40. Jeter TS, Van Sickels JE, Dolwick MF 1984 Rigid internal fixation of ramus osteotomies. A technique article. Journal of Oral and Maxillofacial Surgery 42:270

41. Ellis E III 1994 Condylar positioning devices for orthognathic surgery: are they necessary? Journal of Oral and Maxillofacial Surgery 52:536–552

42. Schendel SA, Epker BN 1980 Results after mandibular advancement surgery: an analysis of eighty-seven cases. Journal of Oral Surgery 38:265

43. Booth DF 1981 Control of the proximal segment by lower border wiring in the sagittal split osteotomy. Journal of Maxillofacial Surgery 9:186

44. Singer RS, Bays RA 1985 A comparison between superior and inferior border wiring techniques in sagittal split ramus osteotomy. Journal of Oral and Maxillofacial Surgery 43:444

45. Moose SM 1964 Surgical correction of mandibular prognathism by intraoral subcondylar osteotomy. Journal of Oral Surgery 22:197

46. Herbert JM, Kent JM, Hines ED 1970 Correction of prognathism by an intraoral vertical subcondylar osteotomy. Journal of Oral Surgery 28:651

47. Hall HD, McKenna SJ 1987 Further refinement and evaluation of intraoral vertical ramus osteotomy. Journal of Oral and Maxillofacial Surgery 45:684

48. Hayward J, Richardson ER, Malhotra SK 1977 The mandibular foramen: its anteroposterior position. Journal of Oral Surgery 44:837

49. Kraut RA 1988 Stabilization of the intraoral vertical osteotomy using small bone blades. Journal of Oral and Maxillofacial Surgery 46:980

50. Steinhauser EW 1982 Bone screws and plates in orthagnathic surgery. International Journal of Oral Surgery 11:209

51. Hohl TH, Epker BN 1976 Macrogenia: a study of treatment results with surgical recommendations. Oral Surgery, Oral Medicine, and Oral Pathology 41:545–576

52. Epker BN, Fish LC 1983 The surgical-orthodontic correction of mandibular deficiency. Part I. American Journal of Orthodontics 84:408–421

53. MacIntosh RB 1974 Total mandibular alveolar osteotomy. Journal of Maxillofacial Surgery 2:210–218

54. Pangrazio-Kulbersh V, MacIntosh RB 1985 Total mandibular alveolar osteotomy: an alternative choice to other surgical procedures. American Journal of Orthodontics 87:319–337

55. Murray RB 1980 Mandibular sagittal subapical osteotomy: a case study. American Journal of Orthodontics 77:469–485

56. Booth DF, Dietz VS, Gainelly AA 1976 Correction of class II malocclusion by combined sagittal ramus and subapical osteotomy. Journal of Oral Surgery 34:630–634

57. Dietz VS, Gainelly AA, Booth DF 1977 Surgical orthodontics in the treatment of class II, division II malocclusions: a case report. American Journal of Orthodontics 71:309–316

58. Frost DE, Fonseca RJ, Koutnik AW 1986 Total subapical subosteotomy – a modification of the surgical technique. International Journal of Adult Orthodontic and Orthognathic Surgery 2:119–128

59. Fitzpatrick B 1977 Total osteotomy of the mandibular alveolus and reconstruction of the occlusion. Oral Surgery, Oral Medicine, and Oral Pathology 44:336–346

60. Peterson LJ 1978 Posterior mandibular segmental alveolar osteotomy. Journal of Oral Surgery 36:454–458

Stability in orthognathic surgery

76

JOSEPH E. VAN SICKELS

INTRODUCTION

When orthognathic surgery is contemplated, one wishes to be able to accurately predict the ultimate outcome for the patient. Although the words predictable and stable are sometimes used interchangeably in the literature, they are two different concepts. 'Predictable' encompasses several facets of treatment: the ability to position the bony skeleton in space, the ability to maintain that position, and the soft tissues' response to the underlying skeletal movement. Predictability can be influenced by surgical and orthodontic planning, intraoperative execution of surgery and postoperative management. The accuracy of a centric relation and face bow transfer can greatly influence the results seen with one- and two-jaw maxillary surgery.[1] Ellis and colleagues,[1] in cases that they studied, noted differences between the maxillary occlusal plane angle on the cephalogram and the articulator. These discrepancies resulted in significant differences in the horizontal position of the maxilla and mandible. Horizontal discrepancies in maxillary position may be secondary to interferences encountered or to failure to seat the condyles appropriately at the time of surgery.[2] Vertical discrepancies in the positioning of the maxillary central incisor may be secondary to parallax errors as a result of using internal reference lines.[3] Van Sickels et al[3] noted that in a group in which an external reference point was employed, the position of the maxillary central incisor was more accurately predicted on both the x and y coordinates than in a group in which internal reference lines were placed.

Stability is one part of predictability. Stability is the ability to maintain skeletal structures in a given position over time. It involves the adaptation of the skeleton and its surrounding soft-tissue envelope to a new equilibrium.[4] The focus of this chapter is stability of commonly performed operations used to correct dentofacial deformities. Specific techniques that can be used to improve stability will be highlighted. The recent literature suggest that fixation appliances, specifically rigid fixation, add to the stability of the osteotomy.[5,6] This chapter is devoted to the concept of stability with commonly used surgical techniques.

Stability or instability varies with the portion or portions of the maxilla or mandible being moved. One cause of instability is excessive micromotion at the osteotomy site,[7] which can result in migration or relapse. At its worse, micromotion can result in a nonunion. Migration is the movement of the bony segments in the direction of the initial move, whereas relapse is movement toward the initial position of the bony segments. Both migration and relapse are seen when analyzing the postoperative stability of maxillary and mandibular osteotomies. Nonunion occurs rarely with osteotomies of either jaw; however, it is most frequently seen with inferior movement of the maxilla.[8]

SEGMENTAL SURGERY

Segmental procedures, whether they are in the maxilla or the mandible, have for years been recognized as being more stable than ramus or total maxillary osteotomies.[9] In 1971, Bell[9] wrote about the correction of anterior open-bites, highlighting the stability achieved with segmental osteotomies. More recently, Rosenquist[10] followed a series of patients who underwent anterior segmental maxillary osteotomies with either the downfracture or the Wunderer method of treatment. Stability was achieved by heavy archwires in all but two of 14 cases. Long-term stability was found to be acceptable except when the osteotomy was used to correct deep overbites. The stability seen following movement of the anterior portions of both jaws is secondary to minimal movement of segments and muscular attachments. Rigid fixation has had little impact on the stability of segmental osteotomies, other than decreasing or eliminating the need for maxillomandibular fixation.

MAXILLARY OSTEOTOMIES

The most commonly performed maxillary osteotomy is the Le Fort I, which allows a great amount of flexibility in correcting discrepancies of the maxilla. Conceptually, it is best to look at the vector of movement when studying the stability of a Le Fort I osteotomy. However, it is recognized that there is frequently more than one vector involved in positioning a maxilla in space. In addition, segmental movement of the maxilla can influence the stability of a move.[11]

ADVANCEMENT

Hoffman & Moloney[12] looked at horizontal stability in 15 patients with an average maxillary advancement of 8.76 mm. Six weeks later, the maxilla had a mean relapse of 0.22 mm and at 1 year 0.61 mm (6.96%). Hoffman & Moloney[12] concluded that, with the use of miniplates and screw fixation, the results were surgically 'predictable' and stable. Several studies have noted that patients who underwent maxillary advancement with rigid fixation have no significant relapse.[13,14] Egbert et al[15] evaluated stability in two groups of patients undergoing maxillary advancement. Those treated by rigid fixation were more stable than those treated by wire osteosynthesis. However, both groups relapsed in a posterior direction.

Rigid fixation has increased the stability seen with maxillary advancements over that seen with wire osteosynthesis, but it has not eliminated relapse. Larger advancements (greater than 5–6 mm) should be considered unstable. Techniques to improve stability in these cases included a period of fixation, or slightly overadvancing the maxilla to compensate for anticipated relapse.

INFERIOR

The least stable move one can make with a maxillary osteotomy is inferior repositioning of the maxilla.[8,16,17] Baker et al[16] followed 19 patients from 12 to 58 months after inferior repositioning of the maxilla. Five patients had relapse of more than 30%. A tendency towards greater relapse was seen in patients with more than 5 mm inferior repositioning, and in patients who had concurrent segmental procedures.

Inferior repositioning of the maxilla is frequently combined with anterior positioning. Chow and colleagues[11] noted a relapse of 27.8% in a vertical position of the upper central incisor following inferior positioning of the maxilla with concomitant forward positioning. Proffit et al[18] evaluated different groups of patients who had maxillary advancements with both wires and rigid fixation. In those where the maxilla was moved down as well as forward, there was a strong tendency for relapse upwards. In addition, they saw no difference in stability between wire osteosynthesis and rigid fixation. This is contrast with the animal study of Ellis, Carlson, & Frydenlund,[19] who compared several types of fixation for inferior movement of the maxilla and found that relapse occurred with all types, but that rigid fixation was the most stable.

It is important to note that in the paper by Ellis et al[19] all groups had relapse. Clinical studies confirm that large inferior movements, especially when segments are involved, are very unstable. When large movements are anticipated, one should consider using a combination of techniques (see the case below).

Vertical and horizontal maxillary-deficient patient

A 36-year-old white female with a history of bruxism presented for evaluation of a maxillary advancement and advancement (Fig. 76.1). Her maxilla was advanced 4 mm and brought down 4 mm. There was no overcorrection built in, nor were any auxiliary techniques used to assist the fixation appliances applied at the time of surgery (Fig. 76.2).

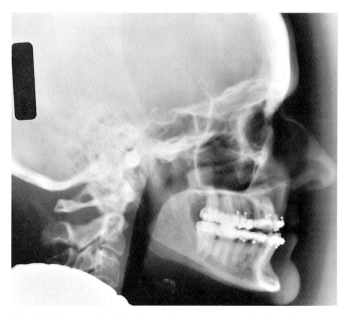

Fig. 76.1 Preoperative lateral cephalogram: horizontal and vertical maxillary deficiency is evident.

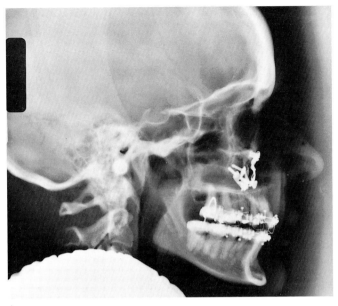

Fig. 76.2 Initially after surgery the maxilla is advanced and brought down 5 mm.

She was stabilized with four 2 mm plates and screws and a simultaneous bone graft. Within 6 weeks the vertical impaction was greater than the amount that had been brought down, and the maxilla had relapsed to a mild end-to-end position (Fig. 76.3). A slight mobility to the maxilla was noted in the evening. The patient was eventually debanded, but it was noted that the maxilla was still mobile. A second operation was carried out using four 2 mm plates and screws, a simulataneous autogenous bone graft, and auxiliary pins secured to the maxilla with an additional screw (Fig. 76.4). The plates have since been removed, but the patient has

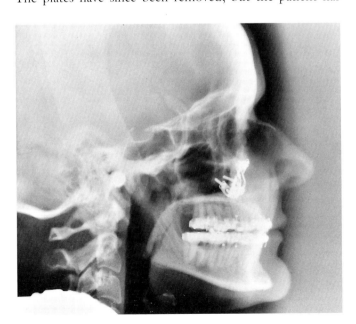

Fig. 76.3 Six weeks after surgery, almost all of the inferior movement has relapsed.

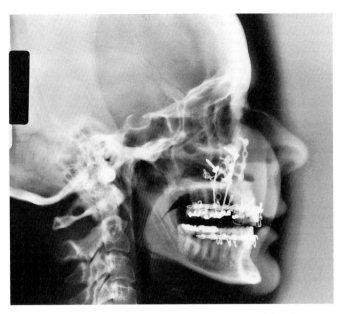

Fig. 76.4 Second operation with auxiliary pins used to stabilize the case.

had chronic sinusitis symptoms on the right side of the maxilla.

This case illustrates how difficult it is to stabilize a maxilla that has been repositioned inferiorly. Patients who have signs of bruxism are particularly troublesome. An alternative therapy that could have been used with the first operation was myotomy of the temporalis and masseter muscles.

IMPACTION

Maxillary impaction, whether fixed by wire osteosynthesis or rigid fixation, is very stable.[20–23] Bishara & Chu[22] compared maxillary impactions to advancements and noted that there was a significant difference in stability between the two groups, with the advancement showing a tendency to move superiorly (migration).

The only advantage that rigid fixation has for isolated maxillary impaction is early mobilization. Smaller plating systems appear to work well for these types of moves. Mogavero et al[24] presented a controversial paper discussing maxillary impaction and advancement in adolescents. They reviewed the results of 48 patients, 23 of whom were stabilized with rigid fixation and 25 with wire fixation. The authors concluded that a Le Fort I osteotomy had little effect on vertical maxillary growth, and that rigid fixation provided superior long-term anteroposterior stabilization compared to wire fixation.

SETBACK

Stability of the maxilla following a maxillary setback has not been reported for a large series of patients. Plates are helpful in preventing impaction of the maxilla when there are bony gaps present.

TRANSVERSE

Stability of the maxilla after correction of a transverse deficiency has shown considerable variability.[25] Transverse discrepancies may exist in isolation or in combination with vertical maxillary excess. Phillips et al[25] evaluated 39 patients who had maxillary expansion, and noted a 49% relapse in the second molar region and 30% at the first premolars. Vertical maxillary excess with an open-bite usually has both a vertical and a horizontal skeletal component. Haymond et al[26] evaluated 38 patients with skeletal open-bite treated with small plate internal fixation: 86% of the sample had a stable result. In those that did not, 50% of the vertical relapse was due to transverse collapse of the expanded maxillary arches.

Suggestions to improve the result with maxillary expansion include overexpansion, maintenance of the occlusal splint for at least 6 weeks, and the use of a lingual or auxiliary labial archwire to maintain molar width.[25] Alternatively, when a transverse deficiency of greater than 6 mm exists in the posterior occlusion, a surgically assisted rapid palatal expansion (SA-RPE) has been shown to be more stable than a multiple segmented maxilla.[27] An SA-RPE is scheduled as the first operation when there is other skeletal dysplasia in the maxilla and mandible. Sequencing the surgery in this fashion allows routine orthodontic procedures to be accomplished while the patient is healing following the SA-RPE.

MAXILLARY AND MANDIBULAR SURGERY

Forssell et al[28] demonstrated that patients who had rigid fixation of the mandible combined with superior repositioning of the maxilla had superior stability to those who underwent the same surgery but with intraosseous wire fixation, skeletal suspension wires and 8 weeks of maxillomandibular fixation.

The influence of the mandibular move on maxillary stability has long been known.[17,29,30] Large advancements of the mandible have a tendency to move in a posterior direction, whereas mandibular setbacks with rigid fixation have a tendency to move forwards. These factors should be considered when evaluating a case for two-jaw surgery (see following sections on mandibular surgery).

CLEFT LIP AND PALATE

The most common skeletal defect seen in patients with cleft lip and palate is maxillary retrusion.[31,32] Ayliffe et al[31] compared rigid fixation to standard fixation techniques, and noted that bone plates were associated with a more stable result. Hochban and colleagues compared patients with idiopathic maxillary deficiency to those with cleft lip and palate, and found that relapse depended on the amount of advancement in both groups; however, the non-cleft group was more stable than the cleft group.[32]

Most surgeons who have carried out orthognathic surgery on patients with cleft lip and palate recognized how difficult it is to achieve the desired skeletal results. Inadequate skeletal positioning can result from an inability to place the maxilla in its desired position at the time of surgery, or may be secondary to relapse seen in the weeks immediately after surgery. The increased instability associated with maxillary advancement in a cleft palate patient suggests that scarring induced by previous surgery limits the amount that one can predictably advance the maxilla in such patients. Choices to improve the stability of a case include the use of maxillomandibular fixation, and 'splitting the difference' when there is a large skeletal discrepancy.

Recent work with distraction osteogenesis to advance the maxilla is encouraging.[33] Guerrero et al[33] presented the results of 10 cases treated by osteogenic distraction using a Hyrax appliance and class III heavy elastics after a corticotomy to promote three-dimensional bone growth. They obtained an increase of transverse expansion of 9.2 mm, with an average advancement of 4.5 mm. Lerner & Lane[34] described a technique of achieving stability for large maxillary advancements in cleft lip and palate patients: they presented a case in which 23 mm of advancement was achieved in such a patient, in whom a Le Fort I osteotomy was performed. The maximum amount of advancement that could be achieved was created and a traction splint inserted. The soft tissue was closed with no attempt made to fix the maxilla. Using an external frame, the maxilla was progressively advanced over the next 4 weeks. The patient was then returned to surgery and corticocancellous iliac bone grafts were used to stabilize the maxilla. Face mask therapy has been shown to be successful in treating children with maxillary deficiency; this same appliance has been used with maxillary corticotomies in older children with cleft lip and palate.[35] The disadvantage of this therapy is its reliance on patient compliance to achieve the desired results. An additional disadvantage is the need for a second operation to remove appliances used to distract the segments of bone.

Further work with this newer form of therapy will help define its use with maxillary deficiency patients, as well as other skeletal deformities.

MANDIBULAR OSTEOTOMY

The most common ramal procedures are the bilateral sagittal split osteotomy (BSSO) and the intraoral vertical ramus osteotomy (IVRO). Stability varies with the fixation appliances used and the technique employed to move the mandible. The stability of the surgical move varies with advancement or retrusion of the mandible.

ADVANCEMENT

Advancement of the mandible by a BSSO is the most commonly used surgical technique for horizontal mandibular deficiency.[36,37] Relapse has been noted for both wire osteosynthesis and rigid fixation.[36–40] Watzke et al[41] evaluated patients who had been treated by a BSSO fixed with either method, and concluded that the stability was comparable between the two groups at 1 year. These findings have been refuted by two recent articles.[5,6] In a retrospective study, Mommaerts[5] found an 11% incidence of sagittal relapse in a group of patients treated by rigid fixation, whereas a group fixed by wire osteosynthesis experienced a 45% relapse after 1 year. The majority of his patients with wire osteosynthesis were fixed with superior border wires. The rigid fixation group had three 3.5 mm stainless steel lag screws on each side. Van Sickels et al[6] reported on a multi-center randomized prospective study comparing rigid fixation (three 2 mm screws per side) and wire osteosynthesis (inferior border wires) for a BSSO advancement. The rigid group was significantly more stable than the wire group at 1 and 2 years after surgery.

Clinical studies have shown excellent stability with miniplates.[38] Blomqvist & Isaksson[42] saw no difference in the stability between two groups of patients who underwent mandibular advancement fixed with either bicortical or monocortical screws and plates. Although rigid fixation has been shown to be more stable than wire osteosynthesis, relapse occurs, especially with larger skeletal moves.[5,6,43] Van Sickels[44] studied two groups of patients undergoing large advancements, both of whom had three 2 mm bicortical screws placed at the osteotomy site. One group had skeletal wires and were kept in fixation for 1 week. The group with bicortical screws and skeletal wires was significantly more stable.

Laboratory studies comparing different appliance designs and configurations of screws and plates have suggested that some types of fixation may be more stable than others.[45] Shetty et al[45] determined that osteotomies stabilized with a combination of miniplates and position screws were more stable than those stabilized exclusively with miniplates or internal screw fixation. Furthermore, miniplate systems alone were the least stable system they tested. Foley and colleagues[46,47] showed that three screws placed in an inverted L pattern were significantly more rigid than those fixed with screws placed in a linear pattern, or one mono-cortical plate. They showed no significant difference in rigidity between compression and bicortical screws placed in identical patterns.

From the preceding sections one can glean the following information. For the average advancement of the mandible (less than 7 mm) rigid fixation will provide adequate stability whether one chooses to use plates or bicortical screws. Compression screws do little to help stability and may increase occlusal discrepancies seen after surgery. For larger advancements one must choose additional technique(s) to ensure stability. Suspension wires in addition to rigid fixation, coupled with 1 week of fixation, have been shown to be efficacious. Alternatively, one may choose to use more rigid forms of fixation, including a combination of plates and screws, and especially screws placed in an inverted L shape. Unfortunately, there are no long-term randomized studies to determine whether these alternative techniques, which show promise in vitro, will be equally effective clinically.

Stability is often viewed as a short-term problem. Once the muscles and connective tissue adapt to a new skeletal position, the results should be stable. However, a small portion of patients who undergo mandibular advancement experience an initial stable result followed by late relapse, the cause of which has been attributed to condylar resorption.[38,48–52] Its incidence has been reported to be between 2.3% and 7.7% of patients treated by a BSSO to advance the mandible.[38,48,53] Most frequently it is diagnosed with the use of radiographs 6–17 months after surgery.[53]

There are several theories as to why this occurs. Kerstens et al[48] postulated that the surgery stimulated a process in the bone by increasing the load on the joint. Others have suggested that an alteration in condylar position may induce remodeling changes in the condyle.[54,55] Condylar resorption has been noted more frequently in females with high mandibular planes, preoperative temporomandibular dysfunction, large mandibular advancement and distal segment counterclockwise rotation.[38,48,50,53,56] Scheerlinck et al[38] noted that progressive condylar resorption was four times greater for advancements of more than 10 mm than for those between 5 and 10 mm.

Late instability due to condylar resorption occurs rarely in clinical practice, but can be problematic. Additional relapse has occurred following second operations.[53,57,58] In considering reoperation in the case of condylar resorption, one should ensure that the resorption has stopped. Splints have been suggested as an interim management.[59] If possible, one should operate in the maxilla to correct occlusal discrepancies.

SETBACKS

Stability with mandibular setbacks must be studied by evaluating two different operations, the IVRO and the BSSO. Traditional management of horizontal mandibular excess was through the use of an extraoral ramus osteotomy. It is still used for some complicated cases; however, the IVRO has gained popularity and is now more commonly used.[60] Movement of the mandible after a vertical ramus osteotomy occurs with a posterior rotation of the mandible (migration), resulting in a further retrodisplacement of the gnathion, an increase in anterior facial height and shortening of the posterior facial height.[61–63] Tornes[64] found no increase in postoperative stability with an increase in the length of the osteotomy cut, nor with increased bony overlap of the segments. Several authors have shown that anterior skeletal wires will prevent downward rotation of the chin.[65–67] Although anterior facial height was maintained, posterior facial height was not.

The IVRO has gained in popularity because it is a quick operation and has a lower incidence of neurosensory injury than the BSSO. Postoperative instability with this operation is in a more posterior direction (migration). There is both a loss of posterior facial height and a gain in anterior facial height. Anterior skeletal wires will prevent the gain in anterior facial height. Rigid fixation has been used with an IVRO in an attempt to improve the stability seen with this surgical procedure.

In 1982, Paulus & Steinhauser[68] reported on their experience with using lag screws versus wire osteosynthesis for vertical ramus osteotomy. The rigid fixation group had two bone screws per side, and they noted that this had a higher incidence of relapse than wire osteosynthesis. Van Sickels et al,[69] in 1990, reported on a technique to facilitate rigid fixation for a vertical ramal type of operation (Fig. 76.5 A,B). Although superior stability has been noted with this technique over wire osteosynthesis, there is a tendency for the anterior facial height to increase. However, posterior facial height has been maintained with this operation. It is probable that anterior skeletal wire and a period of maxil-

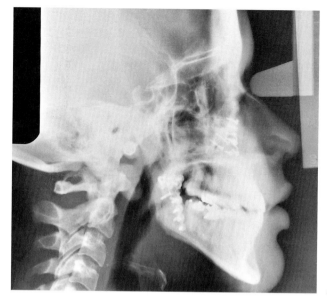

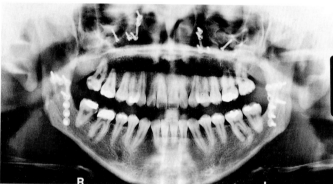

Fig. 76.5 (A) Postoperative lateral cephalogram of a patient with rigid fixation of an inverted 'L' osteotomy. **(B)** Postoperative panorex of the same patient.

lomandibular fixation will prevent an increase in anterior facial height.

The BSSO has also been used for mandibular setbacks.[68] Paulus & Steinhauser[68] noted a decreased incidence of relapse following rigid fixation of a BSSO setback compared to wire osteosynthesis. They found a 7% sagittal relapse and a 5% vertical relapse with rigid fixation, compared to 17.5% sagittal and 15% vertical when wire osteosynthesis was used. Kobayashi et al[70] noted that there was a greater tendency to relapse in cases in which there was a large posterior movement. Franco et al[71] studied 25 cases of mandibular setback fixed with rigid fixation. They noted that two factors accounted for relapse in this group of patients: large posterior movement, and posterior rotation of the proximal segment.

A review of the above shows that there is a fundamental difference in stability between a setback achieved with IVRO and one by BSSO when rigid fixation is used. An IVRO has a tendency for migration in a further posterior direction, whereas a BSSO has a tendency to relapse for-

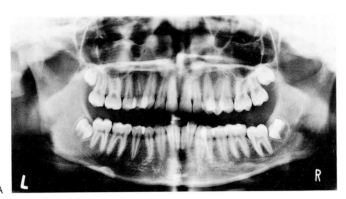

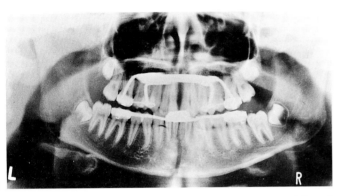

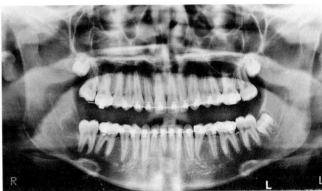

Fig. 76.6 **(A)** Preoperative panorex: note the anterior crowding. **(B)** Appliance in place, expansion begun. **(C)** Postoperative panorex: note the alignment of the anterior teeth.

ward. Techniques to manage forward rotation of the mandible include extensive stripping of the medial aspect and preservation of the proximal segment position.

TRANSVERSE

Recent papers have presented interesting results with widening of the mandible, with tooth-borne appliance utilizing the principles of distraction osteogenesis as an alternative to extraction therapy[72–76] (Fig. 78.6 A,B,C). Preliminary data show that this procedure is very stable.[72–74] In animal studies, Bell et al[75] noted injury to the roots of adjacent teeth and, in a related article, reactive changes in the temporomandibular joints.[76] Clinical studies have not noted these types of problems. The rate and rhythm of distraction differ in the clinical and animal studies. Long-term results with larger samples will resolve some of these questions generated by these early papers.

CONCLUSION

The stability of orthognathic surgery is one part of predictability. Stability varies with the jaw being moved and with the dimension and direction of the move. The hardware

and techniques to fix and stabilize segments should be tailored to the individual case. Distraction osteogenesis may present a favourable alternative for difficult maxillary advancements. Its use with other deficiency states has yet to be fully developed and defined.

REFERENCES

1. Ellis E, Tharanon W, Gambrell K 1992 Accuracy of face-bow transfer: effect on surgical prediction and postsurgical result. Journal of Oral and Maxillofacial Surgery 50:562–567
2. Bays RA 1986 Maxillary osteotomies utilizing the rigid adjustable pin (RAP) system: a review of 31 clinical cases. International Journal of Adult Orthodontics and Orthognathic Surgery 1:275–297
3. Van Sickels JE, Larsen AJ, Triplett RG 1986 Predictability of maxillary surgery: a comparison of internal and external reference marks. Oral Surgery, Oral Medicine, Oral Pathology 61:542–545
4. Ellis E, Carlson DS 1990 Neuromuscular adaptation after orthognathic surgery. Oral and Maxillofacial Surgery Clinics of North America 2:811–830
5. Mommaerts M 1991 Lag screw versus wire osteosynthesis in mandibular advancement. International Journal of Adult Orthodontics and Orthognathic Surgery 6:153–160
6. Van Sickels JE, Keeling S, Tiner BD, Bays R, Rugh J, Clark G 1996 Stability of rigid versus wire osteosynthesis for a BSSO advancement. Journal of Oral and Maxillofacial Surgery 54:106
7. Rosenquist B, Wall G 1995 Mobility of the osteotomy site following Le Fort I osteotomy stabilized by titanium plate osteosynthesis. Journal of Oral and Maxillofacial Surgery 53:1276–1282
8. Van Sickels JE, Tucker MR 1990 Management of delayed union and

nonunion of maxillary osteotomies. Journal of Oral and Maxillofacial Surgery 48:1039–1044

9. Bell WH 1971 Correction of skeletal type of anterior open bite. Journal of Oral Surgery 29:706–714

10. Rosenquist B 1993 Anterior segmental maxillary osteotomy. A 24 month follow up. International Journal of Oral and Maxillofacial Surgery 22:210–213

11. Chow J, Hagg U, Tideman H 1995 The stability of segmentalized Le Fort I osteotomies with miniplate fixation in patients with maxillary hypoplasia. Journal of Oral and Maxillofacial Surgery 53:1407–1412

12. Hoffman GR, Moloney FB 1996 The stability of facial osteotomies. Part 5. Maxillary advancement with miniplate and screw fixation. Australian Dental Journal 41:21–27

13. Luyk NH, Ward-Booth RP 1985 The stability of Le Fort I advancement osteotomy using bone plates without bone grafts. Journal of Maxillofacial Surgery 13:250–253

14. Louis PJ, Waite PD, Austin RB 1993 Long term skeletal stability after rigid fixation of Le Fort I osteotomy with advancement. International Journal of Oral and Maxillofacial Surgery 22:8–86

15. Egbert M, Hepworth B, Mydall R, West R 1995 Stability of Le Fort I osteotomy with maxillary advancement: a comparison of combined wire fixation and rigid fixation. Journal of Oral and Maxillofacial Surgery 53:243–347

16. Baker DL, Stoelinga PJ, Blijdorp PA, Brouns JJ 1992 Long term stability after inferior maxillary repositioning by miniplate fixation. International Journal of Oral and Maxillofacial Surgery 21:320–326

17. de Mol van Otterloo JJ, Tuinzing DB, Kostense P 1996 Inferior positioning of the maxilla by a Le Fort I osteotomy: a review of 25 patients with vertical maxillary deficiency. Journal of Cranio-Maxillo-Facial Surgery 24:69–77

18. Proffit WR, Phillips C, Prewitt JW, Turvey TA 1991 Stability after surgical orthodontic correction of skeletal class III malocclusion. II. Maxillary advancement. International Journal of Adult Orthodontics and Orthognathic Surgery 6:71–80

19. Ellis E, Carlson DS, Frydenlund S 1989 Stability of midface augmentation: An experimental study of musculoskeletal interaction and fixation methods. Journal of Oral and Maxillofacial Surgery 47:1062–1068

20. Proffit WR, Phillips C, Turvey TA 1987 Stability following superior repositioning of the maxilla by Le Fort I osteotomy. American Journal of Orthodontics and Dentofacial Orthopedics 92:151–161

21. Bailey LJ, Phillips C, Proffit WR, Turvey TA 1994 Stability following superior repositioning of the maxilla by Le Fort I osteotomy: five year follow up. International Journal of Adult Orthodontics and Orthognathic Surgery 9:163–173

22. Bishara SE, Chu GW 1992 Comparisons of postsurgical stability of the Le Fort I maxillary impaction and maxillary advancement. American Journal of Orthodontics and Dentofacial Orthopedics 102:335–341

23. Van Sickels JE, Richardson DA 1996 Stability of orthognathic surgery: a review of rigid fixation. British Journal of Oral and Maxillofacial Surgery 34:279–285

24. Mogavero FJ, Buschang PH, Wolford LM 1997 Orthognathic surgery effects on maxillary growth in patients with vertical maxillary excess. American Journal of Orthodontics and Dentofacial Orthopedics 111:288–296

25. Phillips C, Medland WH, Fields HW, Proffit WR, White RP 1992 Stability of surgical maxillary expansion. International Journal of Adult Orthodontics and Orthognathic Surgery 7:139–146

26. Haymond CS, Stoelinga PJW, Blijdorp PA, Leenen RJ, Merkens NM 1991 Surgical orthodontic treatment of anterior skeletal open bite using small plate internal fixation. One to five year follow-up. International Journal of Oral and Maxillofacial Surgery 20:223–227

27. Betts NJ, Vanarsdall RL, Barber HD, Higgins-Barber J, Fonseca R 1995 Diagnosis and treatment of transverse maxillary deficiency.

International Journal of Adult Orthodontics and Orthognathic Surgery 10:75–96

28. Forssell K, Turvey TA, Phillips C, Proffit WR 1992 Superior repositioning of the maxilla combined with mandibular advancement: mandibular RIF improves stability. American Journal of Orthodontics and Dentofacial Orthopedics 102:342–350

29. Turvey TA, Phillips C, Zaytoun HS, Proffit WR 1988 Simultaneous superior repositioning of the maxilla and mandibular advancement. A report on stability. American Journal of Orthodontics and Dentofacial Orthopedics 94:372–383

30. LaBanc JP, Turvey TA, Epker BN 1982 Results following simultaneous mobilization of the maxilla and mandible for the correction of dentofacial deformities: analysis of 100 consecutive patients. Oral Surgery, Oral Medicine, Oral Pathology 54:607–612

31. Ayliffe PR, Banks P, Martin IC 1995 Stability of the Le Fort I osteotomy with cleft lip and palate. International Journal of Oral and Maxillofacial Surgery 24:201–207

32. Hochban W, Ganss C, Austermann KH 1993 Long term results after maxillary advancement in patients with clefts. Cleft Palate–Craniofacial Journal 30:237–243

33. Guerrero C, Bell WH, Contasti G, Rodriguez AM, Gulino D, Vasquez Z 1995 Distraccion osteogenica maxilar intraoral. Odontologica Dia 11:203–218

34. Lerner LL, Lane JA 1992 Orthopedic assisted maxillary advancement in the cleft lip and palate patient, using external headframe traction. In: Bell WH (ed) Modern practice in orthognathic and reconstructive surgery, Vol 3. WB Saunders, Philadelphia, pp 2315–2322

35. Hathaway RR 1992 Orthopedic correction of maxillary deficiency. In: Bell WH (ed) Modern practice in orthognathic and reconstructive surgery, Vol 3, WB Saunders, Philadelphia, pp 2322–2331

36. Schendel SA, Epker BN 1980 Results after mandibular advancement surgery: an analysis of 87 cases. Journal of Oral Surgery 38:265–282

37. Smith GC, Moloney FB, West RA 1985 Mandibular advancement surgery. A study of the lower border wiring technique for osteosynthesis. Oral Surgery, Oral Medicine, Oral Pathology 60:467–475

38. Scheerlinck JPO, Stoelinga PJW, Biljdorp PA, Brouns JJA, Nijs MLL 1994 Sagittal split advancement osteotomies stabilized with miniplates. A 2–5-year follow-up. International Journal of Oral and Maxillofacial Surgery 23:127–131

39. Van Sickels JE, Larsen AJ, Thrash WJ 1986 Relapse after rigid fixation of mandibular advancement. Journal of Oral and Maxillofacial Surgery 44:698–702

40. Van Sickels JE, Larsen AJ, Thrash WJ 1988 A retrospective study of relapse in rigidly fixated sagittal split osteotomies: contributing factors. American Journal of Orthodontics and Dentofacial Orthopedics 94:413–416

41. Watzke IM, Turvey TA, Phillips C, Proffit WR 1990 Stability of mandibular advancement after sagittal osteotomy with screw or wire fixation: a comparative study. Journal of Oral and Maxillofacial Surgery 48:108–121

42. Blomqvist JE, Isaksson S 1994 Skeletal stability after mandibular advancement: a comparison of two rigid internal fixation techniques. Journal of Oral and Maxillofacial Surgery 52:1133–1137

43. Gassamann CJ, Van Sickels JE, Thrash WJ 1990 Causes, location and timing of relapse following rigid fixation after mandibular advancement. Journal of Oral and Maxillofacial Surgery 48:450–454

44. Van Sickels JE 1991 A comparative study of bicortical screw and suspension wires versus bicortical screws in large mandibular advancements. Journal of Oral and Maxillofacial Surgery 49:1293–1296

45. Shetty V, Freymiller E, McBrearty D, Caputo AA 1996 Experimental analysis of functional stability of sagittal split ramus osteotomies secured by miniplates and position screw. Journal of Oral and Maxillofacial Surgery 54:1317–1324

46. Foley WL, Frost DE, Paulin WB, Tucker MR 1989 Internal screw

fixation: comparison of placement pattern and rigidity. Journal of Oral and Maxillofacial Surgery 47:720–723

47. Foley WL, Beckman TW 1992 In vitro comparison of screw versus plate fixation in the sagittal split osteotomy. International Journal of Adult Orthodontics and Orthognathic Surgery 7:147–151

48. Kerstens HCJ, Tuinzing DB, Golding RP, van der Kwast WAM 1990 Condylar atropy and osteoarthritis after bimaxillary surgery. Oral Surgery, Oral Medicine, Oral Pathology 69:274–279

49. Phillips RM, Bell WH 1987 Atrophy of mandibular condyles after sagittal ramus split osteotomy: report of a case. Journal of Oral Surgery 36:45–49

50. Merkx MAW, Van Damme PA 1994 Condylar resorption after orthognathic surgery. Journal of Cranio-Maxillo-Facial Surgery 22:53–58

51. Huang CS, Ross BR 1982 Surgical advancement of the retrognathic mandible in growing children. American Journal of Orthodontics 82:89–95

52. Sesenna E, Raffaini M 1985 Bilateral condylar atrophy after combined osteotomy for correction of mandibular retrusion. Journal of Maxillo-Facial Surgery 13:263–267

53. Moore KE, Gorris PJJ, Stoelinga PJW 1991 The contributing role of condylar resorption to skeletal relapse following mandibular advancement surgery. Journal of Oral and Maxillofacial Surgery 49:448–460

54. Arnett GW, Tamborello JA, Rathbone JA 1992 Temporomandibular joint ramifications of orthognathic surgery. In: Bell WH (ed) Modern practice in orthognathic and reconstructive surgery, Vol 1. WB Saunders, Philadelphia, pp 523–593

55. Ellis E, Hinton RJ 1991 Histologic examination of the temporomandibular joint after mandibular advancement with and without rigid fixation: an experimental investigation in adult *Macaca mulatta*. Journal of Oral and Maxillofacial Surgery 49:1316–1327

56. De Clercq CA, Neyt LF, Mommaerts MY, Abeloos JV, De Mot BM 1994 Condylar resorption in orthognathic surgery: a retrospective study. International Journal of Adult Orthodontics and Orthognathic Surgery 9:233–240

57. Crawford JG, Stoelinga PJW, Blijdorp PA, Brouns JJA 1994 Stability after reoperation for progressive condylar resorption after orthognathic surgery: report of seven cases. Journal of Oral and Maxillofacial Surgery 52:460–466

58. Link JJ, Nickerson JW 1992 Temporomandibular joint internal derangements in an orthognathic surgery population. International Journal of Adult Orthodontics and Orthognathic Surgery 7:161–169

59. Arnett GW, Tamborello JA 1990 Progressive class II development: female idiopathic condylar resorption. Oral and Maxillofacial Surgery Clinics of North America 2:699–705

60. Niebergall CF, Mercuri LG 1985 Intraoral vertical subcondylar osteotomy: a national survey. Journal of Oral and Maxillofacial Surgery 43:450–452

61. Nystrom E, Rosenquist J, Astrand P, Nordin T 1984 Intraoral or extraoral approach in oblique sliding osteotomy of the mandibular ramus. A cephalometric study. Journal of Maxillo-Facial Surgery 12:277–282

62. Tornes K, Wisth PJ 1988 Stability after vertical condylar ramus osteotomy for correction of mandibular prognathism. International Journal of Oral and Maxillofacial Surgery 17:242–248

63. Athanasiou AE, Mavreas D, Touountzakis N, Ritzau M 1992 Skeletal stability after surgical correction of mandibular prognathism by vertical ramus osteotomy. European Journal of Orthondotics 14:117–124

64. Tornes K 1989 Osteotomy length and postoperative stability in vertical subcondylar ramus osteotomy. Acta Odontologica Scandinavica 47:81–88

65. Komori E, Aigase K, Sugisaki M, Tanabe H 1987 Skeletal fixation versus skeletal relapse. American Journal of Orthodontics and Dentofacial Orthopedics 92:412–421

66. Tornes K, Wisth PJ 1988 Stability after vertical subcondylar ramus osteotomy for correction of mandibular prognathism. International Journal of Oral and Maxillofacial Surgery 17:242–248

67. Ahlen K, Rosenquist J 1990 Anterior skeletal fixation as an adjunct to oblique sliding osteotomy of the mandibular ramus. A cephalometric study. Journal of Cranio-Maxillo-Facial Surgery 18:147–150

68. Paulus GW, Steinhauser EW 1982 A comparative study of wire osteosynthesis versus bone screws in the treatment of mandibular prognathism. Oral Surgery, Oral Medicine, Oral Pathology 54:2–6

69. Van Sickels JE, Tiner BD, Jeter TS 1990 Rigid fixation of the inverted 'L' osteotomy. Journal of Oral and Maxillofacial Surgery 48:894–898

70. Kobayshi T, Watanabe I, Ueda K, Nakajima T 1986 Stability of the mandible after sagittal ramus osteotomy for correction of prognathism. Journal of Oral and Maxillofacial Surgery 44:693–697

71. Franco JE, Van Sickels JE, Thrash WJ 1989 Factors contributing to relapse in rigidly fixed mandibular setbacks. Journal of Oral and Maxillofacial Surgery 47:451–456

72. Guerro C 1990 Expansion mandibular quirurgica. Revista Venezolana Ortodontologia 48:1–3

73. Guerrero C, Bell WH, Flores A, Modugno VL, Rodriguez AM 1995 Distraccion osteogenica mandibular intraoral. Odontologia Dia 11:116–132

74. Weil TS, Van Sickels JE, Payne CJ 1996 Early experience and results with rapid symphyseal expansion. Journal of Oral and Maxillofacial Surgery 54(Suppl):92–93

75. Bell WH, Harper RP, Gonzalez M, Cherkaskin AM, Samchukov ML 1997 Distraction osteogenesis to widen the mandible. British Journal of Oral and Maxillofacial Surgery 35:11–19

76. Harper RP, Bell WH, Hinton RJ, Browne R, Cherkashin AM, Samchukov ML 1997 Reactive changes in the temporomandibular joint after mandibular midline osteodistraction. British Journal of Oral and Maxillofacial Surgery 35:20–25

Avoiding surgical complications in orthognathic surgery

77

DAVID RICHARDSON/O. A. POSPISIL

INTRODUCTION

The potential complications of orthognathic surgery are legion.[1,2] Intraoperative prevention and management of the more important complications, relating to the more commonly practiced orthognathic procedures, i.e. Le Fort I osteotomy, sagittal split osteotomy, intraoral vertical subsigmoid osteotomy and genioplasty will be discussed.

Surgical complications will be considered under the following headings:

- Airway
- Maintaining vascularity to the osteotomized segments
- Hemorrhage
- Unfavorable osteotomy patterns
- Neurologic complications
- Correct positioning of jaws and segments
- Temporomandibular joint complications
- Infection
- Teeth and periodontium.

AIRWAY

Nasal endotracheal intubation is necessary to facilitate surgery and the placement of intraoperative intermaxillary fixation.

Accidental damage to the endotracheal tube, the pilot tube, or both, may occur during surgery.[3–7] Care should be exercised in operating in the vicinity of the tube, as damage may require a tube change in difficult circumstances. The anesthetist needs to be aware of the potential for this problem, and to be familiar with techniques designed to facilitate tube replacement.[5–7]

Postoperatively, the airway may be compromised for a variety of reasons, including edema, hemorrhage, change in size and configuration of the upper airway, and the presence of postoperative intermaxillary fixation. Two large studies reported rates of respiratory complications of less than 0.5%,[8,9] and these were unrelated to the type of surgical procedure.[8]

Prolonged postoperative intubation is undesirable:[8,9] fewer complications are encountered with early extubation (less than 8 hours) compared with later extubation.[8] Problems associated with prolonged intubation include accidental extubation, kinking, plugging, tube malposition and patient intolerance.

The use of rigid internal fixation renders immediate postoperative intermaxillary fixation unnecessary.[9,10] Intermaxillary fixation increases airway resistance, reducing peak flow by approximately 50%.[11] This is exacerbated by concomitant nasal obstruction.[12] Intermaxillary fixation is a potential hazard to the airway, which is unnecessary in most cases and should be avoided where possible.

Soft-tissue swelling and hemorrhage may compromise the airway. Careful hemostasis and the use of suction drains where appropriate will reduce hematoma formation. Edema is reduced by the use of perioperative steroids.[13–15] Regimens and doses vary, but 8–16 mg of dexamethasone given intravenously 1 hour before surgery, with one to three postoperative doses at 8-hourly intervals will reduce edema by approximately 50%, with the maximum effect on the first postoperative day.[13]

Management of the obstructed airway includes suction, release of intermaxillary fixation, control of hemorrhage, nasopharyngeal or endotracheal intubation and, in extreme cases, where intubation is not possible, tracheostomy may be required.[9]

MAINTAINING VASCULARITY TO THE OSTEOTOMIZED SEGMENTS

Several studies have demonstrated a marked reduction in blood flow to the jaws following osteotomy.[16-20] However, this is usually transient and has little clinical effect. Vascular compromise may occur and affects both the soft tissues (pulp, periodontium, bone marrow and periosteum) and the hard tissues (bone and teeth).[16]

Mild ischemia can lead to periodontal defects, pulp necrosis, infection and delayed union. Moderate prolonged ischemia can lead to nonunion. Severe ischemia leads to tooth and bone loss.[16] Factors affecting vascularity include the design of the incision, stripping of soft tissues, retraction of soft tissues, placement of bone cuts, mobilization, and the extent of surgical movement.

Avascular necrosis affecting the mandible following sagittal split osteotomy is uncommon,[2,21-24] although undesirable changes in the shape of the mandibular ramus following surgery may, in part, be a consequence of reduced blood supply.[25] The blood supply to the mandible is from the inferior alveolar artery, but predominantly via nutrient vessels in areas of muscle attachments (e.g. masseter, pterygoid and genioglossi), which are derived from the maxillary, facial and lingual arteries.[16,26,27]

In sagittal split osteotomy, stripping of the periosteum and muscles from the proximal segment (ramus) should be kept to a minimum.[15,16,28] With the masseter muscle and periosteum left attached, the blood supply to the proximal segment is preserved on its lateral side, whereas the blood supply to the lingual cortex of the distal segment is derived from its medial side via the attachment of the medial pterygoid muscle. Division of the pterygomasseteric envelope is necessary in order to mobilize the distal segment and avoid major relapse forces, and this should always be performed through the osteotomy cut following bone splitting.

Ischemic problems, such as nonunion, infection and avascular necrosis, have been reported in vertical subsigmoid osteotomy.[29,30] Necrosis of the tip of the proximal segment has been noted. It is suggested that reducing its length by cutting off the most distal (and most ischemic) end may eliminate avascular necrosis.[30] Soft-tissue stripping should be kept to a minimum, although wide periostial stripping of the outer cortex of the ramus is inherent to this procedure.

Genioplasty may also be associated with avascular necrosis,[31] and is preventable by the maintenance of a generous soft-tissue pedicle. Periosteum should not be stripped below the mental triangle, leaving the lower border and lingual tissues attached to the mobilized segment. Combined one-stage genioplasty and ramus osteotomy also has the potential to reduce the perfusion of the body of the mandible caused by excessive buccal soft-tissue stripping, which should be avoided.

The blood supply to the maxilla is derived from the anterior, middle and posterior superior alveolar vessels, the infraorbital artery, the greater palatine arteries, the nasopalatine artery, the palatine branches of the ascending pharyngeal artery, and nutrient vessels derived from the facial artery.[32,33] Following maxillary down fracture the blood supply is derived from the greater palatine arteries, the posterior superior alveolar arteries, and palatine branches of the ascending pharyngeal artery,[20,34] and therefore depends on intact buccal soft-tissue pedicles, soft palate and greater palatine vessels.[19,34]

Although marked reductions in blood flow occur following maxillary osteotomy,[19,34] Bell showed that this is transient,[35,36] even with multiple segmentation, advancement and intentional division of the greater palatine vessels.[20] This applies only to maxillas which have no compromise of blood supply as a result of previous cleft palate surgery.[37] Other studies also suggest that division of the greater palatine arteries is acceptable.[38,39] However, there have been reports of tooth devitalization and loss, periodontal defects and loss of bone segments in maxillary surgery.[40-43] These have been attributed to poor flap design, excessive periosteal stripping or inadvertent detachment, stretching of the palatal pedicle, inappropriate interdental osteotomy cuts, traumatic surgery and compression by palatal splints. Transverse expansion and superior repositioning have higher vascular complication rates than other movements.[19,40]

When utilizing a horseshoe vestibular incision, this should be made high in the sulcus to maintain a thick cuff of labial buccal attached and free gingival tissue, which should not be stripped from the underlying alveolar process. The mucosal incision should be high in the buccal sulcus, and be directed out into the cheek posteriorly (Fig. 77.1). The periosteal incision should be made at a level lower than the mucosal incision, as this prevents prolapse of the buccal fat pad (Fig. 77.2). This reduces the chance of tearing due to excessive retraction of soft tissue, particularly during pterygomaxillary dysjunction. If the incision is too low and turned downwards posteriorly, a tear running along the junction of the free and attached mucosa towards the tuberosity may occur, effectively eliminating the buccal pedicle (Fig. 77.3).

Lanigan[40] has made a number of recommendations to decrease the risk of vascular compromise: Rowes disimpaction forceps should not be used for down fracture, as these may traumatize the palatal mucoperiosteum; the greater palatine vessel should be preserved if possible, especially in segmental procedures. However, they may be divided if

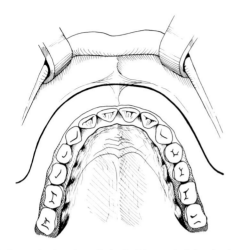

Fig. 77.1 Correctly placed vestibular incision: at height of sulcus and directed into the cheek posteriorly.

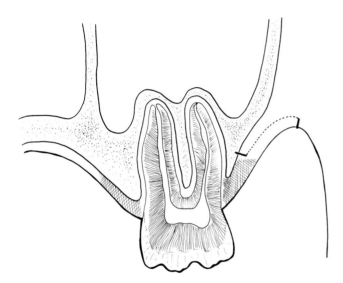

Fig. 77.2 Split-level mucosal and periosteal incision.

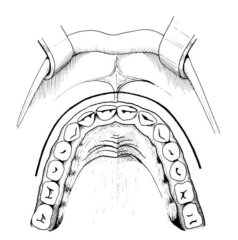

Fig. 77.3 Incorrectly placed vestibular incision: too close to attached gingiva and not directed into the cheek posteriorly.

necessary; segmentalization should be avoided if possible but, if essential, the number of segments should be kept to a minimum. Transverse expansion should be avoided or kept to a minimum, but if necessary should be carried out through a horseshoe-shaped bone cut at the palatoalveolar junction, and not through a midline palatal split. During mobilization of the segments palatal mucoperiosteum should be undermined through the segmental cut from the nasal side, and detached from the segments only to an extent sufficient to allow segment repositioning without tension or tearing of the mucoperiosteum. Detachment from the anterior segment must be minimal, and care should be taken to avoid palatal perforation, particularly tranverse, as this may reduce the blood supply to the anterior dentoalveolar segment.

Circulation may be assessed at operation. Some initial pallor or cyanosis of the gingivae is not uncommon, but should subside quickly following fixation. If pallor or cyanosis persists following reversal of hypotension, then the viability of the jaw or segments may be threatened. In this case, the jaw or segments should be returned to their original position and mobilization and bone movements abandoned. Gradual postoperative movement using orthopedic traction has been shown to have a role in dealing with this situation.

At the end of the operation, care should be taken to ensure that palatal plates do not exert excessive pressure, thereby reducing the palatal blood supply to the maxilla.

HEMORRHAGE

Major hemorrhage associated with orthognathic surgery is uncommon.[9] Maxillary osteotomies carry a higher risk of hemorrhage than do mandibular osteotomies,[9,44–47] and occasionally this may be life-threatening.[46]

Meticulously controlled hypotensive anesthesia reduces blood loss by up to 44% in orthognathic surgery.[48] It may also reduce transfusion requirements and improve the operative field.[49] Some studies, despite showing that the technique is safe, have failed to show significant benefit.[50] For those cases where blood loss can be expected to be high (e.g. extensive midfacial osteotomies or bimaxillary surgery) hypotensive anesthesia may be advantageous.[9,47]

General measures to reduce blood loss from soft tissues include the use of local anesthetic with a vasoconstrictor, dissecting in the subperiosteal plane, and the use of cutting diathermy and bipolar cautery.

The incidence of excessive hemorrhage during mandibular surgery is low, for both sagittal split osteotomy[2,22–24,45,51–53] and vertical subsigmoid osteotomy.[29,30,54] There are a number of vessels at risk during ramus osteotomies, including the maxillary, facial and inferior alveolar arteries, the masseteric vessels, the retromandibular vein and the pterygoid venous plexus.[45] Significant hemorrhage may also follow subapical osteotomies or genioplasty as a result of injury to muscular vessels in the floor of the mouth. This may precipitate acute airway obstruction requiring tracheostomy.[9,45]

During sagittal split osteotomy retractors should be used on the medial side of the ramus to protect the neurovascular bundle and soft tissues. Care should be exercised in completing the split at the posterior border of the ramus, owing to the proximity of the retromandibular vein, which is at risk from laceration by burrs or osteotomes. Similarly, when making the anterior buccal cut a retractor placed beneath the lower border of the mandible will prevent injury to the facial vessels. Identification and preservation of the inferior alveolar neurovascular bundle before completion of the split will reduce risk of hemorrhage from this source.

Excessive hemorrhage during or following maxillary osteotomy may occur from the pterygoid plexus, greater palatine vessels, nasopalatine vessels, the maxillary arteries and the posterior superior alveolar arteries.[47,55] The maxillary artery may be damaged during pterygomaxillary dysjunction, other vessels being vulnerable following osteotomy cuts and down fracture, especially the greater palatine vessels.[47] Despite this, the incidence of excessive hemorrhage is low.[9,41] However, approximately 1% of a series of 1348 maxillary osteotomy patients required transfusion of two or more units of packed cells.[9]

Hemorrhage in maxillary osteotomies can be prevented by exercising care and diligence during a number of surgical maneuvers. On dividing the lateral wall of the nose posteriorly, care should be taken not to damage the descending palatine artery. A definite change in note is heard as the osteotome abuts against the perpendicular plate of the palatine bone, and the osteotomy cut should be stopped at this point. A similar change occurs if completing the posterior end of the lateral cut with an osteotome, and appreciation of this will avert damage to the vessels in the pterygoid region. The osteotomy cut should be kept as low as possible in the region of the tuberosity, for the same reason.

Separation of the pterygoid plates risks injury to vessels in the pterygopalatine fossa, particularly the maxillary artery.[47] There is a 10 mm margin of safety between the vessel and the osteotome if the osteotome is correctly positioned at the lower end of the pterygomaxillary fissure.[56] The use of large curved osteotomes for pterygomaxillary dysjunction can result in extensive and unpredictable pattern fractures of the pterygoid plates.[57,58] These can result in hemorrhage,[55] which may be life-threatening,[46] as well as occasional late vascular, neurologic and ophthalmic complications, if fractures extend to involve the skull base. Ophthalmic complications include blindness due to optic nerve damage or orbital hemorrhage,[59,60] third and sixth nerve palsies, and reduced lacrimation.[59] Vascular complications include arteriovenous fistulae and false aneurysms[61] of the maxillary artery or its branches, especially the descending palatine and sphenopalatine arteries. Carotid cavernous fistulae[62–64] and carotid artery thrombosis[65,66] have also been described.

These complications are uncommon but may occur despite all precautions. When positioning the head, forced hyperextension and rotation should be avoided so as to reduce the chance of indirect trauma to the carotid artery.[67] Pterygomaxillary dysjunction should be carried out with the osteotome low in the pterygomaxillary fissure.[56] Swanneck osteotomes have been designed in order to direct forces more favorably to achieve pterygoid plate separation.[68,69] Avoiding the use of osteotomes has been advocated,[70] although a CT study comparing separation with and without osteotomes showed fractures occurring with both techniques, and neither was associated with clinical problems.[71] Avoidance of the pterygomaxillary fissure altogether, with modification of the osteotomy cut to pass through the tuberosity instead,[72] has also been suggested.

Similar hemorrhagic and vascular problems caused by skull base fractures may result from difficult down fracture, where excessive force has been used. If osteotomy cuts are complete, down fracture of the maxilla should require little force,[58] and can be accomplished by gentle finger pressure anteriorly. If this is unsuccessful the osteotomy cuts should be checked for completeness.

Postoperative hemorrhage may be due to continuing primary hemorrhage, reactionary hemorrhage or secondary hemorrhage. Delayed hemorrhage following maxillary surgery may be the result of rupture of false aneurysms.[61,73,74]

Bleeding from the descending palatine arteries can be controlled following down fracture by ligation with arterial clips or by diathermy. Bleeding from the pterygoid region and pterygopalatine fossa will usually respond to packing. Bleeding is perpetuated by continued manipulation of the osteotomized maxilla, and will usually diminish following internal fixation. Nasal or antral packing, when necessary, should be done against a stable base, following internal fixation of the maxilla, so that adequate pressure may be applied. Ligation of the maxillary or external carotid arteries is rarely necessary, and if bleeding persists consideration should be given to angiography and embolization.[41,47,75]

The management of postoperative bleeding depends on the severity of hemorrhage. If mild, bed rest and light sedation with antifibrinolytic agents may suffice. Anterior and posterior nasal packing may be required and, as discussed, intermaxillary fixation must be released if present. If packing fails to control the hemorrhage, either surgical re-exploration or angiography and embolization should be considered.[41,75] External carotid ligation may be necessary,[55] preferably performed above the linguofacial trunk.[76] Postoperative hemorrhage may compromise the airway and this should be managed accordingly.

UNFAVORABLE OSTEOTOMY PATTERNS

Fractures or undesirable osteotomy patterns may occur in the maxilla or mandible, particularly in sagittal split osteotomy.

Reported rates of untoward osteotomy patterns in sagittal split osteotomies vary, in most reports between 3 and 23%.[2,9,24,51-53] In one report[77] only 13% of splits occurred as planned. Mackintosh[24] outlined untoward fracture patterns in order of frequency. The desired split pattern may be difficult to achieve because of the tenacity of bone, difficulty in placing osteotomes, or anatomical variations.[24] The risk of misdirected splits is reduced by meticulous attention to technique, although problems may occur despite good technical surgery.[24]

Visualization of the medial side of the ramus above the mandibular foramen and the concavity behind the lingula is facilitated by reducing the internal oblique ridge with a large burr.[52] The lingual osteotomy cut can then be made precisely under direct vision. The angulation of the lingual cut is also important. The burr should be angled down posteriorly, especially in patients with a ramus–occlusal plane angle below 70 degrees[78] (Fig. 77.4). If the medial cut is angled superiorly the split may pass upward to the condylar neck, particularly if the Hunscuck modification is being used[79] (Fig. 77.5). This can result in part of the condylar neck remaining on the distal fragment, a condylar neck fracture, or the condyle remaining on the distal fragment.[78]

Following cortical cuts with burrs, the split is initiated at the body of the mandible with osteotomes above the level of the inferior alveolar nerve. The bone segments are then prised apart and, following identification of the neuro-vascular bundle, the osteotomy is completed. Fractures may be related to the use of large osteotomes with a twisting technique.[80] Others consider the angulation[24] and positioning[51] of the osteotome to be important. Still others recommend the use of small fine flexible osteotomes to complete the osteotomy.[53]

Fracture of the lingual plate may occur if pressure is

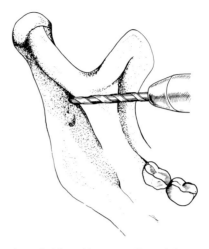

Fig. 77.4 Correctly angled lingual bone cut: directed downwards posteriorly.

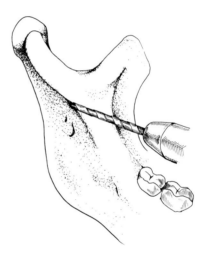

Fig. 77.5 Incorrectly angled lingual bone cut: directed towards the condylar neck.

applied at the ascending ramus between the lingual and buccal plates, especially if any unerupted wisdom teeth are present.[1] These should be removed with care following the split. Removal of wisdom teeth 9–12 months prior to surgery may avoid this problem, particularly where mandibular advancement is planned.[1]

Following splitting, a check should be made to ensure that the condyle is attached to the proximal segment, and to identify any fractures and untoward osteotomy patterns. Management depends on the nature of the lines of fracture and the number of segments. If the fractured segments are small they may be removed. If large, and still attached to periosteum, they should be left in situ and fixed. If a major fracture occurs, or if the condyle is found to be attached to the distal segment, then switching to the other side is recommended before completing the split.[9] If the other side is completed successfully, then at least one side will be stable and a low subcondylar osteotomy on the affected side will allow the planned jaw movement, with the condyle remaining in the fossa. Postoperative intermaxillary fixation will be required in this situation. If the other side seems to be splitting unfavorably the procedure should be abandoned. Once bone healing has occurred, a further osteotomy, using a different technique, can be attempted.[9]

Undesirable bone splits are less frequent in vertical subsigmoid osteotomy than in sagittal split osteotomy. However, inadvertent condylotomy,[77] horizontal ramus osteotomy[2] and division of the gonial angle from the ramus[29] have been described. These appear to be sporadic cases with a low incidence, and some authors do not report any problems of this nature.[30,54]

Undesirable fracture patterns occur infrequently in low-level maxillary osteotomies. However, pterygomaxillary dysjunction, and subsequent down fracture, may result in fractures extending to the cranial base, resulting in bleeding and late vascular, ophthalmic and neurologic problems. If a low fracture of the pterygoid plates leaves the inferior fragment attached to the tuberosity, there may be difficulty in advancing the maxilla and the associated muscle pull will exert a relapsing force, compromising stability. Division of the pterygoid column from the maxilla in this situation is essential.

NEUROLOGIC COMPLICATIONS

Sensory deficit is a major concern, particularly in mandibular sagittal split osteotomy,[23,24,52,81,82] but also in genioplasty[83–85] and vertical subsigmoid osteotomy.[29,30,53] Sensory changes following maxillary procedures tend to be temporary. Occasional facial nerve and other cranial nerve lesions may occur. Nerves are at risk in all stages of surgery, including incision, dissection, retraction, bone cuts, mobilization and internal fixation. Postoperative edema and hematoma may also contribute to nerve damage.

The inferior alveolar nerve is at significant risk during sagittal split osteotomy. Immediate postoperative paresthesia is common, with reports of 85–87% incidence.[23,24,52] A substantial proportion recover sensation,[86] and most reports of the incidence of long-term paresthesia vary between 0 and 24%.[23,24,52,81,82] However, other studies report up to 85% long-term paresthesia.[83,85,87–89] Age is a risk factor for sensory deficit,[24,83,85] patients over the age of 40 being particularly susceptible.[24]

Nerve damage which is apparent at operation during sagittal splitting is reported at 1.3–18%.[9,51–53] The mandibular nerve above the level at the lingula is vulnerable to injury during exposure of the medial side of the ramus, during retraction, and during the lingual osteotomy cut,

when it may be crushed, avulsed from the mandibular canal, or damaged by the burr. Reduction of the internal oblique ridge before making the medial cut allows a direct view of the lingula and the nerve, facilitating its protection.

The anterior vertical cut in the buccal cortex also places the nerve at risk.[90] The neurovascular canal lies approximately 5 mm medial to the buccal cortex at the site of the second molar, with a range of 3–7 mm.[91] Care should therefore be taken to ensure that the burr passes only just through the cortical bone, to prevent encroachment of this cut on to the neurovascular canal. Bleeding from cancellous bone will occur as soon as the buccal cut has passed through the full thickness of the cortex, and when this is seen cutting should be stopped immediately.

In initiating the split, the nerve is at risk when the osteotome is driven into the bone cut on the upper surface of the external oblique ridge. In most cases the nerve is situated between 4 and 11 mm below the surface of the ridge, but in 5% of cases may be between 1 and 4 mm.[91] Some indication of depth may be ascertained from the pre-operative orthopantomogram. Two fundamental techniques exist to complete the split with osteotomes. One uses large osteotomes to initiate the split above the level of the nerve.[51,53] The lingual and buccal cortices are slowly separated, allowing direct inspection of the split for visualization of the neurovascular bundle. Once located, the osteotome is placed beyond the nerve and the split may be completed. If the nerve is seen passing from the buccal to the lingual side, it must be freed from the buccal fragment by removal of the medial wall of the bony canal with a fine osteotome. The nerve can then be delivered from the canal, moved lingually, and the split completed. The nerve is at significant risk during these maneuvers, and the outcome is largely dependent on the skill and experience of the surgeon.

The other technique involves the use of fine thin flexible osteotomes directed toward the buccal plate.[53,92] The tip of the flexible osteotome is driven directly on to the inner aspect of the buccal cortex and slides down it, and therefore should stay lateral to the neurovascular bundle.[80,92] It is claimed that this reduces the risk of fractures and misdirected bone cuts, as well as reducing the incidence of damage to the inferior alveolar nerve.[80,91,92]

The method of fixation may also have an effect on nerve damage.[95] Compression screws should not be used, as compression of the buccal and lingual plates may compress the nerve.[93] Bicortical (non-compression) screws will avoid this,[83,93] as long as they are not over-tightened. In placing bicortical screws care should be taken to avoid damage to the neurovascular bundle.[93] The use of miniplates with monocortical screws could reduce this element of risk.

Intraoral vertical subsigmoid osteotomy carries less

operative risk to the inferior alveolar nerve. Obvious intra-operative nerve damage is uncommon,[29,30,53,54] and long-term sensory disturbance is relatively infrequent, reports varying between 2.3 and 14%.[29,30,54,94] Accurate identification of landmarks and placement of bone cuts is essential to avoid damage to the nerve.[30] Medial displacement of the proximal segment may be associated with paresthesia caused by pressure on the neurovascular bundle.

Any nerve division seen at operation should be repaired where possible. In the authors' experience, one or two epineural sutures will coapt the cut ends without tension in set-back procedures. In advancements this may result in too much tension on the nerve repair, in which case interpositional nerve grafting may be considered.

The mental nerve is at risk during genioplasty, with the long-term incidence of paresthesia between 0 and 20%.[84,85,95,96] Superficial distal fibers may be cut during high labial mucosal incisions with dissection of a mucosal flap, which should be raised superficial to these branches. When bone is exposed the mental nerve requires protection. Separating the mental nerve from its periosteal envelope at its exit from the mental foramen will reduce pull on the nerve, thus reducing the risk of avulsion, and also results in increased access for bone cuts. Placement of the bone cut too close to the lower border of the foramen may result in division of the nerve within its canal. The horizontal bone cut should therefore be kept 3–4 mm below the mental foramen.

Combining genioplasty with a sagittal split osteotomy further increases the risk of altered lip sensation. Two studies have reported the incidence of long-term neuro-sensory deficit at 10% in genioplasty, 30% in sagittal split osteotomy, and 70% in combined procedures.[84,85]

A number of sensory nerves may be damaged during maxillary osteotomies. The nasopalatine nerve and the anterior middle and posterior superior alveolar nerves are inevitably divided during the osteotomy. The infraorbital nerve and greater palatine nerves may be damaged inadvertently. The incidence of long-term infraorbital paresthesia is approximately 1.5–2%,[44,97–99] and nerve damage may occur as a result of direct compression during soft-tissue retraction, mobilization and plating. Because the infraorbital nerve is easily accessible and not directly involved in osteotomy cuts, it should be easily protected. Sensory deficits affecting the teeth, palate and buccal mucosa below the incision gradually resolve over 12–18 months.[97]

Other less common and unpredictable neurologic deficits have been documented following Le Fort I osteotomy. These may be related to unwanted osteotomy patterns or fractures extending to the skull base, or may be the result of late vascular complications (discussed earlier). They include damage to the third nerve,[100] sixth nerve,[101] 10th

and 12th nerves,[46] as well as the fourth nerve, optic and trigeminal nerves.[59,66] Careful technique, particularly in pterygomaxillary dysjunction and down fracture, should reduce the incidence of these already rare complications.

Facial nerve injury is uncommon following intraoral mandibular ramus osteotomies, and the incidence is reported at between 0.4 and 1%.[22–24,102,103] Most cases resolve spontaneously. However, three out of nine cases in one large survey showed only incomplete recovery.[102]

Several potential mechanisms for injury are proposed. The posterior border of the ramus is in close proximity to the proximal facial nerve,[102] and the insertion of retractors at the posterior border may stretch or compress the nerve.[104] Splitting of the posterior border of the ramus may cause crushing of the nerve trunk between the osteotome and the mastoid process.[103] Fracture and displacement of the styloid of the process may impinge on the facial nerve,[104] and pressure from the distal segment of the mandible may occur following mandibular push-backs,[103,104] especially if large. However, facial nerve injuries have occurred in cases of mandibular advancement.[103,105] Postoperative edema or hematoma have also been suggested to have a role.[106]

Care should be taken during manipulations at the posterior border of the ramus and, in mandibular sagittal split osteotomy for push-backs, Hunsuck's modification[79] has been recommended.[103,104] Management of an established facial nerve injury depends on several factors.[106] Incomplete palsies will recover spontaneously. When onset of the weakness is delayed, even if it progresses to a complete palsy the prognosis is good, and a full spontaneous recovery can be expected.[105,106] If onset is immediate and the deficit complete, then early detailed electrodiagnostic testing is indicated, with regular monitoring to assess progress. If these tests indicate that nerve transection has occurred, then exploration and repair by primary suture or nerve grafting is indicated.[106]

CORRECT POSITIONING OF JAWS AND SEGMENTS

Malpositioning of the jaws and segments during osteotomy is uncommon.[9,107] Anterior and inferior repositioning of the maxilla is not difficult, as there are few interferences with movement. However, superior repositioning necessitates the removal of tissues to allow intrusion, particularly if maxillary advancement is not a part of the procedure. Care must be taken that sufficient clearance is made at the point of contact between the maxillary tuberosity and the cranial aspect of the midface, thus avoiding posterior gagging of the maxilla.

Removal of bone at the lateral antral walls, zygomatic

buttress and posterior maxilla (surrounding the greater palatine pedicle) is usually required. In addition, the lateral nasal wall and nasal septum must be reduced and, for larger intrusions (over 5 mm), inferior turbinectomy is desirable. Inadequate reduction of the nasal septum may result in its buckling, with the risk of nasal tip deviation and partial nasal airway obstruction.[41,42]

Undiagnosed posterior interferences may cause distraction of the mandibular condyles from the glenoid fossae during attempts to intrude the maxilla while it is held in temporary intermaxillary fixation, and excessive upward force is applied to the chin point (Fig. 77.6 A,B,C). Following plating of the maxilla and removal of the intermaxillary fixation, the condyles will revert to their normal position, resulting in an anterior open bite. In this case the plates must be removed and interferences removed in order to allow correct maxillary positioning without using excessive upward pressure on the chin, avoiding vertical distraction of the condyles.

In segmental procedures the use of a palatal plate with Adams cribs will allow greater control in the repositioning of segments. In particular, during maxillary arch expansion such a plate will ensure bodily lateral movement of the segments, avoiding their tilting. It also effectively converts multiple mobile segments into a single monoblock, facilitating the removal of interferences to maxillary positioning, and easier internal fixation.

Correct location of the condyles in the glenoid fossae is important when using internal fixation in mandibular procedures.[108] The condyles must be in a passive position, with no excessive seating forces applied. Lateral movement should also be avoided and, particularly in asymmetric movements, some flaring of the distal end of the proximal segment on one side may have to be accepted (Fig. 77.7

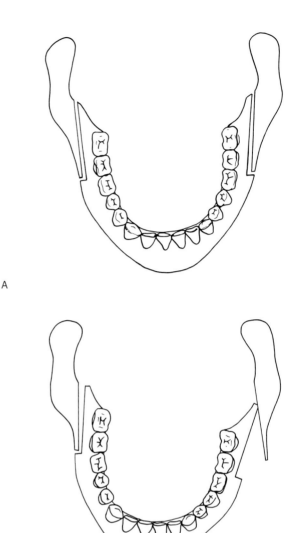

A

B

Fig. 77.7 (A) and **(B)** Assymetric mandibular movement with flaring of proximal fragment.

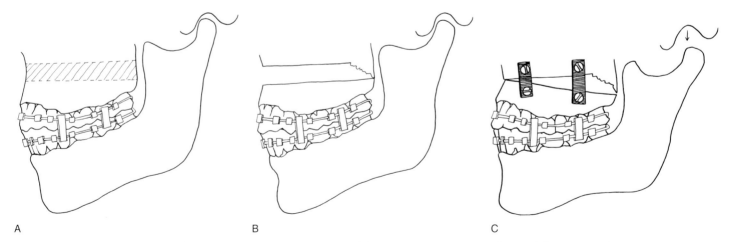

A

B

C

Fig. 77.6 Superior repositioning of the maxilla. **(A)** Planned bone removal. **(B)** Undiagnosed posterior interference. **(C)** Distraction of mandibular condyles on intrusion of the maxilla.

A,B). Various devices have been designed to maintain condylar position during surgery.[109–111] However, in the authors' experience it is possible to achieve acceptable condylar position by gentle posterior pressure without resorting to these mechanical devices.

In vertical subsigmoid osteotomy it is important that the proximal segment is positioned laterally, as medial positioning will allow upward rotation of the proximal segment. Intraoperative displacement is common,[112] and between 3 and 9% have been found to be displaced medially postoperatively.[29,58] Often the displacement is slight and requires no secondary intervention.[29] However, contour defects may be produced with larger displacements, and occasionally malocclusion with anterior open bite may develop due to loss of ramus height (Fig. 77.8).

TEMPOROMANDIBULAR JOINT COMPLICATIONS

Excessive manipulation of the proximal fragment has been reported to cause intra-articular hematoma, leading to pain and limited opening.[113] Inaccurate positioning of the condyle with posterior superior displacement will result in joint compression, with the same effect,[114] particularly if there is a pre-existing internal derangement.[113] This has also been implicated in the etiology of progressive condylar resorption.[115,116] Some degree of condylar displacement is almost inevitable when rigid internal fixation is used, but this is well tolerated in most cases.[109]

Intermaxillary fixation has been shown to lead to reduced mouth opening[114–118] and, if used in situations where the

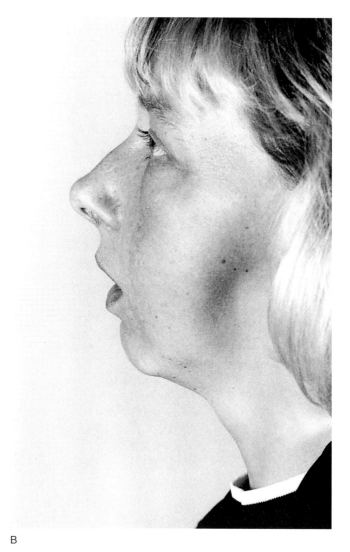

A

B

Fig. 77.8 Outcome following complications of vertical subsigmoid osteotomy. **(A)** Lip incompetence. **(B)** High-angle class II deformity with a visible depression in angle ramus region.

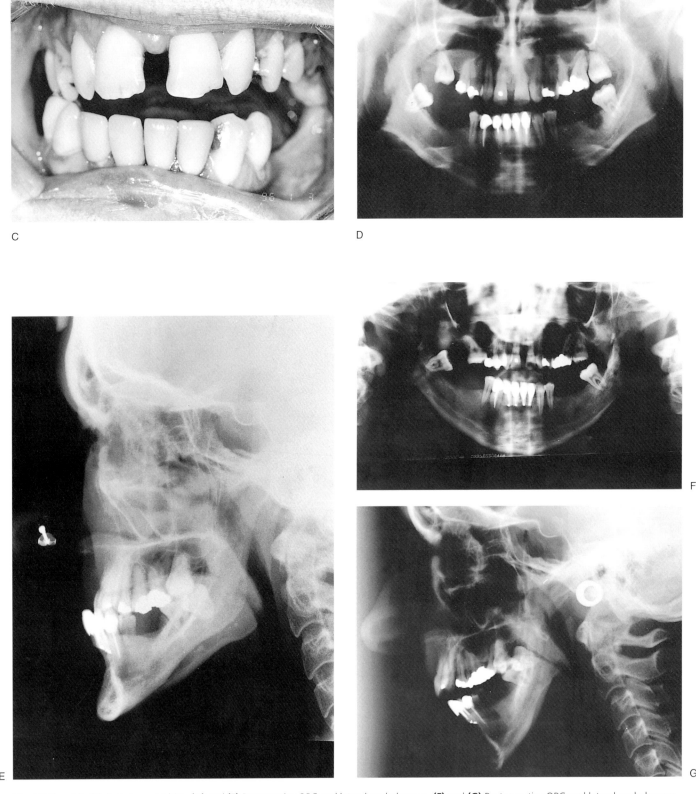

C

D

E

F

G

Fig. 77.8(contd) **(C)** Anterior open bite. **(D)** and **(E)** Preoperative OPG and lateral cephalogram. **(F)** and **(G)** Postoperative OPG and lateral cephalogram.

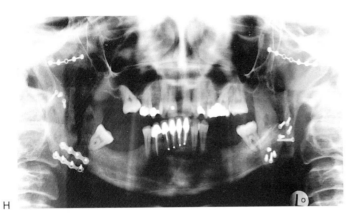

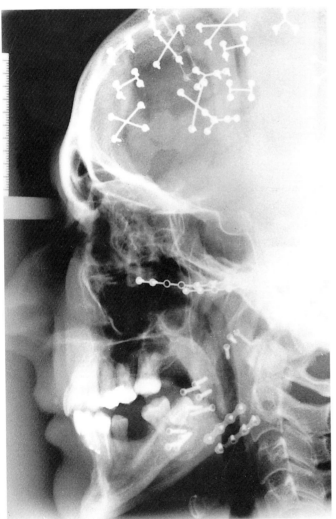

Fig. 77.8(contd) **(H)** and **(I)** OPG and lateral cephalogram following correction with vascularized calvarial bone grafts to restore ramus height.

temporomandibular joint is injured, may result in intra-articular fibrous ankylosis.[113] The use of rigid internal fixation without intermaxillary fixation reduces persistent limitation of mouth opening, with no significant increases in complications.[10]

INFECTION

Postoperative surgical infection in intraoral orthognathic surgery is uncommon,[22,24,29,52,54] with an incidence of less than 1%.[9,23] Risk factors include the duration and type of surgery, the degree of surgical trauma, ischemia, the use of alloplastic implants, and bacterial contamination.[119,120] Most authors advocate the use of prophylactic antibiotics for intraoral procedures.[8,119] These should be commenced just prior to surgery to ensure therapeutic levels at the time of surgery, and continue for 24 hours.[9,119,121] A number of regimens have been described, but penicillin G administered parenterally is considered to be the preferred drug for intraoral orthognathic surgery.

TEETH AND PERIODONTIUM

Both structures are at risk for a number of reasons, particularly during segmental procedures. Vascular compromise may result in tooth mobility, periodontal defects, and necrosis of gingiva and bone with tooth and possibly segment loss. These were discussed in a previous section. The vascularity of the dental pulps is also at risk,[122-124] and bone cuts should be made 5 mm away from tooth apices in order to preserve their blood supply.[97] Loss of response to pulp testing occurs in 90% of teeth in maxillary and subapical osteotomies, but this gradually returns to normal over 18 months.[97]

Periodontal damage is more common in segmental procedures. It is important to create a narrow subperiosteal pocket in the region of the osteotomy in order to prevent tearing of the attached gingiva by the osteotome or on mobilization of the segment. Periodontal bone loss does occur in teeth adjacent to segmental cuts, but this is usually minimal.[125-127]

Mechanical damage to the teeth from saws, burrs and screws should be avoided by careful placement of bone cuts and plates. The tooth roots at either side of a segmental osteotomy cut should diverge (achieved usually by preoperative orthodontics), in order to provide space for the cut without root exposure. Fine osteotomes should be used to complete interdental cuts. Few problems arise as long as teeth and roots are not physically damaged and adequate segmental vascularity is maintained.[41,97,128]

Postoperatively, teeth may be extruded if intermaxillary fixation is used, particularly where preoperative orthodontics was carried out, where incisor teeth are wired on to archbars, and elastics rather than wires being used to maintain intermaxillary fixation. The use of an interdental occlusal wafer extending over the incisor teeth and early postoperative orthodontic management will reduce the occurrence of this complication.

ACKNOWLEDGEMENTS

I would like to thank Julia Blackmore, Medical Secretary, and Jan Hogg, Postgraduate Librarian, Aintree Hospital NHS Trust, for their assistance in the preparation of this chapter.

REFERENCES

1. El Deeb M, Wolford L, Bevis R 1989 Complications of orthognathic surgery. Clinics in Plastic Surgery 16:825–840
2. Behrman SJ 1974 Complications associated with orthognathic surgery. In: Irby WB (ed) Current advances in oral surgery. Mosby, St Louis, pp 109–143
3. Pagar DN, Kupperman AW, Stern M 1978 Cutting of nasoendotracheal tube: an unusual complication of maxillary osteotomies. Journal of Oral Surgery 36:313–314
4. Mosby EL, Messer EJ, Nealis MF, Golden DP 1978 Intraoperative damage to nasotracheal tubes during maxillary surgery. Report of cases. Journal of Oral Surgery 36:963–964
5. Schwartz LB, Sordill WC, Liebers RM, Schwab W 1982 Difficulty in removal of accidentally cut endotracheal tube. Journal of Oral and Maxillofacial Surgery 40:518–519
6. Tsueda K, Carey WJ, Gonty AA, Bosomworth PB 1977 Hazards to anaesthetic equipment during maxillary osteotomy: report of cases. Journal of Oral Surgery 55(1):35–47
7. Peskin RM, Sachs SA 1986 Intra operative management of partially severed endo tracheal tube during orthognathic surgery. Anaesthesia Progress Sept/Oct:247–251
8. Haber-Cohan A, Rothman M 1988 A survey of extubation practices following orthognathic surgery. Journal of Oral and Maxillofacial Surgery 46:269–279
9. Jan P, Van de Perre A, Stoelinga PJ, Blijdorp PA, Brouns JA, Hoppenreijs TJM 1996 Perioperative morbidity in maxillofacial orthopaedic surgery: retrospective study. Journal of Cranio-Maxillo-Facial Surgery 24:263–270
10. Buckley MJ, Tulloch JFC, White RP, Tucker MR 1989 Complications of orthognathic surgery: a comparison between wire fixation and rigid internal fixation. International Journal of Orthodontics and Orthognathics Surgery 4:69–74
11. Kohno M, Nakajima T, Someya G 1993 Effects of maxillomandibular fixation on respiration. Journal of Oral and Maxillofacial Surgery 51:992–996
12. Williams JG, Cawood JI 1990 Effect of intermaxillary fixation on pulmonary function. British Journal of Oral Surgery 19:76
13. Weber CR, Griffin JM 1994 Evaluation of dexamethasone for reducing post operative oedema and inflammatory response after orthognathic surgery. Journal of Oral and Maxillofacial Surgery 52:35–39
14. Gersema L, Baker K 1992 Use of cortico steroids in oral surgery. Journal of Oral and Maxillofacial Surgery 50(3):270–277
15. Schaberg SJ, Stuller CB, Edwards SM 1984 Effect of methylprednisolone on swelling after orthognathic surgery. Journal of Oral and Maxillofacial Surgery 42:356
16. Epker BN 1984 Vascular considerations in orthognathic surgery. 1. Mandibular osteotomies. Oral Surgery, Oral Medicine, Oral Pathology 57:467–472
17. Grammer FC, Carpenter AM 1979 A quantitative histologic study of tissue reponses to ramal sagittal splitting procedures. Journal of Oral Surgery 37:482–485
18. Path MG, Nelson RL, Morgan PR, Meyer MW 1977 Blood flow changes after sagittal split of the mandibular ramus. Journal of Oral Surgery 35:98–101
19. Epker BN 1984 Vascular considerations in orthognathic surgery. II Maxillary osteotomies. Oral Surgery, Oral Medicine, Oral Pathology 57:473–478
20. Bell WH, You ZH, Fin RA, Fields RT 1985 Wound healing after multisegmental Le Fort I osteotomy and transection of the descending palatine vessels. Journal of Oral and Maxillofacial Surgery 53:1425–1433
21. Lanigan DT, West RA 1990 Aseptic necrosis of the mandible: report of two cases. Journal of Oral and Maxillofacial Surgery 48:296–300
22. Behrman SJ 1972 Complications of sagittal osteotomy of the mandibular ramus. Journal of Oral Surgery 30:554
23. Martis CS 1984 Complications after mandibular sagittal split osteotomy. Journal of Oral and Maxillofacial Surgery 42:101
24. MacIntosh RB 1981 Experience with a sagittal osteotomy of the mandibular ramus. Journal of Maxillofacial Surgery 8:151
25. Shepherd JP 1980 Changes in the mandibular ramus following osteotomies – a long term review. Journal of Oral Surgery 18:189–201
26. Castelli WA, Nasjleti CE, Diazperez R 1975 Interruption of the arterial inferior alveolar flow and its effects on mandibular collateral circulation and dental tissues. Journal of Dental Research 54:708–715
27. Hellem S, Ostrup LT 1981 Normal and retrograde blood supply to the body of the mandible in the dog II. International Journal of Oral Surgery 10:31–42
28. Bell WH, Schendl SA 1977 Biologic basis for modification of the sagittal ramus split operation. Journal of Oral Surgery 35:362–369
29. Tuinzing DB, Greebe RB 1985 Complications related to the intra oral vertical ramus osteotomy. International Journal of Oral Surgery 14:319–324
30. Hall HD, Chase DC, Payr LG 1975 Evaluation and refinement of the intra oral vertical subcondylar osteotomy. Journal of Oral Surgery 33:333–341
31. Mercuri LG, Laskin DM 1977 Avascular necrosis after anterior horizontal augmentation genioplasty. Journal of Oral Surgery 35:296
32. Nelson RL et al 1978 Quantitation of blood flow after anterior maxillary osteotomy: investigation of three surgical approaches. Journal of Oral and Maxillofacial Surgery 36:106–111
33. Nelson RL et al 1977 Quantitation of blood flow after Le Fort I osteotomy. Journal of Oral and Maxillofacial Surgery 35:10–16
34. Bellmont JR 1988 The Le Fort I osteotomy approach for nasopharyngeal and nasal fossa tumours. Archives of Otolaryngology Head and Neck Surgery 114:751
35. Bell WH, Fonseca RJ, Kennedy JW, Levy BN 1975 Bone healing and revascularisation after total maxillary osteotomy. Journal of Oral Surgery 33:253–260
36. Bell WH, Phys AM 1973 Biologic basis for maxillary osteotomies. Anthropology 38:279–290
37. Drommer R 1979 Selective angiographic studies prior to Le Fort I osteotomy in patients with cleft lip and palate. Journal of Maxillofacial Surgery 7:264–270
38. Bays RA 1993 Descending palatine artery ligation in Le Fort osteotomies. Journal of Oral and Maxillofacial Surgery 8:142
39. Yu ZH, Zhang ZK, Zhang XE 1991 Le Fort I osteotomy with descending palatal artery intact and ligated: a study of blood flow and quantitative histology. Contemporary Stomatology 5:71
40. Lanigan DT, Hey JH, West RA 1990 Aseptic necrosis following maxillary osteotomies: report of 36 cases. Journal of Oral and Maxillofacial Surgery 48:142–156
41. de Mol Van Otterloo JJ, Tuinzing DB, Greebe RB, von de Kwast WA 1991 Intra and early post operative complications of the Le Fort I osteotomy: a retrospective study on 410 cases. Journal of Cranio-Maxillo-Facial Surgery 19:217–222

42. Westwood RN, Tilson UB 1975 Complications associated with maxillary osteotomies. Journal of Oral Surgery 33:104–115

43. Sher MR 1984 A survey of complications in segmental orthognathic procedures. Oral Surgery 58:537–539

44. Tung-Choin Chung, Yu-Ray Chen, Bendor-Samuel R 1995 Surgical complications of the Le Fort I osteotomy: a retrospective review of 146 cases. Chang Gung Medical Journal 18:102–108

45. Lanigan DT, Hey J, West RA 1991 Haemorrhage following mandibular osteotomies: a reported 21 cases. Journal of Oral and Maxillofacial Surgery 49:713–724

46. Newhouse RF, Schow SR, Kraut RA, Price JC 1982 Life threatening haemorrhage from a Le Fort I osteotomy. Journal of Oral and Maxillofacial Surgery 40:117–119

47. Lanigan DT, Hey JH, West RA 1990 Major vascular complications of orthognathic surgery: haemorrhage associated with Le Fort I osteotomies. Journal of Oral and Maxillofacial Surgery 48:561–573

48. Schaberg SJ, Kelly JF, Terry BC, Posner MA, Anderson EF 1976 Blood loss and hypertensive anaesthesia in orofacial corrective surgery. Journal of Oral Surgery 34:147–156

49. Lessard MR, Trèpanier CA, Baribault JP et al 1989 Isofluorane induced hypotension in orthognathic surgery. Anesthesia and Analgesia 69:379–383

50. Fromme GA, McKensy RA, Gould AB, Blunde BA, Offord KP 1986 Controlled hypotension for orthognathic surgery. Anaesthesia and Analgesia 65:683–686

51. Turvey TA 1985 Intra operative complications of sagittal osteotomy of the mandibular ramus: incidence and management. Journal of Oral and Maxillofacial Surgery 43:504–509

52. Guernsey LH, De Champlain RW 1971 Sequelae and complications of the intra oral sagittal osteotomy in the mandibular rami. Oral Surgery 32:176–192

53. Van Merkesteyn JPR, Groot RH, Van Leeuwaarden R, Kroon FHM 1987 Intra operative complications in sagittal and vertical ramus osteotomies. International Journal of Oral and Maxillofacial Surgery 16:665–670

54. Tornes K 1987 Extra oral and intra oral vertical sub condylar ramus osteotomy for correction of mandibular prognathism. International Journal of Oral and Maxillofacial Surgery 16:617–677

55. Lanigan DT, West RA 1984 Management of post operative haemorrhage following the Le Fort I maxillary osteotomy. Journal of Oral and Maxillofacial Surgery 42:367–375

56. Turvey T, Fonseca R 1980 The anatomy of the internal maxillary artery in the pterygo palatine fossa: its relationship to maxillary surgery. Journal of Oral Surgery 38:92

57. Robinson PP, Hendy CW 1986 Pterygoid plate fractures caused by the Le Fort I osteotomy. British Journal of Oral and Maxillofacial Surgery 24:198–202

58. Renick BM, Symington JM 1991 Post operative computed tomography study of pterygomaxillary separation during Le Fort I Osteotomy. Journal of Oral and Maxillofacial Surgery 49:1061–1065

59. Lanigan DT, Romanchuk K, Olsen CK 1993 Ophthalmic complications associated with orthognathic surgery. Journal of Oral and Maxillofacial Surgery 51:480–494

60. Li KK, Meara JG, Rubin PAD 1995 Orbital compartment syndrome following orthognathic surgery. Journal of Oral and Maxillofacial Surgery 53:964–968

61. Lanigan DT, Hey JH, West RA 1991 Major vascular complications of orthognathic surgery: false aneurysms and arterio-venous fistulas following orthognathic surgery. Journal of Oral and Maxillofacial Surgery 49:571–577

62. Lanigan DT, Tubman DE 1987 Carotid cavernous sinus fistula following Le Fort I osteotomy. Journal of Oral and Maxillofacial Surgery 45:969–975

63. Habel MB 1986 A carotid cavernous sinus fistula after maxillary osteotomy. Plastic and Reconstructive Surgery 77:981–985

64. Hess J, Devan K 1988 Carotid cavernous sinus fistula following maxillofacial trauma and orthognathic surgery International Journal of Oral and Maxillofacial Surgery 17:295–297

65. Brady S, Courtemanche A, Steinbock P 1981 Carotid artery thrombosis after elective mandibular and maxillary osteotomies. Annals of Plastic Surgery 6:121

66. Sanni K, Campbell R, Rasner M et al 1984 Internal carotid artery occlusion following mandibular osteotomy. Journal of Oral and Maxillofacial Surgery 42:394

67. Lanigan DT 1988 Injuries to the internal carotid artery following orthognathic surgery. International Journal of Adult Orthodontics and Orthognathic Surgery 4:215–220

68. Wikkeling OME, Tacoma J 1975 Osteotomy of the pterygo maxillary junction. International Journal of Oral Surgery 4:99

69. Hiranuma Y, Yamamoto Y, Lizuka T 1988 Strain distribution during separation of the pterygo maxillary suture by osteotomies. Journal of Cranio-Maxillo-Facial Surgery 16:13

70. Precious DS, Morrison AB, Ricard D 1991 Pterygomaxillary separation without the use of an osteotome. Journal of Oral Surgery 49:98

71. Precious DS, Goodday RH, Barget L, Skulsky FG 1993 Pterygoid plate fracture in Le Fort I osteotomy with and without pterygoid chisel: a computed tomography scan evaluation of 58 cases. Journal of Oral and Maxillofacial Surgery 51:151–153

72. Trimble LD, Tideman H, Stoelinga PJW 1983 A modification of the pterygoid plate separation in low level maxillary ostotomies. Journal of Oral and Maxillofacial Surgery 41:544–546

73. Bendor-Samuel R, Yu-Ray C, Kho Ting C 1995 Unusual complications of the Le Fort I osteotomy. Plastic and Reconstructive Surgery 96:1289–1296

74. Hemmig SB, Johnson RS, Ferrar N 1987 Management of a ruptured pseudoaneurysm of the sphenopalatine artery following a Le Fort I osteotomy. Journal of Oral and Maxillofacial Surgery 45:533–536

75. Rogers SN, Patel M, Beirne JC, Nixon TE 1995 Traumatic aneurysm of the maxillary artery: the role of interventional radiology. International Journal of Oral and Maxillofacial Surgery 24:336–339

76. Roensburg I, Austin J, Wright P et al 1982 The effect of experimental ligation of the external carotid artery and its major branches on haemorrhage from the maxillary artery. International Journal of Oral Surgery 11:251

77. Jonsson E, Svartz K, Wilander U 1979 Saggital split technique. 1. Immediate post operative conditions: a radiographic follow up study. International Journal of Oral Surgery 8:75–81

78. Stott-Carlton A, Schow SR, Peterson LJ 1986 Prevention of the misdirected sagittal split. Journal of Oral and Maxillofacial Surgery 44:81–82

79. Hunsuck EE 1968 A modified intra oral sagittal splitting technique for correction of mandibular prognathism. Journal of Oral Surgery 26:249–252

80. Simpson W 1981 Problems encountered in the sagittal split operation. International Journal of Oral Surgery 10:81–86

81. Freihofer H, Petresevic D 1975 Late results after advancing the mandible by sagittal splitting of the rami. Journal of Maxillofacial Surgery 3:250

82. Schendel S, Epker B 1980 Results after mandibular advancement surgery: an analysis of 87 cases. Journal of Oral Surgery 38:265

83. Nishioka GJ, Zyssett MK, Van Seckets JE 1987 Neurosensory disturbance with rigid fixation of the bilateral sagittal split osteotomy. Journal of Oral and Maxillofacial Surgery 45:20–26

84. Posnick JC, Al-Qattan MM, Stepner NM 1996 Alteration in facial sensibility in adolescents following sagittal split and chin osteotomies of the mandible. Plastic and Reconstructive Surgery 97:920–927

85. Lindquist CC, Obeid G 1988 Complications of genioplasty done alone or in conjunction with sagittal split ramus osteotomy. Oral Surgery 66:13–16

86. Upton LG, Rajvanakan M, Hayward JR 1987 Evaluation of the

regenerative capacity of the inferior alveolar nerve following surgical trauma. Journal of Oral and Maxillofacial Surgery 45:212–216

87. Walter JM, Gregg JM 1979 Analysis of post surgical neurologic alteration in the trigeminal nerve. Journal of Oral Surgery 37:410

88. Peppersack WJ, Chausse JM 1978 Long term follow up of the sagittal splitting technique for correction of mandibular prognathism. Journal of Maxillofacial Surgery 6:117

89. Broadbent R, Woolf R 1977 Our experience with sagittal split osteotomy for retrognathia. Plastic and Reconstructive Surgery 99:860

90. Flamminghi L, Aversa C 1979 Lesions of the inferior alveolar nerve in sagittal osteotomy of the ramus. Journal of Maxillofacial Surgery 7:125

91. Mercier P 1973 The inner osseous architecture and the sagittal splitting of the ascending ramus of the mandible. Journal of Maxillofacial Surgery 1:171–176

92. Brusati R, Flamminghi L, Sesenna E, Gazzotti G 1981 Functional disturbance of the inferior alveolar nerve after sagittal osteotomy of the mandibular ramus: operating technique for prevention. Journal of Maxillofacial Surgery 9:123–125

93. Lindorf HH 1986 Sagittal ramus osteotomy with tandem screw fixation. Journal of Maxillofacial Surgery 14:311–316

94. Zaytoun HS, Phillips C, Terry BC 1986 Long term neurosensory deficits following transoral vertical ramus and sagittal split osteotomies for mandibular prognathism. Journal of Oral and Maxillofacial Surgery 44:193–196

95. Karas ND, Boyd SB, Sinn DP 1990 Recovery of neurosensory function following orthognathic surgery. Journal of Oral and Maxillofacial Surgery 48:124

96. Nishioka GJ, Mason M, Van Sickets JE 1986 Neurosensory disturbance associated with the anterior mandibular horizontal osteotomy. Journal of Oral and Maxillofacial Surgery 46:107

97. Kahnberg KE, Engström H 1987 Recovery of maxillary sinus and tooth sensibility after Le Fort I osteotomy. British Journal of Oral and Maxillofacial Surgery 25:68–73

98. De Mol Van Otterloo F 1991 Intra and early post operative complications of the Le Fort I osteotomy. A retrospective study of 410 cases. Journal of Cranio-Maxillo-Facial Surgery 19:217–222

99. Jongh M de, Barnard D, Birnie D 1986 Sensory nerve morbidity following Le Fort I osteotomy. Journal of Maxillofacial Surgery 14:10–13

100. Carr RJ, Gilbert P 1986 Isolated partial third-nerve palsy following Le Fort I maxillary osteotomy in a patient with cleft lip and palate. British Journal of Oral and Maxillofacial Surgery 24:206–211

101. Watts PG 1984 Unilateral abducent nerve palsy: a rare complication following a Le Fort I maxillary osteotomy. British Journal of Oral and Maxillofacial Surgery 22:212–215

102. de Vires K, Devriesse P, Huvinga J, Van den Akker HP 1993 Facial palsy after sagittal split osteotomies. Journal of Cranio-Maxillo-Facial Surgery 21:50–53

103. Karabouta-Voulgaropoulou I, Martis C 1984 Facial paresis following sagittal split osteotomy. Oral Surgery 57:600–603

104. Dendy RA 1973 Facial nerve paralysis following sagittal split mandibular osteotomy: a case report. British Journal of Oral Surgery 11:101–105

105. Piecuch JF, Lewis RA 1982 Facial nerve injury as a complication of sagittal split ramus osteotomy. Journal of Oral and Maxillofacial Surgery 40:309–310

106. Jones JK, Van Sickels JE 1991 Facial nerve injuries associated with orthognathic surgery. Journal of Oral and Maxillofacial Surgery 49:740–744

107. Moening JE, Garrison BE, Lapp TH, Bussard DA 1990 Early screw removal for correction of occlusal discrepancies following rigid internal fixation in orthognathic surgery. International Journal of Adult Orthodontics and Orthognathic Surgery 5:225–232

108. Luhe HG 1989 The significance of condylar positioning using rigid internal fixation in orthognathic surgery. Clinics in Plastic Surgery 16:147

109. Merten HA, Halling F 1992 A new condylar positioning technique in orthognathic surgery. Journal of Cranio-Maxillo-Facial Surgery 20:310–312

110. Hiatt WR, Shelkin DM, Moore DL 1998 Condylar positioning in orthognathic surgery. Journal of Oral and Maxillofacial Surgery 46:110

111. Schwestka R, Engelke D, Kubein-Meesenburg D 1990 Condylar position control during maxillary surgery: the condylar positioning appliance and three dimensional double splint method. International Journal of Adult Orthodontics and Orthognathic Surgery 5:161

112. Calderon S, Gal G, Anavi Y, Gonshorowitz M 1992 Techniques for ensuring the lateral position of the proximal segment following intra oral vertical ramus osteotomy. Journal of Oral and Maxillofacial Surgery 50:1044–1047

113. Nitzan DW, Franklin Dolwick M 1989 Temporomandibular joint fibrous ankylosis following orthognathic surgery: report of eight cases. International Journal of Adult Orthodontics and Orthognathic Surgery 4:7–11

114. Argon SB, Van Sickels JE, Dolwick MF et al 1985 The effect of orthognathic surgery on mandibular range of motion. Journal of Oral and Maxillofacial Surgery 43:938–943

115. DeClercq CA, Neyt LF, Mommaerts MY, Abeloos JV, De Mot B 1994 Condylar resorption in orthognathic surgery: a retrospective study. International Journal of Adult Orthodontics and Orthognathic Surgery 9:233–240

116. Moore KE, Gooris PJJ, Stoelinga PJW 1991 The contributing role of condylar resorption to skeletal relapse following mandibular advancement surgery: report of five cases. Journal of Oral and Maxillofacial Surgery 49:448–460

117. Hackney FL, Van Sickels JE, Nummikoski PV 1989 Condylar displacement and temporomandibular joint dysfunction following bilateral sagittal split osteotomy and rigid fixation. Journal of Oral and Maxillofacial Surgery 47:223–227

118. Storum KA, Bell WH 1984 Hypomobility after maxillary and mandibular osteotomies. Oral Surgery 5:7–12

119. Ruggles JE, Hann JR 1984 Antibiotic prophylaxis in intra oral orthognathic surgery. Journal of Oral and Maxillofacial Surgery 42:797–801

120. Gallagher DM, Epker BN 1980 Infection following intra oral surgical correction of dento-facial deformities: a review of 140 consecutive cases. Journal of Oral Surgery 38:117–120

121. Otten JE, Weingart D, Hilger Y, Adam D, Schilli W 1991 Penicillin concentration in the compact bone of the mandible. International Journal of Oral and Maxillofacial Surgery 20:310–312

122. Nader R, Legan HN, Langaland K 1982 Pulp and radicular response to maxillary osteotomy in monkeys. Journal of Oral Surgery 53:624–636

123. Banks P 1977 Pulp changes after anterior sub apical osteotomy in a primate model. Journal of Maxillofacial Surgery 5:39–40

124. Poswillo·DE 1972 Early pulp changes following reduction of open bite by segmental surgery. International Journal of Oral Surgery 1:87–97

125. Kwon HJ, Pihlstrom B, Waite DE 1985 The effects on the periodontium of vertical bone cutting for segmental osteotomy. Journal of Oral and Maxillofacial Surgery 43:952–955

126. Bell WH 1971 Correction of skeletal type of anterior open bite. Journal of Oral Surgery 29:706

127. Dorfman HS, Turvey TA 1979 Alteration in osseous crestal height following intra dental osteotomies. Oral Surgery 48:120

128. Hutchingson D, McGregor AJ 1972 Tooth survival following various methods of sub apical osteotomy. International Journal of Oral Surgery 1:81–86

Revision orthognathic surgery

78

MARK E. MASON/STEPHEN A. SCHENDEL

Studies[1] of individuals who have undergone orthognathic surgery reveal 90–95% of patients are satisfied. A major reason for such high patient satisfaction is that adverse outcomes are rare. Most complications are minor and can be treated conservatively, but some cases need surgical revision. Several surgeons[1–3] have reported small series of patients who required revision orthognathic surgery, but overall data in this area are sparse. Orthognathic surgery has traditionally been revised for functional reasons. In recent years, there has been an increasing awareness on the part of both surgeons and patients of the esthetic aspects of orthognathic surgery. Older individuals are also frequently undergoing treatment. As a result, more patients are having surgery redone for the purpose of improving esthetics.

Surgical revision is necessary after orthognathic surgery because of unacceptable outcomes: these can be broadly classified as functional or esthetic. This chapter will cover the adverse outcomes which most often necessitate surgical revision and emphasize technical points which have proven helpful during revision cases.

MAXILLARY SURGERY

The most common maxillary operation in orthognathic surgery is the Le Fort I osteotomy, either as a single piece or segmentalized. This is the procedure of choice for the correction of vertical facial deformities such as the long and short face syndromes and most skeletal open bites. Obwegeser[4] championed the Le Fort I advancement to correct maxillary retrusion of an idiopathic nature or secondary to cleft lip and palate. However, it was not until Bell[5] demonstrated the biologic basis for the Le Fort I osteotomy and downfracture technique that this procedure became the operation of choice for maxillary deformities. This technique has proved reliable,

and major adverse esthetic and functional outcomes are infrequent.

REVISION FOR ADVERSE FUNCTIONAL OUTCOMES

Occlusal relapse

Occlusal relapse can become evident either in the early postoperative period or much later, and can be dental, skeletal, or both. The tendency for maxillary relapse varies with the attempted movement at the time of surgery. Impaction of the maxilla to correct vertical excess or open-bite deformities is usually very stable and relapse is uncommon.[6–8] Anteroposterior and transverse movements, as well as inferior repositioning of the maxilla, are more prone to skeletal relapse.[7,9–11]

Early relapse, defined as change occurring from the early postoperative period to between 3 and 6 months after surgery, is almost always the result of skeletal instability or incorrect intraoperative jaw positioning. Both of these causative factors are technique driven. Late relapse occurs later than 6 months postoperatively and is the result of complex unbalanced or excessive functional forces. Occlusal changes may be minimal, resulting in minor tooth movement with or without associated periodontal pathology. Conversely, occlusal relapse may be significant and may include skeletal remodeling. Treatment is directed at determining the causes of disequilibrium and correction of these sources.

Maxillary advancement

Revision of maxillary advancement is required if a substantial malocclusion develops because of relapse. Successful maxillary advancement depends on sufficient mobilization of the Le Fort segment to allow passive repositioning and adequate

1321

fixation to promote bony union. Relapse immediately after the release of maxillomandibular fixation is secondary to improper intraoperative positioning of the maxilla, and reoperation is mandatory in most cases. If the occlusal change results in a mild class III tendency, orthopedic protraction forces may be used immediately to correct the maxillary position. Relapse in the early postoperative period occurs when retrusive forces exceed the capacity of the fixation or the fixation is inadequate. Further relapse can sometimes be contained by an anterior orthopedic force device. Interarch elastics can assist in the maintenance of the occlusion but cannot be relied upon as the major retentive factor. Strong elastics can preserve the occlusion while simultaneous movement of the teeth through alveolar bone occurs, further complicating skeletal relapse. Minimal relapse into an edge-to-edge occlusion can be compensated for by postsurgical orthodontic treatment. Late relapse is associated with bone remodeling and tooth movement. Presurgical orthodontic treatment that places the teeth outside of the basal bone will lead to late relapse.[10,12] This most commonly occurs when the maxillary incisors are inclined labially by the presurgical orthodontic treatment. Removal of the fixed orthodontic appliances several months postoperatively allows the teeth to move back to the proper position with a resultant class III malocclusion. This form of dental relapse can be differentiated from skeletal relapse by analysis of postsurgical dental models and cephalometric radiographs. Continued orthodontic force on the maxillary anterior teeth in an attempt to maintain their position will result in periodontal problems and root resorption. Treatment in this scenario may consist of redoing the presurgical orthodontics, placing the teeth over basal bone in the correct angulation, and reoperation of the Le Fort osteotomy.

The maxilla has a tendency to relapse more in a posterior direction with larger anterior movements. Accessory techniques should be employed to ensure stability after revision maxillary advancement, especially when there is a large forward movement. Bone grafting in advancements greater than 6 mm prior to the advent of rigid internal fixation proved advantageous in decreasing the propensity for relapse.[7,9,10] Bone grafting in cases with larger anterior movements is beneficial for the prevention of relapse. Cranial bone is preferred by the authors because of its dense structure and harvest site in the same surgical field. Other surgeons[13] use a period of maxillomandibular fixation after maxillary advancement to diminish the propensity for relapse.

Maxillary setback

Maxillary setback by the anterior maxillary segmental technique is uncommon and has now been superseded by the segmentalized Le Fort I osteotomy. Posterior movement of the maxilla greater than 6 mm using a single piece Le Fort I is difficult technically as bone must be removed from both the tuberosity and the pterygoid areas. Maxillary setback in the range of 6–8 mm is more stable if a Le Fort segmental procedure with extraction of a bicuspid tooth is accomplished. Maxillary setback of this magnitude should be performed with caution however, as the esthetic result of an over-retruded midface is disastrous. Treatment of this adverse outcome is covered in the esthetic section.

Recurrence of a class II malocclusion in the early postoperative period is caused by one of two factors. Seating of the maxilla in preparation for fixation can cause the mandibular condyles to be pulled forward out of the glenoid fossa if insufficient bone has been removed posteriorly. If this is not discovered in the operating room, relapse into a class II malocculsion will ensue immediately in the postoperative period or at the release of fixation. If the pterygoid plates have been fractured during the osteotomies, the maxilla can inadvertently be pushed back farther than anticipated. Rebound will then occur postoperatively and cause a class II discrepancy. Rigid internal fixation has limited this cause of relapse and condylar displacement is now more common. Reoperation for relapse after maxillary setback is straightforward if the etiology of the malocclusion is identified. When the patient is taken back to surgery for maxillary repositioning, four-point rigid fixation is recommended to assure stability.

Maxillary impaction and open-bite

Vertical impaction of the maxilla is very stable and the relapse tendency is most often in the same direction as the desired movement.[7,8,14] Unfortunately, continued upward movement of the maxilla can result in overimpaction. Esthetics more than function will be compromised by overimpaction of the maxilla or excessive surgical retrusion. The most common esthetic problem is the uncontrolled change in the midfacial soft tissues, especially the upper lip and nose. These are covered in the section on esthetic adverse outcomes.

Occlusal relapse after maxillary surgery for the correction of open bite deformities is more common and again can be seen in the immediate or long-term postoperative periods. Immediate open-bite relapse occurs when the mandibular condyles are not seated properly in the glenoid fossae secondary to inadequate posterior maxillary bone resection during the impaction (Fig. 78.1). Reoperation as soon as possible is needed to correct this problem. Late recurrence of the open-bite is most likely dental in nature and not skeletal. Improper presurgical orthodontic treatment or para-

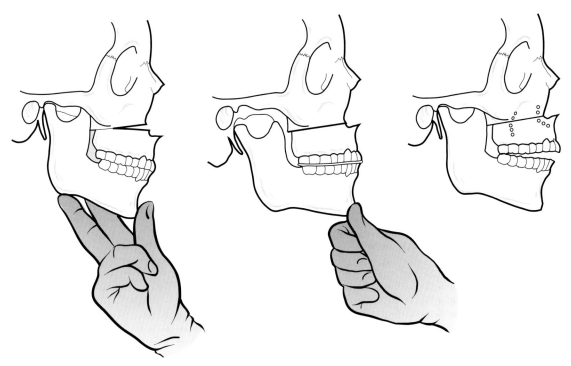

Fig. 78.1 Inadequate reduction of bone from the posterior maxilla can result in distraction of the mandibular condyles from the fossae. If this is not recognized intraoperatively, an open-bite will be present early in the postoperative period. (Reprinted with permission from Bays RA 1997 Complications of orthognathic surgery. In: Kaban LB, Pogrel MA, Perrott DH (eds) Complications in oral and maxillofacial surgery. WB Saunders, Philadelphia)

functional habits are common causes. Preoperative orthodontic expansion of the upper arch when a transverse deficiency is present is a major cause of postoperative relapse.[15] This is usually done in an attempt to prevent the need for segmentalization of the upper jaw. Also, during orthodontic leveling of the maxillary arch in preparation for surgery, the incisors can be excessively extruded resulting in a smaller open-bite deformity. This situation is very prone to relapse, especially after removal of the fixed orthodontic appliances. Parafunctional habits such as tongue thrust also cause late relapse in some patients. Tongue thrust may be eliminated by myofunctional therapy, which usually results in the disappearance of the open-bite. The assistance of an orthodontist may be needed for the fabrication of special appliances. Frolich and co-workers[16] showed diminished tongue pressure after surgical tongue reduction in a group of patients with open-bite deformity, however this should be relegated to cases of true macroglossia only.

Reoperation in patients with an overimpacted maxilla may involve soft-tissue revision only, because a malocclusion is not usually present. Small hardware or even wire osteosynthesis provides adequate fixation for most primary maxillary impactions. If a repeat Le Fort I osteotomy is essential because of an extensive deformity, the surgical movement of the maxilla is the same as for a downgraft procedure. The inferior movement required to lengthen the face at

reoperation necessitates the use of stiffer plates, and bone grafting should be considered.

Maxillary revision in open-bite cases must be done only after the causative factors for relapse have been identified. If distraction of the condyles from the glenoid fossae is not recognized at the time of surgery, reoperation of the maxilla as soon as possible is necessary to properly seat the condyles. Late relapse caused by improper presurgical orthodontics necessitates a more extensive treatment plan including orthodontics prior to returning to the operating room. Preoperative orthodontics must be redone to eliminate excessive extrusion or transverse compensations. Allowing the persistence of extensive orthodontic expansion in an attempt to prevent multiple segmental surgery is setting the patient up for vertical relapse, no matter how rigid the fixation appliances.[15] Myofunctional therapy should be instituted in those with tongue habits.

Inferior repositioning

Inferior repositioning of the upper jaw is the least stable of the maxillary surgical movements. Relapse has been documented[7,8,11] from a minimum of 30% to a maximum of 100% before the introduction of rigid internal fixation. Ellis et al[17] examined the stability of four different fixation techniques after maxillary downgrafting in primates. All groups had relapse, but the most stable in the study had rigid internal fixation of the maxilla. Van Sickels and Tucker[3] demonstrated that, even with rigid fixation, upper jaws surgically repositioned in an inferior direction may undergo vertical impaction after surgery. Factors contributing to this problem include failure to place a bone graft or insertion of an inadequate bone graft, loss of graft, insufficient bone interface, or inadequate fixation. However, there is no doubt that bone grafting and rigid fixation have greatly improved the stability of this procedure. Relapse still remains a problem because of the masticatory forces that drive the maxilla superiorly. Skeletal relapse manifests as vertical shortening of the downgrafted maxilla and may or may not cause an occlusal change. If there is no occlusal change, esthetics will dictate whether a repeat osteotomy is necessary.

Patients who require a second Le Fort I osteotomy to downgraft the maxilla may benefit from bite-opening appliance therapy prior to reoperation. Fixation at the time of revision osteotomy should include rigid plates at four sites combined with bone grafts. Adjunct measures which may assist in maintaining stability include altering osteotomy design, jaw elevator myotomies, periods of maxillomandibular fixation, and the long-term enteral use of muscle relaxants.[8] Botulinum toxin is currently employed for treating facial muscle spasms and masseteric hypertrophy.[18–19] As the use of this toxin becomes more widespread, it may be helpful in temporarily treating the jaw elevator muscles after maxillary downgrafting in those patients who are extremely prone to relapse.

REVISION FOR ADVERSE ESTHETIC OUTCOMES

The final esthetic result after orthognathic surgery is a combination of soft-tissue, skeletal, and dental changes. Adverse esthetic outcomes can be secondary to any one of these factors or a combination of them. Treatment planning is based on the clinical examination, cephalometric radiographs, and dental study models. Over-reliance on cephalometric measurements or concentration only on the malocclusion will result in a less than ideal esthetic result.[12] Whichever cephalometric analysis is used, it should be combined with a soft-tissue analysis. Primary importance should be given to the clinical examination in formulating a sound treatment plan based on esthetic principles. Technical errors in positioning the maxilla result from discrepancies between the prediction tracing (visual treatment objective, VTO) and the actual surgery.[20]

Overimpaction and over-retrusion

The overimpacted maxilla and the over-retruded maxilla are among the most common skeletal base disproportions seen after maxillary surgery. These skeletal discrepancies age the face dramatically.[21,22] The nasolabial angle opens, the nasal tip droops, and widening of the alae occurs. The upper lip is often flat and adynamic. The patient may appear edentulous, with no dental show at rest and very little when smiling. The commonly accepted upper tooth to lip relation is 2–3 mm of anterior tooth show below the upper lip at rest. Overimpaction results when the VTO prediction does not correlate correctly to the soft-tissue changes in the lips. There is a tendency for the upper lip to shorten and lose its normal pout secondary to the facial muscle stripping involved in the Le Fort technique.[22–24] However, these alterations are not predictable, and the variation between cases is large. Thus, in some cases the lip can actually lengthen. Predictable results with maxillary surgery require reconstruction of the lip muscles and perialar muscles simultaneously with the osteotomy (Fig. 78.2). The technique proposed by Schendel[25,26] provides excellent reproducible results by using an alar cinch suture and a V–Y closure of the vestibular incision (Fig. 78.3).

Class II malocclusion and open-bite patients with ver-

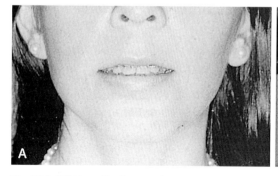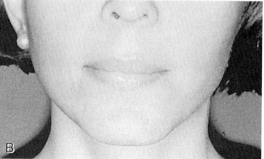

Fig. 78.2 (A) Upper lip changes after Le Fort I osteotomy without adequate muscle reconstruction. The upper lip is thin and flat with loss of vermilion. **(B)** Upper lip after revision with temporalis fascia augmentation and lateral skin triangle excisions at the corners. (Reprinted with permission from Schendel SA, Mason ME 1997 Adverse outcomes in orthognathic surgery and management of residual problems. Clinics in Plastic Surgery 24:489–505)

tical maxillary excess may have discrepancy between centric occlusion (CO) and centric relation (CR) that is not easily determined preoperatively without prior splint therapy. Thus, the preoperative cephalometric radiograph may be accidentally taken with the condyles not seated in the glenoid fossae but rather forward. A VTO based on this radiograph will not be accurate and will underestimate the amount of maxillary retrusion necessary to correct the class II malocclusion. This results in an over-retruded maxilla and a dished-in face postoperatively.

Revision for an over-retruded or overimpacted maxilla in most cases necessitates reoperation with the goal of advancing the maxilla and lengthening it.[1] If the patient at this time has a class I occlusion, then a concomitant mandibular advancement will also be needed. Simple onlaying of the maxilla is not as effective as reversing the primary procedure.[1] The skeletally normal maxilla with no tooth show is a more difficult problem. Minimal lip to tooth disproportions can be corrected or camouflaged by lip surgery. The upper lip lift has been used for shortening the upper lip that has lengthened because of aging.[27–29] A variation of this procedure was used by Jeter & Nishioka[30] for camouflaging iatrogenic vertical maxillary deficiency after orthognathic surgery (Fig. 78.4). This technique provides more

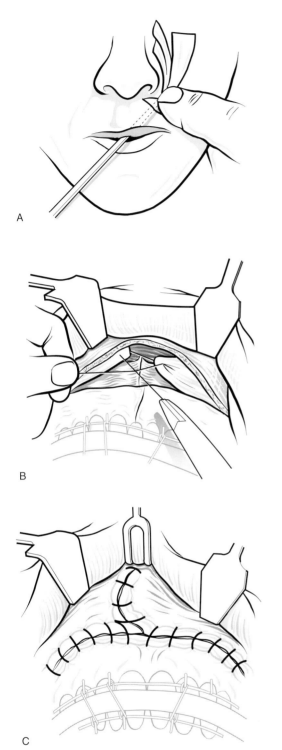

Fig. 78.3 Muscle reconstruction after Le Fort I osteotomy includes an alar cinch suture and V–Y closure of the vestibular incision. **(A)** After the maxilla has been stabilized, the nasolabial muscles detached from the piriform region are retrieved via a skin hook through a vestibular incision. **(B)** The two muscle groups are sutured together with a non-resorbable suture. **(C)** A V–Y closure of the mucosa and underlying muscles is then completed by taking a small bite of mucosa with the needle and a larger bite of the muscle. (Reprinted with permission from Mason ME, Schendel SA 1996 Perioral procedures as an adjunct to orthognathic surgery. Oral and Maxillofacial Surgical Clinics of North America 8:95–110)

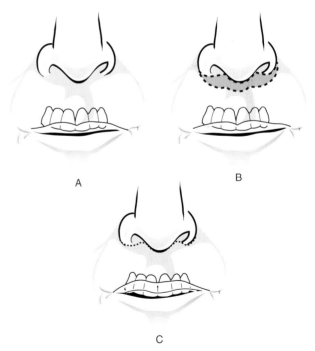

Fig. 78.4 Mild cases of maxillary overimpaction may be treated with a lip lift as described by Jeter and Nishioka. **(A)** Depiction of the upper lip with inadequate maxillary incisor show. **(B)** A wavy ellipse is marked on the upper lip below the nasal base. **(C)** Excision of the soft-tissue ellipse shortens the upper lip and leaves an inconspicuous scar. (Reprinted with permission from Mason ME, Schendel SA 1996 Perioral procedures as an adjunct to orthognathic surgery. Oral and Maxillofacial Surgical Clinics of North America 8:95–110)

exposure of the upper teeth and everts the vermilion, thereby establishing a more youthful appearance to the upper lip. A wavy ellipse is marked on the skin of the upper lip just beneath and following the contours of the base of the nose. The amount of lip lifting is determined by the width of the ellipse. The ellipse of skin is then excised with a slight reverse bevel. Jeter[30] and Cardoso[31] favor excision of skin and orbicularis oris muscle while Austin[27] prefers skin excision only.

Overcorrection by one third is recommended[28] due to 'redroop' of the upper lip postoperatively. This may be necessary with Austin's technique since only skin and no muscle is resected. Mild maxillary retrusion, usually seen as paranasal flattening, can be corrected simply by paranasal maxillary onlay augmentation with either autologous or alloplastic materials.[21]

Open-bite

Occasionally, there are discrepancies between the VTO measured impaction and that on the surgical dental study models.[32] This is most frequently seen in the correction of skeletal open-bite cases using segmental maxillary osteotomies. In some cases, after the correction of an open-bite deformity, an excessive amount of tooth exposure may be seen postoperatively and is associated with bilabial incompetence. In the vast majority of cases, this problem is caused either by an error in treatment planning or by surgical technique. The excessive tooth show and bilabial incompetence may be the result of unpredictable upper lip shortening or actual elongation of the maxilla because of inadequate posterior vertical reduction. Accurate model surgery is essential in avoiding this problem. Reoperation of the maxilla is the treatment when esthetics are severely compromised. Postoperative open bite deformities also necessitate reoperation of the maxilla, and almost every patient must be refitted with orthodontic appliances by the orthodontist.

Adverse soft-tissue changes

Unesthetic facial soft-tissue changes can occur following the Le Fort I osteotomy and may involve the nose, lips, and cheeks.[24] Widening of the alar bases is routinely seen with maxillary surgery and can even be asymmetric with loss of the alar-facial groove (Fig. 78.5). Alar base widening is acceptable in some noses, especially those that were originally thin.[21] With maxillary impaction and advancement, the nasal tip can also turn up, resulting in nasal shortening and a 'Miss Piggy' nose. These changes can be prevented by the alar cinch and V–Y vestibular mucosal–muscular closure described previously by Schendel.[25,26] Alteration of the caudal

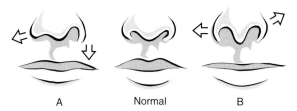

Fig. 78.5 Nasal widening is almost universal after Le Fort I osteotomy if the soft tissues are not reconstructed. **(A)** With maxillary inferior repositioning, the nasal tip and alar bases tend to be pulled down and the change may be asymmetric. **(B)** Asymmetric alar base changes may also occur after maxillary impaction or advancement. (Reprinted with permission from Schendel SA, Mason ME 1997 Adverse outcomes in orthognathic surgery and management of residual problems. Clinics in Plastic Surgery 24: 489–505)

septum, anterior nasal spine, and piriform rims can also prevent the nasal base from turning up.[25] Nasal changes that are unesthetic following a Le Fort osteotomy require a formal rhinoplasty and sometimes alar base reduction.[21]

There are also adverse upper lip changes associated with the nasal changes. These include loss of vermilion border, thinning of the lip, and downturning of the corners of the mouth.[22,26] These are secondary to the lateral movement of the lip muscles when their insertions are elevated during surgery. Again, the best result is obtained if these are reconstructed at the time of surgery. Revision for residual thin lips involves augmentation grafting of the vermilion area. Multiple V–Y or Z-plasties on the lip have little effect on the amount of vermilion show in these cases and should be avoided. Dermal and fat grafts may be used for augmentation but are less predictable because of resorption. Submucosal grafts of temporalis fascia and galea provide a more permanent augmentation (Figs 78.2 and 78.6). After harvesting, the grafts are fashioned to correspond with the areas of the upper lip which need most augmentation. Grafts can be placed through two small upper lip incisions into a tunnel created by blunt submucosal dissection.[33] Temporalis fascia can also be placed through a longer incision such as the upper lip incision made for vermilion advancement.[21] The upper lip fullness obtained with temporalis fascia grafts appears to be long-lasting, with only 15–20% shrinkage reported.[34,35] The corners of the mouth can be elevated by small elliptical skin excisions laterally at the white roll. Austin[28] developed the corner lift to correct the downturned commissures of the mouth which were the result of an overdone lip lift. Patients who have downturned oral commissures as an adverse effect of maxillary surgery also benefit from this procedure. The corner lift is started by making a dot at each commissure and then tracing a triangle with one limb extending medially along the skin–vermilion junction, one limb extending laterally

the resting lip posture is normal, the smile asymmetry is most likely caused by the muscle positions following closure of the vestibular incision or scarring. Revision of the maxillary vestibular scar usually corrects this. Lip asymmetry at rest and during smiling is an indication of a canted occlusal plane and an underlying skeletal asymmetry. Correction of this problem requires a repeat osteotomy, usually of both jaws.

MANDIBULAR SURGERY

Functional adverse outcomes are more common and problematic in the mandible than esthetic adverse outcomes. The temporomandibular joint is the main reason for this difference, since almost all surgery on the mandible involves potential changes to the joint. The most common mandibular osteotomy other than the genioplasty is the sagittal split ramus osteotomy (SSRO) popularized by Obwegeser. This osteotomy has undergone several modifications since its introduction. Intraoral vertical oblique osteotomies are occasionally done for the correction of prognathism. Other procedures such as the inverted-L, extraoral vertical oblique, and body osteotomies are infrequently performed.

REVISION FOR ADVERSE FUNCTIONAL OUTCOMES

Occlusal relapse

Mandibular advancement

Occlusal relapse is secondary to skeletal and dental movements and can occur early or late. Mandibular advancement is the lower jaw procedure most prone to relapse; the rate of relapse ranges from 20–50% in multiple reports.[36–39] The tendency to relapse increases with larger mandibular advancements.[39,40] Rigid internal fixation of SSRO advancement is associated with improved stability and no proven increase in postoperative symptoms.[41,42] Immediate postoperative relapse of the mandible is seen when the condyle has not been properly seated in the glenoid fossa intraoperatively.[36] This can be either unilateral or bilateral, and a revision operation should be done as soon as possible to reseat the condyle correctly in the fossa. Rigid internal fixation allows the surgeon to check the occlusion intraoperatively and thus condylar distraction can usually be avoided. Overseating of the mandibular condyle may lead to excessive postoperative preauricular pain, TMJ clicking,

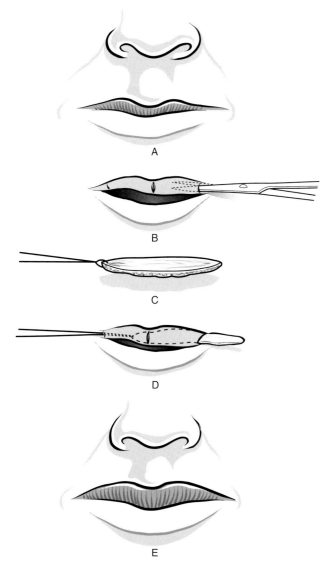

Fig. 78.6 The upper lip can be augmented with temporalis fascia or dermis. **(A)** Thin upper lip. **(B)** Three vertical incisions are made in the vermilion, and submucosal tunneling between them is performed. **(C)** Fascia or dermal grafts should be 20% larger than the desired end result. **(D)** Graft is pulled through the submucosal pocket and the incisions are closed. **(E)** Final result. (Reprinted with permission from Schendel SA, Mason ME 1997 Adverse outcomes in orthognathic surgery and management of residual problems. Clinics in Plastic Surgery 24:489–505)

toward the top of the ear stopping short of the nasolabial crease, and the final limb connecting the two previously drawn ones. The height of the triangle determines the amount the commissure will be lifted. The triangle of skin is then excised and the skin edges closed primarily.

Lateral movement of the central facial musculature results in lateral fullness in the lower cheek area and can accentuate the nasolabial groove. This problem is difficult to correct and may require a facelift or malar fat pad elevation. Occasionally an asymmetric smile may be seen postsurgically. If

and possibly decreased opening if the disk has been dislocated. Overzealous seating of the mandibular condyle can also result in a class III malocclusion, although this is unusual. This condition can usually be managed conservatively by splints and physiotherapy. Unfavorable bony splits are unusual with the SSRO technique, but when they occur it is common to have significant problems stabilizing the osseous segments. An increased propensity for later skeletal relapse may be the end result and necessitate reoperation.

Revision for significant occlusal relapse after mandibular advancement essentially involves repeating the original operation. Old fixation devices must be removed and osteotomies are more difficult because of altered bony anatomy and soft-tissue scar formation. Rigid fixation should be applied and auxiliary techniques should be considered to diminish the chances of relapse.

Mandibular setback

This is less of a problem when the SSRO is used for mandibular setback, however mandibular setback surgery is prone to a type of rebound relapse seen soon after the release of maxillomandibular fixation or guiding elastics. Posterior rotation of the mandibular proximal segments or compression of the condyles into the fossae during fixation are the probable causes. Reoperation is necessary in all cases except those with minimal occlusal changes. Condylar sag can lead to postoperative open-bite when the vertical oblique ramus osteotomy is used for setback of the mandible. Early treatment with interarch elastics in the first 2–5 weeks can usually correct this. Without early aggressive orthodontic treatment, the open-bite will require correction with an osteotomy.

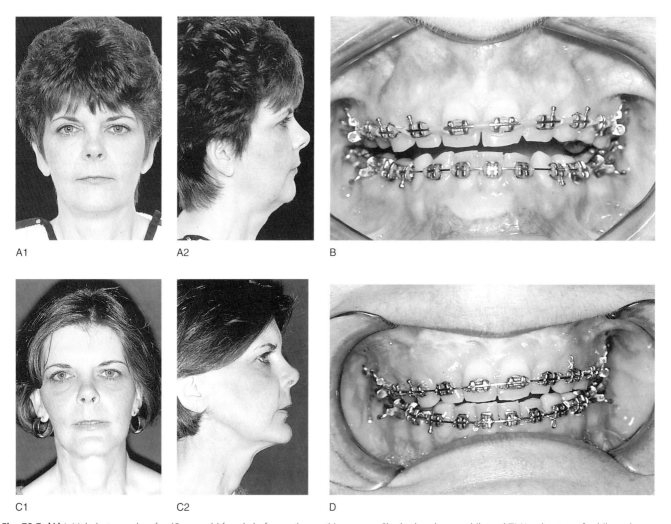

A1   A2   B

C1   C2   D

Fig. 78.7 (A) Initial photographs of a 42-year-old female before orthognathic surgery. She had undergone bilateral TMJ arthrotomy for bilateral internal derangement 17 months earlier at an outside institution. **(B)** Initial preoperative occlusion. **(C)** Postoperative photographs after the patient underwent maxillomandibular advancement and genioplasty twice at an outside institution. Both jaws relapsed after the first procedure and it was repeated 3 ½ months later. Progressive condylar resorption (PCR) developed after the second procedure. **(D)** Occlusion after the second maxillomandibular advancement and genioplasty.

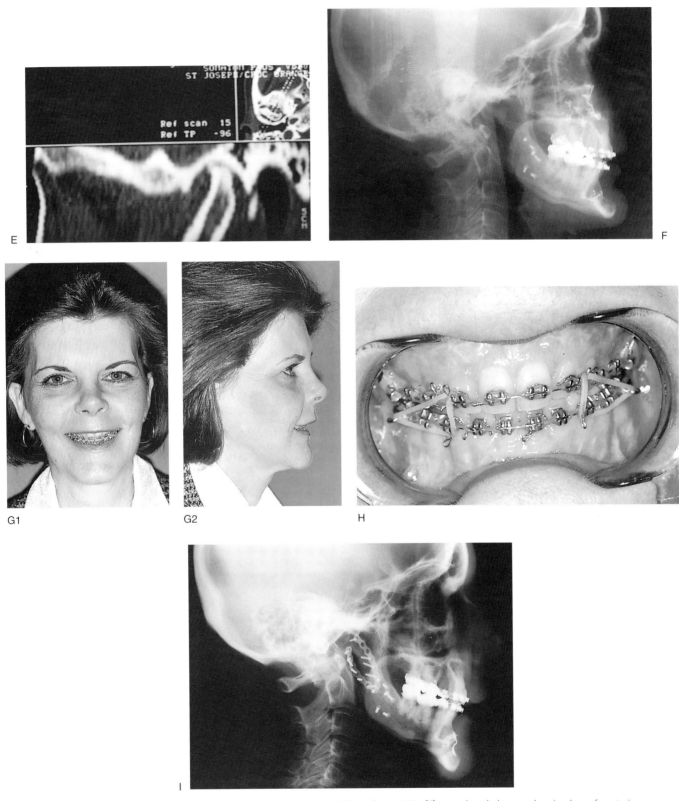

Fig. 78.7(cont'd) **(E)** MRI of the left TMJ showing abnormal condyle morphology due to PCR. **(F)** Lateral cephalogram showing loss of posterior facial height and a developing class II occlusion with anterior open-bite. **(G)** Postoperative photographs 6 months after surgical revision at our institution. The procedure was done nearly 2 years after the previous orthognathic surgery and included bilateral TMJ reconstruction with costochondral grafts placed via an intraoral approach, osteoplasty of left zygoma, removal of maxillary hardware, upper lip augmentation with fascia grafts, rhinoplasty, and revision genioplasty to lengthen and reposition the chin posteriorly. **(H)** Postoperative occlusion was stable at 6 months. Three years after the TMJ reconstruction this patient has maintained a class I occlusion and excellent function. **(I)** Postoperative lateral cephalogram at 6 months shows restoration of posterior facial height and a class I occlusion.

Asymmetry

Rotational movements of the mandible to correct mandibular asymmetry or deviate prognathism can result in a postoperative crossbite or mandibulomaxillary midline discrepancy. Muscle forces are the usual cause, and training elastics or rarely functional appliances are needed to correct the problem. Transverse relapse in the mandible is less problematic than in the maxilla. When transverse relapse is present it is most likely dental and associated with the maxillary arch.

Progressive condylar resorption

Progressive condylar resorption (PCR) following orthognathic surgery is a devastating problem that is very difficult to treat. It has been defined as a change in condylar shape from a normal to a finger-shaped morphology (Fig. 78.7).[43-47] This is accompanied by condylar shortening, a decrease in posterior facial height, and clockwise rotation of the mandible.[43-47] Occlusal relapse and development of an open bite are the end results (Fig. 78.7).[45] The etiology is multifactorial and the process has a predilection for young women with class II malocclusion, high mandibular plane angle, and pre-existing TMJ dysfunction.[44,47,48] Maxillomandibular fixation has also been implicated – Bouwman and co-workers[49] found a 24% incidence of condylar resorption in cases following maxillomandibular fixation and only 11.9% in patients treated without. Merkx & Van Damme[50] re-treated 8 of 329 patients following sagittal split osteotomies while Kerstens and associates[48] found 12 of 206 patients who had what was termed 'condylar atrophy' after mandibular advancement. The term 'aseptic necrosis' is occasionally used for this condition; this term should be avoided as it is too limiting and does not necessarily describe the cause of the deformity. The typical scenario involves the progressive development of a class II malocclusion starting several months after surgery. The postoperative complaints in the study by Merkx et al[50] started 7.5 months after surgery and stabilized at 27 months on average. The condylar resorption is almost always bilateral but may be asynchronous, starting first on one side and then on the other side some time later. The involvement may last one to two years before the joints and occlusion stabilize. The course of PCR is not completely understood because some patients exhibit a continuous resorption which eventually 'burns out' while others show resorption that stops periodically but then recurs. The end-point of PCR occurs when the condyle is resorbed to the sigmoid notch.[46]

A bone scan with technetium-99m methylene diphosphonate has been useful in some patients to determine if the resorptive process is stable or ongoing.[46] Bone scans are not likely to be helpful however in patients who have PCR that stops spontaneously and starts again later. Progressive radiographic changes are also seen in the cephalometric and joint films.

Treatment during the active phase of condylar resorption should be conservative consisting of splint therapy and analgesics. No active fixed orthodontic treatment should be undertaken at this time, especially closure of an open bite. Chasing a developing malocclusion with orthodontics will result in severe periodontal problems, possible root resorption, and an even more unstable occlusion. Unwanted orthodontic movements must be reversed prior to surgical correction. No surgical treatment should be undertaken until the jaw has been stable for a minimum of 6 months. Unfortunately, reoperation for PCR has been generally unsatisfactory. Merkx and co-workers[50] repeated osteotomies on 4 patients because of functional and esthetic complaints. The 3 patients who underwent a repeat sagittal split operation developed renewed TMJ disorders within 3.5 months and eventually had relapse of the overjet. The patient who underwent a Le Fort I had only minor postoperative complaints but did also have some changes in overbite. Arnett & Tamborello[43] reported on an additional 4 patients, 2 of whom had further skeletal relapse secondary to PCR. Crawford et al[44] reported on 7 patients who underwent reoperation for this problem – 5 developed further PCR, although 5 of the 7 had a successful result if occlusion was judged to be the main criterion. Some surgeons prefer maxillary procedures such as the Le Fort I osteotomy as the secondary procedure as they are considered more stable than mandibular procedures. Unfortunately, not all patients are candidates for maxillary surgery to correct the residual occlusal disharmony. The best candidates are those with a mild class II malocclusion and skeletal open-bite. A Le Fort I impaction with anterior autorotation of the mandible should easily correct this mild form of PCR.

Temporomandibular joint reconstruction, instead of/or in addition to orthognathic surgery, may be required in some cases of advanced PCR. Autogenous grafts or alloplastic joint replacements have been used to reconstruct the TMJ. Huang and co-workers[46] studied 22 patients who underwent reoperation for PCR. Five of their patients had condylectomy with costochondral grafting and all showed excellent stability and minimal symptoms at 24 months postoperatively. No study has validated the long-term success of prosthetic joint replacement in cases of advanced PCR.

In summary, some cases of PCR with mild occlusal changes can be treated with orthodontics or prosthetics and have an acceptable result without the risk of reactivating the PCR. Condylar resorption of a lesser magnitude can be successfully treated with orthognathic surgery if the condyles are stable as determined by clinical examination, radiographs, and possibly bone scans.[46] Repeat jaw surgery is best limited to the maxilla when possible. In those patients with advanced condylar resorption with shortened posterior facial height and worsening retrognathism, TMJ reconstruction is usually necessary. Costochondral grafting via an intraoral approach or through extraoral incisions is the treatment of choice for reconstructing the TMJ and restoring posterior facial height (Fig. 78.7).

REVISION FOR ADVERSE ESTHETIC OUTCOMES

The structure of the lower lip and chin is less complex than that of the upper lip and nose. For this reason, adverse esthetic outcomes are less common with mandibular procedures as compared to maxillary procedures.

Skeletal base disproportion

Obwegeser & Marentette[12] emphasized the importance of the three bases of the facial skeletal framework in treatment planning for orthognathic surgery. The profile is a better guide than the occlusion for construction of the VTO. It is important to achieve proper occlusion, but poor esthetics may result if occlusion only is considered and not the skeletal bases.[39] Preoperative orthodontics should align the lower dentition to the mandibular skeletal base and not to the opposing arch.

Mandibular angle and body

Superior rotation of the mandibular proximal segment after SSRO adversely affects esthetics. Many patients undergoing jaw surgery already have a short posterior facial height. Proximal segment rotation leads to the undesirable loss of gonial angle definition. A noticeable notching in the mandibular body area can also develop in thin individuals. These problems are easily prevented by proper positioning and adequate stabilization of the osteotomy segments at the time of surgery.[51] Correction of lost gonial angle definition includes reoperation and repositioning of the proximal segments or alloplastic augmentation for cosmetic improvement.[51] Late treatment of notching in the mandibular body area is difficult and involves placement of a custom alloplastic implant or bone graft. Repeating the osteotomy and repositioning the proximal segment would also correct this problem.

Anterior mandible

Ptosis of the lower lip and chin is the most common esthetic problem of symphyseal surgery or genioplasty.[51] When genioplasty is done via an osteotomy, the anterior mandibular soft tissues are degloved to provide access to the bone. If the anterior dissection is carried below the mandibular inferior border and the mentalis muscles are not reattached at their normal level during closure, lower lip and chin ptosis may occur.[52,53] The normal level for the mentalis muscles is at the junction of the free mucosa and attached gingiva.[51]

Late correction of this problem involves repeating the anterior mandibular degloving through the same vestibular incision and repositioning the mentalis muscles in a more cephalad position. Zide & McCarthy[53] recommend reattaching the mentalis muscles to the anterior mandible by passing non-absorbable sutures through the muscles and then through holes placed in the alveolar bone. Ancillary procedures may also be needed to correct vestibular scarring.

Failure to correct presurgical vertical hyperplasia of the chin may result in lip incompetence after genioplasty.[54] Excessive vertical lengthening of the bony chin yields the same problem. Lip incompetence is obvious when mentalis strain is present during lip closure. A revision genioplasty with vertical shortening of the chin will correct lip incompetency.

Overshortening the chin in the vertical direction or failure to correct a short chin will also adversely affect esthetics. An excessively deep labiomental groove and even lower lip eversion can result (Fig. 78.8). During advancement genioplasty, inadvertent vertical shortening can result as the chin slides forward along the angle of the lateral osteotomies. This is especially true if short bone cuts are made with a steep angle. To help eliminate this vertical shortening and a 'witch's chin' deformity, osteotomies should be made as parallel to the inferior border as possible and should extend posteriorly to at least the first molar region. Long bone cuts will also prevent a noticeable notching along the inferior border that occurs with short, steep osteotomies.[55]

Failure to achieve the desired soft-tissue change after bony chin surgery may be due to poor treatment planning or technical error. With advancement genioplasty, the soft-tissue to bone ratio is approximately 1:1. However, Van Sickels[56] and others[57] found that with advancements greater than 8 mm, the soft-tissue to bone ratio decreased to less than 1:1. They also noted that the soft tissue tends to thicken with vertical shortening of the chin. Conversely, when the chin is lengthened vertically, soft tissues tend to thin.[56] The average thickness of soft tissue overlying the symphysis is greater in males as compared to females, and thickness increases with age.[58] These facts should be remembered during the treatment planning phase.

The versatility of genioplasty using a broad soft-tissue pedicle was emphasized by Bell and Gallagher.[59] Relapse after advancement genioplasty is due to resorption of bone

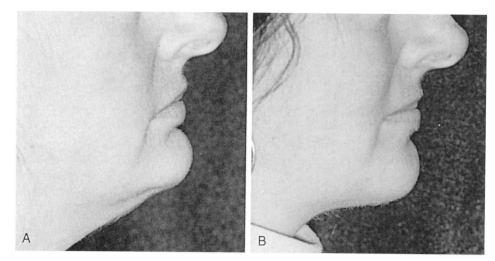

Fig. 78.8 (A) This patient had a sagittal split mandibular advancement for a class II deep bite malocclusion. The chin is overadvanced and vertically short. **(B)** A genioplasty with osteotomy and interpositional bone grafting to lengthen the chin corrected the deformity. (Reprinted with permission from Schendel SA, Mason ME 1997 Adverse outcomes in orthognathic surgery and management of residual problems. Clinics in Plastic Surgery 24:489–505)

rather than fragment instability. Excessive stripping of the soft tissues from the symphysis during the dissection should be avoided as it leads to greater bony resorption along the anterior surface of the genial segment.[56,60] Likewise, excessive or complete stripping of the soft tissues increases the risk of infection and may even result in avascular necrosis of the genial segment.

Asymmetry after genioplasty is usually caused by technical error. Failure to mark the midline of the symphysis may result in asymmetry in the transverse plane. Asymmetry in a transverse and vertical direction may be caused by uneven lateral bone cuts. The mental foramen is commonly used as a landmark for marking the lateral osteotomies. However, the superoinferior position of the mental foramen may vary on each side of the mandible, hence causing asymmetry of the lateral osteotomies. Bony recontouring may be sufficient for the correction of a mild chin asymmetry, however repeating the osteotomy provides a more predictable outcome for significant postgenioplasty asymmetries.

BIMAXILLARY SURGERY

All adverse outcomes possible with isolated maxillary or mandibular procedures may be compounded in bimaxillary surgery. Most of the literature assessing stability in this type of surgery has shown the maxilla to be relatively stable and the mandible to have a greater tendency to relapse.[7,14,52]

A major problem that may develop from simultaneous mobilization of the maxilla and mandible is facial asymmetry which may result from torquing of the maxilla or mandible and canting of the occlusal plane.[51] Uneven mandibular proximal segment rotations and malposition of the inferior fragment of a genioplasty have been discussed above and are also causes of facial asymmetry.

A more obscure form of asymmetry, that is horizontal may develop as a result of inaccurate model surgery. If the posterior maxilla is rotated to one side excessively during maxillary surgery, the mandible will follow because it occludes with the maxilla after mandibular surgery (Fig. 78.9).[32]

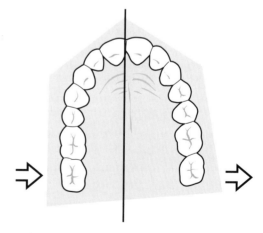

Fig. 78.9 A dental model demonstrates how facial asymmetry can be produced during bimaxillary surgery even though the maxillary and mandibular dental midlines coincide with the facial midline. If the posterior maxilla is rotated to one side, the mandible will follow because of the occlusion. The resultant facial asymmetry is easily noticed as greater fullness on one side of the face. (Reprinted with permission from Schendel SA, Mason ME 1997 Adverse outcomes in orthognathic surgery and management of residual problems. Clinics in Plastic Surgery 24:489–505)

These patients may have preservation of the facial and dental midlines but appear fuller on one side of the face. Commonly, one mandibular angle protrudes laterally more than the other. Ellis[32] described a more accurate method of model surgery which helps to prevent this discrepancy. Late correction may involve recontouring of the more prominent gonial angle from an intraoral approach. A more severe discrepancy might require revision of the osteotomies.

Asymmetry in the vertical plane is made evident by a difference in the vertical position of the maxillary molars on each side. This cant of the maxillary occlusal plane will produce a similar cant of the mandibular occlusal plane. Orthodontics may be able to correct a mild cant of the occlusal plane. Reoperation is necessary if an occlusal plane cant causes significant facial asymmetry.

SUMMARY

Complications after orthognathic surgery that require a revision procedure are rare. Traditionally, revision after orthognathic surgery has been done for functional reasons. In recent years, more patients are having surgery redone to improve esthetics. As a rule, revision orthognathic surgery is more challenging technically and results are less predictable. All factors which might adversely affect the outcome after orthognathic surgery should be eliminated before the initial operation, and a sound treatment plan emphasizing both function and esthetics should be developed. This will minimize the need for reoperation in most patients.

REFERENCES

1. Freihofer HPM 1993 Reversing segmental osteotomies of the upper jaw. Plastic and Reconstructive Surgery 96:86–92
2. Schendel SA, Mason ME 1997 Adverse outcomes in orthognathic surgery and management of residual problems. Clinics in Plastic Surgery 24:489–505
3. Van Sickels JE, Tucker MR 1990 Management of delayed union and nonunion of maxillary osteotomies. Journal of Oral and Maxillofacial Surgery 48:1039–1044
4. Obwegeser H 1969 Surgical correction of small or retrodisplaced maxillae. Plastic and Reconstructive Surgery 43:351–365
5. Bell WH, Fonseca RJ, Kennedy JW, Levy BM 1975 Bone healing and revascularization after total maxillary osteotomy. Journal of Oral Surgery 33:253–260
6. Schendel SA, Eisenfeld JH, Bell WH et al 1976 Superior repositioning of the maxilla: Stability and soft tissue osseous relations. American Journal of Orthodontics 70:663–674
7. Welch TB 1989 Stability in the correction of dentofacial deformities: A comprehensive review. Journal of Oral and Maxillofacial Surgery 47:1142–1149
8. Richardson DA, Van Sickels JS 1996 Stability of orthognathic surgery: A review of rigid fixation. British Journal of Oral and Maxillofacial Surgery 34:279–285
9. Araujo A, Schendel SA, Wolford LM, Epker BN 1978 Total maxillary advancement with and without bone grafting. Journal of Oral Surgery 36:849–858
10. Carlotti AE, Schendel SA 1987 An analysis of factors influencing stability of surgical advancement of the maxilla by Le Fort I osteotomy. Journal of Oral and Maxillofacial Surgery 45:924–928
11. Quejada JG, Bell WH, Hiroshi K, Kawamura K, Zhang X 1987 Skeletal stability after inferior maxillary repositioning. International Journal of Adult Orthodontic and Orthognathic Surgery 2:67–74
12. Obwegeser HL, Marentette LJ 1986 Profile planning based on alterations in the positions of the bases of the facial thirds. Journal of Oral and Maxillofacial Surgery 44:302–311
13. Luyk NH, Ward-Booth RB 1985 The stability of Le Fort I advancement osteotomies using bone plates without bone grafts. Journal of Maxillofacial Surgery 13:250–253
14. Satrom KD, Sinclair PM, Wolford LM 1991 The stability of double jaw surgery: A comparison of rigid versus wire fixation. American Journal of Orthodontics and Dentofacial Orthopedics 99:550–563
15. Haymond CS, Stoelinga PJW, Blijdorp PA, Leenen RJ, Merkens NM 1991 Surgical orthodontic treatment of anterior skeletal open bite using small plate internal fixation. One to five year follow-up. International Journal of Oral and Maxillofacial Surgery 20:223–227
16. Frolich K, Ingervall B, Schmoker R 1993 Influence of surgical tongue reduction on pressure from the tongue on the teeth. Angle Orthodontist 63:191–198
17. Ellis E, Carlson DS, Frydenlund S 1989 Stability of midface augmentation: An experimental study of musculoskeletal interaction and fixation methods. Journal of Oral and Maxillofacial Surgery 47:1062–1068
18. Schantz EJ, Johnson EA 1997 Botulinum toxin: The story of its development for the treatment of human disease. Perspectives in Biology and Medicine 40:317–327
19. Smyth AG 1994 Botulinum treatment of bilateral masseteric hypertrophy. British Journal of Oral and Maxillofacial Surgery 32:29–33
20. Ellis E, Tharanon W, Gambrell K 1992 Accuracy of facebow transfer: Effect on surgical prediction and postsurgical result. Journal of Oral and Maxillofacial Surgery 50:562–567
21. Mason ME, Schendel SA 1996 Perioral procedures as an adjunct to orthognathic surgery. Oral and Maxillofacial Surgical Clinics of North America 8:95–110
22. O'Ryan F, Schendel SA 1989 Nasal anatomy and maxillary surgery. II. Unfavorable nasolabial esthetics following the Le Fort I osteotomy. International Journal of Adult Orthodontic and Orthognathic Surgery 4:75–85
23. O'Ryan F, Schendel S 1989 Nasal anatomy and maxillary surgery. I. Esthetic and anatomic principles. International Journal of Adult Orthodontic and Orthognathic Surgery 4:27–37
24. Schendel SA, Carlotti AE 1991 Nasal considerations in orthognathic surgery. American Journal of Orthodontics and Dentofacial Orthopedics 100:197–208
25. O'Ryan F, Schendel S, Carlotti A 1989 Nasal anatomy and maxillary surgery. III. Surgical techniques for correction of nasal deformities in patients undergoing maxillary surgery. International Journal of Adult Orthodontic and Orthognathic Surgery 4:157–175
26. Schendel SA, Williamson LW 1983 Muscle reorientation following superior repositioning of the maxilla. Journal of Oral and Maxillofacial Surgery 41:235–240
27. Austin HW 1991 Cosmetic surgery of the aging mouth. Virginia Medical Quarterly 118:110–111
28. Austin HW, Weston GW 1992 Rejuvenation of the aging mouth. Clinics in Plastic Surgery 19:511–524
29. Kesselring UK 1986 Rejuvenation of the lips. Annals of Plastic Surgery 16:480–486
30. Jeter TS, Nishioka GJ 1988 The lip lift: An alternative corrective

procedure for iatrogenic vertical maxillary deficiency. Journal of Oral and Maxillofacial Surgery 46:323–325

31. Cardoso AD, Sperli AE 1971 Rhytidoplasty of the upper lip. In: Hueston JT (ed) Transactions of the Fifth International Congress of Plastic and Reconstructive Surgery. Butterworth, Melbourne, pp 1127–1129

32. Ellis E 1990 Accuracy of model surgery: Evaluation of an old technique and introduction of a new one. Journal of Oral and Maxillofacial Surgery 48:1161–1167

33. Lassus C 1992 Surgical vermilion augmentation: Different possibilities. Aesthetic Plastic Surgery 16:123–127

34. Chen PK, Noordhoff S, Chen YR, Bendor-Samuel R 1995 Augmentation of the free border of the lip in cleft lip patients using temporalis fascia. Plastic and Reconstructive Surgery 95:781–788

35. Miller TA 1988 Temporalis fascia grafts for facial and nasal contour augmentation. Plastic and Reconstructive Surgery 81:524–533

36. Schendel SA, Epker BN 1980 Results after mandibular advancement surgery: An analysis of 87 cases. Journal of Oral Surgery 38:265–282

37. Van Sickels JE, Larsen AJ, Thrash WJ 1986 Relapse after rigid fixation of mandibular advancement. Journal of Oral and Maxillofacial Surgery 44:698–702

38. Van Sickels JE, Larsen AJ, Thrash WJ 1988 A retrospective study of relapse in rigidly fixated sagittal split osteotomies: Contributing factors. American Journal of Orthodontics and Dentofacial Orthopedics 93:413–418

39. Will LA, West RA 1989 Factors influencing the stability of the sagittal split osteotomy for mandibular advancement. Journal of Oral and Maxillofacial Surgery 47:813–818

40. Gassmann CJ, Van Sickels JE, Thrash WJ 1990 Causes, location, and timing of relapse following rigid fixation after mandibular advancement. Journal of Oral and Maxillofacial Surgery 48:450–454

41. Flynn B, Brown DT, Lapp TH, Bussard DA, Roberts WE 1990 A comparative study of temporomandibular symptoms following mandibular advancement by bilateral sagittal split osteotomies: Rigid versus nonrigid fixation. Oral Surgery 70:372–380

42. Timmis DP, Aragon SB, Van Sickels JE 1986 Masticatory dysfunction with rigid and nonrigid osteosynthesis of sagittal split osteotomies. Oral Surgery 62:119–123

43. Arnett GW, Tamborello JA 1990 Progressive Class II development: Female idiopathic condylar resorption. Oral and Maxillofacial Surgical Clinics of North America 2:699–716

44. Crawford JG, Stoelinga PJ, Blijdorp PA, Brouns JA 1994 Stability after reoperation for progressive condylar resorption after orthognathic surgery: Report of seven cases. Journal of Oral and Maxillofacial Surgery 52:460–466

45. Moore KE, Gooris PJ, Stoelinga PJ 1991 The contributing role of condylar resorption to skeletal relapse following mandibular advancement surgery: Report of five cases. Journal of Oral and Maxillofacial Surgery 49:448–460

46. Huang YL, Pogrel MA, Kaban LB 1997 Diagnosis and management of condylar resorption. Journal of Oral and Maxillofacial Surgery 55:114–119

47. Cutbirth MA, Van Sickels JE 1995 Condylar resorption after orthognathic surgery in patients with preoperative signs and symptoms of temporomandibular dysfunction. (Abstract). Journal of Oral and Maxillofacial Surgery 53 (suppl 4):128

48. Kerstens HC, Tuinzing DB, Golding RP, van der Kwast WA 1990 Condylar atrophy and osteoarthrosis after bimaxillary surgery. Oral Surgery 69:274–280

49. Bouwman JP, Kerstens HC, Tuinzing DB 1994 Condylar resorption in orthognathic surgery: The role of intermaxillary fixation. Oral Surgery 78:138–141

50. Merkx MA, Van Damme PA 1994 Condylar resorption after orthognathic surgery: Evaluation of treatment in eight patients. Journal of Cranio-Maxillo-Facial Surgery 22:53–58

51. Epker BN, LaBanc JP 1990 Orthognathic surgery: Management of postoperative complications. Oral and Maxillofacial Surgical Clinics of North America 2:901–933

52. O'Ryan F 1990 Complications of orthognathic surgery. Oral and Maxillofacial Surgical Clinics of North America 2:593–613

53. Zide BM, McCarthy J 1989 The mentalis muscle: An essential component of chin and lower lip position. Plastic and Reconstructive Surgery 83:413–420

54. Schendel SA 1985 Genioplasty: A physiological approach. Clinics in Plastic Surgery 14:506–514

55. Posnick JC 1993 Discussion: Rosen HM. Occlusal plane rotation: Aesthetic enhancement in mandibular micrognathia. Plastic and Reconstructive Surgery 91:1241–1244

56. Van Sickels JE, Smith CV, Tiner BD, Jones DL 1994 Hard and soft tissue predictability with advancement genioplasties. Oral Surgery 77:218–221

57. Polido WD, Bell WH 1994 Long-term osseous and soft tissue changes after large chin advancements. Journal of Cranio-Maxillo-Facial Surgery 21:54–59

58. Michelow BJ, Guyuron B 1995 The chin: Skeletal and soft-tissue components. Plastic and Reconstructive Surgery 95:473–478

59. Bell WH, Gallagher DM 1983 The versatility of genioplasty using a broad pedicle. Journal of Oral and Maxillofacial Surgery 41:763–769

60. Ellis E, Dechow PC, McNamara JA, Carlson DS, Liskiewicz WE 1984 Advancement genioplasty with and without soft tissue pedicle: An experimental investigation. Journal of Oral and Maxillofacial Surgery 42:637–645

Indications and patient selection in facial esthetic surgery

79

WILLIAM A. CRAWLEY

INDICATIONS

The primary indications for esthetic surgery of the face are aging of the soft tissues and cosmetic deformities of the facial bones.

The appearance of aging facial skin results from a combination of loss of elasticity, gravity, folding (wrinkles), and atrophy. Although the aging process is frequently thought of as a 'skin only' process, it is obvious that gravity and loss of elasticity affect all of the soft tissues of the face – that is skin, adipose tissue, muscle, and fascia. The skin or fat may show thinning and wrinkling. Pre-existing contour deformities become emphasized when collections of adipose tissue, as well as the muscle and fascial layers, relax over the facial bones. The brow may show horizontal and/or vertical wrinkling and ptosis, with the eyebrow sagging below the level of the supraorbital rim. Asymmetry is frequently noted and may be the result of increased muscle tone on one side of the face compared with the other. The upper eyelids may exhibit excess skin as well as fat herniation in the sulcus of the upper lid. The lower eyelid may demonstrate laxity with poor tone of the lid margin, excess skin, wrinkling, and fat herniation in all three fat tissue compartments. The cheek area may show ptosis of the malar fat pads with an increased prominence of the nasolabial fold. The perioral skin frequently will exhibit increased rhytids with drooping of the oral commissure. Jowling may be present along the inferior border of the mandible. Excess skin in the anterior neck with platysmal banding and perhaps excess fatty tissue may also be seen. Any of the aforementioned facial changes of aging are possible indications for surgical intervention.

Bony deformities of the face (including cartilaginous deformities) may include those of the nose, chin, cheeks, forehead, and gonial angles. It may be that the bony deformities of the face are less obvious than some of the soft-tissue changes seen with aging. Obviously an individual with an overly large nose or microgenia or malar hypoplasia will present a more straightforward indication for surgical correction than an individual with a less obvious deformity. Although knowledge of facial proportions and cephalometric analyses may be of some value, the decision about whether or not a bony deformity exists results from a combination of what is perceived by the patient and the surgeon. Certainly, bony deformities of the face may be indications for esthetic surgery of the facial skeleton or implant correction.

PATIENT SELECTION

Patient selection is more difficult and less predictable than the technical exercise of performing the surgery. Although most individuals can be trained to perform a particular surgical technique, sound surgical judgment in patient selection may require a combination of good common sense, years of experience, and perhaps, some unfortunate experiences derived from selecting the wrong individuals as surgical candidates. An unpleasant outcome may teach a great lesson, despite being painful for the surgeon.

Two of the most important criteria among the many factors in patient selection for facial esthetic surgery are:

1. is there a perceivable deformity?
2. does the patient have realistic expectations?

PERCEIVABLE DEFORMITY

The presence or absence of a perceivable deformity should be the determining factor in deciding whether or not to perform a surgical procedure. Another important aspect of the decision-making process, however, is the surgeon's confidence in his or her ability to fulfill the patient's expectations to improve the perceived deformity. Simply because a patient presents with an obvious deformity does not necessarily make that individual a good candidate for surgery. On the other hand, it may be possible to perform a procedure on an individual with a minor deformity and produce significant satisfaction in that individual. The primary consideration should be the surgeon's confirmation of an actual deformity; the patient's perception that a feature is a deformity must be considered secondary in importance to the surgeon's perception. Further, it would be hard to understand how a surgeon could have the ability to improve a feature of a patient's face without being able to recognize that a problem or deformity is present. If the surgeon does not perceive a deformity, great care and consideration should be taken to discuss this situation with the patient in a very understanding manner. In fact it may be best not to tell the patient that you do not perceive a deformity, but rather that you do not possess the technical skill or experience necessary to give that patient the result that he or she desires. Although the patient may have been referred to you with high praise, and may tell you that he or she believes you to be the very best surgeon to operate on him or her, you as the surgeon still have the last word in determining whether or not to operate on that individual. Persistent adulation of the surgeon by the patient must be considered a relative 'red flag', warning the surgeon that the patient's expectations are high and tolerance for complications low. Do not let your ego get the best of you. If you cannot reliably help the patient, have the courage to say no. It is far better to have the patient upset because you are unwilling to operate rather than to have performed a procedure and 'be responsible' for this individual's unhappiness. An excessive amount of time will be spent with an unhappy patient compared to the amount of time spent with a satisfied patient.

REALISTIC EXPECTATIONS

The second, and equally important criterion in patient selection, is whether or not this individual has realistic expectations. An individual who presents with the desire to look as he or she did at age 18 when they are in fact many years older, or an individual who desires to have the exact nose of a famous personality, clearly has unrealistic expectations.

The patient with an 'extrinsic motivation' who feels that having a specific surgery will lead to a better job or a happier marital relationship or prevent departure of a spouse, also clearly has unrealistic expectations. It is sometimes necessary to arrange for a second or third consultation to 'get a good read' on the patient's expectations and determine whether or not you, as the surgeon, are capable of meeting those expectations.

PATIENT MOTIVATION

Earlier we mentioned the patient with extrinsic motivations (i.e. desire to please an external source, such as to secure a better job, or win back or preserve a relationship). These individuals will most likely be disappointed with the outcome of any surgical procedure because they are focusing on something which cannot be achieved with surgery. On the other hand, an individual who is intrinsically motivated – who simply desires to look better and feel more secure – is more likely to be satisfied and retain a positive attitude after esthetic surgery.

EMOTIONAL INSTABILITY

Although it has been suggested that individuals who are emotionally unstable may possibly benefit from esthetic surgery, it is the experience and advice of most plastic surgeons and mental healthcare providers that these patients not be considered as surgical candidates. Plastic surgeons, as well as other physicians and surgeons have been murdered by emotionally distraught patients; such a given fact should dissuade any surgeon from operating on emotionally unstable patients. It may be worthwhile to carefully suggest to these patients that this particular point in time may not be the best opportunity for this individual to undergo an elective esthetic procedure. The suggestion that it would be fruitful to spend some time working through problem areas with a trained professional is consistently the best course of action for both surgeon and patient.

PSYCHOLOGIC EVALUATION

Each and every time a new patient is seen in consultation for esthetic facial surgery, the surgeon undertakes a psychologic or emotional evaluation as well as a physical evaluation. Routinely, two diagnoses must be made: one physical and one emotional. Patient motivation for elective surgery for reasons such as wanting to please another individual or correcting an imperceptible deformity should immediately indicate the need for psychologic evaluation. A psychologic consultation is often appropriate when trying to arrive at a decision as to whether to operate on this patient. The patient who is obviously depressed or paranoid may also be a good candidate for outside evaluation by a psychiatrist or psychologist. With treatment, this type of patient may eventually become an acceptable operative candidate. The patient who is currently in psychotherapy may also be an acceptable surgical candidate, but caution is advised. It is wise to contact the psychotherapist after requesting the patient's permission. Ideally, the therapist should continue working with the surgeon throughout the pre-and postoperative phase. The decision to proceed with surgery, however, should always rest with the surgeon and not with the psychiatrist.

MALE PATIENTS

The majority of patients seeking cosmetic facial surgery are female. Only 9–24% of patients seeking facial cosmetic procedures such as facelift and eyelid surgery, chin augmentation, cheek implants and rhinoplasty are male. Facial cosmetic surgery is becoming more acceptable for male patients, however concern still lingers among many plastic surgeons for males seeking rhinoplasty. The problem of sexual identity in males seeking rhinoplasty has been the subject of much discussion. The male rhinoplasty patient deserves special consideration, perhaps two or three consultations prior to surgery, to assess precisely the facial anatomic concerns as well as emotional considerations. If the patient has an underlying psychologic problem, this problem will most likely persist after surgery. As the size of the nose has been linked historically with that of the penis, a word to the wise should be sufficient.

CAUTION

There is no reason to rush into any elective esthetic facial surgical procedure. During the course of a typical day in the office, the surgeon may easily spend up to one hour in consultation with a patient trying to arrive at a decision as to whether or not to operate on that particular patient. This relatively small amount of time may be an inadequate amount of time in which to make a good decision. If there is any uncertainty at all, it is far better to see the patient back for a second or third consultation. It is this additional time that may enable the surgeon to get to know the patient better and may confirm an initial impression to proceed with surgery or result in a decision to discontinue

the relationship. In an attempt to better understand the patient it is always a good idea to see a cosmetic surgery patient for an initial consultation and then at least once again for another discussion and/or a preoperative visit. If a situation arises in which you feel uncomfortable proceeding with surgery, the best approach is to simply tell the patient the truth, that you feel uncomfortable in proceeding, and recommend that the patient be seen by someone else. Once an incision has been made, it is difficult to turn back.

THE DISSATISFIED PATIENT

Fortunately, the great majority of plastic surgery patients are pleased following surgery. Unfortunately, there will always be those few patients who are dissatisfied. These may be your patients or those of someone else. That group of dissatisfied patients who are the outcome of your surgical procedure, however small the percentage, may cause you a great deal of stress. Perhaps one of the most important considerations in dealing with the dissatisfied patient is empathy. To become defensive or rude, or to pretend not to know what the patient is talking about will immediately set up a barrier between you and the patient. The dissatisfied patient needs to be listened to and understood. This may require a significant amount of additional office time, or may require meeting with the patient at special times. Time and understanding may often be adequate to get the patient 'over the hump'. If a mistake has been made or an unplanned result noted, the surgeon should accept responsibility and take care of the problem. It is best to have discussed with the patient preoperatively what would happen in case of an untoward result. Generally, patients are not charged a professional fee for an agreed-upon revision, but may well be financially responsible for a facility fee. As some situations improve with time, it is wise not to offer additional surgery unless it is very clearly indicated and the outcome is predictable. It is said that 'time is the great healer', and this certainly can be true in facial esthetic surgery.

When seeing the patient who is dissatisfied with surgery performed by another doctor, it is exceedingly important not to be inflammatory. It is very easy to be critical of others until you are in the same position yourself. Always remember that you may be in that other surgeon's position some day, and try to give every consideration to the other surgeon while being honest with the patient.

If the situation is such that your patient is dissatisfied with his or her outcome, offering a consultation with another surgeon may be a wise decision. In choosing a consultant, of course you would like to have the patient see someone whom you respect and trust even if that individual is not your best friend. It is far better to have a sound and honest opinion, whether it is in your favor or not, than to have a dishonest opinion by a friend, which may ultimately prove to be a disaster.

The imposition of additional financial burden on the dissatisfied patient who needs another procedure has to be dealt with. As previously noted, a preoperative discussion with the patient about financial obligations is most important. I generally tell patients that if they are dissatisfied with some aspect that I feel I could improve on technically, I would be willing to consider performing the additional surgery with no professional fee, however the patient would be responsible for the facility fee. If the dissatisfied patient was the result of someone else's surgery, I do not feel that it is my obligation to assume the financial burden, and charge the patient appropriately.

Successful management of the dissatisfied patient will continue to be a challenge to us all.

SELLING COSMETIC SURGERY

With the advent of advertising, 'free consultations' and computerized imaging, it is easy to forget that you are a physician whose duty it is to help others. As competition and overhead both continue to increase, 'selling' procedures, particularly suggesting additional procedures to a patient, may become tempting. I have had the opportunity to see some patients for a second opinion who were upset that the other doctor told them that a particular facial feature could be improved when the patient thought that feature was perhaps his or her best! There is clearly a fine line between what the patient perceives to be their problem and what surgical procedure the surgeon may feel is necessary in order to get a good result. The difference between the two situations is whether the doctor's behavior is that of a salesman or a caring physician. It is our duty as caring physicians not to let greed and ego overtake our good judgment in the care of the facial esthetic surgical patient.

BIBLIOGRAPHY

Edgerton MT, Langman MW, Pruzinsky T 1991. Plastic surgery and psychotherapy in the treatment of 100 psychologically disturbed patients. Plastic and Reconstructive Surgery 88: 594–608

Gabbard GO, Nadelson C 1995. Professional boundaries in the physician–patient relationship. JAMA 273: 1445–1449

Goin JM, Goin MK 1981. Changing the body: psychological effects of plastic surgery. Williams and Wilkins, Baltimore

Goldwyn RM 1981. The patient and the plastic surgeon, 1st edn. Little, Brown, Boston

Goldwyn RM 1984. The unfavorable result in plastic surgery, 2nd edn. Little, Brown, Boston

Groves JE 1978. Taking care of the hateful patient. New England Journal of Medicine 298: 883–887

Napoleon A 1993. The presentation of personalities in plastic surgery. Annals of Plastic Surgery 31: 193–208

Pertschuk M 1991. Psychological considerations in interface surgery. In: Whitaker LA (ed). Aesthetic surgery of the facial skeleton. Clinics in plastic surgery. W.B. Saunders, Philadelphia

Reich J 1991. The aesthetic surgical experience. In: Smith JW, Aston SJ (eds). Grabb and Smith's Plastic Surgery, 4th edn. Little, Brown, Boston

Surgical techniques – the forehead and brow

80

CLARK O. TAYLOR/JEFFREY S. LEWIS

INTRODUCTION

The advent of forehead/brow lifting for the purpose of facial rejuvenation dates back to the early twentieth century in Europe, as Lexner introduced his approach to the surgical literature in 1910.[1] French and German surgeons offered modifications in the following decades with various incision designs reported by Hunt, Noel, Joseph, and Passot.[2] Approaches to the brow were made through either a coronal or hairline incision with resection of skin, without undermining, until the early 1960s. Extensive undermining and development of a subfrontalis forehead flap was reported by Pangman in 1961,[3] and various modifications including subperiosteal dissection followed shortly thereafter.[4] With the development of more sophisticated technology, endoscopic approaches to facial rejuvenation, including forehead and brow plasty, have been realized in the 1990s.[5-8]

Attention to the impact of brow position and forehead topography among surgeons performing cosmetic procedures has increased dramatically within the past decade. Indeed, one need only study the techniques used by artists and animators to realize the great effect brow position has on facial expression. A change in medial brow position from exceedingly low to high reflects a face that changes from stern or angry to one of surprise. The evenly arched brow with adequate distance from the tarsal crease reflects alertness and composure, while ptosis, even with an appropriate arch, suggests malaise or fatigue.

Important, but less profound in impact on facial expression are the appearance of forehead rhytids. Deep glabellar furrows from chronic procerus and corrugator activation contribute to an expression of seriousness (Fig. 80.1). Noticeable horizontal creases at rest, as a result of frontalis activity during animation, contribute to the appearance of aging. Modern forehead and brow plasty procedures can

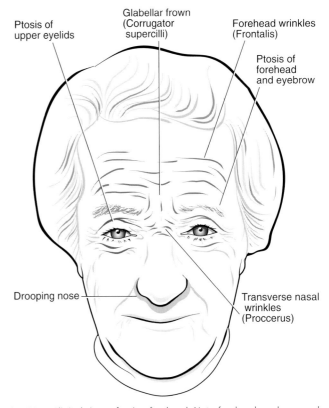

Fig. 80.1 Clinical signs of aging forehead. Note forehead, eyebrow and glabellar ptosis. Forehead and glabellar wrinkles, initially transient, become permanent.

idealize these features. Each technique and surgical approach offers its own advantages and disadvantages.

INDICATIONS/PREOPERATIVE EVALUATION

The rationale for performing a forehead/brow lift is to re-establish the esthetic balance between the upper and middle thirds of the face, and reverse the changes which have occurred secondary to the aging process. The position of the brow at rest is a key anatomic factor in rejuvenation of the upper face. Elimination of vertical and transverse rhytids represents a second important objective of the forehead/ brow rejuvenation procedure. Critical evaluation of post-operative results has shown that the most important effect of forehead/brow rejuvenation is not the magnitude of brow elevation, nor the precise positioning of the brow. Instead, elimination of the 'tense' forehead, which occurs as the brow elevators become increasingly active, results in dramatic rejuvenation even though, in many cases, minimal changes in brow position from the eye-open position have occurred.[9] The brow lift, then, serves to passively establish that brow position normally, actively maintained by hyper-activity of the forehead musculature. This is accomplished by elevation of the brow with proper depressor muscle resection.

The indications for a forehead lift are represented by the clinical changes noted with facial aging. These include brow ptosis, lateral hooding, lateral semilunar 'crow's feet', and hyperactive corrugator, frontalis and procerus activity.[10] The normal descent of tissues that occurs over time can lead to inappropriate or excessive resection of skin in performing upper lid blepharoplasties if the normal brow position is not first established. As this descent continues, the fore-head musculature becomes increasingly hyperactive as it works to maintain a normal brow position and remove the weight of the supraorbital tissues from the upper lid.[9] The dynamic counteraction between the brow elevators (frontalis and corrugator muscles) and the depressors (orbicularis, procerus, corrugator and depressor supercili muscles) leads to the characteristic transverse and vertical rhytids where the above noted muscles attach to the dermis. This 'tense' forehead may result in a normal brow position, however the chronic contraction is a frequently overlooked cause of frontal headaches. Eventually, the vertical distance between the brow and hairline increases, disrupting the balance between the upper and lower facial thirds. The distance between upper eyelid crease and brow is also noted to decrease secondary to gravitational descent of supraorbital tissues.

Evaluation of the patient for forehead/brow rejuvenation requires an understanding of male and female esthetic norms. In females the highest point of the brow arch should occur at the lateral limbus, or canthus of the eye.[6] The medial curvature of the brow should meet the dorsal line of the nose in a smooth arch (Fig. 80.2). The lateral brow should be positioned approximately 1 cm superior to the orbital rim and the medial and lateral extent of the brow should be roughly equal in vertical position. The forehead should exhibit no resting tension and few rhytids.

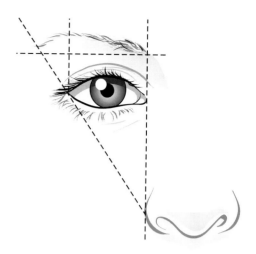

Fig. 80.2 Ideal brow arch position. Note that the highest point of the brow is set along a vertical line running through the lateral canthus of the eye. The lateral end of the brow is either level with or only slightly higher than the medial end.

The male brow in contrast is usually positioned at the orbital rim and is more horizontal in its orientation, with the brow creating a T-configuration with the nasal dorsal line. Variable numbers of forehead rhytids are acceptable. As in females, the medial and lateral brow margin should be roughly at the same level to avoid a surprised, sad, tired, annoyed, or angry appearance.[6]

Sex, age, skin quality, hair quantity and quality, hair pattern, hairline, eyebrow position and shape, presence of forehead, glabellar and nasal rhytids, motor functions of the forehead musculature, and bony architecture must be systematically evaluated. Thorough evaluation leads to identification of specific anatomic problems and selection of the proper surgical approach, and results in improved treatment. Although the literature contains specific criteria for the diagnosis of brow ptosis (less than 2.5 cm from the midpupil to the upper edge of the brow), deficient brow to hairline measurements (less than 5 cm from the top of the brow to the hairline), and deficient upper eyelid crease to brow distance (less than 1.5 cm) (Fig. 80.3), the patient's input before surgery and the surgeon's assessment at the time of the procedure remain critical factors.[7] These measurements can, however, assist the surgeon in determining which areas require treatment and which approach is indicated.

SURGICAL TECHNIQUES

Many different approaches have been described for rejuvenation of the forehead.[6–8] Each clinical situation lends itself most appropriately to a specific procedure according to a number of diagnostic criteria. It is critical that the proper

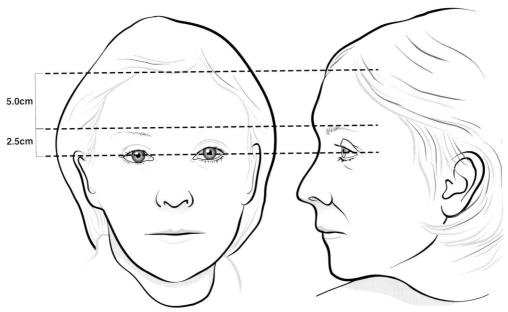

Fig. 80.3 An average of 2.5 cm is found in the esthetic brow. If the distance on a vertical line from the midpoint to the top of the brow is less than 2.5 cm, then brow ptosis exists and the patient may benefit from a brow lift procedure. Measuring on this same vertical line from the top of the brow to the hairline helps the surgeon determine incision placement for the forehead lift. The average measurement here is 5.0 cm.

technique be chosen in order to ensure a satisfactory outcome with minimal risk of complications. The more widely recognized approaches and their indications are discussed below. Many variations are reported for many of these approaches in terms of incision design and layer of dissection. However, the indications for each individual procedure apply to all variations of that procedure. The five basic operations for rejuvenation of the forehead region are:

1. coronal
2. pretrichal
3. midforehead lift
4. direct brow pexy
5. endoscopic.

CORONAL

The coronal approach to forehead rejuvenation has been extensively described in the literature.[6,7,13] It is, historically, the most commonly utilized approach. Other techniques have evolved to overcome some of the disadvantages of the coronal approach. The coronal lift represents the 'workhorse' of forehead rejuvenation and will be described first.

This approach was first described in 1926.[9] Since that time many variations have been reported[6,7,14,15] but the basic technique has remained unchanged.

Indications

The coronal approach is indicated in those patients in whom a visible scar is unacceptable and muscle excision (myotomy) is desired. The procedure is performed in the subgaleal or subperiosteal plane. If the subgaleal plane is chosen, care must be taken in the danger zone of Webster (Fig. 80.4) to leave a mesentery of tissue, thereby avoiding damage to the frontal branch of the facial nerve as it passes from deep to superficial. This 'danger zone of Webster' is delineated by a rectangle beginning 1 cm superior to the lateral brow and continuing posterior to the hairline.

The coronal approach allows full visualization of the forehead/brow region but precise brow positioning, if desired, is difficult because of the distance of the incision from the brow. In addition, the forces of advancement are distributed over a large zone of intervening tissue and relapse can be problematic. This approach does, however, lend itself well to patients who can tolerate posterior displacement of the hairline (brow to hairline distance less than or equal to 5 cm). It is avoided in those patients with forehead heights of greater than 5 cm and also avoided in males as the natural pattern of male hair loss leads to posterior displacement of the hairline over time.

The incision for the coronal brow lift is placed 4–5 cm posterior to the hairline and can connect with a face lift incision or end just superior to the helical attachment of the auricle. In those cases where a face lift is being performed simultaneously, the forehead compartment is in the subgaleal layer with the face lift portion lying in the subcutaneous layer. This is felt to be advantageous in preventing the spread of a hematoma into all areas of dissection.

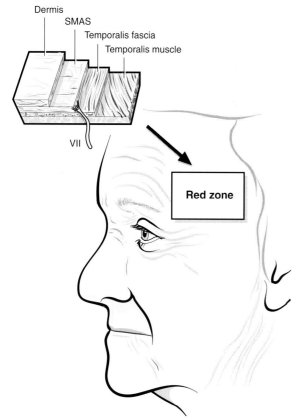

Fig. 80.4 Danger zone or red zone of Webster within which the temporalis branch of the facial nerve changes from deep to superficial in its course. The frontal branch of the seventh nerve at this location runs in the superficial musculoaponeurotic system (SMAS).

With the coronal approach direct access to all of the forehead musculature is possible and alterations to the musculature are readily performed. After all appropriate muscle alteration has been performed, the forehead and scalp tissue is advanced cephalically. Various ratios of amount of excision to brow advancement are quoted in the literature, ranging from 2–2.5 cm of tissue excision for each 1 cm of brow advancement. A 1:1 excision/brow elevation ratio is possible only with direct brow techniques where the incision is placed at the point of elevation. Following excision of the desired amounts of scalp tissue the wound is closed and a light pressure dressing is applied to the forehead region.

Disadvantages to this approach include posterior displacement of the hairline, alopecia, persistent numbness to the scalp posterior to the incision, difficulty in precise brow positioning, excessive blood loss, and length of operation. The above noted complications can be minimized with scrupulous surgical technique, taking care to avoid the supraorbital and supratrochlear neurovascular bundles, as well as beveling the incision parallel to the hair follicles of the scalp.

PRETRICHAL FOREHEAD/BROW LIFT

The pretrichal and modified pretrichal forehead incision is indicated where it is desirable to shorten the forehead visually or to avoid displacement of the hairline posteriorly. This incision is also indicated in patients who exhibit a long forehead and high hairline, and in the female patient who, by virtue of hairstyle, is able to camouflage the incision. Relative contraindications include low hairline and short forehead (brow to forehead distance less than 5 cm), male pattern baldness, thin hair or scar unacceptability. The advantages of the pretrichal technique are similar to those of the coronal in that adequate exposure for performance of myotomies is possible if the procedure is performed in a subgaleal or subperiosteal plane. This procedure has also been described as having been performed in the subcutaneous plane.[16,17] The performance in the subcutaneous plane can be technically difficult and great care must be taken to avoid causing damage to the dermal plexus and thereby compromising vascular supply. Performance of myotomies is difficult as is avoidance of damage to the supratrochlear neurovascular bundles should myotomies be performed in that area. An obvious advantage to the subcutaneous tissue plane is that the main sensory branches are left intact and numbness posterior to the incision is less problematic.

The standard pretrichal incision utilizes an incision placed at the hairline with the incision beveled parallel to the hair follicles as in the coronal technique. This incision frequently leads to an abnormal or obvious scar because of the tendency of the resultant scar to retract anterior to the hairline. If hair loss occurs this tendency is exaggerated. Even in those cases where ideal healing occurs, the patient is often left with an artificial appearance to the hairline. The normal hairline is not an abrupt ending of hair follicles, but is a zone of progressive diminution in hair follicular density 3–4 mm in width. The pretrichal incision often destroys this zone, thus creating an abrupt cessation of hair and mimicking a toupee in appearance. The modified pretrichal incision has been proposed[6] by this author and others to avoid this problem. Essentially, the modified pretrichal incision is beveled posterior to anterior in the zone of decreasing follicular density. This zone is preserved on the 4–5 mm bevel of the superior flap and subsequently allows growth of hair within this zone through the scar with regeneration of a more normal appearing hairline (Fig. 80.5). Closure of this incision is critical in that subcutaneous resorbable sutures must be placed in order to allow maximal advancement of the beveled portion of the incision to retain the normal 3–4 mm zone of decreasing follicular density. If this incision is performed in the subcutaneous plane, preservation of sensory innervation to the posterior

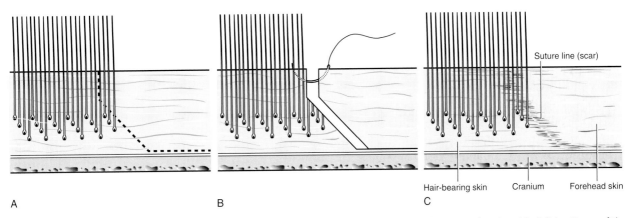

A   B   C

Suture line (scar)

Hair-bearing skin   Cranium   Forehead skin

Fig. 80.5 Skin incision for modified pretrichal forehead approach. **(A)** The incision is beveled posterior to anterior, de-epithelializing 2 mm of the leading edge of the posterior or hairbearing flap to preserve underlying hair follicles. **(B)** Excess skin from the non-hairbearing flap is excised and beveled to allow the leading edge of the flap to match the opposite bevel of the de-epithelialized portion of the hairbearing flap. Careful closure of the incision is performed to prevent damage to hair follicles. The stitches should be positioned so that they do not incorporate hair follicles or strangulate their blood supply. **(C)** Modified pretrichal incision after it has healed correctly. Note how the hair grows through the scar.

scalp is possible with maximal brow repositioning. In addition, any muscle reduction may be performed through a midline inverted V incision in the subperiosteal plane allowing visualization of the supratrochlear as well as supraorbital neurovascular bundles during the resection of corrugator and/or procerus muscles. The supratrochlear and supraorbital nerve are easily identified and avoided with this approach.

MIDFOREHEAD/BROW LIFT

The midforehead approach should be reserved for those patients who will not tolerate posterior displacing of the hairline, and have deep forehead rhytids to camouflage the resultant incisional scar.[18,19] This procedure is mainly indicated in the male population, but female patients with high hairlines and thin hair anteriorly are also candidates. This approach should be avoided in any patient with abnormal scar formation, and in those who show an absence of forehead rhytids, patients with thick sebaceous skin, dark skinned individuals, or in any case where a scar is unacceptable.

The midforehead/brow lift is performed in the subcutaneous plane so that it offers a relatively quick, uncomplicated approach to brow repositioning. In addition, the sensory nerve supply to the forehead is left uninterrupted and numbness of the scalp is avoided. This incision is described as a single incision traversing the forehead or two separate incisions placed in forehead rhytids at differing levels. The disadvantages of this approach include the presence of a scar as well as a lengthy period of scar maturation which the patient must be willing to accept. It has been clearly documented that optimal results take from 9–12 months as the wound matures. During this period,

obvious raised or reddened scar lines may be quite noticeable on the otherwise uninterrupted surface of the forehead.

In developing the flaps for the midforehead/brow lift the inferior flaps are elevated in the subcutaneous plane down to the level of the supraorbital rims. The frontalis muscle can be divided between the supraorbital nerves by connecting both flaps across the midline. A suspension suture of 4–0 nylon is placed from the orbicularis at the point of brow elevation, and secured to the periosteum beneath the superior flap which is not undermined. The skin incision is closed after excision of overlapping tissue and secured with Steristrips for 6–8 weeks postoperatively.

This approach is essential in dealing with certain patients, particularly males with deep forehead rhytids and receding hairlines. Other approaches may be considered in this population if the male patient lacks deep rhytids or scarring is unacceptable.[6]

DIRECT BROW PEXY

Direct brow pexy is rarely the treatment of choice as it may leave a conspicuous scar. It is indicated in patients with significant forehead rhytids and brow ptosis, where correction is primarily for functional reasons and a scar may be acceptable. The incision for the direct brow pexy is placed at the superior brow line or in a transverse crease, if available, just superior to the brow. Advantages to this approach include precise brow elevation and less dissection with minimal edema and ecchymosis. The risk of damage to the main sensory nerves of the forehead is minimized. In addition, this procedure is suited to the typically elderly patient with concomitant medical problems who may need brow elevation for functional reasons and is prepared to accept minor scarring. This procedure should be used with caution, if at all, in patients with thick, oily skin and those who are unwilling to accept a noticeable scar. Those patients with a diffusely ptotic forehead should be treated with other methods since this procedure does not address mimetic function. In addition, patients with extremely low hairlines will undergo visual shortening of the forehead and would benefit from an incision placed posterior to the hairline.

The technique involves the excision of an appropriately sized area of skin directly above the brow and placement of suspension sutures. The placement of the incision within the upper margin of the brow creates a contrast between the distinct superior brow border incision and the natural indistinct inferior brow margin. This contrast between the upper and lower brow margins can be quite noticeable if not camouflaged by cosmetics or epilation. For this reason this approach is generally not recommended for male patients. An additional disadvantage of this approach is the inability to effectively reposition the medial brow. In many cases the selective elevation of the lateral brow leaves the patient with a stern or harsh facial expression, by the creation of a relative medial brow ptosis. Even with these shortcomings, the direct brow lift is a useful tool in every facial surgeon's armamentarium.

ENDOSCOPIC TECHNIQUE

More recently the endoscopic approach has been popularized.[20] The indications for the endoscopic approach are essentially the same as those for traditional approaches. The best candidates are patients 30–50 years of age with limited skin redundancy and early signs of brow ptosis. The endoscopic approach offers the following advantages:

1. no scalp resection
2. minimal risk of sensory/motor disruption
3. less risk of alopecia
4. small camouflaged scars
5. less bleeding
6. improved postoperative comfort.

Relative contraindications are the presence of a high forehead where posterior displacement of the hairline is undesirable, and male pattern baldness where placement of the puncture sites in non-hairbearing areas frequently results in depressed scars which can be quite noticeable.

In essence the technique involves subperiosteal or subgaleal dissection through three sagittal incisions placed 2–3 cm posterior to the hairline. Two additional horizontal incisions down to the deep layer of the superficial temporalis fascia are made in the temporal hairbearing region of the scalp directly over temporalis muscle (Fig. 80.6). Once the

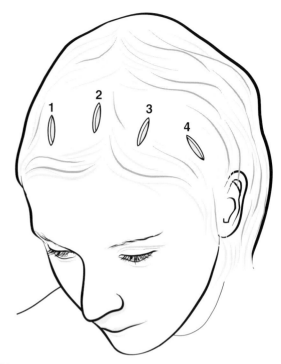

Fig. 80.6 Artist's rendition of the five incisions needed for the endoscopic brow technique. Incisions 1 and 3 are parasagittal, incision 2 is midsagittal, and incisions 4 and 5 are temporal are temporal (incision 5 not shown).

proper layer is encountered, full dissection is undertaken under direct visualization with the endoscope. Using a variety of soft-tissue dissectors, the neurovascular bundles containing the supraorbital and supratrochlear structures are identified. Once the neurovascular bundles are identified, the corrugator supercilii, and procerus muscles are directly visualized through the endoscope and they are either avulsed with a biting instrument or their dermal attachments are transected while taking care to avoid the neurovascular structures coursing through the area. Care is also taken during this portion of the procedure to avoid damage to the subcutaneous or dermal tissues. The temporal dissector is inserted through the temporal incision into the plane just superficial to the deep layer of the superficial temporalis fascia and just under the superficial layer. Under direct visualization, a temporal dissector is used to transect the temporalis fascial attachments along the temporal crest and thus release the scalp flap from the temporal crest region. It is extremely important to maintain a proper tissue plane during this portion of the procedure to avoid damage to the frontal branch of the seventh cranial nerve. The temporalis fascial attachments are released posteriorly until the temporal and frontal flaps are entirely mobile. The scalp is advanced and triangular segments of scalp excised at the puncture site or, more commonly, the posterior scalp is completely undermined blindly in a subperiosteal plane to the attachment of the occipitalis muscles and laterally into the suprahelical areas. The entire scalp is then posteriorly repositioned and secured with unicortical cranial screws. Cutaneous staples or sutures are then placed posterior to the cranial screw, which is placed through the anterior extent of the sagittal incision. The posteriorly positioned flap is thus stabilized directly by means of the transcutaneous unicortical screw and supported with sutures posterior to the screw.

The endoscopic forehead technique is still in its developmental stages; a number of different approaches and techniques have been described, with modifications being incorporated on a trial and error basis. Current areas of controversy include incision design, tissue plane, approach, and the need for disruption of the frontalis muscle and tissue stabilization methods. The endoscopic forehead lift can also be adequately performed through the five incisions previously described. We prefer the straight sagittal incisions and unicortical screw fixations as mentioned previously. T-shaped, chevron and straight sagittal incisional designs have all been described. It is felt that the straight sagittal and perisagittal incisions are preferable to the T-shaped and chevron options as they can be closed with minimal difficulty, are more esthetic and do not require excision of scalp, and carry a lower risk of alopecia.

Although both subperiosteal and subgaleal approaches are described with the endoscopic technique, the subperiosteal plane offers the advantages of safe, quick dissection and excellent hemostasis. In addition, the lymphatic and vascular channels are not disrupted so there is less edema and hemorrhage. The subperiosteal approach allows for the creation of an almost bloodless optical chamber which improves visualization of critical anatomic structures. The periosteum can also be elevated down to, or slightly beyond, the supraorbital rim, aiding in brow repositioning. The periosteum in the subperiosteal plane can be further incised to allow additional relaxation and superior repositioning of the forehead and brow tissue. This incising of the periosteal layer also allows some adherence to the skull to occur during healing, thus aiding in stabilization of the cephalically repositioned tissues. The normal gliding mechanism of the occipitalis – frontalis muscle is preserved by utilization of the subperiosteal plane, therefore maintaining a dynamic and stable brow position.

The use of the endoscopic technique is limited by a number of factors. Significant fronto-orbital bony irregularities that require extensive recontouring and the need for excision of skin preclude the use of the procedure. The presence of an excessively high hairline (greater than 6–6.5 cm from the brow) also precludes any technique that will further lengthen the forehead. The thick or tight skin in prominent frontal and periorbital attachments in patients of Asian, Native American, or Latin descent makes elevation difficult even with open techniques. Other limiting factors include the learning curve required to achieve optimal results, the use of new instrumentation and associated overall investment required for the technology.

There are as yet no long-term studies to document the potential for and rate of relapse of brow ptosis with the endoscopic technique. Early results have been promising in select groups of patients and this technique will continue to undergo further evaluation and modification.

ANESTHESIA

Anesthesia for forehead lifting can be easily performed using intravenous sedation with local anesthesia supplementation. After obtaining adequate intravenous sedation, the supra-orbital and supratrochlear nerve blocks with 2% xylocaine with 1:100 000 epinephrine are accomplished. Tumescent anesthetic solution is then mixed with the following formula.

Tumescent solution using 400 mg of lidocaine (20 ml of a 2% solution) and 1 mg of epinephrine (1 ml of 1:1000 solution) is placed in a 500 ml bag of normal saline. To this solution is added 10 mg of Kenalog (E R Squibb and Sons Inc., Princeton, New Jersey). The McGhan fill kit (McGhan Medical Corporation, Santa Barbara, California), which contains a 10 ml Luer-Lok syringe with automatic spring return and a 108 cm intravenous transfer set with two-way check valve, is used in conjunction with a Byron no. 14 tumescent needle (Byron Medical, Tucson, Arizona). The solution is then inserted into the desired surgical plane and infiltration of the solution is begun. The hydrodissection produced by the infiltrating solution proceeds along the natural tissue planes resulting in less trauma to the associated vasculature.

This solution is injected into the appropriate plane of dissection to a total volume of 50–75 cc and allowed to sit for approximately 10 minutes. The above-noted anesthetic technique provides profound local anesthesia with intense vasoconstriction, thereby minimizing blood loss during the performance of the procedure.

POSTOPERATIVE CARE

Postoperative care involves a light pressure dressing over the forehead region which is left in place for 24 hours. The pressure dressing is then removed and the wound inspected.

An additional 24 hours of a light pressure dressing is recommended, following which a standard tennis headband is recommended for an additional one week to aid in tissue stabilization. Hematoma formation, although extremely rare, tends to form within the first 48 hours after the surgical procedure. The sutures are generally left in place for 7–10 days to allow adequate stabilization and healing prior to their removal.

COMPLICATIONS AND THEIR MANAGEMENT

Forehead/brow lifting techniques are relatively forgiving and major complications are rare.[13,21] Furthermore, the majority of complications from forehead/brow lifts can be either avoided or managed with negligible long-term sequelae if early recognition and intervention takes place. In general, complications can be attributed to violation of blood supply or sensory or motor nerves, excessive flap tension or compression, wound infections, or unrecognized underlying medical conditions.

INFECTION

The extraordinary blood supply to the face and scalp allows the surgeon to incise and perform extensive undermining with little risk of postoperative complications. Infections are rare, even when operating in hairbearing fields. Additionally, the duration of the forehead/brow lifting operating is usually brief, lasting less than two hours—another factor conferring low postoperative infection rates.[22] When infections from these procedures do occur they must be treated expediently, both to minimize local tissue loss and to prevent spread towards the infraglabellar area. Venous drainage in the central midface is via the ophthalmic veins and extended infections in this area can lead to infectious cavernous sinus thrombosis.[21]

In the event of infection, drainage, debridement and antibiotics are indicated. Most wound infections in this region are populated with organisms typically seen in skin infections, and cephalosporins usually offer a favorable spectrum and specificity. The surgeon should make a careful inspection to see if foreign bodies are contributing to the infectious process; extruding suture material can wick skin organisms deeper into the tissues, and inadvertent inversion of scalp hair into the surgical wound can also create a conduit.

Unrecognized or uncontrolled underlying medical conditions may contribute to postoperative infections; examples include diabetes mellitus, the spectrum of immune compromising diseases, and smoking. As forehead/brow lift procedures are elective, the surgeon should avoid these operations in patients likely to experience significant complications. However, patients are not always forthcoming with all aspects of their medical history and it is wise for the surgeon to keep these possibilities in mind if a complication arises and an obvious cause is not found.

TISSUE NECROSIS

Loss of soft tissue following forehead/brow lift surgery occurs because of vascular compromise. Full-thickness tissue loss is extremely rare but can occur. Expanding hematomas can decrease perfusion over wide areas of the forehead flap causing tissue hypoxia or anoxia. The hallmark is rapid onset of severe pain that does not respond even to elevated doses of analgesics or narcotics. Overly tight compression dressings can cause a similar phenomenon. The patient complaining of severe pain postoperatively should be examined immediately. The smooth bony forehead beneath the flap and taut soft tissue following the operation may mean that a clinically significant hematoma does not initially appear obvious in terms of swelling when compared to hematomas seen as a complication after a facelift. Palpation is helpful in making the diagnosis. Immediate evacuation is indicated and can usually be achieved by opening only a portion of the incision, irrigating with iced saline, and re-applying pressure. Bleeding from trauma to the supra-orbital vessels should be evaluated, especially if excessive medial swelling or ecchymosis is noted. Venous bleeding can occur laterally, especially in areas overlying the temporalis.

Partial-thickness tissue necrosis is a more common complication and can result from interruption of the subdermal plexus when overly aggressive resection, cautery or dissection has been performed in the subcutaneous plane. The wound can be managed expectantly with gentle debridement, cleansing and patience, allowing secondary healing to occur. These wounds usually heal quite well, though on close inspection there is often a sheen from loss of sebaceous units.

ALOPECIA

Temporary hair loss following incision in the hairbearing scalp is not uncommon, though often unrecognized by the patient. Even meticulous technique causes some tissue trauma. A period of telogen effluvium in at least some follicles can be expected. When a coronal approach is used, great tension is usually placed on the flap – if stay sutures or staples are left in place, decreased perfusion can occur. Smokers are at greater risk for postoperative alopecia than non-smokers, and should be advised of this.

Alopecia should be managed, at least initially, with patience and encouragement. As the follicles emerge from their telogen phase of growth, areas of alopecia may diminish in size and often disappear completely. This may require months of waiting, but can preclude the need for secondary grafting procedures. Excision and primary closure or micrografting of small persistent areas of alopecia can be effective.

ASYMMETRY

Postoperative brow and forehead asymmetry can occur as a result of asymmetrical elevation and tissue resection, injury to the temporofrontal branch of the facial nerve on one side, or unmasking of a pre-existing underlying asymmetry.

When preoperative asymmetries are clinically significant, they can often be compensated for by intentional asymmetrical surgical manipulation, however it is important to educate the patient about this before the procedure, as even subtle asymmetries are often more noticeable to patients after surgery. To avoid inadvertent asymmetrical tissue elevation, it is helpful to elevate the patient's head during the procedure and inspect from the frontal view after the flap elevation, but before flap resection. When asymmetries are noted postoperatively, revision is necessary.

Injury to the temporofrontal branch of the facial nerve can be avoided by keeping flap undermining deep to the frontalis muscle, and by avoiding frontalis resection beyond the lateral third of the brow when less than 1.5 cm above the supraorbital rim. The majority of nerve injuries in this region are partial and temporary. If paralysis rather than paresis is noted it is first most important to ensure adequate lubrication of the eye. Ocular lubricants and nocturnal taping are early interventions. Early ophthalmologic evaluation is advisable. The need for diagnostic electromyography is controversial, as the small caliber of the temporofrontal branch and the low likelihood of identifying both proximal and distal ends of the nerve branch make it a poor candidate for secondary repair grafting; additionally, the majority of patients will show improvement over time.

LAGOPHTHALMOS

Postoperative lagophthalmos can occur as a result of temporofrontal branch injury, excessive tissue resection in patients undergoing simultaneous forehead/brow procedures and upper lid blepharoplasty, and brow elevation in patients who have previously undergone upper lid blepharoplasty. Careful preoperative planning is essential to avoid this complication in patients who have had previous blepharoplasty. Creating 2–3 mm of lagophthalmos at the time of surgery is acceptable, as some relapse is to be expected. As discussed earlier, prompt ophthalmologic evaluation should be obtained in cases of significant lagophthalmos, and all patients with lid lag should be placed on a regimen to avoid corneal desiccation.

In patients undergoing simultaneous forehead/brow lifting and blepharoplasty, the forehead/brow procedures should be completed first. The upper lids are then treated, planning to create no more than 2–3 mm of lagophthalmos. With the expected tissue relaxation, this minimal amount of lagophthalmos will resolve, usually within two weeks. Reversing this sequence precludes achieving the level of accuracy necessary when combining these procedures.

SENSORY CHANGES

Violation of the supraorbital and supratrochlear nerves causes sensory disturbances of the forehead and scalp to the level of the coronal region. All patients undergoing coronal or pretrichal lifts experience at least temporary anesthesia posterior to the incision line, with return of sensation within weeks to months as long as the main nerve trunks are not transected. Blunt trauma or neuproxia to these nerves can delay return of sensation, but the majority of patients will regain normal sensation over time.

Periods of dysesthesia or pruritis can occur, but these are usually brief and progress to paresthesia. Supraorbital and supratrochlear nerve blocks can be helpful for patients experiencing dysesthesia. Bupivacaine 0.5% with epinephrine 1:200 000 can be injected with a 30 gauge needle at the supraorbital notch, depositing 1–2 cc. The sensory block is usually profound for 12–18 hours and is followed by 24–72 hours of significant analgesia; most patients then describe periods of weeks with less discomfort as sensory function normalizes.

Within 3–6 months, any postoperative nerve morbidity, either motor or sensory, should have resolved and patient is urged for even long periods in certain cases.

CASE STUDIES

CASE STUDY 1
This patient is a 32-year-old female who presented with a chief complaint of a tired, weary appearance. Clinical examination revealed a tense forehead with low, horizontally positioned brows as well as herniation of fat pads on the lower lid. The patient was scheduled for a modified pretrichal (trichophyllic) forehead lift as well as transconjunctival lower lid blepharoplasty (Figs 80.7 and 80.8).

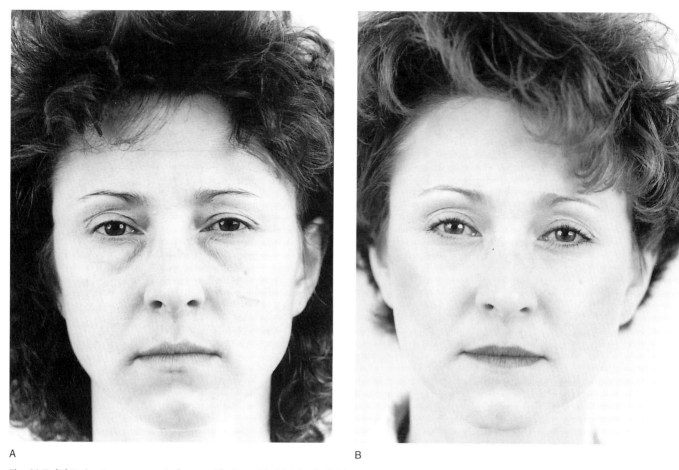

A   B

Fig. 80.7 (A) Patient's appearance before modified pretrichal (trichophyllic) forehead lift as well as transconjunctival lower lid blepharoplasty.
(B) Appearance 6 months after surgery.

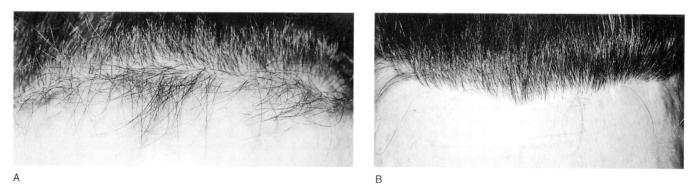

A   B

Fig. 80.8 (A) The modified pretrichal (trichophyllic) incision 3 months postoperatively showing hair growing through and in front of the incision.
(B) Modified pretrichal incision 9 months after surgery showing nearly invisible scar with hair follicles regenerated through and slightly anterior to the incision line.

CASE STUDY 2

This 34-year-old female complained of a tired appearance and presented for evaluation. Initial evaluation revealed a tense forehead with vertical glabellar rhytids consistent with corrugator hyperactivity. The patient was desirous of a minimal incision technique and was treated utilizing an endoscopic forehead lift with corrugator resection (Figs 80.9 and 80.10).

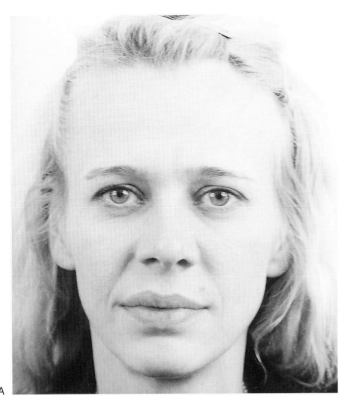

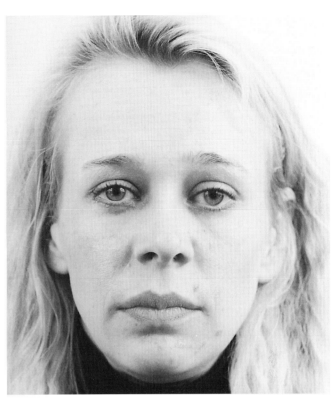

A

B

Fig. 80.9 **(A)** Patient's appearance before endoscopic forehead lift with corrugator resection. **(B)** Six months after endoscopic forehead/brow rejuvenation.

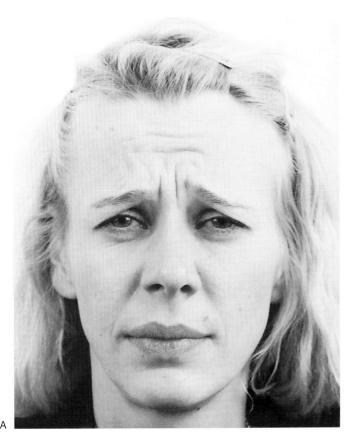

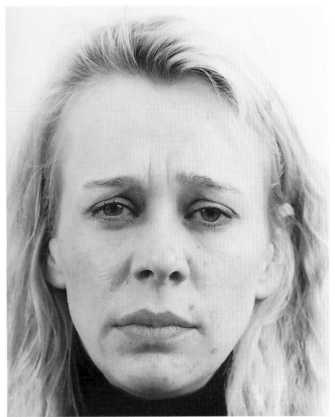

A

B

Fig. 80.10 **(A)** Preoperative frown photo showing reflex contraction of the frontalis muscle with activation of the corrugator supercilii muscles. **(B)** Six months postsurgical frown photo showing diminished corrugator activity with elimination of reflex contraction of frontalis muscle.

REFERENCES

1. Lexner E 1910 Zur Gesichstplastic. Arch Klin Chir 92:749
2. Hunt H L 1926 Plastic surgery of the head, face, and neck. Lea & Febiger, Paris
3. Pangman J W, Wallace R M 1961 Cosmetic surgery of the face and neck. Plastic and Reconstructive Surgery 29:658
4. Friedland J A et al 1996 Safety and efficacy of combined upper blepharoplasties and open coronal browlift: A consecutive series of 600 patients. Aesthetic Plastic Surgery 20:453–462
5. Ramirez O M 1995 The anchor subperiosteal forehead lift. Plastic and Reconstructive Surgery 6:879
6. Toriumi, Dean M, Kerth J D 1990 Management of the aging forehead. Archives of Otolaryngology – Head and Neck Surgery 116:1137–1142
7. Arteaga D M, Taylor C O 1991 Aesthetic evaluation and treatment of the upper one third of the face. Journal of Oral and Maxillofacial Surgery 49:27–32
8. Adamson T A, Johnson C M 1985 The forehead lift. Archives of Otolaryngology 111:325–329
9. Flowers R S, Caputy G G et al 1993 The biomechanics of brow and frontalis function and its affect on blepharoplasty. Clinics in Plastic Surgery 20:2, 255–268
10. Matarasso A, Terino E O 1994 Forehead-brow rhytidoplasty: Reassessing the goals. Plastic and Reconstructive Surgery 93:1378–1389
11. Connell B F, Marten T J 1991 The male forehead-plasty. Clinics in Plastic Surgery 18(4):653–687
12. McKinney P, Mossie R, Zukowski M L 1991 Criteria for the forehead lift. Aesthetic Plastic Surgery 15:141–147
13. Kaye B L 1977 The forehead lift. Plastic and Reconstructive Surgery 60:161
14. Wojtanowski M H 1994 Bicoronal forehead lift. Aesthetic Plastic Surgery 18:33–39
15. Hunt H L 1925 Plastic surgery of the head, face and neck. Lea & Febiger, Philadelphia, pp 163–165
16. Vogel J E, Hoopes J E 1992 The subcutaneous forehead lift with an anterior hairline incision. Annals of Plastic Surgery 28:257–265
17. Benito J 1993 Aesthetic incision in a subcutaneous forehead lift. Aesthetic Plastic Surgery 17:239–242
18. Cook T A, Brownrigg P J 1989 The versatile mid forehead brow lifts. Archives of Otolaryngology – Head and Neck Surgery 115:163–168
19. Johnson C M, Waldman S R 1983 Mid forehead lift. Archives of Otolaryngology 109:155–159
20. Taylor C O, Green J G, Wise D P 1996 Endoscopic forehead lift: Technique in case presentations. Journal of Oral and Maxillofacial Surgery 54:559–577
21. Beeson W H, McCollough G 1985 Complications of the forehead lift. Ear, Nose and Throat Journal 64:27–42
22. Edlich R F et al 1984 Biology of wound repair. Facial Plastic Surgery 1:169

Facelifts

81

STEPHEN A. SCHENDEL

Surgical rejuvenation of the face is not new, yet the facelift techniques of today bear little resemblance to their predecessors.[1,2] The development of these more advanced surgical techniques is based on increasing knowledge of facial anatomy and a desire for perfection. This chapter will review the relevant facial anatomy and more commonly used facelift surgical techniques. At the present time there is no one ideal rhytidectomy and the technique chosen should be based on the surgeon's experience and the patient's anatomy and desires. The reversal of facial aging in addition to the facelift also includes the use of associated procedures such as blepharoplasty, bone sculpting and facial peels.

Aging results in facial skin laxity, fat deposits in the jowls, submental and nasolabial areas, gravitational descent of the muscles and investing fascia and, finally, resorption of the underlying bone support. Changing of the facial skin in aging is generally one of atrophy, particularly in the upper one-third of the dermis.[3–5] Reticular dermis is lost and the total amount of collagen decreased. Actinic damage also causes a decrease in mature collagen and an increase in type III immature collagen.[6,7] Morphologic changes in the face with aging can be summarized as diminished thickness and elasticity of the skin, loss of subcutaneous tissue, decreased skin adherence to underlying layers with gravitational descent and the formation of skin folds along lines of adherence and muscle insertions.[8–10] Skin wrinkles are not all the same and result from several causes as summarized by Barton.[11,12] Animation creases are the result of mimetic muscle insertions and their actions; fine, shallow wrinkles occur due to disruption of the elastic structural network of the skin; and deep wrinkles result from the damage of solar elastosis. Further changes occur from the shifting of tissues such as the malar fat pad, which descends with age, deepening the nasolabial fold among other things.[9] An understanding of the relevant facial anatomy helps to clarify these aging changes and the structures that need to be considered in surgical correction and thus choice of surgical technique.

SOFT-TISSUE FACIAL ANATOMY

The superficial musculoaponeurotic system (SMAS) is the crucial support mechanism for the facial soft-tissue envelope and thus has become an important structure utilized in many of the newer lifting techniques. Deep fixation of the SMAS in addition to its other benefits has been shown to significantly reduce skin tension at the time of closure.[13] Mitz & Peyronie described in detail the anatomy of SMAS in the parotid and cheek area.[14] The concept though is based on the ideas of Skoog & Tessier (Fig. 81.1).[14] The SMAS is continuous with the posterior portion of the frontalis muscle in the upper face and the platysma inferiorly. In Skoog's original rhytidectomy description, the skin and SMAS were elevated in a single unit demonstrating that this fascial layer could aid in skin suspension.[15] However, this technique did not adequately address skin folds in the neck and the nasolabial fold nor did it allow for individual movement of the skin and SMAS.

All facial motor nerve branches run deep to the SMAS in the cheek. Jost & Levet feel that the SMAS is a remnant of the primitive platysma muscle and encompasses four structures: the platysma muscle in the neck, the risorius, the triangularis and the auricularis posterior muscles.[16] They also described a second, deeper layer, which is oriented more vertically. This layer includes the frontalis, periorbital zygomaticus and labii inferioris muscles and, importantly, has direct bony insertions. These authors' description differs from that of the preceding authors, mainly in the fascial anatomy over the parotid. It is described as either a separate SMAS layer or an extension of the primitive platysma which

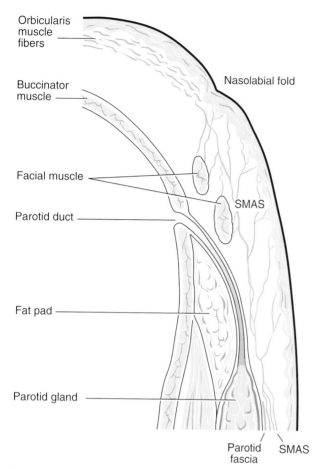

Orbicularis
muscle
fibers

Buccinator
muscle

Facial muscle

Parotid duct

Fat pad

Parotid gland

Nasolabial fold

SMAS

Parotid / \ SMAS
fascia

Fig. 81.1 SMAS according to Mitz and Peyronie. NLF (nasolabial fold), the buccinator muscle; FM, (facial muscles) PD, parotid duct; PG, parotid gland; PF, parotid fascia; OC, oral cavity; PFM, particularis muscle fibers; FP, fat pad; M, maseter muscle. (Reproduced from Mitz & Peyronie.[14])

forms the parotid capsule, thus only one layer. Jost & Levet also feel that the SMAS ends at the zygoma. Gosain and his co-authors have carried out histologic studies and feel that there is a definite SMAS layer separate from the parotid fascia.[17] Clinically, however, in some patients it may be difficult to elevate a separable SMAS flap in these regions and the point is mainly of anatomic interest.

A number of studies have also looked at the SMAS in the anterior face and nasolabial region.[10,12,17–21] The SMAS becomes attenuated in the anterior cheek, eventually becoming the investing fascia of the muscles of the upper lip. Thus mimetic muscle action deepens the nasolabial fold by pulling the actual crease laterally. Lateral to the crease is the actual fold composed of skin and fat of the cheek mass which is in the subdermal plane.[20] In the third decade, the malar fat pad starts to slide forward and downward, increasing the fold. This fat pad is roughly triangular in shape with its base at the nasolabial crease bounded deep by the SMAS and superficially by the dermis. The anchoring effect of the SMAS to the zygomatic muscles limits the

effect of lateral traction of the SMAS on the medial cheek skin and is thus facelifting at this level. In fact traction alone on the SMAS will deepen the fold, while skin traction tends to lessen it. Barton suggests releasing the muscle attachments to the skin while Pessa selectively transects the muscles to allow lateral traction on the facelift flap to be transmitted medially.[12,19] All authors agree that lateral traction on the facelift flap has little effect medially to the nasolabial fold and thus on the nasolabial fold itself, unless adjunctive surgical techniques are employed. Vectors to correct the nasolabial fold are also in a more vertical plane.

Several vertical ligaments also supply fascial support in the face. Furnas has described retaining ligaments from the periosteum to the skin in the region of the zygoma and the mandible near the mental foramen.[22] Others have described supporting ligaments from structures such as the parotid and masseter muscle to the skin that have a similar effect.[23] Attenuation of these ligaments leads to such stigmata of the aging face as deepening of the nasolabial fold and jowls.

The anatomy of the platysma muscle is the key to understanding the neck region in facelifting. Vistnes and Souther described the platysma anatomy based on 14 cadaver and 21 clinical dissections. They found that in 61% of the cases the platysma formed a midline decussation from the hyoid to the mandibular symphysis. In 39% of the cases there was no decussation and the medial borders of the platysma muscles paralleled each other.[24] Cardoso de Castro repeated the study in a larger sample in which he found three types of platysma configures instead of two (Fig. 81.2).[25] Type I, where the platysma decussates for 1–2 cm below the mandibular border, was found in 75% of the cases. In type II, the muscle decussates all the way as described by Vistnes & Souther, while in type III, no decussation was found 10% of the time. Fat in the neck lies both superficial to the platysma or deep. A lack of platysma decussation allows the deep fat to herniate, increasing submental fullness and obliterating the submental angle formed by the neck and mandible. Thus correction of submental fullness depends on the platysmal decussation. Muscle contraction bands are also readily visible in these cases.

An understanding of the facial nerve anatomy is also crucial to present facelifting techniques. The location of the frontal branch is important for safe dissection in the temple. This branch is described as generally running along a line from 0.5 cm below the tragus to 1.5 cm lateral to the end of the eyebrow (Fig. 81.3).[26] However the actual course of the nerve can vary from this guideline.[27] The frontal branch of the facial nerve lies within or on the undersurface of the temporoparietal fascia (remember that

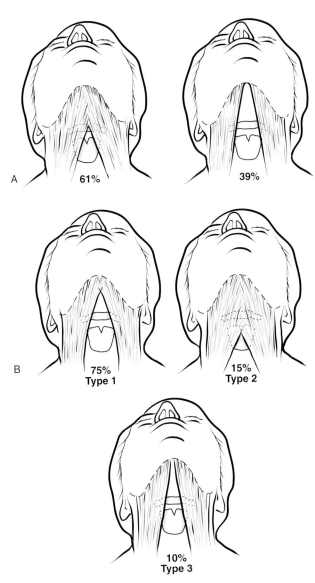

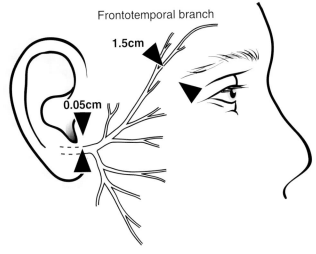

Fig. 81.3 Location of the frontal temporal branch of the facial nerve[31,61].

Fig. 81.2 Platysmal muscle configurations according to **(A)** Vistnes and Souther and **(B)** Cardoso de Castro.

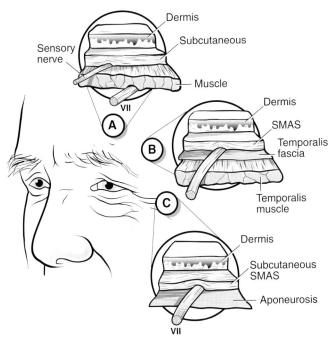

Fig. 81.4 Relationship of the frontotemporal branch of the facial nerve to underlying structures including the SMAS. (Reproduced from Liebman et al.[29])

this is the extension of the SMAS) in the temple. Deep to the temporoparietal fascia lie the superficial and deep layers of the temporal fascia (Fig. 81.4), which becomes progressively more superficial as it approaches the brow.[14,28,29] During facelifting, the dissection should thus be sub-SMAS to the level of the zygomatic arch and then subcutaneous above this to avoid injury to the frontal branch of the facial nerve. The transition area is of critical importance in the cheek – the buccal branches of the facial nerve communicate frequently and are protected by the parotid.[30] Anterior to the parotid, however, the branches lie just under the SMAS which also becomes thinner. The mandibular branch is thus at risk while dissecting along and inferior to the mandibular border.

The great auricular nerve is also an important structure

(Fig. 81.5). This sensory nerve has been studied by McKinney and Katrana, who identified its course in relation to external landmarks.[31] With the head turned 45 degrees to the other side, the nerve crosses the sternocleidomastoid muscle from posterior to anterior, at approximately 6.5 cm inferior to the caudal edge of the external auditory canal. After wrapping around the muscle, the nerve then runs deep into the parotid gland. The postauricular branches of this nerve usually do not extend further than 1.5 cm posterior to the attachment of the ear lobule to the cheek.[32] Based on this

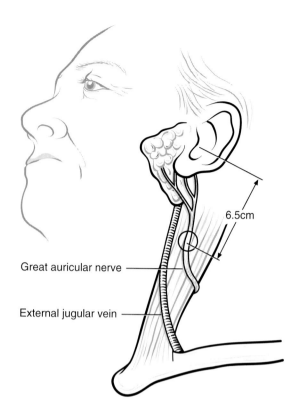

Fig. 81.5 Location of the great auricular nerve in relationship to the tragus.[61] (Reproduced from McKinney & Katrana.[78])

Great auricular nerve

External jugular vein

6.5cm

knowledge, mastoid-tacking sutures should be placed more posteriorly on the mastoid than this and the platysma is most safely penetrated just in front of the sternocleidomastoid muscle.[31]

SURGICAL TECHNIQUE

The patient may be either under general or local anesthesia, with intravenous sedation for the surgical procedure depending on a number of individual factors. After the cutaneous incisions are marked, local anesthetic is first injected along the marks. Marcaine 0.25% or lidocaine 0.25% with epinephrine 1:400 000 can be used. My preference is to infiltrate the entire facelift area by the tumescent technique using the tumescent formula after injecting along the incision lines as above. Liposuction of the neck and facelift flaps can then be performed, followed by completion of the cutaneous incisions. If multiple procedures are planned, the order should be as follows: browlift and upper eyelids, necklift and, lastly, lower lids and facelift.

Cutaneous incisions in facelifting will vary according to the particular anatomy, surgeon preference and whether the patient is male or female. The usual facial incisions may

be combined with coronal incisions, upper and lower eyelid incisions and a submental incision (Fig. 81.6). The coronal incision may be any variation, including a complete classical incision or separate incisions for endoscopic lifting. Neither these incisions nor the eyelid incisions will be covered here because they are discussed in other chapters. If a submental incision is planned, I prefer to do this part of the surgery first. The coronal work with the upper eyelid surgery is also done prior to the facelift incision. Then the lower lid incision is carried out with the face, because work frequently occurs simultaneously in both these areas.

The typical incision in the female patient starts above the ear with a temporal component and then runs in front of the ear following the crus helicus. Depending on the amount and direction of pull, a sideburn component may be necessary to avoid excessive retraction of the hairline (Fig. 81.7). The incision in front of the ear may either run in a skin crease just anterior to the tragus or turn and follow the margin of the tragus, exiting anterior to the lobule above the incisura intertragicus. It then curves around the inferior aspect of the ear lobe and rises superiorly along the back of the ear at the upper aspect of the postauricular sulcus. This incision turns posteriorly at a level corresponding to the superior crus of the antihelix on the front of the ear. It then runs posteriorly into the retromastoid scalp. The incision may be either at the hairline or superior to it and more horizontal. Placement

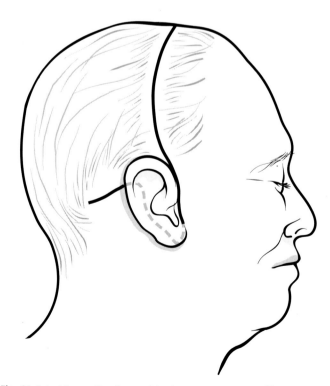

Fig. 81.6 Incision outline for combined coronal and facelift.[38]

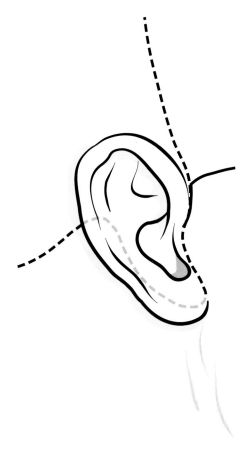

Fig. 81.7 Sideburn incision extension in facelifting.

of the superior aspect of the ear to protect the frontal branch of the facial nerve.[37–39] The skin and subcutaneous tissue is elevated as a flap across the cheek above the level of the SMAS. In a conservative lift, such as for smokers, the flap may be minimally extended. In other cases, especially when the nasolabial fold is deep, the dissection may cross the nasolabial fold and extend into the lip. The zygomatic and mandibular cheek ligaments are severed in this case (Fig. 81.8). The dissection proceeds inferiorly over the mandible and into the neck above the platysma. In some instances the dissection will join the submental dissection near the midline. The ear is next retracted anteriorly and dissection is accomplished in the retroauricular region. This dissection will follow the anterior border of the sterno-cleidomastoid muscle inferiorly. The subcutaneous tissues are very adherent in this area and frequently the dissection must be done with a knife, paying careful attention not to enter into the muscle. The auricular nerve is found at the anterior border of the sternocleidomastoid muscle at 6.5 cm below the external auditory canal, and particular attention should be paid in this region not to injure this structure. Hemostasis is obtained with the electrocautery aided by fiberoptic light retractors. Excess fat is removed from the deep layer just over the SMAS in the jowl or neck areas. The posterior border of the platysma can be sutured under

of the incision depends on the hairstyle and amount of expected skin excision.

The male facelift incision should run in front of the ear at least 1 cm, usually at the junction of the beard and hairless skin.[33,34] Failure to do this will bring the hair-bearing skin into the ear postsurgically making shaving extremely difficult. Other surgeons are not concerned about this and recommend that the incisions be placed in the same position for men and women.[35,36] If this is done, the advanced facial flap should have the hair follicles removed. The temporal incision may also vary if male-pattern baldness is anticipated. In this case, the superior extension should not follow the coronal line but turn transversely at the level of the zygoma. In either case, the flap can be depilated by removing the hair follicles from underneath so that facial hair is not pulled into a non-hair-bearing area.

SUPERFICIAL PLANE FACELIFT

Dissection begins in the temporal region at the subgaleal plane but changes to the more superficial plane at the level

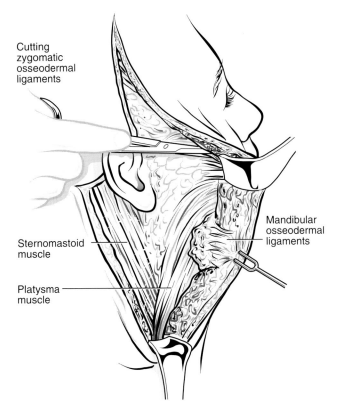

Fig. 81.8 Zygomatic and mandibular cheek ligaments.

tension posteriorly over the sternomastoid fascia. This tightening of the platysmal sling improves the cervicomental angle. The plication is carried superiorly into the SMAS vertically in front of the ear and then horizontally across the zygoma (Fig. 81.9). Non-resorbable sutures are used for this purpose. This side is then packed and a similar procedure is performed on the opposite side. The skin is then redraped posteriorly with the vector extending from the nasolabial crease toward the tragus. A small incision is made and a tack suture or staple is placed above the ear to maintain the appropriate tension. The posterior aspect of the flap is then pulled superiorly and a second tack suture is placed at the top of the postauricular incision. The excess skin is then resected and tailored. Permanent deep sutures are placed above the ear and superiorly behind the ear. A meticulous tension-free closure of the incisions is then performed. I prefer staples in the hair-bearing area, 5–0 chromic behind the ear and 5–0 vicryl buried sutures in front of the ear. Additional sutures of 5–0 nylon are placed just above the ear and above and below the tragus. Drains may be placed prior to closure. Dressings are applied next. Postoperatively, the patient is maintained in a 30 degree head-elevation position without a pillow, which could flex the neck excessively.

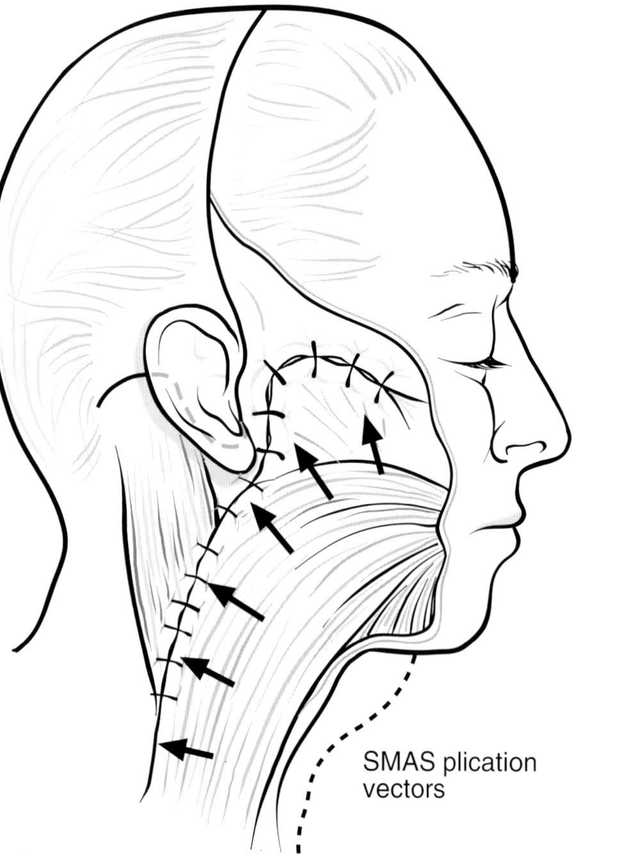

SUPERFICIAL MUSCULOAPONEUROTIC SYSTEM

The SMAS can be added to the superficial plane facelift as a simple plication or as a more extensive dissection and reconstruction. However, most authors feel that a subcutaneous lift with simple plication of the deeper tissues has many shortcomings.[40,41] Addition of this flap is indicated when aging alterations of the lower one-third of the face and neck are significant. The facelift incisions and the subcutaneous underminings are unchanged. The SMAS incision is marked along the zygomatic arch to the malar bone and vertically in front of the ear approximately 1 cm.[42] The vertical component extends into the neck passing behind the mandibular angle to the inferior extent of the subcutaneous dissection. The SMAS flap is then elevated starting in front of the ear either with scissors or a knife. The appropriate level of dissection must be found so that the underlying parotid gland and, anteriorly, the facial nerve are not injured. Once the correct plane is found, the dis-

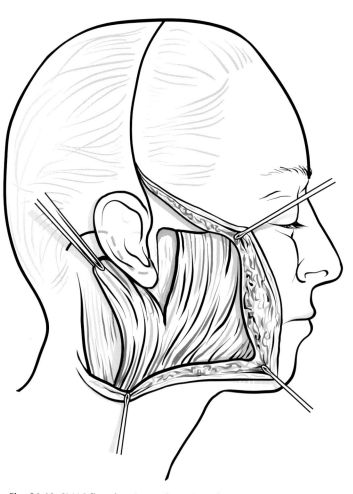

Fig. 81.9 Direction of repositioning for simple suturing of the SMAS.

SMAS plication vectors

Fig. 81.10 SMAS flap elevation and creation of a postauricular vertical component.

section is easy and extends anteriorly by varying amounts depending on the particular anatomy. The flap is dissected sufficiently when posterior traction on the SMAS achieves the desired effect on the face and neck. An average dissection would be about 4 cm. The flap is then pulled supero-posteriorly until the desired effect is achieved (Fig. 81.10). The superior excess is removed while the lateral excess is incised and pulled behind the ear. This small flap will help with the neck suspension and only needs to be as long as the mastoid region where it will be sutured. Any excess is removed to prevent fullness behind the ear. The SMAS flap is sutured with 4–0 vicryl. Occasionally the platysma will need to be horizontally transected posteriorly to aid in the SMAS retraction, but this should be done with care (see Case 1 in Fig. 81.11).

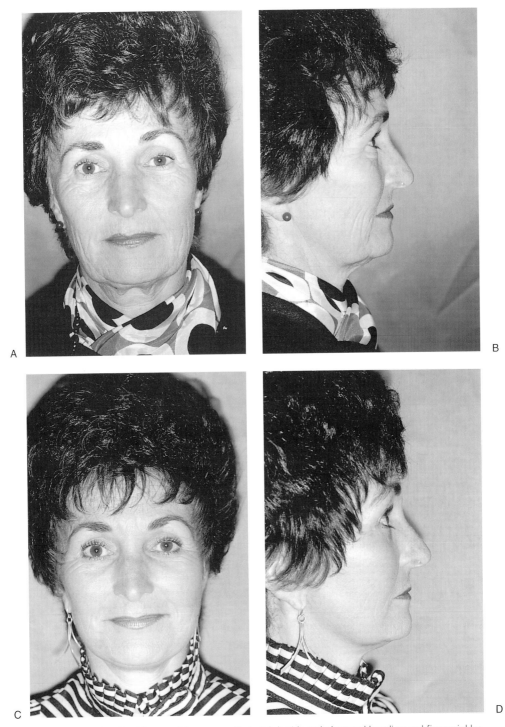

Fig. 81.11 Case 1. **(A,B)** A 52-year-old woman with facial rhytids and platysmal banding and fine wrinkles associated with chronic sun exposure. **(C,D)** One year postoperative result following face and neck lift, including four lid blephorplasties. The SMAS plication was carried out anteriorly in front of the ear, associated with defatting of the neck.

PLATYSMA/NECK

Among the criteria listed by Ellenbogen & Karlin for a youthful neck are: a distinct mandibular border, subhyoid depression, visible thyroid cartilage, visible anterior border to the sternocleidomastoid muscle and a cervicomental angle of 105–120 degrees.[43]

The neck and platysma are approached via an incision in the submental crease. This incision may be as small as several millimeters for liposuction alone to 4 cm for direct exposure of the muscle. Subcutaneous dissection is made along the anterior neck joining with the facelift dissection on either side. The borders of the platysma are identified and dissected free and any decussation repaired by any of several techniques.[44–48] The anterior borders of the platysma are sutured together with a non-resorbable suture from the submental area to the thyroid cartilage. The borders may be repaired edge to edge or overlapped and imbricated, depending on the case (Fig. 81.12). The platysma should not usually be divided transversely from the midline back as submandibular gland ptosis may occur. It is thus safer to vertically resect platysma bands. Feldman corrects the platysma entirely from the front by a platysma corset procedure.[46] Excessive defatting in the midline may also leave a hollow in this area and should be avoided. However,

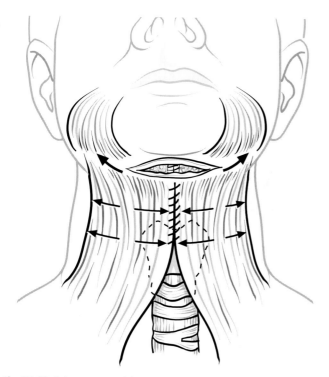

Fig. 81.12 Advancement of the platysma muscle to the midline and plication to tighten the sling and accentuate the cervicomental angle.[38]

excess fat can be removed either directly or by suction cannula.[49–52] The position of the hyoid bone plays an important role in the cervicomental angle, and a low hyoid position makes it difficult to achieve an acute angle.[53] In cases such as this where the cervicomental angle is very obtuse, the use of a suspension suture is advantageous (Gianpappa). The sutures from either side are looped in the anterior midline and woven along the lateral mandibular region in the platysma muscle and tied in the mastoid region. This creates a more definite angle, but the sutures should not be overtightened or simply looped from one side to the other (see Case 2 in Fig. 81.13).

MULTIPLANE AND DEEP PLANE LIFTS

In recent years a number of authors have proposed more extensive dissections and precise repositioning of the anatomic regions of the face to reverse the gravitational changes in aging.[54–59] Skin and deeper anatomic structures are dissected, separated and repositioned independently. These techniques involve more extensive dissection of the SMAS, nasolabial fold, facial musculature and cheek fat pad to permit individual movement vectors as indicated. They also increase the chance for complications and increase the operating time. These different surgical techniques have been called composite rhytidectomy, deep plane facelift, multiplanar or multiple vector facelift. Scientific evidence is still lacking as to whether these techniques produce a result that will last longer than the more classic techniques. Ivy has reported a study where a superficial lift plus incomplete SMAS was done on one side and an extensive SMAS or composite facelift on the other. At 1 year postoperation, no difference could be noted.[39] Rees & Aston also showed no difference in 25 patients who had a platysma sling on one side and a standard subcutaneous lift on the other.[60] The choice of the technique thus remains up to the surgeon based on the individual deformity and his/her experience and familiarity with the different procedures.

Owsley calls his technique the multiple vector biplanar facelift.[56] An upward vector is applied to the SMAS to correct the jowls and re-establish the mandibular border. Superolateral repositioning of the malar fat pad is carried out to reduce the nasolabial crease and the platysma is advanced in order to restore the cervicomental angle. The skin flap undermining is more limited than with the superficial technique, while the SMAS is more extensive. The SMAS flap is bluntly dissected anteriorly into the buccal space and below the mandibular body into the neck. The soft-tissue attachments between the SMAS and mandibular

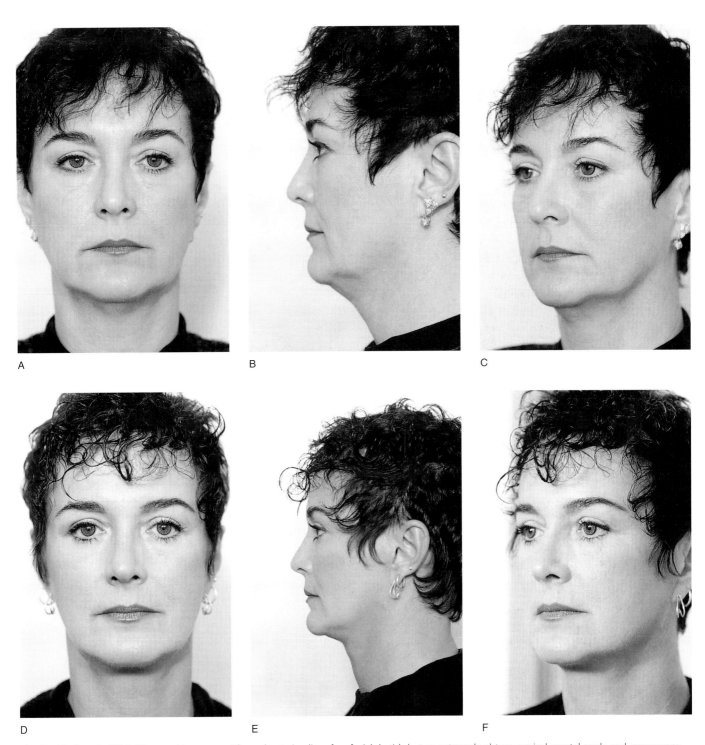

A B C

D E F

Fig. 81.13 Case 2. **(A)** A 46-year-old woman with moderate jowling, few facial rhytids but an extremely obtuse cervical mental angle and appearance of inadequate chin projection secondary to hypodystrophy in this region and hyoid bone position. **(B)** Face profile in three-quarter view following face and neck lift using a SMAS plication with posterior auricular component with associated anterior platysmal defatting and a corset suturing was accomplished, and a Gianpappa suture was also placed to accentuate the cervical mental angle.

body investing fascia are loosened but not severed. The platysma is transected laterally to facilitate upward rotation of the flap. Vertical platysma bands can be cut by extending this transection anteriorly. The subcutaneous flap is carried more medially than usual over the orbicularis oculi muscle to the origin of the zygomaticus muscle. Dissection then follows this muscle to the levator muscles down through the nasolabial fold into the lip. Dissection in this anterior region must be blunt with the finger. The malar fat pad is then elevated along a vector perpendicular to the nasolabial fold and anchored under tension to the underlying SMAS at the malar eminence. Cutaneous irregularities are eliminated by further subcutaneous dissection and the skin flap is then repositioned.

The composite facelift technique of Hamra differs from the above technique in that the orbicularis oculi, malar fat pad and platysma are elevated as a single unit.[55]

MALAR FAT PAD

Identification and repositioning of the malar fat pad is the common denominator in all of these techniques when compared to the SMAS or extended SMAS techniques. Owsley supplements his SMAS dissection with undermining and suspension of the fat pad, as do others.[54–59] Barton has recently described a technique for repositioning the fat pad without undermining.[61] In some cases concomitant malar augmentation may be beneficial, especially when there is underlying bony hypoplasia.

NASOLABIAL FOLDS

The extended SMAS and composite facelift techniques all attempt to address more fully the anterior triangle of the face, that is the cheek and nasolabial fold regions, by dissecting and repositioning of this area followed by independent resuspension. The procedures of Hamra & Barton are particularly relevant in this regard.[11,12,48] Resuspension of the fat pad after dissection is recommended by most surgeons.[62] Robbins recommends an additional vertical SMAS plication just lateral to the nasomandibular fold.[63] Deep folds have also been successfully eliminated by direct excision or augmentation.[64]

SUBPERIOSTEAL FACELIFT

The subperiosteal facelift was first proposed by Tessier and then modified by Psillakis.[65,66] Most of the effect was in the forehead and periorbital areas and the technique was performed via a coronal incision. Injury of the temporal branch of the facial nerve was reported to be 11%.[66] Modifications by Hinderer and others have decreased this complication by carrying the temporal dissection below the superficial layer of the deep cervical fascia.[67–71] A variation of this technique called the supraperiosteal facelift has also

been described.[72] The flap is raised between the periosteum and SMAS, around the zygomatic arch, and then below the obicularis oculi muscle past the infraorbital foramen. Deep tacking and suspension sutures are used in all techniques. These open approaches allow direct visualization and modification of the underlying bony skeleton together with the lifting of the soft tissues.

Endoscopic subperiosteal facelift techniques are based on superior relocation of the deeper planes of the face with limited skin incision and have, in most cases, superseded the open coronal approach.[73–75] These techniques can be combined with the full facelift but are generally best in the younger patient who does not have significant jowls or neck deformities. Development of the endoscope has eliminated the coronal incision and replaced it with multiple small incisions and limited the chance for nerve damage. The endoscopic subperiosteal facelift requires incisions in the scalp, mouth and lower eyelids. Two parasagittal incisions are made in the frontal region posterior to the hairline and an additional midline incision may be made if necessary. Using the endoscope and special instruments, the frontal region is elevated at the subperiosteal level. In the nasofrontal region, the procerus and corrugator muscles can be resected if indicated. The periosteum may also be scored when deep forehead rhytids are present. The dissection is carried towards the temporal region releasing the insertions of the occipitofrontalis muscle and going into the subgaleal plane. One or two additional incisions are made in the temporal scalp region. A vertical incision of 1–2 cm is made above the ear and another may be placed midway between the previous incision and this one if needed. The subgaleal dissection is then continued, passing between the superficial and deep temporal fascia to the zygomatic arch. This is the region of the frontal branch of the facial nerve, thus its anatomy must be kept in mind. The retaining ligament at the lateral brow must be released in order to permit maximum eyebrow elevation. A large communicating vein runs in this area and care should be taken not to transect this structure, this is also the anatomic position of the facial nerve. The zygomatic arch is then dissected at the subperiosteal level, either from a small incision at the triangular fossa of the ear or from an intraoral maxillary vestibular approach. From the intraoral approach, the soft tissues of the midface are elevated in the subperiosteal plane. The two levels of dissection are then joined, being visualized by the endoscope from above. Blunt dissection is performed below the zygomatic arch separating the masseter muscle and SMAS. Suspension of the midface muscles is performed via the lower lid incision. The superficial layer of the deep temporal fascia is suspended from above via the supra-auricular incision using the endoscope to visualize placement of the sutures. Two to three sutures of 4–0 polyglactin or nylon are placed (Fig. 81.14). Suspension of the brow can be done by either of two methods. Posterior dissection from the parasagittal incisions allows suture suspension of the brow to the periosteum. Conversely, two screws can be placed in the frontal bone superior to the brow. Sutures are passed from the medial and lateral brow to the buried screws. All incisions are then closed and a head wrap is placed to exert a posterior pull on the forehead.

Fuente del Campo has categorized facial rhytidosis into four types based on severity. In grade I rhytidosis, the neck is basically unaffected, while in grade II, there is neck laxity which is corrected through a retroauricular incision and a mandibular buccal sulcus incision. Through the sulcus incision, the chin muscles and superior and medial extensions of the platysma are released. Excess skin is removed in the retroauricular area and the neck is suspended. In grade III rhytidosis, skin must also be removed in the perilobular area to avoid a rotational fold (Fig. 81.15). Ramirez also proposes backward rotation of the ear to aid in avoiding this fold or a preauricular incision in mild to moderate cases. A shortened SMAS plication can also be done in the mandibular angle region. Grade IV rhytidosis requires a preauricular incision with 3–4 cm subcutaneous dissection. Depending on the individual anatomy, this approach may be utilized instead of the more traditional facelift techniques,

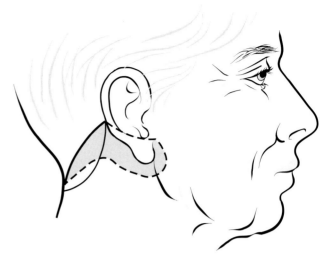

Fig. 81.15 Eliptical skin excision for grade III rhytidosis according to Fuente del Campo.

but its real value lies in correcting brow and malar fat pad ptosis.

RISKS/COMPLICATIONS

Skin flap necrosis and poor wound healing are seen following facelifts in smokers and the flap dissection should thus be very limited. The interval of smoking abstinence in order to avert skin loss has not been determined, but clinical use indicates it is at least 2 weeks. The adverse effects are due to a combination including, but not limited, to nicotine and carbon monoxide.[76] Non-steroidal anti-inflammatory drugs and other drugs that prolong the bleeding time should also be discontinued for at least 2 weeks. Hypertension is another medical condition that needs to be adequately controlled both pre- and postoperatively. The most common complication with facelifting is hematoma formation which is twice as common in men, averaging 8%.[34] Hematomas with subcutaneous dissections run from 0 to 8.1% and in sub-SMAS lifts from 0.2–2.4%.[49,50,51,61] Other than those which are very small, hematomas should be evacuated and an examination for the cause performed. Facial nerve injury occurs most commonly with buccal branch. Most of these injuries resolve with time because of innervation overlap in this area. Temporal and mandibular branch injuries are more noticeable and may be permanent because of the decreased overlap in these areas. Facial nerve injuries have been reported to range from 0 to 4.3%.[77] Skin slough following rhytidectomy ranges from 0 to 14% in the literature.[61] It may be associated with hematomas and infection and is

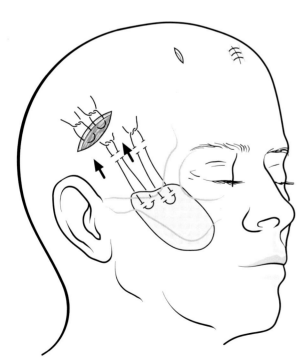

Fig. 81.14 Suspension of the malar fat pad in endoscopic facelifting and suspension of the temporal parietal fascia with endoscopic facelifting.

seen most frequently in the retroauricular area. Areas of skin compromise or frank loss are best treated initially by conservative methods. Many scars that initially look very hypertrophic will, with time, become acceptable or can then be revised. Alopecia may also occur but is relatively infrequent, as are hypertrophic scars, sensory disturbances and parotid injuries.

SUMMARY

This chapter has reviewed the major facelift techniques and their indications. It is obvious that there are several ways to treat many patients. Objective evidence is still lacking to differentiate between techniques, and the multiplicity of these techniques demonstrates that none is applicable in all cases. The final choice of a procedure will depend on the patients' presenting deformities and their desires, combined with the surgeon's experience and familiarity with differing procedures.

REFERENCES

1. Rogers BO 1976 The development of aesthetic plastic surgery: A history. Aesthetic Plastic Surgery 1:3
2. Gonzalez-Ulloa M 1980 The history of rhytidectomy. Aesthetic Plastic Surgery 4:1
3. Gilchrest BA 1982 Age-associated changes in the skin. Journal of the American Geriatric Society 30:139
4. Fenske NA, Lober CW 1986 Structural and functional changes of normal aging skin. Journal of the American Academy of Dermatology 15:571
5. Branchet MC et al 1990 Skin thickness changes in normal aging skin. Gerontology 36:28
6. Montagna W, Carlisle K 1979 Structural changes in aging human skin. Journal of Investigative Dermatology 73:47
7. Sams WM Jr 1989 Sun-induced aging. Clinical and laboratory observations in humans. Clinics in Geriatric Medicine 5:223
8. Gonzalez-Ulloa M, Flores ES 1965 Senility of the face – Basic study to understand its causes and effects. Plastic and Reconstructive Surgery 36:239
9. Yousif NJ et al 1994 The nasolabial fold: a photogrammetric analysis. Plastic and Reconstructive Surgery 93:70
10. Owsley JQ 1993 Lifting the malar fat pad for correction of prominent nasolabial folds. Plastic and Reconstructive Surgery 91:463–474
11. Barton FE Jr 1992 The SMAS and the nasolabial fold. Plastic and Reconstructive Surgery 89:1054
12. Barton FE Jr 1992 Rhytidectomy and the nasolabial fold. Plastic and Reconstructive Surgery 90:601
13. Forrest CR et al 1991 The biomechanical effects of deep tissue support as related to brow and facelift procedures. Plastic and Reconstructive Surgery 88:427
14. Mitz V, Peyronie M 1976 The superficial musculoaponeurotic system (SMAS) in the parotid and cheek area. Plastic and Reconstructive Surgery 58:80
15. Skoog T 1974 Plastic surgery – new methods. WB Saunders Philadelphia

16. Jost G, Levet Y 1984 Parotid fascia and face lifting: a critical evaluation of the SMAS concept. Plastic and Reconstructive Surgery 74:42
17. Gosain AK et al 1993 Surgical anatomy of the SMAS: a reinvestigation. Plastic and Reconstructive Surgery 92:1254
18. Pensler JM, Ward JW, Parry SW 1985 The superficial musculoaponeurotic system in the upper lip: an anatomic study in cadavers. Plastic and Reconstructive Surgery 75:488
19. Pessa JE 1992 Improving the acute nasolabial angle and medial nasolabial fold by levator alae muscle resection. Annals of Plastic Surgery 29:23
20. Yousif NJ et al 1994 The nasolabial fold: an anatomic and histologic reappraisal. Plastic and Reconstructive Surgery 93:60
21. Pensler JM, Ward JW, Parry SW 1985 The superficial musculoaponeurotic system in the upper lip: an anatomic study in cadavers. Plastic and Reconstructive Surgery 75:488
22. Furnas DW 1989 The retaining ligaments of the cheek. Plastic and Reconstructive Surgery 83:11
23. Stuzin JM, Baker TJ, Gordon HL 1992 The relationship of the superficial and deep facial fascias: relevance to rhytidectomy and aging. Plastic and Reconstructive Surgery 89:441
24. Vistnes LM, Souther SG 1979 The anatomical basis for common cosmetic anterior neck deformities. Annals of Plastic Surgery 2:381
25. Cardoso de Castro C 1980 The anatomy of the platysma muscle. Plastic and Reconstructive Surgery 66:680
26. Pitanguy I, Silveira Ramos A 1966 The frontal branch of the facial nerve: the importance of its variations in facelifting. Plastic and Reconstructive Surgery 38:352
27. Ishikawa Y 1990 An anatomical study on the distribution of the temporal branch of the facial nerve. Journal of Craniomaxillofacial Surgery 18:287
28. Stuzin JM et al 1989 Anatomy of the frontal branch of the facial nerve: the significance of the temporal fat pad. Plastic and Reconstructive Surgery 83:265
29. Liebman EP et al 1982 The frontalis nerve in the temporal brow lift. Archives of Otolaryngology 108:232
30. Baker DC, Conley J 1979 Avoiding facial nerve injuries in rhytidectomy. Anatomic variations and pitfalls. Plastic and Reconstructive Surgery 64:781
31. McKinney P, Gottlieb J 1985 The relationship of the great auricular nerve to the superficial musculoaponeurotic system. Annals of Plastic Surgery 14:310
32. Izquierdo R et al 1991 The great auricular nerve revisited: pertinent anatomy for SMAS-platysma rhytidectomy. Annals of Plastic Surgery 27:44
33. Baker TJ, Gordon HL 1969 Rhytidectomy in males. Plastic and Reconstructive Surgery 44:219
34. Sturman MJ 1976 Sideburn relationship in the male face lift. Plastic and Reconstructive Surgery 57:248
35. Baker DC et al 1977 The male rhytidectomy. Plastic and Reconstructive Surgery 60:514
36. Connell BF 1978 Eyebrow, face, and neck lifts for males. Clinics in Plastic Surgery 5:15
37. Duffy MJ, Friedland J 1994 The superficial-plane rhytidectomy revisited. Plastic and Reconstructive Surgery 93:1392
38. Friedland JA 1995 Rhytidectomy: the superficial plane operative technique. Plastic and Reconstructive Surgery 2:84
39. Lassus C 1997 Cervicofacial rhytidectomy: the superficial plane. Aesthetic Plastic Surgery 21:25
40. Aufricht G 1960 Surgery for excess skin of the face. In: Transactions of the Second International Congress of Plastic and Reconstructive Surgery. E & S Livingstone Edinburgh
41. Tipton JB 1974 Should the subcutaneous tissue be plicated in a face lift? Plastic and Reconstructive Surgery 54:1
42. Cardoso de Castro C 1995 The superficial musculoaponeurotic

system in rhytidoplasty. Techniques Operative in Plastic and Reconstructive Surgery 2:91

43. Ellenbogen R, Karlin JV 1980 Visual criteria for success in restoring the youthful neck. Plastic and Reconstructive Surgery 66:826

44. Kaye BL 1981 The extended facelift with ancillary procedures. Annals of Plastic Surgery 6:335

45. Connell BF 1978 Contouring the neck in rhytidectomy by lipectomy and a muscle sling. Plastic and Reconstructive Surgery 61:376

46. Feldman JJ 1990 Corset platysmaplasty. Plastic and Reconstructive Surgery 85:333

47. Lemmon ML 1983 Superficial fascia rhytidectomy. A restoration of the SMAS with control of the cervicomental angle. Clinics in Plastic Surgery 10:449

48. Hamra ST 1984 The tri-plane face lift dissection. Annals in Plastic Surgery 12:268

49. Aston SJ 1979 Platysma muscle in rhytidoplasty. Annals in Plastic Surgery 3:529

50. Lemmon ML 1983 Superficial fascia rhytidectomy. A restoration of the SMAS with control of the cervicomental angle. Clinics in Plastic Surgery 10:449

51. Guerrero-Santos J 1979 Surgical correction of the fatty fallen neck. Annals of Plastic Surgery 2:389

52. Robbins LB, Shaw KE 1989 En bloc cervical lipectomy for treatment of the problem neck in facial rejuvenation surgery. Plastic and Reconstructive Surgery 83:53

53. Marino H, Galeano EJ, Gandolfo EA 1963 Plastic correction of double chin. Importance of the position of the hyoid bone. Plastic and Reconstructive Surgery 31:45

54. Owsley JQ 1993 Lifting the malar fat pad for correction of prominent nasolabial folds. Plastic and Reconstructive Surgery 91:463

55. Hamra ST 1992 Composite rhytidectomy. Plastic and Reconstructive Surgery 90:1

56. Owsley JQ, Weibel TJ 1995 Multiple vector face-lift: SMAS-platysma rotation flap plus midface malar fat pad suspension. Techniques Operative in Plastic and Reconstructive Surgery 2:99

57. Teimourian B, Delia S, Wahrman A 1994 The multiplane face lift. Plastic and Reconstructive Surgery 93:78

58. Teimourian B 1995 Rhytidectomy: the multiplane approach. Techniques Operative in Plastic and Reconstructive Surgery 2:108

59. Byrd HS, Andochick SE 1996 The deep temporal lift: a multiplanar, lateral brow, temporal, and upper face lift. Plastic and Reconstructive Surgery 97:928

60. Rees TD, Aston SJ 1977 A clinical evaluation of the results of submusculo-aponeurotic dissection and fixation in face lifts. Plastic and Reconstructive Surgery 60:851

61. Barton FE 1994 Esthetic surgery of the face. Selected Readings in Plastic Surgery 7

62. Millard DR Jr, Yuan RT, Devine JW Jr 1987 A challenge to the undefeated nasolabial folds. Plastic and Reconstructive Surgery 80:37

63. Robbins LB, Brothers DB, Marshall DM 1995 Anterior SMAS plication for the treatment of prominent nasomandibular folds and restoration of normal cheek contour. Plastic and Reconstructive Surgery 96:1279

64. Guyuron B, Michelow B 1994 The nasolabial fold: a challenge, a solution. Plastic and Reconstructive Surgery 93:522

65. Tessier P 1980 Face lifting and frontal rhytidectomy. In: Ely JF (ed) Transactions of the Seventh International Congress of Plastic and Reconstructive Surgery, Rio de Janeiro, 393

66. Psillakis JM, Rumley TO, Camargos A 1988 Subperiosteal approach as an improved concept for correction of the aging face. Plastic and Reconstructive Surgery 82:383

67. Hinderer UT 1992 The sub-SMAS and subperiostel rhytidectomy of the forehead and middle third of the face: a new approach to the aging face. Fac Plast Surg 8:18.

68. Tapia A, Ferreria B, Blanch A 1991 Subperiostic lifting. Aesthetic Plastic Surgery 15:155

69. Fuente Del Campo A 1993 Face lift without prerauricular scars. Plastic and Reconstructive Surgery 92:642

70. Ramirez OM, Maillard GF, Musolas A 1991 The extended subperiosteal face lift: a definitive soft-tissue remodeling for facial rejuvenation. Plastic and Reconstructive Surgery 88:227

71. Ramirez OM 1992 The subperiosteal rhytidectomy: the third-generation face-lift. Annals of Plastic Surgery 28:218

72. De La Plaza R, Valiente E, Arroyo JM 1991 Supraperiosteal lifting of the upper two-thirds of the face. British Journal of Plastic Surgery 44:325

73. Ramirez OM 1995 Endoscopic forehead and face-lift step by step. Techniques Operative in Plastic and Reconstructive Surgery 2:129

74. Fuente del Campo A 1995 Technique and auxilliary maneuvers for a face-lift without preauricular scars. Techniques Operative in Plastic and Reconstructive Surgery 2:116

75. Isse N 1994 Endoscopic facial rejuvenation: endoforehead, the functional lift. Case reports. Aesthetic Plastic Surgery 18:21

76. Rees TD, Liverett DM, Guy CL 1984 The effect of cigarette smoking on skin-flap survival in the face lift patient. Plastic and Reconstructive Surgery 73:911

77. McGregor MW, Greenberg RL 1972 Rhytidectomy. In: Goldwyn RM (ed) The unfavorable result in plastic surgery – avoidance and treatment. Boston: Little Brown

78. McKinney P, Katranas 1980 Prevention of injury to the great auricular nerve during rhytidectomy. Plastic Reconstructive Surgery 66:675

82

Surgical techniques – the eyes

VISHWANATH S. JIGJINNI/JONATHAN S. JACOBS

INTRODUCTION

The eyes and the periorbital region form one of the most important cosmetic units of the face. The first signs of aging appear in this region.[1] The changes in the eyes and the periorbital area can be corrected with relatively simple surgical procedures and the result can be reasonably predictable. It is no wonder that the blepharoplasty is one of the most common esthetic procedures.

ANATOMY OF THE AGING EYELIDS AND PERIORBITAL TISSUES

The skin, orbicularis oculi muscle, tarsus, orbital septum, periorbital fat and canthal ligaments together form the eyelids. The eyebrows, frontalis, corrugator and procerus muscles and periorbital skin are the significant structures in the vicinity which influence the function and the appearance of eyelids (Figs 82.1–3). The progressive loss of elasticity and the effect of gravity on these structural components are the principal causes of the changes seen in aging eyelids. Although the reduced support of the intraorbital fat causes bulging eyelids ('baggy' eyelids) there may be other causes for the 'baggy' eyelids such as a true increase in the intraorbital fat, edema from renal or cardiac diseases, and endocrine disorders. A careful appraisal of the various factors contributing to the appearance of the eyelids is fundamental to the success of surgery and prevention of the complications associated with the surgery.

The orbital septum in the upper lid fuses with the levator aponeurosis to create a compartment for the preaponeurotic fat. The line of fusion extends inferolaterally.[2] The attachment of the levator aponeurosis to the orbicularis muscle and the skin above the superior margin

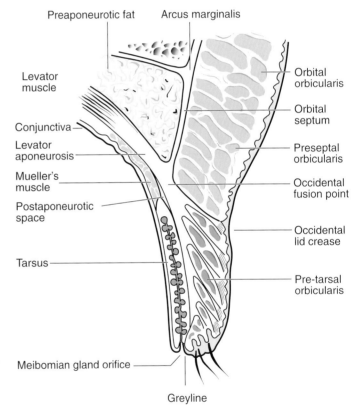

Fig. 82.1 Cross-sectional anatomy of the upper eyelid. Note the attachment of the levator aponeurosis to the orbital septum which creates the supratarsal fold seen in the Caucasian eyelids. This attachment is lacking in oriental eyelids, allowing the preaponeurotic fat to rest in a lower position to give a fuller appearance to the eyelid.

of the tarsus produces the supratarsal fold seen in Caucasians. The upper eyelid crease usually lies 10–12 mm above the lid margin in women and about 7–8 mm in men. This line of fusion is below the superior border of the tarsus in Asian eyelids; this allows the preaponeurotic fat to rest in a lower position, producing a fuller eyelid without a significant eyelid crease.[3]

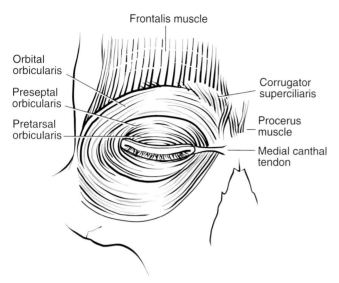

Fig. 82.2 Intrinsic and extrinsic eyelid muscles. In skin and muscle excision blepharoplasty it is important to leave the pretarsal portion of the orbicularis muscle.

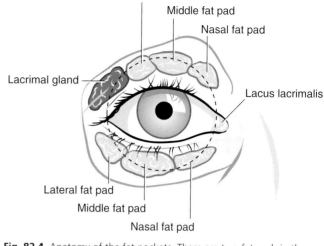

Fig. 82.4 Anatomy of the fat pockets. There are two fat pads in the upper eyelids but the lateral pad may be separated in two. The nasal fat pad is usually at a deeper level. The lower eyelid contains three fat pads. The inferior oblique muscle separates the nasal and the middle fat pads.

Deep to the orbital septum lie the fat pads. Laxity of the septum leads to the bulging seen in aging eyelids. There are normally two fat pads in the upper eyelid; sometimes the lateral fat pad is separated in two. Lying laterally and posterior to the orbital rim is the lacrimal gland, which is paler and firmer than the fat. In the lower eyelid there are usually three fat pads – the nasal and the middle, separated by the inferior oblique muscle, and the lateral.[4]

ESTHETICS OF EYELIDS AND EYEBROWS

Gunther and Antrobus have outlined what constitutes attractive eyes and brows.[5] Attractive eyes have the intercanthal axis tilted slightly superolaterally. The medial portion of the upper lid margin is more vertical than the lateral portion. The upper lid margin overlaps the iris by

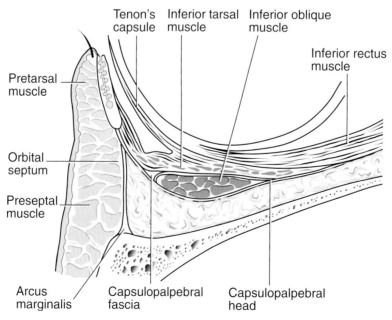

Fig. 82.3 Cross-sectional anatomy of the lower eyelid. The proximity of the inferior oblique muscle to the fat pads potentially exposes it to damage during the resection of fat pads.

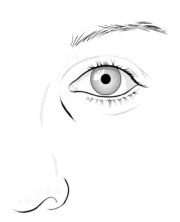

Fig. 82.5 Outline of esthetically attractive eye and eyebrow. In women the medial portion of the eyebrow should be a continuation of the esthetic dorsal line of the nose. The lateral end of the eyebrow is at higher level than the medial end. The periorbital area forms an open oval with the eye in its center. The oval should have its own balance with the rest of the face.

1–2 mm. The upper lid crease extends parallel to the lash margin and does not extend beyond the medial or lateral canthi. There is minimal scleral show between the lower lid margin and the iris. The lower lid margin should bow gently from medially to laterally, with the lowest point falling between the pupil and the lateral limbus.

In women the medial portion of the eyebrow should be a continuation of the esthetic dorsal line of the nose as it curves superolaterally (Fig. 82.5). The medial brow should start approximately above the medial canthus between the most prominent portion of the superciliary ridge and the supraorbital arch. The eyebrow ascends laterally towards the supraorbital notch and continues upwards above the arch to peak somewhere between the lateral limbus and a point just beyond the lateral canthus. The peak of the brow should rarely be more than 10 mm above a horizontal line off the most caudal portion of the medial brow. It should be higher in women than in men. The periorbital area should have its own balance with the rest of the face. It should resemble an oval with an open lateral end. This open-ended oval consists of the eyebrow superiorly, the nasal dorsal line medially and the nasojugal groove inferiorly that fades laterally. The eye should be in the center of this oval, and the size of the oval should balance with the rest of the face. In men the eyebrow is positioned lower than in women and is usually at the level of the supraorbital rim. The shape of the eyebrow is less arched. The lateral end of the eyebrow is more prominent and the upper eyelid fuller than in women.

PREOPERATIVE ASSESSMENT

A detailed history and physical examination are mandatory to assure success of the surgery and also to prevent complications. A systemic inquiry and examination is particularly important in elderly patients because the baggy eyelids could be the result of a systemic illness. Current medications (especially aspirin and anticoagulants) and allergies must be noted.

The eyes are examined in detail. The visual acuity, movement of eyes to detect paralysis of the extraocular muscles, and intraocular tension should be assessed.

ASSESSMENT OF THE EYELIDS

The skin and subcutaneous tissue are examined for thickness and wrinkling. The patient with excessive wrinkling of skin should be warned that the surgery may not eliminate all the wrinkles.

The presence and the position of the supratarsal fold is noted. In many patients with marked ptosis of the upper eyelid skin this fold may be concealed behind the ptotic skin, and in many patients of oriental origin the fold may be absent. The normal height of this fold is 8–10 mm above the lid margin.

The position and the movement of the eyelids is also tested to detect ptosis and absence of blinking.

The involutional changes of the eyelids are examined using different tests. The tension test assesses the laxity of the canthal ligament.[6] The extent of the canthal displacement is examined on digital displacement of the eyelid rim. The snap back test assesses the tonicity and integrity of the supporting structures of the eyelids.[7] The lower eyelid is retracted or pinched off the globe and released to see how quickly the lid repositions against the globe (Fig. 82.6).

ASSESSMENT OF THE LACRIMAL APPARATUS

Ptosis of the lacrimal gland can contribute to the fullness of the upper eyelid. The adequacy of lacrimation and drainage is checked. The Schirmer test is useful to check for potential postoperative dry eyes. A long strip of filter paper is placed in the lateral one third of the unanesthetized lower fornix and the secretion of tear fluid measured in dim light. After an interval of 5 minutes a normal rate of secretion will wet 15–30 mm of the paper. In patients with dry eye less than 5 mm of the paper will be wet.

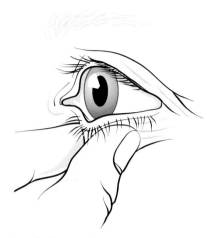

Fig. 82.6 The 'snap back' test. The lower eyelid is pinched off the globe and released to see how quickly the lid repositions against the globe. The aging eyelid would be slower in 'snapping back' in position.

THE EYEBROWS

Lastly the position and contour of the eyebrows is examined as the eyebrows form an integral part of the periorbital anatomy. Ptosis of the lateral end of the eyebrows imparts a sad look while ptosis of the entire length of the eyebrows gives an aged and tired look. Ptosis of the medial end of the eyebrow leads to an angry appearance. More importantly, ptosis of the eyebrows can lead to an apparent fullness of the upper eyelid; inadvertent upper blepharoplasty would accentuate the ptosis and lead to the loss of irreplaceable upper eyelid skin. The position of the supratarsal fold is assessed using Sheen's test (Fig. 82.7).[8] The normal width of skin between the brow and the lid margin at the mid brow position is about 27 mm.[9]

Quantitative measurements are often made with the help of preoperative life-size clinical photographs.[6] The photographs also form important preoperative documentation for future comparison. The points of interest noted from such photographs are:

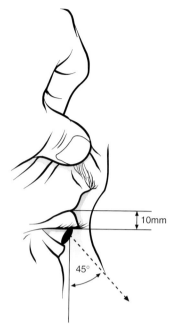

Fig. 82.7 Sheen's test of the supratarsal fold. With the patient's gaze pointed at 45 degrees, the eyebrow is lifted until the redundancy in the upper eyelid skin is compensated. The position of the supratarsal fold can be seen and measured.

1. Scleral show: normal is 0–1 mm.
2. Vertical palpebral fissure: normal is 7–11 mm.
3. Transverse axial lines angle. Transverse axial lines join the medial and lateral canthi of each eye. The lines are extrapolated across the nasal dorsum. The normal angle is positive when the lateral canthus is superior to the medial canthus. This angle also shows the asymmetry between the two sides if the lines do not meet in the midline. The position of the lateral canthus can be compared by measuring the distance between the lateral canthus and the lateral end of eyebrow (Fig. 82.8).

An attempt is also made to quantify excess fat. Lastly, it is important to compare the two sides for symmetry.

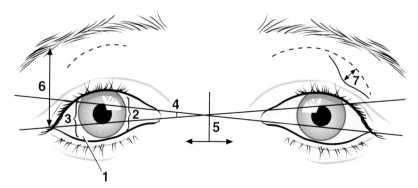

Fig. 82.8 Quantitative measurement of eyelid anatomic landmarks: 1. scleral show; 2. vertical palpebral fissure (medial); 3. vertical palpebral fissure (lateral); 4. TALA – transverse axial lines angle. In symmetrical eyes the axial lines meet in the midline (5). The position of the lateral canthus can be compared by measuring the distance between the lateral canthus and the lateral end of the eyebrow (6).

PSYCHOLOGICAL ASSESSMENT

Psychological evaluation is an integral part of the pre-operative assessment. The patient's motivation for and expectation from the surgery, his or her perceived body image, and the emotional response to the perceived deformity are assessed to determine suitability for surgery.

INFORMED CONSENT

It is important to discuss with patients their areas of concern. A hand-held mirror is useful. The scope and limitations of the surgery should be discussed, together with possible postoperative complications including wound problems, asymmetries, ectropion and even loss of vision.

It is also important to stress that the aim of surgery is to give a more youthful and less tired appearance and not to make the patient 'more beautiful'.

SELECTION OF SURGICAL TECHNIQUE

Upper lid redundancy is treated with *skin and muscle excision*. In those patients with prominent fat pads *fat excision* is carried out. In patients with indistinct supratarsal folds, including Asian patients with absent supratarsal folds, *invagination blepharoplasty* can create a distinct supratarsal fold. Associated ptosis may require *levator shortening* and lacrimal gland prolapse will necessitate additional sutures to fix the gland in position (*adenopexy*).

Redundancy in the lower eyelid can be corrected with *skin and muscle excision*. Raising the skin muscle flap may reduce the postoperative edema as the lymphatic drainage of the lower eyelid skin is preserved. The skin muscle flap does not, however, correct the excess skin redundancy that is seen in some individuals. In such patients skin needs to be dissected off the underlying orbicularis oculi muscle and the excess skin excised separately from the muscle. Laxity of the lower eyelid requires muscle suspension blepharoplasty to provide support to the lower eyelid. Lower eyelid elongation needs wedge excision of the tarsal plate. Canthal laxity requires canthopexy for adequate correction. In young patients with only orbital fat excess, transconjunctival excision of fat can be performed to minimize the morbidity of external scarring. Such procedures can be combined with laser, chemical peel or dermaplaning to tighten the skin excess.

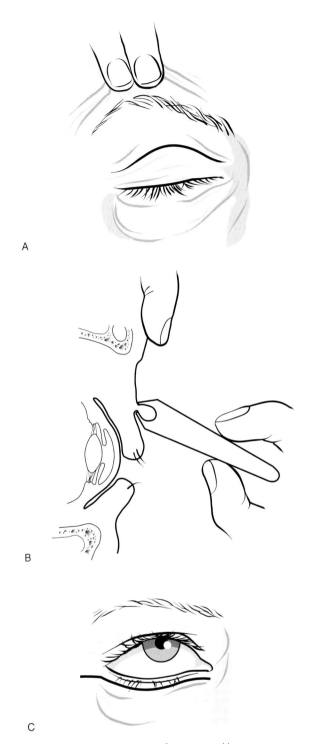

A

B

C

Fig. 82.9 Preoperative skin markings for upper and lower blepharoplasties. **(A)** With the pretarsal skin moderately stretched to eliminate the folds in the eyelid skin, the lower incision is marked about 8–10 mm above the lid margin. **(B)** With the eyebrow positioned in the proper position the excess skin is grasped with non-toothed forceps and pinched in different positions in a medial to lateral direction to mark different points which are joined together to mark the upper margin of excision. **(C)** The lower eyelid blepharoplasty is marked. The upper incision is marked 2–3 mm below and parallel to the lid margin and extends along the natural skin crease at the lateral canthus.

PREOPERATIVE SKIN MARKING

It is important to mark the skin incisions with the patient in the upright position as in the supine position the gravitational pull is in a different direction and masks some of the deformities seen in the upright position.

The sequence of surgery is generally brow/forehead lift, followed by the upper lid blepharoplasty, followed by the lower lid blepharoplasty. The skin marking also follows the same sequence.

For the upper eyelid blepharoplasty the pretarsal skin is stretched moderately to eliminate the folds in the eyelid skin and the lower incision is marked about 8–10 mm above the lid margin (Fig. 82.9). With the eyebrow in the proper position the excess skin is grasped with non-toothed forceps and pinched in different positions in a medial to lateral direction to mark different points which are joined together to mark the upper margin of excision. It is important not to carry the medial extension downward too close to the canthus or this will result in scar webbing. The lateral extension curves slightly up just lateral to the lateral canthus but does not cross the limit of the eyelid skin. This upward diversion is important when lower eyelid blepharoplasty is carried out at the same time so as to preserve a bridge of skin between the two incisions to facilitate lymphatic drainage of the lids.

The lower eyelid blepharoplasty is marked with the upper incision 2–3 mm below and parallel to the lid margin and extending along the natural skin crease at the lateral canthus. The amount of skin to be excised is again determined by the pinching method.

ANESTHESIA

Most blepharoplasties can be carried out under local anesthesia using lidocaine and epinephrine (1:200 000). Sedation with diazepam or neuroleptic anesthesia is useful. The patient is placed in a supine position with the head of the bed raised about 30 degrees. Lubricating eye ointment is instilled into the eye, and an eye shield is used to protect the cornea.

UPPER BLEPHAROPLASTY

SKIN AND MUSCLE EXCISION (Fig. 82.10)

The skin ellipse is excised as marked. Bleeding from subdermal vessels is controlled. A strip of orbicularis is

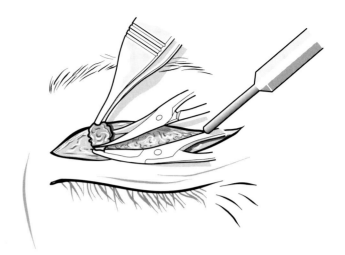

Fig. 82.10 The technique of fat pad excision. The protruding portion of the fat is grasped in the artery forceps, coagulated with diathermy, and excised.

excised; care must be taken not to tent up the muscle as it is cut or the underlying orbital septum may be inadvertently excised with the muscle. Next, the orbital septum is incised if fat removal is planned. The septum is picked up with forceps during the incision to avoid injury to the underlying levator aponeurosis. The septum may be incised through a long incision, or two or three small incisions can be made to gain access to the fat pads. The fat is grasped in tissue forceps and freed of any attachments, allowing the fat to protrude out freely without traction in order to judge the amount to be resected. The fat protruding anterior to the plane of the septum is grasped in cautery forceps, coagulated with diathermy, and excised. Note that the fat in the medial compartment is at a deeper level and is paler than the fat in the lateral compartment. Once the fat excision is complete the hemostasis is checked. The skin is closed with 6–0 nylon as a subdermal running suture with interrupted sutures lateral to the lateral canthus. Narrow bites of skin edges during skin closure ensure good apposition of skin edges and subsequently better healing of the skin. Steristrips are used to reinforce the suture line.

INVAGINATION BLEPHAROPLASTY (SUPRATARSAL FIXATION) (Fig. 82.11)

In this procedure the amount of skin resected is limited so as to leave 30 mm of skin width between the brow and the upper lid margin to achieve proper supratarsal fixation. After resection of the excess skin, a narrow strip of the muscle (1–3 mm) is excised. The orbital septum is exposed and the pocket of orbital fat is opened by incising the septum, remembering that the attachment of the septum

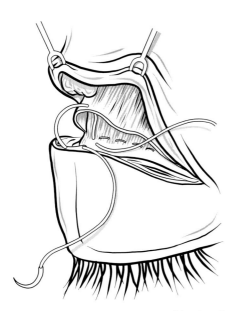

Fig. 82.11 Upper blepharoplasty with supratarsal fixation. Care should be taken to avoid injury to the supratarsal vascular arcade to prevent hematoma.

to the levator aponeurosis extends caudally in the lateral part of the lid. After the desired amount of fat is excised the anterior surface of the tarsus is cleared of excess connective tissue and the pretarsal extension of the aponeurosis. Closure of the wound is carried out by attaching the dermis of the pretarsal skin to the anterosuperior aspect of the tarsus and the superior edge of the aponeurosis. Care is taken to preserve the fine arcade of vessels just superior to the superior margin of the tarsus.[9] Three to four sutures are taken with 6–0 Vicryl. The skin closure is done according to personal preference.

In patients with *ptosis* the levator aponeurosis can be excised in amounts appropriate to the correction of the ptosis. Generally, a 4:1 ratio of excision to lid elevation is seen. In patients with lacrimal gland prolapse, correction can be carried out by taking sutures through the capsule of the gland and the periosteum of the orbital rim and elevating the gland above the orbital rim as the sutures are tightened.

LOWER BLEPHAROPLASTY

SKIN EXCISION

Skin excision was the earliest blepharoplasty technique used and is still indicated in patients with an excess of skin but with adequate muscle tone. The incision is made near the lid margin and the skin is undermined up to the desired level. The excess skin is draped over the lid margin without any tension. The patient is asked to open the mouth and look up. The amount of skin to be excised is determined and excised. It is vital not to pull the cheek skin into the lower eyelid so as to prevent ectropion. The skin is sutured with interrupted 6–0 silk.

SKIN AND MUSCLE FLAP BLEPHAROPLASTY (Fig. 82.12)

The skin is incised near the lid margin. The skin is undermined only in the lateral portion; in the medial portion the skin and muscle flap is raised, working medially from the lateral edge and freeing it from the deeper orbital septum. It is important to preserve the pretarsal muscle. The rationale for preserving the continuity between the skin and the muscle is to facilitate lymphatic drainage of the skin. But the lack of adequate undermining of the skin does not eliminate skin wrinkles. The septum can be opened to excise redundant fat which is commonly contained in three compartments. The excess skin and muscle is draped over the lid margin. A vertical incision is made through the entire thickness of the skin and muscle flap at the level of the lateral canthus and a suture is passed at this level. After this suture has been placed, the excess skin and muscle is trimmed on the medial and the lateral side of the suture. The incision is closed using 5–0 Vicryl for the muscle and 6–0 silk for the skin.

MUSCLE SUSPENSION BLEPHAROPLASTY

The skin excision and the fat removal is done as planned. The muscle suspension is carried out by placing anchoring sutures through the periosteum just lateral to the lateral canthus and taking a bite of the muscle 2–5 mm inferomedial to the periosteal bite. Tying the suture pulls the muscle sling upward and laterally. The amount of the skin to be excised is determined and excised.[12]

In patients with a long, lax lid margin a wedge of tarsus can be excised. The conjunctiva can be sutured with a buried suture of 7–0 catgut, and the tarsus can be sutured with a pull-out type of 6–0 Prolene suture.

TRANSCONJUNCTIVAL LOWER BLEPHAROPLASTY (Fig. 82.13)

The transconjunctival approach leaves the skin, muscle and septum intact, thus avoiding the spectrum of postoperative problems of eyelid retraction. The technique is more suited for younger patients with good muscle tone and minimal excess of skin and muscle. Transconjunctival lower eyelid blepharoplasty can be carried out under local or general

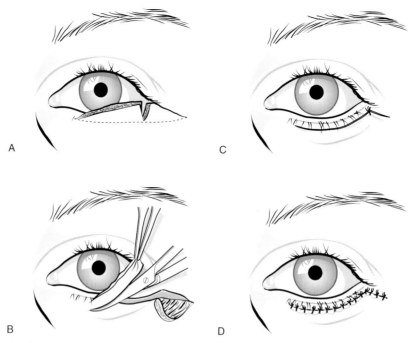

Fig. 82.12 Technique of lower blepharoplasty (skin and muscle excision). After the skin and muscle flap is elevated, the orbital septum is opened and the fat pads excised. **(A)** The lower eyelid flap is draped over the lid margin and a vertical incision is made at the lateral canthus. **(B)** The excess skin and muscle is excised with the patient looking up and with the mouth open to prevent excess skin being excised. **(C and D)** The wound is closed, taking the first suture at the level of the lateral canthus.

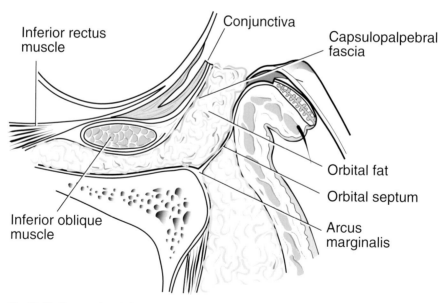

Fig. 82.13 Transconjunctival approach to the lower eyelid fat pads. The capsulopalpebral fascia needs to be incised to gain access to the periorbital fat. It is important to protect the inferior oblique muscle during the fat excision.

anesthesia. After topical instillation of 0.5% tetracaine and protection of the cornea with an eye shield, the lower eyelid is retracted and everted. Transconjunctival injection of 1% lidocaine with 1:200 000 epinephrine is carried out along the length of the lower eyelid. Once the lower eyelid is adequately anesthetized the lid margin is retracted and the palpebral conjunctiva is incised. The incision is carried deeper through the capsulopalpebral fascia. Retraction on the lower wound edge with a Desmarres retractor exposes the periorbital fat and a thin fascia overlying the fat is incised. The fat is grasped with forceps and freed of all adhesions. The fat protruding beyond the level of the infraorbital margin is excised with diathermy coagulation. It is important to protect the inferior oblique muscle that lies between the medial and the central fat pads. Hemostasis is checked; the corneal shield is removed and the eye is irrigated. Conjunctival sutures are avoided and the eyelid is supported externally with a narrow adhesive tape or Steristrip.[13]

ANCILLARY PROCEDURES

CANTHOPEXY

In patients with obvious canthal tendon laxity canthopexy can be carried out. The lateral canthal ligament is identified through the lateral end of the incision. A 4–0 Prolene suture is passed through its substance (often taking a bite through the lateral end of the tarsus and orbicularis muscle in patients with laxity of the lid) and anchored to the periosteum of the lateral orbital wall. Overcorrection ensures that the optimum position is maintained even after relaxation of the repair, which is common. The canthal tendon need not be detached from its insertion prior to its repair. The suture can also be passed through a hole drilled through the lateral orbital rim.

DERMAPLANING

Rhytids in the periorbital area are not always eliminated with the above surgical techniques and additional measures are sometimes necessary to treat these skin wrinkles. Traditionally three techniques have been used for the correction of 'crow's feet':

1. chemical peel
2. dermabrasion
3. surgery.

The effectiveness of a chemical peel in skin resurfacing depends on the chemical used and its concentration. Hypopigmentation and depigmentation are serious side-effects of the procedure. Dermabrasion, although effective in skin resurfacing, is associated with complications such as scarring and pigmentary changes

Laser resurfacing

In recent years pulsed CO_2 laser skin resurfacing has gained in popularity.[14] Laser technology offers advantages over the other methods in the form of 'selective injury'. The amount of tissue removed can be controlled and there is very little residual damage and preoperative bleeding. Several pulsed CO_2 lasers are available (Coherent Ultrapulse, Sharplan Silk Touch).

Briefly, the procedure is carried out under careful sedation as oxygen can not be used during laser surgery. A local anesthetic is given and the eyes (after tetracaine eye drops an eye shield is used) and teeth are protected. Wet towels are used for draping. The relevant esthetic units are treated to an appropriate end-point. It is important to give preoperative antiherpetic prophylaxis. Postoperative care consists of dressings, analgesia, antibiotics and Zovirax. Patients are warned about erythema and advised to use sunscreen creams and hydroquinone for the prevention of hyperpigmentation.

The complications of laser treatment include pigmentary changes, scarring, herpes zoster and eye injury. Long-term results are not available to compare the efficacy of laser treatment with other skin resurfacing methods such as chemical peels.

SURGICAL CORRECTION OF CROW'S FEET DEFORMITY

It is possible to correct crow's feet by selective myotomy of the orbicularis oculi muscle.[15] Through an incision along the temporal hairline, a skin flap is raised in the subcutaneous plane until the lateral margin of the orbicularis is reached. The muscle is incised very carefully in a line drawn directly laterally just deep to the midportion of the cutaneous deformity. The edges of the incised muscle are beveled to smooth out the contours.

POSTOPERATIVE CARE

Antibiotic ointment is instilled into the eyes after the surgery. The patients are advised to lie recumbent with the head end elevated. Cold compresses are applied for 48 hours as tolerated. Patients with dry eyes require methyl cellulose eye drops. Sutures are removed 4–5 days after surgery. Patients are instructed to massage the lids to help control edema.

COMPLICATIONS

The goal of preoperative planning is to prevent complications, nevertheless some complications may be noted.

HEMATOMA

Discontinuation of anticoagulants 2 weeks prior to surgery and meticulous attention to hemostasis help to prevent hematomas. A minor hematoma can be drained up to 10 days after surgery if it persists. A large hematoma needs prompt evacuation.

Retrobulbar hematoma is a dreaded complication of this simple procedure. Bleeding in the soft tissues behind the septum can occur from inadvertent penetration of a blood vessel during injection. Excessive traction on the fat pedicle during the fat excision and inadequate hemostasis can lead to retraction of the bleeding vessel deep into the orbit and formation of a hematoma. Retrobulbar hematoma can lead to blindness from occlusion of the central retinal artery or from the disturbance of retinal blood flow secondary to pressure. Examination of vision in the immediate postoperative period is vital for early detection of this complication. Proptosis, severe postoperative pain and hard consistency of the eyeball should alert the physician to this condition. Reduced vision and pupillary dilatation are late signs. The treatment consists of immediate decompression of the orbit by removal of sutures and opening the orbital septum. An attempt is made to locate the source of bleeding. Lateral canthotomy is useful to decompress the orbital tissues. An ophthalmology consult is advised. Further management consists of reducing extracellular fluid by fluid restriction and intravenous mannitol. Meticulous attention to detail, in particular careful hemostasis, is important in preventing this complication.

BLINDNESS

The exact etiology and incidence are unknown, yet most cases are associated with deep orbital injections and fat removal leading to orbital hemorrhage.[16]

INFECTION

It is rare to see postoperative wound infection because of the excellent blood supply to the eyelids. Orbital cellulitis is a rare but more serious complication. Herpetic eruption around the lids is more common than infection caused by bacterial contamination.

DRY EYE SYNDROME

Patients likely to develop this complication should have been identified during the preoperative evaluation. Dissection near the lacrimal gland should be undertaken with care. The dryness is treated with methyl cellulose eye drops, and the eyes are protected with eye glasses and patching at night until normal lacrimation is established.

PTOSIS

Ptosis is seen in supratarsal fixation, especially if there is hematoma caused by injury to the supratarsal arcade of vessels during the placement of fixation sutures. This is usually self limiting.

DIPLOPIA

Injury to the extraocular muscles can lead to diplopia. The extraocular muscles may also become entrapped in the scar tissue to cause late onset diplopia.

SCARS

The patient is always warned about possible noticeable scarring. The important precautions taken during surgery include leaving an adequate gap between the upper and lower blepharoplasty incisions, and not extending incisions into non-palpebral skin. Hypertrophic scars are managed conservatively with local massage and steroid injections.

ASYMMETRY

Some degree of asymmetry is to be expected and the patients warned accordingly. More severe asymmetry may need further correction.

ECTROPION

Ectropion in the immediate postoperative period is common and is caused by tissue edema. Permanent ectropion is a common problem in the elderly where eyelid supports are weak. It is also a problem commonly seen after excess skin excision. Mild cases can be managed conservatively with massage, but more severe cases require skin grafting to correct the skin deficiency as well as lateral suspension of the lid.

ENOPHTHALMIA

This is seen in patients in whom overzealous fat excision has been carried out. Autologous fat grafting may be required.

RESIDUAL WRINKLES AND FESTOONS

Blepharoplasty may not eliminate fine wrinkles, and the patients should be warned about this limitation. Many residual festoons and gross wrinkles are amenable to local resection.

REFERENCES

1. Gonzalez-Ulloa M 1960 The treatment of palpebral bags. Plastic and Reconstructive Surgery 27:394
2. Flowers RS 1991 Periorbital aesthetic surgery for men – eyelids and related structures. Clinics in Plastic Surgery 18:689
3. Uchida JA 1962 A surgical procedure for blepharoptosis vera and for pseudoblepharoptosis orientalis. British Journal of Plastic Surgery 15:271
4. Smith JW 1973 Cosmetic surgery of the aging face. In: Grabb WC, Smith JW (eds) Plastic surgery – a concise guide to clinical practice, 2nd edn. Little Brown, Boston, p 555
5. Gunther JP, Antrobus SD 1997 Aesthetic analysis of the eyebrows. Plastic and Reconstructive Surgery 99:1808
6. Hinderer UT 1991 Aesthetic surgery of the eyelids and periocular region. In: Smith JW, Aston SJ (eds) Grabb and Smith's plastic surgery, 4th edn. Little Brown, Boston, p 565
7. Rees TD, Tabbal N 1981 Lower blepharoplasty with emphasis on the orbicularis muscle. Clinics in Plastic Surgery 8:643
8. Sheen JH 1974 Supratarsal fixation in upper blepharoplasty. Plastic and Reconstructive Surgery 54:424
9. Flowers RS 1993 Upper blepharoplasty by eyelid invagination. Clinics in Plastic Surgery 20:193
10. Friedland JA, Jacobson WM, TerKonda S 1996 Safety and efficacy of combined upper blepharoplasty and open coronal browlift: A consecutive series of 600 patients. Aesthetic Plastic Surgery 20:453
11. Flowers RS 1993 The biomechanics of brow and frontalis function and its effect on blepharoplasty. Clinics in Plastic Surgery 20:255
12. Mladick RA 1993 Updated muscle suspension and lower blepharoplasty. Clinics in Plastic Surgery 20:311
13. Zarem HA, Resnick JI 1992 Operative technique for transconjunctival lower blepharoplasty. Clinics in Plastic Surgery 19:351
14. Dover JS 1996 Editorial: CO_2 laser resurfacing: Why all the fuss? Plastic and Reconstructive Surgery 98:506
15. Connell BF, Marten TJ 1993 Surgical correction of the crows' feet deformity. Clinics in Plastic Surgery 20:295
16. Stasisor OG 1981 Blindness associated with cosmetic blepharoplasty. Clinics in Plastic Surgery 8:793

83

Rhinoplasty – planning, techniques and complications

KARL HEINZ AUSTERMANN

INTRODUCTION

Corrective nasal surgery is the most frequently requested procedure in esthetic facial surgery. This is not surprising as the nose has a key position in the overall esthetics of the face and even minor changes to it will have major effects on the appearance and the self-confidence of the patient. Although interpersonal communication occurs almost totally 'en face', the profile of the nose and its surrounding area has a greater significance for the subject than the frontal view. From this point of view the patient usually feels that his or her nose is too large and wants a reduction in its size. Only too keen to follow the requests of such patients, a whole generation of rhinoplasty surgeons was faced with poor results. It was the great contribution of Jack Sheen[1] to have researched and demonstrated solutions for the important and hitherto unaccountable causes of these failures.[2] The key to the modern approach to rhinoplasty, therefore, is that although the underlying structure of the nose can be changed freely, the covering skin can not. All the procedures described in this chapter are thus subject to the premise that the extent, thickness and quality of the skin are the limiting elements for rhinoplasty, to which the correction of the skeletal scaffolding must bow.

Another impetus to make the results of rhinoplasty consistent and reduce the risks of secondary deformity came from Tebbetts,[2] who describes how he avoids any kind of measure which weakens cartilage in the tip area and rebuilds through a conservative process. The renaissance of the external approach has effectively been a third milestone on the way to the present state of rhinoplasty.[3–5]

TERMINOLOGY

Since the terms used in the literature concerning rhinoplasty are not used uniformly, those to be used in this chapter are introduced below.

Instructions governing 'direction' are especially problematic: they are not only inconsistently used, but also additionally confusing in that one must distinguish between those relating to the nose and those relating to the skull as a whole, since the nose's main axis stands at an angle to the facial axis. The main footward axis of the nose points *caudally*, that of the skull as a whole *inferiorly*. Accordingly, towards the vertex the main axis of the nose is termed *cranial* (or cephalic) and that of the head *superior*. Perpendicular to the main axis of the nose, the direction towards the nasal dorsum is described as *dorsal* and the opposite direction as *basal*; the corresponding skull axes are *anterior* and *posterior* (Fig. 83.1).

Nomenclature in the tip area, as used in the literature, is a further source of confusion. The concepts of the nasal base and nasal tip are not uniformly defined. In this chapter the *nasal tip* is more narrowly defined, it is reserved for the area between the infratip break (ITB) and the supratip break (STB). All other structures – such as the sides of the nose, columella and nasal entrance basal to the lower breakpoints – are termed the *nasal base*. The nasal tip and nasal base together form the soft tissue of the nose.

The term '*lobulus*', is rarely used in Germany or in the English literature. Two different lobuli must be differentiated: the *tip lobulus* and the *alar lobulus*. The tip lobulus will be designated as the high area between the 'tip defining points'

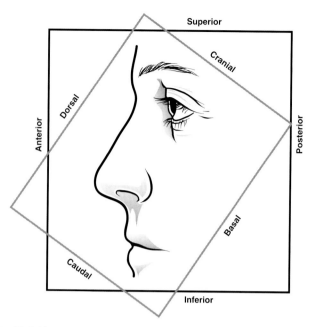

Fig. 83.1 The terms used in this chapter relate to the face and nose.

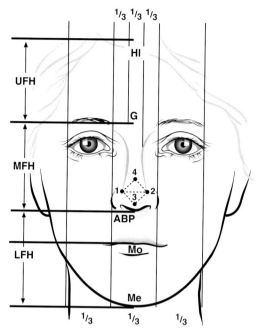

Fig. 83.2 Facial proportions from the frontal view. Horizontally, the shape of the face can be divided into three equal parts: the middle third being the distance between the medial canthi, and the outer thirds being the distances between the medial canthus and lateral canthus of each eye. Vertically, the face is also classically divided into three equal and harmonious thirds: the upper facial height, the midfacial height and the lower face height. The latter can itself be subdivided at the level of the mouth into an upper third and a lower two thirds.
Key: UFH = upper facial height; MFH = midfacial height; LFH = lower facial height; Hl = hairline; G = glabella; ABP = alar base plane; Mo = mouth; Me = menton; 1 = right tip defining point; 2 = left tip defining point; 3 = infratip break; 4 = supratip break.

(T) and the 'infratip break' (ITB), the alar lobulus as the rounded, balloon-like, basal half of the side of the nose.

The term 'dome' is also frequently imprecisely used. In this chapter, in line with common usage in the literature, the highest point of the vestibulum nasi will be called the dome; it is represented by the concavity of the alar cartilage immediately lateral to the point where the crus medial folds over to the crus lateral.

The other terms for anatomic landmarks used in this chapter are to be found in Figure 83.5.

NASAL ANALYSIS AND TREATMENT PLANNING

GENERAL FACIAL ASSESSMENT

It is as a rule perfectly possible to spontaneously assess a nose as esthetic and harmonious in itself and in relation to the face as a whole, but why this is so is difficult to explain in detail. In the same way it is difficult to expound why a less appealing face does not have the effect of beauty and harmony. Esthetics and beauty come in many forms. Therefore, or simply despite this fact, a reliable evaluation of a face cannot be undertaken without precise measurements, from which can be derived a deeper understanding of the interactive proportions within the face.

Symmetry and harmonious proportions are best judged from the frontal view, the face being subdivided vertically into three equally sized parts whose width corresponds to the intercanthal distance (Fig. 83.2).

The vertical proportions can be analyzed in the frontal as well as the side view (Figs 83.2 and 83.5) by dividing the facial height into three parts (Hl–G = G–Sn = Sn–Me). For better definition the subnasal point may be replaced by the alar base plane (ABP). The midfacial height (MFH) then corresponds to the distance G–ABP and the lower facial height (LFH) is the distance ABP–Me. In the lower face a further three-part division can be undertaken through the mouth opening (Mo): a third for the upper lip (ABP–Mo) and two thirds for the lower lip plus chin (Mo–Me). Further combinations for analysis have been described by Legan & Burstone[6] and Powell & Humphreys.[7]

The esthetic facial analysis should always be combined with dentoskeletal investigation so that possible deviations in the latter can be taken into account in the esthetic planning from the very beginning.

RELATIONSHIP OF THE NOSE TO THE FACE

The esthetics of the nose are determined by its surface contour. The preoperative analysis as well as the final esthetic goal are therefore achieved on the cutaneous appearance alone. The superficial appearance itself is determined by the defined anatomic configuration of the nasal structure together with the quality and quantity of the covering skin. The anatomy dictates the operative technique, in that its original state is changed by particular surgical techniques to create a new superficial appearance according to the esthetic goal. To this end the analysis describes the current condition of the superficial morphology, and the planning describes the aim of the final appearance. Analysis and planning are interactive prerequisites in the preparation: the differences between them dictate what needs to be corrected.

Much has been written about how the ideal proportions of the nose can be defined, both in itself and in relation to the face as a whole. Most such procedures fail, however, because the measuring points and angles used and the wide individual variations are hard to define.

The nasal facial angle of approximately 36 degrees of Brown & McDowell[8] is generally accepted as a standard (Fig. 83.3A). However to be applicable, these measurements require a chin prominence (Pg) which fits harmoniously into the facial profile, so that it constitutes a correct reference point on the facial vertical line (G–Pg). Powell & Humphreys[7] give a direct metric relationship between the height of the nose and its projection; they use as the nasal height the distance from the nasion (N) to the subnasal point (Sn) and as the projection the vertical line on N–Sn (intersection point X). The relationship of the thus defined nasal height (N–Sn) to the tip projection (X–T) should be 2.8:1 (Fig. 83.3A). Goode's method appears more valid; the imprecision of the subnasal point is avoided by using a tangent from N to the alar crease junction (ACJ). The perpendicular from T meets this line at point Y. The nasal tip projection (Y–T) corresponds to 0.55–0.6 of the length of the dorsum of the nose (N–T) (Fig. 83.3B). Crumley & Lanser[9] construct a right-angled triangle from the line connecting the nasion (N) to the alar crease junction (ACJ), from a vertical dropped from there at point Y to the 'tip defining point' (T), and from the connecting line N to T. In the ideal case, nasal tip projection (Y–T), nasal height (Y–N) and nasal dorsum length (N–T) are in the relationship 3:4:5 (Fig. 83.3B).

These methods suffer from two serious defects:

1. They have no firm relationship to the proportions of the face as a whole.
2. They use landmarks which have little constancy and are not precisely definable.

These problems may be avoided by using an analysis recommended by Byrd & Hobar,[10] which in our experience

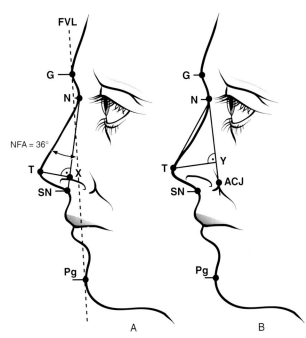

Fig. 83.3 Different methods for evaluating nasal proportions. **(A)** The nasal facial angle (NFA), determined by intersecting a line drawn from G to Pg (= facial vertical line, FVL) with a line tangent to the nasal dorsum (N–T), should be 36° (–40°).[8] The nasal height (N–Sn) should be in the ratio 2.8:1 in relation to the tip projection (X–T).[7] **(B)** The tip projection (Y–T) should be 0.55–0.6 of the length of the dorsum of the nose (N–T). The tip projection (Y–T), the nasal height (Y–N), and the length of the dorsum of the nose (N–T) should be in the relationship 3:4:5.[9] *Key:* FVL = facial vertical line; NFA = nasal facial angle; ACJ = alar crease junction; G = glabella; N = soft-tissue nasion; T = tip defining point; Sn = subnasal point; Pg = soft-tissue pogonion; X = intersection point of the perpendicular from T to N–Sn; Y = intersection point of the perpendicular from T to N–ACJ.

consistently gives harmonious planning results but is not as simple to accomplish as the aforementioned. It is based on the knowledge that on one hand the projection of the nasal tip and that of the nasal root or bony dorsum are correlated with the nasal length, and that on the other hand the nose length is directly correlated with the midfacial height. This correlation follows the acknowledged one third to two thirds proportions in the following relationship (Fig. 83.4):

1. the nasal length (N–T) corresponds to two thirds of the midfacial height (MFH)
2. the nasal tip projection (ACJ–T) corresponds to two thirds of the nasal length (N–T)
3. the nasal root projection (CP–N) corresponds to one third of the nasal length (N–T).

The prerequisites for achieving this relationship are a satisfactory state of the dental occlusion and overall harmony of the vertical facial thirds. If these requirements are not fulfilled, one must consider the need for corresponding corrections to accompany the rhinoplasty.

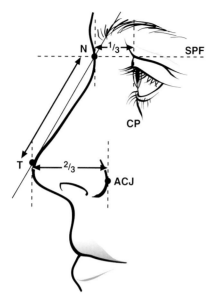

Fig. 83.4 The length of the nose (N–T) has a one third/two thirds relationship with the root projection (N–CP), forming one third, and the tip projection (T–ACJ), forming two thirds.
Key: SPF = superior palpebral fold; CP = corneal plane; N = soft-tissue nasion; ACJ = alar crease junction; T = tip defining point.

A great advantage of Byrd & Hobar's analysis is the consistency of the selected basic measuring points: these are usually not influenced either by the rhinoplasty itself or by accompanying procedures. With the help of these relatively constant landmarks, the stepwise evolution from the current morphology to the eventual ideal position can be planned (Fig. 83.5).

Step 1:
Analysis: Measurement of the midfacial height (MFH) and lower facial height (LFH).
Planning: Measurement of the MFH and LFH. MFH should be equal to LFH; if there are large discrepancies, a skeletal correction must be considered.

Step 2:
Analysis: Measurement of the distance Mo–Me.
Planning: Mo–Me should correspond to two thirds of the lower facial height (LFH); if a large discrepancy exists, a genioplasty must be considered.

Step 3:
Construction: Arbitrary establishment of a constructed nasion (N_H) as a midline point at the level of the superior palpebral fold (SPF) or 6 mm above the internal canthus.

Step 4:
Analysis: Measurement of the current nasal length (N_H–T).
Planning: Estimation of the ideal nasal length N_H–T_H = $0.67 \times$ MFH or = Mo–Me.

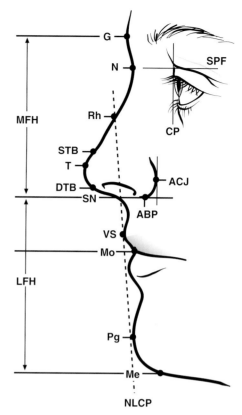

Fig. 83.5 Basal anatomic landmarks for facial analysis and rhinoplasty planning: MFH = midfacial height; LFH = lower facial height; NLCP = nose–lip–chin plane; SPF = superior palpebral fold; CP = corneal plane; STB = supratip break; ITB = infratip break; T = tip defining point; ACJ = alar crease junction; ABP = alar base plane; Mo = mouth; Rh = rhinion; G = glabella; Pg = pogonion; Me = menton; VS = superior vermilion; N_H = hypothetical nasion of Byrd and Hobar (1992); T_H = hypothetical ideal tip defining point of Byrd & Hobar (1992).

Step 5:
Analysis: Measurement of the current tip projection (ACJ–T).
Planning: Estimation of the ideal tip projection ACJ–T_H = $0.67 \times N_H$–Ti.

Step 6:
Analysis: Measurement of the current root projection (CP–N).
Planning: Estimation of the ideal root projection (CP–N_H = $0.28 \times N_H$–T_H).

Step 7:
Analysis: Comparison of the nasal bridge projection with the connecting line N_H–T_H.
Planning: Estimation of the nasal bridge line in line with N_H–T_H.

Step 8:
Analysis: Measurement of the anterior chin projection using the nose–lip–chin plane (NLCP).

Planning: Genioplasty is required if the chin projection lies in front of the nose–lip–chin plane or more than 3 mm behind it.

THE INDIVIDUAL SECTIONS OF THE NOSE

Nasal root (nasion)

In the frontal view the width of the nasal root should constitute about 30% of the intercanthal distance (Fig. 83.2). It should form a smooth curve with the supraorbital rim. These harmonious relationships are present in most cases and seldom need correction in cases with craniofacial dysmorphism. On the other hand, in the profile view, the shape and position of the root exhibit considerable individual variety and have an important influence on the total effect of the face. A sharply angled, too far anteriorly and cranially situated nasal root leads to a serious and severe expression, while a hollowed, dorsally and caudally situated nasal root creates a soft, friendly expression. It is therefore understandable that the planning and correction of the nasal root should play a key role in the rhinoplasty as a whole. The nasal root is also especially suitable for modification because it can be defined against an unmodifiable organ, the eye. The constructed nasion (N_H) should lie at the level of the superior palpebral fold (with a relaxed forward gaze) about one third of the nasal length (approximately 9–14 mm) in front of the corneal plane (Figs 83.4 and 83.5).

Anatomically the nasal root corresponds to the nasofrontal hollow and joins the convex glabella with the straight nasal dorsum. The firm bony structure of the root is formed by the continuity of the frontal bone, the frontal processes of the maxilla, and the paired nasal bones. It is almost always the height alone that requires reduction or augmentation, and very rarely the width.

The dorsum of the nose

The dorsum of the nose joins the nasal root with the nasal tip. In profile the course and the height of the nasal dorsum will be orientated to the connecting line between the level of the tip defining point (T_H) and the constructed nasion (N_H). In women, this line lies 2 mm in front of and parallel to the nasal dorsum, in men the nasal dorsum lies approximately on this line. The length of the nasal dorsum (from N_H to T_H) should ideally be around a third longer than the nasal tip projection (ACJ–T_H) and the same length as the distance between the mouth and menton (Mo–Me) (Figs 83.4 and 83.5).

In the frontal view the side of the dorsum of the nose should continue the curved line of the supraorbital rim over the nasal root to the defining point where it meets the dome on that side. A minor curve in this line at the point where the bony dorsum meets the cartilaginous nasal dorsum because of a slight widening in this area is seldom considered esthetically disturbing.

The nasal dorsum is composed of a cranial bony and a caudal cartilaginous part. The bony nasal dorsum is the continuation of the root and is made up of the paired nasal bones and the two frontal processes of the maxilla, which caudally form a vault. The cartilaginous nasal dorsum is formed by the dorsal prominences of the upper lateral cartilages and the nasal septum. The width of the bony nasal dorsum in the area of the nasofrontal suture is 14 mm and in the area of the nasofrontal angle 10 mm[11]; from there it widens again to 12 mm in the region of the rhinion (Rh), which lies 9–12 mm caudal to the nasofrontal angle and marks the point where the bony and the cartilaginous nose join. In the cartilaginous area the dorsal width lessens only very slightly in the direction of the nasal tips. These values are significant when augmenting the nasal dorsum with cartilage and/or bone grafts.

The upper lateral cartilage is joined along its dorsal edge with the nasal septum; cranially the upper lateral cartilage telescopes under the vault of the bony nasal dorsum and is joined to the bone edge by 2–4 mm of connective tissue.

This anatomic situation can throw up problems when an over-projecting nasal dorsum is being corrected. First, after a reduction, the nasal dorsum skin does not always fit well over the cartilage–bone area, resulting in an unsightly contour especially when the skin is thicker. Second, the continuity between the upper lateral cartilages and the nasal septum is disrupted in resection of the nasal dorsum, and this can have considerable esthetic and functional consequences.

Nasal tip

Esthetic superficial analysis

While the nasal root and nasal dorsum reflect the basic character of a nose, the nasal tip is the decisive measure of the esthetics of the nose. This is determined by three factors:

1. projection and rotation
2. surface contour
3. definition.

Projection and rotation, together with the nasal length, are the decisive relative dimensions for the esthetics of the nose in relation to the face as a whole. The surface contour, by contrast, determines the esthetics of the nose itself.

The tip *projection* refers to a line between the two tip defining points on the nasal tip, which project furthest forward in the profile as well as in the caudal view of the nasal base at its widest (tip-projecting points). Accordingly the tip projection from the subnasal point is better measured in the side view from the alar crease junction (ACJ). The target value, in accordance with the proportions defined in Relationship of the nose to the face, above, corresponds to approximately two thirds of the nasal length (Fig. 83.4).

An ideal nasal tip projection is the central goal in each rhinoplasty and always constitutes a challenge, even for the most experienced surgeon.

For *rotation* of the nasal tip, the degree of cranial movement around an imagined transverse axis in the area of the nasal base is used. It is expressed by the size of the nasolabial angle and to some degree also by the angle of rotation, i.e. the angle between the medial crura and crura intermedia (Fig. 83.6A). Rotation and projection are in close relationship to each other and to the length of the nose: greater rotation increases the nasal tip projection and decreases the nasal length; a lesser degree of rotation decreases the nasal tip projection and increases the nasal length.

The contour of the nasal tip, i.e. its superficial appearance, is of the utmost importance for the esthetic effect of the nose itself, though of course it is of lesser importance to the overall harmony of the face. It is determined by the volume, the width, and the definition of the nasal tip. The *volume* of the nasal tip is determined by the shape and size of the lateral alar crura (Fig. 83.7) and the *width* by the interdomal distance (Fig. 83.6B).

The *definition* manifests itself in the relationship between the thickness of the skin on one hand and the size, form, and supporting effect of the alar cartilage on the other. It describes the clearly defined contours of the nasal tip, which are especially noticeable by their reflection of light and are delineated by four landmarks:[1]

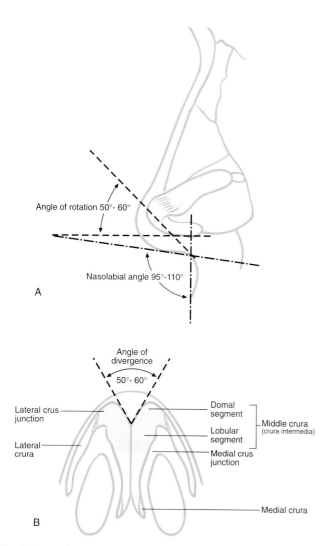

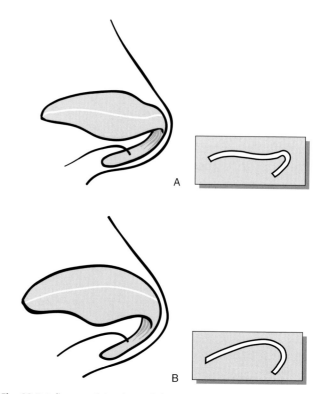

Fig. 83.6 Nasal tip morphology. **(A)** The degree of rotation of the nasal tip is expressed not only by the nasolabial angle but also by the 'angle of rotation'.[1] The 'angle of rotation' is defined as the angle between columella and tip; its structural basis is the angle between the middle and medial cruca (circa 50–60°). **(B)** The lateral angle between the middle crura is defined by the 'angle of divergence' (circa 50–60°). The interdomal distance is determined by this angle.

Fig. 83.7 Influence of the size and shape of the lateral alar crus on the contour and definition of the nasal tip. **(A)** A well contoured and defined nasal tip can be expected if the convex dome segment of the alar cartilage is relatively narrow and takes a sharp curve into the concave lateral crus (inset: section through the alar cartilage). **(B)** A less contoured, rounded nasal tip can be expected if the dome segment forms a wide curve with a large, convex lateral crus (inset: section through the alar cartilage).

1. side projection of the right dome (tip defining point 1)
2. side projection of the left dome (tip defining point 2)
3. transition from the columella to the tip (infratip break, ITB)
4. differentiating point between the nasal tip and dorsum (supratip break, STB).

The first three landmarks correspond to prominent points, the last is a flattened hollow. Together the four points form two isosceles triangles with a common base formed by the connecting line between the projections of the left and right domes (Fig. 83.2). In profile, the middle of this connecting line should be defined as the furthest anteriorly projected part of the nose (T). A nasal tip can only be well defined if the covering skin is not too thick and the cartilaginous skeleton has a sufficient supporting effect to tension the thickness of the skin. An excess of thick skin will always lead to an uncontoured nasal tip (see Fig. 83.12).

Anatomic analysis

The alar cartilage forms the support skeleton for the nasal tip and is responsible for its surface contour. It is described traditionally as a two-part cartilage whose medial and lateral crura join in the dome. Sheen & Sheen[1] further differentiated this structure, in that they described a middle crus forming a bridge between the medial crus and the lateral crus (Fig. 83.6). The shape of this cartilage has far-reaching consequences on the surface contour of the nasal tip. The transitions from the middle crus to the medial and lateral crura have a key influence on the esthetic effect of a nose. The transition from the middle to the medial crus (medial crus junction) is angled cranially (angle of rotation) and thereby forms the esthetically crucial lower break point of the nasal tip (infratip break, ITB). The transition to the lateral crus (lateral crus junction or domal junction) corresponds to the very important lateral light reflection of the dome crus caused by the change in shape between the medial and the lateral crus. The sharper this transition angle and the thinner the covering skin, the more defined the nasal tip appears (Fig. 83.7).

The lateral crus should run with its rim half parallel to the nostril edge, and then turn up posteriocranially. The cranial edge must abut the upper lateral cartilage and is attached to it with closely woven connective tissue. According to Daniel,[12] in approximately 80% of cases convex and concave areas alternate inside the lateral crus. A voluminous nasal tip is not, however, the result only of the shape and size of the lateral crus – it also depends on its position. If the axis of the lateral crus runs more parallel to the nasal dorsum than to the rim, the caudal edge of the alar cartilage forms a bullnosed tip (Fig. 83.8).

Nasal base

The caudal third of the nose consists of the nasal tip and the nasal base; the boundary between these two structures can only be visualized in the caudal view by drawing a line through the tips of the nasal openings (Fig. 83.9). The nasal base includes the following anatomic structures:

- ala or nasal wing (alar lobulus, alar rim)
- nasal openings
- nasal path
- nostril or nasal entrance threshold.

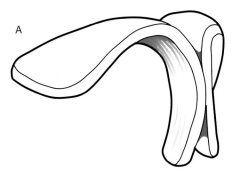
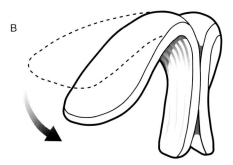

Fig. 83.8 Influence of the position of the lateral alar crus on the morphology of the nasal tip. **(A)** A cranially oriented lateral crus rounds off the dome segment and does not leave a supratip break. **(B)** Repositioning the lateral crus parallel to the nasal alar edge contours the dome segment and makes a supratip break possible.

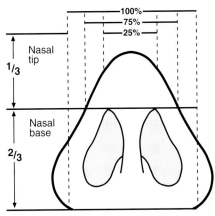

Fig. 83.9 Basal view of the nose demonstrating esthetic proportions.

On the caudal view, the soft-tissue nose resembles an isosceles triangle which the columella divides into two right-angled triangles. The nose is widest in the area of the alar lobuli; in a Caucasian it should not exceed the intercanthal distance by more than 1–2 mm. Towards the tip the nasal base narrows so that at the transition to the tip it is only 75% of its basal width. The nasal openings are pear-shaped and the same length, or at most twice as long as, the tip bulb (Fig. 83.9).

In profile, the columella should be roughly parallel to the alar edges and extend below them caudally by approximately 2–3 mm (columellar show). The transition between the columella and the upper lip forms the nasolabial angle, which to be esthetically appealing should be between 100 and 110 degrees in women and between 90 and 100 degrees in men (Fig. 83.6).

SUPPORT MECHANISM OF THE NASAL TIP

The nasal skin requires support to stretch it and give it contour. A good comparison is a tent, whose tarpaulin is stretched over the tent poles. The tent poles of the nasal tip are the alar cartilages, which form a tripod-like support: a median foot, which supports itself posterocaudally at the nasal spine, jointly formed by the medial crura, and two side feet which drop away over the sesamoid posterocranially opposite the aperture, each of which is formed by a lateral crus.[3] In contrast to a tent, whose poles can be adjusted so that they put the tarpaulin under tension, the alar cartilages in themselves are not solid enough to support the span and the weight of the skin on their own over the nasal spine and/or the aperture. Additional support mechanisms are necessary; these are primarily the connective tissue attachments of the medial crura to the caudal edge of the septum and of the cranial edge of the lateral crura to the caudal edge of the upper lateral cartilage (Fig. 83.10). Alongside these important support structures, there are others that play a subordinate role (Table 83.1). Under pathologic conditions, however, the latter can assume primary support functions, for example the overdeveloped dorsal septum edge in a taut nose.

Both pre- and intraoperatively it is easy to assess the effectiveness of the support apparatus – the recoil forces (elasticity) can be estimated by pressing the nasal tip. At the end of a rhinoplasty one must also ensure that the nasal tip is supported by the alar cartilage (or graft) and that the connective tissue attachments of the alar cartilage to the caudal edges of the septum and upper lateral cartilage are retained or are replaced by suturing.

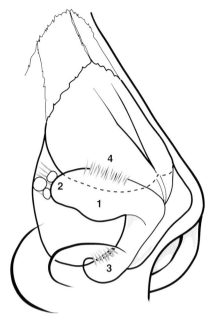

Fig. 83.10 Primary support mechanisms of the nasal tip: 1. size, shape and resilience of the medial and lateral alar crura; 2. support of the lateral alar crura on the piriform aperture; 3. attachments between the medial crura and the caudal edge of the septal cartilage; 4. attachments between the lateral alar crura and the upper lateral cartilage.

Table 83.1 Support structures of the nasal tip

Primary support structures
1. Size, shape and resilience of the medial and lateral crura
2. Support of the lateral crura on the bony aperture
3. Connective tissue attachments between the medial crura and the caudal edge of the septum
4. Connective tissue attachments between the lateral crura and the upper lateral cartilage

Secondary support structures
1. Connective tissue attachments between the crura intermedia (interdomal sling)
2. Connective tissue attachments of the alar cartilage to the skin
3. The sesamoidea between the lateral crura and the aperture
4. The membranous septum
5. The cartilaginous nasal dorsum
6. The nasal spine

SKIN QUALITY AND DISTRIBUTION

Rhinoplasty predominantly involves a correction of the nasal skeleton, in which reducing techniques rather than augmenting techniques generally prevail. The skin and the soft tissues play a rather subordinate role in this scheme of things: they should fit over the reduced overall mass of the scaffold and re-adhere evenly. However, the skin does not always fit or adhere evenly in all areas of the nose because the excess skin contracts and contracted skin thickens. The thicker the skin and the greater the area of excess skin in relation to the reduced supporting skeleton, the more the skin will thicken and lead to loss of contouring. A typical example of this are the results of an over-resection of the scaffolding in relation to the ability of the skin to contract – a rounded-off, contourless nasal tip with a thickened supratip region (Polly beak phenomenon – Fig. 83.47A).

The frequency with which this typical failure occurs depends on the thickness and quality of the skin, which differs not only between individuals but also within a single nose. The skin over the transition of the bony to the cartilaginous nasal dorsum is thinnest; cranially and caudally the skin increases in thickness (Fig. 83.11). After even reduction of the support skeleton the thin skin over the bony part will adjust to the scaffold through contraction; however, the thicker skin in the tip area cannot do this in equal measure and indeed thickens out of proportion. This results in a disproportion between the nasal dorsum and the nasal tip. So an apparent paradox becomes understandable – a voluminous, uncontoured and thick-skinned nasal tip can become esthetically harmonized only through augmentation, and not through reduction of the support skeleton (Fig. 83.12).

The variation in thickness of the skin of the nasal dorsum

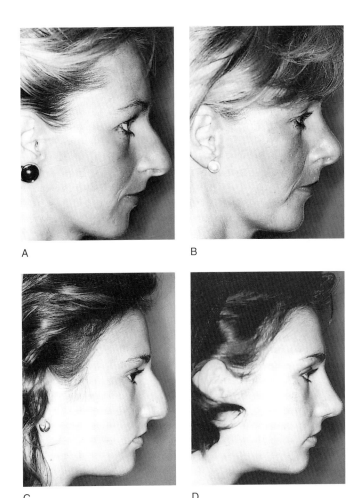

A B

C D

Fig. 83.12 The skin character, which affects outcome. **(A)** Large, prominent hump nose with retrognathic mandible. **(B)** The patient expressly requested a correction consisting mainly of reduction of the nasal hard tissues or 'scaffold' in conjunction with a genioplasty. The excess skin does not fit snugly to the scaffold, resulting in an ill defined and poorly contoured nose. **(C)** Patient with large, prominent hump nose. **(D)** In this case the nose was not reduced, instead being corrected mainly through augmenting techniques (root graft, nasal tip graft as described by Sheen, columellar graft). The nose did not become smaller but gained a more esthetic shape.

and the nasal tip is well demonstrated by X-ray; however, careful palpation and inspection will normally suffice to adequately assess the 'skin element' when forming a strategy for correction. 'Understanding the constraints of the skin is a step toward predictable results.'[1]

ANESTHESIA

After a detailed explanation of the risks involved, the decision between local anesthesia with analgesia and general anesthesia is normally left to the patient. Medically, our preference lies with local anesthesia because of the lower

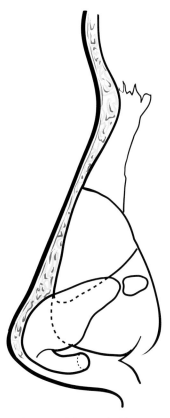

Fig. 83.11 The skin of the nasal dorsum is thinnest over the area where bone and cartilage meet, and increases in thickness cranially and caudally. The nasal dorsum will, therefore, appear straight only if the cartilage–bone junction is slightly convex.

risk of intraoperative hemorrhage, reduced postoperative swelling and quicker recovery time after the procedure.

General anesthesia is undertaken without hypotension with enflurane, N$_2$O and a central analgesic (fentanyl); in addition the patient receives the same local anesthetic as the patient choosing local anesthesia and analgesia. For analgesia the adult patient receives 2.5 mg midazolam orally an hour before induction of anesthesia, followed by 3 mg midazolam and 100 mg tramadol intravenously for induction. Local superficial and infiltrative anesthesia is then given. During the operation midazolam is titrated in 1–2 mg boluses, the frequency depending on the conscious state of the patient and the O$_2$ saturation of the blood. 'Standby', intravenous infusions, permanent O$_2$ insufflation (1.5 l/min) and the facility to intubate must be available.

After induction of the general anesthetic and/or the analgesia, neurosurgical swabs (neurosurgical cotton) saturated with a 5% cocaine solution are inserted along the nasal floor and the nasal dorsum. The cocaine dose is limited to a total of 200 mg (= 4 ml) in a healthy adult.

Infiltrative anesthesia is performed with 1–2% lidocaine solution which contains adrenalin 1:100 000 to 1:200 000. For a complete septorhinoplasty the following nerve branches are blocked:

- supraorbital nerve – bilaterally
- infraorbital nerve – bilaterally
- anterior ethmoidal nerve (endonasally) – bilaterally
- nasopalatine nerve (proximal blockade).

In addition the nasal soft tissues are locally infiltrated in different tissue layers:

- at the bony nasal dorsum – supraperiosteally
- in the area of the upper lateral cartilage – supraperichondrally
- along the intranasal incision lines – submucosally
- on the prepared side of the septum – submucoperichondrally and/or submucoperiostally
- on the unprepared side – submucosally.

Infiltration of the local anesthetic is used simultaneously as hydraulic preparation. The total amount of the local anesthetic is limited to 400 mg lidocaine for adults. If necessary, and if larger volumes are required for the hydraulic preparation, saline or Ringer's lactate solution can be used.

BASIC TECHNIQUE FOR REDUCTION RHINOPLASTY

INCISIONS AND APPROACH

To gain access to the skeletal structures of the nose, an

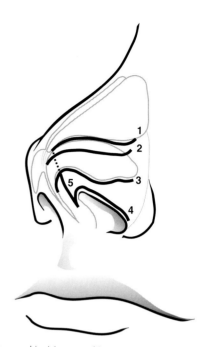

Fig. 83.13 Intranasal incisions used in approaches to the nose: 1. intercartilaginous incision; 2. intracartilaginous incision; 3. infracartilaginous incision; 4. rim incision; 5. hemitransfixion incision.

extranasal or one of a range of different intranasal incisions can be selected (Fig. 83.13):

- intercartilaginous
- intracartilaginous
- infracartilaginous
- rim
- transcolumellar (extranasal) (see Fig. 83.34A)
- transfixion (complete, incomplete)
- hemitransfixion (complete, incomplete).

The *intercartilaginous incision* is generally considered the standard entrance route to the nasal dorsum. It is simple to accomplish and gives excellent access to the support structures of the dorsum. The mucous membrane is directly lateral and parallel to the projecting edge of the caudal edge of the upper lateral cartilage beginning at the septal angle for a length of approximately 1.5 cm (indicated in Fig. 83.14A). The incision is located in the supraperichondral plane of the upper lateral cartilage and the dissection of the dorsum is begun in this layer. It is absolutely essential to avoid leaving this plane of dissection in the direction of the panniculus adiposus, since this can lead to diffuse intraoperative hemorrhages and later to unpredictable scars. The preparation is most successfully carried out using a no. 15 scalpel or fine, pointed preparation scissors (Fig. 83.14B). The extent of the dissection in the area of the upper lateral cartilage depends on the planned extent of the nasal tip rotation and on the condition of the skin. The

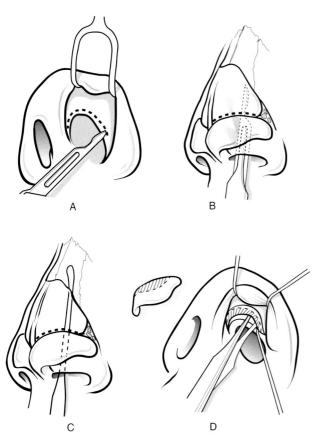

Fig. 83.14 Intercartilaginous incision showing access to the nasal dorsum and the cranial edge of the alar cartilage. **(A)** Intercartilaginous incision (---) with medial extension to the hemitransfixion incision (···). **(B)** Dissection of the nasal dorsum cartilage with a no. 15 scalpel at the supraperichondral level. **(C)** Subperiosteal dissection of the bony nasal dorsum with the sharp edge of a Freer elevator. **(D)** Retrograde view of the cranial edge of the alar cartilage showing planned resection of the lateral crus (insert).

greater the degree of rotation planned and the thicker the skin, the more extensive must be the skeletonizing or exposure – if necessary, up to the aperture.

On the bony nasal skeleton dissection moves from the supraperichondral level to the subperiosteal plane as the periosteum is near the edge. With a narrow, sharp elevator (e.g. Freer's) the periosteum is stripped as far as the naso-frontal suture (Fig. 83.14C). At the side the dissection is only continued as far as is necessary for the planned reduction in height of the nasal dorsum; this ensures the vital attachment of the covering skin on the sloping side of the bony nose. In the case of thin skin in particular, meticulous dissection in the subperiosteal layer is important to avoid unevenness of the bone showing through and scarred adhesions with the skin over the nasal dorsum. After the dissection has been completed on one side of the nose it is repeated in the same way on the opposite side and the dissection planes on both sides are connected.

If it becomes necessary, and has been taken into account

in the preoperative planning, the intercartilaginous incision may be extended to the transfixion incision (or one of its variants – Fig. 83.14A). For this the columella is stretched caudally (e.g. with tweezers or a special columella retractor) and then the columellar skin is separated with scissors or a scalpel directly in front of the caudal edge of the septum. If one considers the alar cartilage to be part of the skin cartilage, the covering skin has now been completely detached from the nasal skeleton. Once this situation has been achieved, correction measures at the septum and nasal dorsum can be undertaken.

The decision to extend the intercartilaginous incision into a transfixion incision must be carefully considered and found justified because although it achieves an entrance it also removes an important support component of the nasal tip (see Fig. 83.10). The tissue adhesion of the medial crura to the caudal edge of the septum, together with the support of the medial crura on the nasal spine, secures the projection of the nasal tip. If excessive projection of the nasal tip is to be reduced, this separation is helpful, otherwise the medial crura must be reattached with non-resorbable sutures to the caudal edge of the septum. In addition to this indication the complete transfixion incision is only indicated if parts of the columellar skin need to be reduced. For all other interventions – such as anterocaudal correction of the septum, correction of the nasal spine, and augmentation of the columella – a lesser degree of exposure will suffice (hemitransfixion incision, incomplete transfixion incision), in which the attachments between the medial crura and the caudal edge of the septum are at least partially retained.

With the intercartilaginous incision not only can the nasal dorsum be modeled but, by working retrogradely, the cranial edge of the lateral crus can be displayed, partially resected, or modeled (retrograde approach – Fig. 83.14D).

An identical result, namely access to the nasal dorsum and to the cranial edge of the lateral crus, is achieved with the use of the *intracartilaginous incision*. Once the width and length of the planned resection of the cranial edge of the alar cartilage have been established and marked, the incisions can be made through the mucous membrane and cartilage (cartilage splitting approach). The detached edge of the alar cartilage can then be excised through these incisions and the incisions are subsequently extended to provide an approach to the nasal dorsum. Both procedures are equally valid as operative approaches to the nasal dorsum and the cranial edge of the alar cartilage, however the tissue trauma caused by the incision for the intracartilaginous approach lies in a functionally less critical area than that for the intercartilaginous (in the proximity of the nasal flaps).

As an approach to the alar cartilage, both previously

described incisions can be summed up as the concept of the 'non-delivery approach'. The opposing concept is the 'delivery approach', in which the *intercartilaginous incision* is combined with an *infracartilaginous incision* which proceeds along the caudal edge of the cartilage. The incision begins in the 'near tip' third of the columella, in the dome area is carried cranial to the soft triangle of the caudal edge of the lateral crus, and ends approximately 15 mm lateral to the dome. The intercartilaginous and infracartilaginous incisions meet between the skin and cartilage in the supraperichondral plane, resulting in a medially and laterally based bridge skin flap that can be delivered out of the nostril (delivery approach). The clearly visualized alar cartilage – including the dome and middle crus – can obviously be much more precisely fashioned than is possible under the conditions of the non-delivery approach (Fig. 83.15).

The non-delivery approach is always preferable because it is less invasive when a simple bilateral resection of the cranial edge of the alar cartilage is the only required measure in the tip area. On the other hand, if there are asymmetries, malpositions and corrections to be made in the dome area, the alar cartilage can be presented clearly by the delivery approach.

In the *external approach* for rhinoplasty (see p. 1402) bilateral infracartilaginous incisions are joined in the middle of the columella through a transcolumellar skin incision. A small inverse V breaks the transverse skin incision, so as to prevent transverse contracture of the scar (see Fig. 83.34). With this incision the skin of the nose is raised directly from the cartilage and the entirety of the skeletal support of the nose is exposed to direct view. The open approach is not a routine method for most rhinoplasty surgeons, but is reserved for special situations, particularly the following:

1. difficult revision rhinoplasty
2. complicated asymmetries of the tip area
3. cleft nose corrections
4. difficult deviated noses
5. voluminous noses with thick skin.

CORRECTION OF THE DORSUM

The projection level of the nasal dorsum results from the root and tip projection. In routine cases the line of the nasal dorsum is adjusted by reduction. The procedure differs in some important points depending on whether only a *mild* or a *considerable reduction* of the nasal bridge is necessary. A maximum reduction in height of 3 mm is considered mild. Up to this extent of resection the connection of the upper lateral cartilage with the septum can be retained (Fig. 83.16); in addition the mucous membrane of the nasal dome can remain intact without mobilization. Both are important factors for undisturbed postoperative nasal ventilation, because if the dome membrane remains intact and so does the fusion between the upper lateral cartilage and the septum (at least partially), the cartilaginous vault in the area of the nose flaps will also keep its previous form and dimensions.

The technique for a slight reduction is as follows. After

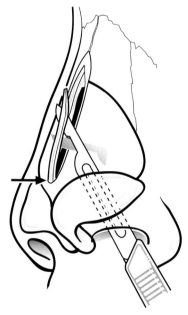

Fig. 83.16 Mild reduction of the bridge of the nose. First the bony hump is reduced with a rasp, then the cartilaginous part with a scalpel. The hump is usually only made up one third to one quarter of bone, the rest is cartilage. The cartilaginous resection comprises the dorsal edges of the upper lateral cartilages where they fuse with the septum. This may result in a narrowed nasal flap angle, a situation which can be avoided by retaining a cartilaginous bridge at the caudal end of the upper lateral cartilage (arrow).

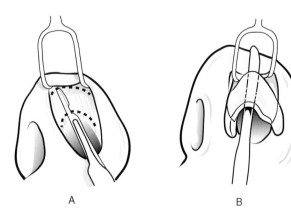

A   B

Fig. 83.15 Delivery approach. **(A)** Inter- and infracartilaginous incision. **(B)** Formation of a chondrocutaneous bridge flap at the supraperichondral level with dislocation of the alar cartilage (delivery approach). The alar cartilage can then be corrected in this position – in this case by resection of the cranial edge.

the dissection the nasal bridge is reduced with a bone rasp without damaging the cartilage. This is achieved by orienting the rasp perpendicular to the nose's main axis rather than in a longitudinal direction. Often it is surprising how little of the bony hump needs to be removed. In a short aquiline nose in particular only a small part of the hump is found in the bony area and by far the larger in the cartilaginous part. After the bony nasal dorsum has been reduced with the rasp to the planned level, the cartilaginous part is then reduced and a corresponding slice of the dorsal cartilage is removed with the scalpel. This should consist of a *single* incision at right angles to the septal base and include the corresponding dorsal areas of the upper lateral cartilage and the septal cartilage. Fine correction by smoothing and modeling is then undertaken.

If a more extensive nasal dorsum reduction is necessary, first of all a bilateral tunnel is formed in the upper nasal vault by lifting the mucoperichondrium of the dorsal septum and upper lateral cartilage as far as is required for the planned resection – the extramucosal procedure[15] (Fig. 83.17A). This tunneling is also carried into the bony area in the subperiosteal plane. In this way the operative site remains isolated from the nasal cavity, even after resection of a large part of the nasal dorsum; this has advantages for later scar formation and especially also in cases in which a nasal dorsum graft will be required. A further advantage is that the excess mucous membrane remaining in the vault then prevents the upper lateral cartilages from forming an over-acute angle with the nasal septum and causing a reduction in the nose flap angle. This advantage can, however, become a disadvantage if the mucous membrane is very thick and its excess prevents sufficient narrowing of the dorsum. After formation of the tunnels with the scalpel, whose cutting edge is directed towards the nasal dorsum, the upper lateral cartilages are separated bilaterally from the septal cartilage. Then the profile line of the dorsum is determined in the cartilaginous area according to the preoperative planning, all three leaves of cartilage being incised from caudal to cranial as far as the transition to the bony dorsum. The stripped cartilage is then removed and the new line of the dorsum examined. The cartilage at the bony hump can be removed (Fig. 83.17). The line of the cartilage incision is then continued into the bony dorsum with a flat osteotome according to the planned profile line. A sharp rasp can be used to remove even a large hump with more precision than the chisel, though this takes much longer. The usual problem that arises is that the cartilaginous dorsum is under-reduced and the bony dorsum over-reduced. In this phase of the operation the different thicknesses of the skin in the cartilaginous and bony areas of the dorsum must be taken into account. Further attention must be paid to

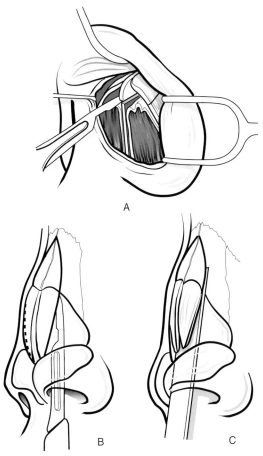

Fig. 83.17 Marked nasal bridge reduction. **(A)** After dissection and raising of the mucoperichondrium on both sides of the nasal bridge vault, a large hump can be reduced without creating a connection to the inside of the nose (extramucosal approach[15]). **(B)** First the cartilaginous part of the nasal dorsum is cut with a scalpel at the planned level. **(C)** The incision is continued over the bony part of the nasal dorsum with an osteotome and the hump is removed in its entirety.

the opening in the nasal roof created by de-humping and the need for osteotomies of the side walls to prevent an 'open roof' which must be closed. In very broad noses this can cause problems if the line of the dorsum has been considerably reduced. In narrow noses it is understandably not a problem.

Alternatively, as part of the dissection, a thin slice of the cartilaginous nasal roof can be left on in continuity with the skin of the dorsum (Fig. 83.18); at the end of the reduction this closes the open roof of the cartilaginous dorsum and holds the upper lateral cartilages in their original transverse relationship, avoiding the need for spreader grafts.[16]

The planned osteotomies which will be required for the dorsal width reduction and the closing of the open roof are associated with brisk bleeding and the rapid onset of swelling. This can complicate the fine correction of the nasal

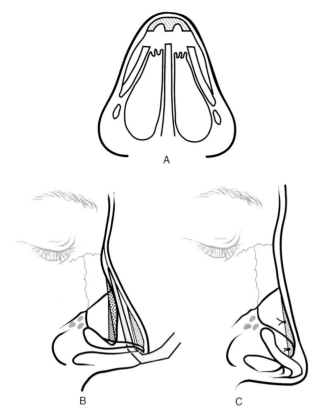

Fig. 83.18 Alternative approach to the nasal dorsum. **(A)** Dissection of the cartilaginous nasal dorsum is undertaken through a transcartilaginous approach by which a thin layer of the dome cartilage remains attached to the skin of the dorsum (hatched area). **(B)** The skin and attached cartilage are raised together by a hook. The hump reduction (dotted area) can then be carried out through this approach. In addition to the hump reduction, a strip of cartilage (cross-hatched area) corresponding in size to the cartilage attached to the skin must be removed from the dorsum. **(C)** Finally, the edges of the upper lateral cartilages are sutured to the repositioned cartilage, thereby preventing transverse collapse of the upper lateral cartilage.

tip. For this reason, after the dorsum reduction has been performed, correction of the nasal tip is undertaken before the concluding action of the osteotomies.

CORRECTION OF THE NASAL TIP

As in reduction of the nasal dorsum, there are correction measures for the nasal tip which can be considered to be basic techniques since they are required in the majority of rhinoplasty procedures. From an esthetic planning viewpoint these include:

1. volume reduction of the nasal tip
2. reduction in the interdomal distance
3. cranial rotation of the nasal tip
4. emphasis of the upper breakpoints.

The large number of techniques for correction of the alar cartilage (excisions, incisions, suture techniques, grafts) is

matched by the wide variation in cartilage and soft-tissue morphology requiring correction; nevertheless the techniques necessary in routine cases can be limited to a few.

It is imperative to have clear concepts about which structures can be changed with what effect and, moreover, which structures can be changed by which techniques; these are described below. It is not so clear, however, to what extent the changes in the structure of the skeleton are transferable to the final superficial esthetic appearance, and, similarly, in which cases this transfer is possible, or only potentially so, by changes in technique. The answer may be found somewhere in the relationship between the firmness of the cartilaginous structure and the thickness of the skin. Sensitive and delicate cartilaginous structures can be ideally modified through the most ingenious technology, but if the skin is thick the only result will be an ungainly nasal tip. It can not be frequently enough emphasized that in these cases a good result can only be achieved, if at all, with augmentation procedures (columellar strut, tip graft, etc.). Following the traditional approach, the cartilage must have sufficient firmness and the skin normal thickness; only then can esthetic goals be achieved by the techniques described below.

In a standard case, the *prominence of the nasal tip* is less the result of its actual size than of the convexity of the lateral alar crus. By proportionate resection of the cranial edge of the alar cartilage (see Fig. 83.14D) the part of the lateral crus principally responsible for this outward effect is reduced and an esthetically pleasing reduction in volume is attained. In certain cases, however, the extent of the convexity is so great that the lateral crus can not be excised without endangering its support function. In these cases an equivalent effect can be achieved without resection through the use of suture techniques which turn the convexity into a concavity. In addition we recommend incising around the relevant part of the cranial edge of the alar cartilage,

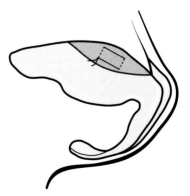

Fig. 83.19 Volume reduction of the nasal tip by suturing. The convex cranial part of the alar cartilage is completely mobilized, weakened, and mattress sutured into a concave shape. The mucoperichondrium remains intact and adheres to the incised cartilage.

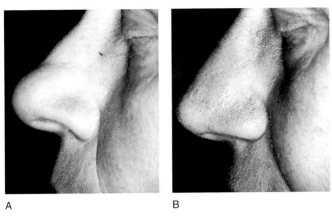

A   B

Fig. 83.20 Volume reduction of the nasal tip. **(A)** A bullnosed tip results mainly from the convexity of the hypertrophic lateral alar crura. Reduction of the tip volume is achieved by cutting around the cranial half of the alar cartilage, weakening the exposed parts, and reforming the convexity into a concavity with mattress sutures. **(B)** Appearance 11 months after correction.

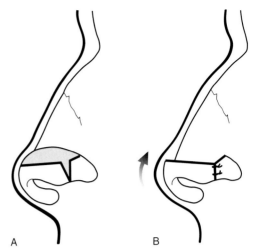

A   B

Fig. 83.21 Marked cranial rotation of the nasal tip by a combination of resection of the cranial edge of the alar cartilage and basal division of the lateral alar crura. **(A)** The resection of the cranial ede of the alar cartilage is planned in such a way that a caudal strip of at least 5–8 mm remains. Basal division of the lateral alar crura consists of removal of a wedge, the angle of this wedge determining the extent of the rotation. **(B)** The cut ends of the lateral alar crura must be repaired by exact end-to-end suturing, avoiding overlapping. Only in this way can the dangers of over-rotation and loss of support by avoided.

leaving the mucoperichondrium intact, weakening it (by scoring or morselization), and then forming it into a concavity by mattress suturing (Figs 83.19, 83.20).

Alongside diminution in its volume, narrowing of the nasal tip, i.e. *a decrease in the interdomal distance*, is frequently also desired. To this end the dome area of the cartilage can be weakened, turning a wide dome region into a narrow one without losing the support function of the cartilage at the same time; this is achieved by making interdigitating partial-thickness incisions. With this technique the narrowing in the tip area can be accompanied by a minimal increase in projection. It is a small step from better malleability to loss of the support function. The increase in projection at the end of the operation may not be able to resist the pull of scar contracture in the postoperative healing phase, leading to loss of projection. The use of suture and grafting techniques avoids this problem (see Suture techniques, p. 1404) and we prefer them.

Resection of the cranial edge of the lateral crus permits a certain degree of *cranial rotation* of the nasal tip (see Ptosis of the nasal tip, p. 1406); this movement is limited by the rigidity of the caudal alar cartilage strip left intact (at least 5–7 mm width) and by the caudal edge of the septum. The rotation can be strengthened in two ways: first of all by shortening the caudal septal edge – perhaps accompanied by shortening of the caudal edge of the upper lateral cartilage – and to a greater extent by severing the basal third of the lateral crus (Fig. 83.21).

OSTEOTOMY

The osteotomies are made at the end of a rhinoplasty, as they are accompanied by brisk bleeding and the rapid onset

of swelling. The *median osteotomy* is commenced with a 3 mm wide osteotome, which is inserted at the cranial end of the acute-angled bony defect created by the hump reduction. The very simple and relatively atraumatic osteotomy extending the dividing line between the septum and upper lateral cartilage is undertaken first of all, swinging approximately 5–6 mm towards the nasal root at an angle

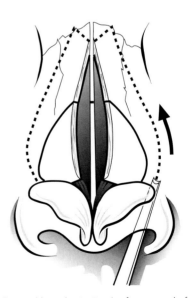

Fig. 83.22 Median and lateral osteotomies for removal of a large nasal hump. A 3 mm wide chisel with a concave edge is used for the lateral osteotomy. During reduction of a large hump the fusion between the upper lateral nasal cartilages and the septal cartilage is always lost.

of approximately 30 degrees (Fig. 83.22). With this swinging movement one bypasses the T-shaped bone mass of the nasal root. In this part of the operation attention must be paid to ensuring that the gap created by the median osteotomy is of equal width on both sides and permits proportionate narrowing of the nasal dorsum. A broad dorsal edge of the septum can impede the narrowing of the nasal dorsum or render it asymmetric. Especially after minor reductions of the nasal dorsum, the T-shaped widening of the dorsal edge of the septum remains and has to be made smaller. Also, care must be taken to ensure that the mucosa does not impede proportionate and sufficient narrowing of the dorsum.

The *lateral osteotomy* is the next step; we prefer a con-

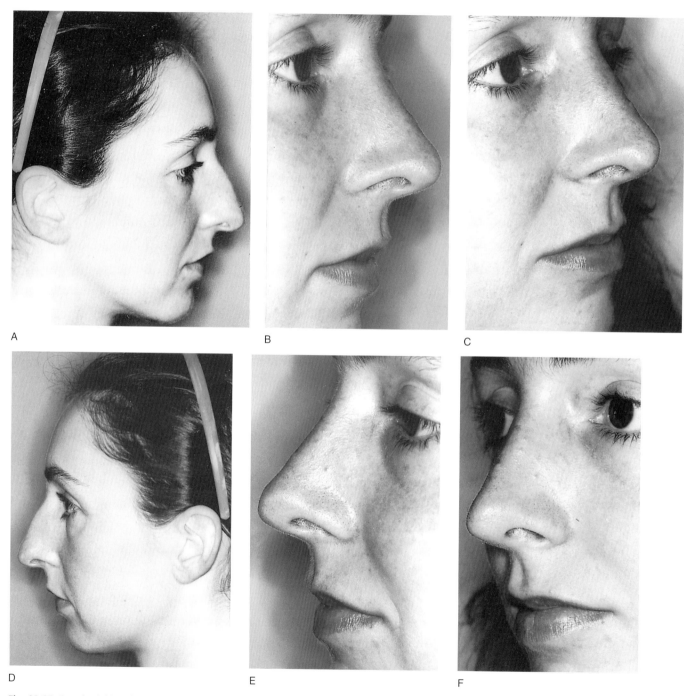

A

B

C

D

E

F

Fig. 83.23 Standard rhinoplasty for the correction of a large hump nose. **(A)** Preoperative right profile. **(B)** 10 months postoperative, right profile. **(C)** 10 months postoperative, right half-profile. **(D)** Preoperative left profile. **(E)** 10 months postoperative, left profile. **(F)** 10 months postoperative, left half-profile. Correction achieved by root graft, reduction of the dorsum and caudal edge of the septum, augmentation of the spine, medial and lateral osteotomies, and spreader graft.

cave 3 mm wide chisel, which is inserted low at the base of the piriform aperture. In the angle between the body of the maxilla and its frontal process the osteotomy is carried in a lateral bow shape to a point between the inner corner of the eye and the nasofrontal angle (Fig. 83.22). The periosteum is not removed for this. Ideally the median and lateral osteotomies should meet so that the bony side walls can be easily shifted inwards by finger pressure. If this is not possible, a broader chisel is inserted again into the median osteotomy and wedged in the frontal bone. By swiveling the chisel outwards the osteotomized bony bridge is fractured at the cranial end. This is facilitated by the fact that the end of the median osteotomy has been swung laterally, as described above.

In every case the fracturing of the bony nasal walls must be complete; leaving even only slightly springy fragments will result in later widening of the nasal dorsum. This danger is particularly great in young patients, necessitating an additional horizontal osteotomy in the area of the nasal root; the required incision of the frontal bone is located either in a cross-fold of the nasal root or between the medial ends of the eyebrows.

The now completely mobilized nasal bones, including the frontal process of the maxilla, can then be moved medially and the open roof of the nasal dorsum closed symmetrically. The upper lateral cartilages are carried along with this movement by their attachment to the nasal bone. If the continuity between the upper lateral cartilages and the septum has been completely disrupted, the upper lateral cartilages are only held laterally by the nasal bones, and their caudal ends swing like doors in the direction of the nasal septum. From the esthetic point of view this can result in the so-called 'inverted V deformity', and its functional consequence is a narrowing of the nasal flaps. In these cases the osteotomy for narrowing the bony nasal dorsum must be combined with spreader grafting and reattachment of the upper lateral cartilages to the dorsal edge of the septum (see Fig. 83.26), or at the outset one can leave a thin slice of cartilage of the nasal roof attached to the skin of the dorsum and reattach the upper lateral cartilages to that (Fig. 83.18).

With thick skin and a very short bony nasal dorsum, consideration should be given to correcting the over-projection of the dorsum indirectly through augmentation in the area of the root and the tip. In order to achieve a stable and functional result one should perhaps be prepared to modify the original plan and accept that it may not be possible to obtain a perfect result (Fig. 83.23).

Osteotomies in combination with spreader grafting are also the method of choice for the correction of transverse anomalies (too broad, too narrow, deviated).

Finally the fine correction of the nasal dorsum takes place; reduction of small errors is mostly undertaken with the rasp and the scalpel, and augmentation with crushed cartilage. Small unevennesses in the nasal scaffolding on outward examination are easily overlooked because of the rapid onset of edema in the soft tissues, only to reveal themselves later to the disappointment of both surgeon and patient.

The nasal dressing has the sole task of compressing the skin against the nasal scaffolding to reduce hematoma, seroma and swelling. It should not in any way be used to give the nose a shape which has not been already gained through operative means.

POSTOPERATIVE CARE

The postoperative phase should be planned long before the end of the surgery itself, in that the patient should be informed orally as well as in writing about the details and possible complications of the procedure and thus have sufficient time to discuss it and familiarize him- or herself with it. The patient also as a rule receives written instructions about conduct after the operation (Table 83.2) several weeks before the scheduled operation; he or she can therefore organize his or her personal life accordingly and adjust psychologically to this time. On the day before the operation; the procedure, the possible complications and the postoperative instructions are explained again and discussed in detail, so that the patient is not confronted with unpleasant surprises later on.

The real postoperative phase begins with the dressing – after a complete septorhinoplasty this consists of internal packs and outer splinting. The internal support tamponade is composed of swabs of neurosurgical cotton which are coated with an antibiotic-containing ointment and inserted in layers in the nasal passages. Threads securing the swabs are tied in front of the columella to ensure that they are not aspirated. The vestibulum is also plugged with small swabs to give the skin in this area an opportunity to re-adapt itself precisely.

For the external splinting an adhesive is first of all sprayed on the nasal skin. Subsequently Steri-strips are affixed under tension so that the skin is adapted as exactly as possible on the underlying scaffold. The first strips are placed like a noose caudally around the nasal tip, supporting the tip in a slightly over-rotated position. The next strips are applied vertically to this, first of all tightly over the supratip region to prevent cavity formation in this area, and then over-lapping over the entire nasal dorsum. For the splint itself we use a pre-prepared aluminum splint which is padded with a thin layer of foam material.

Table 83.2 Patient information: guidelines for behavior after surgery. As used by the author at the Klinik für Mund-Kiefer- und Gesichtschirurgie – Philipps Universtät, Marburg

- If you follow these guidelines you will make an important contribution to the success of the operation.
- Bring this sheet on admission and observe these instructions from the day of your operation. Should you have further questions please contact my colleagues or me.
- Please read the following instructions carefully and become familiar with them before your operation.
- Do not blow your nose within the first four weeks following the operation; if necessary, use clean tissues and/or Q-Tips to dab or carefully wipe. The recommended nose drops (Coldastop®) make cleaning easier.
- If you need to sneeze, open your mouth. The nasal tamponade (plugging of the nostrils) is removed after 24 hours (in certain cases later).
- The external nose splint will be removed after two weeks; sometimes it will be changed in between. Protect this splint from contact and moisture. If it comes loose prematurely it must be replaced.
- The bandange underneath the nose ('nose sling') should soak up blood and nasal secretions during the first few days; this bandage can be changed if necessary. Please do not touch or pull any part of the bandage that protrudes from your nostrils.
- During the first two weeks avoid food that requires excessive chewing; there are no further limitations on diet.
- During the first two weeks avoid physical exertion, long talks, long telephone conversations, as well as close physical and social contact.
- During the first week try to avoid excessive facial movements (e.g. laughing).
- Wash your face carefully to avoid wetting the nose splint.
- Wash your hair only with assistance so that the nose splint does not get damp.
- Bathe rather than shower for as long as you have a nose splint.
- Clean your teeth as usual but avoid strong movements of the upper lip which are transmitted to the nose.
- During the first two weeks wear clothing that can be buttoned at the front or back and does not have to be pulled over your head (no T-shirts, etc.).
- For six weeks avoid strong sunlight and UV rays (sunbeds!).
- For six weeks avoid sports that might involve even minor physical contact (e.g. swimming).
- For three months avoid contact sports (boxing, wrestling, judo, water polo, football, etc.).
- Do not wear spectacles or sunglasses for the first four weeks as they are supported on the bridge of the nose. Spectacle wearers will be told how they can avoid pressure from spectacles on the nose.
- Don't be too worried if, after removal of the splint, the nose and surrounding area are still slightly swollen – this is normal during the healing process and may take 4–6 weeks to subside. In some patients a certain amount of residual swelling may take 12–18 months to subside.
- The biggest risk to the stability of the surgical result occurs during sleep. Wear the nose splint at night for a further four weeks – it will remind you if your nose is pressing too hard into the pillow.
- *Don't take risks!* If anything worries you, contact me, or one of my colleagues, immediately.

The packs are removed after 24 hours; in certain cases where the scaffold is insufficiently stable they may be left in place up to a week after the operation. The external splint is removed after one week. After osteotomies a new splint, depending on the resolution of the swelling, is applied for a further week.

To prevent swelling, 250 mg intravenous prednisolone is prescribed at the end of the operation and a further 250 mg intramuscularly an hour later; the eyelids are cooled with ice compresses for 12 hours. The patient is nursed in the head-up position and liquid food is given for the first 48 hours.

After removal of the nasal tamponade all intranasal crusts are regularly removed and the nasal mucous membrane is tended with nasal oil.

Intranasal stitch removal is necessary only for the transfixion suture on the tenth postoperative day, as we otherwise use resorbable sutures intranasally (6/0 catgut, 5/0 PDS). Any skin sutures after open rhinoplasty or a Weir excision are removed on the sixth postoperative day.

The psychologic wellbeing of the patient is of greatest importance postoperatively. On removal of the splint the patient is cronfronted for the first time with his or her new nose, which is possibly still very remote in appearance from what was discussed in the planning stage and is anticipated by the patient. This situation can be dealt with easily only if the patient has already been carefully prepared for this moment in the preoperative phase.

ADJUNCTIVE TECHNIQUES

CARTILAGE GRAFTS

Autogenous cartilage is unrivaled as a transplant for reconstruction, support and design in the context of rhinoplasty. The following advantages distinguish it in comparison to other transplant materials:

1. constancy of volume even after years in position
2. biomechanical characteristics appropriate for bracing the nose (flexibility and strength)
3. no or only minimal peritransplant soft-tissue reaction
4. easily accessible donor regions, giving adequate volume with minimal morbidity.

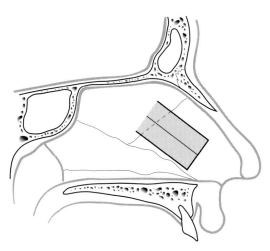

Fig. 83.24 Size and position of the planned septal cartilage removal. Two strips of around 3.5 × 1 cm can be removed without problems or endangering the stability of the supporting framework. The caudal incision is carried out with an angled scalpel, the vertical incision with angled straight scissors. The vertical incisions are taken up to the perpendicular plate of the ethmoid – on the one hand to increase the length of the transplant and on the other to facilitate its removal, the cranial end being simply removed by fracturing it. The residual defect is partly filled with cartilage and bone remnants which are crushed in order to enlarge and straighten them.

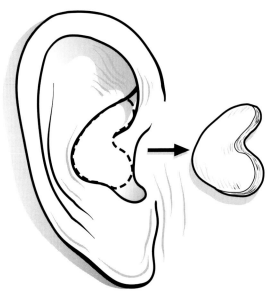

Fig. 83.25 As a donor region for autogenous ear cartilage, the whole of the concha, including the cymba, is available. The caudal end of the crus helicis must, however, be spared. An anterior as well as a posterior approach can be used. Cartilage grafts of up to 3.5 cm in length can be harvested and are suitable for almost all indications in rhinoplasty. With increasing patient age it becomes harder to shape the increasingly brittle cartilage.

Septal cartilage is the first choice. It is easily harvested, particularly in the course of a septoplasty, and can be easily fashioned yet maintains its shape and volume (Fig. 83.24).

If the septum is unsuitable as a donor region because of previous surgery, ear cartilage is the second choice. This site offers easy access for removal and minimal morbidity. As a donor area the entire concha and the cymba are at the surgeon's disposal. In comparison to septal cartilage, however, ear cartilage has the disadvantage that it does not provide a long, straight graft that is relatively rigid and unlikely to deform. This means, for example, that a straight supporting graft for the columella can be achieved only by rolling, and this creates volume problems in the columella. As a 'tip graft' or as a substituting or reinforcing graft for the lateral alar crus, however, ear cartilage is eminently suitable. The simple postauricular approach leaves no visible scars, and as long as the antihelix and the crus helicis are left intact there is no residual deformity (Fig. 83.25).

The use of rib cartilage is only indicated if the aforementioned donor regions can not provide a sufficient amount of cartilage. Apart from morbidity at the donor site, rib cartilage has the disadvantage as graft material that it is not a constant shape. The concept of the balanced design developed by Gibson & Davis,[17] through which distortion can be avoided, is not always possible if the appropriate grafts are not available. Additionally, ossification of the cartilage in older patients creates considerable problems in

shaping it. Nevertheless this graft has to be used sometimes. The cartilaginous ends of the free ribs (10th and 11th ribs) are especially suitable for narrow, oblong grafts such as a columellar strut. If a large dorsal transplant is required, the distortion problem can be limited by selecting a graft that combines bone and cartilage.[18]

The use of autogenous cartilage is established in a variety of shapes and for different indications in the context of rhinoplasty: tip graft, columellar strut, lateral alar crural strut, lateral crural spanning graft, dorsum graft, spreader graft. At this point spreader grafting, columellar grafts and tip grafting need to be discussed in more detail.

Spreader graft

The spreader graft[9] is tremendously important given the wide spectrum of problems in septorhinoplasty; the functional as well as the esthetic result of a rhinoplasty can be decisively influenced by these detailed measures (Fig. 83.26).

To understand the function and indication of a spreader graft, the anatomy and function of the upper lateral cartilage must be reviewed. The upper lateral cartilage forms the cartilaginous nasal dorsum jointly with the septum. The upper lateral cartilages are anchored cranially at the bony aperture and run close to the dorsal edges of the nasal septum. The caudal end forms the cartilaginous basis of the internal nasal valve which must remain patent even

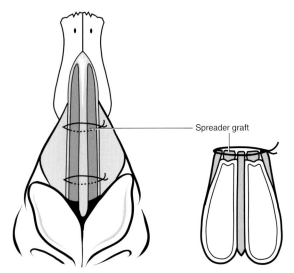

Spreader graft

Fig. 83.26 Spreader grafts. These transplants separate the dorsal edges of the upper lateral cartilages from the septal cartilage after reduction of the dorsum, enabling the physiologic width of the dorsal roof to be maintained.

during vigorous inspiration. The normal angle between the septum and the caudal edge of the upper lateral cartilage is approximately 15 degrees (see Fig. 83.43). On forceful inspiration the air flow is limited by the lower edge of the upper lateral cartilage moving in the direction of the septum and reducing the nasal flap angle. On forceful expiration, on the other hand, the caudal part of the upper lateral cartilage moves laterally, thereby enlarging the nasal flap angle and permitting greater flow. The area of transition between the upper lateral cartilage and the septal cartilage is not actually angular, but plateau-shaped. This plateau is arched bilaterally, resulting in the rounding of the nasal dorsum in this area.

In the course of a rhinoplasty for lowering the nasal dorsum, the plateau between the dorsal edges of the upper lateral cartilage and the dorsal edges of the septum is usually lost; the three dorsal edges of the septum and upper lateral cartilages now lie free from each other at a distance which depends on the original shape of the plateau and the extent of the reduction in height of the dorsum. The position of the upper lateral cartilage is now maintained only by its adhesions to the bony nasal scaffold (see Fig. 83.22). If then, after the osteotomy, the open roof of the bony nasal dorsum is closed by finger compression, the upper lateral cartilages are displaced medially to form an acute angle with the dorsal edges of the septum. This unnatural relationship of the cartilages to each other may not be recognized during or immediately after the operation but will become striking with the decrease in swelling and increase in scar contracture:

- the cartilaginous nasal dorsum becomes disproportionately narrow caudally in relation to the bony nasal dorsum, so that the caudal edges of the bone become visible and form the esthetically unsightly appearance of an inverted V (Fig. 83.27)
- the angle and shape of the medial vault are dramatically changed, with a negative effect on their function.

The shorter the bony nasal dorsum in relation to the cartilaginous, the weaker the cartilage, the broader the original vault and the thinner the covering skin, the more drastic the above problems will be.

The obvious conclusion to be drawn, therefore, is that the vault-shaped support between the upper lateral cartilages and the septum must be restored. Sheen[1] indicated the solution to this in the form of the so-called spreader graft – a 3 mm broad and approximately 2.5 cm long strip of cartilage from the septum inserted bilaterally and extramucosally between the dorsal edge of the upper lateral cartilages and the dorsal edge of the septum. It should be positioned so that it is under the bony vault and caudally level with the upper lateral cartilage, and be fixed at the cranial and caudal ends respectively with sutures to the contralateral graft and the edge of the septum.

A spreader graft is not required in every case of reduction rhinoplasty. For example, after moderate leveling of the nasal hump the plateau-shaped connection between the upper lateral cartilage and the septum in the caudal area remains, and the upper lateral cartilage can not collapse inward because it is reinforced cranially at the bony scaffold and caudally at the remaining cartilage bridge (see Fig. 83.16). Alternatively, it is possible to leave a thin strip of the cartilaginous nasal roof attached to the skin of the nasal dorsum before the reduction and use this as a spreader graft on its reattachment (see Fig. 83.18).

In correction of a unilateral cleft nose the spreader graft has yet another significance in that the upper lateral cartilage on the cleft side is almost always hypoplastic; with a spreader graft the differences between the two sides can be corrected.

The spreader graft has also proved its worth in long-term studies and is a vital component of the armamentarium of every rhinoplasty surgeon.

Columellar graft

A cartilage transplant in the columella can fulfill different functions; predominantly it is inserted within the tripod configuration of the nasal tip[13] as reinforcement of the medial crus (columellar strut). Other indications include correction of the retrusive columella or, less frequently, emphasis of the lower breakpoints.

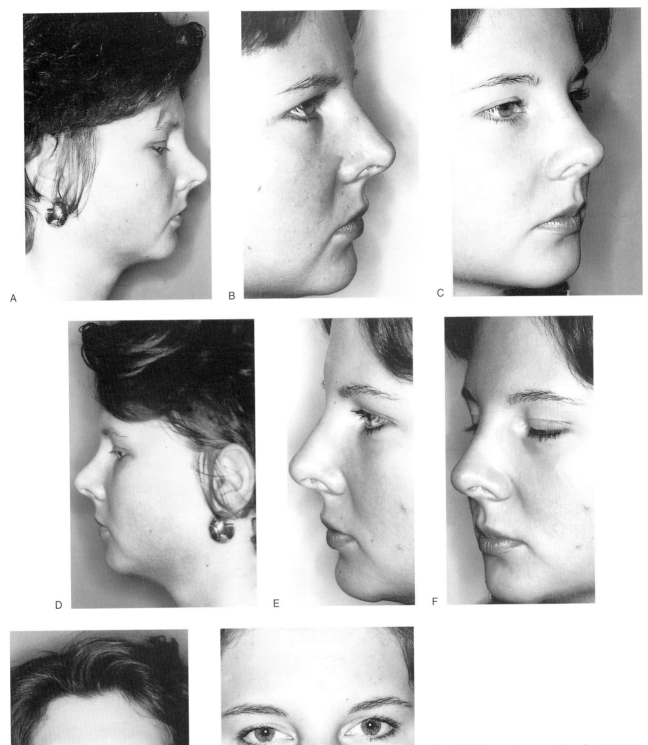

Fig. 83.27 Secondary correction after previous rhinoplasty. There had been relative over-reduction of the bony dorsum in comparison with the cartilaginous dorsum. **(A)** Preoperative right profile. **(B,C)** 9 months postoperative right profile and half profile. **(D)** Preoperative left profile. **(E,F)** 9 months postoperative left profile and half profile. **(G)** Preoperative en face; distinctive inverted V deformity after transverse collapse of the upper lateral cartilage. **(H)** En face 9 months postoperative with reduction of the dorsal septal edge, augmentation of the bony dorsum and root, bilateral spreader grafts, and tip graft as described by Sheen.

As a columellar strut (see also The underprojected nose, p. 1403) the cartilage graft has to improve or completely subsume the supporting function of the medial crura (control columellar strut). If possible, the columellar struts should be taken from a strip of straight septal cartilage; alternatively the free cartilage end of rib 10 and 11 may be used. The strip must be approximately 4–5 mm wide and, according to the extent of the planned tip projection, 30–35 mm long. A cartilage strip of these dimensions and also of sufficient thickness and firmness can really only be obtained from the septum, most likely from the basal part of the quadrilateral cartilage parallel to the edge of the vomer; part of the perpendicular plate of the ethmoid can also be included in the graft if required (Fig. 83.24). The cartilage transplant can be carried out through various operative approaches (transoral, open approach, columellar rim incision, transfixion, hemitransfixion, etc.) to prepare a graft bed between the two leaves of the medial crura. Basally, the graft is supported against the nasal spine of the maxilla, where it must be secured to stop it slipping sideways; this is done in the simplest case by creation of a narrow soft-tissue pocket. We often reinforce this by making a small sagittal bony groove in which the basal end of the graft is fixed by a permanent suture or by vertically splitting the basal end so that it straddles the spine. The graft is fixed to the medial crura of the alar cartilage by non-resorbable sutures placed in the longitudinal direction of the cartilage (Fig. 83.28). Anteriorly the strip is shortened so that it ends posterior to the dome level. If the strip is left too long it can project over the dome and spoil the tip projection by giving the nasal tip an unnatural 'tentpole' effect. In addition it may result in pressure, which in the most unfavorable case can lead to ischemic necrosis and skin perforation. Normally the graft will not protrude caudally between the medial crura. However the possibility exists, by careful positioning in relation to the medial crura and the nasal spine, of accentuating a retrusive columella and/or flattening an over-sharp nasolabial angle. In addition the rotation angle of the tip can be enlarged with a columellar strut so that the lower breakpoint is emphasized.

As desirable as it may be to achieve effective and reliable support for the nasal tip, it should not be overlooked that it is subjected to a relatively unphysiologic process; physiologically, compared to the firm structures of the nasal dorsum and the anterior maxilla, the nasal tip should be highly mobile. However with a columellar strut the mobility in an anteroposterior direction is reduced, that is to say the nasal tip can neither be pulled down through lip-pull nor pressed down through finger pressure. This can create an unnatural appearance, and a blow may dislodge or even fracture the graft. The indications for this procedure must therefore be carefully considered and the execution must be extremely precise. It should always be considered whether a control columellar strut,[2] which does not extend over the medial crura, can not equally fulfill this function.

Tip grafts

Tip grafts provide the nasal tip with greater projection and more contour than can be achieved by surgery to the existing cartilages. In noses with primarily weak support from thin, narrow alar cartilage or possibly in previously operated noses where the alar cartilage has been over-resected, tip grafting can improve the tip projection within the bulb, but not the projection of the nose as a whole. The indication for tip grafts is therefore limited.

Tip graft as described by Sheen

The shield-shaped tip graft described by Sheen[20] solves many problems which onlay grafts can not resolve; it simultaneously produces both strengthening of the projection and a natural surface contour of the tip area. The basic premise underlying this process is very different from what was previously known about tip grafting:[21–23] a cartilage graft is inserted into a soft-tissue pocket in the bulbous tip. This then creates an internal tissue tension which produces an esthetically appealing nose. For this effect it is crucial that the graft itself is anchored properly in the soft-tissue pocket and particularly at the top of the tip–columella junction. Through an additional 35 degree inclination away

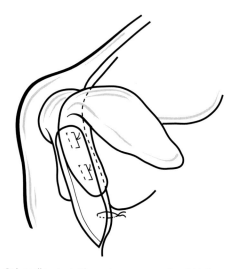

Fig. 83.28 Columellar strut. The autogenous graft, which is usually taken from the septum, is supported basally on the maxilla and fixed between the medial crura with vertical sutures. The graft must not reach as far as the dome, the tip projection being formed by the dome segments of the alar cartilage.

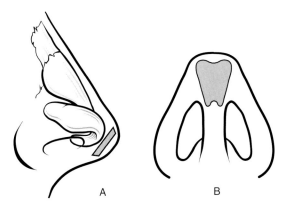

Fig. 83.29 Tip graft as described by Sheen. A cartilage graft shaped like a section through a molar is incorporated in the soft-tissue pocket of the nasal tip. Anteriorly it extends as far as the tip defining points and inferiorly to the point where the columella meets the tip.

from the line of the columella the esthetically vital double-break structure is produced (Fig. 83.29).

In its original design the shape of the graft resembles a longitudinal section through a molar, about 1.2 cm in length and 0.75 cm wide at the anterior edge. A wave-shaped notch is cut into the anterior edge to imitate the surface contour of the twin tip points. Towards the inferior edge the graft is thinned and must remain approximately 0.5–1 mm below the soft tissue at the transition between columella and lobulus. At the inferior edge a sharp notch should be created to support the graft and protect it from undesirable movement.

A unilateral infracartilaginous incision serves as entrance to the nasal tip, beginning at the transition from tip to columella and continuing behind the 'soft triangle' in the dome area. The really important part is less the design of the cartilage than the precise preparation of the graft bed in the nasal tip. Above all, the size of the pocket between the tip/columella dorsally must not extend into the line joining the planned maximum projection anteriorly. The graft must be wedged in this pocket under a certain tension of the covering tip skin. According to the thickness of the skin and the desired effect, the preparation level for the graft bed can be selected to lie more towards the skin surface or further inward towards the level of the cartilage. The dangers of the graft becoming visible through the skin or shifting are essentially determined by the preparation of the soft-tissue pocket. On one hand this pocket must be sufficiently large for the skin to conform with appropriate tension to the graft, on the other it must at the same time be small enough to prevent movement.

With ideal positioning of this tip graft the following effects can be achieved:

• reinforcement of the tip projection

• formation of two tip defining points (analogous to the twin dome projections)
• emphasis of the lower breakpoint between columella and lobulus
• contouring of the surface in the area of the lower triangle (between the twin dome points and the lower breakpoint)
• correction of the proportional length between the tip and the nostril.

After 20 years' experience, Sheen[24] has naturally recognized some of the disadvantages of his technique. The main problem is to find the right relationship between the size of the prepared soft-tissue pocket and the size of the graft. An over-large pocket in relation to a small graft fails to achieve the desired effect, a too-small pocket in relation to an over-large graft can leave edges and corners visible through the skin. Exact, universal recommendations can not be given for solution of this problem, since the quality of skin and cartilage are critical. This fine line between 'too large' and 'too small' relies on the skill and the experience of the surgeon. Sheen[24] in his 20-year report suggested a solution to this problem. He proposed that instead of using one or two large cartilage grafts, it is better to combine several which have been crushed to a variable degree to take out the internal tension.

The Sheen nasal tip graft was modified for open rhinoplasty, and suture fixation of the shield-shaped cartilage to the middle crura was recommended[25] (Fig. 83.30). Whether the unique charm of Sheen's technique – creating the perfect tension on the skin of the tip – is achievable with this method has still to be determined by long-term studies. On the plus side, it does however have the advantage of greater security through direct vision and the open fixation of the graft by sutures.

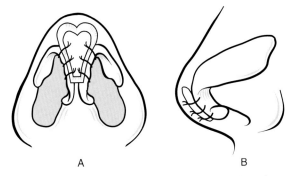

Fig. 83.30 Modified nasal tip transplant as described by Sheen for open rhinoplasty. **(A)** Open rhinoplasty allows accurate retention of the shield-shaped graft in the soft-tissue pocket under the tip; therefore it is sutured to the caudal edges of the middle and medial crura. **(B)** The side view shows the position of the graft in relation to the nasal tip. The graft reinforces the projection and improves the definition of the tip defining points and the infratip break.

Onlay tip graft

The onlay tip graft also enlarges the tip projection through secondary support. For this procedure only autogenous cartilage (septum, concha) should be used, approximately 4 × 9 mm in size and resting directly on the existing dome structure (Fig. 83.31). The onlay must be aligned horizontally with great precision, since even the smallest displacement will later manifest itself in disagreeable asymmetry of the tip. The position of the graft can be secured both by a tailormade preparation of the graft bed and transcutaneous temporary stay sutures. Nevertheless there is a considerable danger that the graft, under the tension of the soft-tissue covering, will slip off over the prominences of the alar cartilages in any direction. Similar problems are encountered with a technique in which the tip defining points on both sides are emphasized by small bilateral slices of cartilage fixed like pillars on the dome segments.[26] An onlay graft can reliably and effectively strengthen the tip projection, however it simultaneously removes the characteristic faceting of the nasal tip and with it its real esthetic refinement.

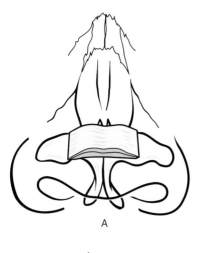

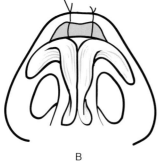

Fig. 83.31 Onlay tip graft. **(A)** The semilunar-shaped graft must be exactly situated transversely and horizontally and sutured over the dome segments of the alar cartilages. **(B)** By W-shaped contouring of its surface the graft can additionally mimic the double tip projection of the alar cartilages. The graft can be kept in position by temporary transcutaneous sutures. In the context of an open rhinoplasty the graft is sutured directly onto the dome segments.

Additionally, with thin skin a circular constriction in the overlying skin frequently becomes visible. This form of tip graft is thus more suitable for cases in which thick skin anyhow veils the finer faceting of the tip contours.

ALAR REDUCTION

The reduction and shaping (sculpture) of the alae forms an element of every rhinoplasty in certain ethnic groups (Asian, negroid), while it is more rarely necessary in the typical Caucasian nose. Like all steps in a rhinoplasty, the alar reduction also requires exact analysis and planning. Before selecting the operative technique to be chosen the following questions must be answered:

a. Should the nostril width be reduced?
b. Should the width of the alar base be reduced?
c. Should the length of the ala be reduced?
d. Should combinations of the above measures be undertaken and, if so, in what relationship to each other?

As a basic rule the 'two surfaces concept'[1] can be enlisted. This says that an excision at the internal surface of the ala brings about a *narrowing of the nostril*, and an excision of the external surface of the ala *reduces the alar base* and/or *shortens the ala*. If the nostrils and the alae are to be reduced together, an internal and external excision are combined.

Depending on the indications the following operative techniques are employed:

For (a), narrowing of the nostrils
For this a superficial rhomboid and deep wedge-shaped excision is made on the floor of the vestibulum nasi (Fig. 83.32A).

For (b), narrowing of the alar base
For this a wedge-shaped excision is taken from the outer surface of the ala near the base, which extends to the lining of the nose without injuring it and keeps the nasal entrance threshold intact. To make it smaller, the axis of the wedge to be taken is directed more vertically (Fig. 83.32A).

For (c), shortening the length of the alar edge
For this a wedge-shaped excision is also taken from the base of the outer ala. The axis of the wedge to be taken for this indication, however, is aligned more horizontally (Fig. 83.32B).

For (d), combinations of a, b, and c
This is the most frequent aim of correction. For this a wedge-shaped excision including the nasal floor (internal surface), the lateral part of the nasal sill, and the outer ala (outer surface) is taken (Fig. 83.32B).

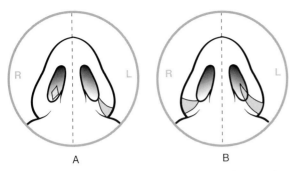

Fig. 83.32 Alar reduction and sculpture. **(A)** Right nostril: narrowing of the nasal entrance with a lozenge-shaped excision on the floor of the vestibulum nasi. Left nostril: narrowing of the nasal base by a vertical wedge-shaped excision. **(B)** Right nostril: shortening of the alar side wall through a horizontal wedge-shaped incision. Left nostril: wedge excision of the internal floor, sill and alar base.

It is obvious that very careful analysis and detailed planning are necessary to find the correct relationship between the external and internal excisions on one hand, and the correct inclination of the axis of the outer wedge excision (more vertical or more horizontal) on the other. In order to keep the external scars as unobtrusive as possible, the following points should be taken into consideration:

- The incision into the nasal entrance is placed as far lateral as possible, possibly with the formation of medial flaps as described by Sheen.[1]
- If possible the nasal entrance should not be affected.[27]
- No incision should be sited directly in the alar fold; it should instead always be placed about 1 mm into the ala.
- The wound edges should be precisely readapted with fine subcutaneous and cutaneous sutures.

MAXILLARY AUGMENTATION

Premaxillary augmentation

Several goals, which are not achievable through the standard rhinoplasty procedure alone, are pursued through premaxillary augmentation:

- protrusion of the nasal base
- protrusion of the cranial third of the upper lip
- basal support for the medial crura (with strengthened projection of the nasal tip)
- enlargement of the nasolabial angle
- paranasal augmentation.

Cartilage grafts (septum, concha, rib) are the first choice for filling material; autogenous bone is not recommended as an onlay material in this region because of resorption. Though the use of alloplastic graft materials is generally not

recommended in the nose, an exception can be made in the premaxillary area. We have found that suitably tailored components of Proplast and hydroxyapatite have proved best. Proplast preformed implants are also available.

If a single surgical approach must be chosen, the incision is made cranial to the nasal entrance at the side of the nose. It is carried from the medial third into the posterior third of the skin of the columella; from here the soft tissues anterior to and at the side of the nasal spine are removed through blunt and sharp dissection, then – according to the extent of the planned side-extension of the augmentation – the graft bed is developed towards the bone of the aperture on that side. If the base of the ala is also deficient then the preparation should be extended to the level of the nasolabial folds. With a unilateral lip, maxilla and palate cleft, the augmentation of the alar base is usually only necessary unilaterally on the cleft side. In connection with a rhinoplasty the sequence is as follows: first of all the premaxillary augmentation is completed, then the rhinoplasty is undertaken on the foundation of the new nasal base and the changed tip morphology.

Spine augmentation

The supporting point for the medial crura is shifted further ventrally by augmentation in the area of the nasal spine and is accompanied by (assuming sufficient stability of the medial crura) strengthening of the nasal tip projection and rotation and increase in the nasolabial angle (Fig. 83.33). The augmentation thus constitutes part of the primary

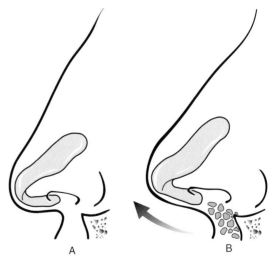

Fig. 83.33 Spine augmentation. **(A)** In a case of caudal rotation of the nasal tip with retrusion of the premaxilla and a small nasolabial angle, augmentation of the spine – especially in conjunction with other measures – can contribute to cranial rotation of the tip. **(B)** Cartilage chips can be used for the augmentation; they should be inserted in a soft-tissue pocket created anterior to the spine.

support of the tip projection. Autogenous cartilage from the septum or the concha is used as graft material.

THE EXTERNAL APPROACH

Although Rethi[3] described it in 1934, the open approach to the nasal skeleton first came to international notice with the publication by Padovan.[4] Through a multitude of papers in the 1980s this previously largely obsolete technique gained a firm foothold in nasal surgery. Meanwhile it is only the range of its indications that remains a matter for debate.

In the individual case the indication for this approach must emerge from the weighing of its advantages and disadvantages compared to those of the endonasal approach. Its advantages are: clear and binocular vision of the operative field, two-handed operating, improved teaching opportunities. In contrast its disadvantages include: visible external scarring, a more difficult and time-consuming surgical approach, and prolonged swelling and anesthesia in the nasal tip area. Goodman & Gilbert[28] observed that in 10% of their patients anesthesia in the nasal tip area after the open approach persisted for a year or longer.

Compared with other authors[29,30] we define the indications of open rhinoplasty quite narrowly, since for the patient looking for perfect esthetics the external scar, even though it is usually scarcely visible, entails a considerable concession. We limit its indications to difficult revision operations, complicated asymmetries in the tip area, lip, maxilla and palate clefts, difficult deviated noses, and prominent noses with thick skin.

Operative procedures

The columella is incised crosswise at mid height, that is to say at its narrowest point. The cross-incision is interrupted by one inverted V-shaped incision so that the suture occlusion relieves and later visually conceals the scar. The incisions begin exactly in the middle between the two medial crura with two stab incisions for the formation of the inverted V. Then the horizontal leg of the incision follows directly horizontally and symmetrically on both sides, and is continued on to the lateral surface of the columella; this is a very delicate stage because the crus medial lies very near the surface of the caudal edge here and must be cut from both sides. Incisions along the caudal edge of the medial crura and the lateral crus follow and are united with each other in the dome area, without injuring the 'soft triangle' (Fig. 83.34A,B).

The incision and the subsequent dissection make severe demands on the precision of the surgeon. The preparation

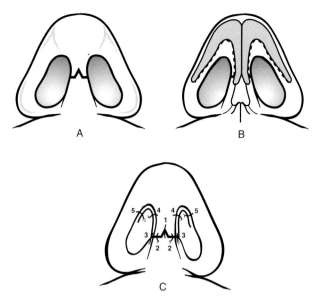

Fig. 83.34 Incision and key suture points for the open approach. **(A)** The mid-columellar incision is broken medially in an inverted V shape. **(B)** The mid-columellar incision is carried laterally on to both sides of the columella by a marginal incision which, in the area of the lateral alar crus, is extended up to the dome of the nostril into an infracartilaginous incision. **(C)** Closure of the wound is started by precise adaptation of the wound edges with 5 key sutures: 1. at the point of the inverted V; 2. at the angle between the inverted V and the horizontal leg of the mid-columellar incision; 3. at the angle between the mid-columellar incision and the marginal incision; 4. medial to the dome segment; 5. lateral to the dome segment.

level for the exposure of the nasal skeleton lies in the supraperichondral plane. Problems with the definition of the preparation plane arise in the 'cartilage-free' areas: (a) between the crura intermedia, (b) between the twin dome tips and the septum, and (c) between the lateral crura and the upper lateral cartilage. Here one performs sharp dissection with scissors in a subcutaneous layer which directly joins the adjacent supraperichondral preparation plane. In the bony area of the nasal dorsum the supraperiosteal preparation level can be continued in a case with thick skin; in a case with thin skin, after incision of the periosteum, the plane is changed subperiosteally. The nasal skin can then be lifted with a hook and the entire nasal skeleton is clearly presented for correction.

The nasal septum can be displayed either caudally or dorsally by this approach. To display the septum caudally, as with the endonasal approach, the connective tissue between the medial crura and behind that the columellar skin can be cleanly cut with the scalpel to the caudal edge of the septum. From there the septum can be displayed in the subperichondral plane. A huge disadvantage of this approach is that, as with the transfixion incision, an important part of the bracing of the nasal tip – namely the adhesion between the medial crura and the caudal edge of the septum

– is partially lost. For this reason we prefer to display the nasal septum dorsally by the open approach once the upper lateral cartilage has been removed from the septal cartilage.

The exact closure of the mid-columellar incision determines how visible or invisible the later scar will be. The first sutures are put in the tip of the V; we always use a two-layer closure (6/0 PDS and 7/0 Prolene) as there is sufficient subcutaneous tissue here to be grasped by the deeper suture and this in turn can take the tension of the skin suture. A skin suture (7/0 Prolene) is then inserted bilaterally at the base of the V and subsequently in the columellar edge on both sides. Then a skin suture (7/0 Prolene) is placed medially and laterally in the dome segments. Thus the key sutures are placed; areas still remaining open extra-nasally are closed with 7/0 Prolene, and intranasally with 6/0 catgut (Fig. 83.34C).

The belief that rhinoplasty becomes simpler through the 'open approach' is false, because the problems of measuring out the individual steps and the difficult evaluation of the potential postoperative changes remain, and a wealth of experience needs to be acquired for this approach. With this restraint in mind, the open approach clearly widens the range of surgical possibilities and is a step in the direction of better and more predictable results.

PARTICULAR PROBLEMS

UNDERPROJECTED NOSES

A central problem in esthetic rhinoplasty is to create an optimal relationship between the projection of the nasal dorsum and the projection of the nasal tip. The esthetic aim is for the nasal tip to form the most prominent projecting point of the facial profile. Simultaneously it should project so far anteriorly from the nasal dorsum that it creates a break in the line from the nasal dorsum. Although the tip projection is only one aspect in the complex esthetic effect of a nose, it plays a significant role in esthetics. Naturally, other factors influence appearance, such as ethnic group, age and sex on one hand and chin projection, depth of the nasofrontal angle, vault of the forehead, length of the nose, etc. on the other. In my own clients underprojection of the nasal tip vis-à-vis the nasal dorsum is the most frequent cause for corrective rhinoplasty, and it is also the most frequent reason for revision surgery after a previous rhinoplasty.

This predominant esthetic significance of tip projection is allied with other, often unpredictable variables related to the healing process. All these factors combine to make surgery of the nasal tip the most complicated and challenging area of rhinoplasty.

That there is still no simple standardized solution to this problem reflects the fundamental question, both in the planning as well as in the execution – whether the level of the hypothetical nasal dorsum should first of all be oriented to the projection of the nasal tip,[1] or whether the projection of the nasal dorsum should be adjusted to the hypothetical nasal tip.[31]

In both these procedures different philosophies are at work in evaluation and above all in the influence of the underlying structures, viz:

- support skeleton of the nasal dorsum
- support skeleton of the nasal tip
- soft-tissue covering.

During planning it is important to consider also what alterations can be achieved by surgery.

Anderson's philosophy proceeds on the assumption that the formation of the nasal tip projection is the part of a rhinoplasty which is realized with most difficulty according to the plan and as such should be treated as the baseline, since surgery is unpredictable. The nasal dorsum is then adjusted accordingly, since the level of the nasal dorsum can be realized much more easily and reliably according to plan. However this also means that the rhinoplasty generally becomes a predominantly reducing process; in other words this procedure implies that the nasal tip projection should be emphasized by relative reduction of the nasal dorsum. The huge disadvantage of this procedure is that the skin element (thickness and adaptation) is not adequately considered, and one proceeds on the tacit assumption that it will fit to the reduced skeleton. It is the sorry experience of every rhinoplasty surgeon, however, that this is not always the case after reduction.

It is primarily for this reason that Sheen[1] advises that the nasal dorsal projection should first of all be determined with regard to the thickness of the skin cover. The nasal tip projection is then adjusted according to this standard. He thereby concedes, as does Constantian,[32] that augmentation measures take precedence over reducing procedures. Naturally this approach can only be adhered to if the nasal tip projection can be precisely controlled. With the development of his excellent method for controlling nasal tip projection by a tip graft, Sheen[20] was to a considerable extent predestined to drive rhinoplasty in this direction. Tebbetts[2] has taken another, similarly successful route in that he preserves the maximum amount of alar cartilage for stabilizing reasons and achieves the desired shape, projection and position of the nasal tip through special suture techniques and invisible 'control' grafts.

Reasons for presentation

There are two categories of patients who complain about too little nasal tip projection: on the one hand are those who are discontented with their natural nasal tip projection, on the other those who have become discontented after a previous rhinoplasty. The loss of tip projection caused by a previous rhinoplasty has its own particularities and is discussed in Secondary rhinoplasty (p. 1414).

Primary underprojection can be put down to multifarious reasons, e.g. ethnic group (black, mestizo, Asian nose), malformation syndrome (e.g. Binder syndrome, cleft lip, maxilla and palate), trauma (e.g. post-traumatic dish face), or individual variation.

The causes of absolute or relative underprojection of the nasal tip can be listed in order of priority:

- high nasal dorsum
- hypoplasia of the maxilla
- lack of support of the alar cartilages
- short columella
- downward rotation of the nasal tip.

An overprojected nasal dorsum, frequently combined with the problem of a 'high bony dorsum', makes the nasal tip appear underprojected in the overall profile. With this starting position and with regard to the complete profile analysis of the face and the skin thickness, it is preferable relatively to strengthen the nasal tip projection. This is done by reducing the nasal dorsum, possibly combined with lowering of the dorsum, without any direct intervention at the tip.

The same applies to underprojection of the nasal tip due to maxillary micro- or retrognathia. In these cases too the nasal tip projection can be improved very effectively without direct intervention at the alar cartilage by anterior augmentation of the maxilla – either through an onlay technique or by a maxillary osteotomy (see Premaxillary augmentation, p. 1401) (Fig. 83.35).

If the cause lies predominantly in insufficient support of the nasal tip, this is when intervention should take place. Projection deficits caused by caudal rotation of the nasal tip (tip ptosis) are discussed in detail in Chapter ••.

Techniques for reinforcing tip projection

Methods for reinforcing the tip projection are divided into three fundamental processes, combinations of which are the rule rather than the exception:

- suturing techniques
- division techniques
- graft techniques.

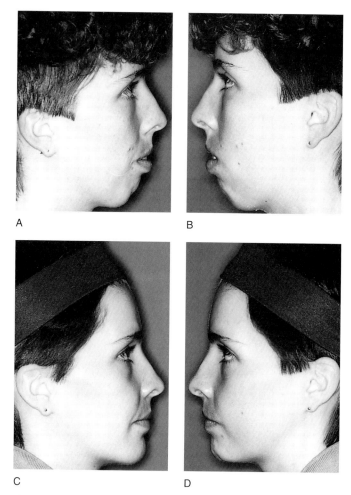

Fig. 83.35 Mandibular and maxillary retrognathia with open-bite (long face syndrome). **(A,B)** Preoperatively tip projection is lacking. **(C,D)** Cranial rotation of the maxilla (with auto-rotation of the mandible) results in stronger tip projection without the need for further corrective measures.

Suturing techniques

Suture techniques, either on their own or in combination with grafts, have largely taken over from division techniques in strengthening the projection of the nasal tip. Tebbetts[2] has developed a logical interdependent system of suture techniques in which maximum retention of alar cartilage allows reliable strength of projection.

Medial crural unification

In this technique the medial crura are joined through two vertical mattress sutures which catch the cranial edges together to form one unit; the anterior suture is placed at the height of the transition between the medial and middle crus (medial crural fixation suture), the posterior one approximately 3 mm anterior to the footplate (flare control suture). The greater the divergence of the medial crura,

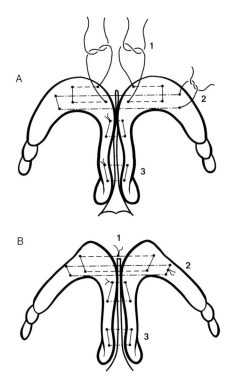

Fig. 83.36 Various suture techniques described by Tebbetts:[2] 1. dome spanning suture, 2. lateral crural spanning suture; 3. medial crural fixation suture.

the greater the projection and strengthening effect there will be (Fig. 83.36). In a case with unstable and badly mis-shaped crura, a cartilage graft which does not project above the medial crura is inserted between the crura and fixed in position by the above sutures (control columellar strut). With the uniting and stabilizing measures at the medial crura variations in projection on both sides can be equalized with strengthening of the projection, the infratip break modified, and the width of the columellar base (flare control suture) influenced.

Reduction of the interdomal distance

A frequent secondary cause of insufficient tip projection is too great a divergence between the crura intermedia ('angle of divergence,'[1]). The projection can be effectively strengthened by inserting mattress sutures close to the dome, usually after weakening the rounded dome region and excising the interdomal connective tissue.[33] There is a great risk of losing the natural shape of the nasal tip with its twin tip-defining points and weakening of the support function. More reliable is the combination of lateral crural spanning sutures and 'dome spanning sutures' ([2]). The lateral crural spanning suture is laid from one lateral crus to that of the other side; by varying the tension of the sutures and their placement a wide range of possibilities exists to adjust the following parameters: convexities of the lateral

crura, interdomal distance, tip projection, and angle of divergence (Fig. 83.36).

For 'dome spanning sutures' horizontal mattress sutures are placed from the deep surface at the upper part of the dome mucosa from the middle to the lateral crus. The effect is to further increase the tip projection with a simultaneous increase in its definition (Fig. 83.36).

Anterior shift of the tip complex

This is the most effective suture technique for strengthening the tip projection; the entire tip complex is fixed anteriorly by a suture inserted between the medial crura and the caudal edge of the septum (Fig. 83.37). With this the part of the suture in the medial crura is placed further dorsally than that in the caudal edge of the septum (projection control suture).[2]

Division techniques

Lateral and medial crura steal

With the 'lateral crural steal' the medial crura are extended at the expense of the lateral crura. In addition the lateral crura must be stripped completely of their external and internal skin covering and after freeing the base they are moved anteriorly so that a new dome can be formed from parts of the lateral crus. The original dome region is 'stretched' and is added to the medial and/or intermedial crus. The resulting gap in the cartilage at the basal end of the alar cartilage must be bridged by a graft and secured against over-rotation by a double suture. This process can be undertaken unilaterally as an important step in correction of a unilateral cleft (Fig. 83.38).

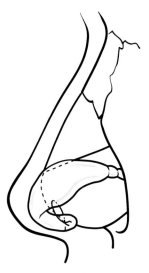

Fig. 83.37 Projection control suture.[2] The medial crura are fixed anteriorly by a suture at the caudal septal edge.

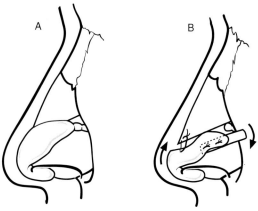

Fig. 83.38 Repositioning of the lateral alar crus. **(A)** On the left side the lateral crus has its dome end shifted caudally and its aperture end shifted cranially. **(B)** After shaping and volume reduction the lateral crus is repositioned with its basal end being brought into a more caudal position. The lateral crus thus runs more parallel to the nose opening. This movement is usually associated with a cranially directed rotation of the dome end. This repositioning must be firmly secured at the upper lateral cartilage by a suture. At the aperture a cartilage graft must be used to bridge the gap with the reconstructed alar cartilage.

In an analogous fashion the medial crus can also be moved anteriorly and used to form a new dome; naturally the support lost by moving the medial crus must be replaced through a columellar strut. This is likewise a standard procedure for us in unilateral cleft nose.

Dome division techniques

Dome division techniques are classically subdivided according to where in relation to the dome tip the removal takes place. In the Goldman technique[34] the tip part of the alar cartilage is cut lateral to the dome, in the Lipsett technique[35] medial to the dome, and in the Safian technique[36] in the dome. Only the Goldman technique is suitable for enlargement of the nasal tip projection; it can lead to an excellent initial outcome but is very controversial because of unpredictable late results. By and large, a technique which involves a near-tip removal of the cartilage is only acceptable if the loss of support of the nasal tip resulting from the removal of the cartilage is otherwise compensated. The nasal skin has also to be thick enough to prevent the inevitable irregularities in the cartilage of the tip area becoming visible through the skin. We do not utilize division techniques for strengthening the projection.

Graft techniques

In all cases in which the tip projection is to be enlarged as much as possible, graft techniques have been the crucial advance and have rendered division techniques largely superfluous.

While some grafts (columellar strut, spine augmentation) involve primary support of the nasal tip projection within the tripod system, others offer secondary support of the nasal tip projection (onlay graft, Sheen graft). The latter can only be effective on the basis of a stable primary support system in which, relying on this support, the tip projection is improved.

Columellar struts

A columellar strut is inserted primarily for the reinforcement and extension of the medial supporting column in the tripod system as well as for correction of a 'hidden columella' or for emphasis of the lower breakpoints. The significance of the medial supporting column, which consists of both the medial crura as well as their support at the nasal spine and adhesions to the caudal edge of the septum, becomes immediately obvious with each rhinoplasty as soon as a complete transfixion incision is undertaken: the nasal tip projection is reduced and the nasal tip rotates caudally, with broadening of the nasal base and decrease in the nasolabial angle. The reason for this is that the medial crura, deprived of support, are pulled towards the nasal spine by the septalis nasi muscle. The same appearances are seen in an old-age defect of nasal tip projection. The columellar strut plays an outstanding role for this indication (see Columellar graft, p. 1396), as do the suturing techniques mentioned earlier.

Tip graft

A multitude of differently shaped and positioned tip grafts to strengthen the tip projection were recommended in past decades; however this method first gained wide acceptance with the pioneering work of Sheen.[20,24] Compared with all other nasal tip grafts, *Sheen's shield-shaped graft* can not only strengthen the tip projection but also give it a more esthetically appealing contour (see Figs 83.27 and 83.29). Sheen[20] achieves this by inserting the tip graft, not as in other methods by applying the alar cartilage as a 'hood', but subcutaneously and under a certain degree of tension in a soft-tissue pocket between the columella–tip angle up to the interdomal line. In this way preparation of the cartilage maintains a special position in which the skin tension produces a skin contour giving a beautifully shaped nose by the tension of the middle crura on the nasal tip skin (see Tip grafts, p. 1398).

PTOSIS OF THE NASAL TIP

The term 'nasal tip ptosis' indicates inadequate nasal tip projection due to caudal rotation of the entire nasal tip complex around an imaginary transverse axis through the ala (Fig. 83.39A). It thus constitutes a particular form of

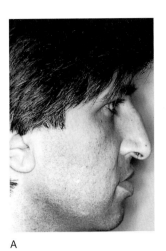 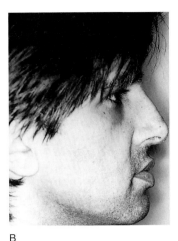

A   B

Fig. 83.39 Tip ptosis. **(A)** Following caudal rotation of the nasal tip the antero-caudal septal angle has become the most anterior projection. **(B)** Two years after correction by a 'complete strip technique' with resection of the cranial edge of the alar cartilage and the caudal edge of the upper lateral cartilage, reduction of the septum by wedge-shaped incision via a 'high septal transfixion incision', columellar strut and projection control suture.

'underprojected nose' (see The underprojected nose, p. 1403) in which the anterocaudal septal angle projects as far as the tip projection.

Apart from the loss of projection compared with the nasal dorsum and the accompanying rounding of the nasal tip, the greatly reduced nasolabial angle (< 90°) is particularly noticeable. Tip ptosis can present as an individual variant which often first manifests itself more clearly with increasing age or also as a sequela of surgical intervention in the nose or septum.

As with the projection of the nasal tip, the effectiveness of the support apparatus of the nasal tip influences the rotation. This is immediately obvious after a complete transfixion incision: on cutting the attachments between the medial crura and caudal septal edge the nasal tip rotates caudally and tip projection is simultaneously lost. A similar effect may be observed in the elderly when the attachments slacken.

Despite the close relationship between tip projection and tip rotation these concepts and their meaning must be clearly differentiated. They deal with two completely different movements which only partially complement each other: reinforcement of the tip *projection* implies a shift of the nasal tip in a sagittal direction anteriorly, reinforcement of the tip *rotation* in contrast entails a cranially directed movement of the nasal tip on an orbit around an axis through the base of the ala.

The different mechanics of these two concepts explain why reinforcement of the nasal tip projection is not inevitably accompanied by rotation; conversely, however, a rotation

of corresponding extent is always associated with strengthening of the projection.

Technically, cranial rotation of the nasal tip is most effectively achieved through surgical modification of the alar cartilage; two fundamental techniques are distinguished:

- rotation techniques without interrupting the continuity of the alar cartilage (complete strip techniques)
- rotation techniques with interruption of the continuity of the alar cartilage (interrupted strip techniques).

Complete strip techniques

A cranially directed rotation of the nasal tip without interrupting the continuity of the alar cartilage (complete strip technique) can be achieved by a resection at the cranial edge of the lateral crus. Since the remaining strip of cartilage prevents extensive rotation, only a slight rotation can be gained with this technique. The resection in any event has to be very limited. If the resection of the lateral crus is too great, the opposite effect threatens – caudal rotation with loss of tip projection. In these cases the elasticity of the lateral crura within the tripod system no longer suffices to resist the soft-tissue pull of the nasal tip – the typical picture of failed tip plasty results (see Fig. 83.47A). It is therefore vitally important to retain a reasonable width of cartilage and the thickness of the skin. This will maintain the firmness of the respective cartilage on the lateral crus – on average 5–8 mm resection is acceptable. The extent of rotation of the nasal tip need not be left just to the pull of the soft tissue if it is defined by a suture between the crura intermedia and the septal angle (tip rotation sutures).[2] This suture can only be effective, however, if the alar cartilage has previously been united to a stable complex (Fig. 83.39).

If, in achieving the planned rotation, one does not want to get too close to the perceived limits of the support function when resecting the cranial edge of the alar cartilage, it is better to revert to a resection and to restore the continuity of the cartilage with sutures after the desired rotation has been obtained (see Fig. 83.21).

One should further take into consideration that a desired reduction in volume of the nasal tip is likewise controlled by the extent of resection of the cranial edge of the alar cartilage (lateral crus), so the individual elements – volume reduction, tip rotation, and support function – must be carefully and judiciously analyzed and then harmonized.

Interrupted strip techniques

With interruption of the alar cartilage's continuity the resistance of the lateral crus to cranial rotation is eliminated and a more extensive degree of rotation becomes possible.

However the support function is also impaired at the same time and there is the potential for overlapping in the lateral crus. These factors may lead, particularly in the long term, to loss of the tip projection as well as visible irregularities at the alar edge. It is thus fundamentally advisable to cut the lateral crus *near the base*, excising the triangular wedge of cartilage formed by the pieces overlapping after the rotation and reattaching the cut edges of the cartilage end-to-end with a double suture (see Fig. 83.21). In this way all the problems associated with an extensive rotation are simultaneously solved:

1. The support function of the lateral crus is retained.
2. The extent of the rotation can be controlled by the width of the resected wedge of cartilage.
3. Possible irregularities at the suture point in the cartilage remain hidden by the thick connective tissue at the base of the ala, even in a case with thin skin.
4. The resection of the cranial edge of the alar cartilage can be specified exclusively according to the requirements of the planned reduction in volume.

Additional measures

Cranial rotation in the form described entails a telescoping of the alar cartilage and the upper lateral and/or septal cartilage, thereby limiting the upward rotation. In order to enable unhindered rotation and also to allow these cartilages to maintain their relationship after the rotation, the caudal edges of the upper lateral cartilage and of the septum must be shortened by an amount corresponding to the extent of the rotation (Fig. 83.40A,B). It does not always follow that this must be done on a 1:1 basis if it simultaneously changes the relationship between the columella and the ala.

To avoid a transfixion incision for the reduction of the caudal edge of the septum and to retain that important element in the support structure of the nasal tip, the use of

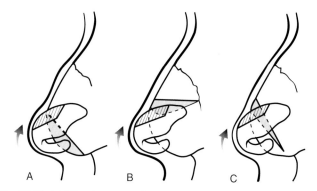

Fig. 83.40 Additional measures for cranial rotation of the nasal tip. **(A)** Resection of the caudal edge of the septum. **(B)** Resection of the caudal edge of the upper lateral cartilage. **(C)** Wedge-shaped resection of the septum through a 'high septal transfixion incision'.

a high septal transfixion incision for shortening the septum is recommended in this situation.[37] For this the transfixion incision is located approximately 3–4 mm cranial and parallel to the caudal edge of the septum, and an appropriately sized wedge of septum and mucoperichondrium cranial to the incision is removed (Fig. 83.40C). After extensive cranial rotations of the nasal tip it is necessary to carefully check whether the resulting excess of mucous membrane will disturb function. If necessary the mucous membrane must be modified according to the new structure of the nasal skeleton.

One can also achieve the illusion of tip rotation by augmentation in the area of the nasal spine (see Fig. 83.33). The premise for this procedure is obviously that the existing nasolabial angle permits enlargement from the esthetic point of view.

THE OVERPROJECTED TIP

It is not difficult to reduce the projection of the nasal tip; indeed this is frequently an unintended consequence of a standard rhinoplasty, though then it is always associated with a loss of contour of the nasal tip. It is difficult, however, to reduce the nasal tip projection and at the same time retain or even improve the nasal tip contour. Here the quality and thickness of the skin are the limiting factors for an esthetically appealing result, as is so often the case in reducing measures in the nose. The length of the columella, the height of the nasal opening, and the volume of the alae also play an essential role. In an overprojected nose with thick skin, a short columella, low nasal openings and voluminous alae it is rather pointless to achieve a decrease of the projection through reduction of the scaffold because it will always be associated with loss of contour of the nasal tip. In such cases an augmenting adjustment of the nasal dorsum is a more promising way of dealing with the overprojecting nasal tip (relative reduction of the overprojection).

If, however, the overprojection of the nasal tip is accompanied by thin skin, a slender nasal base, high nostrils and a long columella, the following four steps for reducing the tip projection have proved themselves in attaining an appealing tip contour (Fig. 83.41).

Strip resection of the cranial edge of the alar cartilage

In comparison with the following techniques only a slight tip reduction can be achieved by resection of the cranial edge of the alar cartilage. With this technique, the more distinctive the convexity of the uncorrected alar cartilage in the dome area, the more perceptible will be the result of

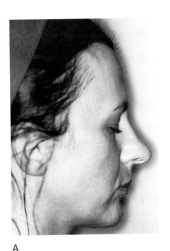 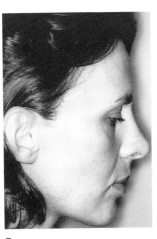

Fig. 83.41 **(A)** Overprojected nose. **(B)** 26 months after correction by: 1. Strip resection of the cranial edges of the alar cartilages; 2. transfixion incision; 3. continuous resection of the base of the lateral alar crura; 4. soft-tissue resection at the base of the nostrils.

reduction. Over-resection must be avoided, however, as this will cause loss of contour. According to the thickness of the cartilage, a cartilage width of around 4–5 mm must always be retained in the dome area, and 6–8 mm in the area of the lateral crus (Fig. 83.42).

Transfixion incision

A complete transfixion incision destroys the connection between the medial crura and the lower edge of the septum, taking with it an important support system for the nasal tip.[14] A considerable reduction in the prominence of the nasal tip is immediately noticeable intraoperatively, and may increase further in the postoperative phase (Fig. 83.42). One should therefore undertake a complete transfixion incision only when a reduction in the prominence of the nasal tip is a desired aim. In many cases in which a transfixion incision is to be undertaken for reasons other than

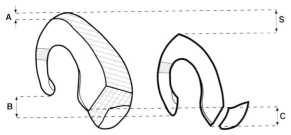

Fig. 83.42 Other reduction methods for an overprojected nasal tip. **(A)** Resection of the cranial edge of the alar cartilage (hatched). **(B)** Complete transfixion incision. **(C)** Continuous resection of the base of the lateral alar crura (cross-hatched). A further option for reduction is to take a segment out of the medial crus (shaded). (S = sum of the effects of A, B, and C.)

reduction of tip prominence, a high septal transfixion incision can be used instead.

Continuous resection of the base of the lateral alar crura

Through continuous resection of the base of the lateral alar crura a further very effective reduction of the nasal tip projection can be achieved, but it is accompanied by the danger of unpredictable results. We prefer the near-base resection of the lateral crus[38] to the resection of the medial crus[35] (Fig. 83.42). We avoid reduction of the nasal tip by excisions in the dome area[36] for fear of causing later irregularities in the area of the nasal tip.

Through the combination of a continuous resection of the lateral crus, excision at the cranial edge of the alar cartilage and a transfixion incision one almost always achieves a sufficient tip reduction. In extreme cases an additional resection of the medial crus[35] may still be necessary.

With all corrections involving resections of the alar cartilage it is absolutely crucial to re-unite the ends of the cartilages end-to-end with double sutures and avoid overlap.

Resection at the base of the ala

The soft tissues of the ala must be adjusted in proportion to the reduction of the tip cartilage through a near-base resection; this avoids disproportion between the base and tips of the nose. For this one of the many variants of alar resection described by Weir[39] is suitable, depending on the initial position (see Alar reduction, p. 1391).

THE 'BOX' NOSE

The principal characteristics of the 'box' nose are the flat, broad nasal tip with a relatively narrow nasal base which, from the caudal view (basal view), results in a square-shaped outline. The broad nasal tip is frequently overprojected in relation to the nasal dorsum and the nasal alae frequently flare in mid point of the sides of a furrow running vertically from cranial to caudal (parenthesis deformation). A characteristic variation of the alar cartilages is responsible for this striking and relatively frequently encountered nasal tip form:

1. a wide angle of divergence[1] of the crura intermedia (see Fig. 83.6)
2. cranial orientation of the lateral crura (Fig. 83.8).

The large divergence in the area of the crura intermedia leads to a far lateral position of the tip-defining points, which then represent the corner points of the 'box', and frequently creates a median notch of the nasal tip.

The axis of the lateral crura, instead of running parallel to the nasal alae, runs more parallel to the nasal dorsum. This causes the dome region to be rounded bilaterally and increases the squareness of the nasal tip. The 'tripod' function of the alar cartilages is impaired at the same time. The vertical furrow formation, sometimes combined with a corresponding creasing of the nasal ala, corresponds to the dorsal edge of the lateral crura.

In response to this striking deviation in shape and position of the alar cartilage the key elements of the operative correction, apart from volume reduction through excision of part of the cranial edge of the alar cartilage, are the following:

1. repositioning of the lateral crura in the direction of the nasal alae
2. reduction of the angle of divergence
3. accentuation of the dome angle.

Repositioning requires the lateral crura to be completely mobilized and sutured into a soft-tissue pocket prepared 3 mm from the nasal alar edge (see Fig. 83.8). In this way the nasal alae regain cartilaginous support and the furrow (parenthesis deformation) is eliminated. The dome region becomes simultaneously narrowed and more sharply accentuated. This phenomenon can be explained by the fact that after correction the crura both take a roughly parallel course.[40] To ensure that there is no loss of support of the lateral crura in the complete mobilization, the crura should be reinforced in their new position with small cartilage strip grafts at the rim[41] (see Fig. 83.38). The angle of divergence is reduced through lateral crural transfixion sutures. The dome tips are accentuated by horizontal mattress sutures placed bilaterally between the crura intermedia and lateral crura (Fig. 83.36). The suture ends can also be left long and then tied to those on the other side, possibly rendering lateral crural spanning sutures superfluous.

THE CROOKED NOSE

The whole nose or just individual segments of it can deviate to one side or other of the medio-sagittal plane. As causes of limited growth, trauma in utero, during birth and during the growth phase are predominant. Trauma occurring after the conclusion of growth can obviously, if left untreated, likewise result in permanent dislocation of the nasal skeleton, usually accompanied by sharp, angular bends with irregular fragmentation of the bone and the cartilage as well as endonasal scar formation.

With *bony deviation* the point of deviation from the medio-sagittal plane lies at the level of the nasion. The nose in itself can therefore be perfectly straight and its individual structures remain in a harmonious relationship with each other.

With a *cartilaginous distorted nose* only the cartilaginous part of the nose is deviated; the bony part of the nasal dorsum remains isolated in its correct position in the medio-sagittal plane. The deviation point lies at the level of the rhinion (Rh) – at the caudal end of the nasal bone. The asymmetry is caused primarily by a vertically directed bow-shaped deviation of the cartilaginous septum.

Cartilaginous and bony deviations can obviously also present in combination; they may complement each other's direction of deviation (C-shaped deviation) or be opposed to it so that an S-shaped deviation results.

From these 'genuine' forms of nasal deviation a pseudo-form must be distinguished: this looks at first glance like a deviation of the nose, but it is not founded in a true side-deviation of the nose. The most frequent causes for this are post-traumatic or postoperative one-sided depressions of parts of the nasal skeleton or endonasal soft-tissue defects with scar contraction.

Correction of the bony crooked nose

The intercartilaginous approach with sparing dissection is used to access the nasal dorsum. The dome region on both sides is undermined and the transition from the septum to the upper lateral cartilage exposed extramucosally. This is followed by bilateral medial and lateral osteotomies, as described in Correction of the dorsum, page 1392 (Fig. 83.43A).

After that, on the side *opposite* to the deviation, which in this example is the right-hand side, the chisel is once more placed in the crack of the medial osteotomy and lodged in the frontal bone by a couple of gentle taps. By swinging the chisel around this anchoring point, the right side (in this example) of the nasal pyramid, including the upper lateral cartilage, is moved outwards. Thus the right half of the nasal skeleton is correctly adjusted; at the same time an open roof results on this side (Fig. 83.43B). A curved 6 mm wide chisel is then inserted in the medial osteotomy on the *right* side with its cutting edge directed to the left, as far as the beginning of the deviation, and here the bony septum is osteotomized (Fig. 83.43C). In this way the medial osteotomies are joined and the chisel arrives in the cranial angled part of the *left-sided* medial osteotomy. Subsequently the nasal skeleton of the deviated side is moved medially through finger pressure and placed in the midline, thus closing the open roof originally created on the right side (Fig. 83.43D). Differences in level often persist in the area of the nasal dorsum; these must be carefully equalized through reducing and/or augmenting procedures.

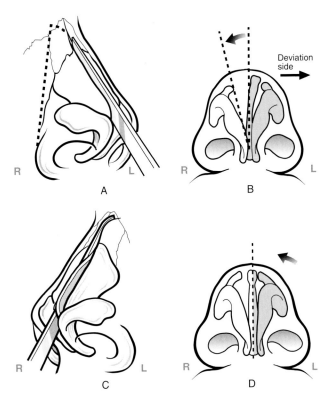

Fig. 83.43 Correction of a left-sided deviated bony septum. **(A)** Standard bilateral medial and lateral osteotomies. **(B)** Shifting of the right half of the nasal pyramid towards the right (arrow), resulting in a unilateral 'open roof'. **(C)** Through the medial osteotomy on the right side the perpendicular lamina is severed to the height of the nasal root with a curved chisel and at this point the median osteotomy on the right side joins that on the left side. **(D)** Finally the left half of the nasal pyramid including the septum is shifted to the right, closing the right-sided 'open roof' and thus medially positioning the nasal pyramid.

If a deviation in the septal part still remains after these measures, it must be straightened with the techniques described below for the cartilaginous crooked nose.

Correction of the cartilaginous crooked nose

The considerable elastic recoil strength of the nasal cartilage makes correction in this area much more problematic than in the bony region. The operative procedure closely follows conventional septal surgery (see above). As a rule a hemi-transfixion incision is used to approach the septum; the caudal edge of the septum including the nasal spine is presented subperichondrally. From here the mucoperiosteum of the septum in the area of the premaxilla and the vomer is lifted bilaterally (lower tunnel), and in addition the muco-perichondrium of the septal cartilage on the left side is prepared (upper tunnel). This preparation is carried dorsally as far as the deviation part of the septum. The septum is incised close to the nasal dorsum and simultaneously a narrow wedge is excised at the deviated part. The muco-

perichondrium of the opposite side should remain intact at the site of the incision. Dorsally the upper and lower tunnels on the left side are joined together from front to back, in that the remaining connective tissue is cut at the transition line between cartilage (quadrilateral cartilage) and bone (premaxilla and vomer). After that the cartilaginous septum can be excised at its transition with the vomer or premaxilla to the extent where it lies without tension or overlap to the bony base in the middle and can be sutured to the nasal spine.

With a more pronounced cartilaginous deviation the cartilaginous nasal dorsum must additionally be exposed through bilateral intercartilaginous incisions and the upper lateral cartilage divided from the septal cartilage. In many instances this is the only way that the nasal tip can be kept in the midline without relapse.

Since with pronounced deviations there is also a size difference between the two upper lateral cartilages, in many cases the caudal and ventral edges on the side opposite to the deviation must be shortened to enable fine adjustment, and the ventral edge of the upper lateral cartilage on the deviation side may require augmentation, possibly with a spreader graft.

THE SADDLE NOSE

In a saddle nose the nasal dorsum lacks adequate ventral projection. The condition is occasionally congenital but more often results from trauma, infection (septal abscess) or excessive resection of the septum (Fig. 83.44). The saddle formation may affect the bone or the cartilaginous nasal dorsum in isolation or include both structures. The guideline for correction may not just be the outer deformity – the internal function of the nasal airway must also be considered in each case. The collapse of the nasal dorsum is always associated with impairment of nasal air flow which is, as a rule, greater the further caudally the saddle formation extends. Apart from the deviations and bulges at the nasal septum, the loss of support of the caudal septum in particular noticeably impairs the function of the nasal valves. The medial crura in this case thus lose an essential element of their support and sink dorsally so that the support of the lateral crura enlarges the nasal base and with this the nasal valve angle increases (ballooning phenomenon) (Fig. 83.44G).

According to the location and extent of the saddle formation, two completely different techniques may be employed – either alone or in combination:

- augmentation of the nasal dorsum
- reconstruction of the nasal septum.

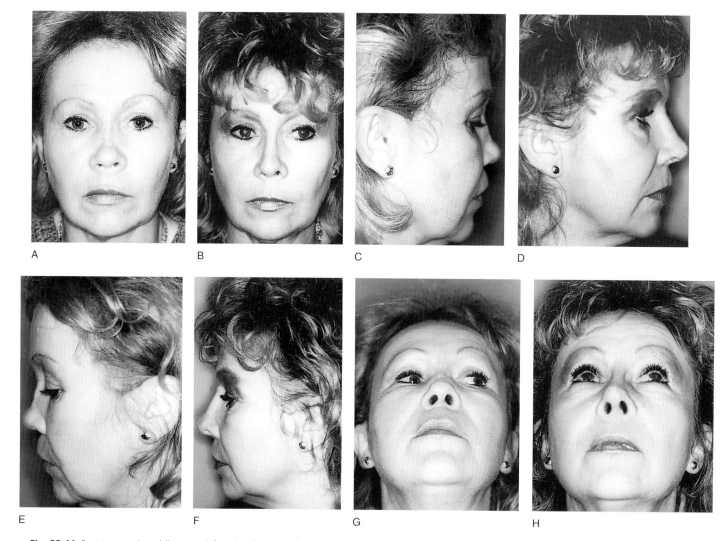

Fig. 83.44 Post-traumatic saddle-nose deformity after several attempts at correction. The reconstruction was performed using an osteocartilaginous rib graft with additional antero-caudal reconstruction of the septum. **(A)** Preoperative en face. **(B)** 19 months postoperative. **(C)** Right profile, preoperative. **(D)** Right profile, 19 months postoperative. **(E)** Left profile, preoperative. **(F)** Left profile, 19 months postoperative. **(G)** Basal view, preoperative. **(H)** Basal view postoperative. The caudal view shows correction of the 'ballooning effects'. As well as the esthetic improvement, good nasal air flow was also achieved.

The relative indications for these two techniques are as follows:

- saddle formation in the bony part alone → augmentation
- saddle formation in the cartilaginous part alone → septum reconstruction
- saddle formation in both areas → augmentation of the nasal dorsum + septum reconstruction.

Augmentation of the nasal dorsum

Four strategic questions must be settled before correcting a saddle formation by augmentation:

- Which approach?
- Which material?

- What shape and size?
- Which fixation?

The intercartilaginous, transcolumellar, and transoral incisions are suitable for access. The open approach, however, offers the widest potential for precision and choice of procedures. Which material to use is unclear. Bone, cartilage and combined grafts are contenders in the category of autogenous materials. With smaller defects and sufficient availability, septal and ear cartilage are definitely the first choice for replacement materials. Larger cartilage grafts must be harvested from the rib.

Cartilage irradiated at high doses (3 000 000 rads) or preserved in Cialit or Methiolat solution is also used as an allogeneic (homologous) or xenogeneic (heterologous) graft.

Unfortunately resorption may be unpredictable,[43] and the risk (however unlikely) of contamination with prions and viruses makes this an unsuitable material. The same also applies to xenogeneic demineralized bones.[44]

The techniques of autogenous cartilage grafting have, however, gained increasing importance in the last decade since the problem of reabsorption was solved by better methods of fixation (e.g. miniscrews) and, furthermore, by careful preparation of the transplant bed.[45] Cranial bone, because of its membranous development in contrast to pelvic bone (formed enchondrally), appears further to reduce the danger of late reabsorption.[46] However difficulties in fashioning and the limited volume available confine its range of indications for use.

Alloplastic implants (Silastic, Proplast, Mersilene mesh, Gore-Tex) are readily available, preformed and easy to use; they do not deform and are, if at all, only negligibly resorbed. On the other hand there exists the lifelong danger of extrusion or infection, so these implants should be inserted only for well-justified indications and with detailed explanation to the patient about these risks.

If the advantages and disadvantages of the different materials are compared, there remain clear advantages for rib grafts and, with large grafts, for a combined bone and cartilaginous segment of the rib. The inherent disadvantages of the two graft components – that is, the tendency of the bone to resorb[47] and the cartilage to warp[17] – are minimized when they are used together. Prerequisites to reduce loss of the bony part through resorption are a good vascular bed for the graft and a stable fixation with one or two miniscrews. The cartilaginous part must, as far as possible, be carefully carved.[17] The 9th and 10th ribs are particularly suitable as donor sites.[1,18]

For the design and measuring of grafts for the nasal dorsum, Sullivan et al[11] took measurements in corpses; on average the nasofrontal suture was the widest point at 14 mm, tapering to 10 mm in the area of the nasofrontal angle. Further caudally, approximately 9–12 mm from the nasofrontal angle, the dorsum reaches a new maximum of approximately 12 mm, then gradually narrows again in the direction of the nasal tip. The dorsal contouring of the graft must take into consideration the different skin thicknesses over the nasal dorsum, and on the underside it should be fashioned concavely in the transverse plane so that it can not be moved out of position by irregularities in the supporting surface (Fig. 83.45).

For all implants and grafts the following guidelines for fixation are valid:

1. custom-made soft-tissue pocket to ensure secured position

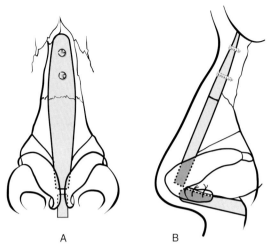

Fig. 83.45 Method for reconstruction of a saddle-nose deformity using an osteocartilaginous graft and columellar strut. **(A)** Anatomical reconstruction with replacement of the bony section of the dorsum with the bone part and the cartilaginous section of the dorsum with the cartilaginous part of the graft. **(B)** The bony part of the nasal dorsum graft must have an extensive and firm foundation on the bony base of the pyramid and be fixed by wire or miniscrew osteosynthesis. Additional nasal tip projection can be achieved with the use of a columellar strut.

2. cranial and caudal support, or
3. vertical stability through one or two lag screws.

Septal reconstruction

If the cartilaginous nasal bridge has caved in, it makes no sense for functional reasons just to augment its shape. Rather the septum should undergo restoration of its form and function simultaneously. For this the two leaves of the septum are separated up to the skin of the septum and further caudally between the medial crura, the section of deformed and worn-out cartilage removed, and a frame of autogenous cartilage inserted to substitute the caudal and dorsal septum edges. This angular cartilage transplant is fixed to the nasal spine and to the remaining septal cartilage. The graft should be of approximately the same thickness, length and height as the septum to be replaced (Fig. 83.46).

The repositioned medial crura and the dorsal edges of the previously mobilized upper lateral cartilages are then fixed to this new septal framework. The nose thereby regains its tip projection and the width of the nasal valve angle normalizes.

In many cases the septum reconstructed in this way does not have enough stability to give the tip cartilage a sufficient hold and to secure the tip projection. This support must then be supplied by a columellar strut; since no septal

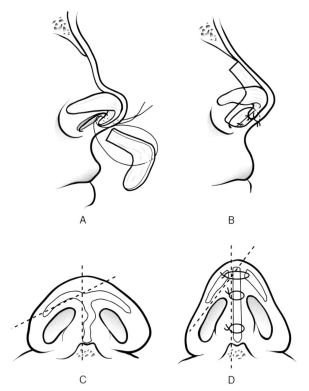

Fig. 83.46 Septal reconstruction of a saddle nose deformity. **(A)** Through a hemitransfixion incision the two septal leaves are separated caudally as far as the skin and cranially up to the lamina perpendicularis; the deformed cartilage is removed and the septum reconstructed with a performed cartilage transplant. The graft is fixed caudally with percutaneous sutures, at the base by attachment to the premaxilla or spine, and dorsally to the rest of the septum. **(B)** Caudally the position is retained with a percutaneous suture. **(C)** In a saddle nose where the support of the septum is lost, the soft-tissue nose spreads and the dorsal roof angle is enlarged to unphysiologic values. **(D)** When the nasal septum is reconstructed and the upper lateral cartilages sutured to the reconstructed septum, the external shape as well as the function are re-established.

cartilage is available in these cases and ear cartilage is less suitable for this indication, a rib cartilage graft must be used. One of the free ribs (10th or 11th) is especially suitable for this indication.

If a nasal dorsum graft is to be combined with a columellar graft, it is important to consider the effects. If possible, the combination of the two should be avoided to give the nasal tip maximum mobility. Only if a tendency to over-rotation of the nasal tip exists do we reinforce the tip of the columellar graft against the tip of the nasal dorsum graft through a 'tongue-in-groove' connection.

Reconstruction of the septal framework with an appropriate tip projection can be considerably complicated by scar-mediated atrophy of the internal soft tissues and by perforation of the septum, in which case more extensive reconstruction becomes necessary, e.g. through free or pedicled mucous membrane grafts or composite grafts.

SECONDARY RHINOPLASTY

Patients who present for revision surgery after rhinoplasty usually exhibit more or less the same basic patterns of deformities:

- saddle formation in the area of the bony nasal dorsum
- swelling in the supratip area
- loss of the nasal tip projection
- loss of nasal tip contour (Polly beak deformity – Fig. 83.47).

These are caused by defects in preoperative planning and treatment which can be summed up respectively as:

1. inadequately balanced reduction of the bony and cartilaginous nasal dorsum
2. inadequately balanced reduction of the cartilaginous nasal bridge in relation to the alar cartilage projection
3. over-resection of the alar cartilage, weakening its support function
4. over-reduction of the support of the nose in relation to the width of the soft-tissue cover.

In reduction of the nasal dorsum it is not generally taken into consideration that the skin over the bony nasal bridge is considerably thinner than that over the cartilaginous area (see Fig. 83.11) and that it can therefore adjust itself to the new, reduced proportions to a greater extent than the remaining, thicker nasal skin. Thus the nasal dorsum may be perfectly straight at the level of the supporting skeleton, but as the nasal skin is thicker it appears as a saddle deformity.

The cartilaginous nasal dorsum – particularly at its caudal end – is often under- or over-resected in relationship to the

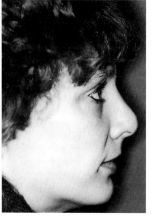
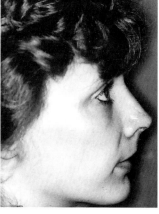

Fig. 83.47 Polly beak deformity. **(A)** Result after reducing rhinoplasty and numerous attempts at correction. **(B)** Final correction by slight reduction of the cartilaginous dorsum and augmentation of the bony dorsum, columellar strut, bilateral lateral crural grafts and tip graft as described by Sheen.[1]

projection of the alar cartilage. Both can lead to a supratip swelling, which is formed either by protruding cartilage or, after over-resection, by scar tissue.

Over-resection of the alar cartilage, usually in efforts to improve the contour, weakens the tripod system and leads to a loss of nasal tip projection and contour. Resection of the alar cartilage must be limited to the extent that the elasticity of the cartilage is the same as the thickness of the covering skin.

Over-resection of the nasal skeleton in relationship to the width of the soft-tissue cover seems to be one of the most frequent errors. How far the skin is capable of conforming to a reduced nasal skeleton is a judgment that comes only from experience and having a 'feel' for the procedure, and is hard to teach didactically. As a rough guide it can only be stated that the thicker the nasal skin, and the further towards the base it is, the less it will conform to a reduction. The common sight of an unsatisfactory rhinoplasty with apparent over-resection of the nasal skeleton in the bony part and apparent under-resection in the cartilaginous area reflects the different adaptive capabilities of the soft-tissue cover in the different regions of the nose (Fig. 83.11). In these cases the temptation to further decrease the volume of the nasal tip through a further resection of the tip scaffolding and thereby give it more contour can end only in disaster. For secondary rhinoplasty augmentation is really almost the only process to be considered (nasal dorsum graft, spreader graft, tip graft) if the skin covering is once again to be put under tension and the contour restored.

COMPLICATIONS

The concept of 'complications' needs to be considered here; from the patient's point of view in particular it is hard to distinguish between inevitable local operative sequelae (side effects), genuine complications and unsatisfactory results. In this respect a rhinoplasty, which is undertaken for esthetic reasons, differs fundamentally from non-elective interventions.

INEVITABLE LOCAL OPERATIVE SEQUELAE

For the patient who was not extensively and sympathetically informed about the postoperative phase (see also p. 1394) it may be hard to distinguish between local operative sequelae and genuine complications. Uninformed patients worry if it is normal, for example, to have postoperative lid swelling and bruising: Is it normal or is it a complication?

The same is true for a hematoma of the sclera, for clots in the nostrils, and for sensory disturbances in the area of the nose or the front teeth. It must made clear to the patient that these consequences (side effects) are unavoidable and that the extent and duration of their resolution can vary considerably.

GENUINE COMPLICATIONS

Under this heading, complications appearing in the early postoperative phase should be distinguished from late complications. The most important complications of the early postoperative phase are epistaxis, hematoma of the septum, infections and skin necrosis. In a few cases serious complications have also been described in the surrounding tissues: intracranial infections after dural tears in the area of the lamina cribrosa, and intraorbital hematoma.[48]

Less important immediate complications are repeated *hemorrhages* from the nose, usually triggered by postoperative fluctuations in blood pressure. The head-up position, calming of the patient with sedative medication, and ice packs on both sides of the nose usually suffice to settle these hemorrhages.

In a supine patient, however, lesser hemorrhages can go unseen as the patient swallows the blood. In this way a vicious circle can be triggered – the swallowed blood leads to sickness and vomiting and the associated blood pressure fluctuations again provoke hemorrhages. Removal of the nasal tamponade may also increase the risk of secondary bleeding.

Persistent hemorrhages which are not controlled by patient positioning and sedation must be resolved by packing the nose. For this, the nose and pharynx are first of all cleared of blood clots under good vision (using a headlamp or endoscope), the nasal mucosa anesthetized with 5% cocaine solution, and an anterior layered pack is placed. The pack is as for the standard postoperative pack. Neurosurgical swabs are coated with Nebacitin ointment. The plug is always inserted to an equal extent on both sides to avoid deviations of the mobilized nasal elements. An additional posterior pack (Belloque tamponade) is hardly ever necessary.

Postoperative *infections* after a rhinoplasty are extremely rare. If an infection appears, it is almost always associated with a hematoma or with a graft. Since hematoma appears most commonly in the septum and this area is particularly infection-prone, a septal hematoma should be suspected. If it is overlooked and not drained promptly, it can present a nidus for infection. Untreated, or not promptly treated, it may result in an infected septal hematoma with necrosis of the septal cartilage and loss of support of the nasal dorsum (saddle nose). Treatment of septal hematoma consists of early incision and drainage. Medication with systemic antibiotics is augmented with local irrigation. Normally antibiotics are commenced, with a presumptive regime, after swabs have been taken. Once the culture and sensitivities have been established microbiologically, the definitive drugs can be used.

Cartilage grafts are more prone to infection the closer they lie to the skin and the greater their tension on the skin. Previous surgery is a further predisposing factor, reducing the circulation and thus the local defenses against infection in the transplant bed. Increasing swelling, reddening and pain are unmistakable warning signs and should occasion a high-dose, presumptive antibiotic regime. If the inflammation is so far advanced that fluctuation is demonstrable, it must either be incised or the wound reopened to relieve the inflammatory exudate and to create an entrance for local irrigation with antibiotic-containing solutions. If these measures to overcome the inflammation are successful the cartilage transplant can often be saved.

Skin necrosis is caused by ischemia and therefore seen either as circumscribed areas of skin pallor or as dark red venous congestion. This extremely rare complication usually affects only skin areas that have been thinned or which have been scarred by previous surgery. Also the skin edges after a columellar incision may suffer from poor blood flow if there is scarring from previous surgery in this area. If skin necrosis develops, the demarcation must be awaited with local treatment using antibiotic-containing ointment and debridement. The size, depth and site of the defect will then determine whether local skin flaps or free skin grafts are necessary. Deep necrosis that exposes the nasal skeleton should be covered as early as possible with a local skin flap to prevent infection of the nasal skeleton.

In the past, disturbances of the nasal air flow were an important late complication. They were observed in about 10% of rhinoplasty patients[49,50] and can be attributed to the then radical techniques. After an esthetic rhinoplasty which is accomplished by modern conservative techniques, no deterioration in nasal air flow is anticipated.[51,52]

UNSATISFACTORY RESULTS

Rhinoplasty is an elective procedure that a patient opts for only after due consideration and careful thought. Accordingly there is a high expectation of a perfect result; even the smallest deviations from the ideal shape will be perceived by the patient as a 'failure'. This can be made worse if video-imaging has given the patient a detailed image of the expected postoperative outcome. It is the task of the preoperative information to make clear to the patient that perfection in the procedure by no means excludes unpredictable scar formation and the appearance of smaller irregularities of contour. These complications are universal and are better termed 'incalculable surgical sequelae'; they occur with a frequency of around 10%. As a rule they can be remedied in small after-corrections under local anesthesia. It must be made clear to the patient before surgery that this may happen. Obviously, these unforeseen operative and planning errors which have led to an unsatisfactory result are not intended, but nevertheless can happen. In the same way the unrealistic ideas that a few patients have, usually the dysmorphic patients, can never be satisfied. It is to be hoped that such obsessional patients can be identified and excluded before surgery.

REFERENCES

1. Sheen JH, Sheen AP 1987 Aesthetic rhinoplasty, 2nd edn. Mosby, St Louis
2. Tebbetts JB 1994 Shaping and positioning the nasal tip without structural disruption: A new systematic approach. Plastic and Reconstructive Surgery 94:61
3. Rees TD 1986 Surgical correction of the severely deviated nose by extramucosal excision of the osseocartilaginous septum and replacement as a free graft. Plastic and Reconstructive Surgery: 78:320
4. Padovan JF 1972 External approach in rhinoplasty (decortication. In: Conley J, Dickinson JT (eds) Plastic and reconstructive surgery of the face and neck. Thieme, Stuttgart, p 143
5. Goodman WS 1973 External approach to rhinoplasty. Canadian Journal of Otolaryngology 2:207
6. Legan H, Burstone C 1980 Soft-tissue cephalometric analysis for orthognathic surgery. Journal of Oral Surgery 38:744
7. Powell N, Humphreys B 1984 Proportions of the aesthetic face. Thieme, New York
8. Brown JB, McDowell F 1951 Plastic surgery of the nose. CV Mosby. St Louis
9. Crumley RL, Lanser M 1988 Quantitative analysis of nasal tip projection. Laryngoscope 202
10. Byrd HS, Hobar PC 1993 A practical guide for surgical planning. Plastic and Reconstructive Surgery 91:642
11. Sullivan PK, Varma M, Rozelle AA 1996 Optimizing bone-graft nasal reconstruction: A study of nasal bone shape and thickness. Plastic and Reconstructive Surgery 97:327
12. Daniel RK 1992 Anatomy and aesthetics. Plastic and Reconstructive Surgery 89:216
13. Anderson JR 1984 Surgery of the nasal base. Archives of Otolaryngology 110:349
14. Jancke JB, Wright WK 1971 Studies of the support of the nasal tip. Archives of Otolaryngology 93:458
15. Robin JL 1979 Extramucosal method in rhinoplasty. Aesthetic Plastic Surgery 3:171
16. Austermann KH 1985 Eine Methode zur Vermeidung der "Supratip"-Schwellung nach aesthetischer Rhinoplastik. In: Schwenzer N (ed) Fortschritte der Mund-Kiefer-Gesichtschirurgie. Thieme, Stuttgart, p 76
17. Gibson T, Davis WB 1958 The distorsion of autogeneous cartilage grafts: Its cause and prevention. British Journal of Plastic Surgery 10:257
18. Daniel RK 1994 Rhinoplasty and its grafts: Evolving a flexible operative technique. Plastic and Reconstructive Surgery 94:597

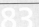

19. Sheen JH 1984 Spreader graft: A method of reconstructing the roof of the middle nasal vault following rhinoplasty. Plastic and Reconstructive Surgery 73:230

20. Sheen JH 1975 Achieving more nasal tip projection by the use of a small autogenous vomer or septal cartilage graft. Plastic and Reconstructive Surgery 56:35

21. Falces E, Gorney M 1972 Use of ear cartilage grafts for nasal tip reconstruction. Plastic and Reconstructive Surgery 50:147

22. Grabb W, Smith JW 1968 Corrective rhinoplasty and augmentation mentoplasty. In: Milliard DR Jr (ed) Plastic surgery. Little Brown, Boston

23. Millard DR Jr 1971 Congenital nasal tip retrusion and three little composite ear grafts: Case report. Plastic and Reconstructive Surgery 48:501

24. Sheen JH 1993 Tip graft: A 20-year retrospective. Plastic and Reconstructive Surgery 91:48

25. Johnson CM Jr, Toriumi DM 1990 Open structure rhinoplasty. WB Saunders, Philadelphia

26. Adham MN 1996 A new technique for nasal tip cartilage graft in primary rhinoplasty. Plastic and Reconstructive Surgery 97:649

27. Gilbert SE 1996 Alar reductions in rhinoplasty. Archives of Otolaryngology and Head and Neck Surgery 122:781

28. Goodman WS, Gilbert RW 1991 External rhinoplasty. In: Krause ChJ, Mangert DS, Pastorek N (eds) Aesthetic facial surgery. Lippincott, Philadelphia, p 111

29. Anderson JR, Johnson CM Jr, Adamson P 1982 Open rhinoplasty: An assessment. Otolaryngology and Head and Neck Surgery 90:272

30. Goodman WS, Gilbert RW 1987 Surgery of the nasal tip by external rhinoplasty. Facial Plastic Surgery 4:277

31. Anderson JR 1971 New approach to rhinoplasty. Archives of Otolaryngology 93:284

32. Constantian MB 1989 An alternative strategy for reducing the large nasal base. Plastic and Reconstructive Surgery 83:41

33. Tardy ME, Cheng E 1987 Transdomal suture refinement of the nasal tip. Facial Plastic Surgery 4:317

34. Goldman IB 1957 The importance of the medial crura in nasal tip reconstruction. Archives of Otolaryngology 65:143

35. Lipsett EM 1959 A new approach to surgery to the lower cartilaginous vault. Archives of Otolaryngology 70:42

36. Safian J 1970 The split-cartilage tip technique of rhinoplasty. Plastic and Reconstructive Surgery 45:217

37. Parkes ML, Brennan HG 1970 High septal transfixation to shorten the nose. Plastic and Reconstructive Surgery 45:487

38. Webster RC 1975 Advances in surgery of the tip. Otolaryngology Clinics of North America 8:615

39. Weir RF 1882 On restoring sunken noses without scarring the face. New York Medical Journal 56:449. Reprinted in: Plastic and Reconstructive Surgery 45:382

40. Hamra ST 1993 Repositioning the lateral crus. Plastic and Reconstructive Surgery 92:1244

41. Gunter JP, Friedman RM 1997 Lateral crural strut grafts: techniques and clinical applications in rhinoplasty. Plastic and Reconstructive Surgery 99:943

42. McCollough EG, English JL 1985 A new twist in nasal tip surgery: An alternative to the Goldman tip for the wide or bulbous lobule. Archives of Otolaryngology and Head and Neck Surgery 111:524

43. Welling DB, Maves MD, Schüller DE et al 1988 Irradiated homologous cartilage grafts: Long-term results. Archives of Otolaryngology and Head and Neck Surgery 114:291

44. Toriumi DM, Larrabee WF Jr, Walike JW, Millard DJ, Eisele DW 1990 Demineralized bone-implant resorption with long-term follow-up. Archives of Otolaryngology and Head and Neck Surgery 116:676

45. Whitaker LA 1989 Biological boundaries: A concept in facial skeletal restructuring. Clinics in Plastic Surgery 16:1

46. Powell NB, Riley RW 1987 Cranial bone grafting in facial aesthetic and reconstructive contouring. Archives of Otolaryngology and Head and Neck Surgery 113:713

47. Wheeler ES, Kawamoto HK, Zarem HA 1982 Bone grafts for nasal reconstruction. Plastic and Reconstructive Surgery 69:9

48. Hunts JH 1996 Orbital haemorrhage during rhinoplasty. Annals of Plastic Surgery 37:618–623

49. Beekhuis GJ 1976 Nasal obstruction after rhinoplasty: Etiology and techniques for correction. Laryngoscope 86:540

50. Goldman JB 1966 Rhinoplastic sequelae causing nasal obstruction. Archives of Otolaryngology 83:151

51. Courtiss EH, Goldwyn RM 1983 The effects of nasal surgery on air flow. Plastic and Reconstructive Surgery 72:9

52. Mertz JS, McCaffrey TV, Kern EB 1984 Objective evaluation of anterior septal reconstructions. Otolaryngology and Head and Neck Surgery 92:302

Ear reconstruction

84

BURT BRENT

Surgical creation of an ear with autogenous tissues is a unique combination of art and science. The outcome is strongly influenced by the surgeon's facility with sculpture and design, but the result will also depend on adherence to sound principles of plastic surgery.

This chapter is meant to present a sound approach to total auricular construction by methods which have evolved through two decades of personal experience with 1100 cases. It focuses on congenital malformation of the auricle to establish basic principles in ear repair, but will also discuss management of acquired ear deformities and the special tissue coverage problems often associated with them.

INITIATING THE SURGERY

In dealing with congenital ear deformity, the age at which one begins surgery is governed by both physical and psychological considerations. It is best to initiate the repair before the child is traumatized by cruel teasing, but the surgeon must not be pressured to begin until rib growth provides substantial cartilage for framework fabrication.[1,2]

In my experience, these children become aware that their ears are different before age 4, but teasing with psychological overtones does not become manifest until ages 7–10. Generally, there is substantial cartilage for the repair by age 6, by which time the child is aware of the problem, usually wants it resolved, and is surprisingly cooperative regarding the surgery. My favorite age to begin surgery is from 7–10, although I have repaired virginal, unoperated microtia in patients as old as 62.

If the opposite, normal ear is large and the child is small, one may have to postpone the surgery for several years. On the other hand, a large child with a small normal ear may permit one to begin by age 5 ½. In my experience, beginning surgery earlier than this merely invites technical handicaps and poor patient cooperation.

SELECTING THE METHOD

In contrast to homologous cartilage, which absorbs,[3] and silicone frameworks, which often fail,[4] autogenous cartilage produces favorable results, experiences few complications and withstands trauma.[5,6] I have seen silicone ear frameworks lost to even minor trauma up to 12 years after implantation. On the other hand, once the tenth postoperative day has safely passed, it would be most unusual to lose an autogenous ear framework. To date, more than 70 of my reconstructed ears have survived major trauma.

For many years there has been considerable interest in creating a 'pre-fabricated' framework from autogenous cartilage in order to circumvent the necessity to fabricate an ear framework during a prolonged reconstructive procedure. Young and Peer first conceived the idea of 'framework pre-fabrication' prior to the actual auricular reconstruction.[7,8] This innovative technique was accomplished by means of 'diced' pieces of autogenous costal cartilage which were placed in a two-piece, fenestrated vitallium ear-shaped mold which in turn was banked in the patient's abdominal wall for approximately five months. However, the results were not consistent, perhaps because contraction of the fibrous tissue surrounding the multiple cartilage islands contributed to distortion of the resultant framework. Recently, interest in this 'pre-fabrication' concept has been rekindled through modern 'tissue engineering' techniques.[9] However, unless a very solid, substantial three-dimensional framework can be produced, it will likely suffer the same consequences as the ears constructed by Peer's method, i.e. flattening out under the restrictive, two-dimensional skin envelope in which the framework must be placed to complete the reconstruction. The other obvious limitation of 'pre-fabricated' ear frameworks is the inability to accommodate the great variation in size and shape that one must produce to match the opposite, normal ear.

PREOPERATIVE PLANNING

The successful grafting of a well-sculpted cartilage framework is the foundation for a sound auricular repair. By accomplishing this as the *first* surgical stage, one takes advantage of the optimal circulation and elasticity of inviolate virgin skin. With this in mind, I avoid initial repositioning of vestige remnants, as the resulting scars can inhibit the circulation and restrict the skin's elasticity and ability to accommodate a three-dimensional framework.[10,11] Secondary procedures such as lobule rotation, tragus construction, and sulcus grafting take place upon sound healing of the 'foundation'. Shortcuts with so-called 'one-stage repairs' are risky and produce ears that inevitably require further detailing to achieve a quality result.[12]

Planning is initiated by first tracing a film pattern from the opposite normal ear; this pattern is reversed and used to plan the new framework. A new pattern is then made several millimeters smaller in all dimensions to allow for the extra thickness which occurs when the cartilaginous framework is inserted under the skin. The framework's inferior pole is greatly reduced to accommodate the earlobe upon its transposition. If the patient has no usable earlobe tissue, the framework's lower end is carved to resemble an earlobe. This is further defined when the ear is separated from the head with a skin graft.

The ear's location can be predetermined in the office by first taping the reversed film pattern to the proposed construction site, and then adjusting its position until it is level to and symmetrical with the opposite normal ear. I trace the pattern on the head, noting the ear's axial relation to the nose, its distance from the lateral canthus, and its lobule's position, which is usually superiorly displaced. The ear's new position is straightforward and easy to plan in a pure microtia, but much more difficult when severe hemifacial microsomia exists. Not only are the heights of the facial halves asymmetrical, but the anteroposterior dimensions of the affected side are foreshortened as well. In these patients, one best plans the new ear's height by lining it up with the normal ear's upper pole – its distance from the lateral canthus is somewhat arbitrary.

In pure microtia, the vestige-to-canthus distance mirrors the helical root-to-canthus distance of the opposite, normal side. However, in severe hemifacial microsomia patients, the vestige is much closer to the eye. If one places the new ear's anterior margin at the vestige site, then the ear appears too close to the eye; if one uses the measured distance of the normal side as a guide, then the ear looks too far back on the head. In these patients, I find it best to compromise by selecting a point halfway between these two positions.

When both auricular construction and bony repairs are planned, then careful, integrated timing is essential. Most often the family pushes for the ear repair to begin first, which helpfully assures the auricular surgeon virginal, unscarred skin. The craniomaxillofacial surgeon argues that by going first he will correct the facial symmetry, thus making ear placement easier.[13] I find this unnecessary when the above described guidelines are followed.

If the bony work is done first, it is imperative that scars are peripheral to the proposed auricular site. When a coronal incision is used to approach the upper face or to harvest cranial bone grafts, special care must be taken that the scar does not lie precariously over the future region of the upper helix.

THE FIRST SURGICAL STAGE

HARVESTING THE RIB CARTILAGE

The rib cartilages are removed through a slightly oblique incision made just above the costal margin. Once the muscle has been divided, the film patterns are used to determine which cartilages will serve best for the framework.

To take advantage of the natural rib configuration, one harvests the cartilage from the side contralateral to the ear being constructed.[14] The first free-floating cartilage tapers favorably to form the helix; the synchondrotic region of ribs 6 and 7 provides an ample cartilage block to form the framework body (Fig. 84.1A). To conserve anesthetic time, my assistant closes the chest wound while I fabricate the framework. Using this approach, the entire operation (rib harvest, framework fabrication, and its insertion beneath the auricular skin) routinely takes me less than three hours.

When grafting cartilage, intraoperative antibiotics are used as a prophylactic measure, and their use is continued for several days after the procedure. In subsequent stages of ear repair, I do not use antibiotics, except when elevating and grafting the ear of an adolescent patient with intractable acne.

FRAMEWORK FABRICATION

The basic ear silhouette is carved from the synchondrotic cartilage block. It is necessary to thin little, if any, of the

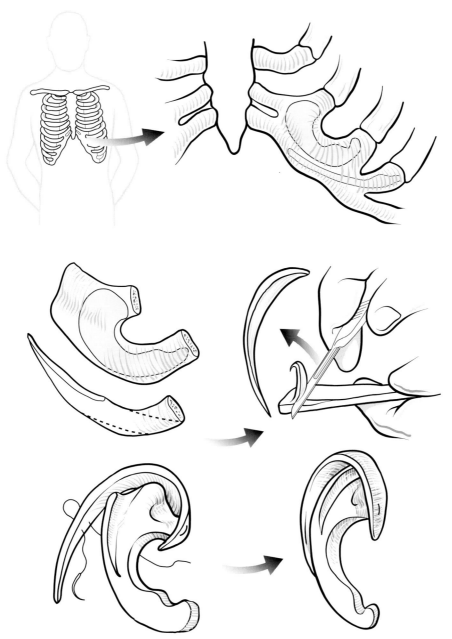

Fig. 84.1 Fabrication of ear framework from rib cartilage grafts. **(A)** Note that the upper border of the sixth cartilage is preserved; this helps to prevent subsequent chest deformity as the child grows. The entire 'floating cartilage' will be used to create the helix. **(B)** To produce the acute flexion necessary to create the helix, the 'floating' rib cartilage is deliberately warped in a favorable direction by thinning it on its outer, convex surface. **(C)** The thinned helix is affixed to the main sculptural block with horizontal mattress sutures of 4–0 clear nylon; the knots are placed on the framework's undersurface.

basic form for a small child's framework, but cartilage thinning is essential for adult frameworks. When thinning is necessary, it is wise to preserve perichondrium on the lateral, outer aspect of the framework (notably the antihelical complex) to facilitate its adherence to and subsequent nourishment from surrounding tissues. When creating the helix, the floating rib cartilage is thinned on its outer, convex surface to cause deliberate warping[15] in a favorable direction (Fig. 84.1B). This allows one to produce the acute flexion necessary to create a helix, which is then fastened to the framework body with horizontal mattress sutures of 4–0 clear nylon; the knots are buried on the framework's undersurface. The helix is stabilized by affixing it to the main cartilage block (Fig. 84.1C).

Through years of observing the healing process, I continue to evolve and modify the framework to achieve optimal helical stability and projection. Presently, I prefer to attach the helical cartilage anterior to the inferior crus first. This creates maximum framework width while maintaining the normal, low projection of the crus helix. Stability is next achieved by wrapping the helix around the superior pole of the helix. Finally, projection can be maximized where it is most needed by affixing the terminal helix on top of the main cartilage block along the framework's posterior border[16] (see Fig. 84.1).

THE CUTANEOUS 'POCKET' AND SKIN COAPTION

A cutaneous pocket is created with meticulous technique so as to provide an adequate recipient vascular covering for the framework. Nearly two hours lapse during the rib harvest and framework fabrication, and the contamination risk can be minimized by prepping and scrubbing the auricular region just prior to beginning the cutaneous dissection.

Using the template and preoperatively determined measurements, the ear's position is marked and a small preauricular incision is made. Upon excising unusable vestigial cartilage, one then develops a thin skin 'pocket', taking great care not to damage the subdermal vascular plexus. To recruit sufficient tension-free skin coverage, the dissection is carried well beyond the marked auricular outline (Fig. 84.2).

Following any necessary adjustments either to the framework height or to the adequacy of the pocket, two small silicone drains are inserted beneath and behind the framework and then into vacuum test tubes (Fig. 84.2). This creates a continuous suction which not only coapts the nourishing skin flap to the carved cartilage but also prevents possible disastrous hematomata.

DRESSINGS AND POSTOPERATIVE CARE

The new ear's convolutions are packed with Vaseline gauze and a bulky, non-compressive dressing is applied. Since the vacuum system provides both skin coaption and hemostasis, pressure is unnecessary and is contraindicated. The first day, the tubes are changed by the ward nurses every few hours, then every 4–6 hours thereafter or when a tube is one third full. Although the patient leaves the hospital in several days, the drains remain in place for another 2–3 days until the test tubes contain only drops of serosanguinous drainage.

Postoperatively, the ear is checked and the protective head dressing is changed several times, and removed after about 12 days. At that time, the patient can resume school, but running and sports should be restricted for another 4–5 weeks while the chest wound heals.

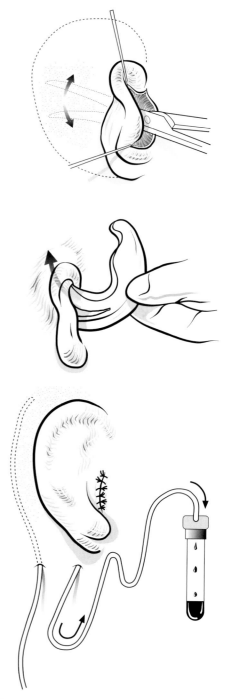

Fig. 84.2 The cutaneous 'pocket' The vestigial native cartilage is excised, then a skin pocket is created. In order to provide tension-free accommodation of the framework, the dissection is carried out well beyond the proposed auricular position. Using two silicone catheters, the skin is coapted to the framework by means of vacuum tube suction.

OTHER STAGES OF THE AURICULAR CONSTRUCTION

To allow for proper healing, a minimum of three months is allowed between the staged surgeries. This extra time allows

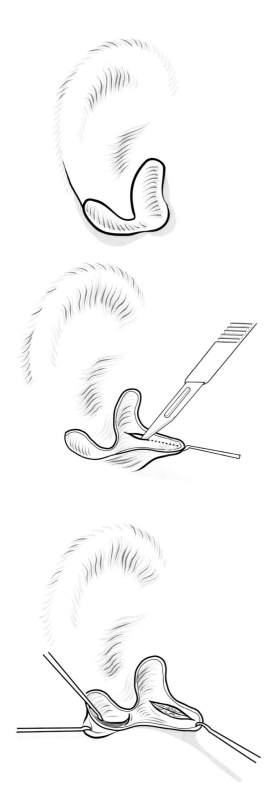

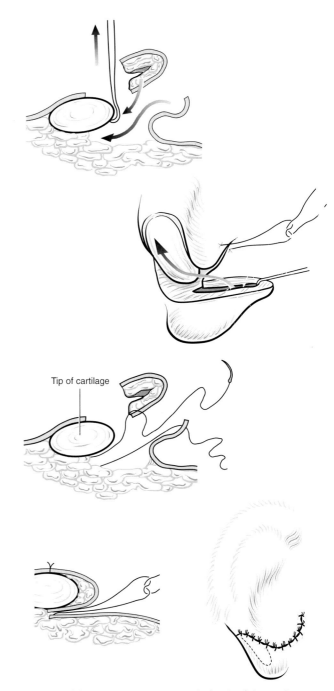

Fig. 84.3 Stage 2, earlobe transposition. By incising around it, the lobule is mobilized as an inferiorly based flap; an incision is outlined at the proposed superior inset margin. The skin overlying the lower ear region is loosened so that it can be slid under the elevated framework's tip to surface the 'floor' beneath it; the lobule is filleted so that it can be wrapped around the cartilaginous framework tip in a two-layered closure (see Fig. 84.4).

Fig. 84.4 Earlobe transposition, continued. The tip of the cartilaginous framework is elevated from its soft-tissue bed, and the filleted earlobe is wrapped around it. In this repair, note that the skin that overlaid the cartilaginous tip is now shifted beneath it to surface the raw bed vacated by the framework.

Tip of cartilage

for the swelling to subside, for circulation to improve, and for the tissues to settle down.

LOBULE TRANSPOSITION

I prefer to perform earlobe transposition as a secondary procedure, because it is easier to 'splice' the lobular remnant into position and to wrap it around the bottom of a well-established, previously constructed auricle. Although it is possible to transpose the lobule while simultaneously placing the framework, I find it safer and far more accurate to transpose the lobule secondarily. This can be accomplished on an outpatient basis several months after the cartilage graft.

Utilizing the lobular remnant can be the most challenging and creative part of the reparative process. Lifting the framework's tip and filleting the lobule to receive it not only enhances the inset (see Figs 84.3 and 84.4) but facilitates the next procedure when the ear is separated from the head with a skin graft.

DETACHING THE AURICLE WITH A SKIN GRAFT

The ear is separated from the head with a skin graft and a sulcus created to define the ear's posterosuperior margin. This improves the ear's appearance by eliminating a cryptotic appearance. This procedure does not project a framework that has been carved with insufficient depth. Frontal symmetry is achieved later during tragus construction, when the contralateral ear can be set back while harvesting grafts for the tragus. Alternatively, one can place a wedge of cartilage behind the elevated ear, but this must be covered with a flap of fascial tissue in order to provide recipient vascularity over the portion of the skin graft which will cover this new cartilage surface. If one is to achieve projection of the ear with this maneuver, then it should be planned from the very start of the reconstructive process, so that extra cartilage can be banked under the chest incision and thus be easily obtained during the elevation procedure.

Beginning with an incision made several millimeters peripheral to its margin, the surgically constructed auricle is lifted from its bed, taking care to preserve connective tissue both on its cartilaginous undersurface and on the bony floor below (Fig. 84.5). The retroauricular scalp is then undermined and advanced towards the newly created sulcus and affixed to the fascia and periosteum with heavy sutures. This not only decreases the size of the graft required, but permits one to advance the hairline so that the graft is invisible from the lateral profile. Since this graft is applied to the back of the ear and color match is no issue, it can be harvested as medium–thick split skin from the side of the hip, hidden beneath the patient's bathing suit region.

TRAGUS CONSTRUCTION

In a single procedure, I form the tragus, excavate the concha, and mimic a canal by inserting a special, arched composite graft through a J-shaped incision in the conchal region.[17] The main limb of the J is placed at the proposed posterior tragal margin; the crook of the J represents the intertragal notch (Fig. 84.6). I excise extraneous soft tissues beneath the tragal flap to deepen the conchal floor. This excavated region looks quite like a meatus when the newly constructed tragus casts a shadow upon it.

To create a realistic tragus with the best curvature, the composite graft is harvested from the anterolateral conchal surface of the normal ear. This technique is particularly ideal when a prominent concha exists, since the donor site closure facilitates an otoplasty, which is often needed to attain frontal symmetry. If the concha is not prominent and/or the projection of both ears is already equal before tragus construction, then I graft the donor concha. This is easily accomplished by harvesting a small ellipse of skin from just in front of the retroauricular hairline.

In a case of bilateral microtia, the tragus can be created by affixing a vertical strut of cartilage from the inferior tip of each framework.

COMBINING SURGICAL STAGES

In creating an ear, one has to use caution when doing more than one surgical stage at one time. Unlike wood carving or clay sculpting, surgical sculpting of tissues depends on good circulation. One should not perilously surround the auricle with incisions and undermining, nor dangerously 'skeletonize' the ear.

I have found it safe to simultaneously elevate the ear and transpose the lobule if the original earlobe vestige is short, because its small wound closure will not compromise the ear's anterior circulation.[6]

BILATERAL MICROTIA

For optimal function and esthetics in bilateral microtia, one must plan to integrate surgical procedures so that one does not compromise the other. In these cases, the auricular construction should precede the middle ear surgery since, once an attempt is made to 'open' the ear, the chances of obtaining a satisfactory auricular repair are severely com-

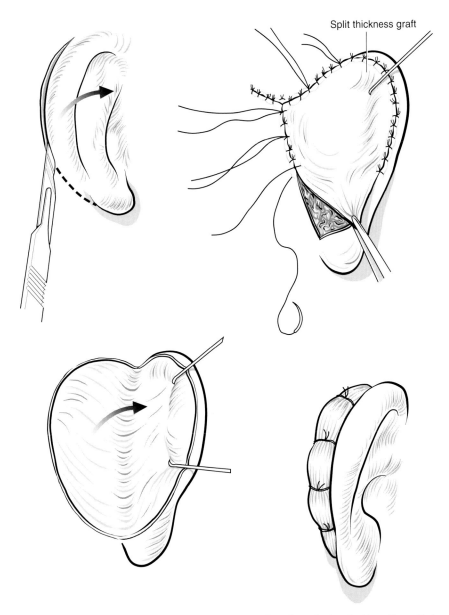

Fig. 84.5 Stage 3, separating the surgically constructed ear from the head with a skin graft. An incision is made several millimeters peripheral to the surgically constructed ear, and the auricle is sharply elevated from its fascial bed. The scalp is advanced to the newly created sulcus to decrease graft requirements and to hide the graft by limiting its placement mostly to the ear's undersurface. Long silk sutures are tied over a bolus dressing.

promised because the invaluable virgin skin has been scarred.

In bilateral microtia, I leave several months between performing the cartilage graft on each side. Each hemithorax contains sufficient cartilage for only one good ear framework, and simultaneous bilateral reconstruction necessitates bilateral chest wounds with attendant splinting and respiratory distress. Furthermore, the first auricular repair might be jeopardized upon turning the head to do the second side. For these reasons, it is preferable to perform the first stage of each ear on separate occasions.

Several months after the second cartilage graft, both earlobes are transposed during a single procedure. Once this stage is healed, one can either separate the ears from the head with skin grafting, do the tragus constructions, or pursue the middle ear surgery.

Middle ear surgery is reserved for cases in which there is high patient motivation and favorable radiologic evidence of middle ear development.[18] It must be thoughtfully planned in a 'team approach'[19] with an otologist who is competent and well-experienced in atresia surgery. Many surgeons presently feel that potential gains from middle ear

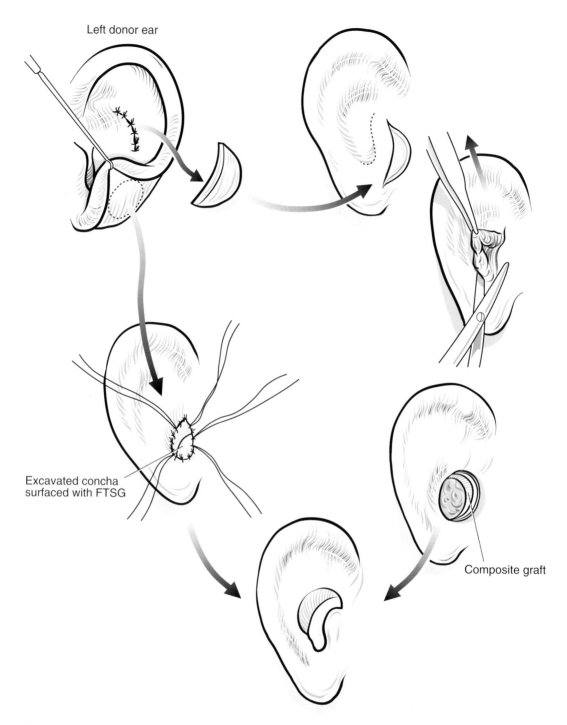

Left donor ear

Excavated concha surfaced with FTSG

Composite graft

Fig. 84.6 Stage 4, tragus construction and conchal excavation. A chondrocutaneous composite graft, harvested from the opposite, normal ear's conchal region, is placed under a thin J-shaped flap to create the tragus. Before surfacing the floor of the tragal region with a full-thickness skin graft (harvested from behind the opposite earlobe), extraneous soft tissues are excised to deepen the region.

surgery in microtia are outweighed by the potential risks and complications of the surgery and that this surgery should be reserved for bilateral cases. It is my conviction that if the otologic surgeon is not qualified to tackle a unilateral case, then he/she certainly shouldn't be operating on the bilateral cases either!

SECONDARY EAR RECONSTRUCTION AND TRAUMATIC DEFORMITY

Total auricular reconstruction after trauma presents special problems not encountered in microtia. These merit special consideration.

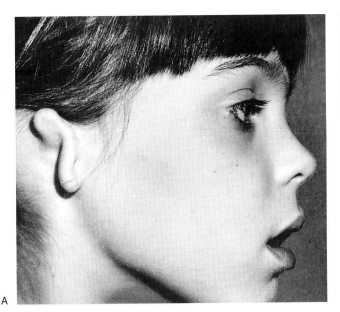
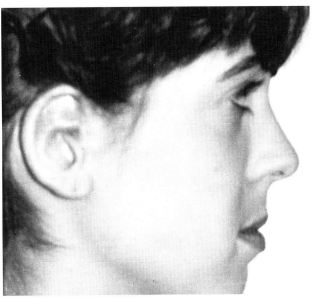

Fig. 84.7 Repair of microtia with sculpted rib cartilage graft. **(A)** A 6-year-old patient with classic microtia. **(B)** Result achieved with sculpted autogenous rib cartilage graft using the author's technique illustrated in Figs 84. 1–6, shown 12 years postoperatively.

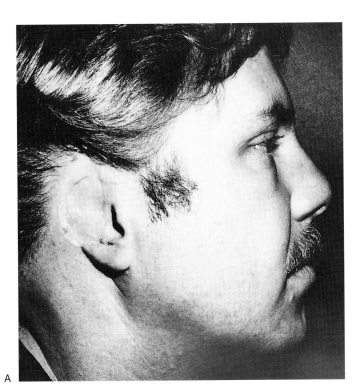
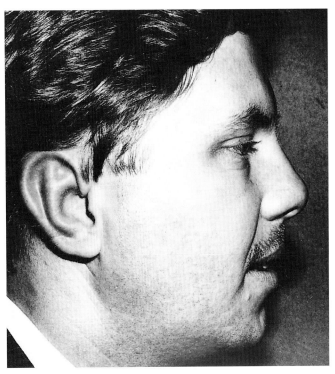

Fig. 84.8 Repair of acquired ear deformity with sculpted rib cartilage graft covered by skin-grafted fascial flap. **(A)** A 33-year-old man with auricular amputation for tumor. The skin-grafted local tissues are too restrictive to accommodate a new ear framework. **(B)** Result achieved with sculpted rib cartilage framework covered by fascial flap and skin graft, one year postoperatively.

The lack of skin coverage is much more critical than in congenital microtia since extra skin, usually gained through removing the crumpled vestigial cartilage, is not available. Furthermore, existing scars are inelastic and compound the skin shortage problem. If the existing skin is of good quality, every attempt should be made to use it, for there is no substitute for the native skin color and protective qualities. If the local cover is good, the cutaneous 'pocket' can be developed through incisions placed above and below the proposed auricular site. If the local tissues are heavily scarred or restrict the development of an ample skin pocket, the repair may be supplemented with fascial flap coverage.

Prior to the innovation of the temporoparietal fascial flap, acquired ear losses and secondary reconstructions were managed by first excising the scar and skin grafting the defect, then waiting for the graft to mature before implanting a new cartilage framework. That method was often beset with compromises in that skin-grafted tissues have limited elasticity as a cutaneous pocket; a detailed framework with depth could not be introduced without significant tension. Use of the fascial flap overcomes this skin coverage dilemma, just as the myocutaneous flap permits the resolution of coverage problems in breast reconstruction, i.e. the temporoparietal fasical flap provides an instantaneous abundance of thin, vascularized tissue which, in turn, permits a framework of any size or thickness to be covered easily[20] (Fig. 84.8).

REFERENCES

1. Tanzer RC 1959 Total reconstruction of the external ear. Plastic and Reconstructive Surgery 23:1
2. Brent B 1974 Ear reconstruction with an expansile framework of autogenous rib cartilage. Plastic and Reconstructive Surgery 53:619
3. Steffenson WH 1955 Comments on reconstruction of the external ear. Plastic and Reconstructive Surgery 16:194
4. Tanzer RC 1974 Discussion of silastic framework complications. In: Tanzer RC, Edgerton MT (eds) Symposium on reconstruction of the auricle. Mosby, St Louis, pp 87–88
5. Tanzer RC 1978 Microtia – a long-term follow-up of 44 reconstructed auricles. Plastic and Reconstructive Surgery 61:161
6. Brent B 1992 Auricular repair with autogenous rib cartilage grafts: Two decades of experience with 600 cases. Plastic and Reconstructive Surgery 90:355
7. Young F 1944 Cast and precast cartilage grafts. Surgery 15:735
8. Peer LA 1948 Reconstruction of the auricle with diced cartilage grafts in a vitallium ear mold. Plastic and Reconstructive Surgery 3:653
9. Cao Y, Vacanti JP, Paige KT, Upton J, Vacanti CA 1997 Transplantation of chondrocytes utilizing a polymer-cell construct to produce tissue-engineered cartilage in the shape of a human ear. Plastic and Reconstructive Surgery 100:297
10. Brent B 1980 The correction of microtia with autogenous cartilage grafts: I. The classic deformity. Plastic and Reconstructive Surgery 66:1
11. Brent B 1980 The correction of microtia with autogenous cartilage grafts: II. Atypical and complex deformities. Plastic and Reconstructive Surgery 66:13
12. Song Y, Song Y 1983 An improved one-stage total ear reconstruction procedure. Plastic and Reconstructive Surgery 71:615
13. Lauritzen C, Munro IR, Ross RB 1985 Classification and treatment of hemifacial microsomia. Scandinavian Journal of Plastic and Reconstructive Surgery 19:33
14. Tanzer RC 1971 Total reconstruction of the auricle. The evolution of a plan of treatment. Plastic and Reconstructive Surgery 47:523
15. Gibson T, Davis WB 1957 The distortion of autogenous cartilage grafts: Its cause and prevention. British Journal of Plastic Surgery 10:257
16. Brent B 1987 Total auricular construction with sculpted costal cartilage. In: Brent B (ed) The artistry of reconstructive surgery. Mosby, St Louis, pp 113–127
17. Brent B 1981 A personal approach to total auricular construction. In: Brent B (ed) Aesthetic aspects of reconstructive surgery. Clinics in Plastic Surgery 8:211
18. Jahrsdoerfer RA, Yeakly JW, Aguilar EA, Cole RR, Gray LC 1992 Grading system for the selection of patients with congenital aural atresia. American Journal of Otology 13:6
19. Brent B 1992 Auricular repair with autogenous rib cartilage grafts: Two decades of experience with 600 cases, Fig. 10. Plastic and Reconstructive Surgery 90:369
20. Brent B, Byrd HS 1983 Secondary ear reconstruction with cartilage grafts covered by axial, random, and free flaps of temporoparietal fascia. Plastic and Reconstructive Surgery 72:141

Skin rejuvenation

85

A.P. HEISE/THOMAS J. LANEY

INTRODUCTION

The last decade has seen major developments in laser treatment of skin problems. This field continues to show rapid change and progress in technology. It is now possible to selectively target and destroy specific cellular and subcellular structures while sparing normal structures. This minimizes scarring and other complications. A range of lasers is now available, each type designed to treat particular conditions such as abnormalities of skin surface topography and texture, vascular lesions, and pigmented lesions. The basic principles of laser operation in clinical applications will be discussed in this chapter.

Current medical therapy for photo aging of the skin involves the use of sunscreens, retinoic acid and alpha hydroxy acids. Retinoids are particularly useful, as they have been shown to downregulate collagenase as well as upregulate messenger RNA. Several investigators have shown that tretinoin results in replacement of the atrophic epidermis with hyperplasia, elimination of dysplasia and atypia, and new collagen formation in the papillary dermis as well as new vessel formation.[1] All of these effects are desirable in reversing photo aging and may be dramatic. These effects are both dose- and time-related and may be profound in sun-exposed as well as non-sun-exposed skin. Much of the clinical improvement has been shown to correlate with new collagen-1 formation. The use of Retin-A (tretinoin) may be complimentary to any surgical resurfacing procedure, and may enhance clinical results as well as prolong the benefits by continued use on a maintenance program.[2] Current surgical rejuvenative therapy for the aged face involves CO_2 laser resurfacing, chemical peels (phenol, TCA and alpha hydroxy acids) and, less commonly, dermabrasion.

LASER PHYSICS AND LIGHT–TISSUE INTERACTIONS

Improved laser therapy has been made possible by combining wavelengths that are selectively absorbed by the target, and pulses short enough to prevent heat transfer to surrounding tissue. Carbon dioxide (CO_2) lasers are useful for treating disorders of skin surface texture and topography, such as wrinkles, scars, sun damage, benign skin appendages and rhinophyma. Vascular lasers, such as the flashlamp-pumped dye laser, are particularly effective for treating port-wine stains, hemangiomas, telangiectasia, rosacea and spider nevi. Q-switched lasers, which allow ultra-short high intensity pulses, are effective for treating most tattoos and some benign pigmented lesions.[3]

All light is part of the electromagnetic spectrum that includes ultraviolet, visible and infrared light. Surgical lasers fall in the zone between the near-infrared and ultraviolet portions of the electromagnetic spectrum and include the visible light spectrum (Fig. 85.1). A solid, gas or liquid is the necessary component for the active medium of the laser. Upon excitation by the absorption of energy, the atom is elevated from its normal ground state to a state of higher energy. Once the energy is absorbed the atom spontaneously returns to its ground state and will then release the absorbed energy. This is called the spontaneous emission of radiation. An atom can be energized to an excited state after interacting with a photon of identical wavelength. The photon that is emitted upon the atom's return to its ground state then travels in the same direction and the same phase with the energizing photon. This is called stimulated emission of radiation. With the appropriate conditions a chain reaction will occur, resulting in an avalanche of energized photons.[4]

A laser consists of a resonator containing an active medium

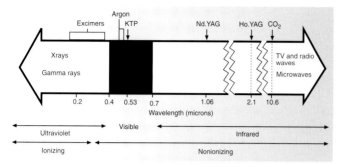

Fig. 85.1 Electromagnetic spectrum. Surgical lasers fall between the near infrared and ultraviolet portions of the spectrum. This portion includes the visible light spectrum. (Courtesy of Coherent, Inc., Palo Alto, CA.)

that is enabled to emit stimulated radiation. Many substances are capable of emitting laser light, including carbon dioxide, argon, neodymium, helium and krypton.[5] The active medium is contained within the laser optical cavity, or resonator. At the end of the resonator there are parallel mirrors. An energizing pump provides thermal, electric, or optical energy which is then absorbed by the active medium. When sufficient energy has been delivered, a population inversion occurs (the majority of atoms are at an upper energy state versus ground state).[6] The majority of the spontaneous radiation is lost to heat, however a sufficient quantity remains in phase and is amplified by reflection between the parallel mirrors. The front mirror is a partial reflector, and so a portion of the energy escapes from the cavity. Energized monochromatic light is columnated and coherent on exit from the cavity.[4] Heating, photochemistry, ionization and other reactions will not occur if a material or substance does not absorb light. This is the underlying principle for the medical use of laser energy. The energy

can be directed to that substance or tissue that absorbs the laser energy without affecting the non-absorbing surrounding tissues.[7]

Laser light can interact with biologic tissue in several ways. It can be reflected, transmitted, scattered or absorbed.[4] These reactions are wavelength dependent and are not mutually exclusive. For light to have any effect, it must be absorbed. Light absorption is wavelength dependent and is determined by the chemical content of the tissue. Each of the components of tissue has its own absorption spectrum and will thus absorb only certain wavelengths of light within the spectrum.[8] This is determined by the chromophore that is present in the tissue.[8] As can be seen in Table 85.1, the absorption characteristics of the various tissue components determine which laser wavelength will be most effective.

The term 'selective photothermolysis' was coined to describe a process whereby thermally-mediated injury was restricted to a site by virtue of the selective absorption of the chromophore at that site.[9] For this to be accomplished, the following criteria must be met: appropriate wavelengths, exposure time and threshold. An appropriate wavelength that is preferentially or selectively absorbed by the target chromophore must be selected. The length of time the tissue is exposed to the light energy should be less than the thermal relaxation time for the target chromophore. The energy density during the exposure time should be equal to or greater than an appropriate threshold: if tissue is being vaporized, this should be the vaporization threshold, whereas if tissue is being coagulated, this should be equal to or greater than the coagulation threshold. If all three criteria are met, precise site-specific damage will take place.

The major chromophores in skin are water, melanin, hemoglobin and collagen[10] (Fig. 85.2). The CO_2 laser at

Table 85.1 Dermatologic laser systems

Emission	Laser system	Wavelength (nm)	Mode of output	Absorption characteristics
Visible (400–700 nm)				
	Argon (blue-green)	488–514	CW	Hemoglobin, melanin
	Dye (pigment)	510	Pulsed	Melanin
	Krypton (green)	521, 530	CW	Hemoglobin, melanin
	Frequency doubled: YAG (green)	532	Q-switched	Melanin, tattoos (recd), hemoglobin
	Copper (green)	511	Pulsed	Hemoglobin, melanin
	Krypton (yellow)	568	CW	Hemoglobin
	Copper (yellow)	578	Pulsed	Hemoglobin
	Dye (vascular)	577, 585	CW, Pulsed	Hemoglobin
	Ruby	694	Q-switch	Melanin, tattoos
	Alexandrite	755	Q-switch	Tattoos, melanin
Infrared (700–100 000 nm)				
	Nd:YAG	1064	CW, Q-switch	Protein, tattoos
	CO_2	10 600	CW, SP	H_2O

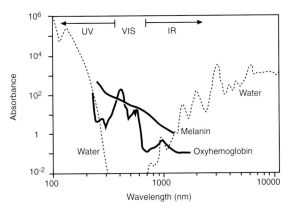

Fig. 85.2 The absorption of light by tissue. UV = ultraviolet light; VIS = visible light; IR = infrared light.

1064 nm will penetrate about 20 µm of tissue, and is therefore excellent for cutting and vaporizing.[11]

STRUCTURE AND FUNCTION OF THE SKIN

Aged skin presents with dryness, wrinkling, pallor, variable pigmentation and thinning, with fragility as well as loss of elasticity and sagging. At a microscopic level this is evident by thinning of the epidermis, flattening of the dermal/epidermal junction, and a decrease in the number of melanocytes and Langerhans cells. A decrease in the capillary plexus with fragmentation of collagen and elastin fibers, as well as development of atypical cells in the epidermis is also observed. These changes are most profound at the surface of this photodamaged skin; removal of the outer layer of badly damaged tissue – combined with stimulation of new collagen, elastin and epidermal regrowth – may result in profound clinical improvement and rejuvenation. The dermis/connective tissue matrix is made up of 70% collagen and 2% elastin fibers. The collagen provides tensile strength, whereas elastin provides elasticity and resilience. In aged skin the collagen matrix is disorganized and the collagen content diminished, decreasing by approximately 1% per year during adult life. Elastin disintegrates in fragments, resulting in an amorphous substance of altered elastic fibers, referred to as elastosis. The elastin content profoundly decreases after age 30 years. The effects of photo aging on the dermis are increased degeneration of elastin, increased destruction of collagen, decreased vascularity, decreased melanocytes, and a decreased number of fibroblasts.

Fibroblasts have a pivotal role in maintaining the dermal architecture. These cells are quiet until they respond to stimuli. Inflammation and wounding stimulate cellular proliferation through pro-collagen production and colla-

Table 85.2 Fitzpatrick sun-reactive skin types

Skin color (unexposed skin)	Skin type	Sunburn	Tan
White	I	Yes	No
	II	Yes	Minimal
	III	Yes	Yes
	IV	No	Yes
Brown	V	No	Yes
Black	VI	No	No

genase inhibition. The overall result is a diminishing ability to maintain the structural integrity of the dermis. The medical treatment of cellular aging involves downregulating proteolytic activity and upregulating structural protein synthesis.

SKIN PHOTOTYPES

Skin color, or constitutive melanin pigmentation, is divided into white, brown and black. Not all persons with white skin have the same capacity to develop tanning. This is the principal basis for the classification of white-skinned individuals into four skin phototypes (SPT)[12] (Table 85.2). The SPT is based on a person's own estimate of sunburning and tanning. One question will permit the identification of the SPT: 'Do you tan easily?' Persons with SPT 1 or 2 will say immediately, 'no'. Those with SPT 3 or 4 will say, 'yes'. Persons with SPT 1 or 2 are regarded as melanocompromised and those with SPT 3 or 4 as melanocompetent, regardless of their phenotypes (hair and eye color). SPT 1 persons sunburn easily with short exposure (30 minutes) and never tan. SPT 4 persons tan with ease and do not sunburn with short exposures. SPT 2 persons are a subgroup of SPT 1 and sunburn easily, but tan with difficulty, while SPT 3 persons have some sunburn with short exposure, but develop marked tanning over time. It is estimated that 25% of white-skinned persons in the United States are SPT 1 and 2. Persons with constitutive brown skin are termed SPT 5, and with black skin SPT 6.

PRESURGICAL TREATMENT

Although some clinicians may advocate no pre- or post-resurfacing treatments, some type of treatment of the skin is generally accepted as being indicated before any resurfacing procedure is undertaken. Skin preconditioning appears to reduce the post-procedure variables of skin resurfacing procedures that may compromise the eventual outcome such as post-inflammatory hyperpigmentation, erythema and scarring. Skin preconditioning can be achieved with various techniques, each of which has its advantages and disadvantages. Currently there is no consensus among practitioners with regard to the best preparation of the skin before and reconditioning of the skin after resurfacing procedures. Described techniques have used various topical preparations such as retinoic acid, alpha hydroxy acid, and bleachers in varying concentrations and schedules of application. At present there is no systematic pre- and post-conditioning protocol that is useful for all types of resurfacing procedures and all skin types.

Preconditioning has several advantages. Full and complete preconditioning minimizes the variables that might otherwise influence the conduct of the procedure; the procedure chosen thus becomes more predictable. Optimum skin management can therefore have a major influence on the outcome. Reduction in variables may also lead to improved postoperative healing with earlier recovery of normal skin function and prompt recognition and minimization of potential complications related to abnormal healing. The major skin conditioning agents are retinoic acid, alpha hydroxy acid, hydroquinone, topical antibiotics and enhancers, such as cleansers and toners, hydrocortisone and moisturizers.

Skin preconditioning ideally promotes an *increase* in:

- The population of well-hydrated keratinocytes and uniform compact well-hydrated stratum corneum. This will increase the evenness of resurfacing procedures.
- Mitotic activity in the basal cell layers of the epidermis and adnexal structures (hair follicles and sweat glands). This leads to enhanced epithelialization after resurfacing, with increased production of epidermal growth factors that enhance keratinocyte migration for faster re-epithelialization and activate dermal fibroblasts for greater collagen and elastin production.
- Restored levels of glycosaminoglycan in the dermis, increasing dermal hydration. Water is the primary chromophore for the CO_2 laser so adequate dermal hydration may reduce the energy requirement for tissue vaporization, the amount of irreversible protein denaturation surrounding the central areas of the operated tissue, and the post-procedural dryness and erythema.
- Regulation of melanocyte function, which will prevent post-inflammatory pigmentation problems and restore normal skin tone faster and more efficiently.

Skin preconditioning also *reduces* inflammatory processes, such as acne, comedones and folliculitis.

These effects result primarily from the use of retinoic acid, and to a lesser extent, alpha hydroxy acids.

FACIAL RESURFACING WITH THE PULSED CO_2 LASER

The theory of selective photothermolysis revolutionized the use of lasers in skin surgery. This concept of confinement of tissue thermal damage by selectively targeting a precise tissue chromophore allows therapeutic intervention with minimal risk of adverse tissue reaction. There are two basic components to this theory. The first is that the wavelength specifically determines the absorption of laser energy in tissue. The second is that the pulse width or exposure time will specifically limit the thermal diffusion time beyond the target tissue if the pulse width is less than the thermal relaxation time or cooling time of the tissue. The net effect of these two refinements in parameters is a very controlled and specific tissue effect without unwanted thermal damage.

The calculated thermal relaxation time for pure water is approximately $325\ \mu s$, whereas that of human skin has been estimated to be around $700\ \mu s$. The thermal relaxation time of the skin is thus approximately 1 ms. When tissue is not vaporized in a single pulse, there is accumulation of the heat delivered to tissue between pulses. To avoid this cumulative tissue heating effect, vaporization needs to occur in a single pulse. Single pulse vaporization allows removal of heat in the steam of vaporization, and there is then little heat conduction into tissue. Tissue temperatures in this situation do not exceed 100°C, and the residual thermal damage has been found to range from 50 to 100 μm.[6] If tissue heating occurs without vaporization, however, tissue temperatures may exceed 600°C and the residual thermal damage may be 300 μm to 1 mm or more, leading to poor wound healing and potential scarring. If the fluence is less than the tissue vaporization threshold, or if the pulse width is longer than the tissue thermal relaxation time, tissue will coagulate, dessicate and carbonize as tissue heat accumulates and unseen thermal damage occurs beyond the site of laser impact. However, when the opposite conditions exist – the fluence being greater than the tissue vaporization threshold and the pulse width less than the thermal relaxation time of tissue – tissue is vaporized with each pulse and no significant thermal damage occurs beyond the site of laser impact.[6]

GENERAL INDICATIONS

Skin types are classified I through VI, according to Fitzpatrick (Table 85.2). Although it is difficult to categorize a skin type based on visual inspection, one should reserve resurfacing with the laser for persons with lighter skin types in the same manner as conventional dermabrasion and deep healing would be restricted to this group. We have treated darker-complected individuals, however, and have found an equally low incidence of hypopigmentation but an increased incidence of hyperpigmentation, with the final outcome taking potentially twice as long as in lighter-skinned individuals. The face is the safest area to treat. At other locations, such as the neck and extremities, scarring and pigmentary changes occur more often. Skin resurfacing with the laser is a form of surgery in which attention to detail is important. The cosmetic surgeon needs to develop a level of skill at which he or she can recognize the landmarks in the epidermis and the dermis to avoid under- or over-treatment. The use of the columnated handpiece or computer-patterned generator is operator-specific, with CPG handpieces being touted as quicker and more accurate in depth of laser penetration.

There are two strategies currently available for selective tissue destruction and laser skin resurfacing: modified or enhanced pulsed light or flash-scanned continuous wave light. At least four companies have rushed to market with different technologies for one of these strategies. Preliminary data comparing pulsed and scanning technologies are equivocal. No histologic difference has been seen, and all data to date suggest there is no clinical difference in the two technologies.[14] It is therefore possible to use either a scanned continuous wave laser or a modified pulse laser for skin resurfacing.

A system of classification has been proposed to assist the cosmetic surgeon in identifying the degree of perioral and periorbital wrinkling, as well as the appropriate choice of treatment. This newly-proposed classification is as follows:[9]

- **Class I**: superficial fine lines with mild surface textural changes
- **Class II**: generalized deep lines with moderate textural changes
- **Class III**: generalized deep lines, occasional furrows, severe dermatoheliosis.

Type I and II wrinkles, with mild laxity of facial skin, respond best to this treatment. Often laser skin resurfacing can achieve superb results as the only treatment. The ablation of wrinkles, together with collagen contraction, gives excellent clinical improvement. Deeper furrows and excessive skin laxity should be treated with rhytidectomy, direct neck lifting and brow lifting. At a later stage after these procedures, laser skin resurfacing will provide additional improvement. One may also consider two consecutive treatments a few months apart for additive clinical effects. The face can be treated fully or in cosmetic units, feathering at the edges to obtain blending of treated and nontreated areas.

Acne scars usually result from mild to severe cystic facial acne, and can be classified into superficial, slightly-depressed or raised scars, and deeper focal icepick scars. Only super-ficial depressed and raised scars will respond to laser skin resurfacing. With deeper scars, excision with punch grafting or subdermal scar release combined with subsequent laser skin resurfacing can achieve acceptable results. As is true for rhytid removal, the combined mechanism of collagen contraction and ablation is responsible for clinical improvement.

Side-lighting with a flashlight and direct magnification are extremely important in aiding the surgeon during the procedure. Often, more passes than are used in rhytid removal are necessary to achieve satisfactory improvement. With the first pass one exposes the widest point of the depressed scar, whereas contouring of the edge of the defect will often require several more passes. The surgeon must recognize the landmarks in the epidermis and the dermis to avoid under- and over-treatment.

For mild dermatoheliosis, with its associated solar lentigines, hypopigmented macules, fine wrinkling and mild telangiectasia, the laser appears to be an attractive alternative to superficial chemical peeling or medical treatment with glycolic acids, synthetic retinoids and bleaching agents such as hydroquinones. A single-pass laser ablation to the full face can achieve good improvement in texture and even out pigmentation changes.

Small facial papular lesions such as syringomas, xanthelasma, sebaceous hyperplasia, fibrous papules, and angiofibromas respond well to laser skin resurfacing with minimal residual scarring. Frequently multiple passes are necessary to bring these lesions into the plane of the surrounding skin. For unwanted pigmentary conditions, such as melasma, a one-pass laser peel is as helpful as trichloroacetic acid peeling of 20–30%. Similarly, for actinic cheilitis, one pass over the lower lip will achieve a high cure rate with minimal healing time when compared to conventional CO_2 laser therapy. Rhinophyma usually presents with gross sebaceous hypertrophy. Although ablation in the initial stages is necessary to debulk the nose, the use of a pulsed mode can be reserved for the final recontouring stages to minimize deep thermal necrosis.

The initial consultation visit with the patient presenting for facial resurfacing should parallel that for other surgical procedures. During our initial consultation with patients we diagnose, discuss surgical options, provide the patient with written information regarding selected surgical options, and lastly, provide financial counseling so that the cost of treatment can be discussed in detail with the patient. The ideal patient is usually between 30 and 80 years old and presents with mild to moderate wrinkling in the perioral and periorbital areas and fine wrinkling or dermatoheliosis of the rest of the facial skin.[15] Deeper furrows can be treated but frequently are only softened and not eliminated. In locations other than facial skin, the outcome might not be as favorable. Realistic expectations should be defined during the consultation period and preoperative interview, as should a willingness to cope with a sometimes difficult postoperative period. A detailed medical and surgical history is obtained, including past allergies to anesthetics, history of herpes infection, keloid formation, recent isotretinoin, and history of unusual pigmentary response to trauma. If patient compliance is questionable, a skin test can be done prior to treating greater surface areas. This has several advantages: it predicts overall outcome, measures patient compliance during the pre- and postoperative phases, and allows one to monitor the patient's coping mechanisms following the surgical skin resurfacing. Past and present sun exposure is discussed, and advice on behavior modification given.

TECHNIQUE

Several safety precautions must be taken when performing CO_2 laser surgery to reduce the risk of injury to the patient, the surgeon and operating room personnel. As with all laser procedures, appropriate eye wear must be worn by all individuals in the operating room. Flammable surgical skin preparation agents, dry surgical drapes and certain types of anesthetic gases must not be used in the laser operating room to avoid the possible hazard of combustion with inadvertent contact with the laser beam. A laser smoke evacuator must always be employed to remove potential infectious particles that are released into the air as a plume. It has now been established that papilloma viral DNA fragments can be recovered from the CO_2 laser plume during the treatment of warts; this is also true for electrosurgical plumes. It has also been shown that bacterial spores can survive CO_2 laser vaporization. The potential risk of transmission of other viral infections, including human immunodeficiency virus (HIV), by laser surgical plumes has not yet been determined. However, no viable simian immunodeficiency virus (FIV) was recovered from the CO_2 laser plumes generated under experimental conditions using different irradiants.[16]

Before surgery the patient is started on acyclovir to prevent perioperative herpetic infection and prescribed an antibiotic regimen to cover skin contaminants.[17] Before the administration of anesthetics, the face is cleansed with Hibiclens. The troughs of rhytids and acne scars are marked with a surgical marking pen. Preoperative marking of the patient becomes important if local anesthetic techniques are used, since the infiltration of the anesthetic solution can obscure the rhytid by the edema of the tissue. In our ambulatory surgery center we tend to use general anesthetic techniques, however a combination of local infiltration, regional blocks and conscious sedation can be used for full-face laser resurfacing. Following the proper degree of anesthesia and draping of the surgical patient, the laser resurfacing is started. The parameters for treatment are set on the control panel of the laser of choice, and the surgical procedure is begun. Many lasers available on the market today are sufficient for surgical laser resurfacing. There are computers which offer collimated handpieces and computer pattern generators, as well as scanner technology. The first laser pass is used to remove the epidermis to reveal the superficial papillary dermis. At this time, residual wrinkle lines can be easily visualized. Use of the computer pattern generator allows slight overlapping (10–40%), and this may be beneficial in achieving a uniform tissue reaction. This allows relatively uniform fluence over the treated area. The entire skin surface to be treated is covered with an even confluent pattern of pulses overlapping. The laser reacts with and vaporizes the intracellular water within the epidermis and leaves behind a white proteinaceous desiccated debris that can be easily wiped away with saline-saturated gauze. Each successive pass needs to be accomplished as an independent procedure. Before the second pass the tissue is examined for further evidence of solar elastosis and wrinkles. If there is a relatively widespread area of sun damage or wrinkles, separated by only 3–4 mm, the entire area is treated again in the same manner as the first pass. If there are isolated wrinkles and papules of solar elastosis, these areas are sculpted selectively by vaporizing the high points of tissue using the same pulse energy as the initial pass. Additional passes are made over the shoulders of each wrinkle line to smooth out the surface of the skin. The second pass will expose the yellowish tissue of the reticular dermis, giving the so-called 'chamois appearance'. No additional passes following this yellow appearance should occur, as this can lead to unfavorable scarring secondary to thermal damage of the tissues. For acne scarring, several passes may need to be done to achieve smoothness over affected areas.[18] More aggressive resurfacing, with its inherent risks such as the chance of permanent scarring, is needed to achieve good clinical improvement. Periorbital rhytids often require fewer passes than do perioral wrinkles. In the periorbital area the upper lid should receive only one pass. The infraorbital tissue often shows remarkable tissue shrinkage from collagen contraction after the first one to two passes. This will not lead to permanent scleral show if it is performed carefully. Temporary ectropion may occur, but it is helped by both time and gentle massage of the area (Fig. 85.3).

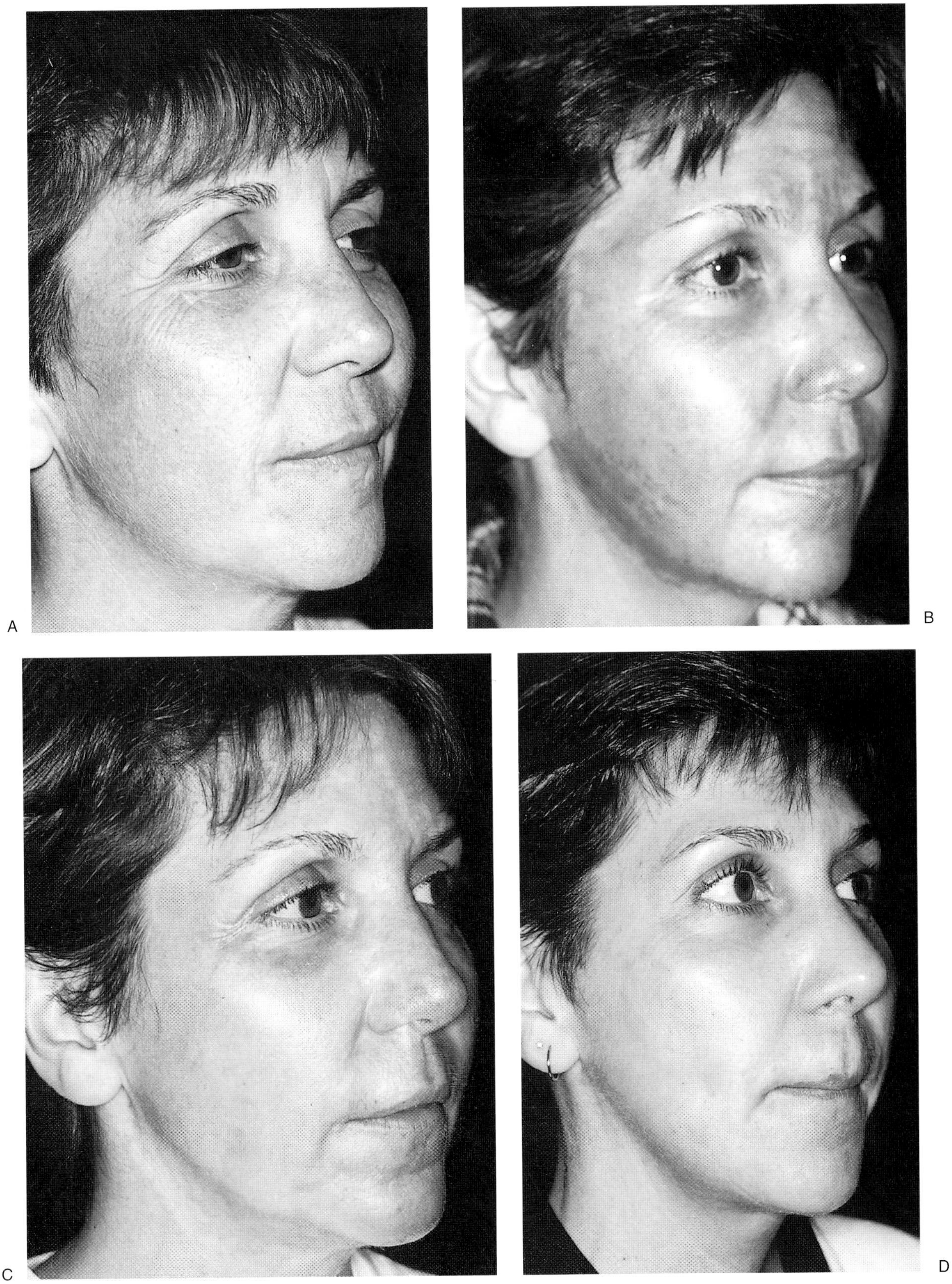

Fig. 85.3 Laser resurfacing: **(A)** preoperative; **(B)** 2 weeks postoperative; **(C)** 4 weeks postoperative; **(D)** 8 weeks postoperative.

The initial effects of vaporizing irregular surface contours will smooth the skin as much as possible. This effect is visible immediately, although there is some secondary beneficial effect from sloughing of thermally damaged areas. The next therapeutic stage involves new collagen formation occurring over the subsequent 6–12 weeks.[19] This new collagen formation will eliminate a significant degree of deeper wrinkling, and should be observed for a period of 2–3 months before consideration is given for retreating areas that have not responded completely.[20]

STUDIES

Weinstein, in a study published in 1997, reported on 643 patients who had undergone facial resurfacing with the UltraPulse CO_2 laser.[21] Weinstein reported good to excellent results in most patients with fine facial rhytids due to actinic damage. The conclusion of this paper stated that lasers have improved the results of skin resurfacing in comparison to other procedures such as dermabrasion and chemical peeling. Other authors, including Fitzpatrick,[9,14] Waldorf,[22] Lowe[23] and Ho[24] have all published papers with similar concluding remarks.

In general, photo damage improves by approximately 50%. Patients take 7–14 days to re-epithelialize, during which time they experience varying degrees of edema, drainage and burning discomfort. We have noted that postoperative discomfort is significantly decreased by a skin surface dressing. Patients with skin types III or IV frequently develop post-inflammatory hyperpigmentation that resolves with hydroquinone and retinoic acid treatment (Fig. 85.4). It is important that the patient be told that this condition can last for months. Scarring and hypopigmentation appear to be uncommon according to the published reports. However, cases of delayed hypopigmentation, first appearing 6 months after treatment, are beginning to be recognized. As more resurfacing procedures are performed, and as longer follow up is achieved, it may become apparent that side effects from this procedure will increase.

POSTOPERATIVE CARE

Postoperatively the acyclovir and antibiotic coverage is continued during re-epithelialization. Initially, when treating postoperative láser resurfacing patients our protocol consisted of using a coverage medium (Bacitracin ointment, Vaseline, zinc oxide ointment, Crisco oil, Calendula cream); following cleansing of the face with a mild soap such as Neutrogena, one of the above ointments was applied to the resurfaced area to keep the skin moist and prevent crusting and/or scabbing formation. We observed moderate patient discomfort in the first three days after surgery if no skin dressing was applied. We now apply a skin dressing immediately after laser resurfacing (Flexan, Silon); this is changed at Day 1 and a second dressing placed for the next several days. Close follow up of the patient in the immediate postoperative period is mandatory to reinforce home wound care and prevent crusting or scab formation at the periphery of the dressing. Following the removal of the dressing at Day 3 to 5, the patients return to a protocol of skin coverage medium such as Calendula cream until their re-epithelialization phase is complete.

Post-conditioning may improve long-term results. Any results achieved by the resurfacing procedure may be short-lived unless followed by a program that maintains the gains accomplished by the resurfacing and prevents further skin deterioration. After healing and re-epithelialization is complete, as evidenced by lessened sensitivity, resolution of oozing and complete eschar separation, post-conditioning should be started. The agents should be reintroduced sequentially, with the most effective and least reactive agents being added first. If the patient has evidence of post-inflammatory hyperpigmentation, hydroquinone should be introduced early. If no post-inflammatory hyperpigmentation is present, retinoic acid should be added in low dosage. If skin tolerance returns, the agents can be increased in dosage and frequency. The duration of treatment is variable, but remodeling of the skin after resurfacing procedures can continue for several months after the procedure.

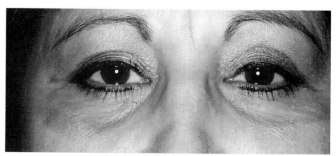

Fig. 85.4 Hyperpigmentation following blepharoplasty with periorbital resurfacing: **(A)** preoperative; **(B)** 8 weeks postoperative.

ALPHA HYDROXY ACID (AHA) PEELS

Recently alpha hydroxy acids (AHA) have been incorporated into a variety of creams, lotions and cleansers in general use. They are also being used as a new modality of chemical peeling. AHAs are a special group of nontoxic organic acids found in natural foods and are often commercially referred to as 'fruit acids'.[25] Members of the AHA group include glycolic acid, occurring naturally in sugar cane, lactic acid occurring in sour milk, malic acid occurring in apples, tartaric acid occurring in grapes, and citric acid occurring in citrus fruits. Glycolic acid represents the smallest alpha hydroxy acid and is composed of a 2-carbon molecule. The exact mechanism of action of AHAs is still unknown, however it has been shown that at low concentrations the AHAs act to diminish corneocyte cohesion at the lower levels of the stratum corneum. AHAs at high concentration can exert profound effects on the skin, dependent on exposure time. Some of these effects include complete epidermal lysis and possibly even some dermal effects such as increased collagen synthesis.[26,27]

Glycolic acid is currently the most common AHA in use. It is a versatile chemical peeling agent and is primarily used by the physician at either a 50% or 70% non-neutralized concentration. Glycolic acid is frequently applied as a series of peels separated by 1–4 weeks. Many of the risks and complications associated with other peeling agents are minimized with the use of glycolic acid. The indications for the use of glycolic acid as a peeling agent are many, and include actinic and seborrheic keratoses, lentigines, melasma, post-inflammatory hyperpigmentation, superficial rhytids, acne and facial rejuvenation to achieve a general improvement in the appearance of the skin. Virtually every patient is a candidate for glycolic acid peels, including Fitzpatrick skin types IV, V and VI.

Ideally, patients should be pretreated with twice-daily at-home applications of glycolic acid appropriate for their skin type, for two weeks prior to the peel.[28,29] Topical tretinoin may also be used concurrently with glycolic acid preparations during pretreatment. Darkly-pigmented patients may benefit from hydroquinone during their pre-peel skin care. Pretreatment glycolic acid use and topical tretinoin enable the patient to better tolerate the glycolic acid peels, as well as partially reducing stratum corneum thickness, and may accelerate healing. Patients are instructed to avoid sun exposure, and daily use of sun protection is encouraged. A recommended 6-month to 2-year rest period after oral retinoids is advisable prior to glycolic acid peels. Chemical peels done immediately after Accutane use have been associated with higher rates of scarring.[30] Prophylactic acyclovir for oral herpes simplex is necessary and is advised prior to glycolic acid peels.

CHEMICAL PEELS

Chemical peeling is performed on sun-damaged skin and is intended to produce a controlled partial-thickness injury to the skin, destroying varying amounts of the epidermis and upper portions of the dermis. The wound healing response following the injury involves removal of actinic keratoses, epidermal regeneration by epithelial migration from adnexal structures, and replacement of new dermal connective tissue. The overall clinical appearance of the skin is usually more homogeneous with fewer wrinkles and fewer pigmentary differences.

Chemical peeling agents are commonly divided into superficial, medium and deep (Table 85.3). This classification is based largely on histologic studies showing the depth of wound produced when they are applied to the skin. It should be emphasized that these classifications are merely guidelines: poor technique can lead to a deeper wound with superficial and medium-depth agents.

To aid in patient selection and classification of clinical photodamage, a relatively simple method was developed to facilitate the discussion of patient types and the appropriate

Table 85.3 Classification of peeling agents

Superficial	Trichloroacetic acid (10–25%) Combes (Jessner's) solution Resorcinol, 14 g Salicylic acid, 14 g Lactic acid 85%, 14 ml Ethanol 95%, 100 ml Alpha hydroxy acids Glycolic acid 30–70% Unna's paste (resorcinol 40 g, zinc oxide 10 g, ceyssatite 2 g, benzoin axungia 28 g) Carbon dioxide snow (± alcohol, ± sulfur)	0.06 (stratum granulosum to superficial papillary dermis)
Medium	Phenol 88% (full-strength) Trichloroacetic acid (35–50%) (± a second keratolytic, e.g. CO_2, Jessner's/Combes', glycolic acid)	0.45 mm (papillary to upper reticular dermis)
Deep	Baker–Gordon phenol formula (occluded/nonoccluded) Phenol 88%, 3 ml Croton oil, 3 drops Septisol, 8 drops Distilled H_2O, 2 ml	0.6 mm (midreticular dermis)

Table 85.4 Glogau photoaging classification

Type 1. 'No wrinkles'
  Early photoaging
    Mild pigmentary changes
    No keratoses
    Minimal wrinkles
  Younger patient, twenties or thirties
  Minimal or no makeup

Type II. 'Wrinkles in motion'
  Early to moderate photoaging
    Early senile lentigines visible
    Keratoses palpable but not visible
    Parallel smile lines beginning to appear
  Patient age, late thirties or forties
  Usually wears some foundation

Type III. 'Wrinkles at rest'
  Advanced photoaging
    Obvious dyschromia, telangiectasia
    Visible keratoses
    Wrinkles even when not moving
  Patient age, fifties or older
  Always wears heavy foundation

Type IV. 'Only wrinkles'
  Severe photoaging
    Yellow-gray color of skin
    Prior skin malignancies
    Wrinkled throughout, no normal skin
  Patient age, sixth or seventh decade
  Can't wear makeup, 'cakes and cracks'

From Glogau RG 1994 Chemical peeling and aging skin. *The Journal of Geriatric Dermatology* 2: 30–35. Copyright © 1994, Health Management Publications, Inc; with permission. Courtesy of Richard G. Glogau, MD.

peeling approaches. The Glogau Photoaging Classification is based on four classifications denoting early, moderate, advanced and severe photoaging of the skin (Table 85.4). Chemical peeling is then directed at type II and III patients, choosing the correct peeling agents from the wide range available. Additionally, during the preoperative assessment the surgeon must also make a determination as to where the patients pigmentary system lies. Fitzpatrick's scale of erythema and tanning responses is the cornerstone for evaluation for chemical peeling. The implication of the Fitzpatrick scale is that there is a range of possible responses of the pigmentary system not only to sunlight but to peeling agents as well. Type I patients will accept a deep chemical peel with less post-inflammatory hyperpigmentation and minimal risk of permanent hypopigmentation, whereas those with type IV skin may develop significant prolonged post-inflammatory hyperpigmentation and are at serious risk for depigmentation from deeper peels. Temporary and permanent alterations in color remain the most significant limiting risk factors in chemical peeling, and are the major driving force behind the preoperative classification schemes.

DEEP CHEMICAL PEELS

Deep chemical face peeling as a primary procedure is indicated for the eradication of heavy wrinkles and lines secondary to chronic photodamage, treatment of superficial premalignant keratoses, and solar lentigines. Deep peels as a class must be compared to phenol in varying concentrations as the primary ingredient. At concentrations greater than 80%, phenol is a keratocoagulant precipitating epidermal proteins and forming a barrier preventing deep dermal penetration. However, when diluted to 50% it is keratolytic, disrupting sulfa bridges and allowing increased phenol penetration and greater dermal destruction.[31] The formula of phenol most commonly used is the phenol peel of Baker's formula in a concentration of approximately 45–50%. The Baker formula is composed of 3 ml phenol 88%, United States Pharmacoperia, 3 drops croton oil, 8 drops Septisol soap, and 2 ml of distilled water. The croton oil is an additional irritant that enhances epidermal destruction by acting as an epidermolytic agent, thus allowing increased penetration of phenol. Septisol liquid soap increases surface tension and may retard phenol penetration.

There are relative contraindications to deep phenol peels, depending on the Fitzpatrick skin type and medical history. The ideal patient for deep phenol peel is a fair complexioned patient with thin, dry skin and fine wrinkles, such as a Fitzpatrick type I or II and a Glogau type III or IV. Pre-existing cardiac, hepatic or renal disease may preclude use of deep phenol peels as the systemic complications of phenol are well documented. Phenol has extensive systemic absorption, is directly cardiotoxic, is inactivated by conjugation in the liver and is 80% excreted by the kidneys. It is therefore contraindicated for use in those patients who have a history of heart, liver or kidney problems.[32] The cardiotoxicity of phenol is well documented and has been shown to occur within the first 30 minutes of application. The use of cardiac monitoring, adequate intravenous fluid maintenance and diuresis, and the treatment of small anatomic units with resting periods will minimize these complications.[33] Absorption of phenol percutaneously has been linked to production of cardiac arrhythmias, usually characterized by the onset of supraventricular rhythm disturbance, which if unrecognized may proceed to ventricular arrhythmia and cardiac arrest.[34]

MEDIUM-DEPTH CHEMICAL PEELS

Medium-depth peeling refers to use of the peeling edge and a combination of agents that will routinely produce an injury that penetrates to the upper reticular dermis.[35] These peels are usually performed as a single therapeutic procedure to treat actinic keratoses, dyschromia and milder forms of rhytids.[36] This group of peels presents the greatest variety of combination of agents and techniques, all advocated with the twin goals of higher efficacy and lower risks and morbidity. The most commonly used agent in this classification is trichloroacetic acid (TCA). As a general rule, most experienced surgeons avoid concentrations of TCA above 40%, since greater concentrations can produce hypertrophic scarring and full-thickness skin loss.

A combination of 35% TCA with prior treatment of the skin with carbon dioxide ice has been described.[29,37] Following the mechanical effect of carbon dioxide ice on the epidermis, causing microvesiculation and disruption of the stratum corneum barrier, 35% TCA achieves deeper penetration of the dermis, whereas such depth is rarely achieved with 35% TCA alone. The technique appears particularly well-suited for acne scarring where individual variation in depth can be achieved by varying the pressure and amount of time that the ice is applied.

A second combination of techniques involves the prior application of Jessner's solution as a keratolytic before application of 35% TCA.[38,39] Histologic depth of injury appears comparable to that achieved by 50% TCA or to the CO_2/35% TCA combination previously discussed. A significant advantage to the TCA regimens over those involving phenol is the lack of potential for cardiac toxicity, and there is therefore no need for intraoperative monitoring. Pre- and postoperative care of the patient is similar to that which has been previously described for laser resurfacing. Intraoperative application and management is the same as has been described for applying phenol.

The end results of a successful chemical peel are dependent on many factors, and knowledge of how to approach the complications of peeling is mandatory. These side effects can include pigmentary changes, prolonged erythema, colloid milia, pustulocystic acne, reactivation of latent facial herpes simplex virus infection, and superficial bacterial infection. Additionally, more significant complications can include hypertrophic scarring, atrophy, and systemic effects such as hepatic, renal and cardiac abnormalities associated with phenol. Procedural side effects and complications of chemical peeling are best controlled by careful preoperative screening, meticulous operative technique, and attentive surgical follow up in the immediate postoperative period.

CAMOUFLAGE THERAPY

Skin pigmentation is altered following laser skin resurfacing and chemical peeling procedures. Postoperative erythema

Table 85.5 Postsurgical pigment alterations

Pigment defect	Postsurgical etiology	Color correction
Red	New blood vessel formation, post-laser erythema	Green
Blue	Acute hematoma, vascular malformation	Orange
Yellow	Resolving hematoma, residual solar elastosis	Purple
Hyperpigmentation	Post-inflammatory, residual melasma, hemosiderin	White
Hypopigmentation, Depigmentation	Post-inflammatory, melanocyte destruction	Brown

can last for 12 weeks after some of these procedures. During this healing phase, patients must return to daily activities and be able to function socially. Patients' re-entry into the social arena following cosmetic dermatologic surgery is greatly aided through the use of camouflaging cosmetics and techniques. Camouflage cosmetics are specially formulated to provide 8-hour waterproof coverage of underlying pigment defects combined with color cosmetics artistically used to minimize contour defects.[40,41] The surgeon should have a basic understanding of the variety of cosmetics manufactured and the theory behind their application (Table 85.5).

There are many companies who manufacture cosmetics specifically for camouflage purposes. Our practice utilizes DermaBlend Corrective Cosmetics, Lakewood, NJ. A good camouflage artist will generally purchase a color palate from at least two different companies to provide the necessary mixture of cosmetic shades required to match a given patient's skin tone.[42] Every attempt should be made to allow the patient to wear as many of their presurgical cosmetics as possible.

REFERENCES

1. Stevens MB, Okagi ZE, Sawaf H 1996 Optimizing the results of your resurfacing procedures by preprocedure and postprocedure skin conditioning. International Journal of Aesthetics and Restorative Surgery 4:133–136
2. Weiss JS, Ellis CN, Headington JT, Tinoff T, Hamilton TA, Voorhees JJ 1988 Topical tretinoin improves photodamaged skin – a double-blind vehicle-controlled study. 259:527–532
3. Goldberg DJ 1996 Treatment of pigmented lesions of the skin with lasers. Facial Plastic Surgery Clinics of North America 4:291–294
4. Waner M 1996 Light–tissue interactions. Facial Plastic Surgery Clinics of North America 4:223–229
5. Grerelink JM 1996 Facial contouring using a flashscanner-enhanced carbon dioxide laser. Facial Plastic Surgery Clinics of North America 4:241–246
6. Dederich DN 1993 Laser/tissue interaction: What happens to laser

light when it strikes tissue? Journal of the American Dental Association 124:47–61

7. Treller MA, David LM, Rigan J 1996 Penetration depth of Ultrapulse carbon dioxide laser in human skin. Dermatologic Surgery 22:863–865

8. Penoff J 1996 Laser skin resurfacing. Annals of Plastic Surgery 36:392–393

9. Fitzpatrick RE 1996 Facial resurfacing with the pulsed carbon dioxide laser. Facial Plastic Surgery Clinics of North America 4:231–240

10. Goodman GJ, Bekhur PS, Richards SW 1996 Update on lasers in dermatology. MJA 164:681–686

11. Hruza GJ 1996 Laser skin resurfacing. Archives of Dermatology 132:451–455

12. Moschella SL, Hurley HJ 1992 Dermatology. WB Saunders, Philadelphia.

13. Lowe NJ, Lask G, Griffin ME 1995 Laser skin resurfacing – pre- and posttreatment guidelines. Dermatologic Surgery 21:1017–1019

14. Fitzpatrick RE, Goldman MP et al 1996 Pulsed carbon dioxide laser resurfacing of photoaged facial skin. Archives of Dermatology 132:395–402

15. Geronemus RG 1995 Laser surgery 1995. Dermatologic Surgery 21:399–403

16. Wheeland RG 1995 Review Series Article: Clinical uses of lasers in dermatology. Lasers in Surgery and Medicine 16:2–23

17. Perkins SW, Sklareu EC 1996 Prevention of facial herpetic infections after chemical peel and dermabrasion: New treatment strategies in the prophylaxis of patients undergoing procedures of the perioral area. Plastic and Reconstructive Surgery 98:427–433

18. Abugel RP, Dahlman CM 1995 The CO_2 laser approach to the treatment of acne scarring. Cosmetic Dermatology 8:33–36

19. Chernoff G, Slatkine M, Zair E, Merd D 1995 Silk Touch: A new technology for skin resurfacing in aesthetic surgery. Journal of Clinical Laser Medicine and Surgery 13:97–100

20. Hruza GJ 1995 Skin resurfacing with lasers. Fitzpatrick's Journal of Clinical Dermatology 3:38–41

21. Weinstein C 1997 Ultrapulse carbon dioxide laser rejuvenation of facial wrinkles and scars. American Journal of Cosmetic Surgery 14:3–11

22. Waldorf HA, Kauhan AN, Geronemus RG 1995 Skin resurfacing of fine to deep rhytids using a char-free carbon dioxide laser in 47 patients. Dermatologic Surgery 21:940–946

23. Lowe NJ, Lask G et al 1995 Skin resurfacing with the Ultrapulse carbon dioxide laser. Dermatologic Surgery 21:1025–1029

24. Ho C, Nguyen Q, Lowe NJ, Griffin ME, Lask G 1995 Laser resurfacing in pigmented skin. Dermatologic Surgery 21:1035–1037

25. Murad H, Shamkan AT, Premo PS 1995 The use of glycolic acid as a peeling agent. Dermatologic Clinics 13:285–307

26. Brody H, Coleman WP, Piacguadio D, Perricone NV, Elson ML, Harris D 1996 Round table discussion of alpha hydroxy acids. Dermatologic Surgery 22:475–477

27. Piacgnadio D, Dolory M, Hunt S, Andree C, Grere G, Hullinbach KA 1996 Short contact 70% glycolic acid peels as a treatment for photodamaged skin. Dermatologic Surgery 22:449–452

28. Newman N, Newman A, Muy LS, Balapour R, Harris AG, Muy RL 1996 Clinical improvement of photoaged skin with 50% glycolic acid, a double-blind vehicle-controlled study. Dermatologic Surgery 22:455–460

29. Peikert JM, Krywonis NA, Rest EB, Zachary CB 1994 The efficacy of various degreasing agents used in trichloroacetic acid peels. Journal of Dermatology and Surgical Oncology 20:724–728

30. Resnik SS, Resnik BI 1995 Complications of chemical peeling. Dermatology Clinics 13:309–312

31. Belinfante LS 1996 Oral and maxillofacial dermatologic procedures. Oral and Maxillofacial Surgery Clinics of North America 8:121–133

32. Brody HJ 1995 Current advances and trends in chemical peeling. Dermatologic Surgery 21:385–387

33. Brody HJ 1992 Update on chemical peels. Advances in Dermatology 7:275–289

34. Forte R, Hack J, Jackson IT 1993 Chemical peeling. Plastic Surgery Nursing 13:194–200

35. Rubin MG 1992 Trichloroacetic acid and other non-phenol peels. Clinics in Plastic Surgery 19:525–536

36. Becker FF, Langford FPJ, Rudin MG, Spielman P 1996 A histologic comparison of 50% and 70% glycolic acid peels using solutions with various pHs. Dermatologic Surgery 22:463–465

37. Mangat DS 1994 Introduction to chemical peeling and dermabrasion. Facial Plastic Surgery Clinics of North America 2:1–20

38. Munheit GD 1996 Combination medium-depth peeling: the Jessner's & TCA peel. Facial Plastic Surgery 12:117–124

39. Munheit GD 1995 The Jessner's trichloroacetic acid peel – an enhanced medium-depth chemical peel. Dermatology Clinics 13:277–283

40. Draelos ZD 1996 Camouflaging techniques and dermatologic surgery. Dermatologic Surgery 22:1023–1027

41. Rayner VL 1995 Camouflage therapy. Dermatology Clinics 13:467–472

42. Draelos ZK 1995 Cosmetics in the postsurgical patient. Dermatologic Clinics 13:461–465

Facial bone sculpturing

86

H. PETER LORENZ/STEPHEN A. SCHENDEL

INTRODUCTION

In order to optimize facial esthetics, a balanced and appropriately shaped skeletal support structure must be present. A beautiful face has a harmonious relation among the different components, including the soft tissues and the skeletal framework. With advances in craniofacial surgery, the facial skeleton can be manipulated safely to provide an optimal platform for the soft-tissue envelope.

Surgery of the facial skeleton can be divided into two major categories: orthognathic and contouring of specific facial bones. Orthognathic surgery not only alters the jaws and occlusion to improve functional deficits, it also alters facial appearance. Sculpturing of facial bones by either reduction or augmentation reshapes the facial skeleton to improve facial appearance. Soft-tissue procedures, such as the facelift, also change facial appearance. Facial bone sculpturing and soft-tissue procedures can be applied in combination, based on the individual needs of a patient, to give a superior and more consistent result.

Proper surgical planning in correcting facial anomalies and esthetic irregularities is complex. An understanding of and familiarity with skeletal shape analysis, including the use of cephalometry, is mandatory. A thorough examination of facial soft-tissue form and knowledge of anthropologic relationships is also necessary. Analysis of skeletal and soft-tissue findings together allows the surgeon to diagnose the basic problem and perform the correct operation.

ESTHETIC FACIAL EXAMINATION

Physical examination of the face should follow a logical order. Routinely, the esthetic examination is performed first. The facial type is determined together with form and shape. The key acceptable and unacceptable features of both the hard tissue and soft tissue are noted, recognizing that these features are inexorably linked. Hard-tissue structures to be examined for esthetic contour include the frontal bone, zygomatic arch, malar eminence, mandibular angle and body, and the chin. Soft-tissue characteristics such as asymmetries, skin texture, color changes, scars, and rhytids are noted.

Vertical, transverse, and anterior–posterior aspects of the face are noted. Anthropologic assessment by facial height in thirds and facial width based on the eyes can be utilized. However, the optimal esthetic determination may vary from these classical cannons, and thus they should be used as aids, not as absolute criteria, in treatment planning. Transversely, esthetic balance has been described as three equal facial partitions: hairline to nasion, nasion to subnasale, and subnasale to menton (Fig. 86.1). In reality, these partitions are not equal, but vary in that the lower facial height is slightly larger than the upper facial height, which in turn is larger than the midface height.[1] These findings hold true for both full face and profile views.

FRONTAL VIEW

In the frontal view, the relative proportions of the facial thirds are noted as discussed above. The widest portion of the face is the bizygomatic distance. The bigonial and bitemporal distances are roughly equal and are 10% less than the bizygomatic distance (Fig. 86.2). The nasal base width is equal to the intercanthal distance, which is slightly greater than one eye width.[2]

The brow position and shape are examined as part of the orbital region. The eyebrow begins medially and arcs upward as it extends laterally. Its highest point is at the junction of the medial two-thirds and lateral one-third of

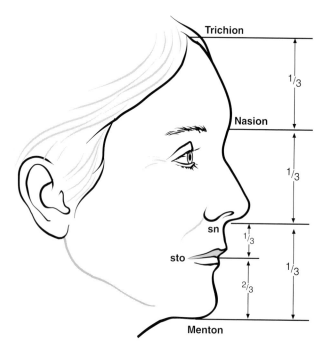

Fig. 86.1 Horizontal facial partitions as shown according to classic artistic cannons.

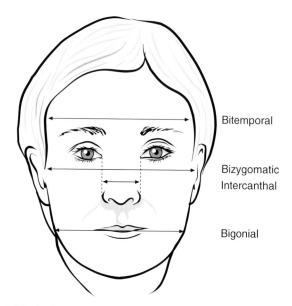

Fig. 86.2 The bizygomatic distance is the maximal width of the face, being 10% wider than the bitemporal and bigonial distances.

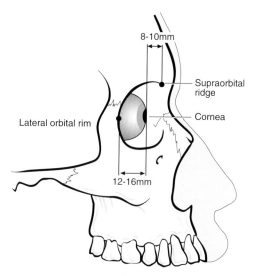

Fig. 86.3 The supraorbital ridge projects 8–10 mm anterior to the cornea. The lateral orbital rim is 12–16 mm posterior to the cornea.

the eyebrow, which is approximately at the lateral canthus.[1] The eyebrow is just above the supraorbital rim in the youthful face. Brow ptosis occurs with age, the eyebrows descending at or below the level of the supraorbital rim. The lower eyelids blend smoothly into the midface. There is no bony or fatty prominence present at the junction of the lower eyelid and cheek.

An evaluation of the intercanthal distance is made. The normal distance is roughly one palpebral width. The inclination of the eye fissure is assessed. The eye normally inclines upward from a medial to a lateral direction. In males, the outer canthus is 2.1 mm higher than the inner. In females, this distance is 4.1 mm. In profile, the supraorbital ridge projects 8–10 mm anterior to the cornea, and the lateral orbital rim lies 12–16 mm posterior to the cornea (Fig. 86.3).[3] Thus, the orbit has a relative setback of its lateral wall.

Nasal morphology is the key to the central face and thus any significant deformities should be noted and discussed with the patient. If rhinoplasty is to be performed, then it must be planned in conjunction with the specific facial bone manipulation under consideration. Any change in the nasal skeletal support will change the nasal appearance regardless of the formal rhinoplasty. In performing facial bone manipulation, the shape of the nose may be altered without a formal rhinoplasty. For example, maxillary impaction will widen the alar base and shorten the nose.[4]

The mid and lower face is examined with particular emphasis on lip-to-tooth relationship and the chin. Burstone reported that up to 3.5 mm of interlabial distance is normal with the lips in repose and the jaws in centric relation.[5] Greater distances signify lip incompetence. Normal maxillary incisal show in repose and with smile is measured. Normal show is 2–3 mm at rest, but can be up to 4–6 mm in some women if mentalis strain is not required to achieve lip competence.[6] The shape and size of the lips are also important. If the upper lip has a thin vermilion, it can worsen with maxillary repositioning and steps to prevent this must be implemented.

PROFILE ANALYSIS

The relative protrusion or retrusion of each facial third is noted in profile. If an abnormality is present in the anterior–posterior relationship of the maxilla and mandible, then one may consider an advancement/setback procedure. Notation of the category of facial type such as vertical maxillary excess or deficiency is helpful for future reference. The mandibular appearance in terms of prognathism and retrognathism is noted.

An evaluation of the forehead is made. The forehead curves gently posteriorly as one proceeds from the glabella to the trichion. This arc is –7 degrees in the female and –10 degrees in the male.[2] In transverse dimension, the bigonial and bizygomatic distances are equal. The forehead curves from glabella to the temporal region with maximal projection at the mid brows.

Chin projection must be studied as it has a significant impact on facial proportion. Retrogenia improvement dramatically improves facial balance and therefore esthetics. Mentalis hyperactivity should be recognized and corrected as part of the treatment plan.

ORAL EXAMINATION

The oral examination is performed after the esthetic examination. This should proceed in the usual fashion, noting the general oral health, state of repair of the dentition, the Angle class of the occlusion, and the crossbite, overjet, and overbite relations. If a significant occlusive abnormality is present, then consideration of surgical repositioning of the maxilla and/or mandible can be entertained and discussed with the patient.

RADIOGRAPHIC ANALYSIS

In patients undergoing genioplasty and/or midface procedures, the next step in preoperative evaluation is analysis with cephalometric and panorex radiographs. Information on the state of the teeth and mandibles is obtained from the panorex. A cephalometric analysis is performed to determine if abnormal skeletal relationships between the facial components exist. These are correlated with the physical examination findings and the patient's desires.

All cephalometric analyses have limitations, and this must be kept in mind. We use the structural and architectural analysis of Delaire, which has correlated best with the senior author's (SAS) experience for 17 years.[7] It relies little on statistical averages and is based on skeletal equilibrium. This technique is valuable in two regards. First, it allows one to visualize the deformity and the ideal position of the skeleton without making numerous measurements and then deciphering them. A step in the analysis is thus saved, and a potential source of variability is removed. Second, analysis of children is easily incorporated and their treatment followed in relation to their growth and development.

PRINCIPLES OF FACIAL BONE CONTOURING

An important paradigm is that increasing the facial soft-tissue envelope by reducing the amount of skeletal support should be avoided. Any increase in the soft-tissue envelope in relation to the facial skeleton results in accelerated aging of the face. This may be acceptable to a young patient in the short term, however it is possible that the patient will appear excessively aged later in life. Surgically-induced premature aging is an undesirable result and a relatively common cause for secondary surgery after retrusive orthognathic procedures.[6]

A second principle of facial bone sculpturing is that surgical procedures should stretch the facial soft-tissue envelope whenever possible. Augmentation of the bony skeleton will fill out to the facial envelope and thereby result in a younger appearance to the face. Rhytids and ptosis of the soft tissue, characteristics associated with age, will be softened with a more robust facial skeleton.

SURGICAL PROCEDURES FOR THE FACIAL BONES

FOREHEAD, SUPRAORBITAL RIDGE, TEMPORAL REGION

The upper third of facial height from nasion to trichion contains the supraorbital ridge, forehead, and temporal region. The relationship of the orbit-globe, location of the brows, and the forehead inclination to the supraorbital ridge are noted prior to procedures in this region. The anthropologic characteristics in this area have been determined by Whitaker et al and should also be reviewed (Figs 86.1–86.3).[3] Variations due to sex are present. The male has extensive supraorbital bossing that forms a plateau prior to rounding to the forehead. In contrast, the female has less bossing with a gradual curve into the forehead.

Procedures are categorized into those producing reduction

and those producing augmentation. Each can be further divided into sculpting through bone burring or with an additional osteotomy. Most patients requesting alteration in this area desire a reduction of the supraorbital bossing. The patient should be young or only a small amount of bone removed in cases of reduction, to prevent brow ptosis and premature facial aging. If ptosis or aging is likely to occur, then a brow lift procedure should be done concomitantly.

Reduction of the supraorbital ridge can be accomplished using a burr with the contouring depth limit at a level where adequate bone remains over the frontal sinus (Fig. 86.4). If thin bone is present over the sinus initially, Ousterhout recommends contouring down to the sinus, without entering, and then applying methyl methacrylate to the concavity above the bossed area.[8] If adequate reduction cannot be achieved without entering the sinus, then sinus osteotomy can be used to set back the anterior sinus wall and supraorbital rim. Fixation of the frontal sinus anterior wall and burr tapering of bony prominences superiorly and laterally is performed. Methyl methacrylate can also be used to smooth the bony rough edges, however it should not be used if the sinus has been entered. Whitaker and others describe similar techniques for forehead reduction.[3] In addition, they have used a pericranial flap with split calvarial bone graft to reshape the anterior sinus wall.

Augmentation of the forehead, temporal region, and

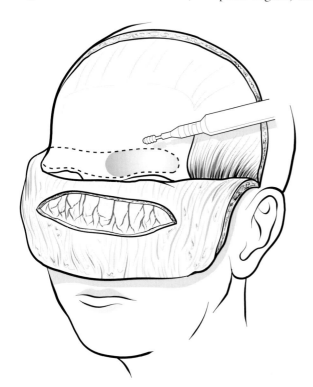

Fig. 86.4 Diagram showing the use of the burr to remodel the supraorbital rim through an endoscopic approach.

supraorbital ridges can be done with local soft tissue, bone grafts, or synthetic material. Soft-tissue choices include local vascularized tissue such as a pericranial flap or a frontalis muscle flap, or free grafts such as dermal fat or temporal parietal fascia. The pericranial flap is useful for the forehead and supraorbital ridge. If a small amount of augmentation at the ridge is needed, then a rolled pericranial flap is sufficient. Bone grafts can be added if more augmentation is required. Cohen et al recommend temporalis muscle advancement flaps to fill anterior temporal fossa depressions.[9] Synthetic material has also been used for augmentation. Methyl methacrylate was used in the past, in part because of the ease of sculpting a desired contour. Its use is currently out of favor because it has a propensity to develop visible ridging at its borders. Recently absorbable hydroxyapatite has become available (Howmedica Leibinger Inc., Dallas, TX). This is slowly replaced with normal bone, thereby potentially eliminating some of the disadvantages of methyl methacrylate such as infection, migration, and edge contour deformity.

The approach for the forehead, supraorbital ridge, and the temporal region depends on the procedure to be performed and the extent of the area at the site that will undergo operation. For burr contouring of the forehead and brow, options include an open approach or endoscopic approach. Available incisions include coronal, hairline, brow, and upper blepharoplasty types. Subperiosteal exposure of the supraorbital ridge is required. Most authors recommend midline and paramedian sagittal incisions and a transverse incision 2.5 cm from the hairline in the temporal region for procedures using an endoscopic approach.[10] These incisions do not desensitize the posterior scalp and result in less scar than does a coronal incision. For larger procedures in which an endoscopic approach is untenable, such as prosthetic contouring of the entire forehead, then a coronal incision is most useful. The best choice of incision is the combination that results in the least visible scar with an adequate amount of exposure to accomplish the goals of the operation.

ZYGOMATIC ARCH AND MALAR EMINENCE

Augmentation

The zygomatic complex may be hyperplastic, hypoplastic, or malpositioned. These deformities are most frequently esthetic but in severe cases they cause functional problems. Congenital or acquired hypoplasia can result in eyelid dysfunction and an unprotected globe. Traumatic malposition can cause diplopia, dystopia, enophthalmos, and restricted mandibular movement. From an esthetic analysis, zygomas in the Caucasian population generally are hypoplastic and require augmentation, whereas in the Asian population they are hyperplastic and reduction is required.[11]

For augmentation in cases of zygomatic complex deficiency, we consider zygomatic osteotomy and repositioning to be generally preferable to onlay techniques with synthetic implant placement. Implant disadvantages of migration and early and late infection severely detract from their usefulness. However, other authors strongly recommend onlay augmentation with alloplastic material in esthetic cases because of the ease of placement and reliable and esthetically pleasing results.[12] The amount of augmentation is determined by the amount of asymmetry in post-traumatic deformities or by esthetic judgment and patient desire in cosmetic cases. For onlay implant augmentation, Whitaker recommends a 6 mm thick implant for most patients. If there is a high degree of hypoplasia or soft-tissue thickness, then 8 mm implants should be used. If there is a thin soft-tissue cover, then a 4 mm implant is adequate or a 6 mm implant can be trimmed (Fig. 86.5).[12] Silicone and polypropylethylene implants are available from several manufacturers and are sold in small, medium, and large sizes.[13] Whitaker emphasizes that the success of implant augmentation is dependent on several important factors: accurate midface anatomic assessment, implant type, implant design, and the surgical technique with attention to detail.

To determine the amount of augmentation necessary, we divide the zygoma into two components. The anterior part is simply classified as the area between the medial and

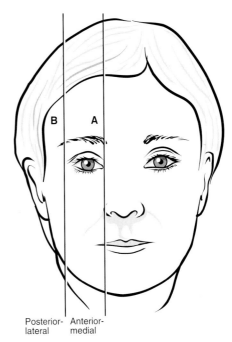

Posterior- Anterior-
lateral medial

Fig. 86.6 Diagram showing zygomatic analysis to assist in the surgical planning of contour changes. Part A determines anterior (malar) projection and part B determines facial width.

lateral canthal tendons (Part A). In reality, this consists of the anterior zygoma laterally and the face of the maxilla medially (Fig. 86.6). From a surgical perspective, this is addressed as one unit. Part A involves mainly the anteroposterior projection in the infraorbital region. Part B is the

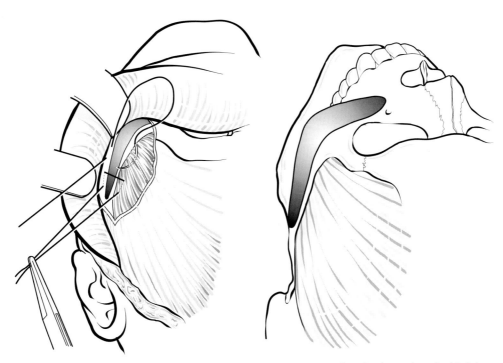

Fig. 86.5 Diagram showing position and shape of malar implant. Distance from implant to lateral orbital rim edge is measured to ensure symmetry.

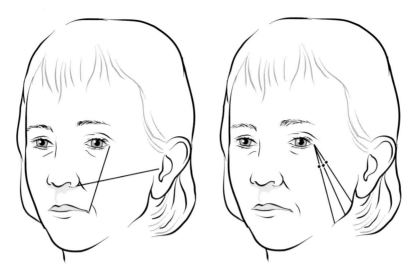

Fig. 86.7 Methods of malar analysis. **(A)** Hinderer analysis: lines drawn from the ala to tragus and from commissure to lateral canthus. The malar eminence lies in the upper triangle in the ideal faces. **(B)** Wilkinson analysis: lines are drawn from the lateral canthus to the mandibular angle. Stars mark the junction of the upper third and lower two thirds of these lines. The malar high point follows the stars.

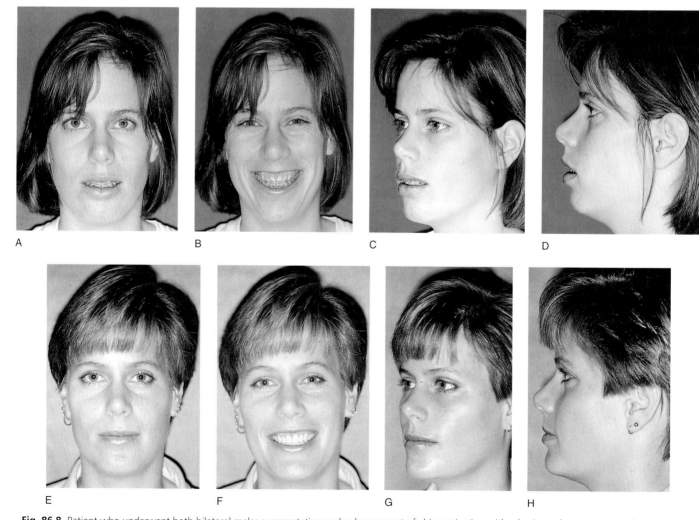

A B C D

E F G H

Fig. 86.8 Patient who underwent both bilateral malar augmentation and enhancement of chin projection with a horizontal osseous genioplasty. Additionally, she had bilateral mandibular sagittal-split advancement osteotomies. **(A–D)** Preoperative. **(E–H)**. Postoperative at 18 months. Note the change in her smile vector due to the malar augmentation **(B & F)**. The malar light highlight is more defined postoperatively **(C & G)**. Improved chin and jaw definition is readily apparent **(D & H)**.

area of zygoma lateral to the lateral canthus. This corresponds to the body and the arch of the zygoma and is important in establishing facial width. As discussed earlier, artistic cannons are useful in assessing this area. Correct placement of the zygomatic prominence is crucial for facial balance and form. This area has the light highlight on the cheek area of the face and is termed the *malar eminence*. It is positioned anterior and medial to the junction of the body of the zygoma and zygomatic arch (Fig. 86.7).[2] All too frequently, this point is placed too low and is too broad, resulting in Neanderthal-appearing cheek bones.

Zygomatic augmentation is indicated for the aging face or for malar hypoplasia (Figs 86.8 and 86.9). A natural appearance of the malar eminence can be achieved by osteotomy of the zygoma at its junction with the maxilla through an intraoral approach. A greenstick fracture is made in the arch and a self-retaining graft is placed in the osteotomy (Fig. 86.10A). Variations in the osteotomy line provide for anterior or lateral projection and are done according to the patient's need. Care is taken to achieve symmetry. In the ideal face, the zygomas are the widest points, with a smooth taper inward to the gonial angles.[12] Augmentation of the zygoma in the older patient can compensate for loss of malar projection occurring with aging. Buccal fat pad removal provides additional projection of the malar eminence. In severe cases of facial aging with malar fat pad ptosis, augmentation alone cannot sufficiently fill the soft-tissue envelope and the malar fat pad should be resuspended, either through a lower lid blepharoplasty or facelift incision.

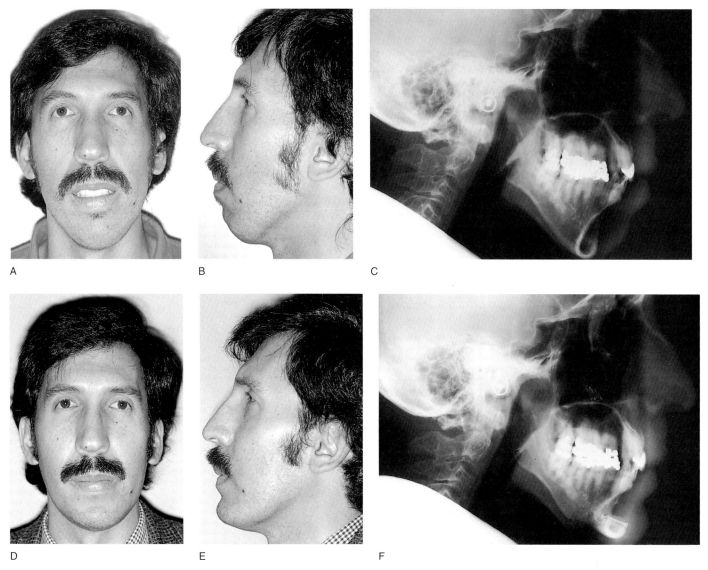

A　　　　　　　　　B　　　　　　　　　C

D　　　　　　　　　E　　　　　　　　　F

Fig. 86.9 Patient who underwent a mm malar osseous augmentation and 8 mm vertical reduction osseous genioplasty. The 8 mm symphyseal bone piece was split in half and used as a graft for the zygomatic osteotomy of the type shown in Fig. 86.10A. **(A–C)** Preoperative. **(D–F)** Postoperative at 6 months.

Surgical technique for facial width augmentation

The distinction must be made between inadequate facial width and inadequate anterior zygomatic (malar) projection. They are different deformities which require specific therapy. Facial width is determined by the zygomatic arch contour whereas malar or cheek projection is determined by the anterior contour of the body of the zygoma. Widening the zygomatic arches increases facial width and can be performed with only autogenous tissue.

An intraoral approach is used with maxillary vestibule incisions bilaterally (Fig. 86.10A). The anterior and lateral faces of the maxilla and zygoma are exposed via a subperiosteal dissection. A reciprocating saw is inserted underneath the arch and brought forward in a vertical fashion. The arch is bowed outward with an elevator, and a bone graft of the desired width is inserted. The graft is self-retained by the inherent recoil from the arch which is not fractured. Thus no prosthetic hard or soft material is used. The graft material may be bone or hydroxyapatite. We recommend autogenous bone because of its lower risks of infection and resorption. Graft width is usually 4–6 mm, depending on the desired movement. Care is taken to achieve symmetry. The wound is irrigated with antibiotic solution and closed with absorbable sutures.

Surgical technique for anterior zygomatic (malar) augmentation

In patients with malar hypoplasia and an inadequate anterior–posterior projection of the zygomatic complex body, a lamellar split osteotomy of the zygoma is recommended. Advantages of this technique include the fact that the osteotomy is favorable and self-retaining. No hardware placement or prosthetic material is required.

Through a combined maxillary vestibular and lower eyelid approach, the zygomatic arch, inferior orbital rim, zygomatic body, and anterior maxilla are exposed subperiosteally. A reciprocating saw is used to cut the lateral zygoma obliquely from an initial point posterior to the arch to a point just lateral to the infraorbital foramen (Fig. 86.10B). The osteotomy is vertically oriented. As in facial width augmentation, a bone graft with adequate surface area to prevent its displacement into the maxillary sinus is wedged into the osteotomy. The graft is held by elastic forces tending to push the osteotomy edges together, and thus no fixation is generally required. The arch may be greenstick fractured as it is bowed outward. The graft width determines the new malar projection: 6–8 mm is usually required. The area is irrigated with antibiotic solution and the wounds closed appropriately.

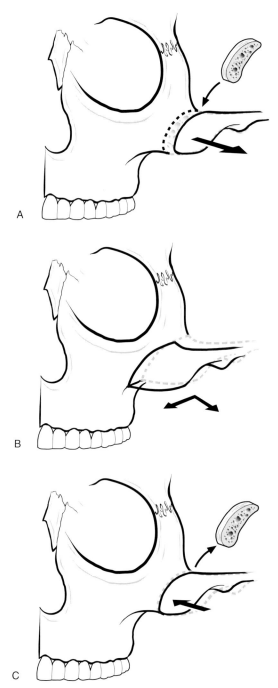

Fig. 86.10 Diagram showing zygomatic osteotomies for augmentation and reduction. **(A)** To augment facial width only, the zygomatic arch is outfractured and either autologous bone graft or allogenic graft material is placed in the intervening osteotomy bone gap. **(B)** To augment both anterior projection and facial width, the osteotomy is curved medially towards the infraorbital foramen. **(C)** For larger zygomatic width reductions in which bur contouring is not possible, the osteotomy is infractured and the arch greenstick fractured inward.

Zygomatic reduction

Excess zygomatic width is a frequently perceived esthetic problem in Asian faces. The area of excess is due to a lateral flare of the inferior half of the arch and the lateral body of the zygoma in the sagittal plane. This results in a lateral increase in facial dimension. Zygomatic reduction can be done either by burr contouring or by osteotomy and infracture. Reduction in projection of up to 6 mm on each side can be performed with a burr providing there is sufficient bone thickness as determined radiographically. Larger reductions, or patients with inadequate bone thickness, require osteotomy and infracture. The arch is greenstick fractured in the opposite direction to the augmentation osteotomy (Fig. 86.10C). The zygoma is wired into its new position. The soft tissue must be resuspended as the fat pad will descend and the soft-tissue envelope will be increased, creating an undesirable result with an aged face.

Surgical technique for zygomatic reduction

A combined minimally-invasive endoscopic forehead, transconjunctival lower eyelid, and intraoral approach is utilized. A lateral canthopexy is performed through the endoscopic approach. Temporal scalp incisions are made bilaterally 2–2.5 cm posterior and parallel to the hairline. Dissection deep to the temporoparietal fascia on the superficial layer of the deep temporal fascia is performed. The temporal crest is crossed and the lateral forehead and orbital wall are subperiosteally exposed. This releases the lateral region for later canthopexy.

A subperiosteal exposure of the anterior maxilla, zygomatic body, and arch is performed through maxillary vestibule and transconjunctival lower eyelid incisions. The zygomatic arch and body can be burred or undergo reduction osteotomy, depending on the desired amount of reduction and the bone thickness. If the bone cortex is thicker than the reduction amount, a pineapple burr reduction is the least difficult technique, especially in obtaining symmetry.

Patients with thin bone or those who need a large reduction generally require an osteotomy. The osteotomy is performed as described above for an augmentation. In many cases, the zygoma can be infractured into the sinus and fixed with either a wire or plate. If the reduction is not sufficient, then a bone wedge is removed prior to infracturing. Impingement on the coronoid and subsequent restricted mandibular movement has not been a problem.

A midface suspension is required after zygomatic reduction because loss of a portion of skeletal support will result in laxity of the overlying soft tissue. This gives the face an aged appearance that may not be evident for several years, but will nevertheless be premature for the patient. To prevent this effect after skeletal reduction, the midface is resuspended. Three sutures are placed in the periosteum overlying the zygomatic complex lateral to the canthus and are fixed to the deep temporal fascia with a vertical vector. Either semipermanent (Maxon or PDS) or nonabsorbable (nylon or polypropylene) suture material can be used. In older patients, nonabsorbable suture material is preferable.

After the midface suspension, a lateral canthopexy is performed. A single hook is placed in the lateral canthus endoscopically from the temporal scalp incision. Again, either semipermanent or nonabsorbable suture is used. The suture is passed through the lateral canthus and then the deep temporal fascia with a vertical vector. As with all components of this procedure, care is taken to ensure symmetry. The incisions are closed and a soft head wrap dressing is placed.

PIRIFORM RIM

The piriform rims are altered mainly to institute a change in the nasal base, usually as an adjunct to another procedure. Reduction of the rim causes the nasal base to rotate down and inward. It can prevent the upturned tip and nostril show that can accompany some cases of maxillary advancement–impaction. Reduction will also close the nasolabial angle.

Augmentation of the rim fills out a depressed paranasal region when normal occlusion is present and a Le Fort-type osteotomy is not indicated. Patients with a retrusion of the upper base of the alveolar process and lower nasal base benefit from augmentation. These patients have a pseudo-prognathic appearance with an acute nasolabial angle and short columella.[14] The skeletal deficiency creates a concave profile and a deep groove in the columella–lip area. Augmentation is useful in increasing upper lip fullness and also aids in the treatment of bone hypoplasia after maxillary advancement.

Surgical technique for piriform reduction/augmentation

The piriform rim and anterior nasal spine are approached through an anterior maxillary vestibule incision from canine to canine. An adequate cuff of mucosa and muscle is left on the inferior aspect of the incision to aid in closure. Subperiosteal exposure of the anterior maxilla and premaxilla is performed, including the anterior nasal spine. The nasal mucosa is freed from the nasal floor and posterior surface of the anterior maxillary wall. The anterior nasal spine and rim can now either be reduced with a burr or augmented with autogenous bone graft or prosthetic material such as hydroxyapatite bone paste.[14] The nasal floor mucosa is protected from injury with a malleable retractor. Closure is begun with an alar cinch stitch of 4–0 clear nylon through the underside of the alar bases. The maxillary vestibule incision is closed in a V–Y fashion with 4–0 absorbable suture.[15] The Y stem component of the closure is 8–10 mm in the midline in a palatal direction. This closure prevents lip thinning associated with excess stretch after augmentation. Suture bites are full-thickness mucosa and muscle.

MANDIBULAR BODY AND ANGLE

Reduction

The mandibular angle has received attention recently as an area on the facial skeleton amenable to change. The prominence of the angle should be in concert with the remainder of the face. Although it is not as central to facial dynamics as the nose or chin, it does have a role in displaying feelings or expressions such as determination, strength, and weakness. When proportions are out of the norm of what is expected, then patients generally do not like what they see and desire change.

Angle reduction is most commonly performed for benign masseteric muscle hypertrophy. This condition is most common in Koreans, Northern Iranians, and Armenians.[11]

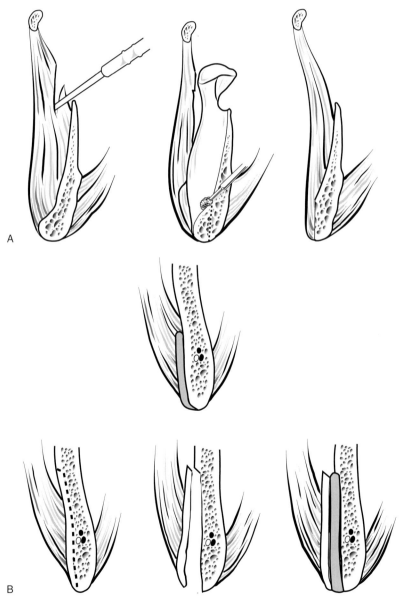

Fig. 86.11 (A) Mandibular angle reduction. The masseter is reduced before the bone. The inferior border of the mandible is subperiosteally exposed and cut with a reciprocating saw or contoured with a bur.
(B) Mandibular angle augmentation. (i) A prosthetic implant can be placed with extreme care to prevent overhang from the inferior border, thus allowing the implant to be perceptible from the mandible. (ii) The angle can also be augmented with an interpositional bone graft placed between the proximal and distal segments of a mandible cut in a sagittal manner. The grafts are cut so that there is greater thickness posteriorly and inferiorly.

Heavy weight-lifting with masseteric stimulation during lifting and neck bracing will also result in this condition. It is usually bilateral, but can be unilateral. The deformity is manifest as excess fullness of the angle. On frontal view, there is a broad-based face. Excess masseter development and lateral flaring of the mandibular angle and inferior margin is present and is best seen on posteroanterior radiographs. In addition, the bizygomatic width is usually enlarged because of the origin of the masseter muscles on the arches. Both the muscle and bone must be modified to treat the condition.

Surgical technique for mandibular reduction

Exposure of the lateral aspect of the angle and proximal body is achieved through an intraoral approach. A mandibular vestibule incision is made from the mid-ramus to the first molar. The insertion of the masseter in the mandible is identified and the masseter's anterior border is exposed (Figs 86.11A and 86.12). This requires exposure of the coronoid, anterior border of the ramus, angle, and proximal body. This dissection is completed on each side and the amount of muscle and bone to be reduced is determined. A conservative resection is advisable, because over-resection can result in too narrow a bigonial distance which can be devastating.

Muscle resection is done with cautery anteriorly. To protect neurovascular structures, scissor dissection is recommended posteriorly. The muscle is removed from the bone. The flared inferior border of the angle and proximal body is now exposed and ready for reduction.

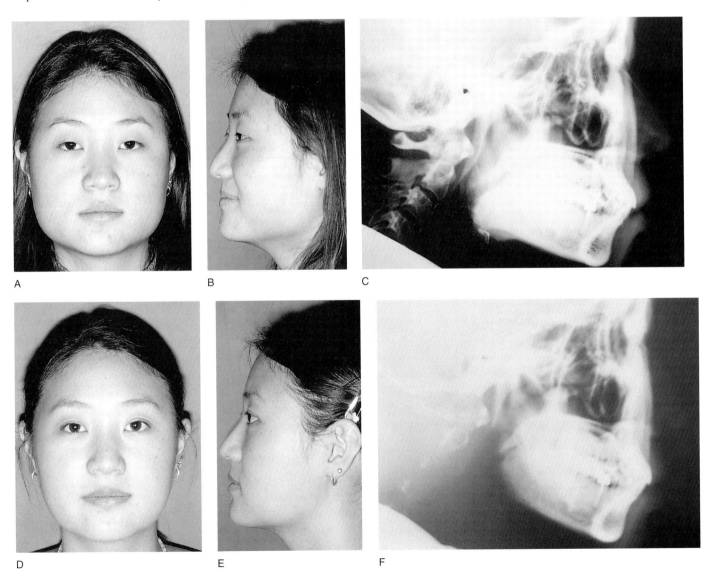

A   B   C

D   E   F

Fig. 86.12 Patient who underwent mandibular angle and masseter reduction. **(A–C)** Preoperative. **(D–F)** Postoperative at 12 months. The amount of bony angle reduction is readily apparent radiographically **(C & F)**.

Protection of the soft tissues is implemented and the excess bone is burred down or alternatively cut with a reciprocating saw and then contoured with a burr. The final adjustments of masseter resection are performed with careful inspection between both sides to ensure symmetry. Again, one must be aware of the location of the facial artery, vein, and marginal mandibular branch of the facial nerve, and adequate steps must be taken to protect these structures. Injury to the nerve has been reported with this procedure.[16]

The wounds are closed with 4–0 chromic or Vicryl suture in a running fashion. We prefer small closed suction drainage for the first 24 hours postoperatively. Patients are kept on a soft diet and instructed to perform no heavy chewing for at least two weeks. Soft-tissue envelope problems are usually not encountered with bone sculpturing in this area.

Augmentation

Increased jaw–neck definition is associated with youthfulness and beauty. It can be accomplished either by soft-tissue alterations such as cervicofacioplasty and buccal fat resection or by augmentation of the bone structure. Onlay and interpositional bone grafts have been used to increase jaw angularity and jaw–neck definition but gave inconsistent results. Onlay calvarial and rib grafts are subject to unpredictable amounts of resorption, making symmetry more difficult to obtain and keep in the long term. Sagittal-split mandibular osteotomies with bone grafts interposed between the segments are technically difficult to perform, particularly in the achievement of symmetry. This has led to the development of implant augmentation.

Whitaker recommends implant utilization for augmentation of the gonial angle.[17] The posterior mandible is augmented from the jowls anteriorly to the angle posteriorly, and superiorly to the zygomatic arch (Fig. 86.11B). Preoperative planning includes assessment of the amount of highlighting desired, the thickness of the soft tissues, and the use of cephalometric and panorex radiographs. The implants are available in 4, 6, and 8 mm thicknesses. The appropriate thickness for a particular patient is determined by the patient's desires, the bigonial, bitemporal, and bizygomatic distances, and the thickness of the overlying soft tissue. The bizygomatic distance should be 10% larger than the bitemporal and bigonial distances at the conclusion of augmentation. A smaller thickness implant should be used if thinner soft tissue is present. An 8 mm implant can be used when the soft tissue is thicker and greater augmentation is necessary. Whitaker stresses that the implant must be positioned precisely on the bone without overhanging it and with no intervening soft tissue.

Surgical technique for mandibular augmentation

A mandibular vestibule incision is made from the ramus down to the second premolar. The entire posterior mandible is exposed subperiosteally on its buccal cortex from the sigmoid notch to the antegonial notch. Once the pocket is dissected and no soft tissue remains on the exposed mandible, the pocket is irrigated with half-strength iodine solution. The carved implant is removed from antibiotic solution and inserted. It must sit freely on the mandible and be checked visually to make certain that there is no folding of edges nor extension of implant beyond the bone border in any direction. The wound is closed in layers using 4–0 Vicryl. The second side is next performed in bilateral cases. The patients are given antibiotic for 5 days. A liquid diet is maintained for 7 days and a soft diet for the next 7 days. Extensive swelling is expected and resolves in 2–3 weeks. Restriction of temporomandibular joint motion lasts 4–8 weeks.

Whitaker reported no infection in 32 Proplast implants in 22 patients. One patient with bilateral implants had a palpable single anterior inferior edge which required revision. An intraoral incision was made directly over the anterior edge and it was trimmed. There were no late displacements, or dysfunction of the masseter muscle.

Additional ancillary procedures may be done simultaneously with augmentation. If cervicofacioplasty is planned, the mandible augmentation should be performed last to prevent infection. It is more difficult at this time because of the new tightness of the skin envelope and postoperative swelling.

CHIN

Genioplasty can be approached in a physiologic fashion in which muscle function and osseous anatomy is restored.[18] The relationship between anterior and posterior chin balance and facial harmony is assessed as part of the facial examination. An abnormal relation is confirmed with the cephalometric analysis. Chin projection is easily assessed in profile; however, vertical dysplasias are commonly missed unless specifically looked for during the examination (Fig. 86.8D, H). In many instances, vertical reduction as well as advancement is required and the two can be done simultaneously (Fig. 86.9C, F). For these patients, an osseous genioplasty will best accomplish both goals. The appropriate advancement and vertical reduction can be done concomitantly with the chin repositioning.

Vertical excess

Vertical excess of the chin necessitates a reduction genioplasty by performing osteotomies and removing a wedge of bone. The excessively long lower facial height is corrected and the different facial thirds are balanced. Removal of bone would appear to violate the facial envelope rule: however, this is not the case with the chin. Most chins that are vertically long are also retrusive to approximately the same extent as if growth was redirected. Thus a vertical reduction with a simultaneous advancement keeps the soft-tissue envelope essentially unchanged.

Vertical hyperplasia of the maxilla and chin are the most common causes of bilabial incompetence in the long face.[19,20] The perioral muscles are unable to sustain lip closure and thus the anterior dentition is not covered. These patients have excessive exposure of the incisor teeth and gingiva, a gummy smile, an everted lower lip, and perioral muscle hyperfunction (Figs 86.8A, C, D, and 86.9A, B). Lip closure is achieved by mentalis strain, which results in an elevation of the soft-tissue menton point and an "orange peel" aspect of the overlying skin. These abnormalities combine to give the patient an unesthetic appearance. In addition, periodontal problems in the anterior dentition are frequent, due to dessication of the gingiva. Surgical reduction of the maxilla and mandible is required in severe cases in which malocclusion is present. In those patients with class I occlusion and isolated chin vertical excess, an osseous genioplasty is indicated.

The amount of vertical bone reduction necessary is determined from the lateral cephalometric radiograph. Normally, the soft-tissue and the bony mentons are on the same horizontal line. In vertical chin excess, the soft-tissue menton, which is the most anterior point on the curve of the soft-tissue chin, is superior to the hard-tissue menton when mentalis strain is present. The vertical distance between these two points is the amount of bone to be resected, with the provision that no maxillary excess is present. If maxillary excess exists, this amount must be deducted from the first measurement if a maxillary procedure is to be performed. In patients without mentalis hyperfunction, the lower lip stomion lies at or just above the level of the mandibular incisors. Any deviation is the amount to be resected. Patients with complex deformities require a thorough cephalometric analysis and prediction tracings to assess possible soft-tissue abnormalities and determine the optimal anteroposterior chin position.

Retrogenia

Most patients who present for esthetic chin surgery will not have a severe dentofacial deformity and will have class I occlusion and retrogenia. These patients desire an increase in chin projection: this can be accomplished with an allo-plastic implant or sliding osseous genioplasty. Implants are suited for small advancements of the order of 4–5 mm, usually as part of a facelift procedure. The sliding osseous genioplasty can be used for shorter as well as longer advancements, and is especially suited for vertical height alterations.

Alloplastic augmentation is advocated because of its simplicity and lesser degree of postoperative pain, edema, and ecchymoses, which leads to a faster recovery (Fig. 86.13). Its supporters emphasize that it gives superb results. Flowers notes that when the implant is designed and placed correctly, it is not palpable.[21] There is none of the perceptible notching or irregularity that can sometimes be present on the lateral mandible after osseous genioplasty. It also combines readily with other esthetic procedures such as blepharoplasty, facelift, and rhinoplasty to impressively enhance results.

The disadvantages of alloplastic implantation have been well described, although its advocates emphasize that many arise from improper technique of the surgeon rather than from the implant methodology itself. The implants are susceptible to infection, more so than the hardware used in osseous genioplasty. Migration and deep bony erosion are complications unique to implants. Erosion can be limited by placing the implant low over the thicker cortex of the inferior mandible, having at least 9 cm of surface area of

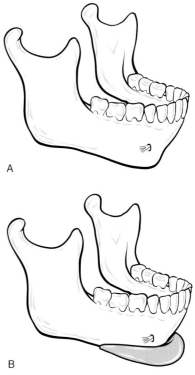

Fig. 86.13 Alloplastic chin augmentation. The implant must be on the inferior border and measure at least 9 cm in length in order to have adequate support and prevent migration.[21]

the base of the implant to disperse pressure, and by placing, at a minimum, the central portion of the implant superficial to the periosteum.

Macrogenia

Chin reduction in the anterior–posterior direction is the most difficult and least indicated technique of facial bone sculpturing. Over-reduction causes a flat chin from the sublabial fold inferiorly, frequently with ptosis of the soft-tissue menton. A posterior sliding genioplasty to reduce the chin also places the inferior component of the chin into the facial view from the anterior, which gives the chin an odd appearance. A reverse wedge osteotomy should be done to avoid this adverse result and still reduce the chin, although the amount of reduction remains limited with this technique.

Chin reductions larger than 7 mm indicate major skeletal disharmony; the patient will require maxillomandibular osteotomies. Shortening the posterior facial height with bimaxillary osteotomies is the most effective way to rotate the pogonion posteriorly and reduce chin over-projection. Although will not alter chin morphology, reductions should be done with caution as this procedure increases the facial envelope.

Horizontal asymmetry

When the inferior border of the symphysis is uneven, the chin point will not be in the facial midline and will be rotated on frontal view. This deformity is readily reconstructed with a sliding horizontal genioplasty. The midpoint of the distal osteotomized segment is placed in the midsagittal plane which corresponds to the facial midline. Vertical asymmetry, if present, is concomitantly corrected by performing a wedge osteotomy on the affected side. This wedge can be transposed to the opposite side if necessary for facial balance. The appropriate dimensions of the horizontal and vertical osteotomies are determined by cephalometric analysis and prediction tracings.

Surgical technique for genioplasty

The sliding horizontal genioplasty is utilized for reduction/advancement of the chin (Fig. 86.14). Periosteal elevation, and thus muscle detachment, is minimized in order to allow precise and predictable soft-tissue repositioning. We have found that with this technique there is a soft-tissue to osseous advancement of nearly 100% and a vertical change of 90%. The 1:1 soft-tissue to bone relationship in part arises from a reduction in stresses when vertical reduction

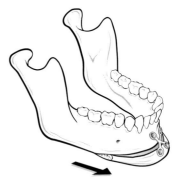

Fig. 86.14 Osseous genioplasty. The osteotomy is made in a plane parallel to the occlusal surface if no vertical height change is desired. To increase vertical height, an interposition bone graft can be placed. To decrease height, a wedge of bone can be removed. See Figs 86.8 and 86.9.

is performed. Long-term radiographic evaluation shows the achieved advancement to be stable, with minimal bone resorption occurring only at the superior edge of the distal segment. Bone deposition occurs near the B point of the alveolus.[18]

This procedure can be done as an outpatient procedure under general anesthesia or with intravenous sedation. The anterior mandibular vestibule is infiltrated with local anesthetic and epinephrine from first bicuspid to first bicuspid. An incision is made from canine to canine on the inner surface of the lip 2–3 mm past the sulcus in order to leave an adequate sewing cuff. The initial cut is perpendicular to mucosa. Then, as muscle is transected, the angle of the cut is altered to perpendicular to the bone and continued through the periosteum. A subperiosteal dissection is performed to just inferior of the planned horizontal osteotomy. At least 5 mm of attached periosteum and muscle is left between the inferior border of the symphysis and the subperiosteal dissection. Detachment of all of the soft tissue from the distal segment results in chin sagging, retraction of the lower lip, and unpredictable soft-tissue changes. Suture closure is assisted by slightly elevating mucosa superior to the incision.

The mental nerves are identified by placing the periosteal elevator at the corner of the incision and the inferior border of the mandible. The periosteum is elevated posteriorly and tented laterally which exposes the neurovascular bundle without causing damage. The mental nerve is superior to this position at the level of the canine apices. Once the mental nerves and foramina are visualized, the subperiosteal dissection is carried posterior and superior to them. If it is necessary to complete the osteotomy without tension on the mental nerves, the incision can be extended posteriorly above the nerves with scissors. The length of incision varies with the individual osseous structure, the type of osteotomy, and the location of the mental nerves. In general, it runs from canine to canine. A subperiosteal dissection is performed beneath the inferior border of the mandible adjacent to the nerves which permits protective retraction for the bone cutting.

The osteotomy must be at least 4 mm below the incisor root apices in order to ensure tooth viability. The incisor length can be measured on the preoperative radiographs and is usually 24 mm from incisal edge to root apex. Calipers are used to mark the incisal midline 27–28 mm from the incisal edge. Bur holes (1–1.5 mm) are made 1 mm above and below the osteotomy line as well in order to keep the distal segment appropriately aligned at the time of fixation.

The osteotomy is made with a reciprocating saw from lateral to medial, with care to protect the nerve. Both the buccal and lingual cortices are cut simultaneously. If the posterior lingual cortex is not cut, then an unfavorable fracture of the cortical plate can occur and prevent later repositioning. In addition, the osteotomy should be 4 mm below the mental foramen because, as it extends posterior to the foramen, it enters the area where the nerve may dip inferiorly prior to its exit from the foramen. If a wedge ostectomy is being done, then the inferior osteotomy should be made prior to the superior osteotomy. This will prevent premature mobilization of the chin, which makes the second (inferior) cut more difficult.

A similar procedure is carried out on the opposite side and mobilization is completed with an osteotome. The osteotomized bone is removed and/or the advancement of the chin is performed next. Calipers are used to measure the advancement from buccal to buccal cortex of the proximal and distal segments.

The inferior segment is fixed with either 26 gauge stainless steel wire, a cancellous screw, or plates and screws. If the advancement is minimal, fixation can be accomplished by two wires passed through the buccal cortex 1.5–2.0 mm from the midline on each side. If the advancement is more substantial, the wires need to be passed through the lingual cortex of the distal segment as well; in these cases, a midline wire or the screw is utilized. For very large advancements that approach the total width of the inferior segment or where a strong pull by the omohyoid muscle rotates the distal segment inferiorly, then a plate system is best utilized. We use the Osteomed semi-rigid genioplasty plate which is X-shaped and pre-made for different advancement distances. Four unicortical 6 mm screws provide fixation (Fig. 86.14).

The surgical site is irrigated, and the incision is closed with a single layer of 4–0 absorbable suture that bites mucosa and muscle simultaneously. Close bone to muscle approximation is obtained with strips of 1/2 inch tape applied to the chin and left in place for 24–48 hours. Patients are kept on a soft diet for one week and given perioperative antibiotics.

SUMMARY

Esthetic surgery of the facial skeleton requires a thorough analysis of facial soft-tissue features and hard-tissue shape, both with physical examination and radiographic studies. Adherence to the general principle of augmenting bone contour and reducing the soft-tissue envelope will maximize youthful appearance and patient satisfaction.

REFERENCES

1. Bartlett SP, Wornom I, Whitaker LA 1991 Evaluation of facial skeletal aesthetics and surgical planning. Clinics in Plastic Surgery 18(1):1–9
2. Farkas LG 1981 Anthropometry of the head and face in medicine. Elsevier, North Holland, New York
3. Whitaker LA, Morales LJ, Farkas LG 1986 Aesthetic surgery of the supraorbital ridge and forehead structures. Plastic and Reconstructive Surgery 78(1):23–32
4. Schendel SA, Carlotti AJ 1991 Nasal considerations in orthognathic surgery. American Journal of Orthodontics and Dentofacial Orthopedics 100(3):197–208
5. Burstone CJ 1967 Lip posture and its significance in treatment planning. American Journal of Orthodontics 53(4):262–284
6. Schendel SA 1997 Chirurgie maxillo-faciale: esthetique et rajeunissement. Orthodontie Francaise 68(1):103–110
7. Delaire J, Schendel SA, Tulasne JF 1981 An architectural and structural craniofacial analysis: a new lateral cephalometric analysis. Oral Surgery, Oral Medicine, and Oral Pathology 52(3):226–238
8. Ousterhout DK, Zlotolow IM 1990 Aesthetic improvement of the forehead utilizing methylmethacrylate onlay implants. Aesthetic Plastic Surgery 14(4):281–285
9. Cohen SR, Kawamoto HKJ, Mardach OL 1991 The impact of craniofacial surgery on facial aesthetic surgery. Advances in Plastic Surgery 8:153–179
10. Isse NG 1997 Endoscopic facial rejuvenation. Clinics in Plastic Surgery 24(2):213–231
11. Satoh K, Ohkubo F, Tsukagoshi T 1995 Consideration of operative procedures for zygomatic reduction in Orientals: based on a consecutive series of 28 clinical cases. Plastic and Reconstructive Surgery 96(6):1298–1306
12. Whitaker LA 1987 Aesthetic augmentation of the malar-midface structures. Plastic and Reconstructive Surgery 80(3):337–346
13. Ivy EJ, Lorenc ZP, Aston SJ 1995 Malar augmentation with silicone implants. Plastic and Reconstructive Surgery 96(1):63–68
14. Hinderer UT 1991 Nasal base, maxillary, and infraorbital implants — alloplastic. Clinics in Plastic Surgery 18(1):87–105
15. Schendel SA, Williamson LW 1983 Muscle reorientation following superior repositioning of the maxilla. Journal of Oral and Maxillofacial Surgery 41(4):235–240
16. Beckers HL 1977 Masseteric muscle hypertrophy and its intraoral surgical correction. Journal of Maxillofacial Surgery 5(1):28–35

17. Whitaker LA 1991 Aesthetic augmentation of the posterior mandible. Plastic and Reconstructive Surgery 87(2):268–275

18. Schendel SA 1985 Genioplasty: a physiological approach. Annals of Plastic Surgery 14(6):506–514

19. Schendel SA, Eisenfeld J, Bell WH, Epker BN, Mishelevich DJ 1976 The long face syndrome: vertical maxillary excess. American Journal of Orthodontics 70(4):398–408

20. Schendel SA, Eisenfeld JH, Bell WH, Epker BN 1976 Superior repositioning of the maxilla: stability and soft tissue osseous relations. American Journal of Orthodontics 70(6):663–674

21. Flowers RS 1991 Alloplastic augmentation of the anterior mandible. Clinics in Plastic Surgery 18(1):107–138

Oral Surgery

Oral surgery

Surgical management of non-malignant lesions of the mouth

87

P. A. REICHART

INTRODUCTION

This chapter describes the surgical management of non-malignant lesions of the mouth, including soft tissues and bone, covering associated clinical and, where relevant, radiographic features. *Non-malignant* has been defined as lesions that do not metastasize; however, they may have locally destructive features, such as the ameloblastoma, or may have the tendency to recur. Non-malignant lesions encompass malformations, hamartomas and neoplasia. Histopathologic features are not described in detail.

BIOPSY PROCEDURE

As an investigational procedure, biopsies are usually straightforward. However, only those who appreciate the fundamental morphologic and biochemical changes in tissues are likely to devise and perform good operations. It is said that 'The best surgeon is a clinical pathologist who performs operations'. Principally, biopsies of a suspicious area are undertaken for objective confirmation of the nature of the lesion but also for assessment of adequacy of excision.

INDICATIONS AND CONTRAINDICATIONS

Biopsy is indicated in practically every oral lesion that cannot be diagnosed clinically or radiographically. However, one argument against the taking of biopsies is that possibly malignant tumors should not be biopsied before definite treatment. It was claimed that surgical manipulation may increase the risk of hematogenous or lymphatic spread or seeding of tumor cells into adherent healthy tissue areas.

However, there seems little evidence to support such arguments for most tumors and as a principle, there is no practical alternative to biopsy for the establishment of a definitive diagnosis. Therefore, an incisional biopsy should always be planned such that, should excision follow, the resection should include the area of previous biopsy. As an exception, salivary gland tumors, particularly pleomorphic adenomas, should be dealt with carefully because myxoid variants have a strong tendency to seed or recur whenever cells are released at biopsy or incomplete enucleation.

Naturally, biopsies are contraindicated in cases of bleeding disorders.

SOFT-TISSUE BIOPSY

Soft-tissue biopsies of the oral cavity are usually taken under local anesthetic. Care should be taken not to inject too close to the area to be biopsied or to crush the specimen with dissecting forceps or artery clips. It is important that a representative piece of the lesion is taken, including normal tissue. Areas of necrosis should be avoided. Further, the incision should include an adequate depth of the underlying connective tissue. Thin biopsies tend to curl up in the fixative. Curling is prevented by orientating the specimens on a square of blotting paper and allowing them to air dry for a minute or so, before placing both into formol saline.

Excisional biopsy

An excisional biopsy is accomplished by removing the entire lesion and submitting it for microscopic examination. This is the approach preferred for small lesions which clinically appear benign. Both diagnosis and treatment are accomplished in one visit. Excisional biopsies are usually taken using a double semilunar incision (Fig. 87.1).

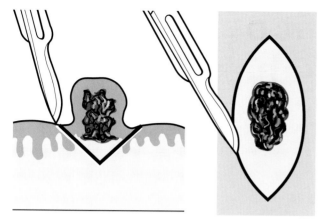

Fig. 87.1 Excisional biopsy. The small mucosal lesion is excised using a wedge-shaped or V-shaped incision. The left side of the figure shows a cross-section of the lesion. The right side shows the view onto the lesion. A semilunar incision with an adequate distance to the lesion is used.

Incisional biopsy

An incisional biopsy implies the acquisition of a representative section from the lesion, preferably including a margin of normal tissue. As with the excisional biopsy, incisional biopsies are usually completed with a scalpel, although other techniques like punch or fine needle aspiration (FNAB) are also employed.

In the case of easily accessible oral lesions the required section of representative tissue is best obtained with a scalpel blade under local anesthesia (Fig. 87.2). The use of ligatures as holding devices is recommended.

All biopsy tissues should be put in fixative immediately because delay can lead to autolysis and drying out. An exception to this would be reactive lymphoid lesions, when markers may be necessary. In those cases fresh material is

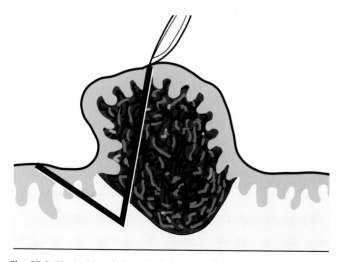

Fig. 87.2 The incisional biopsy includes part of the lesion proper as well as healthy tissue. It should end in such a way that wound margins may easily be adapted to avoid large open wounds.

advised, with rapid transfer to the pathology laboratory. Prior discussion with the pathologist is always advisable as many markers are now used in benign diseases and in general these work much less well on fixed tissues. Completion of the patient details on the pathology request form is mandatory and specimen pots should be clearly labelled if there is any possible risk of infection (for example, AIDS, Hep B, C or TB). Giving as much clinical detail as is known and including radiographs, if available, will always result in a higher quality report.

Other techniques like FNAB, exfoliative cytology or toluidine blue staining tests have been advocated during recent years. Exfoliative cytology and toluidine blue staining are not recommended because they are only applicable to surface lesions. These are, however, accessible to surgical biopsy which has a much lower risk of false-negative results.

FNAB is superficially very attractive for certain lesions, yet often sadly the results fail to justify its use; for example, in parotid swellings it is difficult to obtain clinical evidence of malignancy unless very advanced. Even the presence of facial nerve weakness may be seen in patients with benign lesions. FNAB appears to be a useful tool, yet in most cytologists' hands the results are disappointing. This is partially because over 90% of parotid lesions are benign, but there are other fundamental problems with FNAB. It only samples very small amounts of tissue and the sample is essentially 'blind'. It also may not reflect the architecture of the tissue. So in an area like the parotid where even paraffin sections are difficult to evaluate, FNAB imposes impossible challenges on the cytologist. Despite this, there are experienced operators who claim to provide a valuable service in this field, even in parotid tumors.

Recently, FNAB guided by ultrasound has proved an invaluable tool in evaluating the neck to confirm benign lymphadenopathy. Again, this occurred in a specialized center who have a particular interest in the process.

Frozen-section biopsy has similar but less severe limitations than FNAB. Useful volumes can be harvested and the gross architecture is not destroyed but the microstructure will be atypical, especially in the absence of the normal range of staining agents. In a decision process to distinguish between malignant and benign tumors, it is usually satisfactory but it is not suitable to base histologic opinions on it. Although it has a limited role in the management of benign oral mucosal lesions, it is often used to ensure clearance of locally aggressive lesions on the face, such as basal cell carcinomas.

BONE BIOPSY

For bone biopsies adequate exposure is necessary in order to take representative specimens. These may be obtained using a small punch or a rotating trephine. These techniques result in a solid core of bone. Alternatively, burrs or chisels may be used, depending on whether the clinician needs a fast histologic diagnosis or whether a less aggressive decalcification may be performed, resulting in better morphologic detail.

NON-MALIGNANT MUCOSAL LESIONS

EPITHELIAL TUMORS

HPV-associated lesions

Human papillomavirus (HPV) comprises the largest group of papillomaviruses and 80 types have been identified. HPV gain access by direct implantation through the epithelium and lesions are induced in the skin and oral mucosa. HPV are involved in the etiology of oral squamous cell papillomas, condyloma acuminatum, verrucae vulgares and focal epithelial hyperplasia. Among the HPV types, HPV 1, 2, 4, 6, 7, 11, 13, 16, 18, 32 and 57 have been found in different oral lesions. HPV-13 and HPV-32 seem to be exclusively confined to focal epithelial hyperplasia.[1]

Squamous cell papilloma

Oral squamous cell papillomas are relatively common and occur at any age. They are seen in a wide range of oral sites. Most show wart-associated features on light microscopy, including koilocytes (vacuolated cells) and inclusion bodies. Confirmation requires transmission electron microscopy or immunohistochemistry for HPV antigens, which in most cases is unwarranted. They are simply removed as most are pedunculated and they show no tendency to recur.

Condyloma acuminatum

These have been described particularly in HIV patients. They are usually multiple, small white or pink nodules with a cauliflower-like surface. HPV-6 and 11 but also HPV-2 have been found in 85% of these lesions. Oral warty lesions have been seen in HIV-infected patients containing HPV-7, 13, 18 and 32.

Focal epithelial hyperplasia

FEH is a very rare benign lesion of the oral mucosa mainly found in ethnic groups including Indians from North and South America. FEH appears in the oral mucosa as flat, multiple lesions of the lips, tongue or buccal mucosa. Often children are affected. HPV-13 and/or 32 are found in more than 90% of the biopsies.

Surgical excision is the usual management of HPV-related lesions and the laser is particularly helpful as there is rapid healing with minimal contraction, which is important with extensive lesions. FEH lesions in younger individuals should be left untreated because in many instances they are self-limiting.

NEVI

Nevi are pigmented or non-pigmented lesions of the skin and oral mucosa. Generally, they are more common in younger individuals aged up to 40, are usually small and appear to be static. Several different melanocytic nevi are recognized.

Oral melanotic macule

Pigmented nevi are uncommon in the oral cavity. They are usually well circumscribed, mostly macular or occasionally slightly raised. They can be brown, blue, gray or black, dependent upon the depth of the pigment in the mucosa. The palate is most often affected. Different types of nevi are diagnosed microscopically, of which the compound nevus is most common. Often, non-specialists refer to these lesions as amalgam tattoos. In certain ethnic regions, for example Japan, widespread 'melanosis', which is of course benign lesions, is associated with a higher incidence of malignant melanomas. The transformation is associated with rapid expansion of the lesion, often with bone invasion and lymphadenopathy. This melanosis must be distinguished from changes in pigmentation which occur due to hormonal changes, for example in Addison disease.

Blue nevus

Blue nevi are characterized clinically by color and are histologically distinct. They comprise 35% of oral nevi. Generally a solitary, static lesion in a young person needs no treatment, but if the lesion does not show regression after puberty or has any atypical features or symptoms, then excision biopsy should be carried out.

White sponge nevus (Canon's white sponge nevus)

White sponge nevus is a developmental anomaly inherited as an autosomal dominant trait. The affected oral and occasionally vaginal mucosa is white, soft and appears thickened. It is usually bilateral and variable in distribution but the whole oral mucosa may be involved. Borders are ill defined. Lesions such as traumatic hyperkeratosis, lichen planus and leukoplakia must be considered in differential diagnosis. If the affected area has been abnormal since childhood then clinical features are usually sufficiently characteristic to allow for confident diagnosis, but sometimes patients chew affected areas, leading to 'erosions' and soreness that may justify biopsy. Treatment is unnecessary.

PRECANCEROUS LESIONS AND PRECANCEROUS CONDITIONS

In 1994 oral precancerous lesions and oral precancerous conditions were redefined.[2] A precancerous lesion was defined as a morphologically altered tissue in which cancer is more likely to occur than in its apparently normal counterpart. An example of the precancerous lesion is an oral leukoplakia.

Precancerous conditions have been defined as non-neoplastic disorders associated with a significantly higher risk of cancer. An example of a precancerous condition is submucous fibrosis and squamous cell carcinoma.

Leukoplakia

Oral leukoplakia is defined as a white lesion of the oral mucosa that cannot be characterized as any other definable lesion and may or may not be associated with smoking. Some oral leukoplakias progress to cancer. A provisional diagnosis of leukoplakia is made when a lesion cannot be clearly diagnosed as any other on clinical examination. A definitive diagnosis of oral leukoplakia is made in persistent lesions after elimination of suspected etiological factors by histopathologic examination. It is worth remembering that the time required for white lesions to regress after elimination of suspected etiologic factors may vary from several weeks to months. When no signs of regression are visible within 2–4 weeks a biopsy should be taken. All white lesions for which a local cause can be identified should be classified accordingly and not included among leukoplakias. Common examples are hyperkeratosis associated with friction, dental restorations and cheek biting. There are several clinical variants of white and red lesions of the oral mucosa (Figs 87.3, 87.4). These variants have important implications as sometimes they carry a higher risk of subsequent malignant change. Generally, homogenous leukoplakias have a low risk of malignant transformation whilst non-homogenous forms of leukoplakia and erythroplakia have a higher degree of risk. The following variants should be differentiated:

- homogenous leukoplakia: a predominantly white lesion of uniform flat, thin appearance that may exhibit

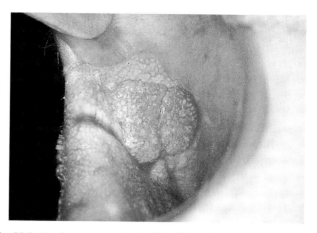

Fig. 87.3 Non-homogenous leukoplakia. The angle of the mouth reveals a non-homogenous leukoplakia of the nodular type, characterized by a red background with numerous small nodules. Ulceration and erosion are also seen. This type of leukoplakia is often suggestive of early malignancy.

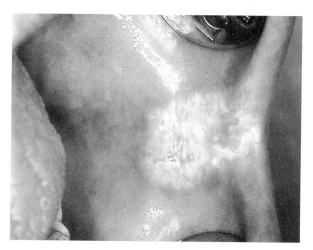

Fig. 87.4 Candida-infected leukoplakia. The retroangular area shows a white and red lesion in a heavy smoker. Smears revealed the presence of candidal hyphae. Antimycotic treatment may change the clinical appearance of this non-homogenous leukoplakia into that of a homogenous leukoplakia.

shallow cracks and has a smooth wrinkled or corrugated surface with a consistent texture throughout;
- non-homogenous leukoplakia: a predominantly white or white and red lesion that may be irregular, flat, nodular or corrugated. The nodular lesions have slightly raised rounded red and/or white excrescences and may also have blunt or sharp projections. This is sometimes referred to as 'speckled leukoplakia'.

Erythroplakia is used analogously to leukoplakia to describe lesions of the oral mucosa that present as red areas and cannot be diagnosed as any other definable lesion.[3] Recently, a staging system for oral leukoplakia including size, clinical aspect and pathologic features has been proposed.[4] This staging system may be helpful in the management of oral leukoplakias.

Management of oral leukoplakia remains controversial. A primary aim should be cessation of tobacco habits, smoking, chewing or in some countries cocktails of tobacco, for example the betel quid, and possible reduction in alcohol intake. It is, however, well noted that a majority of patients with oral leukoplakia continue both smoking and drinking. Management largely depends on the histopathologic diagnosis of the lesion[3] and its site. Lesions showing moderate and severe dysplasia need particular attention and different types of treatment are available. The site plays an important role in predicting its behavior. Floor of mouth lesions, for example, may transform in 20% of cases yet a buccal lesion in only 1%. Surgical excision has been widely recommended, but can be difficult in sites such as floor of mouth where dysplasia may extend to involve sublingual gland duct epithelium. Surgical treatments may result in recurrence rates of up to 20%.[5] Cryotherapy has also been advocated, although some uncertainty about the risk of subsequent invasive carcinomas remains. Carbon dioxide laser ablation has been recommended but recurrence rates of up to 40% have been described. The reasons for the transformation after laser and cryosurgery are speculative. Would the lesions have transformed anyway or is it really due to the surgical modality? Undoubtedly, one of the reasons for the excellent healing after laser is the release of growth factors and it may be these which stimulate the transformation.

In extensive lesions in compliant patients many surgeons rely on a 'wait and watch' policy, accompanied by trying to eliminate tobacco and alcohol abuse. In compliant, well-informed patients this can be very effective. The family dentist and doctor should also be involved in this process.

Probably the greatest problems arise in the Indian subcontinent, where the widespread use of the betel quid (betel leaf, areca nut and quick lime) produces many cases of leukoplakia for the surgeon. Many patients are not well educated and many, not understanding the risks, will go on to develop malignancies.

Treatment with systemic or topical retinoids has also been tried although the toxic effects, particularly with systemic treatment, are unacceptable.

COMMON NEOPLASMS AND NEOPLASM-LIKE LESIONS OF MESENCHYMAL ORIGIN

FIBROMAS

Most soft-tissue swellings in the mouth are connective tissue hyperplasias. True fibromas of the oral cavity are rare. In the majority of cases these lesions are irritation induced, resulting from low-grade trauma. Clinically, fibroepithelial polyps are pink nodules of varying size, often seen on the buccal mucosa or lateral border of tongue. Simple excision biopsy of the lesion is the therapy of choice. It is well recognized that these may recur, especially if the 'irritating factor' is not dealt with. They can grow rapidly sometimes and occasionally contain well-mineralized bone.

DENTURE-INDUCED HYPERPLASIA

Denture-induced fibrous tissue hyperplasia located in the maxillary and, less frequently, mandibular vestibule is characterized by edematous, inflamed, protruding masses of soft tissue. In a number of cases, ulceration may be seen. Ill-fitting dentures are the underlying cause. Denture-induced lesions are generally treated surgically. This should be done after a period of not wearing the dentures, to allow for reduction in size, with reduction in edema and inflammation. This by itself may produce sufficient resolution to obviate surgery. Often primary or secondary vestibuloplasty with mucosal graft is needed, where excision leads to severe contraction. Rebasing of the denture is usually necessary and new dentures should be considered. These lesions often present in old demented patients and removal of the denture from their possession is necessary.

EPULIDES

Epulides are lesions associated with the gingival tissues (Greek *epulides* = on the gums).

Fibrous epulis

The fibrous epulis is another hyperplastic fibrous tissue mass located at the gingiva. It may represent resolving pyogenic granulomas. Usually the fibrous epulis is the same color as the oral mucosa and firm on palpation, though sometimes hard if bone is present within the lesion. Ossification is more common in younger patients. Removal of any irritating factors and excision is the usual treatment. These lesions may, however, recur.

Pyogenic granuloma

Pyogenic granuloma is most commonly observed on the gingiva. It is a red, soft nodule sometimes covered with fibrinoid exudate. It bleeds easily when traumatized. Pyogenic granuloma is common during pregnancy, often showing marked regression postpartum. In all instances, however, there is an initiating factor and this should be sought.

Vascular proliferation may be very active, leading to rapid growth, and distinction from a Kaposi sarcoma should always be considered clinically. Excision is generally curative, but the rich vascular supply should be borne in mind and due attention given to achieving hemostasis after surgery. As poor oral hygiene may be a precipitating factor, the appropriate advice and referral to a restorative dentist may be indicated.

Peripheral giant cell granuloma

This is uncommon and clinically, giant cell granuloma of the peripheral type is more common in the maxilla, with a peak incidence in the second and third decades. It is equally common in males and females. Its surface is smooth and it is sessile. Color can be variable, but is usually purple/red with a brown surface hue. It is soft. Radiographically, bone destruction is often observed. Treatment involves excision, with curettage of the base of the lesion in order to avoid recurrences. It is important, in all cases, to exclude hyperparathyroidism, as histologically these conditions cannot be separated.

FIBROMATOSIS (GINGIVAL, OF TUBEROSITY)

Gingival fibromatosis (Fig. 87.5) is familial or acquired due to treatment with phenytoin, cyclosporine or nifidipine or other calcium channel blockers. In familial gingival fibromatosis large connective tissue masses develop that may cover the teeth. The fibrous hyperplasia is found along the alveolar ridge. Drug-induced gingival fibromatosis is associated with poor oral hygiene. Gingival fibromatosis, including fibromatosis of tuberosity, both thought to be reactive processes, have to be differentiated from fibromatoses which are 'true' proliferative lesions of connective tissue, infiltrating surrounding tissues, often showing a relentless growth pattern and a marked tendency to recur.

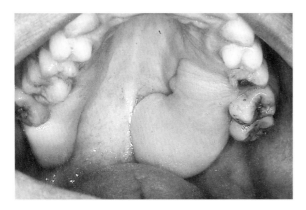

Fig. 87.5 Bilateral fibromatosis of tuberosity. While the left side shows an extensive fibromatosis reaching the midline, the right side is less marked. Surgical reduction of the fibrous masses is indicated.

Different types are recognized in adults and infants. Gingivectomy is the treatment of choice, but it may be necessary to repeat this at intervals. Again, establishing excellent oral hygiene is helpful in reducing the chance and extent of recurrence; however, this may be difficult in some mentally retarded children who are often prescribed some of these drugs, such as epanutin for epilepsy.

TUMORS OF NEURAL ORIGIN

Tumors of neural origin of the mouth are uncommon and may include traumatic neuroma, neurilemmoma (Schwannoma), neurofibroma, plexiform neurofibroma and neurofibromatosis (von Recklinghausen disease). From the clinical point of view most neural tumors have no pathognomonic features. Traumatic neuromas are quite common overlying the mandibular mental foramen in an area covered by a lower denture. They are invariably painful when pressure is applied in the region. Others, however, may occur as superficial or deep small nodules and are often painless. In neurofibromatosis, two genetically distinct forms are known. Type 1 (von Recklinghausen disease) is much more common and is associated with multiple neural tumors and multiple pigmented skin lesions, some of which are *café au lait* spots. The neurofibromas are seen on skin and oral mucosa. Neurofibromas of the head and neck are seen in >75% of the cases and involve the mouth or jaws in >25%. Type 2 is associated with acoustic neuromas, with or without skin tumors, but can also have pigmented skin lesions.

Traumatic neuromas can often be associated with considerable dysesthesia and also, sadly, with impending litigation after third molar surgery. These need to be identified and excised and often need nerve grafts. This is a traumatic experience for the patient and may well be accompanied by loss of all sensation, often permanently, which certainly adds to the drive to take legal action. Unfortunately, neurosensory testing and MRI scanning are not conclusive and surgery is required to explore these lesions.

Neurofibromatosis is particularly difficult to manage if extensive. These lesions may distort and damage by compressing normal anatomic structures. They are, however, infiltrating lesions without clear margins and, often less well appreciated, extremely vascular. Surgical ablation of large lesions may well lead to damage to important nerves and other structures. Caution and good preoperative investigations should be undertaken to decide if real benefits will be gained by removing these lesions.

NEOPLASMS OF FATTY TISSUE

The only benign neoplasm of fatty tissue is the lipoma, a

soft yellowish swelling located submucosally. They may be multiple and are seen in the floor of the mouth or buccal mucosa. They can be 'poorly fluctuant' and often have a distinctive surface vascularity. Distinction from a herniated buccal fat pad is necessary. Excision is curative.

TUMORS OF VASCULAR ORIGIN

Tumors of vascular origin are those hamartomas most often seen in the oral cavity. Hemangiomas are classified as either capillary, cavernous or arterial shunting (AV) lesions. Whilst capillary lesions tend to regress with growth, cavernous lesions may enlarge at puberty. High-flow AV lesions can be extremely difficult to treat and if intra-bony, can lead to fatal hemorrhage, often after dental extractions. Hemangiomas can be flat or prominent red-purplish lesions which characteristically blanch under pressure and bleed when traumatized. Extensive hemangiomas may cause macroglossia (Fig. 87.6). Intraosseous and parotid variants are recognized, with severe and extensive lesions seen in Sturge–Weber syndrome. Some hemangiomas may regress spontaneously due to thrombosis. Small capillary lesions respond

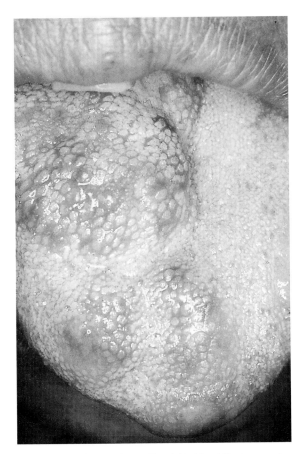

Fig. 87.6 Cavernous hemangioma. The right side of the tongue shows several voluminous hemangiomas. Surgical reduction of this type of hemangioma is complicated and risky.

to cryotherapy or injection of sclerosing agents. Argon laser ablation is also used. Extensive high-flow AV hemangiomas need preoperative angiography to identify the feeding vessels and extent of the lesion. This should be planned as part of a surgical ablation, being embolized at the time of angiography. Within a day of embolization, excision of the malformation should be undertaken. Presurgical ligation of supplying vessels may prevent embolization and these lesions should only be performed by a team with an interest in the angiography and subsequent ablation. Unfortunately embolization by itself is rarely permanently successful.

Lymphangiomas are less frequent than hemangiomas. When superficially located they are pale or pink or even translucent. The surface is often nodular. Deep, large lymphangiomas, called cystic hygromas, can affect the tongue, causing macroglossia. Small lymphangiomas can be completely excised; but those of considerable size need expert treatment. These lesions often spread insidiously into the tissues, making complete excision difficult without damaging important structures like the facial nerve. Unfortunately treatment is often necessary as small infarcts occur, leading to repeated infections within the lesion. They may also distort the normal anatomy to such an extent that removal is required. Again, it is a fine balance between accepting the problems of the lesions and the damage that must occur if they have to be excised. Incomplete excision in the young often leads to regrowth back to the original size.

TUMORS OF MUSCULAR ORIGIN

Extracardiac rhabdomyomas are very rare. The tumor generally occurs in later age and is slow growing and painless. Rhabdomyomas should be fully excised and recurrence is uncommon.

Leiomyoma (angioleiomyoma)

Leiomyomas are rare in the oral cavity and often arise from muscle cells of blood vessels. The tongue is the most common site. Lesions have a non-specific appearance and growth is slow and painless. Clearly, their vascularity needs to be borne in mind when excised.

Granular cell tumor

Granular cell tumors affect the upper aerodigestive tract, but are common on the tongue. Adults in the third to the sixth decades are affected. The lesion may become large. Granular cell tumors are locally excised but recurrent lesions may develop. Whether the granular cell tumor is of neural, muscular or otherwise undifferentiated mesenchymal origin is still debated.

CYST AND CYSTLIKE LESIONS OF THE JAW

Cysts are defined as pathologic cavities having fluid, semi-fluid or gaseous contents, not created by the accumulation of pus. Only the solitary and the aneurysmal bone cyst lack an epithelial lining or fluid contents. The most common odontogenic cyst is the radicular cyst (65–70%), followed by the dentigerous (follicular) cyst (15–18%), the keratocyst (3–10%) and the nasopalatine duct cyst (2–5%). Cysts are non-neoplastic but may rarely show malignant transformation of the cyst epithelium.

The main mechanisms of cyst formation involve in varying degree:

1. proliferation of the epithelial lining and connective tissue capsule;
2. accumulation of fluid within the cyst and the resorption of the surrounding bone;
3. incomplete compensatory repair.

In the early phase of cyst formation active proliferation of epithelium is seen. Radicular necrotic pulpal tissue is the source of irritation. Hydrostatic effects of cyst fluids probably result in enlargement of the cyst in a balloon-like manner. The cyst fluid is usually an inflammatory exudate containing high concentrations of proteins (with the notable exception of keratocysts) with a high molecular weight, cholesterol, hemosiderin, immunocompetent cells, exfoliated epithelial cells and fibrin. In addition to the hydrostatic effects of the cyst fluid, bone-resorbing factors such as prostaglandins affect the growth of cysts.

CLASSIFICATION

Several classifications of jaw cysts have been published based on pathogenic, morphologic, topographical or clinical aspects. The WHO histologic typing of odontogenic tumors including cysts was revised in 1992.[6] This classification is based on the origin of the cyst epithelium. Non-epithelial cysts (pseudocysts) were included under non-neoplastic bone lesions (aneurysmal and solitary bone cyst) (Table 87.1).

There are different management regimes for patients presenting with cysts. In the USA, for example, it is common practice to obtain a histologic diagnosis before proceeding to treatment. This is an attractive option, but may cause the cyst to become infected and the collapse of the cyst

Table 87.1 Classification of epithelial cysts (WHO 1992)

Epithelial cysts
Developmental
Odontogenic
    Gingival cysts of infants (Epstein pearls)
    Odontogenic keratocyst (primordial cyst)
    Dentigerous (follicular) cyst
    Eruption cyst
    Lateral periodontal cyst
    Gingival cyst of adults
    Glandular odontogenic cyst; sialo-odontogenic cyst
Non-odontogenic
    Nasopalatine duct (incisive canal) cyst
    Nasolabial (nasoalveolar) cyst
Inflammatory
Radicular cyst
    Apical and lateral
    Residual
Paradental cyst

Non-epithelial pseudocysts (non-neoplastic bone lesions)
Aneurysmal bone cyst
Solitary bone cyst (traumatic, simple, hemorrhagic bone cyst)

may make its subsequent removal more difficult and incomplete. In the UK and Germany, unless there are any signs or symptoms which might suggest an associated malignancy, the lesion is removed and sent for histology. This policy is satisfactory for most cyst, unless the lesion subsequently is shown to be a locally aggressive cyst like a keratocyst. The lesion may then have been inadequately treated and further surgery may be jeopardized by the initial removal. A useful compromise between these two options is to aspirate fluid from the cyst for both cytology and measurement of the protein content. Cytology is often not helpful because mainly fluid is aspirated, but the protein levels will distinguish between a keratocyst and other cysts. A protein level of >4 mg % is highly suggestive of a keratocyst.

Gingival cysts of infants (Epstein pearls)

These are small cysts arising from epithelial cell rests in the alveolar mucosa of infants.[6] They are white or yellow nodules, located on the alveolar mucosa. They are present at birth and disappear without treatment.

Odontogenic keratocyst

A cyst arising in the tooth-bearing areas of the jaws or posterior to the mandibular third molar and characterized by a thin fibrous capsule and a lining of parakeratinized stratified squamous epithelium, usually about 5–8 cells in thickness and generally without rete ridges.[6]

Keratocysts are frequent in the mandible, particularly

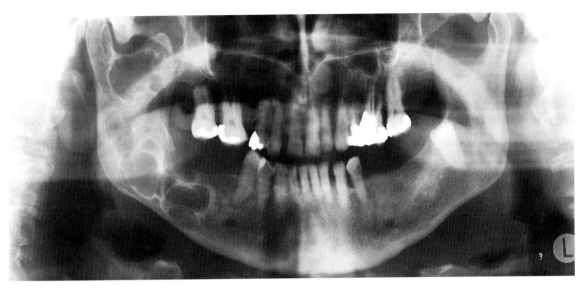

Fig. 87.7 Multilocular keratocyst of body of mandible and ascending ramus of the right side. This 78-year-old patient had experienced a cyst operation in the same region more than 40 years before.

the posterior body and angle (Fig. 87.7). Impacted teeth are seen in about 50% of cases. Keratocysts are more common in men than women and occur more frequently in the second and third decades. Radiographically, spread through cancellous bone in a multilocular pattern is typical. Keratocysts may occur as part of the nevoid basal cell carcinoma syndrome (NBCCS or Gorlin–Goltz syndrome) and commonly recur after treatment, with recurrence rates of up to 60%. This is partly a result of incomplete removal due to the thin, friable wall and partly due to the presence of daughter cysts.

Compared to other cysts of the oral region the surgical management of the keratocyst needs special consideration. Careful enucleation or marsupialization is recommended, with some authorities recommending chemical 'lavage' (with, for example, Carnoy's solution) of the cavity to fix the thin cyst lining in situ. Cryotherapy may also be applied after surgical removal. Of particular importance is the excision of overlying alveolar mucosa, because it often contains numerous daughter cysts. Removal of some bone within the cyst cavity after enucleation seems to reduce the number of recurrences.

Dentigerous (follicular) cyst

This is a cyst which encloses the crown and is attached at the cement–enamel junction of an unerupted tooth. It develops by accumulation of fluid between the reduced enamel epithelium and the crown or between the layers of the reduced enamel epithelium.[6] Dentigerous cysts are commonly found in association with impacted teeth (upper canines and lower third molars) and are asymptomatic,

unless secondarily infected. They are more common in men than women and the second to the fourth decades are most frequently affected. Radiographically, they are unilocular, containing the crown of a tooth (Fig. 89.8). The therapy of choice is removal of the impacted tooth together with the cyst wall.

Eruption cyst

These are rare, follicular cysts that surround crowns of erupting teeth, lie partly outside bone and are lined by non-keratinizing stratified squamous epithelium.[6]

The eruption cyst presenting as a blue swelling on the alveolar crest where a tooth will erupt is a variant of the dentigerous cyst. Many spontaneously rupture, but excision of the covering oral mucosa including the cyst lining will allow the tooth to erupt normally.

Lateral periodontal cyst

Many odontogenic cysts including keratocysts can occur on the lateral aspect or between the roots of vital teeth. However, there appears to be a separate, distinct entity arising from odontogenic epithelial remnants but not as a result of inflammatory stimuli.[6]

The lateral periodontal cyst (LPC) is more frequent in the premolar area of the mandible. Differential diagnosis includes collateral keratocyst, gingival cyst of adults or cysts of inflammatory origin (lateral radicular cyst). Radiographically, LPC is characterized by a round or ovoid radiolucency lateral to or between roots. Often LPC is found

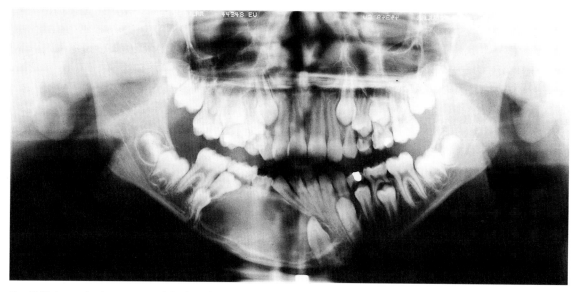

Fig. 87.8 Large dentigerous cyst of the lateral type involving the right lower canine. In some of these cases it may be difficult to differentiate between a dentigerous cyst and a radicular cyst of the deciduous tooth. Marsupialization is the therapy of choice with the aim of integrating the lower right canine into the dental arch.

accidentally on radiographs. Enucleation is the therapy of choice.

Gingival cyst of adults

A cyst of unknown etiology involving the gingiva of adults.[6] Gingival cysts of adults are rare and mainly observed in the canine-premolar area of the mandible. They are well circumscribed and usually less than 1 cm in diameter. There may be no radiographic features or a little superficial bone resorption. Inflammation is usually found in the cyst wall. Enucleation is recommended.

Glandular odontogenic cyst, sialo-odontogenic cyst, polymorphous cyst

This is a rare cyst arising in the tooth-bearing areas of the jaws and characterized by an epithelial lining with cuboidal or columnar cells both at the surface and lining crypts or cystlike spaces within the thickness of the epithelium.[6] Goblet cells are also noted in the lining epithelium or in small crypts in the wall. The glandular odontogenic cyst is rare and has only recently been described. It may reach a considerable size, commonly crossing the midline, and may recur. Long-term follow-up seems to be indicated regardless of the type of therapy.

Nasopalatine duct cyst (incisive canal) (non-odontogenic)

A cyst arising from the epithelial residues in the nasopala-tine (incisive) canal,[6] the nasopalatine duct cyst occurs in the midline of the anterior maxilla. The third to sixth decades are frequently affected and men more frequently than women (4:1). Radiographically, a well-defined round, ovoid or heart-shaped radiolucency is found between the central incisors or along the nasopalatine duct. Pain is common and a 'salty' taste is frequently reported. Enucleation from a palatal approach is the therapy of choice. Recurrence is unusual.

Nasolabial (nasoalveolar) cyst

This uncommon cyst is situated on the alveolar process near the base of the nostril.[6] It is a cyst of the soft tissues, possibly arising from the lower end of the nasolacrimal rod or duct. It may cause resorption of the outer surface of the maxilla. Women are more frequently affected than men with the age peak between the fourth and fifth decades. Radiography may be negative. Enucleation is the therapy of choice. In large lesions an extraoral approach is often used, making the incision in the nasolabial groove.

Other non-odontogenic cysts

Other non-odontogenic cysts of the oral region, so-called fissural cysts such as the median palatine, median alveolar and median mandibular cysts, were not included in the WHO classification of 1992. These were defined as midline cysts of the maxilla and mandible, previously thought to be derived from epithelium entrapped during the fusion of embryonic facial processes. Embryologists and pathologists have now discounted the existence of these cysts. The so-called globulomaxillary cyst was defined as a cyst found within the bone between the maxillary lateral incisor and canine, previously thought to be a fissural cyst arising from non-odontogenic epithelium included at the site of fusion of the globular process of the frontonasal process and the maxillary process. These, however, are now accepted as other cyst variants such as the odontogenic keratocyst or lateral periodontal cyst.

Radicular cyst (inflammatory)

A cyst arising from epithelial residues (rests of Malassez) in the periodontal ligament as a consequence of inflammation, usually following necrosis of dental pulp.[6] Apical and lateral varieties are recognized. The radicular cyst is the most common cyst, is found most frequently in the third and fourth decades and in men rather than women. Maxillary anterior teeth show the highest incidence. Radiographically, periapical granulomas cannot be differentiated from periapical cysts if the lesion is smaller than 5 mm. Radicular cysts appear as unilocular, well-defined round or oval radiolucencies. Infected cysts, however, show less well-defined margins. The cyst lining is usually thick but easily enucleated. Enucleation is the therapy of choice.

Residual radicular cyst

This is a radicular cyst, which is retained in the jaws after removal or root filling of the associated tooth.[6] Residual cysts may sometimes be large but go unnoticed unless facial asymmetry or swelling is present. Without treatment, these lesions will slowly resolve. Radiographically, they are usually well defined but may contain focal calcification.

Paradental cyst

A cyst occurring near the cervical margin of the lateral aspect of the root as a consequence of an inflammatory process in a periodontal pocket.[6] The paradental cyst is associated with a third molar which is partially erupted and has an associated enamel defect. The cyst is attached to the enamel–cemental junction, rarely exceeding 2 cm in diameter. Enucleation is the therapy of choice.

Solitary bone cyst (traumatic, simple, hemorrhagic bone cyst)

An intraosseous cyst having a tenuous lining of connective tissue with no epithelium.[6] The solitary or simple bone cyst (SBC) is a bone cavity without epithelial lining and often no fluid content. It is most often seen during the second decade of life. The SBC is found in the body and symphysis of the mandible. Radiographically, it often appears as a well-defined unilocular radiolucency. Roots of adjacent teeth may be displaced. The terms traumatic or hemorrhagic bone cyst suggest a traumatic cause of the lesion, but there is no evidence that a blow can cause bleeding within the bone. Surgical opening of the cavity confirms the diagnosis. Spontaneous regression normally occurs, after exploration.

Aneurysmal bone cyst (ABC)

A rare intraosseous lesion characterized by bloodfilled spaces of varying size associated with a fibroblastic tissue containing multinucleated giant cells, osteoid and woven bone.[6] ABCs are most often observed in the first and second decades with a slight preponderance in women. The mandible is more frequently affected than the maxilla. Radiographically, a multiloculated radiolucency with ballooning of the cortex is characteristic. ABCs may be associated with other lesions including fibrous dysplasia, ossifying fibroma and cementifying fibroma. Treatment involves curettage, but excision is recommended as recurrences have been described.

PRINCIPLES OF SURGICAL MANAGEMENT

All cysts of the oral region have to be surgically removed with the result of *restitutio ad integrum* of the affected area. Whilst removal of cysts is not essential, they will slowly enlarge and sooner or later they will become infected and painful. Cysts are treated according to two basic principles: enucleation with primary wound closure or marsupialization (decompression). Enucleation (cystectomy) is the complete removal of the cyst lining and primary closure of the incision. Marsupialization (decompression, cystostomy; Greek *ostium* = opening) is a procedure where the cyst is opened by reflecting a mucoperiosteum and a window is made as large as the local anatomy allows. In this way the former cyst cavity becomes an invagination of the oral cavity.[7]

Enucleation (cystectomy, Partsch II)

The principle of enucleation or cystectomy is complete removal of the cyst lining and primary closure of the cavity (Fig. 87.9). Enucleation is recommended for smaller cysts of up to 2 cm in diameter where the cyst cavity is surrounded by bone and no adjacent structures would be damaged. Medium and large cysts may be enucleated in those cases were no neighboring structures would be exposed or injured and where the cavity could be entirely filled by a stabilized blood clot. Finally, enucleation is indicated in the treatment of keratocysts, usually with revision of the bony walls of the cavity, and in solitary and aneurysmal bone cysts. Enucleation has a number of advantages.

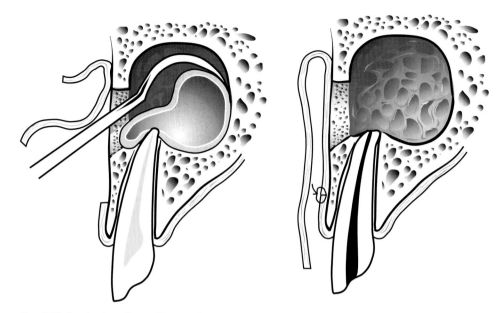

Fig. 87.9 Enucleation of a smaller cyst of an anterior maxillary tooth via a vestibular approach. The cyst is removed in toto; at the same time a root resection with endodontic treatment before or during surgery is performed. Primary closure of the mucoperiostal flap will result in adequate bony healing of the former cyst cavity.

1. The entire period of postoperative care is short (10 days).
2. Bone regeneration takes place spontaneously without the need to, for example, keep replacing packs.
3. Recurrences are rare.
4. The entire cyst lining is available for histologic examination.

Disadvantages of enucleation include the following.

1. Larger cyst cavities may become infected and neighboring structures such as teeth, nerves or vessels may be damaged.
2. The maxillary antrum may be opened.
3. Fracture may ensue in very large cysts, particularly of the mandible.
4. The procedure may require a general anesthetic and in elderly patients with concomitant medical problems, this may be an added risk.

Therefore under certain and infrequent circumstances a two-step procedure may be chosen. First, an initial marsupialization (decompression) is performed. After formation of new bone, the remaining cyst may be enucleated as a second step. Since enucleation has a number of advantages compared to marsupialization, the former method is also applied to cysts. The main problem in larger cysts is contraction of the blood clot and the serum which is then formed; this creates 'dead space' which may become infected. Dehiscence is a consequence of infection. If infection has occurred, the cavity may have to be packed.

Stabilization of blood clot in combination with resorb-able materials can allow the treatment of larger cysts by enucleation.[8] Resorbable denatured gelatinous sponges are used in combination with penicillin and at least 50 NIH/ml of thrombin. The patient's own blood is used and this mixture of blood, gelatinous sponges, penicillin (20–30 000 IE/ml) and thrombin is used to fill the defect. Autogenous bone transplants (particularly spongiotic bone) have also been recommended to fill cavities. This procedure, however, requires an additional surgical step. During the last 15 years, numerous materials, mainly ceramics of different kinds, were used in trials to fill large cystic cavities. In particular, hydroxyapatite and tricalciumphosphate have been used in such cases. Most maxillofacial surgeons currently avoid these techniques. Recently, bone morphogenetic proteins (BMPs) have been recommended for filling bone cavities after enucleation.[9,10]

Marsupialization (cystostomy, Partsch I)

Marsupialization (cystostomy, Partsch I) is a technique relying on incomplete removal of the cyst lining (Fig. 87.10). Opening a window into the cyst forms an invagination of the oral cavity or the maxillary antrum. Decompression halts expansion of the cyst. Appositional growth of bone occurs and the former cyst lumen becomes smaller over time. The surgical technique is easily performed, since it is a kind of trepanation where the oral mucosa and the cyst lining, which remains in the depth of the cyst cavity, are joined by sutures. Marsupialization has some advantages.

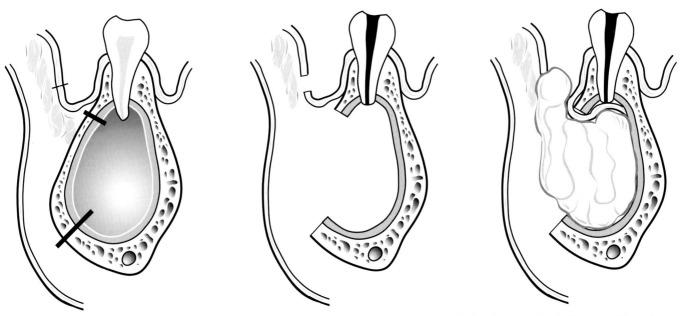

Fig. 87.10 Marsupialization of a mandibular cyst. The cyst is opened using a curved incision in the vestibule. A large window in the cyst wall is made (see marks). The mucoperiostal flap is placed over the resected root and fixed using a sutuare. The cavity is filled with a surgical pack. Most of the cyst membrane remains in place.

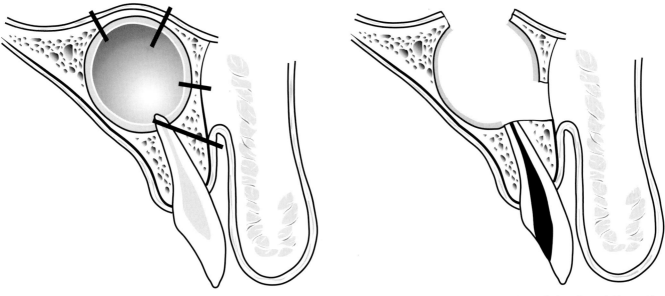

A   B

Fig. 87.11 Rhinomarsupialization. In cases where there is no bony connection between the cyst and the nasal cavity, this technique is used. The cyst is approached via a vestibular incision. The root of the tooth is resected, as is the cyst membrane joining the nasal mucosa. The cavity of the former cyst is covered by cyst membrane to a large extent.

1. The surgical intervention is of short duration and causes little trauma.
2. Swelling and postoperative problems are minimal.
3. Neighboring structures (teeth, alveolar dental nerve, floor of nose, floor of maxillary antrum) are not damaged.

Disadvantages of marsupialization include the following.

1. Postoperative care of up to one year and more is necessary.

2. Complete bony healing will not occur in patients over 20 years old.
3. If no plug or obturator is used a recurrence of the cyst may occur, making a second intervention necessary.
4. The cyst lining is not removed entirely so that only a part of it is examined histologically; ameloblastomas or even carcinomas developing in cyst linings may be missed.

The postoperative care of the open bone cavity involves treatment with surgical packs until all wound margins are epithelialized. This usually takes about 2–3 weeks. After removal of the surgical pack a plug or obturator must be used which keeps the fenestration of the former cyst cavity open until bone apposition has taken place and only a shallow depression is left. The obturator must be reduced regularly (every 8–14 days).

OTHER SURGICAL TECHNIQUES AND METHODS

Several other techniques and methods to treat cysts have been proposed. One variation of enucleation (cystectomy of larger cysts) is the use of suction drainage (Nasteff–Rosenthal). Large mandibular cysts are opened and buccal soft tissues, including masseter muscle, are used to fill the bony cavity. The redon suction drainage will 'suck in' the soft tissue into the bone cavity while wound secretions are continuously removed. There is one specific situation where an anterior maxillary cyst must be joined with the nasal cavity (rhinocystostomy). This technique is used in situations where an oronasal communication has occurred. The surgical principle is that the cyst becomes an invagination of the nasal cavity (Fig. 87.11). Treatment results seem to be good and there is no retention of secretions.

Large cysts of the maxilla which have to be joined with the maxillary antrum are treated with antrocystectomy or antrocystostomy. In principle, the cyst and the maxillary sinus are joined together (Fig. 87.12). In most cases, due to lack of sufficient ventilation of the residual maxillary sinus, a nasal window has to be prepared which should be at least 1 × 3 cm.

ODONTOGENIC TUMORS AND TUMORLIKE LESIONS

CLASSIFICATION

The classification of odontogenic tumors was revised in 1992.[6] Supplementary to all former classifications, the principle of ectomesenchyme was introduced. In addition to those tissues derived from the ectoderm, namely the enamel organ and the mesenchyme proper (mesoderm), the ectomesenchyme is derived from cells of the neural crest during an early phase in embryogenesis. The permutation of different cells of different origin makes the odontogenic tumors a highly complicated group of lesions.[11] The phenomenon of induction which characterizes the normal tooth development is replicated in odontogenic tumors in a more or less perfect way. Odontogenic tumors are not all neoplasms in the strict sense as some are of a hamartomatous or malformation-like nature. The classification includes benign and malignant odontogenic tumors. In this chapter only benign neoplasms and other tumors related to the odontogenic apparatus are summarized (Table 87.2).

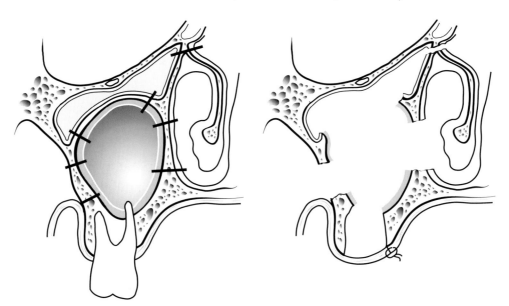

Fig. 87.12 Marsupialization of a large radicular cyst of the maxilla. The cyst is approached via a vestibular incision. The remaining maxillary sinus and the cyst are joined by resection of the cyst wall and the mucous membrane of the maxillary antrum. Also, a nasal window is prepared. The tooth is removed and the resulting oroantral fistula is closed according to standard principles. The major part of the cyst membrane has been removed.

Table 87.2 Benign odontogenic tumors

Odontogenic epithelium without odontogenic ectomesenchyme
Ameloblastoma
Squamous odontogenic tumor
Calcifying epithelial odontogenic tumor (Pindborg tumor)
Clear cell odontogenic tumor

Odontogenic epithelium with odontogenic ectomesenchyme, with or without dental hard-tissue formation
Ameloblastic fibroma
Ameloblastic fibrodentinoma (dentinoma)
Odontoameloblastoma
Adenomatoid odontogenic tumor
Calcifying odontogenic cyst
Complex odontome
Compound odontome

Odontogenic ectomesenchyme with or without included odontogenic epithelium
Odontogenic fibroma
Myxoma (odontogenic myxoma, myxofibroma)
Benign cementoblastoma (cementoblastoma, true cementoma)

Ameloblastoma

The ameloblastoma has recently been reviewed and the biological profile of 3677 cases was described.[12] It accounts for approximately 1% of all oral tumors and is a slow-growing and locally invasive and destructive lesion of odontogenic epithelium. Ameloblastomas occur equally in men and women, with an overall average age of 36 years, though those in developing countries and women patients are affected earlier. The ratio of ameloblastoma of the mandible to maxilla is 5:1. Ameloblastomas of the mandible generally occur 12 years earlier than those of the maxilla.

The molar region of the mandible is most frequently affected. In blacks ameloblastomas occur more frequently in the anterior region of the maxilla. Fifty percent of ameloblastomas appear as multilocular, radiolucent lesions with sharp borders (Fig. 87.13). Histologically, they show a plexiform (irregular and variable epithelial islands and clusters) or follicular (resembling tooth follicle) pattern. Two percent of ameloblastomas are peripheral and 6% appear as unicystic ameloblastomas. Unicystic ameloblastomas have a much less aggressive natural history and occur in patients 15 years younger than those with the multicystic ameloblastoma (Fig. 87.14). It is important that unicystic ameloblastomas should be treated conservatively, except those cases with invasion of epithelium into the cyst walls. Three histologic types of unicystic ameloblastomas are recognized.[13]

Classic ameloblastomas should be treated radically, that is, by resection with a margin of normal tissue around the tumor. This may mean that important structures like the inferior alveolar nerve may be resected en bloc with the tumor. However, ameloblastomas which appear radiologically as unilocular lesions may be treated more conservatively (enucleation or curettage where all areas of the cystic lumen are accessible). Chemotherapy and radiation are contraindicated. The peripheral type of ameloblastoma may be excised because conservative therapy results in low recurrence rates.

The multicystic classic ameloblastoma is characterized by a recurrence rate of up to 50% during the first 5 years postoperatively. Long-term, even lifelong follow-up is indicated. The peripheral ameloblastoma is excised locally and has a low recurrence rate.

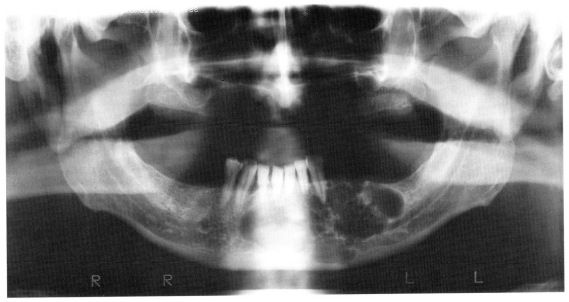

Fig. 87.13 Multilocular radiolucency of the anterior body of the mandible representing a characteristic classic ameloblastoma. Histologically, this ameloblastoma was of the plexiform type.

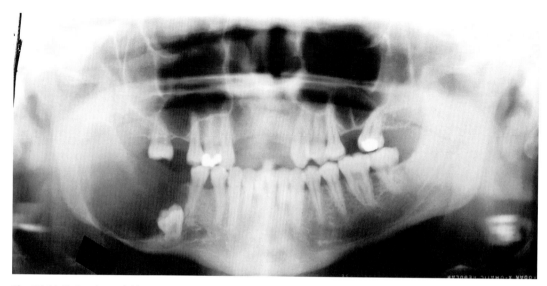

Fig. 87.14 Unicystic ameloblastoma presenting as a dentigerous cyst. In younger individuals these two diagnoses have always to be considered in radiographical situations like this (courtesy M. Shear, South Africa).

Calcifying epithelial odontogenic tumor (CEOT) (Pindborg tumor)

A locally invasive epithelial neoplasm characterized by the development of intraepithelial structures, probably of an amyloid-like nature, which may become calcified and which may be liberated as the cells break down.[6]

The CEOT is found between the second and fifth decades. In 70% of cases the mandible is affected with the premolar and molar areas most often involved. An extraosseous variant has been described. CEOT is often associated with unerupted teeth. Radiographically, an irregular radiolucency with radio-opacities of varying size is seen. The CEOT shows some potential for recurrence and aggressiveness. If the lesion penetrates bone and involves mucosa it can be mistaken for carcinoma. It should be carefully excised with a margin of normal tissue and followed up.

Clear cell odontogenic tumor

A benign but locally invasive neoplasm originating from odontogenic epithelium and characterized by sheets and islands of uniform, vacuolated and clear cells.[6]

The clear cell odontogenic tumor seems to be rare and has only been recently described. It occurs as a central tumor, with an ill-defined radiolucency. The CCOT appears to have a strong potential for local aggressiveness and should therefore be treated radically.

Ameloblastic fibroma and related lesions ('mixed odontogenic tumors')

Neoplasms composed of proliferating odontogenic epithelium embedded in a cellular ectomesenchymal tissue that resembles the dental papilla and with varying degrees of inductive change and dental hard-tissue formation.[6]

The mixed odontogenic tumors have recently been reviewed.[15] They comprise the ameloblastic fibroma, fibro-dentinoma and fibro-odontome as well as the complex/compound odontomes. The tumors develop along two separate lines:

1. the neoplastic line comprising only one tumor, the ameloblastic fibroma, and the closely related ameloblastic fibrodentinoma;
2. the hamartomatous or developing complex odontome line comprising (a) the ameloblastic fibroma (differences in age and biologic behavior indicate that some ameloblastic fibromas are true benign neoplasms whereas others are hamartomas presenting the first stage in the developing odontome line); (b) the ameloblastic fibro-odontome representing the second stage of the developing odontome line; and (c) the fully mineralized odontome.

Ameloblastic fibroma

The ameloblastic fibroma is a rare benign neoplasm in which both the odontogenic epithelial and ectomesenchymal components are neoplastic. The age and time of diagnosis falls within the first two decades. Almost 80% are diagnosed before the age of 20. The ratio between men and women is 1.4:1. The posterior mandible is most often affected. Radiographically, the tumor appears as a well-defined uni- or multilocular radiolucency. Most of the ameloblastic fibroma cases do not recur but recurrences of up to 43.5%

have been reported. Meticulous surgical enucleation with consequent follow-up should be sufficient.

Ameloblastic fibrodentinoma and ameloblastic fibro-odontome

These are lesions similar to ameloblastic fibroma but also showing inductive changes that lead to the formation of dentine and, in ameloblastic fibro-odontome, enamel as well.[6] Few cases of ameloblastic fibrodentinoma have been reported. The tumor appears as a mixed radiolucent and radio-opaque lesion with well-defined borders on radiographs. Conservative enucleation is considered appropriate.

Ameloblastic fibro-odontome

This is an unusual lesion that may be a true mixed tumor. The age and time of diagnosis falls within the first two decades (average age 9 years) and it is more common in males. Most ameloblastic fibro-odontomes are found in the posterior mandible. Radiographically, the tumor appears as a uni- or multilocular radiolucency with a radio-opacity in the center of the lesion. This represents a mostly homogenous rounded calcified mass. Although essentially a benign lesion, increasing numbers of reports describe recurrences unless a margin of sound bone is included.

Adenomatoid odontogenic tumor

A tumor of odontogenic epithelium with ductlike structures and with varying degrees of inductive change in the connective tissue. The tumor may be partly cystic and in some cases the solid lesion may be present only as masses in the wall of a large cyst. It is generally believed that the lesion is not a neoplasm.[6]

Five hundred cases of adenomatoid odontogenic tumor (AOT) were extensively reviewed.[16] The tumor is seen more frequently in girls and occurs in the second decade of life. Radiographically, most cases resemble follicular cysts as they are often associated with an unerupted tooth. The upper canine is involved in most cases. Follicular, extrafollicular and peripheral types are known. The term adenoameloblastoma is discouraged because this tumor is totally benign and should never be treated aggressively. Recurrences are unknown.

Calcifying odontogenic cyst (COC)

A cystic lesion in which the epithelial lining shows a well-defined basal layer of columnar cells, an overlying layer that is often many cells thick and that may resemble stellate reticulum and masses of 'ghost' epithelial cells that may be in the epithelial cyst lining or in the fibrous capsule. The 'ghost' epithelial cells may become calcified. Dysplastic dentine may be laid down adjacent to the basal layer of the epithelium and in some instances, the cyst is associated with an area of more extensive dental hard-tissue formation resembling that of a complex or compound odontome.[6]

COC is commonly found in the second decade of life, presenting as a painless, slow-growing swelling. Radiographically, it shows a well-defined radiolucency containing varying amounts of radio-opaque material and may be associated with an unerupted tooth or denticle.

Complex odontome

A malformation in which all the dental tissues are represented, individual tissues being mainly well formed but occurring in a disorderly pattern.[6] Complex and compound odontomes have recently been reviewed.[15] Complex odontomes occur commonly in the premolar and molar area. Growth is restricted to the formation of dentition. Lesions are usually diagnosed during the first two decades of life. Radiographically, radio-opaque material is seen in close association with teeth (Fig. 87.15). Conservative surgical removal is indicated.

Compound odontome

A malformation in which all the dental tissues are represented in a structured and more orderly pattern than in the complex odontome, so that the lesion consists of many

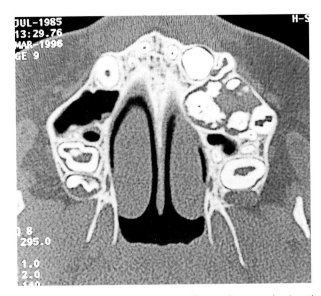

Fig. 87.15 Computed tomography of maxilla revealing a predominantly complex odontome involving the maxillary sinus of the left side. Toothlike structures as seen in the compound odontome are not found in this case.

toothlike structures. Most of these structures do not morphologically resemble the teeth of the normal dentition, but in each one enamel, dentine, cementum and pulp are arranged as in the normal tooth.[6] The compound odontome is very similar in location to the complex odontome and occurs in the same age group. Compound odontomes are painless, non-aggressive lesions and have an even more limited growth potential than the complex odontome. They are often associated with an impacted tooth. Radiographically, the compound odontome appears as a radio-opaque mass of calcified structures with an anatomic similarity to normal teeth. Conservative surgical removal is the therapy of choice. Recurrences are unknown.

Odontogenic fibroma

A fibroblastic neoplasm containing varying amounts of apparently inactive odontogenic epithelium.[6] Several subtypes of odontogenic fibroma have been described depending on the cellularity of fibrous tissue and the amount of odontogenic epithelium.[17] Radiographically, irregular radiolucencies may be seen which are not pathognomonic. The lesion is slow growing and benign and complete removal is curative.

Myxoma (odontogenic myxoma, myxofibroma)

An uncommon, locally invasive neoplasm consisting of rounded and angular cells lying in an abundant myxoid stroma.[6] Radiographically, myxomas are multilocular radiolucencies, similar to ameloblastoma. The tumor is rarely encapsulated and has infiltrative characteristics. Growth may be rapid. Aggressive surgical removal of the odontogenic myxoma is indicated and long-term follow-up is highly recommended.

Benign cementoblastoma (cementoblastoma, true cementoma)

A neoplasm characterized by the formation of sheets of cementum-like tissue containing a large number of reversal lines and being unmineralized at the periphery of the mass or in the more active growth area.[6]

A benign cementoblastoma occurs mostly in the premolar or molar region of the mandible. Most cases are observed in the second and third decades of life. The tumor is closely related to a tooth. Radiographically, a well-defined center of radio-opacity is surrounded by a radiolucent zone. When mature, the tumor shows radio-opacity. The lesion should be enucleated. Recurrence is rare.

NON-ODONTOGENIC TUMORS OF THE JAW

Non-odontogenic tumors of the jaw reflect a wide spectrum of different lesions, such as the ossifying/cementifying fibroma, the osteoma, osteoblastoma, chondroma and various others.[18] The WHO classification of 1992 classifies some of these as neoplasms and other lesions related to bone[6] (Table 87.3).

Cemento-ossifying fibroma (COF)

A well-demarcated or, rarely, encapsulated neoplasm consisting of fibrous tissue containing varying amounts of mineralized material resembling bone and/or cementum.[6] Lesions are well defined radiographically and contain varying amounts of radio-opaque material. Compared to fibrous dysplasia, COF is sharply defined at operation. Hard tissues of the COF do not fuse with the surrounding bone. Management includes meticulous enucleation. Recurrences have been described.

Fibrous dysplasia of the jaws

A benign, self-limiting but non-encapsulated lesion occurring mainly in young subjects, usually in the maxilla, and showing replacement of the normal bone by cellular fibrous tissue containing islands or trabeculae of poorly mineralized bone.[6] This is a common and often difficult condition to treat.

Radiographically, the appearance depends upon the stage of the lesion. During the osteolytic stage there is an ill-defined radiolucency and in the later stages the lesion takes on a ground-glass appearance. Fibrous dysplasia is self-limiting and the affected area will return to normal with time. Usually, fibrous dysplasia of the jaw is solitary or monostotic but a polyostotic variant is known, with a severe form (Albright's) comprising polyostotic fibrous dysplasia, precocious sexual development and skin pigmentation in young girls. Treatment should be limited to minimal cosmetic

Table 87.3 WHO classification of non-odontogenic tumors of the jaw

Osteogenic neoplasms
Cemento-ossifying fibroma
Non-neoplastic bone lesions
Fibrous dysplasia of the jaws
Cemento-osseous dysplasias
Periapical cemental dysplasia
Florid cemento-osseous dysplasia (gigantiform)
Other cemento-osseous dysplasias
Cherubism
Central giant cell granuloma

procedures, preferably after puberty. Occasionally, more aggressive forms are seen in which reactivation occurs after puberty but these cannot be predicted on either clinical or pathologic grounds.

Traditionally, it is said that these lesions should be treated after growth has ceased as the lesion stops growing. Unfortunately unsightly dystopias can develop and surgeons may be pushed by parents into early surgery. Unfortunately the surgical access necessary to remove these large lesions is often as disfiguring as the tumors. Surgically paring away the bony mass may well cover the operating theater floor with bone, but the esthetic results are disappointing. The vascular nature of these lesions makes it hard to close the soft-tissue layers down into the new position. Hematoma formation often occurs even with suction drainage and the final appearance is disappointing. In the growing child results of conservative reductions are poor.

Cemento-osseous dysplasias

There is a variety of jaw lesions characterized histologically by the presence of cementum-like tissue. Both clinically and histopathologically, cemento-osseous dysplasias present in a number of forms and variants. The periapical cementodysplasia, florid cemento-osseous dysplasia and some other similar lesions are rare, some of them self-limiting.

Central giant cell granuloma

An intraosseous lesion consisting of more or less cellular fibrous tissue containing multiple foci of hemorrhage and hemosiderin pigment, aggregations of multinucleated osteoclast-like giant cells and sometimes trabeculae of woven bone forming within the septa of more mature fibrous tissue that may traverse the lesion.[6] Giant cell granuloma may occur in either jaw at any age. It is more common in the third decade of life. Radiographically, there is an area of bone destruction showing slender bony septa, resulting in a multilocular appearance. The histologic pattern varies considerably. Very cell-rich areas of a lesion may resemble a giant cell tumor. Histologically, giant cell granuloma cannot be differentiated from cherubism and the brown tumor of hyperparathyroidism. Treatment consists of curettage; some of these tumors are more aggressive.

LESIONS OF SALIVARY GLAND TISSUE ORIGIN

MUCOCELE

Apart from the benign tumors of salivary gland origin,

which will not be dealt with here, mucoceles and ranula are the common lesions which need surgical intervention. A mucocele results from damage to the duct or obstruction to the drainage of a minor salivary gland. As such, it may be a retention or an extravasation cyst. The lower lip opposite the upper canine is most often affected. History often involves a trauma or bite into the area which later develops into a non-tender swelling. Mucoceles may spontaneously rupture but will commonly recur without surgical removal. A linear incision through the overlying mucosa will allow removal of the lesion and its associated minor gland. Recurrence is therefore prevented.

RANULA

A ranula is a site-specific mucous extravasation cyst in the floor of the mouth usually caused by damage to the submandibular gland or duct or, less commonly, the sublingual gland. A ranula (Latin *rana* = frog) is located above the mylohyoid muscle with a diameter of 3 or 4 cm. In rare circumstances it may push between the mylohyoid and genioglossus muscle and present as a swelling in the submandibular triangle, the so-called plunging ranula. Children or young adults are usually affected. Excision, in some cases including the sublingual gland, is recommended. This can be a difficult procedure as the cyst lies between the submandibular duct and the lingual nerve. It is better not to suture the wound as healing is very fast and it prevents any tension in the floor of the mouth from hematoma.

REFERENCES

1. Scully C 1996 New aspects of oral viral diseases. In: Seifert G (ed) Oral pathology – actual diagnostic and prognostic aspects. Springer, Berlin
2. Axèll T, Pindborg JJ, Smith CJ et al 1996 Oral white lesions with special reference to precancerous and tobacco-related lesions: conclusions of an international symposium held in Uppsala, Sweden, May 18–21, 1994. Journal of Oral and Pathological Medicine 25:49–54
3. Pindborg JJ, Reichart PA, Smith CJ, van der Waal I 1997 Histological typing of cancer and precancer of the oral mucosa, 2nd edn. Springer, Berlin
4. Schepman KP, van der Meij EH, Smeele LE, van der Waal I 1996 Prevalence study of oral white lesions with special reference to a new definition of oral leucoplakia. Oral Oncology, European Journal of Cancer 32:416–419
5. Vedtofte P, Holmstrup P, Hjøting-Hansen E, Pindborg JJ 1987 Surgical treatment of premalignant lesions of the oral mucosa. International Journal of Oral and Maxillofacial Surgery 16:656–664
6. Kramer IRH, Pindborg JJ, Shear M 1992 Histological typing of odontogenic tumours, 2nd edn. Springer, Berlin
7. Horch H-H 1995 Chirurgie der Zysten im Kiefer- und Gesichtsbereich. In: Hausamen J-E, Machtens E, Reuther J (eds) Mund- Kiefer-, und Gesichtschirurgie. Springer, Berlin

8. Schulte W 1969 Zentrifugiertes Eigenblut zur Füllung großer Knochendefekte – eine Modifikation der Eigenblutmethode. Deutsche Zahnärztliche Zeitschrift 24:854

9. Kübler N, Urist MR, Reuther J 1992 Subperiostale Knochenneubildung durch Knochenmatrixproteine (bone morphogenetic protein). Deutsche Zeitschrift für Mund-, Kiefer- und Gesichtschirurgie 16:265

10. Urist MR 1989 Bone morphogenetic protein induced bone formation and the bone–bone marrow consortium. In: Aebi M, Regazzoni P (eds) Bone transplantation. Springer, Berlin

11. Reichart PA, Ries P 1983 Considerations on the classification of odontogenic tumours. International Journal of Oral Surgery 12:323–333

12. Reichart PA, Philipsen HP, Sonner S 1995 Ameloblastoma: biological profile of 3677 cases. Oral Oncology, European Journal of Cancer 31b:86–99

13. Ackermann GL, Altini M, Shear M 1988 The unicystic ameloblastoma: a clinicopathological study of 57 cases. Journal of Oral Pathology 17:541–546

14. Philipsen HP, Reichart PA 1996 Squamous odontogenic tumour (SOT): a benign neoplasm of the periodontium. A review of 36 reported cases. Journal of Clinical Periodontology 23:922–926

15. Philipsen HP, Reichart PA, Praetorius F 1997 Mixed odontogenic tumours and odontomas. Considerations on an interrelationship. Review of the literature and presentation of 134 new cases of odontomas. Oral Oncology, European Journal of Cancer 33:86–99

16. Philipsen HP, Reichart PA, Zhang KH, Nikai H, Yu QX 1991 Adenomatoid odontogenic tumour: biological profile based on 499 cases. Journal of Oral Pathology and Medicine 10:149–158

17. Gardner DG. 1996 Central odontogenic fibroma – current concepts. Journal of Oral Pathology and Medicine 25:556–561

18. van der Waal I 1991 Diseases of the jaws – diagnosis and treatment. Munksgaard, Copenhagen

Pathological perspectives of non-malignant lesions of the mouth

88

GERNOT. JUNDT

INTRODUCTION

The mouth is divided into several topographic regions: *lips* with vermilion border of the upper and lower lip and commissures, *buccal mucosa* with cheek mucosa, retroalveolar areas, upper and lower buccal sulci (vestibulum of the mouth), both *upper* and *lower alveolus* and *gingiva* (upper and lower gum), *hard palate, tongue* with dorsal surface including lateral borders and inferior surface, and *floor of the mouth*.[1] The surface is covered by stratified squamous epithelium that in the mouth is more intensely connected with the underlying soft tissues by elongated rete ridges

than with the normal skin (Fig. 88.1). The epithelial surface is mainly of non-keratinizing type in the more mobile parts (lips, cheeks, floor of the mouth) while a parakeratotic (gingiva) or orthokeratotic keratinization (hard palate, upper and lower gum) is found in areas closely fixed to bone and exposed to mastication.[2] Because of local defense mechanisms (e.g. secretory immunoglobulin A and other immunoglobulins, subepithelial lymphocytes and plasma cells, antibacterial effects of saliva, competitive suppression of pathogens by low-virulence organisms) the oral mucosa is very resistant to infectious agents.[3]

Out of the large number of congenital, inflammatory, tumorlike and neoplastic diseases, the following discussion

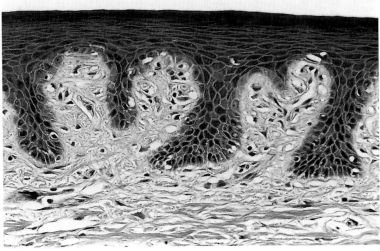

B

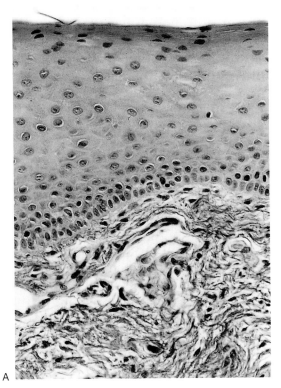

A

Fig. 88.1 (A) Normal (locolabile) mucosa of cheeks, floor of the mouth or lips. Stratified non-keratinized squamous epithelium with prominent basal cell layer and flattened rete ridges. **(B)** Normal (locostable) mucosa, mastication type, of gingiva and hard palate. Stratified squamous epithelium with para- or orthokeratotic keratinization, elongated rete ridges and collagenized submucosal connective tissue.

only deals with the more common lesions, especially those predisposing to or imitating oral cancer. In this context the value of clinical information provided by the clinician to the pathologist cannot be overemphasized.

CONGENITAL ABNORMALITIES

DERMOID CYSTS AND HETEROTOPIAS

Dermoid cysts and heterotopias can give rise to cyst formation in the oral cavity.

A *dermoid cyst* is a rare congenital malformation derived from ectodermal tissue. It is usually found in the midline of the tongue. Clinically, the dermoid cyst presents as a slow-growing painless nodule and may reach diameters from a few millimeters up to more than 10 cm, leading to difficulties in speaking and eating. Such cysts are usually found in younger people. Being a true cyst, the wall is lined by stratified squamous epithelium and may contain adnexal structures of the skin like sebaceous glands or hair follicles (Fig. 88.2). Sometimes an inflammation is superimposed. When centrally located, the differentiation of (traumatic) epithelial inclusion cysts – purely consisting of epidermal elements without adnexal structures and lined by a stratified squamous epithelium – from dermoid cysts is not always possible.

Histologically, the dermoid cyst must be differentiated from the exceptionally rare mature true craniofacial teratomas that contain tissue from all three germ layers. These congenital lesions usually originate in the hypophyseal region and extend through a cleft palate to the oral cavity.

Heterotopic tissue, mainly gastrointestinal epithelium or neural tissue, may also be found in the oral mucosa. Sometimes gastrointestinal epithelial proliferations lead to cyst formation. These heterotopic oral gastrointestinal cysts (enterocystomas) are regarded as choristomas, i.e. normal tissue in an abnormal site. Heterotopic nerve tissue, containing nodule-forming glial and ependyma-like elements, may be found in the hard palate and parapharyngeal tissues. Neoplasms arising from these nodules have been reported.[4,5]

WHITE SPONGE NEVUS

The rare white sponge nevus is an inherited autosomal dominant disease of the oral mucosa, especially affecting the buccal mucosa bilaterally, but may be found in other intra- (and extra-) oral sites. Recent data suggest an inherited mutation of keratin genes for cytokeratins 4 or 13.[6,7]

The lesion is present at birth or in early childhood but progresses during adolescence. If one does not pay attention to the symmetrical distribution and the age of the patient, it clinically can be mistaken for leukoplakia.[1]

Histologically, a prominent acanthosis is seen accompanied by a marked intraepithelial edema leading to clear cell change (Fig. 88.3). There are no atypical cells or dysplastic disturbances of the epithelial architecture. The pathognomonic eosinophilic perinuclear condensations, especially of the spinous layer (consisting of condensed tonofilaments[8],) are not always present and best visible on Papanicoulaou-stained smears. As the lesion is harmless, no therapy is necessary when

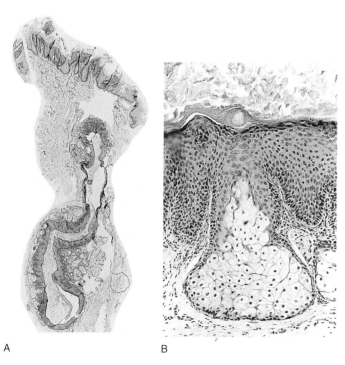

A   B

Fig. 88.2 (A) Dermoid cyst of the tongue with sebaceous glands near to the cyst wall, lined by stratified keratinized squamous epithelium **(B)** with granular cells and desquamation of the cornified layer into the lumen of the cyst. Sebaceous glands (center, lower half) are in close connection to the epithelial lining.

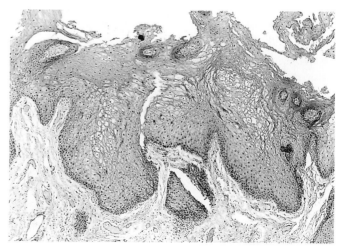

Fig. 88.3 White sponge nevus. Acanthotic squamous epithelium with clearly visible basal cells and light-appearing keratinocytes of spinous layer due to intraepithelial edema. No cellular atypia.

the diagnosis is established. Differentiation from leukedema, a thickening of the epithelium with striking edema of the spinous layer prevailing in smokers, may be difficult.

FORDYCE GRANULES

Histologically, *Fordyce granules* or *Fordyce disease* consist of normal sebaceous glands appearing in an abnormal location, the oral mucosa, thus representing a true choristoma (Fig. 88.4). Clinically, yellow to white, sometimes confluent papules are seen mainly on the buccal mucosa or the vermilion border of the upper lip. Rarely the glands can enlarge and present as discrete nodules.[9] They are more common in adults than in children, probably reflecting hormonal stimuli during puberty. These granules may be found in 80% of the population. As they are asymptomatic and harmless, no treatment is required.

JUXTAORAL ORGAN (ORGAN OF CHIEVITZ)

Near to the internal pterygoid muscle in the buccotemporal space adjacent to the fascia buccotemporalis and innervated by the buccal nerve, a normal, constantly present anatomic structure can be found (Fig. 88.5) that may give rise to the

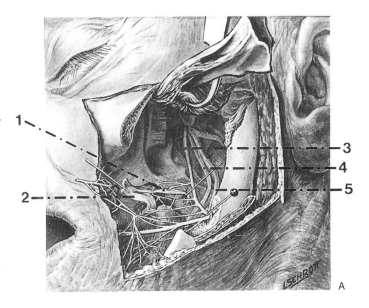

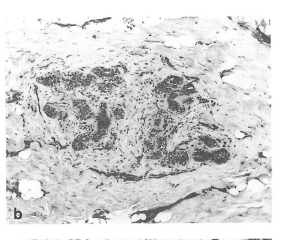

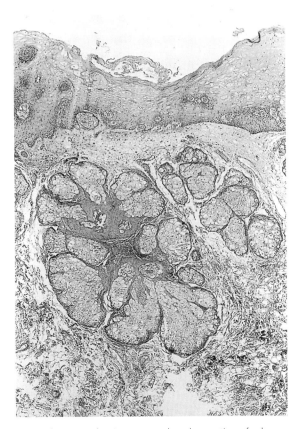

Fig. 88.4 Fordyce granules. Intramucosal agglomeration of sebaceous glands underneath the buccal epithelial surface.

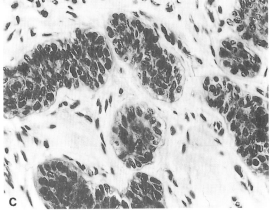

Fig. 88.5 (A) Juxtaoral organ (organ of Chievitz). Topographic localization of the juxtaoral organ (1) in the spatium buccotemporale close to the fascia buccotemporalis (2) and innervated by the buccal nerve (3) that is located next to the lingual (4) and inferior alveolar nerves (5). **(B)** Juxtaoral organ at low power surrounded by a perineurium-like stratum fibrosum (upper half). At higher magnification (lower half) epithelial cells arranged in small nests or trabecular structures are clearly visible (with permission from Zenker W 1982 *The Juxtaoral Organ*. Urban & Schwarzenberg, Baltimore).

erroneous diagnosis of perineural invasion of a squamous cell carcinoma.[10–12] This so-called *juxtaoral organ*, first described by Chievitz erroneously as a kind of parotid appendage only present during embryonic life, was investigated in detail by Zenker.[13] It represents small epithelial nests in sensory nerve endings[13,14] that might undergo nodular hyperplasia.[15] The typical setting should help the pathologist to avoid the confusion with a carcinoma.

INFLAMMATORY AND OTHER NON-NEOPLASTIC DISEASES

GENERAL REMARKS

Inflammation is a localized complex tissue reaction to injury. Its morphologic appearance in oral mucosa is influenced by the endogenous or exogenous cause and the immunologic

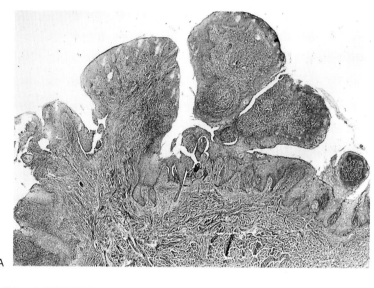

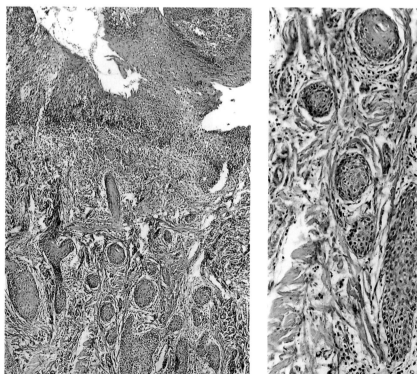

Fig. 88.6 Inflammatory papillary hyperplasia. **(A)** Acanthotic stratified squamous epithelium with papillary projections and elongated rete ridges. **(B)** Pseudoepitheliomatous hyperplasia mimicking invasion of epithelial cells into submucosa. **(C)** Absence of cellular atypia and dysplastic changes helps in distinguishing pseudoepitheliomatous hyperplasia from invasive squamous cell carcinoma.

defense mechanisms of the human organism. Common causes are viral, bacterial or fungal infections, ill-fitting dentures and – mostly ill-defined – (auto)immunologic disturbances. Additional factors like smoking and alcohol may also contribute to the clinical picture. Macroscopically, vesiculo-bullous lesions are separated from erosive-ulcerative conditions and white lesions. While the first group is mainly related to viral infections and immunologic disorders, bacterial and fungal infection or immunologic disturbances (as well as neoplasms) are found in the second group. The third group comprises hereditary conditions, reactive and immunologic related lesions, fungal infections, precancerous states and invasive carcinomas.[16]

In the following text, those lesions that histologically – especially without provided clinical information – may be mistaken for carcinoma are briefly discussed.

INFLAMMATORY PAPILLARY HYPERPLASIA

Predominantly on the hard palate of denture-wearing patients, a soft, non-removable, bright red-colored papillary overgrowth of the oral mucosa may be present. This condition, termed *inflammatory papillary hyperplasia*,[17] is strongly associated with ill-fitting dentures, permanent denture wearing and poor dental hygiene. Often, an additional candida infection is found but its role in the pathogenesis is controversial. Histologically, multiple mucosal projections covered by thickened stratified squamous epithelium are found. At the base of the lesion pseudoepitheliomatous hyperplasia may be seen, leading to the erroneous diagnosis of cancer in small biopsies without accompanying clinical data (Fig. 88.6). However, the lack of atypical cells and the absence of epithelial dysplasia should lead to the right diagnosis. In addition, a chronic inflammatory infiltrate of lymphocytes and plasma cells is common. In long-standing cases subepithelial fibrosis may predominate and give rise to an *irritation fibroma*.

CANDIDA-RELATED LESIONS

Candidiasis, almost exclusively caused by *C. albicans*, is the most common infective disease of the oral mucosa. As *C. albicans* is found in high frequency in the normal healthy population additional factors are necessary to cause overt clinical symptoms, e.g. alterations of the immunological status of the host, endogenous or exogenous endocrine disturbances, pathogenicity of the respective strain or changes in the composition of the normal bacterial flora of the mouth. A weak inflammatory response in an adequate biopsy should raise the suspicion of an underlying immunocompromised state. Most Candida infections are diagnosed clinically in combination with exfoliative cytology.

Sometimes the usually removable white patches cannot be scraped off. It is not clear whether this rare form, termed *chronic hyperplastic candidiasis*, represents leukoplakia in combination with fungal infection or fungal-induced hyperkeratosis of the underlying epithelium. The lesions are found in the anterior buccal mucosa and have to be biopsied if antimycotic therapy is unsuccessful. Histologically, a parakeratotic hyperplastic epithelium superficially invaded by Candida hyphae can easily be demonstrated by a PAS or silver (Grocott) stain. Inflammatory cells, especially neutrophil granulocytes, are found throughout the epithelium and in the lamina propria. Elongated, plump rete ridges may mimic the appearance of verrucous carcinoma.

Closely related to chronic hyperplastic candidiasis is *median rhomboid glossitis*, a benign, usually painless red and elevated lesion anterior to the foramen cecum. It may reach a size from a few millimeters to several centimeters. Formerly it was thought to be a developmental abnormality but some studies point to a relation with Candida infection.[18] Microscopically, there is loss of the filiform papillae, acanthosis and sometimes hyperparakeratosis. A mild infiltrate of lymphocytes and plasma cells is present in the lamina propria, together with superficial Candida hyphae. The rete ridges are elongated, plump and show pseudoepitheliomatous hyperplasia. Mitoses or atypical cells are absent (Fig. 88.7). Although squamous cell carcinoma only rarely occurs in the center of the tongue, tissue from a superficial biopsy may be misdiagnosed as carcinoma.

SYPHILIS

On rare occasions, syphilis presents with a primary oral manifestation. This veneral infectious disease, caused by *Treponema pallidum*, passes through three different stages when left untreated. In recent years an increase has occurred, primarily in immunocompromised patients. Histologically, a plasma cell-dominated granulomatous infiltrate with giant cells is found typically in a perivascular location with obliterative endarteritis. Spirochetes can be visualized by silver impregnation techniques or immunofluorescence microscopy. In stage III an atrophic glossitis develops ('*syphilitic glossitis*') that seems to predispose to leukoplakic changes which may undergo malignant transformation.[1] However, some reports question this association.[19]

LICHEN PLANUS

The etiology of *lichen planus*, a dermoepidermal disease with oral manifestations, is still unknown. Immunologic factors seem to play an important role in this mucocutaneous disease that is rare in children and more common in

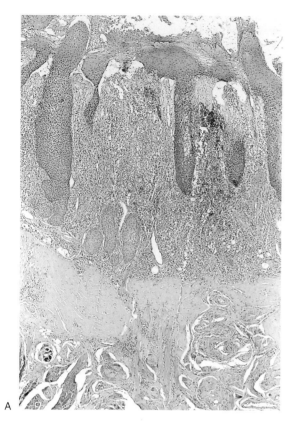

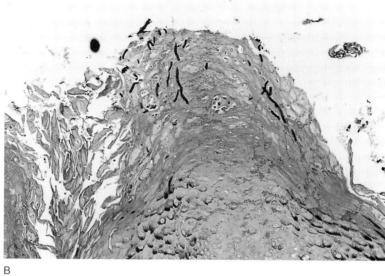

Fig. 88.7 Median rhomboid glossitis. **(A)** Epithelial acanthosis with marked elongated rete ridges and pseudoepitheliomatous hyperplasia accompanied by a moderate lymphoplasmacytic inflammation. Skeletal muscle of the tongue is visible at the bottom. **(B)** Superficial hyperparakeratosis with cellular desquamation and black-colored intraepithelial Candida hyphae.

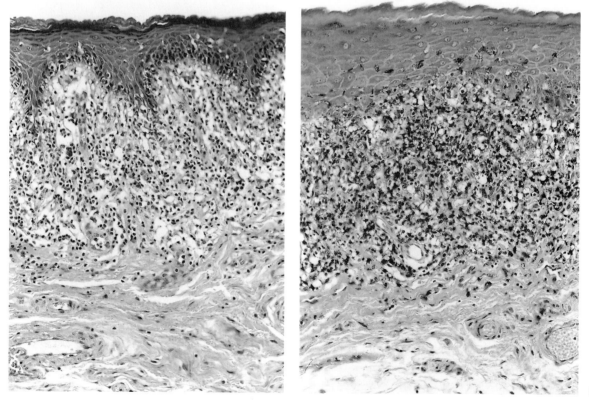

Fig. 88.8 Lichen planus. **(A)** Saw-tooth-like configuration of rete ridges partly obscured by a dense band-like lymphocytic infiltration of the basal epithelial parts and bordering subepithelial mesenchyme. **(B)** Inflammatory cells predominantly react with T-cell antibodies, e.g. UCHL 1/CD 45RO.

middle-aged female adults.[20,21] Additionally, an association between hepatitis C infections and lichen planus is reported.[22,23] Lichen planus has to be differentiated from lichenoid-like drug reactions or contact reactions to amalgam and lichenoid dysplasia.[24,25] Clinically, there are different forms of oral lichen planus: the most common, often asymptomatic *reticular variant* produces the characteristic white streaks ('Wickham striae'), plaquelike or papular lesions reminiscent of leukoplakia but with a multifocal distribution and *atrophic, erosive or bullous variants*, with dark red, sometimes ulcerated areas. Usually the lesions are located in the posterior buccal mucosa.

Histologically, epithelial hyperplasia with acanthosis, hyper-para- or -orthokeratosis or atrophy is present. Characteristically, the rete ridges have a sawtooth appearance. There is basal cell degeneration with hyaline bodies ('Civatte bodies') accompanied by a dense and pure lymphocytic infiltrate obscuring the epithelial–mesenchymal interface (Fig. 88.8). Epithelial atypia or dysplastic changes are usually absent but may be induced by concomitant Candida infection. Long-standing erosive and atrophic forms are thought to undergo malignant transformation but this is still controversial[26,27] and the risk seems to be low.[28–30]

BENIGN EPITHELIAL TUMORS AND TUMORLIKE LESIONS

HPV-ASSOCIATED EPITHELIAL PROLIFERATIONS

Some of the most frequent papillary epithelial proliferations in the oral mucosa are *squamous papillomas*. They are nearly always related to a human papillomavirus (HPV) infection. HPV is a double-stranded DNA virus of the papova group capable of completely integrating into the host genome. More than 70 subtypes are known. Their identification is facilitated by in situ hybridization and more recently by the polymerase chain reaction.[31,32] There has been increasing suspicion that HPV is implicated in some premalignant and malignant oral lesions.[33] Some subtypes are linked to papillomas (type 6 or 11), other benign lesions like verruca vulgaris, condyloma acuminatum, focal epithelial hyperplasia (type 2, 4, 6, 11, 13, and 32) or neoplastic changes (type 16, 18) of the epithelium.[34]

Papillomas are most often found on the vermilion border of the lip, the tongue or the soft palate, presenting as an exophytic lesion with fingerlike projections. They are most often found in middle-aged patients but may occur at any age. Histologically, a fine fibrovascular core is covered by regular proliferating squamous epithelium showing para-keratotic or orthokeratotic keratinization. This may lead to a macroscopically visible white colorization but only rarely raises suspicion of carcinoma. Dysplastic changes are usually absent or, when they occur, are always mild. A typical finding are the so-called 'koilocytes' (epithelial cells with pyknotic nuclei surrounded by a clear halo) that indicate HPV- induced alterations.

Another HPV-related lesion that appears with increasing frequency in the oral mucosa is *condyloma acuminatum*. It is regarded as a sexually transmitted disease and often found in immunocompromised patients. HPV can nearly always be demonstrated, usually types 2, 6, 11, 16 and 18. Microscopically, there is pseudopapillomatous epithelial proliferation with broad acanthosis and blunted epithelial downward projections. Koilocytes are commonly seen and keratinization is usually missing (Fig. 88.9).

Verruca vulgaris is a third HPV-related lesion (mainly type 2[35,36]) that is very common on the skin but also occurs in the anterior parts of the mouth, obviously by autoinoculation. It is usually found in children but may also be seen in adults. Morphologically, the epithelium shows a broad-based cauliflower-like proliferation with hyper(para)keratosis, acanthosis and a broad granular layer containing basophilic keratohyaline granules and koilocytes. The plump rete ridges tend to bend to the center of the lesion. If an inadequate or tangentially orientated biopsy is performed the separation from well-differentiated squamous cell carcinoma may be difficult.[1]

Focal epithelial hyperplasia (Heck's disease) has only recently been linked to HPV (type 13, 32) infection.[37,38] In early studies the disease was described in native Americans in both South and North America, and Inuits (Eskimos) but it is increasingly found in other areas as well. Preferentially, the disease occurs in children but is also found in patients of older ages. Mostly, the tongue, the labial and the buccal mucosa are affected. On macroscopic examination there are single or multifocal well-demarcated aggregates of wart-like lesions, sometimes covering a larger area, usually without discoloration.

Histologically, there is often abrupt acanthosis, mainly by enlargement of the stratum spinosum, with thickening, clubbing and fusion of rete ridges (Fig. 88.10). Characteristically, mitotic-like figures ('mitosoid cells') may be found in the superficial epithelial layers in addition to koilocytes. The presence of mitosoid cells may lead to the misdiagnosis of carcinoma in situ. The lesion is perfectly benign, readily diagnosed from its clinical aspect and usually needs no therapy as it regresses spontaneously.

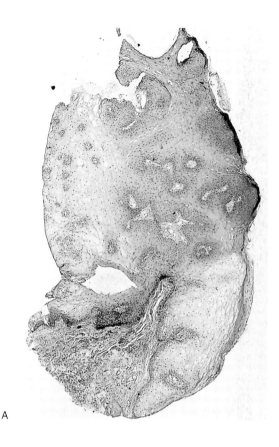

A

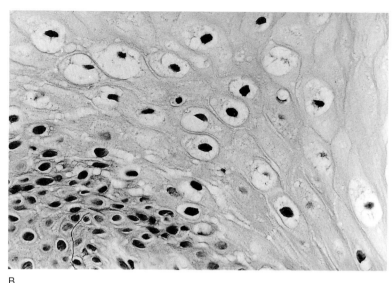

B

Fig. 88.9 Condyloma acuminatum. **(A)** Pseudopapillomatous acanthotic epithelial proliferation. **(B)** Koilocytes, i.e. epithelial cells with perinuclear halo and condensed nuclear chromatin, in spinous layer.

VERRUCIFORM XANTHOMA

The etiology of *verruciform xanthoma* is still unknown but is linked to localized epithelial trauma or damage. Recent studies point to an immunologically mediated pathogenesis.[39] It is an uncommon benign oral lesion, mainly of the gingiva, most often found in middle-aged patients, preferentially in women. Usually sharply circumscribed and small, it may reach up to 4 cm in diameter.[40] The lesion may be clinically mistaken for a verrucous carcinoma.

On histology, there is an epithelial proliferation with acanthosis, hyperparakeratosis and prominent papillomatosis. The elongated rete ridges are of a nearly uniform length.

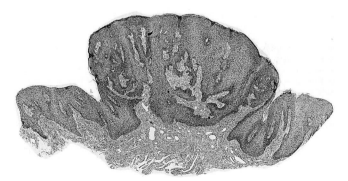

Fig. 88.10 Focal epithelial hyperplasia (Heck's disease). Abrupt epithelial thickening with marked acanthosis, absence of cellular atypia and fusion of rete ridges.

They are in close contact with accumulations of large xanthoma cells, i.e. vacuolated histiocytes, containing lipids and diastase-resistant PAS-positive granules. Underneath the epithelium a dense inflammatory infiltrate is found, consisting mainly of T cells. Dysplastic changes are absent. Recurrences after surgical removal are rare.

EPITHELIAL DYSPLASIA AND CARCINOMA IN SITU

The terms *leukoplakia* and *erythroplakia* are commonly used as synonyms for precancerous lesions of the oral mucosa. However, according to the WHO, both terms should only be used for those clinical findings (white or red lesions of the oral mucosa) that cannot be otherwise characterized, histologically or clinically.[1] Therefore, all other diseases with a similar appearance have to be ruled out before a clinical diagnosis of leukoplakia can be made, e.g. lichen planus, frictional keratosis, nicotine stomatitis, white sponge nevus or erythematous candidiasis, and mucositis associated with infections, etc.

Macroscopically, leukoplakias can be divided into the (more common) *homogenous* and the (rare) *inhomogenous* types. The latter have a greater risk for developing cancer. This risk is increased at certain sites like floor of the mouth, tongue and lip.[41]

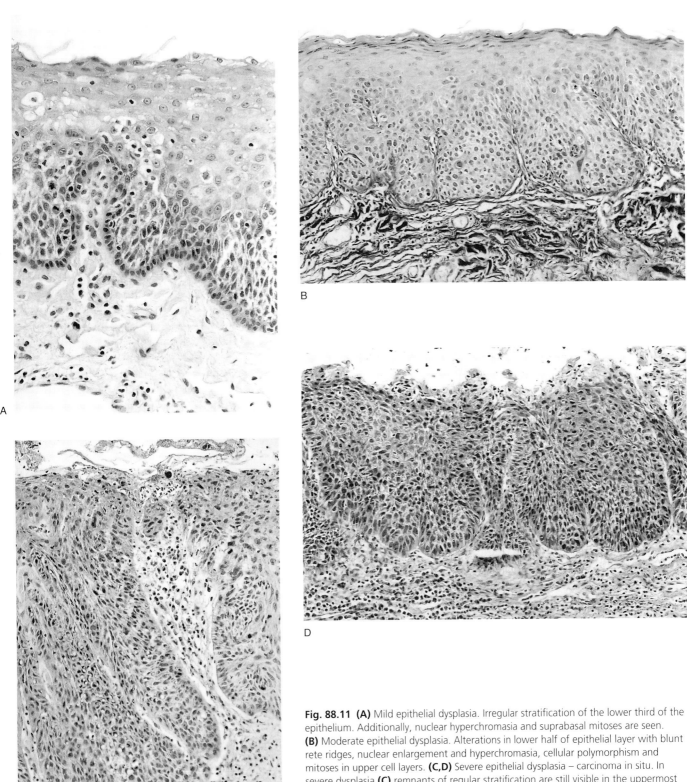

Fig. 88.11 **(A)** Mild epithelial dysplasia. Irregular stratification of the lower third of the epithelium. Additionally, nuclear hyperchromasia and suprabasal mitoses are seen. **(B)** Moderate epithelial dysplasia. Alterations in lower half of epithelial layer with blunt rete ridges, nuclear enlargement and hyperchromasia, cellular polymorphism and mitoses in upper cell layers. **(C,D)** Severe epithelial dysplasia – carcinoma in situ. In severe dysplasia **(C)** remnants of regular stratification are still visible in the uppermost cell layer in addition to atypical mitoses, loss of cell polarity, nuclear polymorphism and hyperchromasia. In carcinoma in situ **(D)**, alterations comprise the whole epithelial thickness, however tumor cells do not cross the basal lamina. All dysplastic changes are usually accompanied by chronic inflammation.

To achieve a definitive diagnosis a biopsy is necessary to determine the grade of dysplastic change that runs parallel to the development of overt cancer. For biopsy, that part of the lesion should be chosen in which the most extensive dysplastic alterations usually occur. With ascending frequency these are nodular, verruciform, ulcerated, erythroleukoplakic or pure erythroplakic areas.

The histologic findings should be termed keratosis and are graded to assess the severity of dysplastic changes.[42] Usually, epithelial dysplasia is classified as mild, moderate, severe and carcinoma in situ (Fig. 88.11). Severe dysplasia and carcinoma in situ seem to carry a similar high risk for cancer development.[1] Almost 7% of all leukoplakias are severe forms or carcinomas on histologic examination.[43]

Microscopically, leukoplakias show acanthosis and hyperortho- or -parakeratosis, sometimes combined with mild chronic inflammation of the lamina propria. Dysplastic changes are not seen in all cases. These sometimes subtle alterations typically begin in the basal epithelial layer and involve the whole epithelial thickness with progressive disease.[44] They include:

- enlargement of nuclei
- altered nuclear:cytoplasmic ratio
- cellular and nuclear pleomorphism
- nuclear hyperchromasia
- dyskeratoses (i.e. abnormal keratinization of single cells in deeper epithelial layers)
- increased and/or abnormal mitotic activity
- mitoses above the basal layer
- irregularity of normal epithelial stratification
- loss of cellular maturation
- coarse or blunt rete ridges

In *mild dysplasia* these changes are present in the basal third of the epithelial layer. *Moderate dysplasia* is confined to the lower half of the epithelium whereas in *severe dysplasia* more than half of the epithelium demonstrates alterations. In *carcinoma in situ* dysplastic changes are found throughout the whole epithelial thickness but invasion of the lamina propria is absent. As the true risk of leukoplakias or erythroplakias developing cancer can obviously only be estimated, all lesions with dysplastic changes should be removed or at least thoroughly controlled.

ACTINIC CHEILITIS

Similar to actinic keratosis of the skin, *actinic cheilitis* represents a premalignant lesion of the vermilion border, especially of the lower lip, due to alterations induced by the ultraviolet components (UV-B) of sunlight. Actinic cheilitis is found especially in light-complexioned persons with a tendency to sunburn.[45] Most patients are older than 50 years.

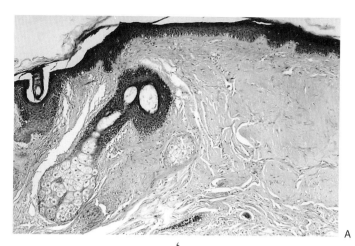

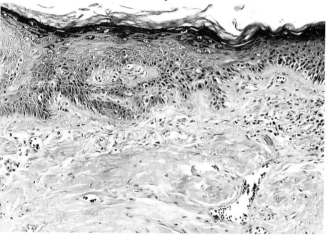

Fig. 88.12 (A) Actinic elastosis. Homogenization of subepithelial collagen with fragmentation of elastic fibers and epithelial atrophy ('solar elastosis'). In actinic cheilitis **(B)** these changes are accompanied by a mild to moderate chronic inflammation with or without epithelial dysplasia.

Outdoor workers or sun worshippers are at particular risk for developing actinic lesions. After prolonged exposure, squamous cell carcinomas develop in about 9% of actinic cheilitis.[46]

Histologically, the epithelium shows atrophy and often hyperkeratosis associated with varying degrees of dysplasia. Additionally, the underlying tissue demonstrates damage to elastic fibers and collagen ('solar elastosis'). A mild chronic inflammation is usually present (Fig. 88.12). As in other forms of epithelial dysplasia, the risk of progression to malignancy increases with the grade of dysplastic changes.

BENIGN SOFT-TISSUE TUMORS AND TUMORLIKE LESIONS

ORAL SUBMUCOUS FIBROSIS

Oral submucous fibrosis is generally seen in India or south east Asia and is obviously associated with betel quid chewing, although it may rarely be found in other patients as well.[39,47,48] It can also be found in immigrants from this geographical region. There is evidence from experimental data that betel nut components increase collagen production enormously.[43] Chewing of pan masala/gutkha, a mix of tobacco and a less moist form of betel quid lacking the betel leaf, seems to be associated with an earlier age of onset of oral submucous fibrosis.[49] The lesion is mostly found in young persons and the soft palate and the buccal mucosa are mainly affected. Usually the patients complain of pain when eating spicy food. An increased stiffness and a whitish palor of the affected area are found.

Histologically, hyalinized, poorly vascularized collagen depositions are visible in the submucosa while the epithelium is atrophic. In 10–15% dysplastic changes occur, leading to the development of squamous cell carcinoma.

EPULIS GRANULOMATOSA, GIANT CELL EPULIS, EPULIS FISSURATA, OSSIFYING FIBROID EPULIS

Strictly speaking, the term 'epulis' derives from the Greek and denotes any lesion that develops on the gingiva or alveolar mucosa, irrespective of its histology. In general, only reactive lesions in tooth-bearing areas leading to localized tumor formation are diagnosed as epulis with the exception of epulis congenita, a benign (myofibroblastic?) soft-tissue tumor of the newborn.[50] However, some authors prefer to abandon the term 'epulis' and to diagnose these lesions descriptively.[51] Additionally, one should bear in mind that some intraoral malignant tumors may present in an epulislike fashion so histologic examination seems advisable.[52]

Histologically, four different types may be discriminated:

- epulis granulomatosa (pyogenic/telangiectatic granuloma)
- giant cell epulis (peripheral giant cell granuloma)
- epulis fissurata (denture epulis, inflammatory fibrous hyperplasia)
- epulis fibromatosa/ossifying fibroid epulis (peripheral ossifying fibroma).

As *epulis granulomatosa* is also found in parts of the mouth other than the gingiva, the more descriptive term *telangiectatic or pyogenic granuloma* should be preferred for lesions of the lips, tongue or buccal mucosa. All these lesions are obviously related to trauma or minor injuries presenting an exuberant tumorlike tissue reaction. Although occurring at any age, epulis granulomatosa mainly presents in adolescents and young adults, especially females. Obviously, hormonal stimuli play an important role as these lesions

often develop during pregnancy ('*epulis gravidarum*'). Macroscopically, they present as painless, at times rapidly growing red-blue lesions covered by normal-appearing mucosa that is sometimes ulcerated and may raise the suspicion of malignancy. On histology, an often lobulated, highly vascularized type of granulation tissue is seen infiltrated by neutrophil granulocytes, plasma cells and lymphocytes. In older lesions there is a tendency towards fibrosis (Fig. 88.13). If the lesion is removed and underlying etiologic problems are eliminated, there is only rarely a tendency for recurrence.

The *giant cell epulis* or *peripheral giant cell granuloma* develops exclusively on the gingiva or edentulous alveolar ridges. It can be seen at any age but mostly occurs in females between 40 and 60 years. Giant cell epulis is also probably reactive in nature, perhaps due to bleeding, as erythrocytes or siderin deposits are very often found close to giant cell clusters. On visual inspection it cannot be differentiated from epulis granulomatosa/pyogenic granuloma. As in its intraosseously located counterpart ('central giant cell granuloma'), the histologic hallmark of giant cell epulis are groups of giant cells with 5–20 nuclei scattered around the whole lesion, often accompanied by fresh bleeding or hemosiderin deposits in macrophages. The stroma has the aspect of a granulation tissue with a mixed infiltrate of inflammatory cells and sometimes with collagen production or scarce reactive bone formation. Mitoses are always found but atypical forms are absent. After surgical removal recurrences may occur. Although extremely rare, a 'brown tumor' of hyperparathyroidism should be ruled out by laboratory tests as its histology is almost identical to central or peripheral giant cell granuloma.

The *epulis fissurata* (*denture epulis, inflammatory fibrous hyperplasia*) represents a reactive tissue alteration that is obviously related to persistent traumatization by ill-fitting dentures. As the clinical situation implies, it is most commonly found in elderly patients, with a female predominance. The lesion presents as single or multiple firm folds mostly of the anterior alveolar mucosa. At times ulcerations are seen. On histology fibrous connective tissue is covered by hyperparakeratotic squamous epithelium with irregular, elongated rete ridges and sometimes pseudoepitheliomatous hyperplasia. A sparse infiltrate of chronic inflammation may be present. Rarely, osseous or chondromatous metaplasia may occur,[53] leading the pathologist to the suspicion of an underlying sarcoma. This mistake can be avoided by providing sufficient clinical data.

The *epulis fibromatosa/ossifying fibroid epulis (peripheral ossifying fibroma)* is regarded by some authors as a development stage of a pyogenic granuloma. In favor of this assumption are the occurrence in younger age groups and

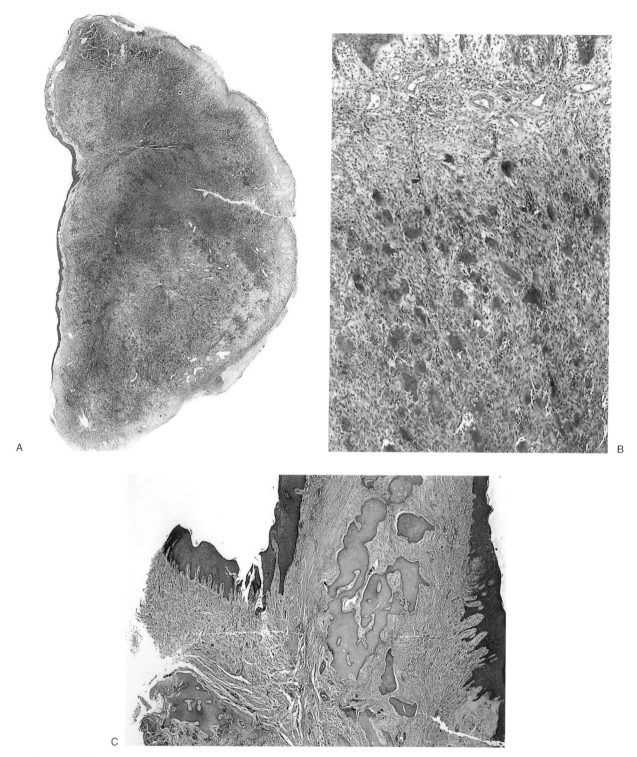

Fig. 88.13 (A) Epulis gigantocellularis. Low power view of a completely excised giant cell epulis covered with normal stratified epithelium and many dot-like dark inclusions representing giant cells. **(B)** Multiple foreign body giant cells are scattered throughout the subepithelial stroma. **(C)** The stroma of ossifying fibroid epulis is characterized by incorporation of bony trabeculae or cemental masses.

the prevalence in females. However, in contrast to pyogenic granuloma, it almost exclusively occurs in the gingiva and mainly on the interdental papillae.[54] Very often the surface is ulcerated. On histology a cellular fibroblastic proliferation predominates with intermingled inflammatory cells and capillaries. Additionally, calcifications and mineralizations are found, sometimes appearing as bone trabeculae or cementum-like depositions. At times newly formed unmineralized osteoid is visible. The lesion is connected to the periosteum which should also be excised, otherwise a high recurrence rate has to be expected.

EPULIS CONGENITA

In contrast to the aforementioned lesions, *congenital epulis* is a true soft-tissue neoplasm that occurs exclusively on the alveolar ridges of newborn children.[55] It presents as a fleshy prolabial mass lateral to the midline and more often in the maxilla than in the mandible. The lesion is about ten times more common in females than in males. Although on light microscopy there is great similarity to the granular cell tumor of the adult (see below), immunohistochemical and ultrastructural findings point to a myofibroblastic differentiation.[50] The tumor is characterized by large polygonal cells with abundant eosinophilic granular cytoplasm and small, round, dark-staining nuclei. Mitoses are rare. In contrast to the adult granular cell tumor, the overlying epithelium never shows pseudoepitheliomatous hyperplasia but shortened rete ridges (Fig. 88.14). The tumor is totally benign. Even after incomplete excisions recurrences are not seen.[55] In rare cases spontaneous regression occurs.[56]

FIBROMA, GIANT CELL FIBROMA AND FIBROMATOSIS

Most probably the so-called *fibroma* of the oral mucosa is reactive in nature and represents a scarlike endstage of a mucosal injury. The lesion is often found along the row of the teeth in the buccal mucosa, representing the local tissue response to biting the cheek ('*irritation fibroma*'). True tumors may exist but lesions without an identifiable cause are extremely rare. Fibromas are sessile, seldom pedunculated and bear the color of the surrounding mucosa. They are usually found in adults.

On histology dense collagenous connective tissue is covered by squamous epithelium often with atrophic rete ridges. A mild inflammatory infiltrate consisting of some lymphocytes and plasma cells may be present. Although atypical cells or dysplastic changes of the epithelium are always absent and the fibromas are usually diagnosed clinically, complete excision and histologic examination are recommended to rule out other benign or malignant tumors.

A rare type of fibroma occurs from childhood to early adulthood and presents as a nodule on the gingiva. The

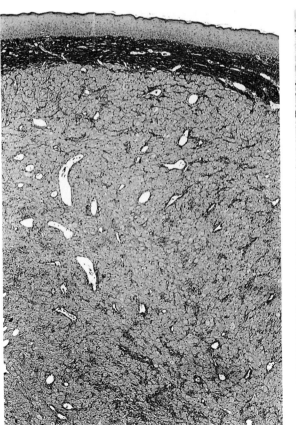
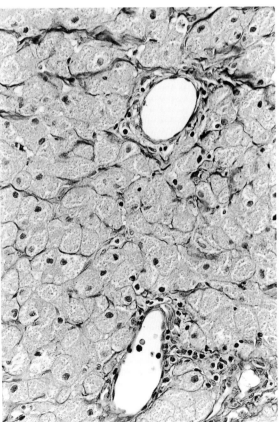

A   B

Fig. 88.14 (A) Congenital epulis with cell-rich lesional tissue that compresses subepithelial collagen leading to completely flattened epithelial rete ridges. **(B)** The tumor cells are well delineated, rich in granulated cytoplasm and possess small, dark-staining nuclei.

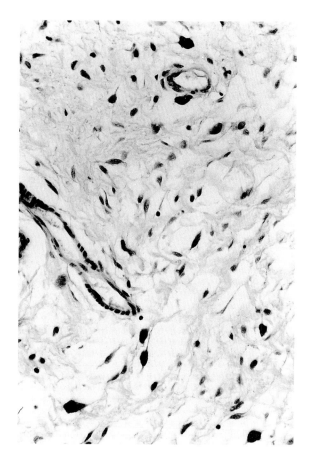

Fig. 88.15 Giant cell fibroma. Loosely arranged connective tissue with some enlarged cells containing dark-staining irregular shaped nuclei.

tongue or the palate may also be involved. This lesion is characterized microscopically by loosely arranged vascular connective tissue with numerous large stellate fibroblasts, some of them containing several nuclei. Therefore the lesion is termed *giant cell fibroma* (Fig. 88.15). The treatment consists of excision. Recurrences are rarely seen.[57]

Fibromatosis or *extra-abdominal desmoid* is an aggressive fibrous proliferation that occurs mainly in adolescents and young adults but may also be seen during childhood. Usually found in the trunk and shoulder, the head and neck may also be involved, especially the perimandibular connective tissue.[58] On histologic examination highly differentiated fibroblasts with innocent-appearing nuclei infiltrate into the surrounding connective tissue, skeletal muscle and even bone. The lesion never metastasizes. Numerous mitoses or atypical mitotic forms should raise the suspicion of fibrosarcoma. Treatment consists of wide excision with safe margins but recurrence rates are very high.

MYOFIBROMA AND MYOFIBROMATOSIS

These rare hamartomatous lesions are seen in a more common solitary form (*myofibroma*) or as multiple nodules (*myofibromatosis*).[59,60] They may also occur in bone and internal organs.[61] Neonates and infants are affected but some lesions have also been reported in adults.[62] The nodules are composed of spindle-shaped myofibroblastic cells and collagen and are richly vascularized. Usually a zonal arrangement is present with more eosinophilic elongated cells in the periphery and hemangiopericytoma-like areas in the center of the lesion. Centrally located necroses may lead to the erroneous diagnosis of sarcoma. Immunohistochemistry is of help in differentiating the lesion from hemangiopericytoma, smooth-muscle or neurogenic tumors (Table 88.1). A marginal resection is sufficient and spontaneous regressions

Table 88.1 Immunohistochemical findings in soft-tissue tumors

	Vim	Act	SMA	Des	Myo	S-100	EMA
Fibroma	+	–	–	–	–	–	–
Fibromatosis	+	–	–	–	–	–	–
Myofibroma	+	+	+	–	–	–	–
Leiomyoma	(+)	+	+	+	–	–	–
Rhabdomyoma	–	+	–	+	+	–	–
Palisaded encapsulated neuroma	+	–	–	–	–	+	+
Mucosal neuroma	+	–	–	–	–	+	+
Neurilemoma	+	–	–	–	–	+	+
Neurofibroma	(+)	–	–	–	–	(+)	–
Granular cell tumor	+	–	–	–	–	+	–
Epulis congenita	+	–	–	–	–	–	–

Vim, vimentin; Act, human muscle (α, γ) actin (clone HHF 35); SMA, α-smooth muscle actin (clone 1A4); Des, desmin; Myo, myoglobin; S-100, S-100 protein; EMA, epithelial membrane antigen

occur. Multifocal involvement including the viscera worsens the prognosis, especially in infants and small children.

MYOGENIC TUMORS

Leiomyoma and rhabdomyoma

Tumors of smooth-muscle differentiation in the oral cavity are rare. These lesions may present as leiomyomas, angioleiomyomas or as epithelioid leiomyomas.[63] Although frequently found in the gastrointestinal tract, *epithelioid leiomyomas* (leiomyoblastomas) are extremely rare in the oral cavity.[64] Most *leiomyomas* occur in middle-aged adults. The lips, tongue, palate and cheeks are the main locations in the oral cavity. Usually the tumor is painless. Histologically, leiomyomas are composed of spindle-shaped cells with eosinophilic cytoplasm and blunt-ended or cigar-shaped nuclei, showing almost no nucleoli or atypia. Necroses are absent and mitoses are rare. More than five mitoses per ten high-power fields warrant the diagnosis of leiomyosarcoma. The cells are arranged in interlacing bundles. Special stains may highlight intracellular longitudinal striations and immunohistochemistry (positive for smooth-muscle actin, muscle actins, or desmin; negative for S-100 protein) will confirm its leiomyomatous nature (Fig. 88.16).

Oral *angioleiomyomas* present as small and well-circumscribed nodules of smooth muscle intermingled with thickwalled vessels.[65] While the inner layer of the vessel's musculature is regularly arranged, the outer layer blends into the surrounding tumor tissue. Myxoid change, calcifications and incorporated fat are seen in this always benign lesion.[64]

Rhabdomyomas are benign tumors of skeletal muscle.[66] In contrast to other soft-tissue tumors, they are far outnumbered by their malignant counterparts, the various forms of rhabdomyosarcoma. The very rare *fetal type* of rhabdomyoma is preferentially found in infants not older than 1 year but may also occur in older children and even in adults.[61] In contrast and important for the differential diagnosis with rhabdomyosarcoma, these lesions are well circumscribed, confined to the submucosa and may be pedunculated. Microscopically, they contain relatively uniform spindle-shaped cells with mild pleomorphism intermingled with myofibrils and sometimes embedded in a myxoid stroma. Cross-striations may be found. Mitoses are rare or absent (Fig. 88.17). The *adult type* of rhabdomyoma is more common in men between 40 and 60 years. Intraoral lesions are found in the floor of the mouth, soft palate or base of the tongue. About 20% are multifocal and usually confined to the neck.[67] The tumor is well demarcated and consists of tightly packed cells with enlarged granular eosinophilic cytoplasm. Cross-striations can be identified at least in some cells. One or two small nuclei are peripherally placed. In general, no mitoses are found. Because of fixational and processing artifacts resulting in loss of glycogen, the cyto-

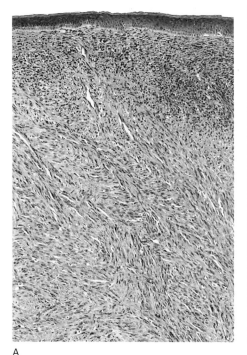 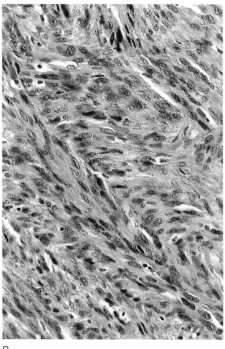 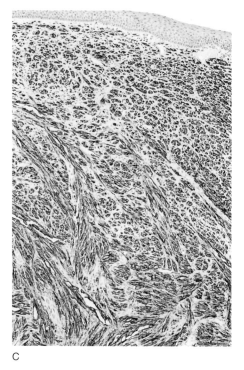

A   B   C

Fig. 88.16 (A,B) Subepithelial leiomyoma composed of spindle-shaped cells with inconspicuous nuclei arranged in intersecting bundles at right angles. **(C)** Immunohistochemically, the tumor cells are positive for desmin and smooth-muscle actin (not shown). Epithelium (top) is negative.

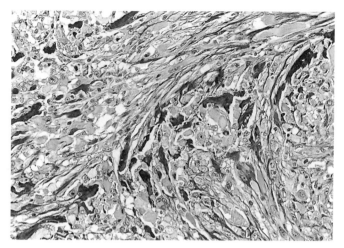

Fig. 88.17 Rhabdomyoma with remnants of dark-staining collagen fibers (van Gieson stain). The tumor cells are rich in cytoplasm, polygonal to spindle-shaped with only moderate nuclear irregularities and no mitoses.

plasm is vacuolated and might be retracted from the cell membrane, leading to a 'spider web' appearance of the tumor cells. The lesion is benign although recurrences may occur even after several years.

NEUROGENIC TUMORS

Multiple mucosal neuroma syndrome

Not infrequently, *oral mucosal neuromas* are the first clinical sign of the inherited autosomal dominant syndrome of multiple endocrine neoplasia (MEN) type 2b/III. This disease, that also shows a high rate of cases with new mutations, leads to the development of pheochromocytomas, medullary thyroid cancer and oral mucosal neuromas.[68] The latter are mainly located in the lips and anterior tongue but also in the cheeks or the palate. They present as painless nodules and show histologically irregular nerve bundles with prominent perineurium in the loosely arranged connective tissue of the submucosa (Fig. 88.18). Their detection should prompt the clinician to search for other manifestations of this life-threatening disease and the pathognomonic disturbances of the *ret* oncogene.[69]

Palisaded encapsulated neuroma

Usually occurring on the facial skin of middle-aged adults, the *palisaded encapsulated neuroma (solitary circumscribed neuroma)* may also affect the oral cavity as a single dome-shaped nodule.[70] Most commonly, it is found on the hard palate. Affected patients do not suffer from neurofibromatosis or MEN. Microscopically, these well-circumscribed tumors show interlacing bundles of spindle cells with wavy nuclei but without atypia. Sometimes a plexiform growth pattern is seen.[71] With special stains or by immunohistochemistry and in contrast to schwannomas or neurofibromas, axons are demonstrated throughout the lesion.[72]

Neurofibroma and neurilemoma

Although frequently found in the head and neck region, *neurilemomas (schwannomas)* are relatively rare in the mouth. Young adults are most often affected. The tumor is localized in the tongue, hard palate, buccal mucosa and, exceptionally, within the mandible.[73] It is an encapsulated nerve sheath tumor in close association with a peripheral nerve and exhibits two histologic components on microscopy: highly cellular ordered areas with wavy nuclei (Antoni A pattern – Fig. 88.19) and loosely arranged myxoid fields (Antoni B pattern). A palisaded arrangement of tumor cells bordering

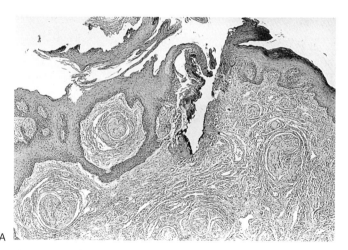

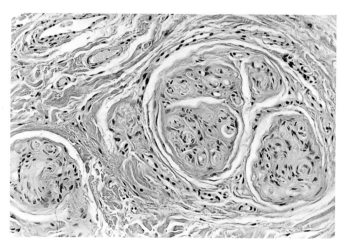

A   B

Fig. 88.18 Oral mucosal neuromas. Subepithelial neuromas leading to pseudopolypoid or nodular mucosal conformation **(A)**. The neuromas contain axonal and schwannian elements and are covered by a perineurium **(B)**.

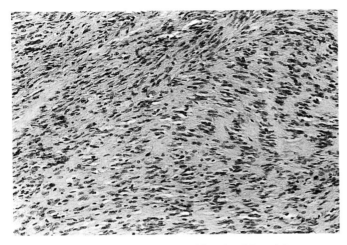

Fig. 88.19 Neurilemoma/schwannoma with ordered Antoni A areas, spindle-shaped cells and slender nuclei arranged in a parallel fashion.

an acellular eosinophilic area (Verocay body) is also characteristic. Neurites may only be seen in the periphery.

Neurofibromas may present as solitary lesions or in the setting of neurofibromatosis type I. They consist of fascicles of spindle-shaped cells with wavy, dark-staining nuclei, strands of collagen and mucin (Fig. 88.20). They also contain tiny neurites throughout. Their reaction with antibodies to S-100 protein is not as strong as in neurilemomas. For information on the forms of neurofibromas and details of neurofibromatosis, the reader is referred to specialist texts.[64]

Granular cell tumor

Although in the early descriptions this was linked to muscle ('granular cell myoblastoma'[74]), recent evidence supports a neural differentiation of *granular cell tumor*.[75]

These tumors are twice as common in females as in males and are predominantly found in the oral cavity and the skin.[76] The tongue is the most often affected intraoral site followed by the buccal mucosa and the lips.[77] Usually the tumor presents as an asymptomatic nodule of less than 2 cm that has been noted for months to years. On histology the poorly circumscribed tumor is composed of rather uniform, large, pale eosinophilic cells with granulated cytoplasm, small nucleoli and practically no mitotic figures. Sometimes a slight nuclear pleomorphism may be seen but in the absence of mitoses this should not be mistaken for malignancy (Fig. 88.21). However, two or more mitoses per ten high-power fields should raise the suspicion of malignancy, particularly since there is a striking histologic similarity between the benign and the very rare malignant variants of granular cell tumor.[78] The cells are arranged in sheets, nests or small groups. Additionally, the overlying squamous epithelium may very often show a pseudoepitheliomatous hyperplasia that occasionally, in superficial biopsies with few or no granular cells, may be erroneously mistaken for well-differentiated carcinoma.[79]

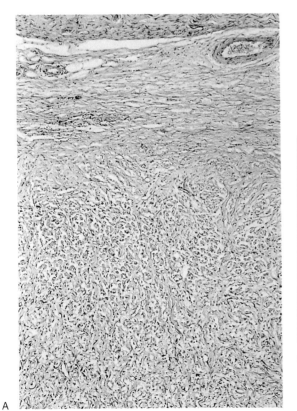

A

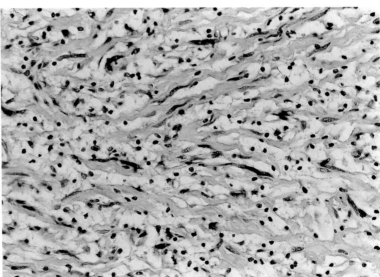

B

Fig. 88.20 Neurofibroma without capsular delineation **(A)**, with loosely textured tissue and 'wavy' or comma-shaped nuclei **(B)**.

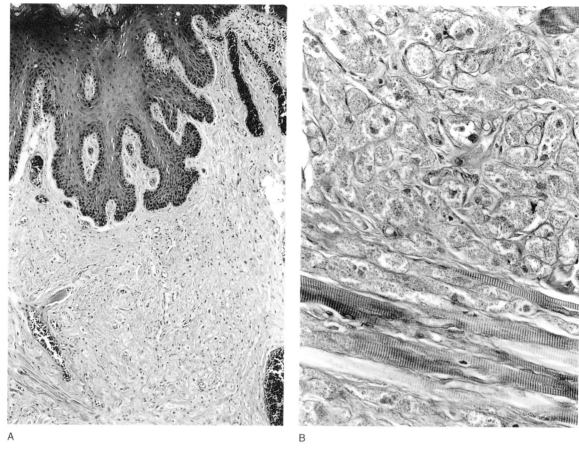

A   B

Fig. 88.21 Granular cell tumor with pseudoepitheliomatous hyperplasia of covering epithelial layer **(A)**. Tumor cells are rich in granulated cytoplasm, and infiltrate between skeletal muscle fibers **(B)**. Mitoses are absent.

VASCULAR TUMORS

By definition, benign tumors of blood or lymph vessels, that are commonly found in the oral mucosa, do imitate their normal counterparts. However, the discrimination between true neoplasms, hamartomas and malformations is often arbitrary. Hemangiomas and lymphangiomas are primarily tumors of childhood and preferentially occur in the head and neck area.[80] On histologic grounds several forms can be discriminated.[81]

Capillary hemangiomas, the most common, are found in the oral cavity, especially in the tongue, the buccal mucosa and the lip. They present as enlarging, bluish-red spots or nodules that are often detected at birth or during the first weeks of life. Females are more often affected than males. Histologically, they are composed of densely packed capillaries without atypia but may show moderate mitotic activity. They may show a polypoid growth pattern, presenting as 'epulis' on the gingiva (see above). Immature, highly cellular hemangiomas with prominent endothelial cells are termed *juvenile (cellular) hemangiomas*. Capillary hemangiomas regress spontaneously over the years and may involute completely.

Cavernous hemangiomas posess dilated thin walled vessels, are less circumscribed and do not regress spontaneously. Furthermore, they tend to involve deeper structures. Sometimes oral hemangiomas may be part of the Sturge–Weber syndrome that is characterized by hamartomatous vascular proliferations involving the brain and the face. These patients are born with a facial capillary hemangioma (nevus flammeus) in one or more segments of the trigeminal nerve and meningeal hemangiomas leading to seizures, glaucoma and mental retardation.[82] Surgery in an affected area may be accompanied by severe bleeding.

Lymphangiomas are most often found in the head and neck region of infants and newborn children.[83] Although some authors divide them into capillary, cavernous and cystic forms, this seems only of academic interest since all three types may be found in the same lesion. Capillary types of lymphangioma are predominantly located in the neck while cavernous ones are more often found in the mouth, especially the tongue, where they may lead to macroglossia.[84] Characteristically the surface of the tongue appears 'blebby' or 'frog-egg' like. On the microscope one sees cystic dilated spaces with thin endothelial-like lining cells and occasionally intraluminal lymphocytes. Erythrocytes should be absent but may be visible because of hemorrhage. However, this makes the diagnosis uncertain. Endothelial cell markers like factor VIII or CD 31, however, are immunohistochemically negative. These lesions may extend into the deeper connective tissue and skeletal muscle.

BENIGN TUMORS AND TUMORLIKE LESIONS OF THE MINOR SALIVARY GLANDS

Principally, the same pathologic conditions are found in the major and the minor salivary glands. The following text will concentrate on those lesions that preferentially affect the minor salivary glands.

MUCOCELE, EXTRAVASATION AND RETENTION TYPE

Mucoceles are one of the most common minor salivary gland lesions. Two types are recognized: the *extravasation type* (mucus escape reaction) and the *retention type* (salivary duct cyst, sialocyst). The retention type, being most common in the major salivary glands and by far outnumbered by the extravasation type, is a true cyst with an epithelial lining. Although some cases may represent pure duct dilatation, it seems likely that they also may form by epithelial proliferation due to partial duct obstruction.[85] The extravasation type is related to trauma with rupture of a duct and spillage of mucin into the surrounding tissue, leading to a mild inflammatory reaction of the connective tissue and the respective gland. The formation of the cavity, that is covered by macrophages, may be promoted by locally released proteolytic enzymes.[86] An epithelial lining is lacking (Fig. 88.22).

Nearly 70% of the *extravasation type mucoceles* are located on the lip, especially the lower lip, followed by the buccal mucosa, floor of the mouth and the tongue. Most patients are children or young adults and both sexes are equally affected.[87] Clinically, these lesions appear as painless swellings, being present for some days to a week. They may rupture but often recur within a month. Large lesions of the floor of the mouth are called ranulas. With some exceptions, they are related to the sublingual gland and typically found lateral to the midline. They fluctuate on palpation. If this type of mucocele is located inferior to the mylohyoid muscle it may be palpable below the mandible. The differential diagnosis includes lymphangioma, hemangioma, adenomas of salivary gland and, especially on

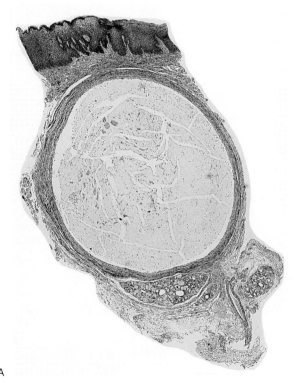

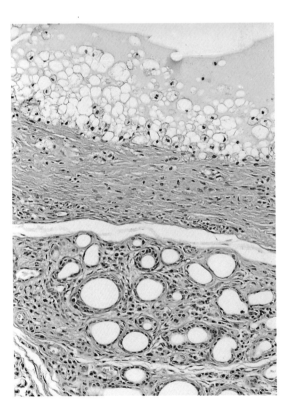

A   B

Fig. 88.22 (A) Mucocele, extravasation type, with subepithelial pseudocystic cavity surrounded by compressed connective tissue. Remnants of partly dilated salivary glands are visible in lower third. **(B)** The pseudocyst is filled with mucin and its wall is lined by macrophages that also spill out into the cyst lumen.

histology, mucoepidermoid carcinoma and low-grade adeno-carcinoma, the latter appearing in an older age group and presenting at least some epithelial structures.

More than 90% of *retention-type mucoceles* are found in the parotid, submandibular or sublingual gland, with descending frequency. They occur usually after the age of 20 years with a slight male preponderance, presenting as a slowly enlarging and persisting painless mass that may be present for years. Microscopically, the presence of a squamous epithelial lining is the leading diagnostic feature. Again, the differential diagnosis includes lymphangioma, hemangioma, cystic salivary gland tumors and extravasation mucocele.[87]

BENIGN LYMPHOEPITHELIAL LESIONS AND SJÖGREN'S SYNDROME

Although *benign lymphoepithelial lesions* as well as manifestations of *Sjögren's syndrome* are mostly found outside the minor salivary glands, their involvement in these conditions is of diagnostic importance.

In 1892 Mikulicz published his classic paper on a symmetrical swelling of the lacrimal and major salivary glands unrelated to any detectable cause.[88] In 1952 Godwin sug-gested the designation lymphoepithelial lesion for this special type of gland enlargement that was also known as Mikulicz's disease.[89] Shortly thereafter, Morgan & Castleman present-ed evidence for an overlapping of the pathologic findings in Sjögren's syndrome and benign lymphoepithelial lesions.[90] Furthermore, it became obvious that patients with benign lymphoepithelial lesions with or without Sjögren's syndrome were at increased risk for developing intra- or extrasalivary gland non-Hodgkin lymphomas predominantly of B-cell type.

On histology, lymphoepithelial lesions consist of a dense lymphocytic infiltrate that destroys the acini while the salivary ducts persist. The surrounding myoepithelial cells and the ductal epithelium proliferate by forming the so-called 'epimyoepithelial islands'. However, these islands are only rarely found in the small salivary glands. Here, small lymphocytic infiltrates predominate consisting of more than 50 cells (Fig. 88.23).

In Sjögren's syndrome patients are suffering from the so-called 'sicca syndrome'. This autoimmune disorder affects salivary and lacrimal glands leading to xerophthalmia (dry eyes) or keratoconjunctivitis sicca and xerostomia (dry mouth). It may be associated with other autoimmune diseases

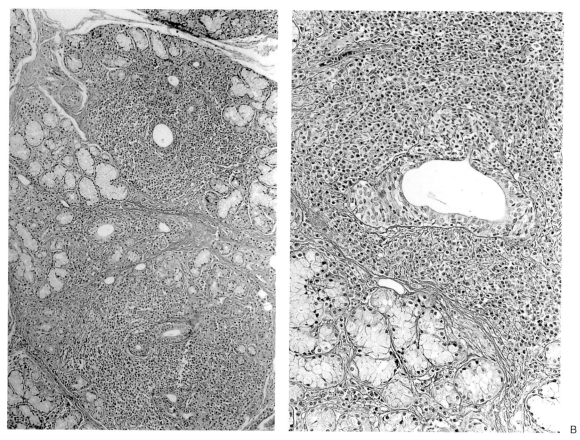

Fig. 88.23 Benign lymphoepithelial lesions. Lobulated small salivary gland (**A**) with a dense lymphocytic infiltration obscuring the glandular tissue. Proliferation of epithelial ductal cells and myoepithelial cells leads to the characteristic epimyothelial islands (**B**; center).

like primary biliary cirrhosis, vasculitis or interstitial lung fibrosis ('secondary Sjögren's syndrome'). The reduced tear production can easily be measured by the Schirmer test, using sterile strips of filter paper placed over the margins of the lower lids. Additionally, autoantibodies, antinuclear antibodies and a positive rheumatoid factor may be found together with an increased blood sedimentation rate and elevated immunoglobulin levels. If a biopsy of the minor salivary glands of the lip is performed in patients with these clinical and laboratory findings, few to multiple foci of glandular lymphocytic infiltrations with acinar destruction are found. Although not specific, these findings strongly support a suspected diagnosis of Sjögren's syndrome.[91,92] According to follow-up studies, patients with primary Sjögren's syndrome are at particular risk of developing malignant lymphoma.[93] The treatment depends on the patient's symptoms. Because of reduced saliva production antifungal therapy for secondary candidiasis and daily fluoride administrations for preventing caries are necessary. Patients should be informed about their increased risk of developing malignant B-cell lymphomas.

NECROTIZING SIALOMETAPLASIA

Necrotizing sialometaplasia is predominantly found on the hard and soft palate.[94] Most commonly, it develops in male adults, sometimes following injuries or surgery, injections, radiation, ill-fitting dentures or adjacent tumors, especially in extrapalatal sites.[95] It is assumed that local factors are responsible for circulatory disturbances leading to ischemic conditions and subsequent infarction of salivary gland tissue.[96]

Clinically, patients present with an asymptomatic ulcer, 1–5 cm in diameter, that develops within a few weeks. The lesion is sometimes preceded by a submucosal tumorlike swelling accompanied by mild pain or burning sensations. Characteristically, the pain stops after ulcer formation. A biopsy is usually performed to exclude a carcinoma.

On histology an acinar necrosis is found but typically the lobular architecture of the gland is still preserved (Fig. 88.24). Additionally, mucin pools are seen accompanied by a mild lymphocytic infiltration. Subsequently squamous metaplasia of ductal remnants develops that may be mistaken for squamous cell or mucoepidermoid carcinoma. However,

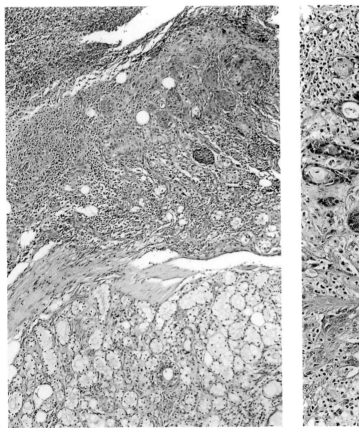
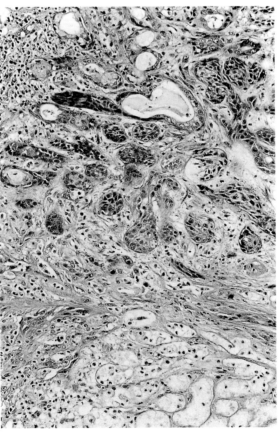

Fig. 88.24 Necrotizing sialometaplasia. **(A)** Lobular arrangement of a small salivary gland with intact acini and mild inflammation (lower half). In the upper part the glandular tissue is mainly necrotic and its architecture obscured by lymphoplasmacytic inflammation. Small epithelial islands are visible, e.g. upper right. **(B)** At higher magnification remnants of ducts with metaplastic squamous epithelium are seen (upper half) simulating infiltrative carcinoma. Note the absence of cellular atypia.

the still discernible lobular arrangement in the absence of atypia should lead to the correct diagnosis. Sometimes pseudoepitheliomatous hyperplasia of the surface epithelium and regenerative changes in areas of necrosis may complicate the picture. If the diagnosis is established, no further therapy is necessary as the lesion resolves spontaneously within a few weeks.[95]

ADENOMAS AND PAPILLOMAS OF THE MINOR SALIVARY GLANDS

The minor salivary glands are the second most common site of salivary gland neoplasms.[97] Unfortunately, nearly half of the tumors are malignant, mainly consisting of mucoepidermoid carcinoma and acinic cell carcinoma. As in the major glands, the pleomorphic adenoma is the most common benign tumor followed by various other adenomas, e.g. canalicular adenoma, basal cell adenoma and ductal papillomas.[98] Although very rare, the *canalicular adenoma* predominantly occurs in the upper lip followed by the buccal mucosa. It usually gives rise to a palpable soft swelling similar to mucocele but these lesions are rare on the upper lip. As a rule, the tumor is found in elderly female patients. Under the microscope, columnar cells are seen arranged in parallel bilayered rows (Fig. 88.25). Sometimes cystic spaces are formed containing papillary projections. The stroma is loosely textured and devoid of metaplastic changes, e.g. chondroid material.

The most common locations of *basal cell adenoma*, following the parotid gland, are also the upper lip and buccal mucosa. Basal cell adenoma, constituting not more than 2% of all salivary gland tumors, shows a female preponderance as well and may occur at any age but predo-

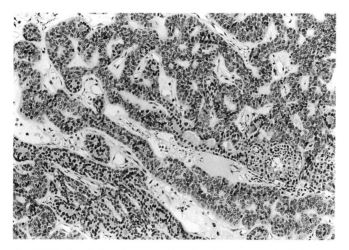

Fig. 88.25 Canalicular adenoma with trabecular pattern, cuboidal to columnar cells and dark-staining nuclei that grow in parallel rows forming bilayered cords of tumor cells, occasionally including cystic spaces. No stromal tumor components are present.

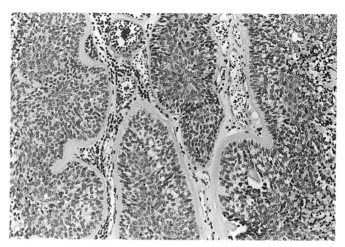

Fig. 88.26 Basal cell adenoma of salivary glands, membranous subtype, with islands of tumor cells and peripheral cellular palisading similar to basal cell carcinoma of the skin. Characteristically, tumor complexes are surrounded by a thickened hyalinized eosinophilic band-like lining consisting of basement membrane material.

minantly in older adults. Presenting as a slow-growing mass, the tumor is usually encapsulated and composed of isomorphic basaloid cells with a prominent basal layer. These cells are arranged in solid nests or trabecular cords surrounded by a prominent basement membrane (Fig. 88.26).

Ductal papillomas, presenting as painless swellings or nodules, are extremely rare and arise from the excretory ducts of the minor salivary glands, predominantly of the lip. An *intraductal variant* is distinguished from an *inverted type*. While the former consists of intraductal papillary projections lined by one or two layers of cuboidal to squamous epithelial cells, the latter shows extensions into the surrounding connective tissue that are still in connection with the ductal epithelium.

A third form of papilloma, the *sialadenoma papilliferum*, has its most common location on the palate. In contrast to the aforementioned papillomas, this lesion is predominantly found in older male patients. It presents as an exophytic papillary lesion similar to viral papillomas but in contrast to these exophytic projections, ductlike structures covered by a double-layered epithelium are found beyond the epithelial surface down to the submucosa.

All three lesions are treated by excision. Recurrences are very rare.

BENIGN PIGMENTED LESIONS OF THE ORAL CAVITY

Although the oral mocosa contains as many melanocytes as the normal skin, pigmented lesions of the oral cavity are very rare.[99] Some lesions are caused by exogenic agents like tobacco smoking or trauma. The latter especially is responsible for the development of *melanoacanthoma*, a lesion that is almost exclusively seen in young female black adults.[100] On histology an epithelial and melanocytic proliferation is visible, leading to acanthosis, spongiosis and a diffuse intra-epithelial distribution of dendritic melanocytes. Since this lesion is rapidly growing a biopsy will usually be performed to rule out melanoma.

Oral melanosis or *oral melanotic macules*, the most common melanocytic lesion of the mouth, are similar to cutaneous ephelides or freckles. They are flat, small (usually < 2 mm), tan to dark brown and occur on the vermilion border of the lips, the labial and buccal mucosa. If their number is increased and perioral freckles are also visible, Peutz–Jeghers syndrome (multiple freckle-like lesions in conjunction with intestinal polyposis) should be excluded.[101] Usually, melanotic macules do not increase in size once having been discovered. Histologically, as in the skin, an increased amount of melanin pigmentation of the basal cell layer is seen, sometimes together with melanin incontinence and storage of pigment in subepithelial macrophages (Fig. 88.27). In general, no therapy is necessary; however, since an early

melanoma may have the same clinical appearance excision and histopathologic examination are recommended. The same holds true for all the other lesions mentioned below.

Very rarely a pigmented lesion clinically similar to oral melanosis may exhibit the histologic findings of *lentigo simplex*, showing elongated rete ridges and an increased numbers of melanocytes.

Acquired melanocytic nevi sometimes develop in the oral mucosa. As in the skin, nevus cells are located in the epithelial layer, at the epithelial–mucosal junction or sub-epithelial layer, giving rise to a smooth and sharply defined, slightly elevated, tan to dark-brown but sometimes amelanotic papule. About two-thirds of the lesions are found in women. According to Buchner[102] intramucosal nevi, corresponding to the intradermal nevi of the skin, are the most common type and represent nearly two-thirds of all nevi while compound and junctional nevi are rare (Fig. 88.28). They are found preferentially at the buccal mucosa, the gingiva, the lips and the palate but are nearly absent on the tongue.[102]

The second most common nevus is the *blue nevus* that predominantly affects the hard palate. It is not composed of nevus cells but of dendritic melanocytes that are located deep in the subepithelial connective tissue. This deep location is responsible for the sometimes blue coloration as the longer wavelengths of the light reflected from the lesions tend to be more absorbed by the intervening tissue than the short-waved blue. Most of the lesions are smaller than 1 cm. Under the microscope, elongated melanocytes with dendritic extensions are seen within the lamina propria. Usually the cells are oriented more or less in parallel to the epithelial surface (Fig. 88.29).

Congenital, combined (blue nevus and melanocytic nevus) or intraoral Spitz nevi are exceptional findings.[103–105]

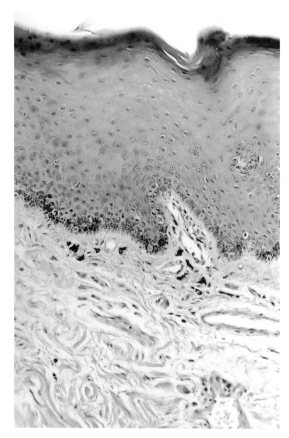

Fig. 88.27 Oral melanosis with increased pigmentation of the basal cell layer and melanin droplets in subepithelial macrophages ('pigment incontinence'). Notice normal number of melanocytes (i.e. enlarged cells with clear perinuclear halo scattered throughout the basal cell layer).

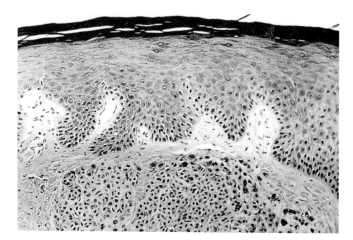

Fig. 88.28 Subepithelial or intramucosal nevus-cell nevus showing typical decrease in cell size with increasing distance from the epithelial surface.

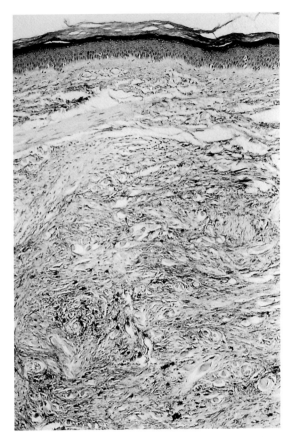

Fig. 88.29 Blue nevus with intramucosal black pigmented slender dendritic melanocytes separated by collagen fibers.

REFERENCES

1. Pindborg JJ, Reichart PA, Smith CJ, van der Waal I 1997 Histological typing of cancer and precancer of the oral mucosa, 2nd edn. Springer, Berlin
2. Strachan DS 1994 Histology of the oral mucosa and tonsils. In: Avery JK (ed) Oral development and histology, 2nd edn. Thieme, Stuttgart
3. Cotran RS, Kumar V, Robbins SL 1994 Robbins pathological basis of disease, 5th edn. WB Saunders, Philadelphia
4. al-Nafussi A, Hancock K, Sommerland B, Carder PJ 1990 Heterotopic brain presenting as a cyst mass in the palate. Histopathology 17:81–84
5. Bossen EH, Hudson WR 1987 Oligodendroglioma arising in heterotopic brain tissue of the soft palate and nasopharynx. American Journal of Surgical Pathology 11:571–574
6. Richard G, de Laurenzi V, Didona B, Bale SJ, Compton JG 1995 Keratin 13 point mutation underlies the hereditary mucosal epithelia disorder white sponge nevus. Nature Genetics 11:453–455
7. Rugg EL, McLean WHI, Allison WE et al 1995 A mutation in the mucosal keratin K4 is associated with oral white sponge nevus. Nature Genetics 11:450–452
8. Morris R, Gansler TS, Rudisill MT, Neville B 1988 White sponge nevus: diagnosis by light microscopic and ultrastructural cytology. Acta Cytologica 32:357–361
9. Daley T 1993 Pathology of intraoral sebaceous glands. Journal of Oral Pathology and Medicine 22:241–245
10. Lutman GB 1974 Epithelial nests in intraoral sensory nerve endings simulating perineural invasion in patients with oral carcinoma. American Journal of Clinical Pathology 61:275–286
11. Krammer EB, Zenker W 1974 Comments on oral neuroepithelial structures. American Journal of Clinical Pathology 62:571–574
12. Tschen JA, Fechner RE 1979 The juxtaoral organ of Chievitz. American Journal of Surgical Pathology 3:147–150
13. Salzer GM, Zenker W 1962 Das juxtaorale Organ. (Chievitzsches Organ). Karger, Basel
14. Mandl L, Nerlich A, Pankratz H, Huebner G 1993 Das juxtaorale Organ (Chievitz-Organ) – ein sensibles Organ in der Buccotemporalregion? Pathologe 14:205–209
15. Leibl W, Pflüger H, Kerjaschki D 1976 A case of nodular hyperplasia of the juxtaoral organ in man. Virchows Archiv (Pathological Anatomy and Histology) 371:389–391
16. Regezi JA, Sciubba J 1993 Oral pathology, 2nd edn. WB Saunders, Philadelphia
17. Bhaskar SN, Beasley JDI, Cutright DE 1970 Inflammatory papillary hyperplasi of the oral mucosa. Journal of the American Dental Association 81:949–952
18. van der Waal I, Beemster G, van der Kwast WA 1979 Median rhomboid glossitis caused by candida? Oral Surgery, Oral Medicine and Oral Pathology 47:31–35
19. Meyer I, Abbey LM 1970 The relationship of syphilis to primary carcinoma of the tongue. Oral Surgery, Oral Medicine and Oral Pathology 30:678–681
20. Eversole LR 1997 Immunopathogenesis of oral lichen planus and recurrent aphthous stomatitis. Seminars in Cutaneous Medicine and Surgery 16:284–294
21. Jungell P 1991 Oral lichen planus. A review. International Journal of Oral and Maxillofacial Surgery 20:129–135
22. Imhof M, Popal H, Lee JH, Zeuzem S, Milbradt R 1997 Prevalence of hepatitis C virus antibodies and evaluation of hepatitis C virus genotypes in patients with lichen planus. Dermatology 195:1–5
23. Carrozzo M, Gandolfo S, Carbone M et al 1996 Hepatitis C virus infection in Italian patients with oral lichen planus: a prospective case-control study. Journal of Oral Pathology and Medicine 25:527–533
24. Krutchkoff DJ, Eisenberg E 1985 Lichenoid dysplasia: a distinct histopathologic entity. Oral Surgery, Oral Medicine and Oral Pathology 60:308–315
25. Eisenberg E, Krutchkoff DJ 1992 Lichenoid lesions of oral mucosa. Diagnostic criteria and their importance in the alleged relationship to oral cancer. Oral Surgery, Oral Medicine and Oral Pathology 73:699–704
26. Batsakis JG, Cleary KR, Cho KJ 1994 Lichen planus and lichenoid lesions of the oral cavity. Annals of Otology, Rhinology and Laryngology 103:495–497
27. Eisenberg E 1992 Lichen planus and oral cancer: is there a connection between the two? Journal of the American Dental Association 123:104–108
28. Lozada-Nur F, Miranda C 1997 Oral lichen planus: epidemiology, clinical characteristics, and associated diseases. Seminars in Cutaneous Medicine and Surgery 16:273–277
29. Barnard NA, Scully C, Eveson JW, Cunningham S, Porter SR 1993 Oral cancer development in patients with oral lichen planus. Journal of Oral Pathology and Medicine 22:421–424
30. Voute AB, de Jong WF, Schulten EA, Snow GB, van der Waal I 1992 Possible premalignant character of oral lichen planus. The Amsterdam experience. Journal of Oral Pathology and Medicine 21:326–329
31. Miller CS, Zeuss MS, White DK 1994 Detection of HPV DNA in oral carcinoma using polymerase chain reaction together with in situ hybridization. Oral Surgery, Oral Medicine and Oral Pathology 77:480–486
32. Zeuss MS, Miller CS, White DK 1991 In situ hybridization analysis of human papillomavirus DNA in oral mucosal lesions. Oral

Surgery, Oral Medicine and Oral Pathology 71:714–720

33. Scully C, Prime S, Maitland N 1985 Papillomaviruses: their possible role in oral disease. Oral Surgery, Oral Medicine and Oral Pathology 60:166–174

34. Garlick JA, Taichman LB 1991 Human papillomavirus infection of the oral mucosa. American Journal of Dermatopathology 13:386–395

35. Eversole LR, Laipis PJ, Green TL 1987 Human papillomavirus type 2 DNA in oral and labial verruca vulgaris. Journal of Cutaneous Pathology 14:319–325

36. Padayachee A 1994 Human papillomavirus (HPV) types 2 and 57 in oral verrucae demonstrated by in situ hybridization. Journal of Oral Pathology and Medicine 23:413–417

37. Carlos R, Sedano HO 1994 Multifocal papilloma virus epithelial hyperplasia. Oral Surgery, Oral Medicine and Oral Pathology 77:631–635

38. Padayachee A, van Wyk CW 1991 Human papillomavirus (HPV) DNA in focal epithelial hyperplasia by in situ hybridization. Journal of Oral Pathology and Medicine 20:210–214

39. Iamaroon A, Vickers RA 1996 Characterization of verruciform xanthoma by in situ hybridization and immunohistochemistry. Journal of Oral Pathology and Medicine 25:395–400

40. Nowparast B, Howell FV, Rick GM 1981 Verruciform xanthoma: a clinicopathological review and report of fifty-four cases. Oral Surgery, Oral Medicine and Oral Pathology 51:619–625

41. Waldron CA, Shafer WG 1975 Leukoplakia revisited. A clinicopathologic study of 3256 oral leukoplakias. Cancer 36:1386–1392

42. Burkhardt A 1985 Advanced methods in the evaluation of premalignant lesions and carcinomas of the oral mucosa. Journal of Oral Pathology 14:751–778

43. Bouquot JE, Gorlin RJ 1986 Leukoplakia, lichen planus, and other oral keratoses in 23,616 white Americans over the age of 35 years. Oral Surgery, Oral Medicine and Oral Pathology 61:373–381

44. Krutchkoff DJ, Eisenberg E, Anderson C 1991 Dysplasia of oral mucosa: a unified approach to proper evaluation. Modern Pathology 4:113–119

45. Picascia DD, Robinson JK 1987 Actinic cheilitis: a review of the etiology, differential diagnosis, and treatment. Journal of the American Academy of Dermatology 17:255–264

46. Awde JD, Kogon SL, Morin RJ 1996 Lip cancer: a review. Journal of the Canadian Dental Association 62:634–636

47. Seedat HA, van Wyk CW 1988 Submucous fibrosis in non-betel nut chewing subjects. Journal de Biologie Buccale 16:3–6

48. Kaugars GE, Burns JC, Gunsolley JC 1988 Epithelial dysplasia of the oral cavity and lips. Cancer 62:2166–2170

49. Shafer WG, Waldron CA 1975 Erythroplakia of the oral cavity. Cancer 36:1021–1028

50. Damm DD, Cibull ML, Geissler RH et al 1993 Investigation into the histogenesis of congenital epulis of the newborn. Oral Surgery, Oral Medicine and Oral Pathology 76:205–212

51. Anneroth G, Sigurdson A 1983 Hyperplastic lesions of the gingiva and alveolar mucosa. A study of 175 cases. Acta Odontologica Scandinavica 41:75–86

52. Raess T, Prein J 1992 Differential diagnosis of epulis-type changes in the mouth. Swiss Dentistry 13:21–27

53. Cutright DE 1972 Osseous and chondromatous metaplasia caused by dentures. Oral Surgery, Oral Medicine and Oral Pathology 34:625–633

54. Buchner A, Hansen LS 1987 The histomorphologic spectrum of peripheral ossifying fibroma. Oral Surgery, Oral Medicine and Oral Pathology 63:452–461

55. Lack EE, Worsham GF, Callihan MD, Crawford BE, Vawter GF 1981 Gingival granular cell tumors of the newborn (congenital 'epulis'): a clinical and pathologic study of 21 patients. American

Journal of Surgical Pathology 5:37–46

56. O'Brian FV, Pielou WD 1971 Congenital epulis: its natural history. Archives of Disease in Childhood 46:559–560

57. Magnusson BC, Rasmusson LG 1995 The giant cell fibroma. A review of 103 cases with immunohistochemical findings. Acta Odontologica Scandinavica 53:293–296

58. Fowler CB, Hartman KS, Brannon RB 1994 Fibromatosis of the oral and paraoral region. Oral Surgery, Oral Medicine and Oral Pathology 77:373–386

59. Jones AC, Freedman PD, Kerpel SM 1994 Oral myofibromas: a report of 13 cases and review of the literature. Journal of Oral and Maxillofacial Surgery 52:870–875

60. Lingen MW, Mostofi RS, Solt DB 1995 Myofibromas of the oral cavity. Oral Surgery, Oral Medicine, Oral Pathology, Oral Radiology and Endodontics 80:297–302

61. Sugatani T, Inui M, Tagawa T et al 1995 Myofibroma of the mandible. Clinicopathologic study and review of the literature. Oral Surgery, Oral Medicine, Oral Pathology, Oral Radiology and Endodontics 80:303–309

62. Beham A, Badve S, Suster S, Fletcher CD 1993 Solitary myofibroma in adults: clinicopathological analysis of a series. Histopathology 22:335–341

63. Baden E, Doyle JL, Lederman DA 1994 Leiomyoma of the oral cavity: a light microscopic and immunohistochemical study with review of the literature from 1884 to 1992. European Journal of Cancer B Oral Oncology 1:1–7

64. Enzinger FM, Weiss SW 1995 Soft tissue tumors, 3rd edn. Mosby, St Louis

65. Anastassov GE, van Damme PA 1995 Angioleiomyoma of the upper lip: report of a case. International Journal of Oral Maxillofacial Surgery 24:301–302

66. Willis J, Abdul Karim FW, di Sant' Agnese PA 1994 Extracardiac rhabdomyomas. Seminars in Diagnostic Pathology 11:15–25

67. Kapadia SB, Meis JM, Frisman DM et al 1993 Adult rhabdomyoma of the head and neck: a clinicopathologic and immunophenotypic study. Human Pathology 24:608–617

68. Schenberg ME, Zajac JD, Lim Tio S et al 1992 Multiple endocrine neoplasia syndrome – type 2b. Case report and review. International Journal of Oral Maxillofacial Surgery 21:110–114

69. Goodfellow PJ 1994 Inherited cancers associated with the RET proto-oncogene. Current Opinion in Genetics and Development 4:446–452

70. Magnusson B 1996 Palisaded encapsulated neuroma (solitary circumscribed neuroma) of the oral mucosa. Oral Surgery, Oral Medicine, Oral Pathology, Oral Radiology and Endodontics 82:302–304

71. Argenyi ZB, Cooper PH, Santa Cruz D 1993 Plexiform and other unusual variants of palisaded encapsulated neuroma. Journal of Cutaneous Pathology 20:34–39

72. Chauvin PJ, Wysocki GP, Daley TD, Pringle GA 1992 Palisaded encapsulated neuroma of oral mucosa. Oral Surgery, Oral Medicine and Oral Pathology 73:71–74

73. Krolls SO, McGinnis JP Jr, Quon D 1994 Multinodular versus plexiform neurilemoma of the hard palate. Report of a case. Oral Surgery, Oral Medicine and Oral Pathology 77:154–157

74. Abrikossoff A 1926 Über Myome ausgehend von der quergestreiften willkürlichen Muskulatur. Virchows Archiv (Pathology and Anatomy) 260:215–233

75. Weber Chappuis K, Widmann JJ, Kapanci Y 1995 [Histologic and immunohistochemical profiles of benign granular cell tumors. Report of 41 cases.] Annals of Pathology 15:198–202

76. Lack EE, Worsham GF, Callihan MD et al 1980 Granular cell tumor: a clinicopathologic study of 110 patients. Journal of Surgical Oncology 13:301–316

77. Stewart CM, Watson RE, Eversole LR, Fischlschweiger W, Leider AS 1988 Oral granular cell tumors: a clinicopathologic and

immunocytochemical study. Oral Surgery, Oral Medicine and Oral Pathology 65:427–435

78. Simsir A, Osborne BM, Greenebaum E 1996 Malignant granular cell tumor: a case report and review of the recent literature. Human Pathology 27:853–858

79. van der Wal N, Baak JP, Schipper NW, van der Waal I 1989 Morphometric study of pseudoepitheliomatous hyperplasia in granular cell tumors of the tongue. Journal of Oral Pathology and Medicine 18:8–10

80. Coffin CM, Dehner LP 1993 Vascular tumors in children and adolescents: a clinicopathologic study of 228 tumors in 222 patients. Pathology Annual 1:97–120

81. Weiss SW 1994 Histological typing of soft tissue tumors, 2nd edn. Springer, Berlin

82. Sujansky E, Conradi S 1995 Outcome of Sturge–Weber syndrome in 52 adults. American Journal of Medical Genetics 57:35–45

83. Gimeno Aranguez M, Colomar Palmer P, Gonzalez Mediero I, Ollero Caprani JM 1996 [The clinical and morphological aspects of childhood lymphangiomas: a review of 145 cases.] Anales Españoles de Pediatria 45:25–28

84. Penna KJ, Verveniotis SJ 1995 Lymphangiomatous macroglossia. Medical and surgical treatment. New York State Dental Journal 61:30–33

85. Chaudry AP, Reynolds DH, LaChapelle CF, Vickers RA 1960 A clinical and experimental study of mucocele (retention cyst). Journal of Dental Research 39:1253–1262

86. Azuma M, Tamatani T, Fukui K et al 1995 Proteolytic enzymes in salivary extravasation mucoceles. Journal of Oral Pathology and Medicine 24:299–302

87. Koudelka BM 1991 Obstructive disorders. In: Ellis GL, Auclair PL, Gnepp DR (eds) Surgical pathology of the salivary glands. WB Saunders, Philadelphia

88. Mikulicz J 1892 Ueber eine eigenartige symmetrische Erkrankung der Tränen- und Mundspeicheldrüsen. Beiträge zur Chirurgie: Festschrift für Theodor Billroth 610–630

89. Godwin JT 1952 Benign lymphoepithelial lesion of the parotid gland. Cancer 5:1089–1103

90. Morgan WS, Castleman B 1953 A clinicopathologic study of 'Mikulicz's disease'. American Journal of Pathology 29:471–503

91. Daniels TE, Whitcher JP 1994 Association of patterns of labial salivary gland inflammation with keratoconjunctivitis sicca. Analysis of 618 patients with suspected Sjogren's syndrome [see comments]. Arthritis and Rheumatism 37:869–877

92. Vitali C, Bombardieri S, Moutsopoulos HM et al 1993 Preliminary criteria for the classification of Sjögren's syndrome. Results of a prospective concerted action supported by the European Community. Arthritis and Rheumatism 36:340–347

93. Kruize AA, Hene RJ, van der Heide et al 1996 Long-term follow up of patients with Sjögren's syndrome. Arthritis and Rheumatism 39:297–303

94. Brannon RB, Fowler CB, Hartman KS 1991 Necrotizing sialometaplasia. A clinicopathologic study of sixty-nine cases and review of the literature. Oral Surgery, Oral Medicine and Oral Pathology 72:317–325

95. Jensen JL 1991 Idiopathic diseases. In: Ellis GL, Auclair PL, Gnepp DR (eds) Surgical pathology of the salivary glands. WB Saunders, Philadelphia

96. Shigematsu H, Shigematsu Y, Noguchi Y, Fujita K 1996 Experimental study on necrotizing sialometaplasia of the palate in rats. Role of local anesthetic injections. International Journal of Oral and Maxillofacial Surgery 25:239–241

97. Auclair PL, Ellis GL, Gnepp DR, Wenig BM, Janney CG 1991 Salivary gland neoplasms: general considerations In: Ellis GL, Auclair PL, Gnepp DR (eds) Surgical pathology of the salivary glands. WB Saunders, Philadelphia

98. Seifert G 1991 Histological typing of salivary gland tumors, 2nd edn. Springer, Berlin

99. Barrett AW, Scully C 1994 Human oral mucosal melanocytes: a review. Journal of Oral Pathology and Medicine 23:97–103

100. Goode RK, Crawford BE, Callihan MD, Neville BW 1983 Oral melanoacanthoma. Review of the literature and report of ten cases. Oral Surgery Oral Medical and Oral Pathology 56:622–628

101. Kitagawa S, Townsend BL, Hebert AA 1995 Peutz–Jeghers syndrome. Dermatology Clinics 13:127–133

102. Buchner A, Leider AS, Merrell PW, Carpenter WM 1990 Melanocytic nevi of the oral mucosa: a clinicopathologic study of 130 cases from northern California. Journal of Oral Pathology and Medicine 19:197–201

103. Ficarra G, Hansen LS, Engebretsen S, Levin LS 1987 Combined nevi of the oral mucosa. Oral Surgery, Oral Medicine and Oral Pathology 63:196–201

104. Nikai H, Miyauchi M, Ogawa I et al 1990 Spitz nevus of the palate. Report of a case. Oral Surgery, Oral Medicine and Oral Pathology 69:603–608

105. Allen CM, Pellegrini A 1995 Probable congenital melanocytic nevus of the oral mucosa: case report. Pediatric Dermatology 12:145–148

Orofacial pain

89

STEPHEN R. PORTER/R. GEIR MADLAND/RODERICK CAWSON

Table 89.1 Causes of orofacial pain

Local causes
Dental (e.g. pulpitis, dentine hypersensitivity, periapical periodontitis)
Gingival (e.g. primary herpetic gingivostomatitis, acute necrotizing ulcerative gingivitis, desquamative gingivitis)
Mucosal (e.g. ulceration)
Salivary gland (e.g. bacterial sialadenitis)
Temporomandibular joint (dysfunction and others)
Maxillary sinuses (sinusitis, malignancy)

Neurologic disease
Trigeminal neuralgia and variants
Glossopharyngeal neuralgia
Ramsay Hunt syndrome
Post-herpetic neuralgia

Vascular
Migraine and variants
Cluster headache, chronic paroxysmal hemicrania and others
Giant cell arteritis and variants

Psychogenic
Atypical facial pain
Burning mouth syndrome and variants

Referred pain

INTRODUCTION

Pain is the most likely symptom that a patient will complain of. There are many causes of facial pain; these can be broadly split into five categories (Table 89.1), there being considerable overlap with headache-type disorders.

This chapter will focus on common orofacial pain not otherwise detailed in other sections of this text.

TRIGEMINAL NEURALGIA

Trigeminal neuralgia (TN) typically manifests as a unilateral sharp, lancinating pain, elicited by touching a superficial 'trigger point', and radiating from that point across the distribution of a branch of the trigeminal nerve. The pain lasts for a few seconds but may recur with variable frequency. Occasional patients report a dull background ache in addition to the lancinating pain, and hence there can be some confusion with local causes of orofacial pain.

Trigeminal neuralgia is rare, arising in about 4 in 100 000 persons. It is a disorder of middle to late life with a slight female predisposition.[1]

Trigeminal neuralgia typically arises in otherwise well persons with no neurologic deficit. It can, however, be a feature of early multiple sclerosis, especially in young adults,[2] HIV disease[2], Lyme disease, and neoplasia or vascular malformations in the central and peripheral distribution of the trigeminal nerve.

A prodromal phase, sometimes termed pre-trigeminal neuralgia, comprising pain similar to local pulpitis or sinusitis, but without evident pathology, has been detailed; this is unlikely to be of notable help as the diagnosis is made after the onset of typical trigeminal neuralgia.

ETIOLOGY OF TRIGEMINAL NEURALGIA

The etiology of idiopathic trigeminal neuralgia is well described elsewhere.[3] Current evidence suggests that local microcompression, altered neuronal processing and/or demyelinating processes may be involved.

MANAGEMENT

The management of trigeminal neuralgia always includes detailed clinical assessment to exclude neurologic deficit. Referral to an appropriate specialist is warranted when the presentation is atypical and/or there is evidence of other neurologic or related disease, particularly multiple sclerosis.[3]

Non-surgical therapy is the mainstay of treatment of

Table 89.2 Some medical therapies of trigeminal neuralgia[3]

Drug	Dose-related effects	Idiosyncratic effects	Chronic effects
Carbamazepine	Ataxia, dizziness, double vision, nausea, vomiting	Rash, reduced white blood cell count	Folate deficiency, hyponatremia
Phenytoin	Ataxia, lethargy, nausea, headache, involuntary movements, behavioral change	Rash, pseudolymphoma, hepatitis	Gingival hypertrophy, dysarthria, hirsutism, coarsening of facial features, folate deficiency, intellectual blunting, mood and behavioral changes, cerebellar syndrome
Baclofen	Ataxia, lethargy, fatigue, nausea, vomiting		
Clonazepam	Lethargy, fatigue, dizziness	Rash, thrombocytopenia	
Lamotrigine	Ataxia, diplopia, dizziness, headache, irritability, somnolence	Rash	Not yet known
Oxcarbazepine	Ataxia, lethargy, diplopia, nausea, vomiting, hyponatremia	Rash	Not yet known
Valproic acid	Irritability, restlessness, tremor, confusion, nausea, vomiting	Gastric irritation, rash	Alopecia, weight gain

trigeminal neuralgia – typically with anticonvulsant agents such as carbamazepine and, less commonly, phenytoin, baclofen, sodium valproate and others (Table 89.2). In patients refractory to medication, or for whom such drugs are contraindicated, surgical procedures are available.

Medical management

Carbamazepine remains the main drug used in medical management of trigeminal neuralgia. Therapy typically commences at doses of 100 mg three times daily and is increased gradually to a maximum of 1600 mg per day until pain relief is achieved.[3] Proportionally more of the drug should be taken at night, so that there are adequate drug levels in the morning when most pain tends to occur. Up to 20% of patients develop side effects such as tremor and ataxia that may limit therapy. Other side effects include hepatic enzyme induction, hyponatremia, bone marrow suppression and folate depletion.

Skin rashes can develop up to three months after commencing carbamazepine therapy; the rash may be accompanied by pyrexia and lymphadenopathy and may represent an increased risk for the development of lymphoma.[4]

Patients require careful monitoring of clinical and relevant hematologic parameters when receiving carbamazepine therapy – up to 17% can develop folic acid deficiency and megaloblastic anemia, without peripheral neuropathy, and hyponatremia may occur at high doses of therapy in the elderly. The dose of carbamazepine in slow-release preparations may require to be highest, and there can be variation in the availability of carbamazepine between different slow-release agents.[3]

Although no appropriate trials have been undertaken, phenytoin is a commonly employed alternative therapy to carbamazepine. In addition, phenytoin may be given in combination with carbamazepine. The typical dose of phenytoin is 100 mg three times daily up to a maximum of 600 mg per day. Aside from the well-detailed side effects of phenytoin, there can be some cross-reactive hypersensitivity between phenytoin and carbamazepine.

The antispasmodic baclofen, particularly L-baclofen, may be an effective adjunct to carbamazepine therapy, but supporting data is lacking.

Other agents, albeit often formally untested, that may be of benefit in the management of trigeminal neuralgia include clonazepam, sodium valproate and oxcarbazepine.[5] Newer agents that may be of some promise in the management of trigeminal neuralgia include lamotrigine.[3]

Surgical management

A number of peripheral surgical procedures are available for the management of trigeminal neuralgia recalcitrant to therapy or for the treatment of patients in whom anticonvulsants may be contraindicated.[3] These procedures are *generally* safe but disadvantages include the transient response of cryotherapy (and the need for repeated and increasingly complicated local surgery), permanent anesthesia following alcohol and glycerol injections, and the risk of local tissue damage.

Surgical management – central

Central surgical management is indicated for trigeminal neuralgia recalcitrant to both non-surgical and local surgical therapies, and usually for patients in whom the pain is significantly affecting their quality of life.[6] A variety of surgical techniques has been described, with variable clinical outcome and associated morbidity and mortality. A detailed discussion of these methods is beyond the scope of the present text, however this area is well reviewed elsewhere[3].

GLOSSOPHARYNGEAL NEURALGIA

Glossopharyngeal neuralgia (GN) is an uncommon disorder characterized by lancinating pain of the oropharynx or neck, sometimes triggered by swallowing, coughing or talking. The pain is usually unilateral and may radiate to the ear and/or mouth. Syncope can be a feature. Rarely there can be other cardiac arrhythmias due to vagal stimulation, and other rare accompanying features include xerostomia or excess salivation.

Glossopharyngeal neuralgia is much more uncommon than trigeminal neuralgia. The disease usually arises in middle to late life and occurs equally in males and females. An identifiable cause is rarely found, although glossopharyngeal neuralgia can be associated with multiple sclerosis, and benign and malignant CNS tumors.[7]

As in trigeminal neuralgia there is usually a clustering of pain attacks, these lasting weeks to months. The pain attacks usually occur during the day but can wake the patient from sleep.

The management of glossopharyngeal neuralgia typically parallels that of trigeminal neuralgia. Carbamazepine is the mainstay of therapy. Phenytoin may not be an effective adjunct, although baclofen may be of benefit.

Local measures such as cryotherapy or injections of alcohol or glycerol are rarely possible, although surgical section of the glossopharyngeal nerve and upper rootlets of the vagus can be of benefit.[8] Central surgical methods such as microvascular decompression can produce complete resolution of symptoms in over 75% of treated patients, but are not without risk of morbidity and mortality.[9]

POST-HERPETIC NEURALGIA

Post-herpetic neuralgia (PHN) represents pain in the area of a previous episode of infection by varicella zoster virus that persists for more than one month after cessation of the accompanying vesicular rash.[10] Orofacial PHN typically affects the ophthalmic division of the trigeminal nerve, and less commonly the maxillary and mandibular divisions. The pain is a deep-seated, burning or throbbing sensation, sometimes with an accompanying lancinating nature that may mimic trigeminal neuralgia. Allodynia arises in 90% of affected individuals and the pain may interfere in activities of daily living such as speech, eating, washing and sleep. Post-herpetic neuralgia usually arises late in life; there is a female predominance. Patients may have evidence of herpetic scarring in the site of the orofacial pain and there can be hypoesthesia, hyperesthesia and/or hypoalgesia. The pain persists for months to years, and unlike trigeminal neuralgia does not have periods of remission.

The severity of pain of PHN has been found to correlate with preservation, not loss, of thermal sensory function, which suggests that rather than being due to deafferentation and central reorganization, a significant component of the pain in allodynic PHN is generated by activity in preserved primary afferent nociceptors.[11]

A PHN patient was found to have decreased contralateral thalamic activity on positron emission tomography,[12] suggesting a central functional alteration. It is hypothesized that PHN is multideterminate. The acute pain of shingles might set the stage for the chronic pain of PHN, for example, by the initiation of nociceptor-evoked central hyperexcitability and the production of axonal damage which may lead to ectopically discharging nociceptor sprouts.[13]

In some but not all studies, oral acyclovir (800 mg five times daily) given not more than 72 hours after the onset of the herpetic rash significantly hastened healing and reduced acute pain and the likelihood of PHN development; hence acyclovir may lessen the duration of established PHN in some, but not all, affected patients. The efficacy of newer antiviral drugs – including valaciclovir, famciclovir, sorivudine and BW882C87 – is being evaluated.

High dose systemic corticosteroids given at the time of an attack of shingles can reduce the incidence of PHN from 73% to 30%, however there remains the risk of disseminated herpes, which can be fatal.

Amitriptyline and nortriptyline can reduce the symptoms in up to two thirds of patients with PHN. Pain relief is independent of any effect on mood and is probably unrelated to serotoninergic action, since a specific serotoninergic antidepressant, zimelidine, has proved to be ineffective in the management of PHN. Amitriptyline or nortriptyline should be administered by slow upward titration, beginning with a small nightly dose of 25 mg (10 mg in the elderly) and rising in similar increments weekly. Patients must be warned of potential side effects, including sedation, anticholinergic effects and postural hypotension.[14] Patients able to tolerate higher doses (up to a maximum of 150 mg/day) tend to report more pain relief than those on lower doses of these antidepressants.

Intravenous morphine can provide effective pain relief, although intravenous ketamine produced greater pain relief than morphine in a randomized double-blind cross-over study of 8 PHN patients.[15]

Topical aspirin/diethyl ether mixture or aspirin in chloroform can provide some pain relief; topical capsaicin may also be of some clinical benefit for some, but not all patients, as can topical lignocaine gel.

Local anesthetic blockage with bupivacaine of the stellate ganglion, via an anterior paratracheal approach, may produce short-term relief of PHN in up to 75% of affected patients. Although this procedure can be repeated, there is a risk of transient recurrent laryngeal nerve palsy.

TEMPOROMANDIBULAR JOINT (TMJ) DYSFUNCTION

Temporomandibular joint dysfunction is the most common noninfective pain disorder of the orofacial region. It is clinically characterized by pain within and around the temporomandibular joint(s) and adjacent muscles of mastication, clicking of the joints, sometimes limitation of mouth opening, and rarely locking of the joint in opening or closing.[16]

There is considerable disagreement between authorities on the precise clinical features, and hence the diagnostic criteria of TMJ dysfunction. Indeed, the terminology used to describe this group of symptoms varies widely. As a consequence of these problems, the literature is often confusing and difficult to interpret accurately.

In general, up to 67% of groups of children, young adults and semiselected and randomly selected patients have experienced at least one painful symptom of the temporomandibular joint and associated structures, the majority of complaints being minor and transient. Clinical examination can detect associated signs in up to 69% of examined persons, and these signs can often be found in asymptomatic individuals. Studies of US households suggest that as many as 8.8% of interviewed persons had had TMJ or facial pain more than once in the last 6 months,[17] but the intensity of the associated pain may vary considerably with time and may be recalled inaccurately.

Symptoms and signs of TMJ dysfunction can arise in children as young as 3 years of age. The prevalence of TMJ dysfunction has been suggested to increase towards middle age and then gradually fall but this is not a consistent finding. Although a female predisposition has long been suggested, the frequency of symptoms and signs may be similar in both genders; however females, particularly those in the third and fourth decades, may have more severe clinical upset (particularly headache, joint and muscle tenderness and joint clicking), recognize painful symptoms better than males, and more readily seek professional therapy than affected males.

Despite the apparently high frequency of symptoms and signs of TMJ dysfunction, perhaps only 2–7% of patients actually seek, and perhaps warrant, treatment.

ETIOLOGY OF TEMPOROMANDIBULAR JOINT DYSFUNCTION

Parafunctional habits

Parafunctional habits such as biting foreign objects, pressing the tongue against the teeth, lip biting, clenching and grinding may have a variable and possibly minor association with TMJ dysfunction. The assessment of parafunctional habits may be complicated and influenced by the self-reporting of patients and/or the abilities of the attending clinician.

Occlusal anomalies

Occlusal anomalies are not a common feature of patients with TMJ dysfunction. Anterior open-bite is uncommon in symptomatic patients and is not significantly associated with disk displacement, with or without reduction. Likewise no notable association has consistently been demonstrated between degree of overbite or overjet and TMJ dysfunction, and most studies report no greater prevalence of crossbite in adults with TMJ dysfunction compared with healthy control subjects, although an association between contralateral crossbite and reducing disk displacement may exist.

Some, but not all studies of TMJ dysfunction patients have suggested an association between molar loss and painful symptoms, joint clicking and progression to locking, but there is little correlation between loss of molar support and TMJ symptoms in randomly selected individuals.

Some studies have suggested that an asymmetric retruded contact position (RCP) can cause abnormal TMJ sounds and masticatory muscle tenderness, but there is not always a significantly increased frequency of asymmetric RCP in TMJ dysfunction, although an abnormal retruded contact position may be a feature of some patients with uncommon, specific joint derangements.

There may be a higher frequency and severity of TMJ dysfunction in patients with restored dentitions compared with those with intact dentitions, but the precise contribution such factors make to the etiology of TMJ dysfunction is unclear.

Skeletal factors and orthodontic treatment probably play little role in the etiology of the majority of patients with TMJ dysfunction. Similarly the long-term effects of orthognathic surgery upon TMJ dysfunction are not clear.

Trauma

Trauma from eating, wide opening and dental treatment have all been cited as possible etiologies of TMJ dysfunction but there is little objective evidence to support this.

Previous head and neck injury may be a feature of patients with TMJ dysfunction; such trauma may precipitate TMJ pain and may underlie the arthroscopic findings such as synovitis, fibrillar organization and adhesions. It is unclear if a specific injury gives rise to a particularly increased frequency or type of TMJ injury, but since only mild to moderate dysfunction occurs in patients with previous mandibular condyle fracture it seems unlikely that this local trauma is of notable etiological significance. There are inadequate data to suggest that whiplash injuries are a likely precipitant of most instances of TMJ dysfunction.

While there may be an increased frequency of generalized joint hypermobility in some affected patients, and children with generalized joint hypermobility may have an increased liability to painful TMJ symptoms,[18] it seems unlikely that joint laxity is significant in the etiology of TMJ dysfunction.

Life events

Stressful life events may be more frequent in groups of patients with TMJ dysfunction than in non-affected control subjects. However, this association only exists for patients with muscle-related symptoms, and it is worthy of note that bruxism and/or myofascial pain may adversely affect quality of life.[19] An association with post-traumatic stress disorder has been suggested but remains to be confirmed.

While there is still some equivocal evidence of an association between psychiatric illness and TMJ dysfunction, many dental surgeons are of the belief that the two are linked.[20]

Anxiety neuroses, other affective disorders (particularly depression), somatoform disorders and personality disorders may be more frequent in groups of TMJ dysfunction patients than suitable control groups. Forty percent of one US patient study group had the diagnostic criteria for at least one personality disorder, the most common being paranoid or obsessive-compulsive personalities. Minnesota Multiphasic Personality Inventory (MMPI) scores of another group of US patients revealed significantly higher levels of hypochondriasis, depression, hysteria, psychopathic deviation, paranoia, schizophrenia and social introversion than in control subjects. Patients with muscle symptoms alone may be more likely to have higher MMPI scores than those also having internal derangement.[19] Older TMJ dysfunction patients are more likely to be anxious or depressed than are younger patients.

Most patients with the chronic pain of TMJ dysfunction can bear their condition adequately. Nevertheless, a cohort of affected patients may be unable to cope well and have higher levels of depression, somatization and healthcare attendance compared with other patients with the same degree of symptoms.[21] Finally, patients with TMJ dysfunction may have increased sensitivity to anxious stimuli.

DIAGNOSIS OF TEMPOROMANDIBULAR JOINT DYSFUNCTION

The clinical diagnosis of TMJ dysfunction has been well reviewed recently.[22]

Radiologic assessment is almost always undertaken, supposedly to exclude primary joint disease.[22] Plain radiologic methods, for example oblique lateral transcranial projections, do not always represent the mandibular condyle position in the glenoid fossa, indeed these views may not accurately demonstrate joint surfaces. Similarly, serial plain sagittal tomographs are not always fruitful and may require rotation of the patient's head, correction for the vertical angulation of the condyle, or additional submentovertex views. Panoral tomography is used routinely for screening for TMJ disease, but this does not accurately delineate bony morphology and, like other plain radiographic techniques, it can be difficult to interpret and is open to widely different interpretation by different examiners.

Scanning with technetium diphosphonates is not reliable, and arthrography has largely been superseded by computer tomography and magnetic resonance imaging.

Computed tomography (CT) may be unable to delineate adequately the position of the meniscus, and together with the relatively high radiation dose exposure, this technique may not be routinely undertaken.[22]

Magnetic resonance imaging is probably the technique of choice; it is noninvasive and it can detect internal derangements of the TMJ, and delineate disk morphology, the horizontal angle of the mandibular condyle and details of the muscles of mastication and the local blood supply. Magnetic resonance imaging may be the principal radiologic method of detecting bilateral joint derangement in children and adults with TMJ dysfunction and can possibly detect areas of increased vascularity in painful joints.[23,24]

Nevertheless, even MRI does not accurately detect all internal derangements of the TMJ. Indeed MRI may detect supposed disk displacements in the contralateral asymptomatic joint of patients with unilateral joint pain.

Assessment of joint sounds is not a reliable diagnostic tool.[22] Thermography,[25] vibration analysis,[26] and jaw tracking devices are not of proven benefit in the diagnosis of TMJ. Likewise analysis of the electromyographic activity of the masticatory muscles is rarely helpful in the diagnosis or monitoring of treatment of TMJ dysfunction.

TREATMENT OF TEMPOROMANDIBULAR JOINT DYSFUNCTION

The non-surgical treatment of TMJ dysfunction will be considered in this chapter.

Homecare practices

Homecare practices are favored by most clinicians, however there is a lack of data concerning their precise clinical benefit in the treatment of TMJ dysfunction. Commonly employed homecare procedures may include avoidance of excess chewing, use of a soft-consistency diet, limited talking, avoidance of wide yawning, and use of physical therapy such as local application of ice for acute pain or heat for low grade chronic pain, muscle massage, hot showers, saunas or steam baths.

Passive or active jaw exercises have been recommended for joint clicking, restricted opening, irregular mandibular movements, muscle incoordination and recurrent anterior dislocation of the condyle, but there are no objective data as to the efficacy of such procedures in the management of TMJ dysfunction, though the results of one study suggested that exercises and physiotherapy successfully reduced pain and improved mouth opening in 53% of patients with reciprocal TMJ clicking.

Analgesia

Pain, and possibly inflammation may be controlled by non-steroidal anti-inflammatory drugs (NSAIDs). There do not, however, appear to be any documented trials of the efficacy of specific NSAIDs in the management of TMJ dysfunction.

Occlusal readjustment

As noted above, there is only equivocal evidence that occlusion plays any role in the etiology of TMJ dysfunction. Nevertheless occlusal readjustment continues to be cited as a useful therapeutic method for TMJ dysfunction, particularly when myalgia is a major symptom. Occlusal readjustment involves repositioning the mandible in a centric position by prosthodontic or orthodontic means and/or occlusal equilibration. Most studies have only assessed short-term outcome, but one study of a small number of patients with TMJ dysfunction associated with abnormal condyle–disk relationship reported significant reduction in painful symptoms and locking for up to 3 years after occlusal correction by prosthodontic and/or orthodontic therapy. Patients with asymptomatic clicking of the TMJ may benefit from replacement of any lost posterior teeth but this assumes, probably incorrectly, that loss of posterior teeth causes TMJ clicking and that patients with asymptomatic TMJ sounds require therapy.

Splint therapy

A variety of different occlusal splints has been reported to be of value in the management of TMJ dysfunction. Hard acrylic plane splints may be effective in reducing muscle and joint pain in up to 87% of studied patients but are unlikely to reduce joint clicking and limited opening. Nocturnal splint therapy may be effective in reducing the symptoms of myogenous pain, but arthrogenous pain requires continuous splint use – at least in the short term. In the long term, patients often have a return of painful symptoms after cessation of use of the splint. Flat plane splints may rapidly reduce nocturnal bruxism and sometimes, but not always, effect a decrease in maximum masticatory muscle activity.

Despite the lack of detailed, well designed studies, current evidence suggests that anterior repositioning splints are more effective than flat plane occlusal splints in eliminating reciprocal clicking and tenderness of the TMJ and may also sometimes be more effective in reducing muscle tenderness. However clicking often returns and anterior repositioning splints are only likely to obtain long-term recapture of the disk in one third of all treated patients.

Only about 50% of clicking, painful joints may be suitable for repositioning therapy, hence clinical benefit is unlikely in all treated cases, and the success of therapy may not be dependent on the precise malposition of the disk. A further disadvantage of anterior reposition splints is that after the mandible has been maintained in an anterior position it must be stepped back to the original occlusal position; at this time a posterior open-bite may develop because the condyle has not completely returned to its original position within the fossa, necessitating later orthodontic therapy or complex occlusal adjustment.

The reduction in pain may (theoretically at least) be due to the forward positioning of the disk allowing the retrodiskal tissues time to repair, but if the retrodiskal tissues have not adequately repaired when the condyle returns to the fossa there will be further inflammation.

Soft splints may lessen TMJ dysfunction related headache and clicking, but their effect is not always significant, particularly in the long term, and they can cause a worsening of pain in up to 26% of patients.

Available, limited data suggest that pivot splints may be of benefit in reducing the pain of TMJ dysfunction, but additional data are required. Buccal separators are not effective for TMJ dysfunction.

Passive eruption

Passive eruption of posterior teeth has been suggested to be an effective method of treatment for 30–98% of symptoms associated with TMJ dysfunction, but this suggestion must be treated with extreme caution as the data collection of the relevant study did not involve clinical examination of patients and the study contained no control group.

Psychiatric intervention

Psychiatric referral for assessment and suitable therapy is an important component of the management of TMJ dysfunction.

A number of psychotropic agents have been suggested to be of value in the management of TMJ dysfunction, of which dothiepin hydrochloride has probably received the greatest attention.

Dothiepin hydrochloride in daily doses of between 25 and 225 mg can significantly reduce the painful symptoms of TMJ dysfunction after 9 weeks' therapy, but it may not reduce any associated depressive symptoms and thus requires long-term therapy. A study of Australian patients found that both occlusal splint therapy and doxepin therapy were required to reduce TMJ symptoms in those patients with depression, while non-depressed patients responded poorly to splint therapy alone and had an intermediate response to doxepin therapy alone.

Other suggested medical therapies include amitriptyline or trifluoperazine hydrochloride in addition to dothiepin; fluphenazine with nortryptyline may be useful for nocturnal use, and flupenthixol 0.5–1.5 mg twice daily may be of benefit for resistant cases. Diazepam (2–5 mg up to three times daily) may reduce the painful symptoms of TMJ dysfunction and recently clonazepam has been found to reduce painful TMJ and head and neck symptoms at nocturnal doses of 0.25 mg to 1 mg. Alprazolam, a much more potent anxiolytic than diazepam, has been found to increase mandibular movement and decrease local pain and muscle tenderness, but does not significantly reduce joint sounds. Therapy with a flat plane occlusal splint may be as effective as alprazolam, and combined drug and splint therapy does not significantly positively influence clinical outcome.

Complementary therapies

Acupuncture therapy may produce some reduction in local pain and tenderness, but this benefit lasts less than six months. Mandibular manipulations of various types have been suggested to be of benefit in the management of TMJ dysfunction, but consistent supportive data are required to determine if such manipulation has any long-term benefits and what additional treatment may be warranted.

Ultrasound may benefit some individuals with TMJ dysfunction but there appear to be few, if any, controlled studies. Similarly the benefit from phonophoresis is not known.

Studies of transcutaneous electrical nerve stimulation (TENS) have often lacked suitable control groups, have included small sample sizes, or have used inappropriate methods of assessment. Electromyography (EMG) has been extensively used in conjunction with relaxation and biofeedback therapy and current data suggest that, while nocturnal EMG biofeedback may provide some control of nocturnal bruxism, the beneficial effect seems to be of short duration. Diurnal biofeedback relaxation techniques are not effective in reducing nocturnal bruxism.

Injection therapies

Intra-articular corticosteroids are probably of little long-term benefit. Intra-articular injection of sclerosant may be a useful technique in the very rare patients with TMJ dysfunction secondary to joint hypermobility. The benefits of denervation of the TMJ via injection of a sclerosant or surgical procedures are not known.

ATYPICAL FACIAL PAIN

Atypical facial pain (AFP) is essentially a diagnosis by exclusion and no longer included in the International Association for the Study of Pain's *Classification of Chronic Pain*,[27] nevertheless it is a clinically useful diagnosis. The pain is usually a continuous dull ache with intermittent severe episodes, primarily affecting areas of the face other than joints and muscles of mastication, such as the zygomatic maxilla. Pain may be bilateral and will often have been present for several years. Analgesics are ineffective. Atypical odontalgia (AO) has a similar character but is localized to one or more premolar or molar teeth, simulating pulpitis. There may be a history of inappropriate dental treatment, including extraction, and subsequent recurrence of symptoms apparently from another tooth.

Almost all patients with AFP complain of other symptoms, including headache, neck and back pain, dermatitis or pruritis, irritable bowel and dysfunctional uterine bleeding. Confusingly, 50% of patients may be diagnosed as having TMJ dysfunction.

Differentiation of AFP from trigeminal neuralgia (TN) can be difficult.[28] The vague distribution, constancy and lack of trigger points contrast with trigeminal neuralgia, but the latter may be complicated by a background ache.[29] It has been suggested that patients can be identified by their differing responses to the McGill Pain Questionnaire. With trigeminal neuralgia, patients tend to choose words such as 'flashing', 'terrifying' and 'blinding' to describe their pain, while those with AFP choose 'vicious', 'diffuse' and 'excruciating'.

There are no detailed epidemiologic studies of AFP. However, 1.9% of women and 0.9% of men in a large US adult population study reported 'a dull, aching pain' across the face or cheek ('excluding sinus pain') more than once in the previous six months.[17] The mean age of onset of AFP is probably in middle to late life.[30]

ETIOLOGY OF ATYPICAL FACIAL PAIN

Atypical facial pain probably has an association with neuroses, particularly depression; however, as with other chronic pain conditions, the prevalence of depressive symptoms neither establishes depression as a cause of AFP, nor vice versa. Studies of depression in chronic pain disorders including AFP are hampered by methodologic problems such as disparate diagnostic methods (e.g. a lack of specific diagnostic criteria), poor methods of pain assessment, inadequate patient selection, overlap in symptoms of pain and depression, and lack of prospective studies.

Like other chronic pain disorders, there would appear to be no empirical support for traditional psychodynamic models of AFP being a conversion reaction, a pain-prone disorder or a masked depression.

Some possible predisposing factors for AFP have been identified. One study has found a reduced tyramine conjugation (an established trait marker for endogenous unipolar depression) in orofacial pain patients, with the greatest deficit in the never-depressed subjects.[31] These findings were considered suggestive of a common underlying metabolic vulnerability to idiopathic facial pain and endogenous depression. However, the authors did concede that the probability of false-positive tests (0.33) precluded the recom-

mendation of tyramine conjugation deficit as a diagnostic screening test. The basis of the deficit is not understood.

Another study, using positron emission tomography, has demonstrated an increased contralateral cingulate cortex activity (and decreased prefrontal cortex activity), in response to both heat and nociceptive stimuli, in AFP patients relative to controls.[32] This is suggestive of an exaggerated perception of pain in response to peripheral stimuli but how this might develop remains a matter for speculation. The authors suggested that the mechanism for the observed differences is related to anxiety and attention and therefore that the pain might be brought under conscious control.

Approximately 50% of AFP patients attribute their pain to an antecedent event such as an endodontic or exodontic procedure, or minor trauma to the face. Despite the notorious unreliability of such retrospective reports, it has been suggested that AFP may be a deafferentation syndrome, also labeled 'Phantom tooth pain' (PTP).[33] One retrospective study found the incidence of PTP to be 3% in a sample of 256 women who had undergone endodontic therapy. Similarities between AFP and postamputation pain include the burning quality, the self-reported description as severe despite lack of sleep disturbance, poor localization, and delay between injury and incidence. The lack of response to nerve block is also a common feature.

Unilateral increase in facial blood flow, as measured by increased heat loss, and tenderness over the site of pain have been reported in two small studies of AFP patients, possibly suggesting an inflammatory component.

Rarely, AFP-like symptoms are secondary to CNS malignancy[34] or vascular anomalies.

MANAGEMENT OF ATYPICAL FACIAL PAIN

As a consequence of the belief that AFP has a psychogenic basis, antidepressant therapy is the main mode of treatment.

Forty-three percent of a group of patients with different chronic orofacial pains who had initially participated in a double-blind trial of dothiepin, and received further courses of the drug and counseling sessions, became pain-free; however, those with AFP were the least responsive.

Pain relief with tricyclic antidepressants such as dothiepin may be independent of the antidepressant effect of the agent. Instead these drugs may alter the sensory discriminative component of pain. The possibility of interference with serotonin re-uptake in the brainstem has been proposed. However, short-term therapy with the serotonin antagonist iprazochrome was of equivocal benefit in a group of patients with AFP.

Various other therapies have been tried. Salmon calcitonin is not effective and frequently causes side effects;

ketamine probably only has a placebo action, although TENS may be of some benefit. Sphenopalatine ganglion blocks have been suggested to be of benefit,[35] but additional data are required to confirm this notion.

In general, dental surgery and other surgical procedures such as neurectomy or even small neurodestructive procedures lead to a worsening of the pain.

BURNING MOUTH SYNDROME

Burning mouth syndrome (BMS; oral dysesthesia; glossodynia; glossopyrosis) presents as a variety of symptoms including pain, burning or itching in the tongue, lips, denture-bearing areas and/or elsewhere in the oral mucosa, and is generally bilateral. There may be an alteration in taste and subjective dryness.[36] Symptoms may be relieved or exacerbated by eating or drinking. Some workers subclassify BMS: Type 1 – burning is absent on waking but develops as the day goes on; Type 2 – the burning is present on waking and persists throughout the day; Type 3 – the symptoms are intermittent.

Intraoral examination reveals a normal, healthy mucosa and patients are otherwise well.

Burning mouth syndrome has a reported prevalence of 2.6–5.1%; it is about 3 times more common in females than males and has its onset in middle to late life.

ETIOLOGY OF BURNING MOUTH SYNDROME

As with other chronic orofacial pain conditions, the precise etiology of burning mouth syndrome is unknown. Local, systemic and psychologic factors have been suggested.

Local factors

Many patients with BMS attribute the onset of their symptoms to an antecedent dental procedure, particularly the fitting of dentures. Ill-fitting dentures have been suggested to give rise to BMS symptoms but, since BMS is not limited to denture wearers, this etiology seems unlikely. Hypersensitivity to the denture base material, methyl methacrylate, was found in 23% of 22 patients, yet affected patients had atypical symptoms limited to the denture-bearing area and restricted to periods of denture wearing.[37]

Burning mouth syndrome is neither a consequence of tobacco smoking nor of lingual atherosclerosis, ill-defined hypersensitivity reactions are also unlikely to be of significance. While the intraoral prevalence of Candida species and coliforms may be increased in BMS, patients do not have clinical evidence of infection, and patients with severe candidal infections do not complain of BMS. Curiously, fusospirochetal infection that responded to metronidazole therapy was suggested to be the cause of BMS in one small group of patients.

Systemic factors

There is little consistent evidence that alterations in female sex corticosteroids are important in the etiology of BMS. Hormone replacement therapy is of limited efficacy, and affected patients do not have notably altered age-related levels of relevant hormones. Parodoxically BMS has been described in a patient with a secretory ovarian tumor.

The symptoms of BMS can only rarely be attributed to an underlying undiagnosed diabetes mellitus.

Iron, folic acid and vitamin B_{12} deficiencies are rare in BMS. It is of note that 40% of 70 Scottish BMS patients were deficient in vitamins B_1, B_2, and/or B_6. Twenty-four of this group of 28 patients had resolution of BMS following replacement therapy and at 3-month follow up, while 2 had some improvement. However, a subsequent study failed to show any improvement with replacement therapy in 15 B_1 and/ or B_2 deficient BMS patients from a group of 16, and others have also found that vitamin B supplementation is not of benefit. It is unlikely that zinc deficiency is of significance in the etiology of BMS.

Psychologic factors

Between 44% and 92% of BMS patients have symptoms of anxiety or depression.[35,38] Nevertheless, the relevant studies have not always used standardized methods.

Several studies have identified subgroups of BMS patients with and without psychiatric disorder.[37,39] However, no longitudinal study has been undertaken to establish the nature of the temporal relationship between psychologic factors and BMS symptoms. There are conflicting data regarding the relevance of previous life events in the etiology of BMS.[38]

MANAGEMENT OF BURNING MOUTH SYNDROME

Chlordiazepoxide and dothiepin have been suggested to be of use. Cognitive therapy may also be of benefit in the management of BMS, lending further support for the importance of psychological factors in the maintenance of BMS symptoms, if not their development. Recently 27% of a group of 15 BMS patients had resolution while the remainder had some lessening of symptoms following 12–15 one-hour weekly cognitive therapy sessions, compared with a placebo control group who showed no resolution.[40]

The management of BMS initially entails the exclusion of potential local causes such as local trauma, infection or profound xerostomia. However, these are present only in a minority of affected patients. Screening for underlying hematologic or endocrine disease is unlikely to be of notable benefit, except in those patients with an atypical presentation and/or signs or symptoms of underlying systemic disease.

Local application of agents such as lignocaine in carboxymethylcellulose,[36] or benzydamine hydrochloride spray or mouthrinse can provide some transient relief, but to date there are no formal studies of the efficacy of this approach. Antifungal agents are unlikely to be of clinical benefit.

REFERENCES

1. Barker F, Jannetta P, Bissonette D et al 1996 The long-term outcome of microvascular decompression for trigeminal neuralgia. New England Journal of Medicine 334:1077–1083
2. Porter SR, Scully C 1994 HIV disease: the surgeon's perspective 2:diagnosis and management of non-malignant oral manifestations. British Journal of Oral and Maxillofacial Surgery 32:231–240
3. Zakrzewska J 1995 Trigeminal neuralgia. WB Saunders, London
4. De Vriese A, Philippe J, Van Renterghem D et al 1995 Carbamazepine hypersensitivity syndrome: report of 4 cases and review of the literature. Medicine 74:144–151
5. Remillard G 1994 Oxcarbazepine and intractable trigeminal neuralgia. Epilepsia 35:S28–29
6. Walchenbach R, Voormolen JH 1996 Surgical treatment for trigeminal neuralgia. British Medical Journal 313:1027–1028
7. Greene K, Karahalios D, Spetzler R 1995 Glossopharyngeal neuralgia associated with vascular compression and choroid plexus papilloma. British Journal of Neurosurgery 9:809–814
8. Taha JM, Tew JM 1995 Long-term results of surgical treatment of idiopathic neuralgias of the glossopharyngeal and vagal nerves. Neurosurgery 36:926–930
9. Resnick D, Jannetta P, Bissonnette D, Jho H-D, Lanzino G 1995 Microvascular decompression for glossopharyngeal neuralgia. Neurosurgery 36:64–69
10. Lee JJ, Gauci CA 1994 Post herpetic neuralgia: current concepts and management. British Journal of Hospital Medicine 52:565–567, 570
11. Rowbotham M, Fields H 1996 The relationship of pain, allodynia and thermal sensation in postherpetic neuralgia. Brain 119:347–354
12. Iadarola M, Max M, Berman K, Byas-Smith M, Coghill R, Gracely R, Bennett G 1995 Unilateral decrease in thalamic activity observed with positron emission tomography in patients with chronic neuropathic pain. Pain 63:55–64
13. Bennett G 1994 Hypotheses on the pathogenesis of herpes zoster-associated pain. Annals of Neurology 35:S38–41
14. Watson C 1993 The medical treatment of postherpetic neuralgia: antidepressants, other therapies, and practical guidelines for management. In: Watson C (ed) Herpes zoster and postherpetic neuralgia. Elsevier, Amsterdam, pp 205–219
15. Eide P, Jorum E, Stubhaug A, Bremnes J, Breivik H 1994 Relief of post herpetic neuralgia with the N-methyl-D-aspartic acid receptor antagonist ketamine: a double-blind, cross-over comparison with morphine and placebo. Pain 58:347–354
16. Porter SR 1996 Aspects of non-surgical therapy of temporomandibular joint dysfunction. In: Porter SR, Scully C (eds) Innovations and developments of non-surgical management of orofacial disease. Science Reviews, Northwood
17. Lipton J, Ship J, Larach-Robinson D 1993 Estimated prevalence and distribution of reported orofacial pain in the United States. Journal of the American Dental Association 124:115–121
18. Adair SM, Hecht C 1993 Association of generalised joint hypermobility with history, signs, and symptoms of temporomandibular joint dysfunction in children. Pediatric Dentistry 15:323–326
19. Bush FM, Harkins SW 1995 Pain-related limitation in activities of daily living in patients with chronic orofacial pain. Journal of Orofacial Pain 9:57–63
20. Glaros AG, Glass EG, McLaughlin L 1994 Knowledge and beliefs of dentists regarding temporomandibular disorders and chronic pain. Journal of Orofacial Pain 8:216–222
21. Dworkin SF, Massoth DL 1994 Temporomandibular disorders and chronic pain: disease or illness? Journal of Prosthetic Dentistry 72:29–38
22. Mohl ND, Dixon C 1994 Current status of diagnostic procedure for temporomandibular disorder. Journal of the American Dental Association 125:56–64
23. Sano T, Westesson PL 1995 Magnetic resonance imaging of the temporomandibular joint. Increased T2 signal in the retrodiskal tissue of painful joints. Oral Surgery, Oral Medicine, Oral Pathology, Oral Radiology and Endodontics 79:511–516
24. Laskin DM 1993 Diagnosis of pathology of the temporomandibular joint. Radiological Clinics of North America 31:135–147
25. Gratt BM, Sickles EA 1993 Thermographic characterisation of the asymptomatic temporomandibular joint. Journal of Orofacial Pain 7:7–14
26. Ishigaki S, Bessette RW, Maruyama T 1993 Vibration analysis of the temporomandibular joints with meniscal displacement with and without reduction. Journal of Craniomandibular Practice 11:192–201
27. Merskey H, Bogduk N 1994 Classification of chronic pain, 2nd edn. IASP Press, Seattle, pp 59–60
28. Turp J, Gobetti J 1996 Trigeminal neuralgia versus atypical facial pain. Oral Surgery, Oral Medicine, and Oral Pathology 81:424–432
29. Loeser J 1994 Tic douloureux and atypical facial pain. In: Wall P, Melzack R (eds) Textbook of Pain. Churchill Livingstone, London, pp 426–434
30. Allerbring M, Haegerstam G 1993 Characteristics of patients with chronic idiopathic orofacial pain. A retrospective study. Acta Odontologica Scandinavica 51:53–58
31. Aghabeigi B, Feinmann C, Glover V et al 1993 Tyramine conjugation deficit in patients with chronic idiopathic temporomandibular joint and orofacial pain. Pain 54:159–163
32. Derbyshire S, Jones A, Devani P et al 1994 Cerebral responses to pain in patients with atypical facial pain measured by positron emission tomography. Journal of Neurology, Neurosurgery and Psychiatry 57:1166–1172
33. Marbach JJ 1993 Is phantom tooth pain a deafferentation (neuropathic) syndrome? Part I: evidence derived from pathophysiology and treatment. Oral Surgery, Oral Medicine, and Oral Pathology 75: 95–105
34. Huntley TA, Wiesenfeld D 1994 Delayed diagnosis of the cause of facial pain in patients with neoplastic disease: a report of eight cases. Journal of Oral and Maxillofacial Surgery 52:81–85
35. Peterson JN, Schames J, Schames M, King E 1995 Sphenopalatine ganglion block: a safe and easy method for the management of orofacial pain. Cranio 13:177–181
36. Schulten EAJM, van der Waal I 1996 Burning mouth syndrome. In: Porter SR, Scully C (eds) Innovations and developments in non-invasive orofacial health care. Science Reviews, Northwood, pp 27–38

37. Lamey P-J, Lamb A, Hughes A, Milligan K, Forsyth A 1994 Type 3 burning mouth syndrome: psychological and allergic aspects. Journal of Oral Pathology and Medicine 23:216–219

38. Eli I, Kleinhauz M, Baht R, Littner M 1994 Antecedents of burning mouth syndrome (glossodynia) – recent life events vs. psycho-pathological aspects. Journal of Dental Research 73:567–572

39. Rojo L, Silvestre F, Bagan J, De Vicente T 1994 Prevalence of psychopathology in burning mouth syndrome: a comparative study among patients with and without psychiatric disorders and controls. Oral Surgery, Oral Medicine, and Oral Pathology 78:312–316

40. Bergdahl J, Anneroth G, Perris H 1995 Cognitive therapy in the treatment of patients with resistant burning mouth syndrome: a controlled study. Journal of Oral Pathology and Medicine 24:213–215

Surgical treatment of TMJ internal derangement

90

M. FRANKLIN DOLWICK/ALAN W. WILSON

INTRODUCTION

Temporomandibular disorders (TMD) are common problems that occur in about 33% of the general population.[1] It has been estimated that 75% of the population have symptoms and 33% have signs of TMD. Approximately 5% of the population will require treatment of TMD[2] and about 5% of all patients being treated will undergo surgery.[3] Surgery of the temporomandibular joint (TMJ) therefore has a small, but nonetheless important role in the management of specific temporomandibular disorders.[4]

Historically, interest in TMJ surgery has been cyclical with periods of high enthusiasm followed by periods of skepticism. Invariably, enthusiasm for various procedures waned because they failed to achieve the expected results. The rediscovery of TMJ disk derangement by Farrar in 1971,[5] followed by the reintroduction of TMJ arthrography by Wilkes in 1978,[6] stimulated renewed interest in TMJ disk derangement and its surgical treatment. Clinical, anatomic, imaging and surgical studies focused on the importance of disk displacement and deformity as the cause of TMJ pain and dysfunction.[7-11] Open joint surgery (arthrotomy) procedures were introduced to reposition and reshape the displaced, deformed disk.[7,12,13] Old procedures such as diskectomy[14] (meniscectomy) and condylotomy[15] received new interest.[16-19] Because disk repositioning and diskectomy procedures failed to consistently achieve the desired results, surgeons continued to search for alternative procedures.

The introduction of TMJ arthroscopy revolutionized the surgical management of internal derangement of the TMJ.[20-22] The observations that arthroscopic lavage and lysis of adhesions in the upper joint space resulted in reduced pain and improved joint function raised serious questions about the significance of disk displacement as the cause of TMJ pain and dysfunction.[23,24] More recently, observations made following a conservative form of TMJ lavage, arthrocentesis, have added to the doubts about the significance of disk displacement.[25]

Today, the TMJ surgeon has several options for the treatment of TMJ internal derangement. While each procedure has its enthusiastic supporters, each procedure also has its critics. It is impossible to select the appropriate surgical procedure based on scientific evidence since randomized prospective studies have not been performed. Selection of the surgical procedure must therefore be based on the currently available clinical data and each surgeon's experience. It seems prudent to select the procedure that has the highest probability of a favorable outcome with the lowest probability of morbidity for each patient's specific problem.

The succeeding sections of this chapter will discuss clinical evaluation, indications, surgical techniques, outcomes and complications associated with currently utilized surgical procedures for the treatment of TMJ internal derangement. This chapter will not discuss other TMJ entities such as ankylosis, pathologic conditions, or trauma.

CLINICAL EVALUATION

HISTORY

The most important part of the clinical evaluation of temporomandibular disorders is the history. The role of the clinician is to establish a diagnosis from the clues provided by the patient and to formulate a treatment plan that will address the patient's chief complaint(s). At the most basic level, the surgeon should determine whether the patient's complaints are caused by a muscular or a joint condition.

The chief complaint may be pain, joint noise, restricted mouth opening or a combination of these; there may in addition be other less specific problems such as headaches, neck pain, and earaches. Pain should be carefully evaluated in terms of onset, nature, intensity, site, duration, aggravating and relieving factors and, especially, how the pain relates to other features such as joint noise and restricted mandibular movements.

The history of the presenting complaint is basically a timetable of the onset and duration of the symptoms and a record of the treatment that the patient has undergone for the condition in the past. Generally speaking, the prognosis for each case appears to be a function of the duration of the symptoms and the number and outcomes of previous treatments. That is to say, the longer the duration of the symptoms, and the greater the number of treatments, in particular 'failed treatments' (and especially failed surgical treatments), the less likely it is that the patient will respond favorably to further treatment.

During the history-taking, the clinician should be able not only to establish a rapport with the patient, but also to determine the patient's reliability as a historian. Unfortunately the indications for surgery are not objective and are often dependent on the patient's ability to report his or her symptoms, as well as the surgeon's ability to interpret them. Equally, an impression of the patient's personality is vital to the overall understanding of the disease process. Underlying influences, such as stress, anxiety, depression or significant life events, must be elicited during the history, so that a clearer understanding of how TMD affects the patient is made possible. The history provides most of the important clues that determine subsequent management and prognosis.

It is important, however, that the clinician involved in the management of TMD cultivates the essential skill of listening and gently directs the verbal interaction through simple questioning to steer the patient to a point where the diagnosis becomes apparent. Most importantly, the clinician must appear to be empathetic to the patient's 'suffering' otherwise a poor patient–doctor relationship will most likely compromise the prognosis, no matter what the treatment.

CLINICAL EXAMINATION

A comprehensive physical examination of the patient involves observation, palpation, auscultation, and measurement of the range of mandibular motion. Additionally, the patient's occlusal function should also be thoroughly evaluated.

The TMJ should be evaluated for tenderness in those areas accessible to palpation at rest and during function. Palpation is accomplished by placing the finger tips at the lateral condylar poles and exerting medially directed force. The patient is then asked to open the mouth and the finger tip will fall into the depression left by the translating condyle. Pain on loading of the TMJ may be evaluated by having the patient bite on a tongue blade placed in the cuspid/biscuspid areas, which will serve to load the contralateral joint. Joint sounds and their location during opening, closing and lateral excursions of the mandible may be detected with a stethoscope. It must be kept in mind, however, that joint noises such as clicking are a common finding in the general population and may not be related to the patient's complaint.

Mandibular function may be evaluated by observation and measurement of the free range of mandibular movement. One should note whether the line of vertical opening is straight and smooth or deviates with jerky movements. Joint locking due to intracapsular mechanical interference is evidenced by limited or guarded mandibular movement. The range of painless maximal vertical opening (normal range is 42–55 mm), protrusive (>7 mm) and lateral excursions (>7 mm) should be recorded. Limitations of the mandibular range of motion may be caused by intracapsular pathology or muscle dysfunction, or a combination of both. It is essential to determine the cause of the decreased mandibular movements so that the most appropriate course of management may be undertaken.

Examination of the masticatory musculature may be accomplished by digital palpation. Areas of tenderness, trigger points and pain referral patterns should be noted. The patient is asked to rate levels of tenderness as mild, moderate or severe. Direct palpation of the lateral pterygoid muscle is not possible so provocation testing of this muscle may be accomplished by having the patient protrude the mandible against the mild to moderate resistance of the clinician's fingers placed against the patient's chin.

Although malocclusion is not a recognized etiologic factor in TMD, it may play a contributory role as an exacerbating and maintaining factor in the pathophysiology of TMD.[26] The relationship of the teeth in centric relation, occlusal guidance in excursive movements and the condition of the supporting structures are assessed in terms of the degree of structural adaptation of the TMJ that may have occurred to accommodate the malocclusion. Discrepancies between centric relation and centric occlusion should be noted. Occlusal conditions thought to affect adversely the health of the stomatognathic system include: balancing side contacts in excursive movements, protrusive guidance on posterior teeth, dual bite (>2 mm anterior–posterior difference between centric relation and centric occlusion), mandibular retrognathia, and crossbites. Most importantly, the clinician should note evidence of parafunctional behavior such as faceting, fractures and craze lines on teeth. Pain during clenching may initiate or exacerbate the patient's chief complaint if the cause is of a myofascial nature resulting from bruxism.

IMAGING STUDIES

Imaging studies are adjunctive measures which serve to provide additional information that cannot be obtained by history and physical examination alone. In the overall assessment of TMD, investigations play a relatively minor role, since the majority of the pertinent information should already have been provided by the history and physical evaluation. One of the most useful roles for imaging studies, however, is to eliminate the possibility of other pathologic processes that may mimic TMD symptoms.

Plain radiographs of the TMJ serve a somewhat limited role in the diagnosis of TMD. Despite the limitations, high level orthopantomograms and transcranial projections are useful as baseline studies for identifying any gross pathologic, degenerative or traumatic changes in the bony component of the TMJ complex. In addition, panoramic radiographs will screen for any gross tooth, periodontal, mandibular or maxillary pathology. Although the majority of plain radiographs of the TMJ will show no abnormalities, nonetheless the X-rays not only eliminate the possibility of any gross pathology but also act as a permanent record of the pretreatment condition of the TMJs, especially if surgery is planned.

In recent years, magnetic resonance imaging (MRI) has increasingly been used in the study of TMD, in particular internal derangements of the TMJ.[27,28] MRI has gradually been replacing arthrography as it is a painless, noninvasive, non-ionizing radiation alternative with expanded capabilities of imaging not only the articular soft tissues but also surrounding muscles, vasculature and neural structures without the need for contrast media. Various pulsing sequences are used to accentuate differences between tissue types. 'T$_1$-weighted' pulse sequencing best delineates disk position and morphology, whereas on 'T$_2$-weighted' pulse sequencing free water and tissue inflammation show high signal intensity (Figs 90.1, 90.2).[29,30] The significance of this finding has been attributed to joint effusion. Bone appears black regardless of the pulse sequence.

MRI imaging has proven reliable in depicting disk anatomy and position[28] but has been disappointing in differentiating symptomatic TMJ patients from asymptomatic TMJ patients.[31,32] Over-reliance on the diagnostic value of imaging may lead to over-diagnosis of internal derangement and

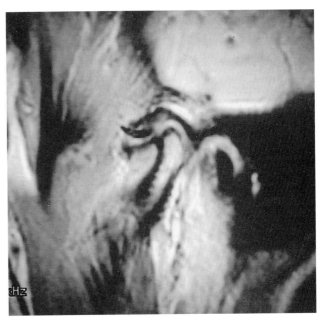

Fig. 90.1 T$_1$-weighted MRI showing a deformed anteriorly displaced disk.

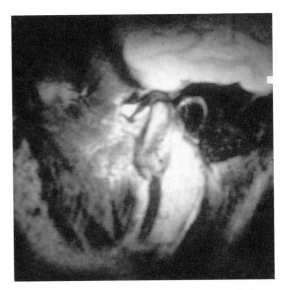

Fig. 90.2 T$_2$-weighted MRI showing a large effusion in both the upper and lower joint spaces. The disk is also anteriorly displaced.

hence to over-treatment. MRI findings should, therefore, always be correlated with the history and clinical findings.

The use of TMJ arthrography has for the most part been replaced by MRI. Arthrography is more accurate than MRI in identifying the presence of adhesions and disk perforations but, because the technique is invasive and uncomfortable to the patient, its use has diminished. Other imaging techniques such as scintigraphy, CT and ultrasound have limited value in diagnosing TMJ internal derangements and therefore are generally not recommended.

DIAGNOSIS

An accurate diagnosis is the key to planning the most appropriate course of treatment.[33]

Myofascial pain and dysfunction generally presents with diffuse pain that is cyclic and distributed in multiple sites in the head and neck, particularly the muscles of mastication. It is frequently worst in the morning and the patient will often report sore teeth and clenching. There is often a history of stress and difficulty in sleeping. Clinically the patient presents with diffuse muscle tenderness and a decreased range of mandibular movements with occasional joint noises and wear facets on teeth. Other features – such as abnormal jaw posturing, or chewing only on one side as an avoidance mechanism to a sore tooth, or a large centric relation and centric occlusion discrepancy – may be found. Imaging findings generally do not contribute to the diagnosis apart from ruling out other possible diseases.

Internal joint derangement on the other hand presents with continuous pain which is localized to the TMJ and exacerbated by jaw function. Mechanical interferences in the joint such as clicking and locking will often result in deviation of mandibular movements during opening and closing. The TMJ is tender to palpation and painful on loading. Reciprocal clicking and grating (crepitus) is often present. A decreased range of mandibular movements is another common feature, secondary to pain and mechanical joint interferences. Imaging findings are sometimes helpful in determining the source and extent of the disease process.

Other less common temporomandibular disorders present with clinical features that reflect abnormalities in the structural integrity of the TMJ complex. Developmental or neoplastic conditions of the TMJ result in changes to the occlusion and/or lower facial symmetry. Chronic severe limitation of mouth opening may indicate ankylosis, whereas acute changes in occlusion with painful limited opening usually follow a traumatic incident involving the TMJ. In these instances, imaging plays a more significant role in the definitive diagnosis.

TREATMENT PLANNING

The treatment selected should aim to alleviate the pain, decrease adverse joint loading, restore mandibular function, reduce or eliminate joint noise, and allow the patient to return to normal daily activities. A well-designed treatment schedule not only treats the physical and/or psychologic disorder(s), but also eliminates all contributing factors that serve to maintain or nurture the disease process.

The most important point to consider is that signs and symptoms of TMD are often transient and self-limiting and tend to resolve with time and with no long-term effects.[34–36] With this in mind every effort should be made to avoid aggressive, irreversible therapy such as occlusal adjustments or surgery as a first line of treatment. Simple, conservative and reversible therapy must always take first priority in treatment planning for TMD, no matter how significant the initial presentation may appear. All contributing factors, such as nocturnal bruxism or depression, must be resolved and the symptoms stabilized prior to undertaking even the simplest of irreversible treatments, otherwise aggressive therapy in an unstable TMD patient will most likely exacerbate their problems.

SURGERY

INDICATIONS FOR SURGERY

The indications for TMJ surgery are very rare, but can be divided into general indications for surgery and indications specific to each surgical technique. TMJ surgery is indicated for the patient diagnosed as having an internal derangement when there is severe chronic TMJ pain and/or dysfunction which are refractory to non-surgical treatment. The indications specific to each surgical technique will be presented in association with the technique.

Diagnosis presents the greatest dilemma to the surgeon because there are no objective tests for diagnosing internal derangement. The diagnosis is made on the basis of the history and clinical examination. The clinical criteria for diagnosis of internal derangement are subjective and therefore highly dependent upon the patient's ability to accurately report them and then the surgeon's ability to interpret them. Based on the history and clinical examination, the surgeon must be convinced that the patient's symptoms primarily arise within the TMJ if surgery is to be considered. The best surgical candidate specifically localizes the pain and/or dysfunction to the TMJ, has a tender TMJ to palpation, and experiences an increase in TMJ pain when the joint is loaded. The more localized the pain and dysfunction is to the TMJ, the better the prognosis; conversely, the more diffuse the symptoms the worse the prognosis.

While MRI findings should not be used as the primary diagnostic criteria, they may be helpful in confirming the presence of internal derangement and in identifying the specific anatomic derangement. MRI is therefore generally recommended prior to surgery, especially open surgery.

Experience has shown that most TMJ patients benefit from appropriate non-surgical treatment; TMJ surgery should therefore be rarely, if ever, performed before non-surgical treatment has been attempted and found to be ineffective.[34,35] The patient considering TMJ surgery should understand that while TMJ internal derangement may progress anatomically, the pain and dysfunction frequently decrease even in the absence of treatment.[36]

TMJ surgery is not without significant risks,[37] and it is not known whether or not the progression of the anatomic derangement is altered, either favorably or unfavorably, by surgery. The decision to perform TMJ surgery should therefore be predicated not on the basis of anatomic derangement but on the severity of the patient's symptoms and the inability of the patient to manage and tolerate the existing symptoms. TMJ surgery should not be performed for preventive reasons because it is not known whether the surgical treatment is, in fact, better than the natural course of the disorder. Some patients with diagnosed internal derangement may also have psychologic disorders and/or muscular disorders such as myofascial pain and dysfunction.[38] When these problems exist, they must be evaluated and their management included in the overall treatment plan. It is also possible to have an internal derangement which causes no pain in association with myofascial pain or another painful disorder.[33] Surgery should be considered only for the treatment of refractory TMJ pain and/or dysfunction and not for pain and/or dysfunction of myofascial origin.

ARTHROTOMY

TMJ arthrotomy includes several surgical procedures which are performed through an open incision into the TMJ. There are two basic procedures – disk repositioning (diskoplasty) and disk removal (diskectomy) – which may be used in the treatment of internal derangement. TMJ arthrotomy procedures are indicated for all stages of internal derangement, especially patients who have mechanical interference in the joint, e.g. hard clicking or intermittent locking. TMJ arthrotomy is also indicated for patients who have failed previous surgical procedures.

SURGICAL ACCESS

The most commonly used approach to the TMJ is the preauricular approach.[39] There are several variations of skin incisions used, including the standard preauricular, extended preauricular, and the endaural. While there are stated advantages and disadvantages to each location of the skin incision, these are minor in importance and therefore the location of the incision is determined by the surgeon's choice based on personal experience. The facial nerve is avoided using the Al Kayat and Bramley modification.[40]

The preauricular region is prepared and draped so that the ear and lateral canthus of the eye are exposed. The hair in the temporal region can be shaved although we have not found this to be necessary unless the extended incision is utilized. The external acoustic meatus should be occluded to prevent coagulum adhering to the tympanum; it is wise to perform a visual inspection of the tympanum at the end of the operation and irrigate if necessary to avoid this complication. The skin incision is marked according to the preferred flap design. Local anesthetic with vasoconstrictor is injected along the incision line to aid hemostasis.

The skin incision is executed, starting superiorly through the scalp, and the temporalis fascia is identified. Development of the flap in this plane is carried out antero-inferiorly to a point where the fat is visible through the superficial layer of temporalis fascia. This appears at about 2 cm above the zygomatic arch. The skin is dissected off the tragus and the cartilaginous external acoustic meatus (Fig. 90.3). This plane is avascular but the operator should take care not to dissect too vertically as this risks entry into the external acoustic meatus. This part of the dissection ends with exposure of the post-glenoid tubercle, which is at the same level as the fascial plane sited above. The superficial layer of temporalis is incised from the root of the arch 45 degrees antero-superiorly to avoid the facial nerve.

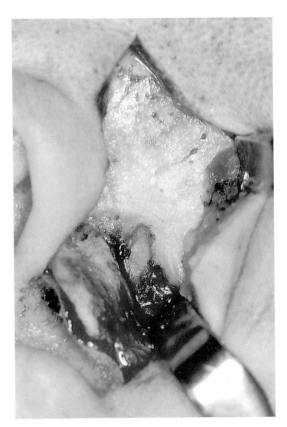

Fig. 90.3 Endaural skin incision with the temporalis fascia identified.

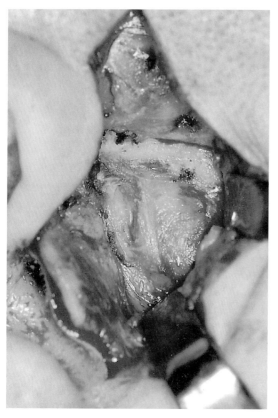

Fig. 90.4 Endaural skin incision with superficial temporal fascia and periosteum reflected to expose the joint capsule.

Deep to this layer the periosteum of the arch is identified and incised and raised as one flap with the outer layer of temporalis fascia. Periosteum may be incised as far forward as is deemed necessary to gain good exposure of the joint capsule inferiorly (Fig. 90.4). The superficial temporal vessels and their branches may require ligation or diathermy during the course of the dissection. Bipolar diathermy is preferable to monopolar and great care is needed with retraction of the tissues lest the assistant induce a traction palsy of the facial nerve. Tissues should be kept moist at all times as desiccation will affect healing. Blunt dissection of the tissues off the capsule is performed. The capsular exposure should extend to the height of the articular eminence. With the condyle distracted inferiorly, pointed scissors are used to enter the upper joint space anteriorly along the posterior slope of the eminence. The opening is extended antero-posteriorly by cutting along the lateral aspect of the eminence and fossa. The capsule is reflected laterally, opening the upper joint space. The disk and its attachments can now be visualized and inspected as to position, movement and integrity. After completion of the intra-articular procedure the wound is closed in layers. Drains are rarely needed if hemostasis is fastidious.

DISK REPOSITIONING

Disk repositioning surgery was introduced in 1979 by McCarty and Farrar.[7] It is performed when the disk can be repositioned to a normal anatomic relationship with the condyle and fossa and is not under tension in the position, is essentially normal as to shape and thickness, and is normal in appearance, i.e. white, firm, glistening and not erythematous or soft.

The surgical approach for disk repositioning is by the preauricular incision as previously described. Once the upper joint space has been opened, the disk and its attachments are inspected as to position, movement and integrity. Usually the disk is displaced anteriorly and medially (Fig. 90.5). If the disk can be reduced, demonstrating that it can be repositioned correctly, then a partial thickness plication as described by Hall is performed (Fig. 90.6).[12] If the disk cannot be repositioned with entering the lower joint space, a full-thickness plication as described by Dolwick and Sanders is performed.[13] Recontouring of the lateral third of the articular eminence is generally performed in order to improve visualization and access into the upper joint space. Reduction of the lateral eminence also redistributes the joint load during function more medially. If the disk position is satisfactory with the teeth in occlusion and during function, the surgical site is closed in layers.

Postoperative treatment is directed at reducing joint load-

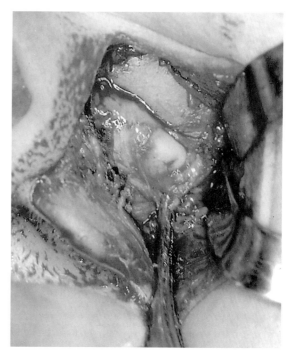

Fig. 90.5 The capsule is reflected laterally exposing the upper joint space. The disk is displaced anteriorly.

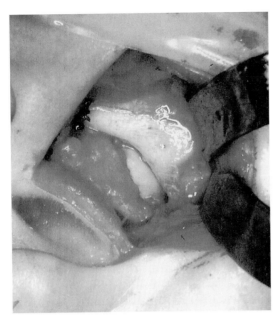

Fig. 90.6 The disk is repositioned posteriorly and laterally to its correct position.

ing and re-establishing a normal range of motion. While the exact magnitude of joint load during function and dysfunction is not known, it seems important to minimize it during the healing phase following surgery. This is accomplished by restricting the patient to a soft diet and controlling bruxism. The patient is restricted to a soft non-chew diet for about three months. The diet is then gradually increased as determined by the patient's ability to chew without discomfort. Bruxism can be difficult to control. The postoperative management of bruxism is the same as that for bruxism in general, i.e. medications for sleep and an occlusal appliance. Movement of the TMJ is started immediately following the surgery. Initially, the range of motion is limited to opening and excursive movements that are not painful, e.g. 10–20 mm opening, 2–5 mm excursive movement. These movements should be performed as frequently as possible without causing prolonged discomfort. Approximately two weeks postoperatively the range of motion is increased in order to re-establish normal opening and excursive movement. Reasonable goals are 40 mm opening and greater than 5 mm excursive movement. While the use of continuous passive motion is theoretically good, on a practical basis it is difficult to perform for the TMJ.

Results

The results of disk repositioning surgery have been favorable on the one hand and disappointing on the other. Clinical studies indicate that 80–90% of the patients have had a decrease in pain and improvement in their range of motion and masticatory function.[7,12,13,41,42] The results have been disappointing in that 5–10% of the patients are either not improved or in some cases worse after the surgery. Dolwick and Nitzan evaluated 152 patients who underwent TMJ disk surgery between the years 1980 and 1988 and found that about 90% of the patients reported 70–80% improvement after disk repositioning surgery.[43] The data indicated that improvement was maintained for the eight years evaluated and was not simply a short-term improvement related to the post-surgical anesthesia of the auriculotemporal nerve. Excellent results were reported by 51.5% of the patients and good results by another 28%. Disappointingly, 4.5% of the patients reported that they were worse and another 5.3% reported no change. They also observed that the majority of patients who were improved continued to have symptoms of pain, joint noise and decreased range of motion.

Complications

The most common complications following TMJ arthrotomy have been continued pain and the development of fibrous adhesions within the joint.[37] These frequently occur together. Facial nerve weakness occurs in less than 5% of patients and has been generally temporary and limited to the temporal branches. Significant malocclusions occur rarely, but many patients have minor changes in their occlusion. Infection occurs in less than 1% of patients.

DISKECTOMY

Diskectomy is one of the oldest TMJ surgery procedures, first described in 1909 by Lanz. It is performed when the disk cannot be repositioned because of deformity or degeneration. Instability of the disk from perforation, fragmentation or loss of elasticity necessitates disk removal. Persistent pain and dysfunction after disk repositioning is also an indication for diskectomy. After the joint components have been exposed the disk is excised, leaving as much synovium as possible. After removal of the disk the articular surfaces are inspected for osteophytes or irregularities; if these are present they are recontoured conservatively, taking care to protect intact articular cartilage. Until recently the disk was replaced with an alloplastic implant material. The high occurrence of foreign body reaction to these alloplastic materials militates against their continued usage.[44-47] At the present time the excised disk is generally not replaced. Various autogenous tissues – i.e. auricular cartilage, dermis and temporal flaps – have been advocated as replacement tissues for the disk.[48–51] The advantages, if any, of using these tissues for replacement of the disk are unclear at the present time.

Postoperative treatment is similar to that for disk repositioning and is directed at reducing joint load and re-establishing the range of motion. When bilateral diskectomy is performed there may be a tendency for the mandible to shift posteriorly, resulting in heavy posterior occlusal contacts and a slight anterior open bite. This can usually be prevented by using inter-arch elastics for 6–8 weeks postoperatively.

Results

The results of diskectomy with replacement using alloplastic materials have been uniformly bad. Foreign body reaction and detritic synovitis to Silastic implants were first reported in 1985.[44] Subsequently, numerous studies reported foreign body reaction and osseous degeneration associated with the use of alloplastic implants.[45–47] Interpositional alloplastic implants are no longer indicated for use in the TMJ because of these complications.

The perception of significant complications associated with diskectomy has caused surgeons to be reluctant to accept the procedure in spite of generally favorable results with diskectomy without replacement. Short-term studies report a success rate of about 80% for relief of pain and improved masticatory function.[52] Long-term follow up of almost 30 years in one study reported excellent results.[53,54] In fact, the results were better than the reported short-term results.[54] Ericksson & Westesson evaluated 15 patients who had diskectomy performed between 1947 and 1960. On clinical examination all patients were free of pain, none had subjectively experienced dysfunction and all but one could open their mouths more than 39 mm. Radiographic changes after diskectomy occur primarily in the condyle and seem to stabilize after one and a half years.[55] These radiographic changes most likely represent adaptation of the condyle and fossa to each other.

Complications

Complications after diskectomy are uncommon, but can be significant.[37,56] As with any arthrotomy procedure, facial nerve paresis can occur. It occurs in less than 5% of cases and usually temporarily affects the temporal branches. Heterotopic bone formation may occur, resulting in ankylosis; this is more likely if extensive articular surface recontouring is done. Condylar degeneration or resorption can occur, particularly in the patient who has had multiple operations.

Changes in the occlusion are common following diskectomy but can usually be corrected by occlusal adjustment. Infection is rare and usually is not difficult to manage if it occurs.

ARTHROSCOPIC SURGERY

TMJ arthroscopy was described by Ohnishi in 1975,[20] but did not gain popularity until the late 1980s.[21,22] The application of arthroscopy to the TMJ revolutionized the treatment of internal derangement. More importantly, the clinical observations made on arthroscopy raised significant questions as to whether or not there is absolute necessity to relocate the disk to resolve pain and treat dysfunction.[23,24]

The increasing use of arthroscopic techniques in the TMJ has followed logically from usage in other larger joints. Access, interpretation, high initial capital demands and a steep learning curve have limited its widespread adoption. An in-depth knowledge of the anatomy of the joint is essential for arthroscopic techniques as the pathologic joint space can be difficult to interpret, if not navigate. The optical distortions inherent in such fine instruments compound the difficulty. Attendance at a recommended arthroscopic course is a minimal requirement, as is a good image database to refer to. Not everyone has an aptitude for such techniques. Preoperative imaging of the joint is essential. Images convey much more than the written word so we will rely on these in this section of the chapter to demonstrate important anatomy.

An arthroscopic intervention beyond that of simple lysis and lavage is undoubtedly time consuming. Proponents of arthrotomy contend that the preauricular approach is not only safe and swift but also allows a greater flexibility of therapeutic intervention. Such approaches allow access to all parts of the joint, not just the superior joint space. Endoscopic access, however, is invariably less traumatic and recovery after such a procedure is quicker. The ability to visualize the anatomy and record its nature is invaluable in surgical and medicolegal terms. Arthrocentesis is arguably just as effective for lavage and lysis but needle position within the joint space remains a matter of educated guesswork. The way in which either of these techniques produces its effects remains in the realm of conjecture. Research into synovial fluid components has been extensive, yet the algesic factor(s) responsible for TMJ pain has not been identified.[57,58] There is no significant correlation between mediators and symptoms.

The applications of the arthroscope include adhesiolysis, lavage, debris removal, biopsy, debridement, scarification, tissue ablation, retrodiskal coagulation, prediskal section, and meniscal plication.[59] More recently such techniques have been supplemented by the use of lasers, in particular the neodymium-Yag. A bare Nd:Yag quartz fiber can be introduced to the joint space via a double cannula or a separate port to divide adhesions and/or coagulate the retrodiskal tissues.[60] Coagulation seeks to aid retraction of the meniscus by the formation of scar tissue. This can be supplemented by the insertion of a suture to the auditory canal.

Arthroscopic lysis and lavage is more effective than arthrocentesis in management of chronic closed lock. This presumably relates to the fact that adhesions can be more readily freed under direction vision. Acute closed lock responds to either measure but arthrocentesis may be simpler to perform. Some have attributed its efficacy to the fact that suction effects rather than adhesions are the source of the locking. However, it should be kept in mind from earlier discussion that there is no clear relationship between radiologically demonstrable derangement and symptoms. Without visualizing the internal workings of the joint, one cannot be sure of what is being treated and to what effect.

TMJ arthroscopy is indicated in only two instances: articular pain and limited range of jaw opening. It is reasonable to proceed with arthroscopy once all conservative and medical treatments have failed and the above criteria have been met. A careful review of the minority of cases that fail following such interventions is absolutely essential: there is plenty of evidence to show that the law of diminishing returns applies to this group of patients. The use of other techniques may have proportionally less success in this situation. Weaknesses in the size and design of studies continue to hamper progress in this, as in all other areas of TMJ intervention.

Many varieties of needle arthroscope are available for imaging and therapeutic intervention. The choice of system largely depends on the individual surgeon's needs, preference and pocket – Olympus, Efer, Leibinger, Wolf, Dynonics and Storz are among a growing number of manufacturers. In addition to the scope, a variety of different view angles may be needed including forward, forward oblique and lateral viewing systems. A light source, TV equipment, sheaths, a laser and a variety of instruments are necessary, along with sterilization equipment.

Simple arthroscopy is possible under local anesthetic but in all other instances a general anesthestic is preferable. The approach to the joint may be anterolateral, posterolateral or endaural.

Once the surface anatomy has first been marked out, the upper joint space is expanded by injecting local anesthetic solution via a 16 or 18 gauge needle or vascular catheter. The needle can subsequently be used as a guide for the insertion of the scope trocar. In the case of the posterolateral approach the cannula is introduced using a sharp trocar through a 2 mm skin incision anterior to the local

anesthetic needle with a 30 degree upward and anterior angulation to the skin to enter the superior joint space. Needless to say, it is crucial to avoid the deepest point of the glenoid fossa and Hugier's canal: anatomic studies place these as little as 7.4 mm and 13.9 mm, respectively, from the lateral rim of the fossa.[61] The use of a sharp trocar and avoidance of excessive force should limit such complications. A second cannula is introduced approximately 15–20 mm anterior to the first puncture site using a sharp trocar (Fig. 90.7). The endaural route involves inserting the trocar behind the tragus in the external acoustic meatus in a plane parallel to the tragocanthal line. The articular tubercle and an increased risk of facial nerve damage complicate the anterior approach. Whatever the direction of insertion, it should be remembered that peppering the capsule with untamponaded perforations is likely to result in fluid ballooning out the superficial tissues when irrigation is initiated.

Once in the joint cavity, a familiar landmark is sought and exploration begun. By 'scanning', 'rotational' and 'pistoning' maneuvers, the anatomy of the space can be mapped out (Figs 90.8–10). During these movements the assistant may have to perform various mandibular manipulations to optimize the view. Therapeutic and diagnostic intervention is then possible. The selection of arthroscopic techniques at this stage depends on the intra-articular findings.

Arthroscopy is followed by aggressive physical therapy to improve joint mobility. It is also important to reduce joint load by using a soft diet for one to three months and by controlling bruxism.

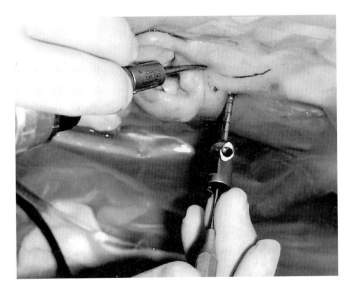

Fig. 90.7 This view demonstrates the correct positions of the posterior and anterior cannulas. The arthroscope is placed into the posterior cannula.

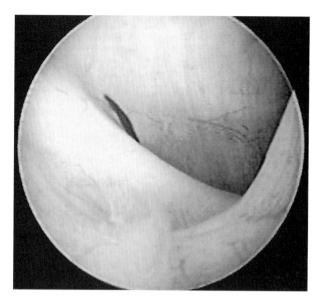

Fig. 90.8 Arthroscopic view in upper joint space of the posterior recess demonstrating posterior attachment, oblique protuberance and medial capsule wall.

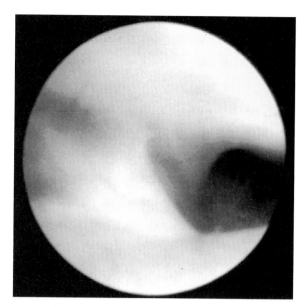

Fig. 90.10 Arthroscopic view in the upper joint space demonstrating dense fibrous adhesions between the disk and articular eminence.

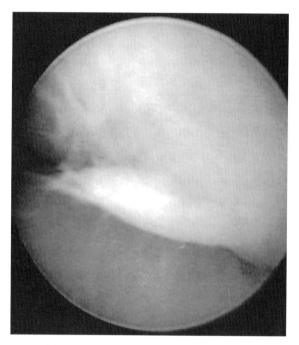

Fig. 90.9 Arthroscopic view in the upper joint space demonstrating the disk below and articular eminence above. The lateral aspect of the articular eminence shows fibrillation of the articular surface.

Results

The results with TMJ arthroscopic surgery have been very good. Success, as determined by decreased pain and improved range of motion, has varied from 79% to 93%.[21–23,59,60,62,63] The best results are obtained using arthroscopic lavage and lysis of adhesions for the treatment of painful limited opening (closed-lock).[21] Retrospective studies indicate that arthroscopic lavage and lysis of adhesions is as effective as arthrotomy for the treatment of closed-lock. This procedure may not be as effective for the treatment of the reducing disk. The outcomes of more complex operative techniques are unclear at the present time.

Complications

When arthroscopy was first introduced there was a sense that it was a safe procedure which might help, but could not hurt, the patient. This has not proven to be true: significant complications can occur with TMJ arthroscopy.[37,56] However, complications with arthroscopic lavage and lysis of adhesions are rare and usually temporary. Possible complications include facial nerve injury, hemorrhage, infection, changes in hearing and altered occlusion. Extravasation of fluid and broken instruments within the closed joint space are potential complications unique to arthroscopy. Clearly, complications with arthroscopic lavage and lysis of adhesions occur less commonly than with arthrotomy procedures.

ARTHROCENTESIS WITH JOINT LAVAGE AND MANIPULATION

Arthrocentesis with joint lavage is the simplest form of surgical intervention into the TMJ as it was recently described by Nitzan.[25] Arthrocentesis is indicated for the treatment of painful limited opening caused by TMJ derangement of acute onset. The technique is simple to perform in the office under local anesthesia alone or in combination with con-

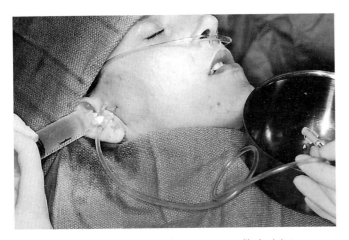

Fig. 90.11 Arthrocentesis of the right temporomandibular joint.

scious sedation. A 19 gauge needle is placed into the upper joint space approximately 1 cm in front of the tragus. Hydraulic pressure is created by injecting about 2 cc of Ringer's lactate into the space. A second 19 gauge needle is placed approximately 1 cm anterior to the first needle (Fig. 90.11). The joint is then lavaged with 50–100 cc of Ringer's lactate. The outflow needle is periodically occluded in order to create hydraulic pressure within the joint space. At the termination of the procedure 1 cc of betamethasone is injected into the upper joint space. After removal of both needles, the mandible is gently manipulated in order to evaluate the joint movement.

Postoperative therapy is primarily directed at re-establishing and maintaining an increased range of motion. The patient is started immediately on opening and excursive movement exercises. It is also important to control bruxism when present.

Results

Arthrocentesis with joint lavage has both diagnostic and therapeutic benefits. Patients who have normal, smooth opening during mandibular manipulation following arthrocentesis with joint lavage generally do well postoperatively, whereas patients who continue to have limited opening or increased opening but with mechanical interference (hard click) do not do well. Short-term results with this procedure have been good in effectively establishing increased opening, improving function and relieving pain.[25,64–66] Intra-articular injection of sodium hyaluronate into the TMJ has been shown to be effective in reducing TMJ pain and improving function.[67,68] Currently, there is interest in using sodium hyaluronate as the irrigating solution during arthrocentesis. Whether this will improve the results is not yet known.

Complications

Complications are rare and consist of temporary swelling secondary to extravasation of injected fluid or hemorrhage from a damaged blood vessel.

MODIFIED CONDYLOTOMY

The condylotomy procedure was first introduced by Ward in 1957 using a Gigli saw to make a closed subcondylar cut through the neck of the condyle for the treatment of the painful TMJ.[15] While reported results were good, the procedure was not widely accepted, probably because of its significant potential for complications in facial nerve injury and hemorrhage. Nickerson modified the condylotomy procedure by converting it to a variation of the transoral vertical ramus osteotomy.[18] The primary indication for condylotomy is the treatment of chronic refractory TMJ pain associated with a reducing disk.

The procedure is performed under general anesthesia and usually as an outpatient procedure. Through a transoral incision the lateral aspect of the mandibular ramus is exposed. A vertical cut extending from the sigmoid notch to the angle is made parallel to the posterior border of the mandible (Fig. 90.12). The teeth are placed in maxillomandibular fixation and the incision closed.

Postoperatively the patient is maintained in fixation for about two to six weeks depending upon the surgeon's preference. After release of fixation, training elastics are used for six weeks to prevent malocclusion. Exercises are performed to maintain and/or increase the range of motion. TMJ loading is reduced with the use of a soft diet from about three months. It is also important to control bruxism.

Results

The results of modified condylotomy have been excellent –

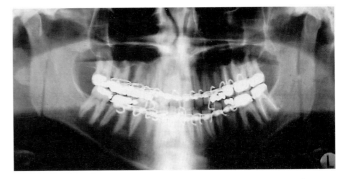

Fig. 90.12 Postoperative panographic X-ray demonstrating vertical cuts extending from the sigmoid notch to the mandibular angle.

about 90% of patients have reduced pain and increased mandibular motion.[18,19,69] Hall has reported that condylotomy frequently results in a normal disk position and is the only surgical procedure which consistently does so.[69] The procedure seems to be effective because the condyle sags slightly, thus increasing the joint space. The major disadvantage of condylotomy is that the condylar sag can be excessive, resulting in a malocclusion.

Complications

Complications of modified condylotomy include infection, damage to the inferior alveolar nerve and malocclusion.[37] Although minor malocclusion has been reported to occur in only 1–2% of cases, our experience indicates that it is more common than this.

CONCLUSION

Surgical treatment of TMJ internal derangement, although infrequently used, has proven effective for reducing pain and increasing range of motion in about 80% of the patients operated, regardless of the technique used. The results are based on short-term retrospective studies. Long-term studies are lacking, as are randomized prospective studies. While one reports surgical results, it must be realized that the results are, in fact, the results of comprehensive treatment plans of which surgery was only a part.

The surgeon has several surgical procedures available for the treatment of internal derangement. While each procedure has its enthusiasts, clinical observations and reported studies suggest that each procedure has a specific stage of internal derangement for which it is most effective. The prudent surgeon should select the operative procedure that has the highest potential for success with the lowest potential complications for each patient's specific problem. Obviously, the choice of procedures will be influenced by the surgeon's experience.

TMJ surgery has not only proven effective in treating patients but has also resulted in elucidation of the pathology of internal derangement. The observations that simple procedures in the upper joint space not only reduced pain but also increased range of motion without repositioning the disk raised serious questions about the importance of disk position. The intriguing question is 'why are lavage and lysis of adhesions of the upper joint space therapeutic'? If one accepts the premise that the location of the disk is only a conditional factor and of less importance than is generally believed, then the apparent dilemma can be explained. Any impediment in the upper joint space results in a more restricted motion than does similar pathology in the lower joint space. Thus, lavage and lysis of adhesions in the upper joint space may improve range of motion.

If disk position is not the critical factor in dysfunction and pain of the TMJ, one must look elsewhere. Synovitis in the upper joint space of the TMJ has been observed during arthroscopy. Clearly, inflamed synovium may cause joint pain. Alterations in the constituents of the synovial fluid may also affect lubrication of the joint with resultant stickiness and decreased movement. This may also adversely affect the articular surfaces of the joint components and ultimately lead to degenerative changes. Conversely, degenerative changes within the articular surfaces or disk may release chemical substances into the synovial fluid, altering its viscosity and engendering pain.[57,58,70] These comments are highly speculative and much further research is needed to elucidate the pathologies associated with TMJ pain and dysfunction.

In summary, the good news is that 80% of operated patients benefit from TMJ surgery. The bad news is that 20% do not benefit. Surgeons must temper their enthusiasm about the patient who has a successful outcome with the disappointment and consequences for the patient who does not have a successful outcome. Both the patient and surgeon must realize that TMJ surgery may make the patient worse; thus the decision to operate must be carefully made.

REFERENCES

1. Rugh JD, Solberg WK 1985 Oral health status in the United States. Temporomandibular disorders. Journal of Dental Education 49:398–404
2. Solberg WK, Woo MW, Houston JB 1979 Prevalence of mandibular dysfunction in young adults. Journal of the American Dental Association 98:25–34
3. McNeill C (ed) 1993 Temporomandibular disorders – guidelines for classification, assessment and management, 2nd edn. Quintessence, Chicago
4. Dolwick MF, Dimitroulis G 1994 Is there a role for temporomandibular joint surgery? British Journal of Oral and Maxillofacial Surgery 32:307–313
5. Farrar WB 1971 Diagnosis and treatment of anterior dislocation of articular disc. New York Journal of Dentistry 41:348–351
6. Wilkes CH 1978 Arthrography of the temporomandibular joint in patients with TMJ pain dysfunction syndrome. Minnesota Medicine 61:645–652
7. McCarty WL, Farrar WB 1979 Surgery for internal derangement of the temporomandibular joint. Journal of Prosthetic Dentistry 42:191–196
8. Dolwick MF, Katzberg RW, Helms CA, Bales DJ 1979 Arthrotomography of the temporomandibular joint. Journal of Oral Surgery 37:793–799
9. Isberg AM, Westesson P-L 1982 Movement of the disc and condyle in temporomandibular joints with clicking. An arthrographic and cineradiographic study on autopsy specimens. Acta Odontologica Scandinavica 40:151–164

10. Solberg W, Hanson T, Nordstrom B 1984 Morphologic evaluation of young adult TMJs at autopsy. Journal of Dental Research 63:228

11. Westesson P-L, Rohlin M 1984 Internal derangement related to osteoarthritis in temporomandibular joint autopsy specimens. Oral Surgery, Oral Medicine, and Oral Pathology 57:17–22

12. Hall MB 1984 Meniscoplasty of the displaced temporomandibular meniscus without violating the inferior joint space. Journal of Oral and Maxillofacial Surgery 42:788–792

13. Dolwick MF, Sanders B 1985 TMJ internal derangement and arthrosis – surgical atlas. CV Mosby, St Louis

14. Lanz AB 1909 Dictis mandibularis. Zentralblatt für Chirurgie 36:289–291

15. Ward TG, Smith DG, Sommar M 1957 Condylotomy for mandibular joints. British Dental Journal 103:147–148

16. Ericksson L, Westesson P-L 1985 Long-term evaluation of meniscectomy of the temporomandibular joint. Journal of Oral and Maxillofacial Surgery 43:263–269

17. Hall HD, Link J 1989 Diskectomy alone and with ear cartilage in joint reconstruction. Oral and Maxillofacial Surgery Clinics of North America 1:329–340

18. Nickerson JW, Veaco NS 1989 Condylotomy in surgery of the temporomandibular joint. Oral and Maxillofacial Surgery Clinics of North America 1:303–327

19. Upton LG, Sullivan SM 1991 The treatment of temporomandibular joint internal derangement using the modified open condylotomy. A preliminary report. Journal of Oral and Maxillofacial Surgery 49:578–584

20. Ohnishi M 1975 Arthroscopy of the temporomandibular joint. Japanese Journal of Stomatology 42:207–213

21. Sanders B 1986 Arthroscopic surgery of the temporomandibular joint: Treatment of internal derangement with persistent closed lock. Oral Surgery, Oral Medicine, and Oral Pathology 62:361–372

22. McCain JP 1988 Arthroscopy of the human temporomandibular joint. Journal of Oral and Maxillofacial Surgery 46:648–655

23. Nitzan DW, Dolwick MF, Heft MW 1990 Arthroscopic lavage and lysis of the temporomandibular joint: A change in perspective. Journal of Oral and Maxillofacial Surgery 48:798–801

24. Nitzan DW, Dolwick MF 1991 An alternative explanation for the genesis of closed-lock symptoms in the internal derangement process. Journal of Oral and Maxillofacial Surgery 49:810–815

25. Nitzan DW, Dolwick MF, Martinez A 1991 Temporomandibular joint arthrocentesis. A simplified treatment for severe, limited mouth opening. Journal of Oral and Maxillofacial Surgery 49:1163–1167

26. Droukas G, Lindee C, Carlsson GE 1985 Occlusion and mandibular dysfunction: A clinical study of patients referred for functional disturbances of the masticatory system. Journal of Prosthetic Dentistry 53:402–406

27. Schellhas KP 1989 Imaging of the temporomandibular joint. Oral and Maxillofacial Surgery Clinics of North America 1:13–26.

28. Westesson P-L, Katzberg RW, Tallents RH, Sanchez-Woodworth RE, Svensson SA 1987 CT and MR of the temporomandibular joint: Comparison with autopsy specimens. American Journal of Roentgenology 148:1165–1171

29. Westesson P-L, Brooks SL 1992 Temporomandibular joint: Magnetic resonance evidence of joint effusion relative to joint pain and internal derangement. American Journal of Roentgenology 159:559–563

30. Murakami M 1996 MRI evidence of high signal intensity and temporomandibular arthralgia and relating pain. Does the high signal correlate to the pain? British Journal of Oral and Maxillofacial Surgery 34:220–224

31. Kircos LT, Ortendahl DA, Mark AS 1987 Magnetic resonance imaging of the TMJ disc in asymptomatic volunteers. Journal of Oral and Maxillofacial Surgery 45:397–401

32. Raustia AM, Phyhtinen J, Pernu H 1994 Clinical, magnetic resonance imaging and surgical findings in patients with temporomandibular joint disorder: A survey of 47 patients. Rofo Fortschritte auf dem Gebiete der Rontgenstrahlen und der Neuen Bildgebenden Verfahren 160(5):406–411

33. Dolwick MF 1989 Clinical diagnosis of temporomandibular joint internal derangement and myofascial pain and dysfunction. Oral and Maxillofacial Surgery Clinics of North America 1:1–6

34. Green CS, Laskin DM 1983 Long-term evaluation of treatment of myofascial pain–dysfunction syndrome: Comparative analysis. Journal of the American Dental Association 107:235–238

35. Mejersjo C, Carlsson GE 1983 Long-term results of treatment for temporomandibular pain and dysfunction. Journal of Prosthetic Dentistry 49:809–815

36. Nickerson JW, Boering G 1989 Natural course of osteoarthritis as it relates to internal derangement of the temporomandibular joint. Oral and Maxillofacial Surgery Clinics of North America 1:27–46

37. Dolwick MF, Armstrong JF 1997 In: Kaban LB, Pogrel MA, Perrot DH (eds) Complications of temporomandibular joint surgery. WB Saunders, Philadelphia, Ch 7, pp 89–103

38. Harris MD 1987 Medical versus surgical management of temporomandibular joint pain and dysfunction. British Journal of Oral and Maxillofacial Surgery 25:113–120

39. Rowe NL 1972 Surgery of the temporomandibular joint. Proceedings of the Royal Society of Medicine 65:383–388

40. Al Kayat A, Bramley PA 1979 A modified pre-auricular approach to the temporomandibular joint and malar arch. British Journal of Oral Surgery 17:91–103

41. Marciani RD, Zeigler RC 1983 Temporomandibular joint surgery: A review of 51 operations. Oral Surgery, Oral Medicine, and Oral Pathology 56:472–476

42. Piper MA 1989 Microscopic disc preservation surgery of the temporomandibular joint. Oral and Maxillofacial Surgery Clinics of North America 1:279–392

43. Dolwick MF, Nitzan DW 1990 TMJ disk surgery: 8 year follow-up evaluation. Fortschritte der Kiefer- und Gesichts-chirurgie 35:162–167

44. Dolwick MF, Aufdemorte TB 1985 Silicone induced foreign body reaction and lymphadenopathy after temporomandibular joint arthroplasty. Oral Surgery, Oral Medicine, and Oral Pathology 59:449–452

45. Westesson P-L, Ericksson L, Lindstrom C 1987 Destructive lesions of the mandibular condyle following discectomy with temporary Sialastic implants. Oral Surgery, Oral Medicine, and Oral Pathology 63:143–150

46. Kaplan PA, Tu HK, William SM 1988 Erosive arthritis of the temporomandibular joint caused by Teflon-Proplast implants: Plain film features. American Journal of Roentgenology 151:337–340

47. Ryan DE 1989 Alloplastic implants in the temporomandibular joint. Oral and Maxillofacial Surgery Clinics of North America 1:427–441

48. Witsenberg B, Freihofer HPM 1984 Replacement of the pathological temporomandibular disc using autogenous cartilage of the external ear. International Journal of Oral Surgery 13:401–404

49. Hall HD, Link J 1989 Diskectomy alone and with ear cartilage in joint reconstruction. Oral and Maxillofacial Clinics of North America 1:329–340

50. Meyer RA 1988 The autogenous dermal graft in temporomandibular joint disc surgery. Journal of Oral and Maxillofacial Surgery 46:948–954

51. Feinberg S, Larsen P 1989 The use of a pedicled temporalis muscle – pericranial flap for replacement of the TMJ disc: Preliminary report. Journal of Oral and Maxillofacial Surgery 47:142–146

52. Ericksson L, Westesson P-L 1992 Temporomandibular joint diskectomy. Oral Surgery, Oral Medicine, and Oral Pathology 74:259–272

53. Silver CM 1984 Long-term results of meniscectomy of the temporomandibular joint. Journal of Craniomandibular Practice 3:46–57

54. Ericksson L, Westesson P-L 1985 Long-term evaluation of meniscectomy of the temporomandibular joint. Journal of Oral and Maxillofacial Surgery 43:263–269

55. Agerberg G, Lundberg J 1971 Changes in the temporomandibular joint after surgical treatment. A radiological follow-up study. Oral Surgery, Oral Medicine, and Oral Pathology 32:865–875

56. Vallerand WP, Dolwick MF 1990 Complications of temporomandibular joint surgery. Oral and Maxillofacial Surgery Clinics of North America 2:481–488

57. Aghabeigi B, Henderson B, Hopper C, Harris M 1993 Temporomandibular joint fluid analysis. British Journal of Oral and Maxillofacial Surgery 31:15–20

58. Aghabeigi B, Haque M, Wasil M, Hodges SJ, Henderson B, Harris M 1997 The role of oxygen-free radicals in idiopathic facial pain. British Journal of Oral and Maxillofacial Surgery 35:161–165

59. McCain JP, Humberto R 1989 Principles and practice of operative arthroscopy of the human temporomandibular joint. Oral and Maxillofacial Surgery Clinics of North America 1:135–152

60. Ohnishi M 1989 Arthroscopic surgery for hypermobility and recurrent mandibular dislocation. Oral and Maxillofacial Surgery Clinics of North America 12:153–160

61. Sugisaki M, Ikai A, Tanube H 1995 Dangerous angles and depths for middle ear and middle cranial fossa injury during arthroscopy of the temporomandibular joint. Journal of Oral and Maxillofacial Surgery 53 (7):803–810

62. Holmlund A, Hellsing G, Wredmark T 1986 Arthroscopy of the temporomandibular joint: A clinical study. International Journal of Oral and Maxillofacial Surgery 15:715–726

63. Moses JJ, Poker I 1989 TMJ arthroscopic surgery: An analysis of 237 patients. Journal of Oral and Maxillofacial Surgery 47:790–794

64. Dimitroulis G, Dolwick MF, Martinez A 1995 Temporomandibular joint arthrocentesis and lavage for the treatment of closed lock: A follow-up study. British Journal of Oral and Maxillofacial Surgery 33:23–27

65. Nitzan DW 1994 Arthrocentesis for management of the severe closed lock of the temporomandibular joint: Current controversies in surgery for internal derangements of the temporomandibular joint. Oral and Maxillofacial Surgery Clinics of North America 6:245–257

66. Murakami K, Hosaka H, Moriya Y et al 1995 Short-term treatment outcome study for the management of temporomandibular joint closed lock: A comparison of arthrocentesis to nonsurgical therapy and arthroscopic lysis and lavage. Oral Surgery, Oral Medicine, and Oral Pathology 80:253–257

67. Kopp S, Wenneberg B, Haraldson T, Carlsson GE 1985 The short-term effect of intra-articular injections of sodium hyaluronate and corticosteroid on temporomandibular joint pain and dysfunction. Journal of Oral and Maxillofacial Surgery 43:429–435

68. Bertolami CN, Gay T, Clark GT, Rendell BS, Vivek S, Changrui L, Swann D 1993 Use of sodium hyaluronate in treating temporomandibular disorders: A randomized, double blind, placebo controlled clinical trial. Journal of Oral and Maxillofacial Surgery 51:232–242

69. Hall HD, Nickerson JW, McKenna SJ 1993 Modified condylotomy for treatment of the painful temporomandibular joint with a reducing disc. Journal of Oral and Maxillofacial Surgery 51:133–142

70. Quinn JH 1990 Identification of prostaglandin E2 and leukotriene B4 in the synovial fluid of painful, dysfunctional temporomandibular joints. Journal of Oral and Maxillofacial Surgery 48:968–971

Trigeminal neuralgia

91

ALISTAIR JENKINS

EPIDEMIOLOGY

Trigeminal neuralgia is a truly agonizing condition which has received much attention during the past century but surprisingly little prior to this. Although early manuscripts, including the Bible, mention many medical conditions familiar to us today, and graphic medieval accounts may be found of other neurologic conditions such as subarachnoid hemorrhage, epilepsy, and facial palsy, the first recognizable descriptions of trigeminal neuralgia are not found until the 17th and 18th centuries.[1]

The reasons for this are unknown. It is usually a disease of middle-aged to elderly patients, and has an association with atherosclerosis and therefore with a 'developed' diet, but even given the life expectancy and diet of earlier generations the lack of early documentation is surprising.

The incidence is difficult to ascertain, as recognition of the condition is still not as good as it might be. An estimate of 1/70 000/year is a reasonable approximation.

CLINICAL FEATURES

Trigeminal neuralgia is characterized by episodes of usually excruciating pain in a constant position on the face. The pain is most frequently confined to one part of one division of the trigeminal nerve – almost always the maxillary or mandibular – but may occasionally spread to an adjacent division or rarely all three. Between attacks there is usually no pain although some patients, particularly those in whom symptoms are severe, complain of a background ache. In the most severe cases, attacks are so frequent as to render the pain more or less constant.

The character of the pain is virtually diagnostic. It is usually agonizing and of sudden onset, rarely lasting for more than an instant or a few seconds. It is frequently brought on by touching the face in a particular site, often near the nasolabial fold or beside the mouth – the trigger spot. It may be brought on by chewing or even by speaking or smiling. In extreme cases, the patient will have a motionless face – the 'frozen face' – and will talk little for fear of triggering an attack; serious weight loss is not unknown. For reasons which are unknown, but which may be simply to do with posture, attacks rarely occur at night. Spontaneous remission may occur, sometimes for prolonged periods, but if untreated the pain almost always returns.

Neurological examination is most commonly normal. Mild hypo- or hyperesthesia is sometimes found, particularly in patients on anticonvulsant medication, but more profound sensory loss or the presence of other cranial nerve deficits – including the trigeminal motor root – should raise the suspicion of other pathology.

It will be seen from this description that the clinical picture of trigeminal neuralgia should be almost impossible to confuse with any other type of facial pain. Nevertheless, it is only the exceptional patient who receives adequate treatment for this extremely painful condition within a reasonable time scale. Whether because of unfamiliarity with the condition, confusion with other conditions or ignorance of the effective treatments available, many patients are allowed to continue for years with a very poor quality of life. Some will have wholly inappropriate treatment such as dental extraction, peripheral nerve avulsion, opiate analgesia, etc. It is by no means uncommon for patients finally to be referred to a neurosurgeon having had all the teeth on one side removed in an effort to track down the one 'causing the pain'. A moment's reflection, however, will tell the clinician that trigeminal neuralgia is wholly unlike any other type of facial pain, and in particular is difficult to confuse with dental causes.

ETIOLOGY

The discovery of the etiology of trigeminal neuralgia came surprisingly late in the history of its treatment and is still not appreciated by many. Only after nearly fifty years of open surgical procedures for the condition was it noticed that in most cases an arterial branch – usually of the superior cerebellar artery,[2,3] but occasionally of others – could be seen in close relation to the nerve root as it entered the pons. In most cases the nerve has a pronounced groove in it at the site of contact, and it may even be appreciably thinned. Electron microscopy has shown areas of demyelination in affected nerves.

It would be fair to say that acceptance of this association was slow and incomplete in spite of the excellent results obtained by simple separation of the nerve from the vessel at operation (see below). Sceptics pointed out the frequent finding of root–vessel contact in asymptomatic cases at postmortem, and suggested that cure was due to manipulation and damage to the nerve during surgery – the basis of treatment hitherto.[4] However Miles et al, in an elegant study, have shown actual improvements in sensory perception thresholds following surgery, concluding that damage to the nerve root is not present in successful cases and is not necessary for relief of symptoms.[5,6]

In cases where no arterial compression is found, veins are often seen compressing the root entry zone and may be responsible for generation of pain. In a small minority of cases, no identifiable cause can be found.

Other pathologies causing irritation or demyelination of the trigeminal nerve at the root entry zone may cause the syndrome (see below), and in the younger or otherwise atypical patient every effort must be made to exclude a space-occupying lesion or multiple sclerosis.

DIAGNOSIS

The diagnosis is made principally from a well-taken history. The absence of physical signs is indeed a hallmark of trigeminal neuralgia, and all cranial nerves should be examined to exclude involvement. In severe cases sensation may be marginally reduced on the affected side, particularly if the patient is on large doses of carbamazepine, but significant sensory impairment should be treated with suspicion. Involvement of the trigeminal motor root in simple trigeminal neuralgia is not recorded. If the history is diagnostic, the finding of one or more carious teeth is likely to be coincidental.

All patients should ideally have MRI scanning, or at least a CT scan. Certainly those who are refractory to medical treatment should be imaged prior to any surgery: a competent surgeon might be expected to deal with an unexpected tumor at open operation, although its limits would be difficult to ascertain, but unwitting placement of a wide-gauge needle into such a lesion percutaneously could create serious problems.

The development of high-field, high-definition MRI and special imaging sequences has led to an increasing emphasis on preoperative localization of compressive vessels at the root entry zone.[7] Such sequences highlight vascular structures while giving recognizable images of the pons and trigeminal nerve, and it is likely in future that 'negative' explorations will be avoided by use of such technology (Fig. 91.1).

Response to treatment with carbamazepine is almost universal in trigeminal neuralgia but unusual in other types of facial pain. Many physicians therefore use this response,

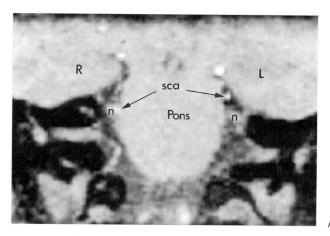

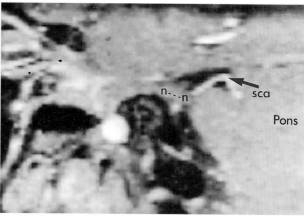

Fig. 91.1 MRI time-of-flight images taken in the coronal plane **(A)** and in the plane of the trigeminal nerve **(B)** of a patient with right-sided trigeminal neuralgia. The superior cerebellar artery (SCA) is clearly seen compressing the trigeminal nerve (N) at the root entry zone on the right. On the left, seen only in (A), it is well clear of the nerve. Images courtesy of Mr J B Miles, Walton Hospital, Liverpool, UK.

even if incomplete, as the final step in definitive diagnosis of the condition. Failure to obtain any improvement with this treatment should bring the diagnosis into question.

DIFFERENTIAL DIAGNOSIS

1. Multiple sclerosis. A plaque of demyelination at the root entry zone of the trigeminal nerve can cause a syndrome indistinguishable from idiopathic trigeminal neuralgia. Usually such patients will have an established diagnosis of multiple sclerosis, but in some this is the first symptom or arises amidst other confusing neurological symptoms before the diagnosis is clear. As idiopathic trigeminal neuralgia is mostly a disease of the middle-aged to elderly, symptoms arising in the younger patient should alert the clinician to the possibility of this disease. Similarly, neuralgia due to multiple sclerosis is occasionally bilateral, or becomes so with the passage of time, while this is very rare in the idiopathic type. The condition is most easily diagnosed now by magnetic resonance imaging. T_2-weighted images will show the characteristic plaques in the cerebral hemispheres in most established cases, although it is uncommon for definite evidence of demyelination to be seen at the root entry zone.

2. Post-herpetic neuralgia. This unpleasant condition is usually easy to diagnose from a preceding history of facial herpes zoster, usually confined sharply to one division of the trigeminal nerve and often leaving residual scarring. The pain is constant, intense, and burning in quality. It starts during or immediately after the active infection and unless promptly treated remains permanent and refractory to medical or surgical intervention.

3. Neoplasia. Intracranial neoplasms at the cerebello-pontine angle may cause facial pain if they irritate or compress the root or the ganglion of the trigeminal nerve. This may be episodic and indistinguishable from idiopathic trigeminal neuralgia, and is usually termed 'symptomatic trigeminal neuralgia'. This is the main reason for imaging patients with facial pain of any type, particularly when progressive. Usually careful examination will show other cranial nerve or cerebellar features in such patients, for instance unilateral deafness with acoustic neuroma. Other mass lesions occasionally discovered include chordomas, meningiomas, aneurysms, arteriovenous malformations or extensive pituitary tumors. In Asia, for reasons which are unknown, intracranial epidermoid tumors are comparatively common and often occur at this site. Neoplasms of the skull base, often malignant, may invade or compress the trigeminal nerve.

4. Inflammatory/infective conditions. Dental or temporomandibular joint problems can give rise to pain which is episodic, but its relationship to occlusion or jaw movement is usually obvious. Pain in such conditions usually lacks the agonizing quality seen in trigeminal neuralgia. More usually, dental infection or sinusitis causes constant throbbing or aching pain. An inflamed pulp may cause stabbing pain early on but usually becomes constant and can be characterized as 'toothache' by the patient.

5. Glossopharyngeal neuralgia is very rare and is likely to have the same cause as trigeminal neuralgia, i.e. vascular compression of the nerve root. The quality of the pain and its severity are similar also, but it is felt unilaterally in the throat and base of the tongue on one side, sometimes radiating to the ear. The pain is often precipitated by swallowing and indeed the patient may be scared to swallow. Carbamazepine and other anticonvulsants are less likely to be effective, but microvascular decompression of the root entry zone is usually curative. The offending vessel may be the vertebral artery or one of its branches.

6. Cluster headache. This is a variant of migraine and is usually confined to the upper part of the face but may radiate into the maxilla. It is most commonly centered behind the eye, and during attacks the eye may water or become suffused. The nose may also become congested, and occasionally there are color changes in the affected area of the face as well. The name 'cluster headache' arises from the tendency of attacks to come in runs or clusters with periods of several weeks' relief in between. Pain is often present at night, unlike trigeminal neuralgia, and may last for half an hour or more. Treatment with beta-blockers or antimigraine preparations is usually successful although some cases remain refractory.

7. Depression, for reasons which are unknown, is not infrequently associated with facial pain. This is usually a background ache of variable severity with more acute exacerbations; in patients with no psychiatric history the diagnosis may be difficult to make. The diagnosis should be considered in patients with atypical pain, particularly when ill-defined and constant, but it must be remembered that chronic pain in any site can be associated with depression.

8. Atypical facial pain. Ultimately a small group of patients will evade an effective diagnosis and fall into this category. The pain in these patients is seldom well localized or easy to define. It may be bilateral; it often radiates in a non-anatomic fashion; it is usually constant and severe; and it is almost always refractory to medical or surgical treatment. As with many pain syndromes, psychiatric problems may play a part, but it must be remembered that chronic pain itself alters the psyche and such pain can gradually become the whole focus of a patient's existence. It is of vital importance that a diagnosis of atypical facial pain is backed up by normal or negative examination and investigations and that a potentially serious condition is not missed.

It is equally important that the clinician is not driven by the patient's or his/her own desperation into performing destructive surgery.

TREATMENT

The pain of trigeminal neuralgia is refractory to treatment with most analgesics including opiates. It was not until 1962 that Blom[8] showed a response to anticonvulsants in experimental models of the condition and it became possible for medical treatment to be successful.

Carbamazepine has now become the first-line drug for this condition[8] and should be tried as soon as the diagnosis is suspected. Not only is it extremely effective, often removing the need for other therapies, but a response to carbamazepine is almost diagnostic of trigeminal neuralgia. If the frequency of attacks is not affected by adequate doses of the drug, the diagnosis should be seriously questioned.

The adequacy of the dose is an important point. A starting dose of 200 mg twice a day may be rapidly raised in the face of a poor response up to the maximum dose tolerated by the patient. This is likely to be in the region of 1500 mg per day although there is considerable variation. When side effects appear a reduction of 200 mg will often eliminate them. Such side effects include visual blurring, dizziness, and somnolence; skin rashes are occasionally seen. All patients on carbamazepine should have regular blood counts and liver function tests performed in the first year or so of treatment as aplastic anemia and liver disturbances are rare but important complications of what is generally a very safe treatment. Plasma levels are generally meaningless as it is response and side effects that matter; unlike epilepsy, where a significant proportion of patients do not comply fully with their treatment for various reasons, the intensity of the pain in trigeminal neuralgia makes this much less likely.

If carbamazepine does not control symptoms adequately, another anticonvulsant such as sodium valproate may be added, but significant improvement is unlikely. A few patients will achieve further response with amitryptiline.

Failure of acceptable control with medical treatment should lead to immediate consideration of surgery. All too often incomplete response or a progressive reduction in response is followed by a prolonged period of inactivity by the medical attendants and increasing pain for the patient when surgery is the only possible solution. Age should not be a barrier; advances in anesthesia have dramatically improved safety over the past years, and some procedures can be performed using only sedation or local anesthesia.

Surgical procedures for trigeminal neuralgia have undergone a fascinating process of evolution during this half century,[1,9] and have in themselves contributed significantly to understanding of the pathologic processes involved in the condition. They may be divided into three groups: peripheral procedures, percutaneous ganglion procedures, and open operations.

PERIPHERAL PROCEDURES

One of the interesting and unexplained features of trigeminal neuralgia is its ability to be modulated by interruption of any part of the trigeminal pathway, from peripheral sensory nerves to nerve root entry zone. Thus local anesthetic blocks of peripheral nerves in the region of the perceived pain can be used as an emergency measure in some cases of virtually continuous pain, although the response will be very short-lived. Peripheral nerve destruction – usually by cryotherapy, alcohol injection or nerve avulsion – has been and still is used extensively by maxillofacial specialists to achieve a response of variable duration. The supraorbital, infraorbital or mental nerves are most commonly approached. This should generally be discouraged where there is access to neurosurgical evaluation, except again as a first-aid measure.

GANGLION PROCEDURES

Around 1900 the first operations were performed on the trigeminal ganglion for neuralgia. These were open procedures and although hazardous were effective in abolishing pain at the expense of sensation. About ten years later Harris, Tapatas and Hartel separately introduced percutaneous approaches to the ganglion via the foramen ovale. Alcohol was the neurolytic agent most commonly used, and a surprising degree of specificity could be achieved as to the nerve divisions affected, sparing the important ophthalmic division in many cases and the motor root in most. Since then, many different percutaneous procedures have been proposed, but three main techniques remain in common use: thermocoagulation, glycerol injection, and balloon compression.

The technique of needle placement is common to all of these. Although the pioneering operations were done freehand, image intensification or hard-copy X-ray are almost universally employed now for visualization first of the position of the foramen and then for confirmation of the depth of penetration and the position of any contrast medium used.

The anterior approach is the more commonly used. The patient lies on a radiolucent table with the neck well extended. The foramen ovale is best visualized with the X-ray tube placed for a submento-vertical projection. The entry point for the needle is about 15 mm lateral to the angle of the mouth. It is best to infiltrate the skin and cheek with local anesthetic even if the procedure is done under general anesthesia, as the needle is less likely to penetrate the buccal mucosa if the cheek is swollen. The needle is initially directed slightly laterally for the same reason, and then towards the foramen. The position of this is determined from surface markings: it lies in the base of the skull at the intersection of a sagittal plane through the inner canthus of the ipsilateral eye and a coronal plane through the zygoma 2.5 cm anterior to the tragus. The lateral pterygoid plate is close to the path of the needle in this trajectory but is usually just medial to the correct line.

A lateral route, introduced by Harris in 1910, has the needle pass from the cheek below the midpoint of the zygomatic arch, over the sigmoid notch of the mandible in the coronal plane, to enter the foramen ovale laterally. Further passage of the needle will lead the operator from the mandibular to the ophthalmic division. The foramen is entered rather obliquely by this method and therefore presents a smaller target than the anterior route. This route is not suitable for balloon compression.

Engagement of the needle in the foramen is best confirmed by biplanar radiology, but some clinical signs may be apparent. If insufficient local anesthetic is used in local anesthesia cases, penetration of the mandibular nerve will be extremely painful. Even careful local anesthetic administration at this point does not usually make the remainder of the procedure painless. In general anesthesia cases, fibrillation of the ipsilateral masseter may be apparent as the nerve is entered, as may bradycardia. The latter is occasionally profound enough to give some concern to the anesthetist. Once in the entrance to the foramen, subsequent manipulation varies with each procedure.

Radiofrequency thermocoagulation

The needle used here has an insulated shaft and a bore sufficient for the passage of a radiofrequency electrode. It is reusable and therefore must be kept well sharpened. An indifferent electrode is usually a simple hypodermic needle inserted obliquely into the skin of the forehead. Once the radiofrequency needle is in the foramen ovale it is advanced into the trigeminal ganglion. When it is correctly placed, cerebrospinal fluid should emerge on removal of the stylet as the ganglion contains CSF. The electrode is inserted just beyond the tip of the needle and a low amplitude current is applied using a lesion generator. The patient, who by this stage must be awake and cooperative, is asked to indicate where on the face the stimulation is felt. A picture of a face

held in front of the patient is useful here. The position of the electrode is adjusted sequentially until stimulation is felt in the normal distribution of the patient's trigeminal neuralgia. When the patient and surgeon are quite happy that this is the case, a short-acting intravenous anesthetic is given and the radiofrequency lesion made.[10-16]

Glycerol injection

This procedure may be done entirely under local anesthesia – indeed it is very difficult without the cooperation of the patient as the position on the operating table has to be changed and the head kept still and flexed for some time afterwards. A 16 g spinal needle is used and is inserted through the foramen ovale into the ganglion until CSF is obtained on withdrawal of the stylet. The patient is then sat up, supported with the head flexed. A modified dental chair is useful. In this position an injected fluid with a higher specific gravity than CSF will lie within the ganglion or in Meckel's cave. Contrast medium is injected to check the position of the needle. The contrast should either pool in Meckel's cave or outline the inside of the ganglion, the latter being preferable. Adjustment of the needle will be required if the contrast is extradural or if it diffuses rapidly away from the cave. The contrast is evacuated and replaced with 0.5–0.75 ml of pure glycerol. The patient is transferred back to the ward with the head to be maintained in the same position for at least two hours.[11,17-21]

Balloon compression

This is technically the easiest of the three procedures but once again requires general anesthesia. A 4 FG Fogarty catheter is used, the balloon being primed with X-ray contrast medium from a 1 ml syringe. A 12 g spinal needle is required. In this case, it is advanced only just into the foramen ovale and the balloon catheter passed through it. This should be discernible on image intensification. If the needle is passed too far, the balloon will pass intracranially rather than into the ganglion, and if not far enough it will be extradural or will not pass. When inflated, the balloon should take on the shape of Meckel's cave and should appear pear-shaped. No more than 0.75 ml of contrast should be injected, and prior to full inflation the needle should be withdrawn slightly to prevent the balloon bursting on it. If the balloon takes on a regular oval shape, it is not within the cave and should be repositioned. The balloon should remain inflated for 1 minute (Fig. 91.2).[11,22-25]

Hazards common to all percutaneous procedures relate to hemorrhage caused by inappropriate placement of the needle, usually in the foramen lacerum and thus the basal

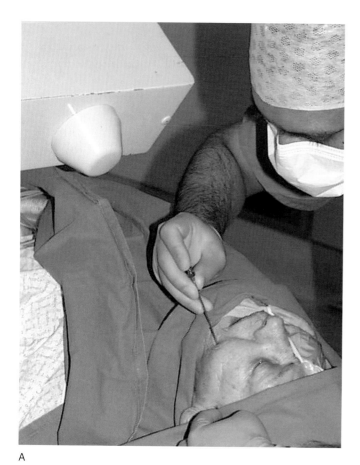

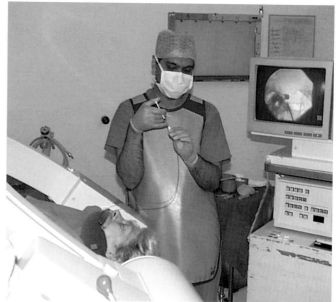

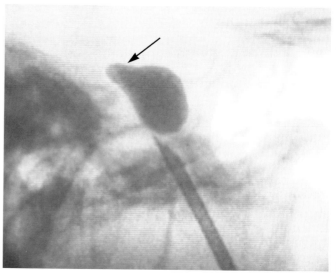

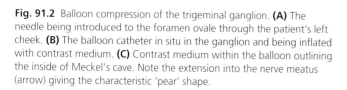

Fig. 91.2 Balloon compression of the trigeminal ganglion. **(A)** The needle being introduced to the foramen ovale through the patient's left cheek. **(B)** The balloon catheter in situ in the ganglion and being inflated with contrast medium. **(C)** Contrast medium within the balloon outlining the inside of Meckel's cave. Note the extension into the nerve meatus (arrow) giving the characteristic 'pear' shape.

carotid artery, or by the needle transgressing a vessel in its appropriate trajectory. Extracranial bleeding may cause facial swelling or bruising but is not serious. Intracranial bleeding is rare but may cause all the symptoms and complications of subarachnoid hemorrhage. Progressive and gentle manipulation of the needle, particularly once the foramen ovale is entered, with frequent radiologic checks, will help to reduce the incidence of untoward events. Infective complications are so rare that few surgeons use antibiotic prophylaxis.

Radiosurgery

Stereotactically focused radiotherapy – provided either by an adapted linear accelerator or by the so-called 'Gamma Knife' – has increasingly found a place in the treatment of vascular lesions and tumors. The mechanism of action here is clear. When directed at the root entry zone of the trigeminal nerve, however, radiosurgery has also proved effective in reducing or abolishing the symptoms of trigeminal neuralgia.[26] It is not yet clear for how long this effect will last or what is its rationale, although like many of the procedures above it presumably causes focal damage to the root and interrupts the 'short-circuits' generating neuralgia.

OPEN OPERATIONS

Microvascular decompression

This has virtually replaced all other open procedures and in many centers is the first-line treatment in patients whose pain is refractory and who are able to tolerate surgery.

Technique

The patient is placed in the lateral position and a 5–6 cm retromastoid incision is made on the affected side. A small craniotomy or craniectomy is made up to the confluence of the transverse and sigmoid venous sinuses. This represents the junction of the tentorium and the petrous temporal bone. An opening is made in the dura up to this junction and the cerebellum is retracted gently while cerebrospinal fluid is aspirated. Under the microscope the right-angled corner between tentorium and petrous is identified and followed medially. The petrosal vein is encountered next and may be safely divided. Just medial to this, the trigeminal nerve root will come into view.

The root is examined closely and arachnoid adhesions divided. In most cases, a compressing vessel will be seen medial to the nerve at the root entry zone – the area where its rootlets enter the pons. This is usually a branch of the superior cerebellar artery. Any artery encountered in this region must be treated with the utmost respect as most are end-vessels and obstruction or division will result in a stroke. The offending vessel is carefully dissected away from the nerve, upon which a groove is often then seen where it has been compressed. If it is possible to displace the vessel permanently – if for instance it is a loop and may be displaced lateral to the nerve – this is done, but more commonly the vessel is merely dissected off the nerve and then separated permanently from it by the interposition of an inert material such as Teflon wool. It is important to avoid kinking the artery as this may obstruct or compromise blood flow. Before this is done, a thorough search of the length of the nerve must be carried out to ensure that there are no other compressive vessels. If no artery is found but a vein is compressing the nerve, this should be treated similarly although the chances of cure of symptoms are less good. After meticulous hemostasis, retraction is withdrawn and the craniotomy closed. The patient is closely observed overnight and may usually be discharged within 3–5 days.[3,27–35]

Trigeminal root section

This is rarely used now, although it enjoyed popularity as the standard operation for trigeminal neuralgia from its introduction in the early 1900s by Frazier and Ferrier until the 1950s.[1] This operation was originally performed via a subtemporal, extradural route, exposing the ganglion and dividing the sensory root – sparing the motor root – as close to the brainstem as possible. Although this inevitably caused facial numbness, often involving the ophthalmic division of the nerve and rendering the patient liable to keratitis, particularly when the greater superficial petrosal nerve was damaged, it was nevertheless extremely successful at relieving neuralgia. In 1932 Walter Dandy published data recommending an approach to the root in the posterior fossa, dividing it only partially and affording pain relief with considerable preservation of sensation. More importantly, he later suggested that pain might be caused by compression of the root at its entry zone by an aberrant artery – the basis of trigeminal neuralgia as it is understood today.

In cases refractory to percutaneous techniques or microvascular decompression, partial root section is still occasionally used. It is important to be sure of the diagnosis of trigeminal neuralgia, however, when considering this move, as other types of facial pain may be made worse or will at best not respond. It is most frequently performed when a re-exploration for recurrent neuralgia reveals no vascular compression.

Potential hazards of posterior fossa surgery include cranial nerve damage (5th, 7th or 8th)[30] from excessive retraction or manipulation; vascular damage, particularly to perforating vessels; and postoperative hemorrhage causing cerebellar or brainstem compression. These are extremely rare in experienced hands.

CENTRAL LESIONS

Surgical lesions of the brainstem or sensory tracts have an uncertain place at present in the treatment of facial pain, and probably no place in trigeminal neuralgia. Tractotomy[36] and dorsal root entry zone (DREZ) lesions[12,37] have been performed for desperate patients and in careful hands have produced some good results, but potential complications are many and pain relief unpredictable. Electrical stimulation of central target areas rather than destruction, is currently being evaluated and has had some success in otherwise intractable facial pain.

POSTOPERATIVE CARE

All surgical procedures carry a risk of sensory loss. While this may be inconvenient when affecting the second or third trigeminal divisions, anesthesia of the first division and thus of the cornea is potentially highly dangerous as unrecognized scarring can lead to blindness. All patients should therefore have an eye shield applied until they are cooperative enough for corneal sensation to be tested. If sensation is absent and fails to return, special glasses with side panels should be worn and the patient instructed about appropriate eye care.

Routine clinical observations are sufficient for patients following percutaneous procedures, and they can usually be allowed home the same or the following day. Open procedures carry more serious risks: observation in an intensive care or high dependency unit is recommended as the development of a posterior fossa hematoma, while exceedingly rare, is a life-threatening emergency. The patient will often have headache or be dizzy or nauseated for a day or two, and will not usually be discharged until the third or fourth postoperative day.

If pain is abolished by the procedure, medication may be withdrawn immediately although some patients prefer a gradual withdrawal.

OUTCOME

Medical treatment with adequate doses of anticonvulsants may be sufficient to control symptoms in many patients and, given the relapsing and remitting nature of the disease, may only need to be administered as intermittent courses. It is, however, unusual for a patient to be successfully treated in this way in the long term, and increasing pain or intolerable drug side effects should quickly lead to neurosurgical referral. Even at first treatment around 10% of patients will not be able to tolerate anticonvulsant therapy and this rises with time.

All surgical procedures have a reported immediate success rate in excess of 85%. Carefully selected patients undergoing microvascular decompression will have a >95% rate of immediate relief of pain with a total complication rate of <2%. This is without doubt the most effective procedure, but must be recommended with circumspection in the elderly.

The main differences between the procedures are in rates of recurrence, with reported relapse rates at 2 years varying from 2 to 47%.[10,11,15,18,24,27,28,33,35] A recurrence rate of around 7% per year has been quoted for microvascular decompression, but many authors report substantially lower rates.

Whatever the initial method used, recurrence should stimulate serious consideration of a repeat operation. Even when thorough exploration of the nerve and root entry zone has been undertaken, compression by a new or overlooked vessel can occur or material interposed between nerve and vessel may become dislodged. Complication rates are higher for repeat open procedures, however, and a percutaneous approach may be preferred. Primary percutaneous procedures may be readily repeated with reasonable expectation of success; early failure, however, may prompt consideration of an alternative approach.

REFERENCES

1. Wilkins RH 1990 Historical perspectives. In: Rovit RL, Murali R, Jannetta PJ (eds) Trigeminal neuralgia. Williams & Wilkins, Baltimore, pp 1–25

2. Hardy DG, Rhoton AL Jr 1978 Microsurgical relationships of the superior cerebellar artery and the trigeminal nerve. Journal of Neurosurgery 49:669–678

3. Janetta PJ 1967 Arterial compression of the trigeminal nerve at the pons in patients with trigeminal neuralgia. Journal of Neurosurgery 26:159–162

4. Adams CBT 1989 Microvascular compression: an alternative view and hypothesis. Journal of Neurosurgery 70:1–12

5. Bowsher D, Miles JB, Haggett CE et al 1997 Trigeminal neuralgia: a quantitative sensory perception threshold study in patients who had not undergone previous invasive procedures. Journal of Neurosurgery 86:190–192

6. Miles JB, Eldridge PR, Haggett CE, Bowsher D 1997 Sensory effects of microvascular decompression in trigeminal neuralgia. Journal of Neurosurgery 86:193–196

7. Meaney JFM, Miles JB, Nixon TE et al 1994 Vascular contact with the fifth cranial nerve at the pons in patients with trigeminal neuralgia: detection with 3D FISP imaging. American Journal of Roentgenology 163:1447–1452

8. Blom S 1962 Trigeminal neuralgia: its treatment with a new anticonvulsant drug (G-32883). Lancet 1:839–840

9. Mullan S, Brown JA 1996 Trigeminal neuralgia. Neurosurgery Quarterly 6:267–288

10. Broggi G, Franzini A, Lasio G, Giorgi C, Servello D 1990 Long-term results of percutaneous retrogasserian thermorhizotomy for 'essential' trigeminal neuralgia: Considerations in 1000 patients. Neurosurgery 26:783–787

11. Fraioli B, Esposito V, Guidetti B, Cruccu G, Manfredi M 1989 Treatment of trigeminal neuralgia by thermocoagulation, glycerolization, and percutaneous compression of the gasserian ganglion and/or retrogasserian rootlets: Long-term results and therapeutic protocol. Neurosurgery 24:239–245

12. Sampson JH, Nashold BS Jr 1992 Facial pain due to vascular lesions of the brain stem relieved by dorsal root entry zone lesions in the nucleus caudalis. Journal of Neurosurgery 77:473–475

13. Sweet WH 1990 Treatment of trigeminal neuralgia by percutaneous rhizotomy. In: Youmans J (ed) Neurological surgery. W B Saunders, Philadelphia, pp 3888–3921

14. Sweet WH, Wepsic JG 1974 Controlled thermocoagulation of trigeminal ganglion and rootlets for differential destruction of pain fibres. Part 1: Trigeminal neuralgia. Journal of Neurosurgery 40:143–156

15. Taha JM, Tew JM Jr 1996 Comparison of surgical treatments for trigeminal neuralgia: re-evaluation of radiofrequency rhizotomy. Journal of Neurosurgery 38:865–871

16. Tew JM Jr, Keller JT 1977 The treatment of trigeminal neuralgia by percutaneous radiofrequency technique. Clinical Neurosurgery 24:557–578

17. Arias MJ 1986 Percutaneous retrogasserian glycerol rhizotomy for trigeminal neuralgia; A prospective study of 100 cases. Journal of Neurosurgery 65:32–36

18. Fujimaki T, Fukushima T, Miyazaki S 1990 Percutaneous retrogasserian glycerol injection in the management of trigeminal neuralgia: Long-term follow-up results. Journal of Neurosurgery 73:212–216

19. Lunsford D, Bennett M 1984 Percutaneous retrogasserian glycerol rhizotomy for tic douloureux: Part 1 – Technique and results in 112 patients. Neurosurgery 14:424–430

20. Saini SS 1987 Retrogasserian anhydrous glycerol injection therapy in trigeminal neuralgia: Observations in 552 patients. Journal of Neurology, Neurosurgery and Psychiatry 50:1536–1538

21. Young RF 1988 Glycerol rhizolysis for the treatment of trigeminal neuralgia. Journal of Neurosurgery 69:39–45

22. Brown JA, Hoeflinger B, Long PH et al 1996 Axon and ganglion cell injury in rabbits after percutaneous trigeminal balloon compression. Neurosurgery 38:993–1004

23. Brown JA, McDaniel MD, Weaver MT 1993 Percutaneous trigeminal nerve compression for treatment of trigeminal neuralgia: Results in 50 patients. Neurosurgery 32:570–573

24. Lichtor T, Mullan JF 1990 A 10-year follow up review of percutaneous microcompression of the trigeminal ganglion. Journal of Neurosurgery 72:49–54

25. Lobato RD, Rivas JJ, Sarabia R, Lamas E 1990 Percutaneous microcompression of the gasserian ganglion for trigeminal neuralgia. Journal of Neurosurgery 72:546–553

26. Rand RW, Jacques DB, Melbye RW et al 1993 Leksell gamma knife treatment of tic douloureux. Stereotactic and Functional Neurosurgery 61(suppl 1):93–102

27. Barker FG II, Jannetta PJ, Bissonette DJ et al 1986 The long-term outcome of microvascular decompression for trigeminal neuralgia. New England Journal of Medicine 334:1077–1083

28. Burchiel KJ, Clarke H, Haglund M, Loeser JD 1988 Long-term efficacy of microvascular decompression in trigeminal neuralgia. Journal of Neurosurgery 69:35–38

29. Cho DT, Chang CGS, Wang YC, Wang FH, Shen CC, Yang DY 1994 Repeat operations in failed microvascular decompression for trigeminal neuralgia. Neurosurgery 35:665–670

30. Fritz W, Schafer J, Klein HJ 1988 Hearing loss after microvascular decompression for trigeminal neuralgia. Journal of Neurosurgery 69:367–370

31. Jannetta PJ 1976 Microsurgical approach to the trigeminal nerve for tic douloureux. Progress in Neurological Surgery 7:180–200

32. Janetta PJ 1990 Microvascular decompression of the trigeminal nerve root entry zone. Theoretical considerations, operative anatomy, surgical technique, and results. In: Rovit ML, Murali R, Jannetta PJ (ed) Trigeminal neuralgia. Williams & Wilkins, Baltimore, pp 201–211

33. Kondo A 1997 Follow-up results of microvascular decompression in trigeminal neuralgia and hemifacial spasm. Neurosurgery 40:46–52

34. Naraghi R, Gaab M, Walter GF, Kleineberg B 1992 Arterial hypertension and neurovascular compression at the ventrolateral medulla. Journal of Neurosurgery 77:103–112

35. Rath SA, Klein HJ, Richter H-P 1996 Findings and long-term results of subsequent operations after failed microvascular decompression for trigeminal neuralgia. Neurosurgery 39:933–940

36. Hitchcock ER 1970 Stereotactic trigeminal tractotomy. Annals of Clinical Research 2:131–135

37. Nashold BS Jr, Lopes H, Chodakiewitz J et al 1986 Trigeminal DREZ for craniofacial pain. In: Samii M (ed) Surgery in and around the brainstem. Springer Verlag, Heidelberg, pp 54–59

Management of orofacial infections

92

ALISTAIR G. SMYTH

INTRODUCTION

Clinical symptoms and signs of infection may present within the orofacial region because of a localized infection such as a bacterial abscess or as part of the overall presentation of a systemic generalized infection. Infections presenting within the orofacial region are common and account for the largest single reason for referral to a maxillofacial surgery department.

The spectrum of presentation of infections can usually be categorized into one of the following groups:

- Infection due to a mixture of nonspecific micro-organisms that are normally found within the oral and facial region – *endogenous commensal organisms*. Dento-alveolar infections and acute submandibular sialadenitis are examples of this group. A characteristic is that the infection is usually caused by a small number of organisms rather than by a single pathogenic species.
- Infection due to a single specific micro-organism that is normally found within the oral and facial region – *endogenous opportunistic organism*. Certain local or systemic conditions are required which favor the development of this type of infection. Examples are candidal infections of the mouth or actinomycosis of the face and jaws.
- Infection due to a single specific organism which is not normally part of the local oral flora – *exogenous pathogenic organisms*. The majority of the viral infections and specific bacterial infections such as tuberculosis and syphilis fall into this category.

Infections within the orofacial region cause pain and debility and are a common source of lost working days. Occasionally they can be life-threatening, when early and accurate diagnosis is required followed by aggressive treatment and careful monitoring.

Untreated, many initial acute infections will enter a chronic phase with persistence and further morbidity.

APPLIED ANATOMY

Blood supply

The orofacial region is richly vascularized by branches of the external carotid artery system; this greatly assists the defense against infection. It is surprising how infrequently infection arises after trauma such as following a tooth extraction, compound fracture of the mandible, or contaminated facial lacerations. Under these circumstances, the rich network of blood vessels is an important barrier against infection. Conditions which impair this vascularity such as radiotherapy or diabetes mellitus increase the risk of infection after tissue trauma.

The venous drainage from the face runs into the jugular venous system, however anatomic connections between the intracranial and extracranial venous systems also exist and therefore there is a potential route for the spread of infection from the facial area to the brain. These connections arise predominantly around the orbits, between the angular vein which drains inferiorly into the facial vein and the superior and inferior ophthalmic veins which pass posteriorly through the superior oblique fissure into the cavernous sinus (Fig. 92.1). The facial vein is valveless and therefore infected venous thrombi resulting from a localized infection in the vicinity of the facial vein can pass retrogradely and reach the dural venous sinuses. Other connections also exist, such as between the pterygoid venous plexus and the cavernous sinus. Although the clinical spread of infection intracranially by this route is uncommon, the consequences

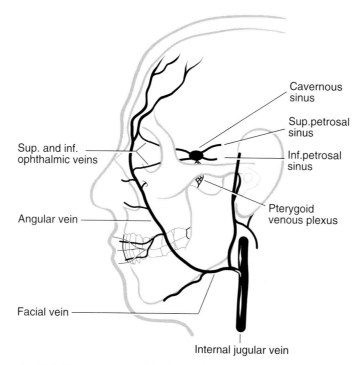

Fig. 92.1 Venous drainage of the face and intracranial connections.

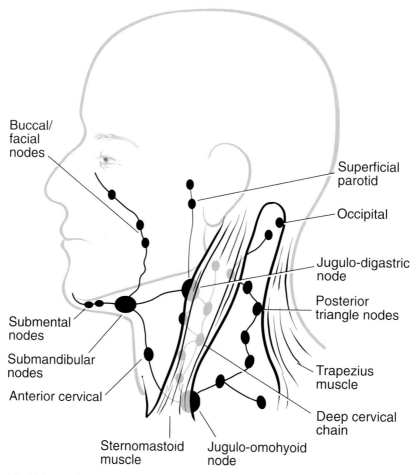

Fig. 92.2 Lymphatic drainage of the head and neck.

– such as the development of cavernous sinus thrombosis or cerebral abscess – are serious and life-threatening.

Lymphatic drainage

Infections within the orofacial region often involve the draining lymph nodes, which are arranged in recognized groups (Fig. 92.2), resulting in a regional lymphadenitis. Knowledge of the pattern of drainage is essential to understand the likely pathway of spread of infection and direct the treatment accordingly. The pattern of lymphadenitis may also indicate the likely source of local infection if this is not readily apparent.

The most frequently involved nodes are the submandibular and upper cervical (jugulodigastric) as the lymph vessels from the forehead, anterior face, mouth and jaws follow the facial vessels into the submandibular nodes and then into the deep jugular chain of lymph nodes. Lymph drainage from the lateral part of the face including the eyelids and temporal scalp drains into the superficial parotid nodes and then into the deep cervical nodes. The deep parotid nodes within the parotid gland also drain into the upper deep cervical nodes. Infection arising within the midportion of the lower lip, chin, lower incisor teeth and anterior floor of mouth may spread via the local lymphatics to involve the submental nodes, from which the lymph may drain directly to the inferior deep cervical nodes (jugulo-omohyoid) or via the submandibular nodes to the upper cervical chain.

Tissue spaces and compartments

Infection may spread from the original focus; for example, a dento-alveolar infection may spread along tissue spaces and lead to a facial cellulitis, a rapidly developing acute infection of the subcutaneous tissues which can spread through tissue spaces and deeper fascial planes. The tissue spaces are potential spaces bounded by muscles, bone and actual fascial layers. The tissue spaces and fascial compartments can be described on anatomic grounds and infection may often be contained within one or more of these compartments. The compartments communicate with each other and therefore allow the spread of infection beyond a single compartment. The following classification attributed to Scott[1] is frequently used:

- *Superficial compartment.* This compartment is contained within the superficial aspect of the face between the overlying skin and the underlying mandible and maxilla covered by the masseter and buccinator muscles. The space extends from the zygomatic arch above to the lower border of the mandible below. Posteriorly the space is limited by the fascial covering of the parotid gland. It communicates with the pterygoid space medial to the ramus of the mandible. Contents include the muscles of facial expression, the facial nerve, buccal pad of fat, blood vessels and facial lymph nodes.

- *Floor of mouth.* This compartment can be subdivided by the mylohyoid muscle into the sublingual space above and the submental and submandibular spaces below (Fig. 92.3). The *sublingual space* extends from the mylohyoid muscle below up to the tongue and mucosa of the floor of the mouth. It communicates posteriorly with the submandibular space and contains the sublingual salivary glands and the deep lobes of the submandibular salivary glands. The *submental space* lies between the two anterior bellies of the digastric muscle and extends between the mylohyoid muscle above and

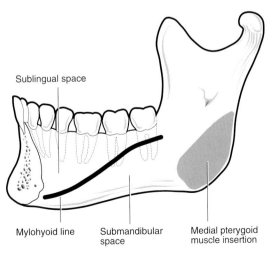

Sublingual space

Mylohyoid line

Submandibular space

Medial pterygoid muscle insertion

Fig. 92.3 Floor of mouth divided by mylohyoid muscle into sublingual space above and submandibular space below (note relationship of mylohyoid line to apices of mandibular teeth).

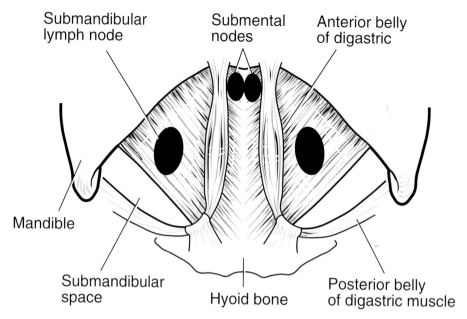

Submandibular lymph node

Submental nodes

Anterior belly of digastric

Mandible

Submandibular space

Hyoid bone

Posterior belly of digastric muscle

Fig. 92.4 Inferior view of floor of mouth beneath mylohyoid muscle showing central submental space and lateral submandibular spaces.

the deep cervical fascia and overlying platysma below (Fig. 92.4). It contains the submental lymph nodes and communicates directly with the submandibular spaces. The paired *submandibular spaces* are bounded laterally by the mandible below the mylohyoid line, medially by the mylohyoid muscle, and below by the deep cervical fascia and overlying platysma and skin. The submandibular space contains the superficial parts of the submandibular salivary glands and associated lymph nodes and communicates with the sublingual, superficial facial and deep pterygoid spaces.

- *Masticator space*. This space is bounded laterally by the temporalis fascia, zygomatic arch and the masseter muscle, while the medial border is formed by the lateral and medial pterygoid muscles (Fig. 92.5). The intervening presence of the ramus of the mandible and the attached temporalis muscle divides this compartment up into superficial and deep temporal spaces above and the submasseteric and superficial pterygoid space below. The deep cervical fascia splits to contain and surround the masseter and pterygoid muscles and forms part of the actual boundary. The superficial pterygoid space between the inner ramus of mandible and the fascia overlying the medial pterygoid muscle is sometimes known as the pterygomandibular space and communicates with the deep pterygoid space.

- *Parapharyngeal space*. The parapharyngeal space is a gutter which runs from the base of the skull above to the base of the neck and mediastinum below. It is bounded anteromedially by the pharyngeal wall and posteriorly by the carotid sheath and prevertebral fascia. Laterally, the space is bounded by the deep cervical fascia on the deep aspect of the medial pterygoid muscle and the styloid process and attached muscles and ligaments (Fig. 92.6). The superior portion of the space is known as the deep pterygoid space and communicates with the superficial pterygoid space and the floor of the mouth. Infection may arise within these sites and spread along the parapharyngeal space down the neck to the mediastinum and thorax.

- *Parotid space*. The superficial layer of the deep cervical fascia splits to envelop the parotid gland. The fascial boundary is thin on the medial aspect of the parotid gland but thickens laterally and superiorly where it forms the stylomandibular ligament. The space contains the parotid gland, the superficial and deep parotid nodes, facial nerve, external carotid artery and retromandibular vein.

- *Paratonsillar space*. This space contains the palatine tonsil and lies between the faucial pillars medially and the superior constrictor muscle laterally. It communicates with the deep pterygoid space and the remainder of the parapharyngeal space.

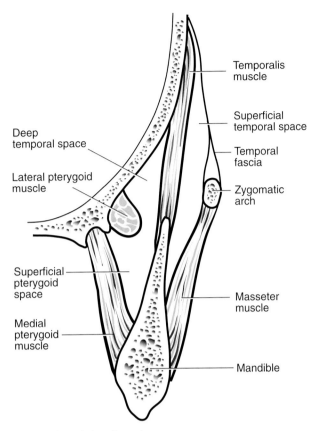

Temporalis
muscle

Superficial
temporal space

Temporal
fascia

Zygomatic
arch

Masseter
muscle

Mandible

Deep
temporal space

Lateral pterygoid
muscle

Superficial
pterygoid
space

Medial
pterygoid
muscle

Fig. 92.5 Anatomic boundaries of masticator space.

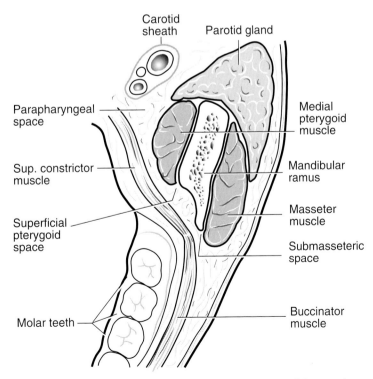

Carotid
sheath

Parotid gland

Parapharyngeal
space

Medial
pterygoid
muscle

Sup. constrictor
muscle

Mandibular
ramus

Superficial
pterygoid
space

Masseter
muscle

Submasseteric
space

Molar teeth

Buccinator
muscle

Fig. 92.6 Axial section through ramus of mandible showing relationships of the parapharyngeal space.

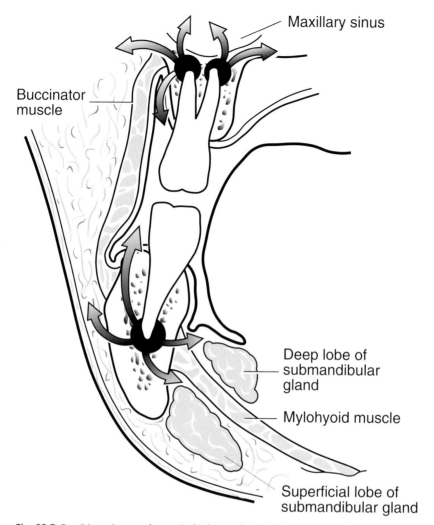

Fig. 92.7 Possible pathways of spread of infection from maxillary and mandibular molar teeth.

Teeth and jaws (Fig. 92.7)

Acute infection arising from the teeth frequently spreads in a predictable manner due to the location of the teeth within the jaws and the attachments of the muscles such as buccinator and mylohyoid. Periapical infection arising from the upper teeth often spreads labially or buccally into the sulcus. Buccal spread of infection from the maxillary molar teeth may track below the attachment of the buccinator muscle and present intra-orally within the buccal sulcus or may spread above the attachment and into the superficial facial space. The root of the upper lateral incisor tooth is often more palatally inclined and therefore periapical infection may preferentially point into the palate. The canine root is long, and so apical infection may either present within the labial sulcus or track superiorly to the side of the nose and up to the inner canthal area of the eye. Occasionally, infection arising from a palatal root of an upper premolar or molar tooth can also present in the palate.

Infection arising from the lower incisor teeth roots often presents in the labial sulcus as a localized swelling. Sometimes the infection tracks between the two bellies of mentalis muscle to present on the point of the chin where it may be misdiagnosed as a local skin abscess or folliculitis (Fig. 92.8). Periapical infection arising from a mandibular canine may present within the superficial facial compartment as this tooth root is longer than the adjacent teeth and consequently does not often present in the labial sulcus. Infection arising from the mandibular premolars and molars may present buccally within the vestibular sulcus although the roots of the second molar are situated nearer the lingual plate and therefore infection tracking from this tooth is more likely to spread lingually. Buccal spread of infection from the molar teeth may pass below the mandibular attachment of buccinator muscle to present in the superficial

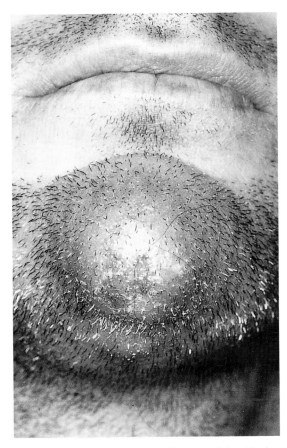

Fig. 92.8 Abscess formation within the soft tissues of the chin due to spread of infection from the roots of the lower incisor teeth.

facial compartment. Lingual spread of infection may occur from any of the lower teeth when the infection may involve the sublingual space or the submandibular space. If the incisors, canine, premolar or first molar teeth are implicated then the infection is more likely to pass into the sublingual space as the apices of these teeth are above the mylohyoid line. Conversely, the apices of the second and third molar teeth are below the mylohyoid line and therefore lingual spread of infection would tend to present within the submandibular space.

INFECTIONS OF THE MOUTH AND FACE

BACTERIAL INFECTIONS

Periapical abscess

This common bacterial infection arises from a nonvital tooth which is often the result of dental caries or trauma. The infection arises within the necrotic pulp tissues and spreads beyond the confines of the pulp canal to the peri-

apical tissues of the jaw bone to present as an acute periapical or dento-alveolar abscess. This infection is usually due to a mixture of predominantly anaerobic bacteria[2] commonly found as part of the oral flora. *Bacteroides* species and anaerobic streptococci are commonly isolated. Clinical features include severe, constant, localized throbbing pain, swelling overlying the apical region, and tenderness to percussion of the causative tooth which is nonvital and often discolored, carious or fractured. A soft fluctuant tender swelling may also be present within the sulcus, or occasionally the subperiosteal abscess may present within the palate. Signs of local spread may be present with trismus or regional lymphadenopathy and systemic signs of toxicity such as pyrexia, flushing, rigors or tachycardia. The basis of treatment is to establish drainage of the abscess; this can be accomplished by tooth extraction, incision and drainage of an intraoral swelling, or open drainage of the tooth pulp chamber depending upon the clinical circumstances.

If the acute infection is untreated or inadequately treated then the infection may become chronic with persistent sinus formation, intermittent purulent discharge and attempts at periapical healing with the development of a periapical granuloma. This is usually accompanied by an improvement in the symptoms although the chronic phase can revert to an acute infection if drainage is impeded. Early radiographic changes include loss of the lamina dura and later the development of a periapical radiolucency (Fig. 92.9).

Periodontal abscess

This acute infection arises within a periodontal pocket and can present with the same symptoms as a periapical infection. The swelling is usually situated over the root of the tooth nearer the gum margin rather than over the apical region as in periapical abscess. Evidence of chronic periodontal disease is often widespread, and the associated tooth is nearly always mobile and may retain vitality on testing. Pus may drain from the orifice of the periodontal pocket or may extend through the alveolar bone to the overlying gingiva via a sinus. Similar mixed organisms are implicated as occur in periapical infection such as *Bacteroides* species, fusobacteria, α-hemolytic streptococci and anaerobic streptococci. Treatment usually requires the extraction of the associated tooth.

Pericoronal infection

Infection may arise within the soft tissues surrounding a partially erupted tooth; it usually resolves following full eruption. If full eruption does not occur then conditions

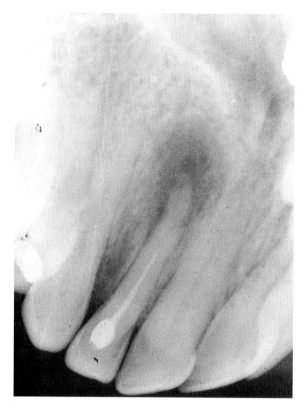

Fig. 92.9 Periapical radiolucency consistent with apical abscess arising from upper right lateral incisor tooth (maxillary occlusal radiograph).

may exist for the development of acute or chronic pericoronitis. This infection is most frequently associated with the lower third molar tooth which may be partially erupted and impacted. The same mixed endogenous organisms are involved as in periapical and periodontal abscesses. Acute pericoronitis may present with acute pain and swelling around the wisdom tooth associated with trismus and lymphadenitis. Spread of infection may occur into the paratonsillar space, parapharyngeal space or submandibular space. Infection may also track laterally into the buccal sulcus or into the submasseteric space. Chronic pericoronitis may result with intermittent episodes of localized tender painful swelling associated with occasional discharge and bad taste. An associated intrabony pocket may be seen on radiographic examination of the impacted tooth.

Treatment of the acute infection may require surgical drainage of the abscess in addition to systemic antibiotics and general supportive treatment. Removal of the impacted tooth is generally required to prevent further episodes of infection.

Facial cellulitis and fascial space infections

Infection arising within the mouth, face or jaws can extend into the subcutaneous tissue, resulting in a facial cellulitis, or more deeply into the fascial compartments with spread to the floor of mouth and neck. The most common source of infection is from the teeth with an associated periapical, periodontal or pericoronal infection. The same anaerobic organisms are implicated as before, although occasionally *Staphylococcus aureus* may be isolated.

The clinical features of facial cellulitis (Fig. 92.10) include a tense painful swelling of the face which is red, hot and tender. There is often considerable periorbital edema on the affected side due to the lax nature of the tissues in this region, and the eye may be closed as a result. Regional lymphadenitis, although likely to be present, is often difficult to palpate because of the tense nature of the facial swelling. The patient is unwell, pyrexial and anorexic. The history of the infection may be short with rapid spread of infection occurring within hours, although often a localized dento-alveolar infection has been previously inadequately treated or ignored by the patient over the last 5–10 days, with marked deterioration occurring within the last 12–24 hours marking the onset of the cellulitic spread of infection. Facial cellulitis resulting from an upper tooth, particularly the canine or premolar teeth, presents on the cheek alongside the nose which is often distorted by the

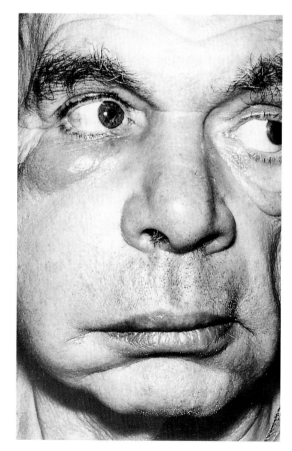

Fig. 92.10 Facial cellulitis secondary to periapical infection.

soft tissue swelling and the possible presence of a sub-periosteal abscess collection which lifts up the alar base. Cellulitic infection arising from the lower anterior teeth presents on the chin, while the posterior teeth cause a marked inflammatory diffuse swelling over the ramus and angle of the mandible. Examination includes careful inspection of the mouth for a possible source of infection, radiographic examination for retained roots, carious or impacted teeth, periapical infection, etc., and blood investigations which often reveal a neutrophil leukocytosis. It is also good practice to include a blood sugar estimation to exclude an acute presentation of diabetes mellitus. If the patient is pyrexial with rigors then blood cultures should be performed to search for aerobic and anaerobic organisms.

The patient should be hospitalized and supportive treatment commenced with rehydration, antipyretic analgesics and systemic antibiotics. The antibiotic of choice is a combination of penicillin and metronidazole given intravenously in adequate dosage. Alternatively, metronidazole may be administered as a suppository, providing similar blood levels. Suitable alternatives to penicillin include erythromycin or clindamycin. The antibiotic regime should be reviewed following microbiological culture and likely antibiotic sensitivities although significant changes in the antibiotic regime may not be necessary if the infection appears to be responding well. Surgical drainage can sometimes be avoided in the early stages of the cellulitic process as long as the patient is carefully observed. If the patient does not show signs of improvement or the cellulitic process is seen to extend then surgical exploration should be urgently carried out. Abscess cavities should be drained and the likely source of infection treated – this frequently requires tooth extraction. Alternatively, if the patient presents with an established infection, which often includes a brawny swelling and a high swinging temperature, then surgical treatment with drainage of the superficial facial space and removal of the causative tooth should not be delayed.

If the infection has spread into the deeper fascial compartments other symptoms and signs may be present depending on the actual compartments involved. In addition to the symptoms described above, the patient may complain of difficulty in opening the mouth and in swallowing with pooling of saliva. Spread of infection into the floor of the mouth and the parapharyngeal space can be complicated by impairment of the upper airway; constant vigilance is required to observe for early signs of impending airway compromise which will require urgent intervention. Particular attention should be paid to the patient who will not lie back in bed and prefers to sit forward with salivary secretions running out of the mouth as this may be due to swelling within the floor of the mouth pushing the tongue

upwards and backwards and thereby compromising the airway. Severe trismus is not uncommon and therefore the clinician may find it difficult to examine the floor of the mouth for swelling or the pharyngeal wall for the possible presence of a peritonsillar abscess (quinsy). Infection within the submandibular space often presents with a brawny diffuse swelling within this area and the patient often adopts a head tilt away from the affected side to avoid pressure on the swelling from clothing or against the shoulder. Needle aspiration of the swelling frequently results in a sample of pus which can be sent for microscopy and culture (Fig. 92.11). A lateral skull radiograph may show the elevated position of the tongue if the sublingual space is involved. Fiberoptic nasal endoscopy is a useful adjunct in doubtful cases to examine the lateral pharyngeal walls and upper larynx for evidence of swelling due to a collection of pus or edema. If required, a CT scan will help to localize the position of a deep cervical collection and thereby direct appropriate drainage.

Management of a fascial space infection

Consideration must be given primarily to the patency of the airway and possible compromise. These patients require close observation as they can deteriorate rapidly; timely intervention can be life-saving. Indicators of airway compromise include open mouth breathing, use of accessory muscles of respiration, dilation of the nares and tachypnea. Late signs include stridor, hypoxia and cyanosis due to a marked reduction in airway space and impending complete obstruction. A high level of suspicion is required. If airway compromise is present then intervention such as endotra-

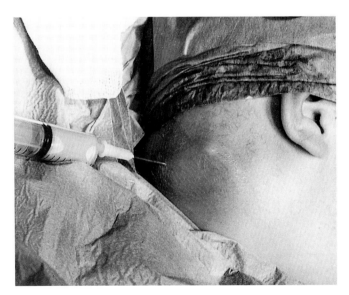

Fig. 92.11 Needle aspiration of pus for microbiologic Gram-stain film and culture.

cheal intubation is required to protect the airway. There is no place for a fasciotomy-like procedure to release the deep cervical fascia with incision across the neck as in a compartment compression syndrome. The potential consequences if this surgical procedure is unsuccessful are too great. The presence of airway compromise indicates intervention by endotracheal intubation or tracheostomy.

An expectant policy with systemic antibiotics can also be fraught with danger unless a very careful examination has been possible including examination of the oropharynx and indirect laryngoscopy. Otherwise, if a fascial space collection is deemed present, drainage should be urgently established. Intravenous antibiotics should be started with intravenous fluid therapy. Surgical drainage is frequently carried out under general anesthesia; the anesthetist should be informed of the nature and location of likely swelling and also the presence of any trismus. The trismus can be difficult to overcome even after muscle paralysis and therefore orotracheal intubation can be hazardous. A gaseous induction is often used or, more frequently, fiberoptic assisted intubation. Inadvertent rupture of a pharyngeal collection can also occur during intubation with further risk to the airway and possible aspiration of pus.

After examination of the neck and particularly the mouth and pharynx under anesthesia, the involved fascial spaces are explored through a submandibular skin crease incision. Sharp dissection through the skin, platysma and deep cervical fascia is followed by blunt dissection with sinus forceps into the submandibular space, submental space and sublingual space, if required (Fig. 92.12). Insertion of the index finger is very useful for breaking down loculated abscess cavities, particularly in the region of the deep pharyngeal space. Drainage of free pus is usually establish-

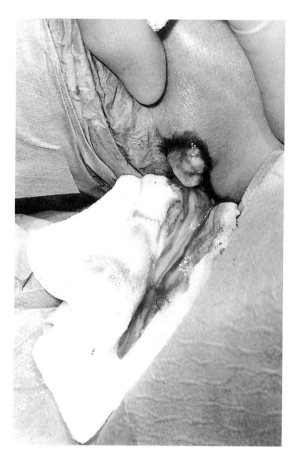

Fig. 92.13 Free drainage of pus established prior to placement of open surgical drain.

ed (Fig. 92.13); a sample should be collected in a sterile container and also on a swab to be transported in nutrient media. Specimens of pus should be sent to the microbiology department without delay.[3] Drainage within the mouth may also be required with incision in the buccal sulcus to gain access to the submasseteric space or within the floor of the mouth to gain access to the sublingual space. the parapharyngeal space can be drained through an incision just medial to the ascending ramus of the mandible. After incising through the mucosa only, the parapharyngeal space is explored with sinus forceps or curved Spencer Wells forceps to establish drainage. Again, blunt dissection with a finger is very helpful. The source of the infection is dealt with, such as the removal of a carious tooth or roots, or the removal of an impacted wisdom tooth. The fascial spaces are drained externally with the insertion of corrugated or Yates drains to allow continuing drainage for a further 24–48 hours. A decision must also be made regarding the airway; if compromise is deemed likely or is indeed already present then endotracheal intubation should be continued on return to an intensive care facility or elective tracheostomy performed if transfer to an ITU is

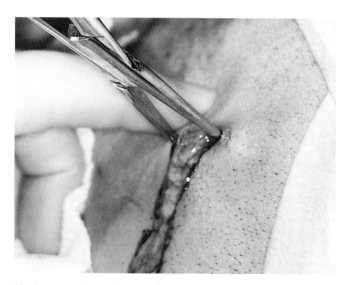

Fig. 92.12 Drainage of submandibular space infection using blunt dissection with sinus forceps.

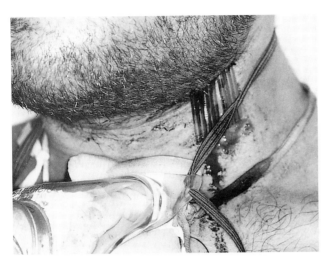

Fig. 92.14 Tracheostomy to secure and protect airway. Drains sutured in position to allow continuing drainage of pus.

not possible (Fig. 92.14). Early indicators of a satisfactory outcome are a return to normal of the temperature and pulse rate and a decline in the neutrophil white cell count. The swelling and trismus often takes 2–3 weeks to resolve completely.

Ludwig's angina

This acute cellulitic infection is described as involving the tissues of the floor of the mouth on *both* sides. The infection is dental in origin in about 90% of cases, other less common sources being infected mandibular fractures or submandibular sialadenitis. The teeth most commonly implicated are the second and third mandibular molars. The clinical features are those of systemic toxicity with a board-like swelling across the upper neck from angle to angle within the suprahyoid region and swelling within the floor of the mouth which raises the position of the tongue. The skin is red and inflamed; pitting edema may be present. Oral commensal bacteria are frequently the cause – especially mixed infection with *Bacteroides* species, *Fusobacterium* and anaerobic streptococci – although bacterial culture may be negative in a substantial proportion of cases.[4] Before antibiotics, the mortality was around 75%; aggressive early treatment with surgical drainage and intravenous antibiotics has reduced this to around 5%. The infection may spread down into the neck with edema around the laryngeal glottis causing respiratory obstruction. There is a need for vigilance and management of the airway as described previously. Adequate drainage of both submandibular spaces is required through bilateral upper cervical incisions and also intraoral incisions if necessary. Any dental focus of infection should be eradicated by tooth removal. The submental and sub-

lingual spaces are explored and drained. Intravenous penicillin and metronidazole in combination is usually effective against the causative organisms.

Acute ulcerative gingivitis (AUG)

This acute infection of the gingiva is due to a synergistic infection by a fusospirochetal complex in a susceptible host. It is likely that associated factors such as emotional stress, heavy smoking, malnutrition or recent infection, especially with measles, results in a depression in host defenses and immunity, thereby allowing the increased development of fusobacteria and the spirochetal organisms. The clinical features include an acute inflammation of the attached gingiva with irregular shaped ulcers appearing initially on the tips of the interdental papillae. The painful ulcers enlarge to involve the marginal and attached gingiva. The ulcers are often covered by a gray or yellow slough which can be readily detached. The breath has an unpleasant odor and the patient may complain of a metallic taste in the mouth. Systemic upset is usually mild and local lymphadenitis may arise in the submental or submandibular nodes. Diagnosis is usually clinically based, however the diagnosis can be confirmed by microscopic examination of a Gram-stained smear prepared from a scraping of the ulcerated area. The infection responds rapidly to systemic treatment with oral metronidazole, and a chlorhexidine mouthbath is also helpful. Resolution of the infection should be followed by local debridement and cleaning and oral hygiene instruction.

Cancrum oris (Noma)

This condition is characterized by a gangrenous necrosis of the gingiva which continues to involve the oral mucosa and subsequently may spread rapidly to include the perioral tissues and face. Cancrum oris is predominantly seen in children in underdeveloped countries in association with malnutrition, dehydration and epidemic infections.[5] It is occasionally seen in developed countries in patients with underlying immunosuppresion from leukemia, chemotherapy or infectious disease such as measles. The majority of patients are children; the condition is rarely seen in adults. It is believed that AUG may be the precursor of cancrum oris and that the presence of a concurrent infectious disease such as measles or typhoid promotes the spread of the gangrenous condition by further impairment of the immune system. The acute lesion consists of a brawny, erythematous swelling, often around the commissure of the mouth. This has a glossy appearance with surrounding edema and an advancing area of necrosis in the center. The tissue necrosis is caused by a mixed syner-gistic infection of the fusospirochetal complex, which can be seen on a Gram-stained smear. The foul odor of the necrotic tissue also suggests the presence of anaerobes and indeed *Bacteroides* species are frequently isolated.

Immediate treatment requires hospitalization with re-hydration and correction of any electrolyte imbalance. Antimicrobial treatment with penicillin and metronidazole is appropriate. Extensive surgical debridement is not necessary and local wound care is restricted to removal of loose slough, mobile teeth and any bony sequestra. A chlor-hexidine mouthbath is also beneficial. Subsequent orofacial reconstruction is delayed until at least 3 months after the cancrum oris has responded to treatment, some have advised delaying reconstruction for up to a year.[6]

Necrotizing fasciitis

This polymicrobial soft-tissue infection is characterized by necrosis of fascia and subcutaneous tissue. The condition more commonly involves the groin, perineum or abdominal wall, however the head and neck region can also be affect-ed. The mortality of necrotizing fasciitis is about 40%[7] despite early recognition and aggressive treatment. Cervical necrotizing fasciitis is nearly always the result of a spread-ing infection from a dental focus. The causative organisms are a mixed bacterial infection of aerobes and obligate anaerobes[8] such as a Group A β-hemolytic streptococcus acting in synergy with *Bacteroides asacharolyticus* (formerly *B. melaninogenicus*). Patients often have an underlying systemic disease such as diabetes mellitus, alcoholism, mal-nutrition or chronic renal failure.[7]

The condition needs to be distinguished from cervico-facial cellulitis as the condition can spread very rapidly if appropriate treatment is delayed. In necrotizing fasciitis the skin is often pale and mottled rather than erythematous. With further thrombosis of skin vessels the skin may have a purple hue and develop fluid-filled blisters which ulcerate. The skin may also become paresthetic or anesthetic in the later stages. The rapid spread of the skin changes is also a dominant feature and the white cell count is frequently markedly elevated. Misdiagnosis and delay in treatment can result in severe systemic toxicity, carotid artery erosion, jugular vein thrombosis, lung abscess, mediastinitis and cranial neuropathies.[9] The necrosis is limited to the fascia and subcutaneous tissue; the presence of muscle necrosis, foul odor or gas production may indicate a co-infection with clostridial organisms. Necrotizing fasciitis requires emergent treatment with surgical drainage, antibiotics, air-way protection and occasionally hyperbaric oxygen. At operation, a wide and extensive fasciotomy with exposure

and exploration of all the involved fascia is required.[10] Necrotic tissue is debrided and the wound irrigated freely with dilute hydrogen peroxide. The wounds are drained and the incision margins only loosely approximated. Signs of further deterioration indicate the need for urgent surgical re-exploration to locate any necrotic tissue; this is removed, followed by further irrigation and multiple simple drains. Successful outcome is dependent on early recognition and immediate aggressive surgical management.

Scarlet fever

This acute infection is caused by the Group A hemolytic *Streptococcus pyogenes* which produces a specific exotoxin causing a widespread punctate erythematous rash. The primary site of infection is usually the pharynx and tonsils. Scarlet fever occurs most commonly in children and in more severe cases presents with sore throat, pyrexia, head-ache and nausea. The pharynx is inflamed and the tonsils enlarged with a covering slough. The tongue is initially furred with prominent red fungiform papillae giving an appearance known as 'white strawberry' tongue (Fig. 92.15). The erythematous rash is generalized but may be more pronounced and confluent on the limbs. The face is not affected by the rash but the face is usually highly flushed except around the mouth giving a typical appearance of perioral pallor (Fig. 92.16). Treatment is with penicillin and most cases respond rapidly.

Tuberculosis

Tuberculosis is a chronic granulomatous infection caused by *Mycobacterium tuberculosis*, an acid- and alcohol-fast

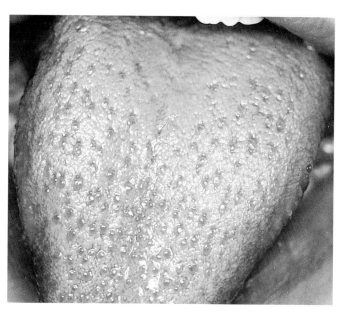

Fig. 92.15 White strawberry tongue of scarlet fever.

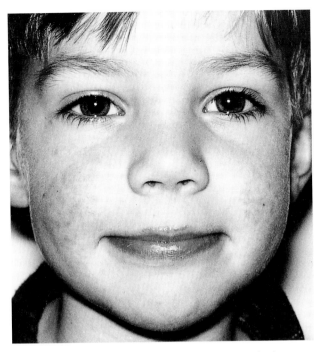

Fig. 92.16 Flushed cheeks with perioral pallor seen in scarlet fever.

bacillus. The incidence of tuberculosis is rising in developed countries because of a combination of increased migration, the spread of human immunodeficiency virus infection, and decreased commitment to disease control.[11,12] At present, HIV infection is the most potent risk factor known for tuberculosis resulting from reactivation and progression of recent infection.[13] Oral lesions of tuberculosis are usually secondary to a primary pulmonary infection. The active organism present in sputum may enter the oral mucosa through a minor abrasion or injury to produce a tuberculous ulcer. The tongue is most commonly affected followed by the buccal mucosa and the remainder of the oral cavity. The ulcer is usually painful and persists as a well-defined stellate ulcer, classically with an undermined edge; it may be mistaken for an aphthous or herpetic ulcer. Tuberculous lymphadenitis may also be present within the neck in association with pulmonary disease. Initially the nodes are separate, firm and mobile, however later they become fixed and matted. A tuberculous abscess may develop followed by sinus formation over the lower border of the mandible or occasionally on the face.

In children, tuberculous cervical lymphadenopathy is more often due to an atypical organism such as *Mycobacterium avium-intracellulare*. Investigations should include a chest X-ray and sputum samples for bacteriological examination. Blood examination often shows a raised plasma viscosity and a lymphocytosis. Surgical excision of the node is the mainstay of treatment.[14] Histopathologic examination reveals the granulomatous inflammation and the central caseating necrosis. A portion should also be sent dry to the bacteriology department for the preparation of a slide (acid- and alcohol-fast bacilli) and culture.

Lupus vulgaris is a primary tuberculous infection of the skin which often presents on the face or neck. The typical lesion is a reddish-brown nodule which is said to have an 'apple-jelly' appearance when compressed and viewed through a glass slide. The disease usually starts in adolescence and can involve the nasal septal cartilage leading to collapse and nasal deformity.

Treatment of tuberculosis requires combination chemotherapy with antituberculous drugs such as isoniazid, ethambutol and rifampicin.

Syphilis

Syphilis is a systemic disease caused by infection with the spirochete *Treponema pallidum*; it can present with features in the orofacial region during the primary, secondary or tertiary stages of the disease. The most frequent presenting group is homosexual men.

Primary syphilis

The typical lesion is a chancre which arises at the point of entry of the organism about 3 weeks following infection. The chancre is a painless ulcerated lesion with a regular bevelled edge and indurated base. The lip is the most common extragenital site and the chancre often appears at the corner of the mouth. Other, intraoral, sites include the tongue and gingivae. The lesion is infectious and heals spontaneously within a mouth. Regional lymph nodes are often enlarged.

Secondary syphilis

The second stage of syphilis occurs about 6 weeks later with a macular or papular skin rash, generalized lymphadenopathy, fever, headache and malaise. The oral manifestations are mucous patches appearing as slightly raised grayish-white patches on the mucosa of the cheek, tongue or soft palate which may coalesce to form 'snail-track' ulcers. These lesions are also highly infectious. Cervical lymph nodes are frequently enlarged and are rubbery in consistency.

Tertiary syphilis

The disease may enter a latent phase and later become active as the third stage of syphilis. Reactivation occurs usually between 5 and 10 years after the initial infection. The characteristic lesion is the gumma which can develop in the skin, mucous membranes or bone. The usual site within the mouth for gummatous formation is the hard palate although the soft palate, lips and tongue can also be affected. The lesion begins as a small pale nodule which ulcerates and rapidly enlarges creating a large area of necrosis. The palatal lesion usually occurs in the midline and can perforate the palate through to the nose. The gumma is painless and is not particularly infectious. Syphilitic glossitis is also a feature of the tertiary stage and is often associated with areas of leukoplakia which are premalignant. Neurosyphilis with general paralysis of the insane is a feature of late syphilis.

Congenital syphilis

Infection of the fetus in utero produces congenital syphilis; the patient may present within the first few months of life as a snuffly child with weight loss, a generalized macular rash and the presence of linear scars or rhagades at the corners of the mouth. Hypoplasia of the permanent teeth may occur, most commonly affecting the maxillary central incisors: these so-called 'Hutchinson's incisors' are peg-shaped with a notch on the incisal edge. The first molars may also be affected, with rounded ill-formed cusps described as 'mulberry' molars. In early adolescence, gummatous destruction of the nasal complex may occur resulting in a saddle nose deformity.

Diagnosis of syphilis requires serological confirmation including the venereal disease research laboratory (VDRL) test and the *Treponema pallidum* hemagglutination assay (TPHA).

The most effective drug for treatment is penicillin.

Actinomycosis

Actinomycosis may occur in the abdomen or lung, but the most common site is within the cervicofacial region. The infecting organism is *Actinomyces israelii*, a common inhabitant of the mouth, and the etiology is thought to involve a degree of trauma to the jaws such as a tooth extraction or a fracture of the mandible, thereby providing a route of access for the organism. Ingress of the organism may also occur through an exposed necrotic tooth pulp with subsequent access to the periapical area. It is not clear why the infection is therefore so uncommon and undoubtedly other factors are also involved. Acute actinomycosis can be clinically indistinguishable from an acute dento-alveolar abscess. Drainage of pus may reveal the presence of 'sulfur granules' which can be quite soft. Chronic infection is characterized by the development of multiple discharging sinuses surrounded by areas of brawny induration, and the sulfur granules, if detected, have more of a gritty con-

sistency. The most common site is the submandibular region although other sites such as the maxillary sinuses, salivary glands and the masseter muscle have been described.[15] The most common form of presentation is an acute painful swelling associated with soft-tissue abscess secondary to a dental infection.[16] A sample of pus should be collected by needle aspiration if possible to reduce the chance of contamination and also collected within a dry container if external drainage is performed. The microbiologist should be informed of the possibility of actinomycosis as specific requirements and prolonged culture are necessary.

Treatment of an acute infection requires incision and drainage and eradication of any suspected etiologic focus such as an infected tooth. Antibiosis with penicillin is continued for 3 weeks. Chronic infection requires a similar approach except that the antibiotics are continued for longer – up to 6 weeks. Erythromycin or clindamycin are satisfactory alternatives.

Cat scratch disease

This is a common cause of cervical lymphadenopathy in children; it has a widespread geographic distribution as the disease is spread by the domestic cat.[17] The head and neck regions are frequently affected. The causative organism is probably a Gram-positive bacterium and the organism *Rothia dentocarisoa* is present in up to 66% of cases. The infection presents as a primary skin lesion at the site of the cat scratch or bite with regional lymphadenopathy. The nonpruritic erythematous skin papule appears 3–7 days after the injury and persists for up to 3 weeks. Regional lymphadenopathy occurs approximately 1 week after the appearance of the skin papule. Diagnosis is based on the history and clinical findings and occasionally histologic examination of an excised lymph node. Treatment is symptomatic with occasional aspiration of necrotic lymph nodes. Antibiotics are not of any value.

VIRAL INFECTIONS

Herpes simplex

Primary herpetic gingivostomatitis is caused by a herpes virus type 1 infection. Primary infection arising in childhood is usually subclinical or mild whereas the primary infection in adults is more severe. The virus is transmitted by direct contact with infected lesions or from saliva which may remain infectious for several months. The clinical features include fever, lymphadenopathy and painful mouth and throat followed by the appearance of multiple vesicles throughout the oral mucosa and lips. The vesicles rupture

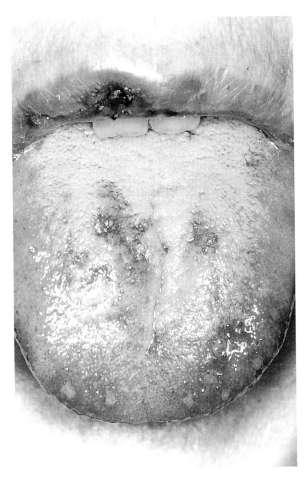

Fig. 92.17 Primary infection with herpes virus type 1 showing vesiculation and ulceration of lips and tongue.

to form painful ulcers with yellowish-gray bases and a surrounding erythema (Fig. 92.17). The infection is self-limiting and the lesions resolve in about 10 days. More severe cases should be treated with oral and topical acyclovir; supportive treatment includes adequate hydration, analgesia and chlorhexidine mouthbaths.

Secondary herpetic infection may occur in about 30% of patients due to later reactivation of the latent virus. The virus remains dormant in the trigeminal ganglion until it is reactivated by a stimulus such as exposure to sunlight, recent dental treatment or febrile illness. The secondary lesion or 'cold sore' commonly develops on the lips although the perioral skin and nasal mucosa can also be affected. Prodromal symptoms of prickling or burning of the lip are quickly followed by the vesicular stage and subsequent ulceration and crust formation. The lesion heals within 10–14 days without scarring.

Herpes zoster

Primary infection with the varicella zoster virus causes chickenpox; reactivation in later life presents as shingles, which is an eruption of vesicles on an erythematous base arising within a skin dermatome supplied by the sensory ganglion within which the virus lay dormant. The trigeminal nerve is involved in about 15% of cases and the ophthalmic, maxillary and mandibular divisions are involved in that order of precedence. Pain and paresthesia within the sensory nerve distribution precedes the rash for several days. The lesions are infectious and a susceptible host can acquire chickenpox from transmission of the varicella zoster virus. Lesions may also be found in the mouth as well as the skin when either the maxillary or mandibular division are affected. Reactivation within the geniculate ganglion results in the Ramsay Hunt syndrome with ipsilateral facial paralysis, vesicular eruption on the ear, and ipsilateral combined loss of taste and tearing of the eye. An unpleasant sequela is the development of a post-herpetic neuralgia within the site of the previous eruption which may remain for many months.

Infectious mononucleosis (glandular fever)

This acute infection of children and young adults is caused by the Epstein–Barr virus. The majority of patients affected are between 15 and 25 years of age and the virus is transmitted directly via oropharyngeal secretions by kissing. The disease is characterized by sore throat, pharyngeal inflammation, fever and lymph-node enlargement due to lymphoid hyperplasia. During the course of the infection an exudative membrane may develop within the mouth and pharynx, especially on the tonsils. Occasionally the disease may be misdiagnosed as an acute pericoronitis. Hematological investigations may show a lymphocytosis and atypical mononuclear cells, a rapid serological diagnosis is possible with the Monospot test or Paul–Bunnell test which demonstrate a rising antibody titer.

Hand, foot and mouth disease

This common infection is caused by the Coxsackie A virus (predominantly A16), an enterovirus. Children are most often affected and the diagnosis is straightforward due to the nature of the distribution of the signs. The oral lesions begin as bright red macules up to 5 mm in diameter which form small vesicles with a surrounding erythematous ring. The vesicles quickly rupture and are not commonly seen, however the resulting ulcers persist for up to about a week. Similar lesions develop on the palms of the hands and soles of the feet, and in young children lesions may also appear on the buttocks. The oral mucosal and skin lesions are accompanied by mild headache, sore throat and malaise. If necessary the virus can be isolated from saliva, vesicular fluid or the feces.

Herpangina

This infection is also due to the Coxsackie virus (A2, A4, A5) and again is more common in children. Acute onset of fever and sore throat is followed by the appearance of multiple pinhead-sized vesicles surrounded by a red areola. The lesions predominate at the back of the mouth over the soft palate and pharynx. The infection lasts for 3–5 days and the lesions heal without scarring. Occasionally the systemic upset can be quite severe and require hospitalization. The oral lesions do not usually affect the gingivae or buccal mucosa which helps to differentiate this infection from herpetic gingivostomatitis. Virus samples for culture can be collected from vesicular fluid, by swabbing an ulcer, or from a stool sample.

Measles

Measles is a highly infectious disease which occurs in small epidemics every 2–3 years. Transmission is by droplet spread; patients are infectious during the prodromal phase and remain so for about two days following the appearance of the rash. The initial *catarrhal* stage is similar to a common cold with conjunctivitis and photophobia. The buccal mucosa is erythematous and on the second day of the illness small white pinpoint spots surrounded by red areolae appear, usually opposite the molar teeth – Koplik's spots. These oral lesions remain for only a day or so. The skin lesions appear on the third or fourth day as a discrete macular rash during the *exanthematous* stage. The rash first appears on the back of the ears and at the junction of the forehead and the hair. Within hours the rash has spread to the rest of the skin and the spots fuse to form the blotchy appearance typical of measles. After 2–3 days the rash fades to a light brown color and then disappears. The illness is accompanied by fever and malaise.

Orf (ecthyma contagiosum)

This viral skin infection is contracted from the saliva of infected sheep and goats, especially young lambs. The lesions frequently occur on the hands, arms, or face and neck. The lesion commences as a raised painless papule which increases in size up to 1–3 cm in diameter and is covered with small vesicles which rupture and crust over. The lesion heals without scarring in about 6–8 weeks.

Papilloma

Viral warts occasionally occur in the mouth, particularly on the tongue and occasionally the gingiva. They are caused by the same papilloma virus which causes the more common skin wart.

FUNGAL INFECTIONS

Candidiasis

Fungal infection of the mouth with *Candida albicans* is very common. This fungus is a normal commensal organism of the mouth in about 40% of humans and causes clinical infection when local or systemic factors promote the growth of the fungus. It is therefore an opportunistic infection and the predisposing factors include age (the young and the old), antibiotic therapy, corticosteroids, dentures, anemias, dry mouth and immunosuppresion (leukemia, chemotherapy and HIV infection). While candidal infection is usually confined to the mucosa, the organism can disseminate in the immunocompromised to produce a fungemia and septic shock and may be rapidly fatal.

Acute pseudomembranous candidiasis (thrush)

This is an infection which occurs most frequently in the young, particularly neonates, and the elderly due to immature or impaired immune responses. Thrush may also occur in fit adults following a course of antibiotics. The infection appears within the mouth as a creamy-white pseudomembrane covering most of the mouth and pharynx. The membrane is easily wiped off leaving a red, raw area. Symptoms are often mild, however the patient may complain of sore mouth and throat. A swab of the lesions can be taken for culture and a scraping of the membrane can be prepared on a slide to demonstrate the fungal hyphae. The infection may also involve other mucosal sites such as the vagina. Treatment is with an antifungal agent such as nystatin, amphotericin B, or an imidazole such as miconazole.

Acute atrophic candidiasis

This form of candidiasis generally affects the tongue which becomes depapillated and sore. Other areas of the mouth such as the palate and cheeks may also be affected. This candidal infection occurs in response to prolonged steroid therapy such as steroid inhalers or following broad spectrum antibiotics. Small areas of white pseudomembrane may be located. Treatment requires elimination of the predisposing drug or long-term treatment with antifungals.

Chronic atrophic candidiasis (denture associated stomatitis)

This is the most common form of candidiasis. It is always associated with an upper denture and the mucosal inflammation is restricted to the denture bearing site. Most affected patients admit to wearing the denture throughout the day and the night. The condition is asymptomatic although long-term infection leads to the development of hyperplastic nodules which may be noticed by the patient. The condition is usually accompanied by candidal infection at the corners of the mouth – angular cheilitis. Occasionally, an underlying systemic disease may be present such as diabetes, iron deficiency anemia, or xerostomia. Treatment is dependent on denture hygiene instruction, leaving the denture out at night, and topical antifungal medication such as amphotericin lozenges or nystatin pastilles and miconazole gel applied to the palate, denture and the corners of the mouth.

Chronic hyperplastic candidiasis

Persistent candidal infection within the mouth can lead to the development of areas of leukoplakia, often within the cheeks or on the tongue. The lesions have a firm white surface which can not be readily wiped off. Many such patients are smokers and the leukoplakia is often stained brown. These lesions are recognized as premalignant and biopsy is indicated. A speckled appearance due to adjacent white and red areas – speckled leukoplakia – has a higher malignant potential. Some of these lesions resolve with long-term antifungal therapy.

Histoplasmosis

This infection, which is endemic in the United States, is caused by the yeast *Histoplasma capsulatum*. The primary infection is usually pulmonary, however oral lesions can occur with the formation of indurated ulcers.

Other rare systemic fungal infections such as South American blastomycosis, coccidioidomycosis and cryptococcosis can involve the mouth with ulceration in addition to other systemic features.

INFECTIONS OF THE JAWS

Local osteitis

This painful infection is an occasional complication following tooth extraction. It may occur when the blood clot is lost from the extraction site; anaerobic bacteria in particular may cause this by their fibrinolytic activity. The lower molar region is the most frequent site. The 'dry socket' is acutely painful and tender and the patient may also complain of a bad taste. Regional lymphadenopathy may

also be present. The condition responds well to local measures such as irrigation, sedative wound dressing, and antibiotic treatment especially with metronidazole.

Suppurative osteomyelitis

This acute or chronic infection of the medullary cavity of the jaws, more often the mandible, is a rare infection since the introduction of aseptic technique and antibiotics. Osteomyelitis presenting in developed countries is usually associated with an underlying predisposing condition such as diabetes, alcoholism,[18] immunosuppresion and local radiotherapy, but the disease remains relatively common in underdeveloped countries such as Nigeria.[19] Although the infection begins in the medullary cavity, the cortical bone and periosteum are involved in the later stages. Previously, many reports have commented on the importance of *Staphylococcus aureus* as the causative organism, however it is now widely accepted that anaerobic bacteria such as *Bacteroides* species and anaerobic streptococci are more often implicated. The source is usually a dentoalveolar infection although occasionally cases of true hematogenous spread occur. Other organisms are occasionally implicated such as *Klebsiella*, *Proteus* species, and *Pseudomonas aeruginosa*.

Early clinical features include severe constant pain, usually in the mandible, associated with mild fever and possible altered sensation within the distribution of the inferior alveolar nerve. Later features include swelling, sinus formation, tooth mobility, trismus and pathologic fracture. Pyrexia is often marked, along with regional lymphadenopathy. Areas of bone necrosis occur which separate from the remaining viable bone to form a bony sequestrum. If the infection becomes chronic then attempts at bony healing may occur with new bone – termed an involucrum – surrounding the dead bone.

Radiographic examination may show no abnormalities in the early stage except for perhaps a carious tooth or periapical infection. Later on, the gradual resorption of the mandible gives rise to a 'moth-eaten' appearance. A subperiosteal bone reaction may also be seen.

If at all possible, a sample of pus should be collected aseptically before commencing antibiotic treatment although this should not be delayed as early treatment with antibiotics can cure an acute osteomyelitis. A combination of benzylpenicillin and metronidazole is a suitable choice. Flucloxacillin should be included if *Staphylococcus aureus* is isolated. Clindamycin is a suitable alternative to penicillin when hypersensitivity is reported. Antibiotic therapy should be continued for a period of 2 weeks following clinical resolution of the infection. Any presumed focus of infection such as a dead tooth should be removed and drainage of contained pus achieved. Once the acute infection is under control, any bony sequestra which have not separated spontaneously should be removed. Following complete resolution of the infection, reconstruction of significant bony defects may be required and the transfer of vascularized bone with microvascular anastomosis is preferable. While acute or chronic suppurative osteomyelitis is usually due to a mixed infection of nonspecific bacteria, occasionally osteomyelitis can be due to other single organisms such as *Actinomyces israelii* and *Mycobacterium tuberculosis*.

Suppurative arthritis of the temporomandibular joint

Acute bacterial infection of the temporomandibular joint is uncommon, however cases have arisen following a penetrating wound or direct extension into the joint from a neighboring infection in the middle ear cavity, mastoid cavity or parotid gland. The most frequently implicated organisms are *Staphylococcus aureus*, *Neisseria gonorrhoeae* and streptococci, accounting for up to 95% of all cases. *Haemophilus influenzae* is also important, especially in children, who account for the greatest proportion of cases.[20] The affected acutely painful joint shows signs of acute inflammation and the joint space may be widened on plain films or CT scan. Aspiration of pus from the joint space confirms the diagnosis. Treatment consists of intravenous benzylpenicillin and flucloxacillin; surgery is directed toward the source of the infection such as the middle ear which requires treatment by the ENT surgeon. Aspiration and lavage of the infected joint is useful and may obviate the need for open surgical drainage.

INFECTIONS OF THE PARANASAL SINUSES

Viral, bacterial and fungal infections of the paranasal sinuses may occur. In essence, acute bacterial maxillary sinusitis is the most common, followed by chronic bacterial sinusitis and fungal infections.

Acute maxillary sinusitis

The usual infecting organisms are *Haemophilus influenzae*, streptococci, pneumococci and staphylococci. The infection is usually mixed and often also includes anaerobic organisms such as anaerobic streptococci. Acute bacterial sinusitis may complicate acute viral rhinitis because of middle meatal obstruction and stagnation of mucous secretions which become secondarily bacterially infected. Recurrent acute maxillary sinusitis should indicate the possibility of an underlying source such as an adjacent dento-alveolar infection arising from the maxillary premolar or molar teeth. Symptoms usually include acute throbbing pain within the cheek which is worse on bending forwards or lying down. Edematous inflammatory swelling may be noticed over the cheek, and the anterior maxillary wall may be tender on palpation. The maxillary teeth are often tender to percussion on the affected side and occasionally sensation of the infra-orbital nerve may be impaired. Radiographic examination with an occipitomental film may reveal diffuse radiopacity of the affected sinus (Fig. 92.18). The majority of cases will quickly settle with a broad spectrum antibiotic such as amoxycillin or augmentin. Any associated dental infection should be treated once the acute infection has subsided.

Chronic maxillary sinusitis

Chronic bacterial infection of the sinus is uncommon since the widespread use of antibiotics and the reduction in environmental pollution in towns and cities. Patients presenting with chronic sinusitis may have an underlying abnormality such as a primary ciliary dyskinesia, immune deficiency or cystic fibrosis.[21] Primary ciliary dyskinesia

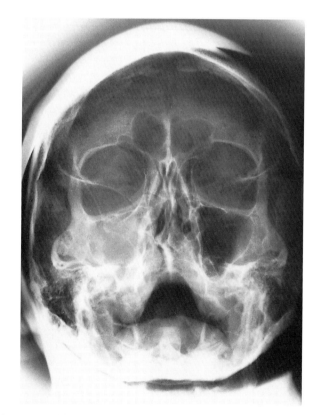

Fig. 92.18 Diffuse radiopacity of right maxillary antrum in acute suppurative maxillary sinusitis.

occurs in Kartagener's syndrome which consists of bronchiectasis, sinusitis and situs inversus. Chronic sinusitis is frequently associated with antral and nasal polyps although the bacterial infection is generally thought to be secondary.[22] Again, a dental focus of infection should be excluded as this is a frequent finding. A careful search should also be made for a possible previously unrecognized oro-antral fistula following a previous tooth extraction. Plain radiographic films have a limited role except to search for periapical or other dental infection (Fig. 92.19); CT or MRI is more useful to show the extent of the disease, air–fluid levels, soft-tissue masses and possible bone erosion. Up to 40% of all CT and MRI scans of the head have been reported as showing coincidental disease in the paranasal sinuses.[23] Conventional surgical treatment consists of antral washout and intranasal antrostomy and occasionally Caldwell–Luc antrostomy and removal of the infected sinus lining. In recent years, a more conservative approach to sinus surgery has been promoted with the advent of functional endoscopic sinus surgery.[24]

Fungal sinusitis

Chronic fungal sinusitis may arise spontaneously in other-

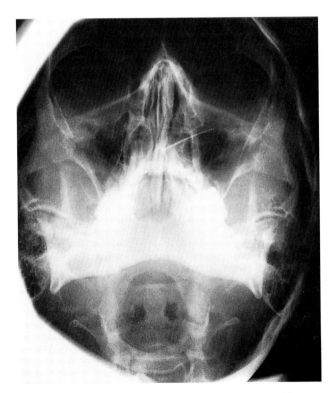

Fig. 92.19 Occipitomental radiograph of patient presenting with symptoms of chronic maxillary sinusitis due to a displaced gutta percha point lost during molar endodontics. The GP point is seen lying within the left maxillary antrum and at antrostomy was located within the ostium of the sinus.

wise healthy patients. The two most common fungi involved are aspergillus and mucosporidium. The saprophytic mould *Aspergillus fumigatus* is the most common fungal pathogen of the paranasal sinuses. It is thought that the spores may be inhaled directly from the air into the antrum, where they propagate in the anaerobic conditions. The infection may take the form of a localized ball of fungus (mycetoma) or a diffuse infiltrative/invasive form. Although the majority of patients affected are fit and healthy, a careful search should be made for an underlying systemic disease causing immunosuppression[25] such as diabetes, leukemia or HIV infection. A link between chronic aspergillus sinusitis and zinc-containing endodontic obturating pastes[26] has also been postulated. The condition presents as a unilateral chronic sinusitis with occasional pain, nasal obstruction and rhinorrhea. Late features may include ocular or neurologic signs. The clinical picture can therefore be similar to that of malignant disease.[25] The radiographic features include a unilateral homogenous opacification of the sinus with foci of increased radiodensity. CT scan examination is more sensitive and may detect areas of increased radiodensity from the concretions present within a mycetoma. CT is also more likely to visualize any bony destruction, indicating the infiltrative/aggressive form of the disease. A fulminant form of the disease is recognized in immunocompromised patients; this is rapidly progressive and leads to bony destruction, dissemination of the disease to the brain and lungs, and often death if not treated promptly.[27] Treatment consists of surgical debridement of the sinus, antifungal drugs being reserved for the invasive or fulminant form of the disease. A Caldwell–Luc approach to the maxillary sinus with removal of the mycetoma and a draining intranasal antrostomy is the surgical procedure of choice.

INFECTIONS OF THE SALIVARY GLANDS

Viral and bacterial infections of the salivary glands are common. The parotid gland is most frequently affected by infection, followed by the submandibular salivary gland. Infection arising within the sublingual gland or minor salivary glands is virtually never seen.

Mumps (endemic parotitis)

The most frequently encountered infection of the salivary glands is mumps, caused by a paramyxovirus. It generally occurs in childhood and is more common in winter and spring. Transmission of the virus is by droplet spread or directly from saliva. A prodromal period of pyrexia and sore throat is followed by painful swelling of the parotid glands, frequently bilateral, occasionally unilateral or sequential. An early sign which may be seen is inflammation with localized swelling of the parotid duct opening. The parotid gland swelling can be quite marked and the submandibular glands can also become enlarged. The infection runs a course of about 10 days with subsequent complete recovery of the patient and salivary function. Complications may occur from involvement of other tissues such as meningoencephalitis (30%) or orchitis (25%) in males which are more common following infection in adults. The white cell count is raised with a differential profile of a lymphocytosis. The diagnosis can be confirmed serologically by demonstrating the rising titer of IgM antibodies to the mumps virus antigen.

Other viruses such as cytomegalovirus (salivary gland inclusion disease), parainfluenza, echo and Coxsackie are occasionally implicated in a non-suppurative sialadenitis.

Acute suppurative sialadenitis

This acute infection most commonly arises in the parotid gland; acute infection does occur in the submandibular gland but is usually associated with a predisposing obstruction such as a sialolith. Acute suppurative parotitis was a frequently seen complication in postoperative patients in the past. Nowadays it is less common due to better preparation of patients for surgery, improved fluid balance and prophylactic antibiotics. The infection is still occasionally seen in surgical wards postoperatively and in debilitated patients with dehydration or Sjögren's syndrome. The widespread use of diuretics in the elderly also facilitates infection which ascends from the mouth into the parotid duct. Common isolates of bacteria include α-hemolytic streptococci and *Staphylococcus aureus*. Organisms less commonly implicated are *Haemophilus* species, *Bacteroides* species and anaerobic streptococci.

The acute infection is usually unilateral and occasionally bilateral. The patient may present with a high fever, rigors and leukocytosis though occasionally no systemic upset may be apparent. The parotid gland is tense, swollen and tender and pus may be seen at the parotid duct, especially on 'milking' the gland. A large number of bacterial organisms may be involved, so a sample of pus should be collected wherever possible on a swab at the duct orifice or by percutaneous needle aspiration prior to commencing antibiotic therapy. When there is doubt about the diagnosis ultrasound examination of the area can be useful to confirm the parotid swelling and possibly localize collections of pus.

Treatment consists of ensuring adequate hydration of the patient and combination intravenous antibiotics of benzylpenicillin and flucloxacillin or augmentin. Clindamycin

is a suitable alternative to penicillin, however the antibiotic regime should be reviewed following satisfactory bacteriological culture and guidance obtained from the microbiologist. Needle aspiration of pus also helps to relieve pain by decompressing the tight parotid capsule. Open surgical drainage may be required for abscesses which have spread into the superficial facial space or which reaccumulate after needle aspiration. Drainage should also be considered in patients who show no signs of improvement after 24–48 hours and the antibiotic regime should be reviewed. The incision should be sited in a skin crease below and behind the angle of the mandible followed by blunt dissection with sinus forceps into the superficial parotid region. Drainage should be continued with the insertion of a Yates drain.

Chronic obstructive sialadenitis

Chronic infection of the salivary glands is always associated with an underlying cause such as obstruction (calculi, mucous plug, tumor, stricture) or persistently reduced salivary flow (diuretics, Sjögren's syndrome, irradiation). The infection is usually low-grade with no systemic features. The submandibular gland is more frequently affected because of the higher incidence of calculi within the gland, however strictures, Sjögren's syndrome, tumor and radiotherapy frequently involve the parotid gland. Occasionally, calculi may also form within the parotid ductal system.

The underlying cause can often be diagnosed following investigation with sialography and CT scan. Patients with chronic obstruction due to stricture or mucous plugs often describe an improvement in symptoms or indeed complete resolution after sialography, which in these instances is therapeutic. Definitive treatment is dependent on the general condition of the patient, the location and severity of the symptoms, and the cause of the obstruction; it may include dilatation of stricture, removal of calculus, occasional salivary stimulants, or excision of the affected gland.

Uncommon bacterial infections of the salivary glands include tuberculosis, actinomycosis, syphilis and infection with *Neisseria gonorrhoeae*.

Recurrent parotitis of childhood

This recurrent infection of the parotid gland occurs in children usually over the age of 3 months, presenting with a history of recurrent episodes of pain and swelling within the gland. Both glands can be affected although not usually at the same time. Signs of systemic toxicity are infrequent and lymphadenopathy is not significant. The infecting organism is often *Streptococcus viridans* or *Staphylococcus aureus*. Occasionally a Gram-negative bacillus may be isolated such as *Escherichia coli*. Individual episodes can be treated with a broad spectrum antibiotic; surgical intervention is rarely necessary as the condition tends to remit completely during puberty.

OROFACIAL INFECTIONS IN IMMUNOCOMPROMISED HOSTS

The number of immunocompromised patients is rapidly increasing with advances in transplant surgery, chemotherapy and, especially, HIV infection. These patients have an increased susceptibility to infection as a result of the impaired immune response; any of the infections mentioned so far may affect such a host, and other atypical infections may also arise. These latter infections may be fungal, viral or bacterial, and the presence of an unusual 'atypical' organism or an uncharacteristically severe infection or poor response to treatment should raise the possibility of an underlying immunodeficiency.

Patients with AIDS frequently present with orofacial manifestations of infection and occasionally they may be the only presenting signs.

Fungal infections

Oral candidiasis (thrush) is present in about 75% of AIDS patients. The development of oral thrush during HIV infection is an indicator of transformation from AIDS-related complex (ARC) to full-blown AIDS. The infection usually persists for months and only temporarily responds to antifungal treatment. An atrophic variety of candidiasis may also occur, particularly on the palate and dorsum of the tongue. Chronic hyperplastic candidiasis and candidal-associated angular cheilitis are also commonly present. The candidal infection may disseminate to produce a candidal fungemia and septic shock. While *Candida albicans* accounts for over 85% of candidal infections in HIV patients, other candidal species such as *C. kruseii* and *C. tropicalis* are occasionally responsible.

Aspergillus infection may commonly infect the paranasal sinuses with occasional destruction of the bony walls and extension of the disease. Other occasional fungal pathogens include mucor, fusarium, cryptococcus and histoplasmosis.

Viral infections

Severe and persistent infections caused by the herpes group of virusus are common in ARC and AIDS due to the reduced activity of the T-cell lymphocyte population. Herpes simplex infection can occasionally disseminate; the infection frequently responds to acyclovir, but further relapses are common with herpetic ulcers appearing in the mouth and sometimes on the face. The ulcers frequently become secondarily infected with bacteria. Orofacial shingles (herpes zoster) presenting in a young adult should also raise suspicion of possible immunodeficiency as should local infection with cytomegalovirus (CMV) causing chronic oral ulceration or infection within the salivary glands. Lesions caused by the papilloma virus, such as papillomatous warts within or around the mouth, are commonly seen in HIV infected patients as are verruca vulgaris and condylomata accuminata. Hairy leukoplakia is a distinct clinical entity described in HIV infected patients (Fig. 92.20). It is particularly characteristic in HIV infected homosexual men and is strongly associated with full-blown AIDS. The appearance is of raised white striated patches on the lateral borders of the tongue; the dorsum of the tongue can also be affected. Initially, hairy leukoplakia was thought to be pathognomonic of HIV infection, however it is now clear that similar lesions can be seen in patients with other causes of severe immunocompromise.[28] The lesion is thought to be virally induced and at present it is thought that Epstein–Barr virus is the likely cause. Candidal infection is commonly associated with the lesions, however they do not respond to antifungal therapy.

Bacterial infections

HIV-associated gingivitis and periodontitis are characterized

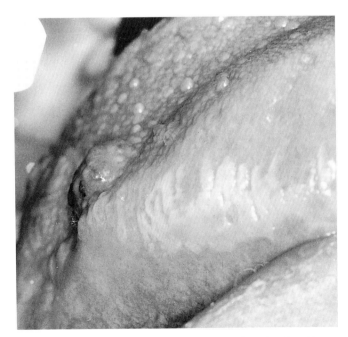

Fig. 92.20 Hairy leukoplakia of tongue in an HIV infected patient. The raised lesion seen on the lateral border of the tongue is a Kaposi sarcoma.

by their severity and aggressive nature with widespread involvement and periodontal destruction. Acute ulcerative gingivitis may also occur but differs from the usual condition in that it tends to recur and the destruction of tissue including bone is often more extensive, reminiscent of cancrum oris. Oral lesions from mycobacterial infection can arise, especially due to atypical mycobacteria such as *M. avium-intracellulare*. Cervicofacial actinomycosis may also occur in association with HIV disease.

Sinusitis is particularly common and is often severe and recurrent. A pansinusitis may be apparent and recalcitrant organisms involved such as *Pseudomonas aeruginosa*.

Orofacial infections will continue to challenge the oral and maxillofacial surgeon through the continuous development of micro-organisms and, in particular, increasing bacterial resistance to antibiotics and the development of pathogenic organisms such as methicillin-resistant *Staphylococcus aureus* (MRSA). The exponential increase in immunocompromised patients has produced an increase in the number of unusual or atypical infections which challenge the diagnostic skills of the clinician. Viral infections are also increasingly implicated in the etiology of head and neck malignancy and in the future an infective association with other common mucocutaneous diseases of the head and neck will undoubtedly be found.

REFERENCES

1. Scott JH 1952 The spread of dental infection – anatomical considerations. British Dental Journal 92:236–240
2. Lewis MA, MacFarlane TW, McGowan DA 1986a Quantitative bacteriology of acute dentoalveolar abscesses. Journal of Medical Microbiology 21:101–104
3. Smyth AG, McDowell DB, Stassen LF 1993 An in-vitro study of the comparative viability on different swab types of simulated specimens of bacteria commonly present in orofacial infections. British Journal of Oral and Maxillofacial Surgery 31:161–164
4. Iwu CO 1990 Ludwig's angina: report of seven cases and review of current concepts in management. British Journal of Oral and Maxillofacial Surgery 28:189–193
5. Nash ES, Cheng LH, Smart K 1991 Cancrum oris-like lesions. British Journal of Oral and Maxillofacial Surgery 29:51–53
6. Adekeye EO, Ord RA 1983 Cancrum oris: principles of management and reconstructive surgery. Journal of Maxillofacial Surgery 11:160–170
7. Valko PC, Barrett SM, Campbell JP 1990 Odontogenic cervicofacial necrotising fasciitis. Annals of Emergency Medicine 19:568–571
8. Steel A 1987 An unusual case of necrotising fasciitis. British Journal of Oral and Maxillofacial Surgery 25:328–333
9. Balcerak RJ, Sisto JM, Bosack RC 1988 Cervicofacial necrotising fasciitis: report of three cases and literature review. Journal of Oral and Maxillofacial Surgery 46:450–459
10. De Backer T, Bossuyt M, Schoenaers J 1997 Management of necrotising fasciitis in the neck. Journal of Cranio-maxillofacial Surgery 24:366–371.
11. Cotton MM 1996 Tuberculosis: a growing problem. British Journal of Hospital Medicine 56:193–194
12. Bagg J 1996 Tuberculosis: a re-emerging problem for health care workers. British Dental Journal 180:376–381
13. Corbett EL, De Cock KM 1996 Tuberculosis in the HIV-positive patient. British Journal of Hospital Medicine 56:200–204
14. Akhtar J, Howatson AG, Raine PA 1997 Atypical mycobacterial infection in childhood: a 'surgical disease'. Journal of the Royal College of Surgeons of Edinburgh 42:110–111
15. Barnard NA, Magennis JP 1992 Intra-masseteric actinomycosis: report of a case. British Journal of Oral and Maxillofacial Surgery 30:190–191
16. Samuels RH, Martin MV 1988 A clinical and microbiological study of actinomycetes in oral and cervicofacial lesions. British Journal of Oral and Maxillofacial Surgery 26:458–463
17. Premachandra DJ, Milton CM 1990 Cat scratch disease in the parotid gland presenting with facial paralysis. British Journal of Oral and Maxillofacial Surgery 28:413–415
18. Davies HT, Carr RJ 1990 Osteomyelitis of the mandible: a complication of routine dental extractions in alcoholics. British Journal of Oral and Maxillofacial Surgery 28:185–188
19. Adekeye EO, Cornah J 1985 Osteomyelitis of the jaws: a review of 141 cases. British Journal of Oral and Maxillofacial Surgery 23:24–35
20. Bounds GA, Hopkins R, Sugar A 1987 Septic arthritis of the temporomandibular joint – a problematic diagnosis. British Journal of Oral and Maxillofacial Surgery 25:61–67
21. MacKay I, Cole P 1987 Rhinitis, sinusitis and associated chest disease. In: MacKay I, Bull T (eds) Scott Brown's Otolaryngology, 5th edn. Vol 4. Rhinology. Butterworths, London, pp 61–92
22. Dawes P, Bates G, Watson D, Lewis D, Lowe D, Drake-Lee A 1989 The role of bacterial infection of the maxillary sinus in nasal polyps. Clinical Otolaryngology 14:447–450
23. Drake-Lee A 1996 Sinusitis. British Journal of Hospital Medicine 55:674–678
24. Swift AC 1996 Functional endoscopic sinus surgery. British Journal of Hospital Medicine 55:554–558
25. Falworth MS, Herold J 1996 Aspergillosis of the paranasal sinuses. Oral Surgery, Oral Medicine, and Oral Pathology 81:255–260
26. Theaker ED, Rushton VE, Corcoran JP, Hatton P 1995 Chronic sinusitis and zinc-containing endodontic obturating pastes. British Dental Journal 179:64–68
27. Weir N 1987 Acute and chronic inflammations of the nose. In: Mackay I, Bull T (eds) Scott Brown's Otolaryngology, 5th edn. Vol 4. Rhinology. Butterworths, London, pp 115–141
28. Porter S, Scully C 1994 HIV: the surgeon's perspective. Part 2. Diagnosis and management of non-malignant oral manifestations. British Journal of Oral and Maxillofacial Surgery 32:231–240

Oral implantology

93

M. STEPHEN DOVER

Osseointegration has had a fundamental impact on the reconstruction of oral and facial structures. This has resulted in renewed interest in all forms of implantology, with current research being directed towards utilizing the concept in joint, digit and limb replacement. Within the mouth, osseointegrated implants offer the means to predictably reconstruct the dentition, rehabilitate the patient, and improve quality of life. Many of the alternative pre-prosthetic techniques developed within the past 30 years are now obsolete.

HISTORY AND BACKGROUND

The replacement of missing teeth has long been a goal of both patients and clinicians. A Honduran skull from pre-Columbian times is cited as showing one of the first known dental implants.[1] A mandibular incisor had been replaced with a black stone; this was covered with calculus, and would therefore have been inserted during life. Between the 16th and 20th centuries, attempts at replacing the dentition with homologous teeth, gold-wire baskets, iron posts and china pegs were reported,[2] although the results invariably were not. More recently, various implant designs have been developed, all based on an increasing understanding of biocompatibility, tissue healing and functional requirements.

Schroeder recognizes four methods of oral implantation:

- transfixation or endodontic implants
- submucosal implants
- subperiosteal implants
- endosteal implants.

Transfixation involves the use of a metal pin inserted down the root of a tooth, through the apex and into the surrounding bone. The root length is increased, the root and periodontal membrane are retained, and the implant is isolated from direct contact with the mouth.

Submucosal implants provide retention by sinking into surgically created holes in the palate. The male attachment is fitted into the denture, and the mucosa acts as the female component. They are associated with underlying bone resorption, and may exacerbate bone loss in an already atrophic maxilla.

Subperiosteal implants were devised 50 years ago by Muller (1937) and Dahl (1943) (Fig. 93.1). They are designed to rest on the bone and under the periosteum, distributing masticatory forces over a wide area. These implants usually require a two-stage surgical approach. At the first operation, the subperiosteal flaps are reflected and an impression taken of the underlying bone. The implant is produced on the model cast from this impression. It is placed into the mouth at a second operation. The use of computerized tomography (CT) and computer aided design, computer aided manufacture (CAD/CAM), enables the creation of an accurate model of the jaw from CT scans.

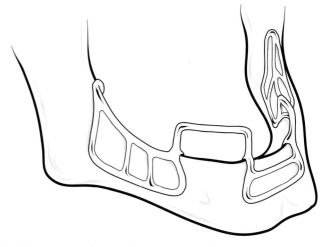

Fig. 93.1 Diagram of a mandibular subperiosteal implant.

The implant can be produced on this computer generated model, and inserted in a single surgical procedure, thereby avoiding an impression and the need for the first operation.

Subperiosteal implants are connected to the bone by fibrous tissue, although some exhibit direct bony contact in places. The transmucosal abutment posts are an integral part of the implant and are used to retain a denture.

The facility to coat the implants with hydroxyapatite, the refinement of the substructure design, and the development of accurate CAD/CAM derived models have resulted in renewed interest in this implant type in recent years. Subperiosteal implants remain of value in selected edentulous cases where narrow ridges or deep undercuts and severe angulations preclude endosteal implants.[3] They can be produced quickly and can be specifically designed to avoid anatomic structures or localized defects. Loading is possible immediately after soft-tissue healing. They may be less expensive for the patient. The denture is very stable, and can be removed by the patient to maintain oral hygiene.

Subperiosteal implants are not appropriate in the very atrophic jaw.[3]

Endosteal implants are surgically placed into bone as a means of retaining a prosthesis. This type of implant has been tried with limited success for centuries. A variety of materials have been used, including platinum–iridium, vitallium, stainless steel, aluminium hydroxide, chrome cobalt and titanium.

Until recently, few designs had been based on thorough research and development. The Swedish and Swiss groups working in the 1950s and 60s provided the foundation for the current explosion of interest in dental endosseous implants. These implants broadly fall into three groups: root form, blade form and transmandibular.

Root form implants are the most commonly used, and many companies produce a number of differing designs. The implants are either threaded for screw insertion, cylindrical for push-fit insertion, or a combination of both.

Surfaces are either smooth or roughened. The former are usually threaded to mechanically lock with the bone and achieve primary stability. Roughened implants have a pitted surface or a titanium plasma sprayed surface, both of which are secondary processes in the implant manufacture. They can be threaded but also rely on surface roughness and an implant diameter slightly larger than that of the drill to achieve primary stability. The roughened surface increases the surface area and promotes increased bone–implant surface contact once integrated.[4] These implants can therefore be produced in smaller lengths, typically 6–12 mm, and do not require bicortical engagement for reliable prosthetic reconstruction. Smooth-surfaced implants tend to be longer (up to 20 mm or so in length).

Some implants are coated with hydroxyapatite to form ionic bonds with the bone and greater bone – implant contact. They have been advocated for use in the cancellous bone of the maxilla. Some concerns have been expressed over the durability of the coating.[5]

All implants come prepackaged and most come presterilized. This avoids potential contamination prior to implant placement either by metal contamination from nontitanium instruments or by organic contamination from tissue contact. Both have been reported as interfering with healing.[6]

Recent innovations include the development of wide-bodied implants. They are available in shorter lengths and are primarily designed for use in the posterior regions where the greater surface area improves their load carrying abilities. The increased implant head diameter corresponds well to molar dimensions, and improved emergence profile esthetics can be achieved. The shorter implants can be used to avoid the inferior dental (ID) nerve or the maxillary sinus. They may also be used where primary stability of the normal diameter implants cannot be achieved and to engage more cortical bone between the buccal and lingual cortices, thereby improving primary stability and osseointegration.

Linkow's name is associated with blade implants. He introduced a design in 1966[7] designed to maximize masticatory load spreading and to accommodate the majority of anatomic variations encountered in both jaws. These and similar designs remain in use today.

Transmandibular implants require placement via an extra-oral submental approach. Endosseous threaded posts transfix the mandible and emerge into the mouth. They are secured to a baseplate that is in turn screwed to the lower border of the mandible. The intraoral parts of the posts are joined with a laboratory custom-made bar soon after surgery. This achieves a very stable box-girder type design.[8] The design of the prosthesis, with contact on the implants and retromolar regions only, is crucial. Bosker has demonstrated that this design causes tensile forces to be distributed along the upper border of the mandible, inducing bone growth in that area.[9] This has obvious advantages in the atrophic jaw. The technique also allows for a submental lipectomy and chin contouring at the same time as implant insertion. There is an immediate improvement in the soft-tissue profile of the lower face.[10] The technique has not found universal favor because of the need for an external approach and (usually) general anesthesia. However, in selected cases, particularly the mandible with the very atrophic body, this implant design has considerable value (Figs 93.2 and 93.3).

One area of difficulty with all implant types is that terminology varies between each manufacturer. Some compo-

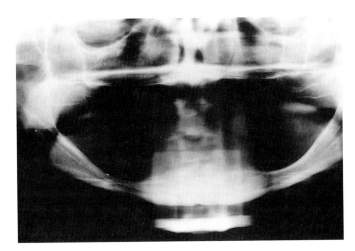

Fig. 93.2 Tomogram of an atrophic mandible.

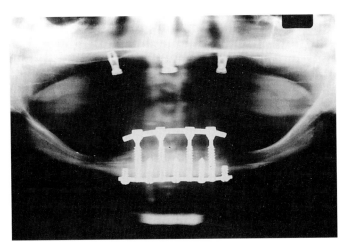

Fig. 93.3 Same case after transmandibular and Branemark implant insertion.

nents are interchangeable, but most are not, and new developments add to the range of products each system offers. Chapters such as this can only give general information. Reputable companies provide implant instruction courses and manuals to which the reader is referred for specific details. These are constantly being updated.

OSSEOINTEGRATION

The ideal tooth replacement should be surrounded by a periodontal ligament. To date, implants have been either in contact with fibrous tissue (fibrous encapsulation), or bone (osseointegration). Implants that are surrounded by fibrous tissue have an increased failure rate.[11] The most predictable long-term success rates are associated with osseointegration, defined as a direct structural and func-

tional connection between ordered living bone and the surface of a load-carrying implant.[12] This is the basis upon which most root form implants are now produced.

The concept of osseointegration is based on work undertaken by Dr Per-Ingvar Branemark in the 1950s and early 1960s. Optical chambers made out of titanium were implanted into rabbit tibias to study in vivo bone and marrow function. Once healed, these chambers could not be removed because the bone had grown directly against the titanium frames. Animal models were developed to investigate the potential of these findings.[12]

Early studies evaluated titanium splints in the reconstruction of bony defects in the canine mandible. From these results, titanium implants were developed to replace the dentition. The success and longevity of this technique, together with ongoing research and development, clinical trials, meticulous documentation and worldwide usage have resulted in Branemark fixtures being recognized as the gold standard against which other systems are compared.

Predictable osseointegration requires the gentle and minimally traumatic placement of a biocompatable implant into bone.[12] The implant should not be mobile at the time of insertion – it should exhibit primary stability.[13] A period of undisturbed healing should take place prior to loading with a prosthesis. Recent work has suggested that implants can be loaded immediately in certain situations.[14] However, preliminary results suggest that this approach may be associated with a higher failure rate.

THE IMPLANT–TISSUE INTERFACE

The precise mechanism of osseointegration remains unknown, although the physiology of bone healing with which it is intimately associated is well documented.[13,15,16]

The implant material is important. Direct bone–implant contact, i.e. osseointegration, is not restricted to titanium or titanium alloys. Aluminium oxide ceramics, tantalum, stainless steel, and cobalt and nickel based alloys have all been shown to osseointegrate.[16] However, titanium remains the material of choice. It is a reactive metal that spontaneously forms a surface oxide layer on exposure to air. This titanium oxide is inert, practically insoluble and very resistant to body fluids.[4] Titanium can be easily machined into shapes that are small enough to be placed in the jaws, and yet it is strong enough to withstand masticatory loads. Of fundamental importance is that bone predictably grows on the surface of a titanium implant.

The surgical placement of an implant into bone causes bleeding and an acute inflammatory response in the tissues immediately adjacent to the implant. A blood clot forms between the implant and the bone. This gradually organizes into an increasingly dense procallus, with mesenchymal cells differentiating into osteoblasts and fibroblasts.[15] The osteoblasts produce fibers that have the potential to calcify. The fibrocartilaginous callus that develops matures into woven bone by the third week. After 7 weeks, lamellar bone is being laid down. This is more mineralized and further stabilizes the implant. Any bone rendered nonvital by the surgery is gradually replaced by living bone.

On a molecular level, at the interface between the titanium oxide layer and the environment, water molecules are split into hydroxyl ions. Depending on where these are in relation to the adjacent titanium ions, either a basic or an acidic polarity exists. Photoelectron spectroscopy has demonstrated that amino acids having a bipolar characteristic can form a strong bond with titanium oxide. These amino acids build together to produce the proteoglycan glue that binds cells together, and would appear to form the substructure onto which bone is built.[6] The fibers produced by osteoblasts are intimately associated with this glue. A very thin layer of proteoglycan exists between the bone and the implant surface of all osseointegrated implants. In effect, the body fails to recognize the implant as a foreign body and it becomes incorporated into bone as part of the wound healing process.

The final stages of healing involve maturation of the bone at the implant interface. There is an increase in bone hardness and density that is associated with loading and functional use, and which is ongoing even a year after implant placement. This correlates with Wolff's law.[4]

The soft-tissue interface between the gingivae and the implant is equally important. It consists of both epithelium and connective tissue. A rough implant surface has been demonstrated to promote connective tissue fiber attachment.[13] However, as maintenance of good oral hygiene and avoidance of plaque accumulation is impossible on this roughened surface, endosseous implants are designed with smooth transgingival components. This facilitates mechanical plaque removal. The connective tissue fibers run parallel to the implant surface in this situation, forming a tight cuff rather than a direct attachment.[17] A peri-implant sulcus is formed and lined with nonkeratinized epithelium during soft-tissue healing. The sulcus disappears farther apically, such that the epithelial cells are in direct contact with the implant. This is analogous to the junctional tissue of the normal periodontium. As in all clinical situations epithelium does not contact bone, and a layer of connective tissue exists just above the bony ridge.[18] Where submerged, two-stage implants are used, the placement of the abutment results in epithelium growing down to the implant abutment junction. If this is at or below the bone level, some resorption occurs as connective tissue always separates the epithelium from the bone. In practice, this apparent shortcoming does not compromise long-term success.

The integrity of the soft-tissue cuff around the neck of an implant is easily disturbed. Probing to assess pocket depth is therefore not recommended.

Inflammation and excessive loading can cause bone resorption.[19,20] Where peri-implant disease develops, the sulcal epithelium desquamates, exposing the underlying connective tissue which becomes inflamed. This inflammation induces osteoclast activity and chemical mediator release from cells adjacent to the implant surface.[15] As this tissue is less well differentiated than that around teeth, progression can be more rapid. Within the bone, premature loading or overload (as can occur in occlusal trauma) cause areas of pressure concentration, osteoclastic activity and angular bone loss at the implant site. This is particularly damaging during the healing phase, when osseointegration has not fully developed, and the bone resorbs easily.

The combination of inflammation and overload is particularly harmful but, separately or together, the end is the same as osseointegration is progressively lost and the implant fails.

ANATOMICAL CONSIDERATIONS

Bone density varies throughout the jaws, and between individuals. Various classifications have been suggested.[21,22] Most trials recognize that the greater the proportion of cortical bone to cancellous bone, the better the long-term results. This is cited as one reason why mandibular implants have better success rates than maxillary implants. However, care is required in the preparation of dense bone where the risk of overheating during drilling is greatest.

The presence of adequate bone volume is a prerequisite for the successful placement and subsequent osseointegration of an implant. However, bone resorption is ongoing after tooth loss or in the presence of active periodontal disease such that function and esthetics become compromised. These patterns of bone loss are well established and have been classified.[23] It is usually those patients who are most in need of implants who have the least volume of bone into which any can be inserted.

MAXILLA

In the upper jaw, bone density is poorer, and the proximity of the nasal floor, maxillary sinuses, and the incisive foramen can all have an impact on implant placement.

Alveolar bone supports the roots of the teeth. In the

dentate upper jaw, this bone is rarely sufficient to enclose all the root surfaces. Some parts of the roots invariably lie outside the bone, either through a buccal fenestration or dehiscence or into the floor of the maxillary sinus. Tooth loss and bone resorption exaggerate this deficiency and bone stock becomes concentrated between the nasal wall and the maxillary sinus. This canine buttress, running up towards the pyriform rim, is the most predictable bone for implant placement in the upper jaw. On occasions, it is the only site available in the edentulous maxilla, as there is a relative increase in the size of the maxillary sinuses with advancing age.[24]

The tuberosity can be used for implant placement. It consists of cancellous bone but often the site is too posterior for use. Osseointegration is most suspect in this low density bone.

Buccal and vertical bone resorption narrow the arch width and increase the intermaxillary distance respectively. If the dental arches are to occupy the original form the implants have to be angled away from the sagittal plane, resulting in greater lateral load on the implants. The greater the intermaxillary distance, the greater the prosthesis: implant length ratio. These factors have to be taken into account when planning the number of implants to be used in the reconstruction. Taken together, more implants are required.

The incisive foramen comes to lie on the anterior ridge with ongoing resorption. It is most evident when the edentulous upper jaw is opposed by a dentate mandible. The prominence of the incisive nerve can interfere with implant placement in the central incisor position. However, avulsion of the nerve and bone grafting of the foramen can create a site for implant placement.[25]

In the atrophic upper jaw, maxillary ridge width and height is reduced. Additional techniques may be required such as ridge expansion, guided tissue regeneration using membranes, and bone grafting of the ridge, sinus floor, and nasal floor. These procedures and others will be discussed later.

MANDIBLE

Bone quality in the mandible is predominantly cortical, especially in the interforaminal region. The genial undercut should be taken into consideration when assessing the depth of bone available near the mandibular symphysis. The true depth is frequently less than the apparent depth. A lateral cephalogram will demonstrate this feature and allow accurate measurement of the available bone (Fig. 93.4).

The genial tubercles can lie above the level of the ridge in the very atrophic mandible (Cawood and Howell VI),[23]

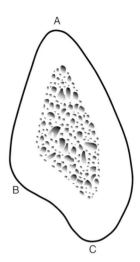

Fig. 93.4 Diagram of a cross-section of the mandibular symphysis. Real height = A–B, apparent height = A–C. Note the undercut B–C.

where they can compromise implant placement, and surgical removal of the prominences may be required.

The mylohyoid ridge creates a lingual undercut in the molar regions (Fig. 93.5). Avoidance of lingual perforation through the cortical plate is important, as hemorrhage into the floor of the mouth can have life threatening consequences.[26] In practice, this may preclude using the full height of bone available above the inferior dental nerve. Clinical assessment at the time of patient evaluation can be supplemented with CT scans, coronally reformatted to demonstrate the relevant anatomy.

The inferior dental nerve runs a variable course from the lingula to the mental foramen and influences implant placement.[27] Bicortical engagement is only possible proximal to the mental foramen, unless the implants are inserted either buccal or lingual to the nerve, or the nerve itself is

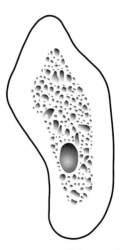

Fig. 93.5 Diagram of a cross-section of the mandibular body, second molar region. Note the mylohyoid undercut.

transposed laterally at the time of implant placement. An alternative is to use shorter implants and place them above the nerve. It is prudent to leave at least 2 mm of bone above the nerve when estimating implant length. Where possible, the use of shorter, wide-bodied implants is to be recommended, rather than risk damage to the nerve itself.

Prior to emergence from the mental foramen, the nerve loops anteriorly to a variable extent.[28] This is often apparent on a panoral tomogram. Care is required when placing an implant immediately in front of the mental foramen, so that this anterior loop is undamaged and lip sensation preserved.

In the very atrophic mandible, the mental foramen may lie on or lingual to the alveolar ridge. In this position the nerve is at risk during any crestal approach to the implant site and careful dissection in this area is required if the nerve is to remain uninjured during the reflection of a buccal subperiosteal flap.

A cuff of healthy, non-mobile, keratinized mucosa of adequate width is required around an implant neck if hygiene is to be maintained and a hyperplastic response avoided. Only the narrowest band of keratinized gingivae may remain over the crest of an atrophic ridge as soft-tissue atrophy follows bone resorption, particularly in the mandible. The surgical management of this situation is dealt with later.

TREATMENT PLANNING

Many late implant failures can be traced back to poor preoperative assessment. Time spent in the early planning and evaluation of a case pays dividends later on in the treatment. This is particularly important when more than one clinician is involved in providing care.

Assessment of the suitability of a patient for implants is based on general and local factors. Absolute contraindications to implant treatment include immunosuppression (either by disease or drug therapy) and psychiatric disorders, including those associated with abnormal perceptions of body image. patients with susceptibility to infective endocarditis or those with prosthetic joint replacements need special consideration. Discussion with the clinicians managing these conditions is appropriate. In view of the radiographs needed, it is prudent to avoid implant placement during pregnancy.

Radiotherapy to the head and neck does not preclude implant placement, but failure rates approach 50%.[29] Hyperbaric oxygen therapy, both before and after implant placement, should be used to minimize the onset of osteoradionecrosis and subsequent late implant loss.[30] Twenty dives before, and 10 dives after surgery at 2 atmospheres is recom-

mended as a minimum. This usually restricts the management of these patients to the hospital setting. Failure rates are reduced to less than 10%.[31]

Diabetes should be well controlled before any elective surgery is considered. Osteoporosis in our experience is not a problem, although longer healing times and careful loading of the implants is appropriate.[32]

Local factors of influence include the presence of poor oral hygiene, ongoing periodontal disease, caries and dental neglect. The presence of epithelial or connective tissue disease within the mouth such as erosive lichen planus, pemphigus and pemphigoid is a contraindication. In these conditions, poor wound healing and loss of soft-tissue integrity around the implant are likely to compromise the overall outcome.[32]

Smoking has a detrimental effect on implant osseointegration and long-term survival.[33–35] Patients should be warned of this during the pre operative assessment. Where it is decided to undertake the treatment, consideration should be given to over-engineering the reconstruction so that the increased risk of failure is built in to the treatment plan and sufficient implants remain to support any superstructure.

Once a patient has been screened for contraindications to implant placement it is important at the outset to establish what the patient wants. This has to be balanced against that which is clinically achievable and appropriate. Where more than one clinician is involved in the treatment it is particularly important that all parties have a clear understanding of each other's role, and a common purpose. Many medico-legal claims relating to implant cases can be traced back to errors and misunderstandings during the preoperative assessments.

A diagnostic setup is essential for most implant cases. The clinician can use it to determine the reconstructive options (fixed or removable) and the ideal sites for implant placement. The patient can assess the setup for appearance. All parties should agree on this diagnostic setup before continuing with treatment. The position of the lip line at rest and in function should be noted for esthetic purposes. In the patient with a high smile line and showing tooth and gum, achieving an acceptable appearance may be very difficult.

Skeletal and occlusal influences on treatment are dealt with in prosthodontic texts.

Once approved, the setup should be retained and duplicated in clear acrylic. Should problems later arise with the construction and appearance of the superstructure then the original setup is still available to refer back to. The clear acrylic setup can be used as an accurate template or stent, from which the implant sites and angles of insertion can be transferred from the study casts directly to the patient's mouth during the operative phase.

Where the intermaxillary distance is increased, it should be remembered that it is much easier to achieve acceptable esthetics with a removable denture than with a fixed prosthesis. This former option is cheaper and requires fewer implants. If a fixed prosthesis is used the teeth are very long unless disguised with pink porcelain, or a buccal acrylic mask or veneer is applied. Patients are less accepting of 'oil rig' type fixed prostheses in recent years, even where a low lip line hides the gap between the prosthesis and gum. These factors must be addressed at the planning stage.

The site of implant placement is determined according to superstructure design, patient requirement, and radiographic findings. All patients should have a panoral tomogram and periapical radiographs of existing teeth as a minimum. Where concerns exist about other anatomic structures or defects then computerized tomography, particularly when software-enhanced to produce 1:1 3D images, is to be recommended. Where surgical experience is limited, a CT scan can provide information that should avoid the embarrassment of abandoning a procedure after starting it.

A stent can be produced containing radiopaque markers over the proposed implant sites. This is placed in the patient's mouth prior to the scan and is also used to ensure that the scan is taken at right angles to the occlusal plane. Correct vertical distances between the ridge and underlying structures are then achieved. The resulting pictures allow an accurate assessment of the underlying ridge (Fig. 93.6).

If a patient is wearing a metal-based partial denture it should be replaced with an acrylic-only prosthesis. These are much more easily adjusted during the healing phase so as to avoid loading the implant and operative sites. They can also be used as a guide for reconstructive intentions and patient appraisal.

Implant cases can be time-consuming, difficult and expensive. Estimates should be carefully worked out to include all components, clinical time, review appointments and laboratory costs. Mistakes at this stage are costly.

Meticulous records should be kept throughout treatment and thereafter, to form the basis for prospective and retrospective analysis, appraisal of success or failure, and to support a defense against litigation. Patients should be well aware of the implications of implant treatment in terms of oral hygiene and recall appointments. Anything less than meticulous cleaning and regular attendance for review can jeopardize the long-term success of the case. The treatment plan, alternatives, possible complications and cost should be documented and signed by the patient as part of the consent for treatment before commencing any implant case.

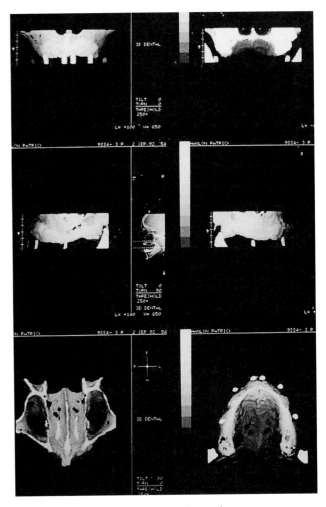

Fig. 93.6 Maxillary CT scan with diagnostic template.

SURGICAL PROCEDURE

Surgery can be undertaken under local anesthetic, with or without sedation, or general anesthetic. Local anesthetic alone can be advantageous. During implant placement, even using a template, difficult interarch and opposing tooth relationships need continuous intraoperative assessment. This is best achieved by maintaining full patient cooperation.

Antibiotics are recommended during the surgical phase. A single, 3 g dose of amoxycillin given orally one hour preoperatively (or 600 mg of clindamycin with a second dose 6 hours later) is effective. For routine implant placement, an extended antibiotic course is not necessary.

The use of a surgical template has been discussed. Where possible it should be self-retaining in the mouth and allow visualization of the operative site from all angles. There should be no interference with the flow of irrigation to the operative site during drilling. Various designs have been

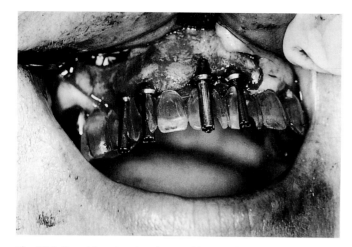

Fig. 93.7 Buccal face template in use with ITI implants.

advocated; the buccal face template is shown in use in Figure 93.7.

The essence of implant surgery is a precise surgical technique with minimal soft and hard-tissue trauma. The careful manipulation of the bone during preparation of the implant site is crucial to long-term success. The use of an incision in the buccal sulcus, thereby avoiding wound closure over an implant site, has been superseded by the incision over or close to the crest of the ridge. Exposure of the implant sites is improved, soft-tissue dissection is reduced, and osseointegration is not compromised.[36]

The incision line is planned using the surgical template. This is placed in the mouth, and at the planned implant site, a hole is drilled through the mucosa into the underlying bone. The holes can then be joined up as a crestal incision. Where esthetics are important, especially in the anterior maxilla, a more palatal approach is recommended. This results in a longer buccal flap which can be contoured to give the best possible soft-tissue appearance during the reconstructive phase. It is particularly useful where a high lip line may reveal the junction between the crown, implant and gum.

Flaps are raised in the subperiosteal plane and any relieving incisions placed remote from the implant site. Flap reflection is undertaken only to allow adequate access and assessment of the bony architecture. Any concavities that may result in fenestration or dehiscence of the implant body are noted. Where possible the implant should be inserted at an angle that will place it entirely within bone. However, this should not compromise abutment position, emergence profile, or construction of the prosthesis. The alternatives of choosing another implant site, or considering the use of guided tissue regeneration or bone grafting are dependent on local factors, the type of reconstruction planned and the experience of the surgeon.

In an edentulous mouth, the stent must be accurately positioned so that the centerline line is correct. It can be secured in place with a 2 mm miniscrew into the palatal vault or mandibular symphysis. Freehand placement is acceptable if implant position is not crucial. A long drill, inserted in the midline of the jaw at the correct angulation, can also be useful as a guide to implant alignment. However, even in these circumstances, a template ensures parallel implant placement.

Irrespective of the implant system used, a series of drills is used to enlarge and deepen the implant site. Continuous irrigation and cooling of the burs is essential if overheating of the bone is to be avoided.[37] The use of chilled, normal saline as the irrigant is recommended. It is relatively easy to exceed the 47°C temperature that causes bone necrosis, particularly when drilling in dense bone at increasing depths. Sharp drills are essential and single use instruments are therefore preferred. An intermittent drilling technique clears the cutting end of the drill of bone debris, allows the irrigant to reach the depth of the hole, and promotes heat dissipation.[38] Internally irrigated burs have an advantage in this respect.

The depth of implant placement is predetermined during the planning stages and can be checked at the time of surgery with the depth gauges supplied with each implant system. Assessment of the local anatomy at the time of surgery may result in modification of the depth. Where a CT scan has been used, implant width can also be predetermined. Ridge mapping is advocated by some authors, but in practice, whether using probes or ridge calipers, it is at best inaccurate and at worst misleading. CT scans, direct exposure of the ridge, and sufficient surgical experience to deal with unforeseen eventualities are the best solutions. Intraoperative radiographs are taken if there are any concerns about adjacent anatomic structures such as the inferior dental nerve or maxillary sinus.

Once prepared to the correct length, the implant site can be irrigated to clear any remaining debris. Where a screw implant is to be used, a thread is tapped into the bone if it is too dense for a self-tapping implant. Pushfit implants do not require tapping, and in less dense bone, implants can be used as a self-tapping instrument. In some circumstances, only the cortical plate may require tapping, thereby allowing easier insertion of the threaded implant with reduced local trauma.

Whether to bury or expose the implants during the healing phase is a matter of great debate. The validity of the ITI system and the transmucosal approach is well documented.[39] Many systems that previously adopted a submerged healing period with secondary exposure after osseointegration are increasingly being assessed using the transgingival technique. This technique does not adversely affect osseo-integration and confers some advantages,[40] namely:

- single operative procedure
- continuous implant assessment during the healing period
- soft-tissue maturation equal to that of the bone
- easier placement of the abutments under direct vision (although with progressively deeper implant placement for esthetics, this is less valid)
- the junction between the implant and abutment may be above the soft tissues
- better leverage conditions exist where the abutment–implant junction is closer to the crown.

After implant insertion, the wounds are closed meticulously with a nonirritant suture material that will remain clean within the mouth. The use of silk or catgut is not recommended as they encourage debris to collect around them and detrimental local inflammatory reactions can result.

The avoidance of direct pressure over the implant site during the healing period is important. This is best achieved with tooth-supported bridges or dentures that remain completely free of the underlying soft tissue and implants. Where practical, dentures that rest on the soft tissues or implants during the healing phase should not be worn. This is not always possible, and any prosthesis that is borne by the soft tissues must be well relieved over the operative site.

Written instructions to eat a soft diet, to leave the denture out whenever possible, and to return immediately if there is any suggestion of it touching the mucosa or the implant should be verbally emphasized. This is especially important if a metal denture is still used: direct loading of the implants will interfere with osseointegration and rapidly result in implant loss.

Healing time varies between 3 and 6 months depending on the operative site, quality of bone, age of patient, and implant system used. Throughout this time, meticulous attention to oral hygiene and the provision of an intermediate oral reconstruction that does not impinge on the healing area are essential.[41]

In the first 2 weeks postoperatively, normal oral hygiene techniques can be used on the existing dentition. Over the operative sites cleaning with a cotton wool pledget soaked in aqueous chlorhexidine is sufficient. Once the sutures have been removed at about 7 days, tooth brushing can gradually commence, taking care not to scrub at the gingival margin of an implant. This can cause recession. Review appointments are recommended on days 7, 14, and 28 after implant placement, and then monthly thereafter to check on healing. This is particularly important if a membrane has been used.

Once an adequate time for osseointegration has passed, implants that are buried are uncovered, and the transmucosal components placed. Great care is needed to ensure correct alignment of these components. There should be no visible gap between the implant and abutment, either clinically or radiographically. This is particularly true of those implants that employ an hexagonal head rather than an internal taper. Soft-tissue maturity 2 weeks after second-stage surgery is usually sufficient to allow prosthetic reconstruction to commence.[19]

The need for progressive loading is contentious.[42] It would seem prudent in grade 3 and 4 bone to gradually increase the loading exerted on the implant and therefore allow the bone to be loaded gradually. Physiologically, this meets with Wolff's law of bone remodeling. In practice, many reconstructions are placed immediately after osseointegration has been confirmed without any obvious detriment to the implants.

Although the prosthetic reconstruction of implants is a specialist field beyond the scope of this chapter, certain points are worthy of emphasis:

- The prosthesis should determine the position and number of the implants and not the reverse. All too often, the prosthesis is only considered once the implants are in place, to the detriment of the overall reconstruction.
- Implant-retained overdeptures are less demanding than fixed prostheses.
- The provision of a retrievable fixed prosthetic superstructure has advantages if there is any doubt about an implant, and allows direct assessment and treatment of any problems at the earliest opportunity. Screw-retained prostheses are more expensive, and the use of cement-retained prostheses confers theoretical advantages in passive fit of the superstructure.[43] The use of temporary cement enables easy retrievability and avoids the access holes in the occlusal surfaces of screw-retained prostheses.
- Occlusal factors can have a considerable bearing on long-term function and success, and readers are directed towards texts dealing with these issues by prosthodontists with experience in this area.

MAINTENANCE

The long-term maintenance of implants is essential for success. Patients should be made aware of their responsibility for implant care as part of the informed consent.[41,44]

Regular review appointments to assess soft-tissue health, and radiographic examination of marginal bone levels, initially on an annual basis, are recommended. Standardized film techniques are required, with thread configuration clearly visible. Recalls 3-monthly, 6-monthly and then annually over a period of 3 years in the first instance are usual. However, an individual's needs cannot be determined until the final occlusal state is achieved, up to 18 months after completion of treatment. Recalls can be extended or reduced in accordance with clinical need. The patient should be instructed in oral hygiene methods appropriate to the prosthesis. Tooth brushing of fixed prostheses is in itself inadequate, and should be supplemented with interdental and peri-implant cleaning using floss single tufted brushes, or gauze.[45]

ADVANCED TECHNIQUES

The patients who most benefit from implants are frequently those with the least bone. They are therefore invariably the most difficult to treat.

Methods devised to overcome these difficulties range from local manipulation of tissues to extensive grafting with bimaxillary osteotomies and free vascularized tissue transfer. Distraction osteogenesis will no doubt become increasingly important in the future.

Bone and soft-tissue deficiencies may be localized or generalized throughout the mouth. Bone resorption increases the impact of adjacent anatomic structures on implant placement. The superficial migration of muscle attachments with respect to the atrophic ridges, when combined with aging, leads to facial collapse.[46] The reduction in keratinized mucosa and the proximity of the maxillary cavities and the inferior dental nerves all impact on implant placement in the atrophic jaw. There is a corresponding increase in the complexity of implant-based reconstructions for both the patient and the clinician.

Local buccal deficiencies at the site of implant placement, particularly in the upper anterior, single tooth situation can be overcome by a number of means. Positioning the implant rather more to the lingual, or ridge expansion are simple methods of addressing small deficiencies.

The development of expanders such as the Summers' osteotomes allows bone manipulation.[47] The central cancellous bone is gradually compacted against the buccal and palatal walls. These walls gradually expand under careful pressure using increasing sizes of the osteotomes. Microfractures develop in the bone surrounding the expanded implant site. This technique is only suitable in the maxilla

where cancellous bone predominates. The technique is usually possible with hand pressure alone although the use of a mallet is occasionally necessary. The implant is placed directly into the expanded site, in a self-tapping manner, and allowed to heal for 4–6 months. The use of a drill at the expanded implant site is to be avoided. The stress fractures within the walls weaken them such that they can shear off if vibrated with an implant drill (Figs 93.8–93.10).

Disguise of the buccal deficiency can be achieved either with the use of a connective tissue graft taken from the

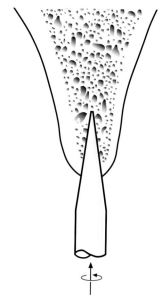

Fig. 93.8 Ridge expansion – narrow ridge.

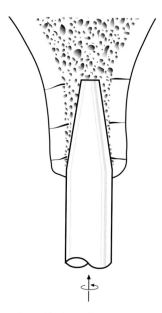

Fig. 93.9 Ridge expansion widening ridge.

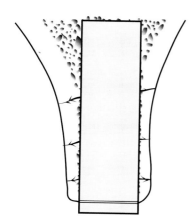

Fig. 93.10 Ridge expansion with implant in place.

palate[48] or with the insertion of a few nonresorbable hydroxyapatite granules placed under the buccal flap to plump out the contour.

Larger defects require the production of an environment conducive to bone growth or the placement of bone grafts. To date, guided bone regeneration with membranes achieves the former point most predictably.

The key element in bone augmentation of any defect is the soft-tissue envelope. The closure of the mucoperiosteal flap over the site of bone manipulation is a fundamental requirement for success. Adequate mobilization of the soft-tissue flaps, and tension-free primary closure over the grafted or augmented site is important. Consequently, the degree to which the area can be enlarged is determined by the soft tissues. In turn these can be increased initially either by tissue expansion[49] or by the introduction of new tissue. A free keratinized graft taken from the palate,[50] rather than a non-keratinized local pedicled flap, is preferred.

Guided tissue regeneration (GTR) is the use of a membrane to selectively exclude gingival tissues from the wound site, thus allowing the migration of bone or periodontal ligament progenitor cells into the area. This favors bone regeneration when dealing with osseointegrated implants,[51] but was first described around teeth.[52] Better results have been achieved around implants[53] than teeth, probably because the former are sterile when placed and the oral health has been optimized.

GTR can be used:

- immediately, at the time of tooth extraction
- at recent sites, after soft-tissue healing of the extraction socket at delayed sites, when GTR is used after extraction and before implant placement
- at delayed sites when GTR is used after extraction and before implant placement
- at mature sites, when GTR is needed at the site of previous, healed extractions.[54]

The technique of directing tissue regeneration dates back to the 1950s when microporous cellulose acetate filters were used for tendon and neural regeneration.[55] Barrier membranes are placed to seal off an anatomical site and prevent soft-tissue ingress from interfering with osteogenesis. Membranes currently in use are either resorbable – e.g. Resolut, Vicryl, collagen sheets, lamellar bone sheets – or nonresorbable, e.g. Goretex (ePTFE), titanium mesh. Dahlin demonstrated that isolating a bony defect from fibrous tissue invasion using ePTFE allowed bony healing within the defect.[56] Those defects not isolated were filled with fibrous tissue with very little bony ingrowth. An absence of tissue reaction to the membranes is essential if bone healing is to be promoted with minimal interference.

Membranes can be used to optimize a site for implant placement, or to encourage bone ingrowth to an area of deficiency around an existing implant. This can either be at the time of implant placement or after osseointegration, if evidence of bone loss becomes apparent.

Membranes should be larger than the defect to be augmented. They are cut to shape, placed passively over the defect, and all sharp corners removed. To prevent collapse of the membrane into the defect and loss of augmentation volume, it should be supported from below. This can be achieved with a bone graft, taken from an adjacent area, or the use of augmentation pins such as the Memfix or Frialit systems (Figs 93.11, 93.12). Any periosteal release required for tension-free closure is best undertaken remote from the membrane. The membrane should be kept clear of adjacent teeth, as flap dehiscence can occur, with detrimental effects on healing.

Tension-free, soft-tissue closure over the implanted membrane is essential to avoid premature exposure of the membrane, which may result in infection with loss of any regeneration gained. In the event that the material becomes exposed during the first 6 weeks the wound can be cleaned with aqueous chlorhexidine.[57] The membrane should be removed if there is any clinical evidence of inflammation present during the healing phase.

Wherever possible, the membrane is left in place for 9 months. This allows adequate time for bony regeneration and maturation. Removal earlier than this leaves an augmented site with soft immature tissue that tends to resorb. Resorbable membranes do not need to be removed unless infected.

There are concerns that bone formed under a membrane is of poor quality and resorbs easily. Indeed, the benefit of small crestal augmentations is open to debate as there is evidence that local bone dehiscences with threads visible above the marginal bone crest do not compromise implant survival.[58] However, successful long-term osseointegration in membrane regenerated bone has been reported.[59]

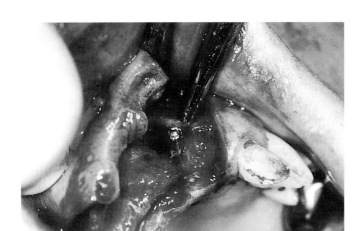

Fig. 93.11 Guided tissue regeneration with Goretex and Memfix pin insertion, stage 1.

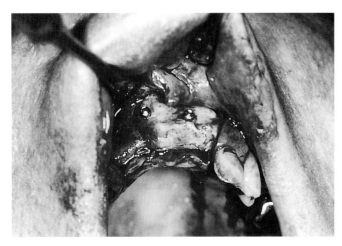

Fig. 93.12 Guided tissue regeneration with Goretex and Memfix pin removal, stage 2.

Where significant bony deficiencies exist then the use of barrier techniques alone is not appropriate and bone grafts are needed. The best grafting material is autogenous bone. The local supply of this in the mouth is most deficient in those patients who most need it. To overcome this deficiency, extraoral sites may be used such as the iliac crest, tibia or cranium. An alternative is to use bone graft substitutes.

Various bone graft substitutes have been advocated. All should be used in the knowledge that they are second best alternatives to autogenous bone. They can be divided into osteoconductive and osteoinductive materials. Osteoconduction implies bone apposition on to and into a material and occurs from existing bone or bone progenitor cells. Osteoinductive materials can convert undifferentiated cells into osteoblasts or chondroblasts, in areas remote from bone. Autogenous bone is capable of both of the above as well as osteogenesis, the production of bone in the absence of undifferentiated cells.[60]

Most osteoconductive materials are synthetic alloplasts, usually ceramics. The two main groups of ceramics used in conjunction with implants are tri-calcium phosphate (TCP) and hydroxyapatite (HA) derived from a variety of sources. They are highly biocompatible substances that bond strongly to bone. By providing a matrix suitable for new bone deposition, ceramics encourage bone growth into areas that it would otherwise not occupy.[61] They may maintain bone bulk where resorption normally occurs. These materials are well tolerated by the soft tissues with no adverse reactions. However, the ingrowth of gingival tissue into nonresorbable ceramics results in tethering. Sharp dissection is then required to raise a soft-tissue flap in these areas.

TCP is much more soluble than HA and is at least partially resorbable. This occurs at a rate equivalent to the ingrowth of normal bone, and is related to the manufacturing process of the TCP.

HA is the major inorganic component of bone. It has good compressive but poor tensile strength, and in these respects is similar to bone. The porous type of particulate HA is most frequently used with osseointegrated implants. The pore size determines the type of tissue ingrowth. Pore sizes greater than 150 μm facilitate ingrowth of mineralized bone.[62]

Osseoinductive materials are in the main allografts derived from human sources. All donors are carefully screened for diseases that could affect the health of the recipient. Demineralized freeze-dried bone is most frequently advocated. The manufacturing process activates bone morphogenic proteins (BMP) that are present in the bone collagen matrix. These have been purified and isolated as a number of different osseoinductive substances and are predominantly present in cortical bone. The use of synthetically produced BMP in the future may overcome increasing reticence to use human derived bone by both patients and clinicians.[63]

These materials have applications in the management of extraction sockets, localized ridge defects, sinus augmentation and the treatment of peri-implant deficiencies, either at the time of placement or later during salvage surgery. Wherever possible autogenous bone should supplement the use of these osseoinductive and osseoconductive materials.

ADJUNCTIVE IMPLANT TECHNIQUES

Where local factors adversely affect conventional implant placement, a number of procedures have been developed to modify the local anatomy and aid implant placement. In the upper jaw, where atrophy and sinus enlargement can preclude conventional implant surgery sinus grafting, tuberosity placement and pterygoid plate placement have all been advocated. In the anterior region, the use of ridge expansion, vestibuloplasty, nasal floor and onlay grafting may be required.

The management of the atrophic posterior maxilla requires augmentation of the available bone between the alveolar ridge and the sinus floor to correct the vertical deficiency. In severely resorbed maxillae, onlay grafting to correct buccal bone deficiency may also be required.

There has been a gradual evolution in sinus grafting procedures, with current techniques offering predictable success rates. Implant placement into augmented sinuses is associated with at least 80% long-term osseointegration in most series.[64]

Early attempts at onlay grafting of the posterior maxillary ridge with rib grafts were unsuccessful as the bone grafts rapidly resorbed. Deliberately placing implants through the maxillary sinus lining has been associated with a higher failure rate.[65] Where sufficient bone exists to provide primary stability for the implant, careful elevation of the sinus lining, either with osteotomes or the implant itself, results in predictable osseointegration.[24] Tatum developed a modified Caldwell–Luc procedure, elevated the sinus mucosa, and placed bone grafts into this area.[66] Autogenous marrow has been used,[67] together with a variety of osseoinductive and osseoconductive materials, in attempts to avoid extraoral donor site morbidity.[68]

Grafting is undertaken prior to implant placement with a healing period of at least 6 months. Where primary stability is achievable then grafts can be placed around stable implants. A third alternative is the use of the implant as a lag screw to retain a block of corticocancellous bone within the maxillary sinus.[69]

The techniques can be undertaken with local anesthetic, using an infraorbital block and infiltrations. Where more extensive bone harvesting and grafting is needed, general anesthesia is preferred.

The lateral wall of the maxillary sinus is approached via a buccal flap. Crestal incisions, to coincide with those used for later implant placement, rather than palatal incisions are recommended. The suture line will still lie on bone. The buccal flap is raised in a subperiosteal plane to expose the lateral wall. The antrostomy is undertaken adjacent to the area to be grafted. This is predetermined at the planning stage and coincides with the proposed implant positions. The template can be used to confirm the correct position. Grafting should be confined to the area to be implanted. Extensive sinus grafting is unnecessary and increases postoperative morbidity.

Using a small, round bur in a contra-angled handpiece, with the shank held parallel with the lateral wall, a pilot hole is made. The shank of the bur acts as a stop to prevent it falling through the sinus lining once the bone has been breached. Gradually altering the angle of approach allows the hole to be deepened if the wall is thicker than the radius of the bur. The procedure is carried out at high drill speed with copious irrigation.

Using either a postage stamp technique or gentle strokes, a channel can be cut in the bone that exposes the antral lining without perforating it. A window is developed of a size determined by the area to be grafted. The inferior edge of the window should be about 3 mm above the floor of the sinus, so that a lip will be present once the antrostomy has been completed. Tatum advocates infracturing the antral wall and carefully elevating the sinus lining so that the antral wall lies parallel to the alveolar ridge and forms the roof of the sinus graft.[66] Smiler advocates removing the window completely.[24] This has the advantage of easier manipulation of the sinus lining, and allows placement of the window back over the antrostomy after the grafting procedure.

In practice, both techniques should be mastered. The infracture method can impinge on the medial antral wall, causing difficulty with mobilization and a tendency to tear the lining while, in some cases, the window almost falls into the sinus thereby dictating the preferred technique.

Elevation of the antral lining in the subperiosteal plane requires careful dissection through the antrostomy. Specific instruments have been developed for this, but in practice dental excavators and a Mitchell's trimmer work equally well. The lining should only be elevated over the area to be grafted. Septa within the antrum can be seen on preoperative radiographs. An antrostomy either side of the septum provides the best access to these structures and facilitates elevation of the lining without tearing.

Once elevated, the lining is inspected for tears. Movement of the sinus lining with respiration is not reliable as a sign of an intact lining. Where a tear occurs, it should be covered to minimize graft displacement into the antrum. A collagen sheet or piece of Surgical is adequate. Attempts to suture the tear are unnecessary and usually increase the size of the defect.

The cavity to be grafted is bounded by the antral lining and bony window above, the medial and lateral sinus walls, and the floor of the sinus. To achieve axial loading, the maxillary implants are buccally inclined. The graft should therefore be placed more towards the medial wall (Fig. 93.13). Care should be taken not to stenose the osteum draining into the middle meatus. The bony window is replaced or a collagen sheet used to cover the antrostomy, and the mucosal flaps closed without tension. A denture can still be worn unless implants have been placed simul-

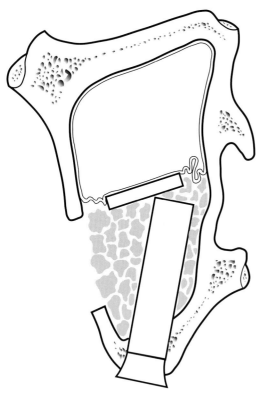

Fig. 93.13 Diagram of sinus graft with implant placement to show position of graft, implant and bone window.

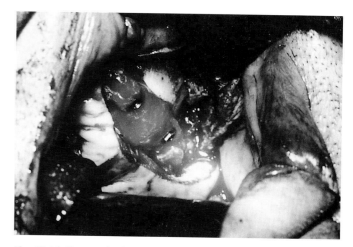

Fig. 93.14 Sinus grafted with bone block and immediate Branemark lag screw implant.

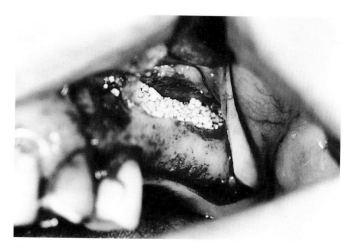

Fig. 93.15 Sinus lift with hydroxyapatite graft in place.

taneously. Antibiotics are continued for 5 days. Nasal decongestants are not routinely used.

Where adequate primary stability is possible the implants are placed simultaneously and the graft packed around them. The single-stage procedures (where implants lag screw a block of corticocancellous bone)[69] require meticulous implant placement (Fig. 93.14). The position of the implant with respect to the ridge, angulation and lag screw effect must all be compatable with reconstruction. This can be difficult to achieve.

While autogenous bone is the ideal, in practice the volume that can be collected intraorally is limited. The volume can be supplemented with a bone substitute. Good results have been achieved with hydroxyapatite (Fig. 93.15), de-mineralized freeze-dried bone, glass derivatives and hard-tissue replacement.[24,64,68] In the author's experience, with informed consent, patients prefer to avoid human derived bone if possible.

A similar approach can be adopted in the atrophic pre-maxillary region, where the nasal floor can be elevated and a bone graft placed to allow anterior implant placement. This area is difficult to anesthetize reliably and may require surgery under a general anesthetic.

Where there is considerable buccal deficiency, the use of grafts not only widens the arch and restores normal inter-maxillary anteroposterior relationship, but it also allows for vertical ridge augmentation. This decreases the intermaxillary distance and improves the ratio between crown length and implant length. Where a volume of bone is needed, then the iliac crest is preferred.[70] It offers an easily accessible site and adequate volumes of cortical, cancellous or cortico-cancellous grafts, which can be cut to shape for insertion at the recipient site.

An example is shown in Figure 93.16, where implant placement through onlay grafts was undertaken with osseo-integration and subsequent reconstruction of all implants. In this case, the bone grafts were retained with 2 mm mini screws, and the implants lag screwed through the buccal onlay grafts into the residual bone of the maxilla.

Where this approach is adopted, the implants should always be submerged, and a stepped palatal approach with extensive periosteal release on the buccal side prior to implant placement ensures maximum flap mobility and

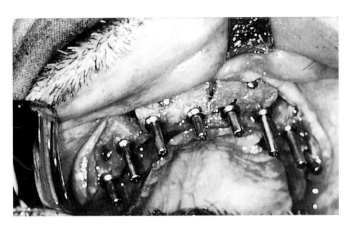

Fig. 93.16 Onlay bone grafting with immediate ITI implant placement and guide screws in place.

tension-free closure. Exposure of the implants, prior to bone union, usually results in premature loss of the graft and the associated implants.

In the anterior maxilla the narrow ridge can be treated by osteoplasty.[71] A horseshoe type osteotomy, extending from the crest to the nasal floor, with anterior advancement creates a gap into which bone graft can be placed for subsequent implant placement. The result is a widened alveolar ridge with improved facial contour and good quality bone suitable for osseointegrated implants.

Where the maxilla is very atrophic, the skeletal and bone volume deficiency is best corrected with a Le Fort I osteotomy, advancing the maxilla downwards and forwards, and grafting the sinus floor and nasal floor with autogenous bone.[72,73] Both solid graft blocks and cancellous mush mixed with hydroxyapatite have been used with success. Delayed implant placement is recommended as graft consolidation can be variable.[74] Implant placement can then be predetermined in the optimum site after bone healing has occurred.

The onlay grafting of a block of iliac crest directly on to the maxillary ridge has the advantage of decreasing the intermaxillary distance, but soft-tissue closure is difficult. If the graft is lag screwed into place with implants, there is a significant risk of losing both the graft and the implants. The latter are rarely in the ideal position for optimal prosthetic reconstruction.

Placement of implants into the pterygoid plates has been reported.[75] In practice this usually results in a prosthetic reconstruction that extends much further back than is required. However, where no other bone stock exists, the dense bone of the pterygoid plate of the sphenoid bone and the pyramidal process of the palatine bone provide excellent stability if sufficient width is available. CT scanning is essential for assessment. The surgical approach is difficult and requires long instrumentation to overcome the poor

access. Oblique insertion of the implant is required if the plates are to be engaged. Nonaxial implant loading results. The technique appears to be of most value in the reconstruction of maxillary defects after ablative surgery.

A simpler approach is to use the tuberosity for implant insertion. The volume of bone is often adequate, but the quality is poor. Careful assessment of healing and progressive loading of the implants in this area give predictable results. Roughened surface implants which maximize bone–implant contact should be used.

In the atrophic mandible interforaminal implant placement enables reconstruction of the dentition in most cases. Posterior cantilever prostheses fixed to anteriorly placed implants can provide full arch restoration of the lower jaw. In some cases, however, implant placement proximal to the mental foramen is indicated. Wherever possible, the avoidance of nerve repositioning is to be recommended as sensory changes in the lower lip after nerve manipulation are almost inevitable, ranging from transitory to permanent.[76] Shorter, wide-body implants, the use of roughened surface implants designed to be used in shorter lengths, or placement of implants lingual to the inferior dental nerve taking care of the mylohyoid undercut, are all possible with careful planning. Where insufficient bone is available above the inferior dental nerve, consideration should be given to repositioning procedures.[77] Appropriate consent should specifically include changes in nerve function postoperatively.

The procedure can take place under general or local anesthetic. Using a template, the implant sites are marked, through the mucosa, into the underlying bone. A crestal incision with extension up the external oblique ridge, and relieved well anterior to the mental foramen, allows for the elevation of a large subperiosteal flap gaining access to the lateral mandible and exposing the mental foramen. A window of bone is removed around the mental bundle, gaining access through the cortex to the cancellous bone. Using a probe or Sailor retractor within the inferior dental canal the lateral cortical wall of the bone overlying the nerve is carefully removed with burs and hand instruments. Sufficient proximal bone needs to be removed to allow tension-free displacement of the nerve laterally. The less manipulation required, the lower the chances of long-term anesthesia, paresthesia, or dysesthesia.

Preservation of the incisive branch of the inferior dental nerve minimizes nerve trauma and may decrease altered sensation in the lip. However, where mobilization of the nerve is compromised, division of the incisive branch may be required.

After conventional implant placement, the nerve is allowed to lie passively within the groove that has been cut. Bone mush taken from the bone trap connected to the suction can be placed between the implants and the inferior dental nerve to cushion the nerve and maintain direct bone–implant contact around the implant. The use of a bone trap on the suction aids bone collection for later use.

Where the mandible is very atrophic, the inferior dental nerve can be dissected out through the alveolar crest (Fig. 93.17). This retains the strong lateral wall of the mandible, eases surgical exposure, and allows safe implant placement under direct vision. In this situation the nerve remains outside the mandible. Care with further soft-tissue surgery is needed if the carefully dissected nerve is not to be damaged during subsequent incisions over the crest of the ridge proximal to the original mental foramen. Where this technique is adopted, engagement of the lower border of the mandible is essential if primary stability is to be achieved. The channel cut in the crest of the ridge can be filled with bone dust and bone chips removed during nerve exposure.

Severe atrophy of the interforaminal zone can be addressed with short, wide-body implants, transmandibular implants or onlay grafting. Onlay grafting alone has been associated with rapid resorption and disappointing results.[78] When combined with osseointegrated implants, onlay grafting is more predictable and long-term reconstruction of the atrophic mandible is possible. Onlay grafting allows the placement of longer implants and reduces the risk of mandibular fracture.[79] The anterior iliac crest is the usual donor site. Implants can be placed at the same time as the bone

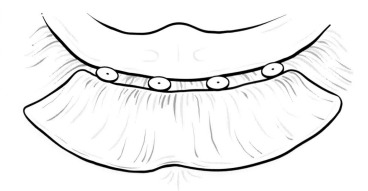

Fig. 93.18 Diagram of a free mucosal graft.

grafts or after bone healing. The latter requires a second procedure but correct implant placement is easier and complete loss of the graft during healing does not also result in loss of the implants.

Holes drilled in the basal bone encourage bleeding and open the cancellous bone and marrow spaces prior to graft placement. The graft should be contoured to shape and secured rigidly to the mandible with wires, screws or plates. Careful mobilization of the soft-tissue flaps is needed for a tension free closure over the bone graft. Removal of prominent genial tubercles can be undertaken at the same time and eases the prosthetic reconstruction. Vestibuloplasty after graft union may be required if soft-tissue closure compromises the depth of the buccal sulcus. This can be combined with delayed implant placement.

In the atrophic mandible, the keratinized gingiva often shrinks to a thin band overlying the ridge. This is frequently inadequate to give a non-mobile soft-tissue margin around the implant, and soft-tissue surgery to the local area is required. A vestibuloplasty with mucosal graft gives predictable results. Previously reported complications such as mental nerve sensory changes, chin ptosis and circumoral muscle hypotonia can be overcome with contemporary techniques.[80] Care should be taken to avoid the mental nerves and retain mentalis attachment. Supraperiosteal dissection, with suturing of the buccal flap to the depth of the newly formed sulcus, ensures a vascularized bed on to which the graft can be laid. The graft can be taken from the buccal mucosa, palate or skin. A stent sutured into place maintains sulcal depth and pressure on the graft but is not strictly necessary (Fig. 93.18).

IMPLANT SALVAGE

Peri-implant infections are relatively uncommon and usually develop gradually. Regular reviews enable early assessment

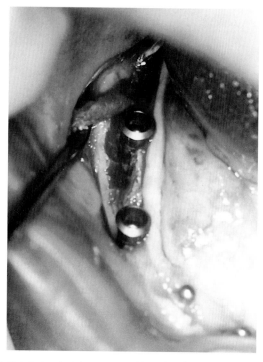

Fig. 93.17 Inferior dental nerve repositioned and ITI implants in place.

of inflammation around an implant. The occlusion and the abutment–implant junction should always be checked if this situation presents. Most infections are treatable, but the longer they remain, the greater the volume of bone lost resulting in eventual loss of the implant. Metronidazole is an appropriate antibiotic for most peri-implant infections and is prescribed at 200 mg tds for 10 days. When this is combined with an aqueous chlorhexidine mouth rinse and irrigation of the peri-implant tissues using a fine syringe most acute infections will resolve. Where bone loss is apparent, surgical salvage is required. The implant is exposed and the surface smoothed and mechanically cleaned with fine diamond and stone burs to achieve a macroscopically smooth surface. This surface is disinfected with topical chlorhexidine gel or citric acid. The soft tissues can be recontoured and sutured around the implant, or guided tissue regeneration with a membrane attempted.[81] The latter requires meticulous technique and careful follow-up if the membrane is not to get infected and aggravate the situation.

If bone loss is extreme, implant removal is required. The removal of the superstructure allows access to the implant. Various trephines have been devised to enable implant removal with minimal surrounding bone loss. Ideally the defect is then cleaned, allowed to heal, and an implant replaced for incorporation into the existing superstructure in due course. Membranes help to maximize the ridge height in these cases. Where very long implants have been used in the mandible and explantation is planned, consideration should be given to sectioning the implant at the level of the remaining bone. This avoids weakening the mandible unduly. Fractures have been reported in this situation.[82]

CONCLUSIONS

Osseointegrated implants provide the means to reconstruct and rehabilitate. Case selection is important, and indefinite review and maintenance is essential if long-term benefits are to be maintained. With appropriate planning and careful execution implant-borne prostheses may last the lifetime of the patient.

REFERENCES

1. Schroeder A 1996 The ITI system. In: Schroeder A, Sutter F, Buser D, Krekeler G (eds) Oral implantology, 2nd revised edn. Thieme, New York
2. Watzek G, Blahout R 1996 Historical review. In: Watzek G (ed) Endosseous implants: Scientific and clinical aspects. Quintessence, Chicago
3. Misch CE 1993 Mandibular complete subperiosteal implants. In: Contemporary Implant Dentistry. Mosby, St Louis
4. Steinmann S 1996 The properties of titanium. In: Schroeder A, Sutter F, Buser D, Krekeler (eds) Oral implantology, 2nd revised edn. Thieme, New York
5. Dalton JE, Cook SD 1995 in vivo mechanical and histological characteristics of HA-costed implants vary with coating vendor. Journal of Biomedical Materials Research 29(2):239–245
6. Albrektsson T, Branemark P-I, Hansson H-A et al 1983 The interface zone of inorganic implants in vivo: Titanium implants in bone. Annals of Biomedical Engineering 11:1–27
7. Linkow LI 1968 The blade-vent – a new dimension in endosseous implants. Dental Concepts 11:3–10
8. Small IA 1975 Metal implants and the mandibular staple bone plate. Journal of Oral and Maxillofacial Surgery 33:571–588
9. Bosker H, Jordan DJ, Sindet-Pedersen S et al 1991 The transmandibular implant: A 13 year survey of its use. Journal of Oral and Maxillofacial Surgery 49:482–492
10. Powers MP, Bosker H 1996 Functional and cosmetic reconstruction of the facial lower third associated with placement of the Transmandibular Implant System. Journal of Oral and Maxillofacial Surgery 54:934–942
11. Brunski JB, Moccia AF, Pollack SR, Korostoff E, Trachtenberg DI 1979 The influence of functional use of endosseous dental implants on the tissue – implant interface. II. Clinical Aspects. Journal of Dental Research 58:1053–1069
12. Branemark P-I 1985 Introduction to osseointegration. In: Branemark P-I, Zarb GA, Albrektson T (eds) Tissue integrated prostheses. Quintessence, Chicago
13. Schroeder S, Buser D 1996 Tissue response. In: Schroeder A, Sutter F, Buser D, Krekeler G (eds) Oral implantology, 2nd revised edn. Thieme, New York
14. Tarnow DP, Emtiaz S, Classi A 1997 Immediate loading of threaded implants at stage 1 surgery in edentulous arches: ten consecutive case reports with 1 to 5 year data … International Journal of Oral and Maxillofacial Implants 12(3):319–324
15. Hobo S 1990 Biological considerations for osseointegration. In: Hobo S, Ichida E, Garcia LT (eds) Osseointegration and occlusal rehabilitation. Quintessence, Tokyo
16. Plenk H, Zitter H 1996 Material considerations. In: Watzek G (ed) Endosseous implants: Scientific and clinical aspects. Quintessence, Chicago
17. Branemark P-I 1983 Osseointegration and its experimental background. Journal of Prosthetic Dentistry 50:399–410
18. Buser D, Weber HP, Donath JP et al 1992 Soft tissue reactions to non-submerged unloaded titanium implants in beagle dogs. Journal of Periodontology 63:225–235
19. Adell R, Lekholm U, Rockler B, Branemark P-I 1981 A 15 year study of osseointegrated implants in the treatment of the edentulous jaw. International Journal of Oral Surgery 10:387–416
20. Adell R, Lekholm U, Rockler B et al 1986 Marginal tissue reactions at osseointegrated titanium fistures. I.A three-year longitudinal prospective study. International Journal of Oral Surgery 15:39–52
21. Lekholm U, Zarb A 1985 Patient selection and preparation. In: Branemark P-I, Zarb GA, Albrektson T (eds) Tissue-integrated prostheses. Quintessence, Chicago
22. Misch CE 1990 Density of bone: effect on treatment plans, surgical approach, healing and progressive bone loading. International Journal of Oral and Maxillofacial Implants 6:23–31
23. Cawood JI, Howell RA 1991 Reconstructive preprosthetic surgery. 1. Anatomical considerations. International Journal of Oral and Maxillofacial Surgery 20:75–82
24. Smiler DG, Johnson PW, Lozada JL et al 1992 Sinus lifts grafts and endosseous implants. Treatment of the atrophic posterior maxilla. Dental Clinics of North America 36(1):151–182

25. Rosenquist JB, Nystrom E 1992 Occlusion of the incisive canal with bone chips: A procedure to facilitate insertion of implants in the anterior maxilla. International Journal of Oral and Maxillofacial Surgery 21(4):210–211

26. Mason ME, Triplett RG, Alfonso WF 1990 Life threatening hemorrhage from placement of a dental implant. Journal of Oral and Maxillofacial Surgery 48:201

27. Carter RB, Keen EN 1971 The intra-mandibular course of the inferior alveolar nerve. Journal of Anatomy 108:433–440

28. Rosenquist B 1996 Is there an anterior loop of the inferior alveolar nerve? International Journal of Periodontology Research in Dentistry 16(1):41–45

29. Jacobsson M, Tjellstrom A, Thosen P, Albrektsson T, Turesson I 1988 Integration of titanium implants in irradiated bone. Histologic and clinical study. Annals of Otology, Rhinology, and Laryngology 97:337–340

30. Marx RE 1984 Osteoradionecrosis of the jaws: review and update. HBO Rev 5:78–126

31. Granstrom G 1992 The use of hyperbaric oxygen to prevent implant loss in the irradiated patient. In: Worthington P, Branemark P-I (eds) Advanced osseointegrated surgery. Applications in the maxillofacial region. Quintessence, Chicago

32. Misch CE 1993 Medical evaluation. In: Contemporary implant dentistry. Mosby, St Louis

33. Haas R, Haimbock W, Mailath G, Watzek G 1996 The relationship of smoking on peri-implant tissue. Journal of Prosthetic Dentistry 76(6):592–596

34. De Bruyn H, Collaert B 1994 The effect of smoking on early implant failure. Clinical Oral Implant Research 5(4):260–264

35. Bain CE, Moy PIC 1993 The association between the failure of dental implants and cigarette smoking. International Journal of Oral and Maxillofacial Implants 8(6):609–615

36. Hunt BW, Sandifer JB, Assad DA, Gher ME 1996 Effect of flap design on healing and osseointegration of dental implants. International Journal of Periodontology Research in Dentistry 16(6):583–593

37. Eriksson RA, Albrektsson T 1983 Temperature threshold levels for heat-induced bone tissue injury. A vital microscopy study in the rabbit. Journal of Prosthetic Dentistry 50:101–107

38. Sutter F 1996 Preparation of the implant bed. In: Schroeder A, Sutter F, Buser D, Krekeler G (eds) Oral implantology, 2nd revised edn. Thieme, New York

39. Sutter F, Schroeder A, Buser DA 1988 The new concept of ITI hollow-cylinder and hollow-screw implants: part 1. Clinical engineering and design. International Journal of Oral and Maxillofacial Implants 3:161–172

40. Buser DA, Schroeder A, Sutter F, Lang NP 1988 The new concept of ITI hollow-cylinder and hollow-screw implants: part 2. The clinical aspects, indications and early clinical results. International Journal of Oral and Maxillofacial Implants 3:173–181

41. Lekholm U 1983 Clinical procedures for treatment with osseointegrated implants. Journal of Prosthetic Dentistry 50:116–120

42. Misch CE 1993 Progressive bone loading. In: Contemporary implant dentistry. Mosby, St Louis

43. Misch CE 1993 Principles of cement-fixed prosthodontics and implant dentistry. In: Contemporary implant dentistry. Mosby, St Louis

44. Henry PJ 1992 Maintenance and monitoring. In: Worthington P, Branemark P-I (eds) Advanced osseointegrated surgery. Applications in the maxillofacial region. Quintessence, Chicago

45. Krekeler G 1996 Follow up care and recall. In: Schroeder A, Sutter F, Buser D, Krekeler G (eds) Oral implantology, 2nd revised edn. Thieme, New York

46. Stoelinga PJW 1992 Preprosthetic reconstructive surgery. In: Principles of oral and maxillofacial surgery. JB Lippincott, Philadelphia

47. Summers RB 1994 Maxillary implant surgery. Compendium of Continued Education in Dentistry 1520:152–162

48. Silverstein LH, Kurtzman D, Garnick JJ et al 1994 Connective tissue grafting for improved implant esthetics: clinical technique. Implant Dentistry 3(4):231–234

49. Quayle AA, McCord JF 1992 Current status of tissue expanders in alveolar ridge augmentation: a review. Implant Dentistry 1(3):177–181

50. Parel SM 1989 Restorative options – compromised fixture locations. In: Parel SM, Sullivan DY (eds) Esthetics and osseointegration. Taylor, Dallas

51. Wilson T Jr 1993 Guided tissue regeneration. In: ITI dental implants planning, placement, restoration and maintenance. Quintessence, Chicago

52. Nyman S, Linde J, Karring T et al 1982 New attachment following surgical treatment of human periodontal disease. Journal of Clinical Periodontology 4(4):290–296

53. Dahlin C, Sennerby L, Lekholm U et al 1989 Generation of new bone around titanium implants using a membrane technique. An experimental study in rabbits. International Journal of Oral and Maxillofacial Implants 4(1):19–25

54. Wilson TG, Weber HP 1993 Classification and therapy for areas of deficient bony housing prior to dental implant placement. International Journal of Periodontal Restorative Dentistry 13:5–19

55. Hurley AL, Stinchfield FE, Bassett CAL et al 1959 The role of soft tissues in osteogenesis. Journal of Bone and Joint Surgery 41A:1243

56. Dahlin C, Linde A, Gottlow J et al 1988 Healing of bony defects by guided tissue regeneration. Plastic and Reconstructive Surgery 81:672–681

57. Becker W, Becker BE 1994 Bone promotion around e-PTFE augmented implants placed in immediate extraction sockets. In: Buser D, Dahlin, C, Schenk RK (eds) Guided bone regeneration in implant dentistry. Quintessence, Chicago

58. Lekholm U, Sennerby L, Roos J et al 1995 Soft tissue and marginal bone conditions at osseointegrated implants that have exposed threads: a 5 year retrospective study. International Journal of Oral and Maxillofacial Implants 11(5):599–604

59. Buser D, Dula K, Lang NP et al 1996 Long-term stability of osseointegrated implants in bone regenerated by membrane technique. Five year results of a prospective study with 12 implants. Clinical Oral Implants Research 7:175–183

60. Misch CE 1993 Residual ridge augmentation. In: Contemporary implant dentistry. Mosby, St Louis

61. Jarcho M 1989 Biomaterial aspects of calcium phosphates. Dental Clinics of North America 30(1):25–43

62. White E, Shors EC 1989 Biomaterial aspects of Interpore 200 porous hydroxyapatite. Dental Clinics of North America 30(1):49–66

63. Boyne PJ, Marx RE, Nevins M et al 1997 A feasibility study evaluating rhBMP/absorbable collagen sponge for maxillary sinus floor augmentation. International Journal of Periodontology Research in Dentistry 17(1):11–25

64. Dover MS 1994 A prospective study of sinus lift and sinus grafting techniques. Abstracts BAOMS meeting April 1994

65. Branemark P-I, Adell R 1984 An experimental and clinical study of osseointegrated implants penetrating the nasal cavity. International Journal of Oral and Maxillofacial Surgery 42:497–501

66. Tatum OH 1986 Maxillary and sinus implant reconstruction. Dental Clinics of North America 30:207–229

67. Boyne PJ, James RA 1980 Grafting of the maxillary sinus floor with autologous marrow and bone. Journal of Oral Surgery 38:613–616

68. Chanavaz M 1990 Maxillary sinus: anatomy, physiology, surgery and bone grafting related to oral implantology – Eleven years of surgical experience (1979–1990). Journal of Oral Implants 16:199–209

69. Raghoebar GM, Brouwer ThJ, Reintsema H et al 1993 Augmentation of the maxillary sinus floor with autogenous bone for

the placement of endosseous implants. Journal of Oral and Maxillofacial Surgery 51:1198–1203

70. Keller EE, Triplett WW 1987 Iliac bone grafting: review of 160 consecutive cases. Journal of Oral and Maxillofacial Surgery 45:11–14

71. Richardson D, Cawood JI 1991 Anterior maxillary osteoplasty to broaden the narrow maxillary ridge. International Journal of Oral and Maxillofacial Surgery 20:342–348

72. Bell HW, Buche WA, Kennedy JW et al 1977 Surgical correction of the atrophic alveolar ridge. A preliminary report on a new concept of treatment. Oral Surgery 45:485

73. Sailor HF 1989 A new method of inserting endosseous implants in totally atrophic maxillae. Journal of Cranio-maxillofacial Surgery 17:299–305

74. Keller EE, Van Roekel NB. Desjardins RP et al 1987 Prosthetic-surgical reconstruction of the severely resorbed maxilla with iliac bone grafting and tissue-integrated prostheses. International Journal of Oral and Maxillofacial Implants 2:155–165

75. Tulasne JF 1992 Osseointegrated fixtures in the pterygoid region. In: Worthington P, Branemark P-I (eds) Advanced osseointegration surgery applications in the maxillofacial region. Quintessence, Chicago

76. Davis WH, Rydevik B, Lundborg G et al 1992 Mobilization of the inferior alveolar nerve to allow placement of osseointegrated fixtures. In: Worthington P, Branemark P-I (eds) Advanced osseointegration surgery applications in the maxillofacial region. Quintessence, Chicago

77. Rosenquist B 1994 Implant placement in combination with nerve transpositioning: Experience with the first 100 cases. International Journal of Oral and Maxillofacial Implants 9(5):522–531

78. Wang JH, Waite DE, Steinhauser E 1976 Ridge augmentation: and evaluation and follow up report. Journal of Oral Surgery 34:600

79. Astrand P 1992 Onlay bone grafts to the mandible. In: Worthington P, Branemark P-I (eds) Advanced osseointegration surgery applications in the maxillofacial region. Quintessence, Chicago

80. Huybers AJM, Stoelinga PJW, De Koomen HA et al 1984 Mandibular vestibuloplasty using a free mucosal graft. A 2–7 year evaluation. International Journal of Oral Surgery 14:11–18

81. Jordanovic S, Spiekermann H, Richter E-J et al 1992 Guided tissue regeneration around dental implants. In: Laney WR, Toman DE (eds) Tissue integration in oral, orthopaedic and maxillofacial reconstruction. Quintessence, Chicago

82. Buser D, Maeglin B 1996 Complications with ITI implants. In: Schroeder A, Sutter F, Buser D, Krekeler G (eds) Oral implantology, 2nd revised edn. Thieme, New York

Oral implants: what the restorative dentist needs

94

CLARK M. STANFORD

INTRODUCTION

The use of dental implants to replace missing teeth has become a standard of care in treating patients. Following the introduction of an endosseous cylindrical-style implant design that coupled retrievability with long-term clinical success, dental implants have assumed a major role in dental rehabilitation.[1–2] Crucial to the predictable esthetic and functional outcome is the complete diagnostic treatment planning by the restorative dentist prior to implant placement.[3] Following placement, a healing period of 3–6 months is allowed for biologic integration. During this period, the inflammatory matrix scaffold is replaced with an unorganized woven bone.[4] For long-term success, this needs to occur around an implant that has immediate rigid fixation (i.e. minimal micromotion).[5] Depending on the implant system, some advocate a 'two-stage' surgical approach with an initial implant placement (stage I) followed by a second uncovering and abutment connection (stage II). Alternatively, other systems advocate a 'one-stage' approach in which the head of the implant is allowed to remain exposed within the oral cavity but in a relatively 'unloaded' state.

Dental implant treatment is essentially a bioengineering technique that follows an engineering design theory (Fig. 94.1). The objective of implant treatment is the controlled delivery of functional loads (i.e. the occlusion) for the long-term osseous and mechanical stability of an esthetic prosthesis. In order for this objective to be achieved, the restorative dentist and the surgeon must work together as a team to create a design strategy. This strategy must include the impact of the patient's medical condition, the concerns of the patient, the anatomic status of the tissues and the application of osseous and soft-tissue augmentation in using the respective implant system and restorative options. Indeed, we are now in the era when the restoration dictates the implant position rather than the osseous anatomy alone. Finally, it is important that the surgeon evaluate the role of implant position, shape, healing time and the provisional restoration in helping the restorative dentist to achieve the objectives of implant treatment: a long-term stable, esthetic restoration. This chapter discusses treatment planning issues for the complete, partially edentulous and single-tooth restorative approaches in the skeletally mature patient.

IMPLANT TREATMENT PLANNING FOR THE EDENTULOUS ARCH

For any patient, an initial assessment of the medical and dental history is an important part of understanding the etiological causes for the edentulous state, the patient's attitudes towards treatment, his/her ability to undergo treatment and the economic impact of treatment.[1] Assessment of key factors such as a history of bruxism, periodontal disease, smoking, uncontrolled diabetes mellitus and metabolic diseases of bone is vital.[6] Informed consent with verbal and written reinforcement of what this means is critical throughout the multiple stages of implant treatment.

A key to predictable treatment outcome is a design of the proposed prosthesis (fixed detachable or overdenture) made during the diagnostic phase by the restorative dentist. Planning will dictate the number of implants, their position and angulation. Using this diagnostic information,

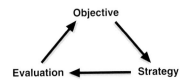

Fig. 94.1 Implant design theory.

a surgical guide or denture is then used to indicate the desired implant position, angulation and need for hard/soft-tissue augmentation prior to or at the time of implant placement.

The restoration of the mandibular arch is commonly performed with a fixed-detachable screw-retained cast gold framework having a prosthetic acrylic resin occlusion.[1] Alternatively, an overdenture utilizing attachments to implants for full support and retention or a combination mucosa/implant-borne prosthesis is used in certain cases.[7–9] The maxillae can be restored with a porcelain fused-to-metal restoration only if there has been little bone resorption.[10] Evaluating the smile line (i.e. the anterior and posterior occlusal planes) and comparing this to a mounted diagnostic set-up is vital in maxillary implant treatment planning. Diagnostic evaluation of the patient with and without the denture in place (having removed the facial denture flange) provides clues as to the degree of lip support needed.[11,12] The anterior smile line (relaxed and exaggerated) demonstrates the degree of tooth exposure anticipated, providing clues as to the expected crown length with a proposed fixed-detachable design. The maxillary fixed-detachable design has greater incidences of esthetic, phonetic and oral hygiene problems.[11] Consequently, an overdenture is often more successful by providing predictable esthetics, lip support and prevention of air escape (e.g. superior to the prosthesis or through exaggerated gingival embrasures). An overdenture is considered the treatment of choice for patients with moderate to severe resorption.[7]

The use of a mandibular fixed-detachable prosthesis has demonstrated a high success rate,[1] with excellent function and patient acceptance.[12–15] The advantages and disadvantages of the fixed-detachable versus an overdenture must be discussed with the patient during the initial diagnostic phases (Table 94.1). When discussing the treatment options, the patient should be warned that the final design cannot be decided, *and no promises should be made*, until the implant position, number and angulation are evaluated following stage II surgery. For the fixed-detachable design, the positions of the 5–6 implants needed to support this prosthesis are evaluated with a diagnostic denture set-up. Clinical examination must include identifying the mental foramina and transferring their location to the diagnostic denture, and sounding the soft-tissue thickness (commonly 1 mm) followed by an evaluation of the position of attached mucosa relative to the labial and buccal fenum attachments. Using the denture set-up, a radiographic stent is fabricated with radio-opaque markers (e.g. lead foil or round balls) within the denture. This denture is used to evaluate the height and position of the prosthetic teeth relative to the symphyseal cross-sectional anatomy.[16,17]

Table 94.1 Advantages and disadvantages of various implant restorative options

Fixed-detachable prosthesis
Advantages
1. Rigid fixation (non-removable)
2. Dramatic improvement in function
3. Prospective study validation of long-term success
4. Psychological benefits (improved self-image)

Disadvantages
1. Difficult to establish proper phonetics and esthetics in the maxillae
2. Accelerated occlusal wear and excessive loading of the opposing dentition
3. Difficult to clean in patients with limited dexterity
4. High cost and technically sensitive

Removable overdenture prosthesis
Advantages
1. Good control of esthetics and phonetics
2. Improved function with enhanced retention
3. Prospective study validation of long-term success
4. Adaptation of existing prosthetic procedures with initially less expensive and shorter surgical procedures

Disadvantages
1. A removable prosthesis with costly and frequent maintenance
2. Technical difficulties in moderately resorbed ridges
3. Requires adequate salivary flow rates to maintain healthy tissues
4. Component wear (clips, attachments, etc.)

Lekholm & Zarb[18] correlated implant success with the radiographic appearance of the remaining cross-sectional bone by classifying the amount of remaining cortical to cancellous bone (Table 94.2). Implants placed in bone types 1 and 4 have a lower success rate due in part to excessive heat formation (type 1) and insufficient immediate fixation (type 4).[18,19] Since approximately 1 mm of peri-implant bone is rapidly replaced during healing, an implant should be positioned 2 mm or more (measured from the edge of the implant) from living structures (neurovascular bundle, teeth, etc.) and a minimum of 3 mm apart. To insure immediate fixation and long-term stability, an implant length (typically >10 mm) should be selected to engage the inferior cortical plate or the sinus floor. Finally, depending on the implant system chosen, the patient needs to be able to open >35 mm or more at the site of interest in order to allow surgical access for the osteotomy and implant placement.

Table 94.2 Cross-sectional radiographic classification of bone quality[18]

Type 1	Greater than 75% cortical/cancellous bone
Type 2	Thick cortical bone surrounding dense cancellous bone
Type 3	Thin cortical bone surrounding dense cancellous bone (<25% cortical/cancellous bone by volume)
Type 4	Thin cortical bone surrounding low-density cancellous bone

Using the radiographic information, the diagnostic set-up is evaluated for tooth position relative to the remaining bone. Skeletal class I and II relationships with minimal resorption will allow normal contours and lip support with occlusal loading down the long axis of the implants. Prognathic class III relationship can result in increased prosthetic problems (e.g. fractured screws and teeth) along with increased bone loss under the opposing maxillary denture due to an excessive amount of anterior loading. The diagnostic set-up will also determine the degree of anterior–posterior (A–P) spread in implant position.[20–22] The most distal implant is located 2 mm anterior (edge to edge) of the mental foramen on each side and a third is located in the midline. The remaining two are then located equally on both sides. The radiographic analysis should also evaluate the position of the neurovascular bundle as it passes both mesial and then facial before exiting through the mental foramen.[23] The A–P spread is the distance between a line connecting the two most distal implants and a line bisecting the three anterior implants. Due to the fulcrum effect of a cantilever extension, its length is limited to 1–1.5 times the A–P spread.[20] In the class I and II patient, this is typically about 15 mm or less. In contrast, the class III patient commonly has a square-shaped arch resulting in a much smaller A–P spread. This occurs since the distance between the midline implant and the most distal implant on each side is limited by the more anterior position of the mental foramens.[23] The class III situation is more predictably approached with an overdenture to provide posterior occlusion to stabilize the maxillary denture.[7]

The overdenture approach provides significant treatment flexibility for the patient. Two implants spaced 12–16 mm apart (edge to edge) in the canine region can be connected with an occlusogingival 'L'-shaped bar (e.g. Hader bar) with a plastic clip attachment in the denture. Alternatively, free-standing attachments (e.g. system-specific balls or magnets) can be used. In order to provide rotation around the bar upon posterior mucosal contact, the occlusogingival position of the implant should be as equal as possible to allow a horizontal bar that parallels the retromolar pads.[6] Alternatively, where the osseous anatomy is uneven, different abutment heights can be used to accomplish a parallel bar.[6] For biomechanical reasons, cantilevering bar extensions, either off the posterior implant or mesial to the incisal region, should be avoided. This creates a large bending moment on the bar/implant system which can lead to screw and/or bar fracture. In the maxillary arch, full palatal coverage is needed when two implants are used while an open palate design necessitates four or more implants connected with a bar and clip.[12]

IMPLANT TREATMENT PLANNING FOR THE PARTIALLY EDENTULOUS AND SINGLE-TOOTH RESTORATION

Implant-retained fixed partial dentures (FPD) provide patients with an excellent alternative to removable partial dentures while a single-tooth implant is an alternative to a conventional fixed partial denture. The implant FPD must be esthetic for the complete success of this treatment option. This necessitates preoperative planning by the restorative dentist. In the initial evaluation of the patient a number of critical factors must be considered (Table 94.3). As part of informed consent, consideration must be given to the ability to control esthetics and function with a conventional FPD, an adhesive resin restoration or a removable partial denture.

During the diagnostic phase, the number of endosseous-style implants to be used must be determined. High-strength implant and implant components (e.g. type IV commercially pure titanium or Ti-6A1-4V alloy) should be used. This will provide fatigue durability of the materials. In order to provide sufficient load transfer and to avoid overloading the mechanical limits of the implant components, using one implant per replaced posterior tooth has been recommended.[6,24] In the anterior maxillae, replacing four incisors can be accomplished with two implants, one placed in the position of each respective lateral incisor. In the anterior mandible, it is possible to replace two incisors with one fixture. In the posterior maxillae and mandible with sufficient mesiodistal space, a high-strength wide-diameter implant (5–6 mm) can provide increased surface area for osseointegration, greater cortical bone contact, higher frac-

Table 94.3 Factors to consider for implants in the partially edentulous patient

Optimized tooth/teeth position
Resorptive clefts, undercuts, etc. that necessitate preimplant onlay grafting
Trauma-induced bone loss
Anatomic limitations (sinus, neurovascular bundle)
Facial–lingual position of the adjacent teeth
Mesial–distal tooth size/arch length discrepancies
Form and position of the teeth during speech
Smile line, anterior incisal and posterior occlusal plane
Need for lip support
Hard- and soft-tissue periodontal architecture
Periodontal status
Restorative status of the adjacent teeth
Ability to control lateral forces on the prosthesis (canine guidance?)
Signs of parafunctional wear
Prosthesis design (framework design, screw retained versus cemented)
Access for oral hygiene

ture strength and better emergence profile for molar-shaped restorations.[25,26]

Preoperative consideration must be given to the resorptive pattern following tooth extraction. The dentition tends to be positioned facial to the central axis of the alveolar ridge, resulting in a thin facial plate of bone that unevenly resorbs in a palatal and apical direction in the maxillae. In the mandible, this pattern has an uneven rate such that greater bone loss in the thin superior regions results in a wider ridge with high muscle attachments.[27] Using a diagnostic set-up, the optimal tooth position for functional and esthetics purposes is used to determine the potential need for ridge augmentation. In this wax-up, the occlusal scheme must be planned. The occlusion should consist of tooth contacts in centric relation that provides vertical loading down the long axis of the implant(s). Lateral sliding contacts will create large bending or torsional loads which lead to premature failure of mechanical components.[28] In addition, eccentric contacts may have the potential for alteration of the integrated status of the implant(s).[5,6] If external hexed implants are used, they should be positioned in a slightly staggered or tripod arrangement to decrease horizontal bending moments.[11,24,29]

It has been controversial to connect teeth to implants with fixed partial dentures. Patient desires to avoid a removable partial denture with insufficient bone for multiple implants can result in a terminal abutment tooth being connected to a single implant placed in the distal region.[30] In cases where this connection has been with a non-rigid connector, unpredictable incidences of intrusion of the natural tooth have been reported.[11,30–33] This appears to be unrelated to bruxism, periodontal disease or tooth position but has been related to situations where the tooth is non-rigidly connected to the implant.[11] This impaction phenomenon has been suggested to be due to disuse atrophy of the tooth (since the rigid implant conducts most of the load to the osseous interface) or ligament impaction, although the cause is not known.[11,31] Since connecting natural teeth to implants increases the complexity of care and creates a situation where complications with either the tooth (endodontic, periodontal and caries) or the implant (mechanical overloading, screw fracture, etc.) lead to costly remakes, it is generally considered that a completely free-standing implant-retained restoration is the best option. This may mean placing additional implants (one/tooth), using onlay bone or sinus lift grafting and/or using wider diameter implants.[3,6,33]

Implant position in the partially edentulous or single-tooth situation is critical for a predictable esthetic outcome. The proposed site must be evaluated in three dimensions for hard and soft tissue contours using clinical observations in combination with mounted diagnostic casts and a diagnostic wax-up. An implant is the apical extension of the restoration, essentially designed from the 'top down' rather than from the 'bottom up'. Osseous contours can be evaluated by palpation and sounding with anesthesia (e.g. with an endodontic explorer and stopper) coupled with a radiographic exam using a stent containing reference markers (e.g. gutta percha) positioned within a drilled channel(s) parallel to the desired angulation of the implant(s).

At the same time, soft-tissue contours should be evaluated for shape, quantity, texture and color. Notations of these observations can be made directly on the diagnostic wax-up so that the radiographic and surgical stent reflects these critical issues. The periodontal tissues must be in optimal health prior to and during all stages of implant placement. Upon visualization of the soft tissues in the proposed region, compare contours, height and thickness to the contralateral side. The periodontium can be classified into two general groups: a relatively thick, pale, opaque fibrous tissue covering relatively thick flattened osseous plates or a thin, erythematous, translucent tissue covering a thin, scalloped alveolar crest.[34,35] Evaluate the gingiva on the contralateral tooth/teeth for the size, shape and color of the interdental papillae, the arcuate form of the free marginal gingiva, the relative root shape and size (i.e. the emergence profile), the width of attached gingiva and the facial root prominence. The thin, friable periodontium is sensitive to facial and interproximal recession and unesthetic discoloration.[34,36] Thickened fibrous tissue, in contrast, can be sculpted since it forms a deepened sulcus by perirestorative coronal growth following placement of a provisional restoration.[34] These characteristics can obviously have a significant esthetic impact on the final result. Papillae 'saving' incisions have been advocated to help improve the predictability of implant soft-tissue management (Fig. 94.2). Unfortunately, the

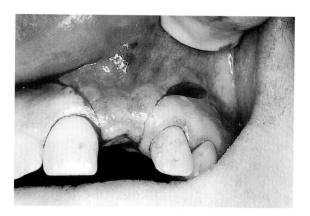

Fig. 94.2 Incision made to preserve interproximal papillae for a screw-retained single-tooth implant placement on the maxillary left central incisor. Wide facial-releasing incisions maintain blood supply to the flap.

gingival response is very difficult to predict preoperatively. For the patient with a thin periodontium and high esthetic expectations, a more predictable restoration may be a conventional or adhesive resin PFM fixed partial denture.

Logically, the placement of implants in the partially edentulous and single-tooth situation demands the use of a surgical stent. During the osteotomy, the stent is a visual statement of the restorative dentist's treatment plan; it is literally a prescription. The particular stent design is often the result of communication, collaboration and familiarity between the surgeon and the restorative dentist. In some cases a simple vacuum matrix (e.g. Omni Vac form) with the occlusal surface removed is sufficient to indicate facial and lingual contours. In cases where the implant position is absolutely critical (e.g. in the esthetic zone or adjacent to vital structures) a hard acrylic resin stent can be made with the implant position(s) and desired angle programmed into it (Fig. 94.3). When a radiographic stent is used for computed tomography (CT scan), radio-opaque gutta percha in the desired implant locations will provide a reference for the desired implant angle and position. Analysis of the individual tomographic images will then provide a means to convert the radiographic stent into a surgical stent.[16] The surgeon uses this stent coupled with his/her clinical skills to prepare the surgical site. One advantage of using the surgical stent made from a diagnostic wax-up is the ability to determine if augmentation (e.g. ramal onlay grafting) is needed to prevent fenestration or dehiscence during implant placement.[3,37] Therefore, the stent should be designed not only with the desired tooth position, contours and angulation, but with the expected soft- and hard-tissue contours necessary for a balanced esthetic gingival profile.

The implant position and angle are dictated in part by the final restoration selected by the restorative dentist (Fig. 94.4). A screw-retained restoration necessitates a more

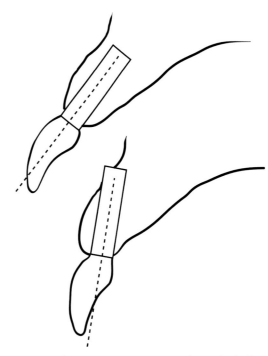

Fig. 94.4 Impact of cement versus screw-retention on implant angulation. If a cement retained restoration is selected the implant can be positioned at a greater angle to the incisal plane (45–65°). If a screw-retention is selected, the implant needs to be in a more perpendicular position to the incisal plane. This can increase the potential for apical fenestration of the implant when there is a thin facial cortical plate.

vertical implant orientation to the occlusal plane which usually results in a more palatal position of the implant head. If the implant is placed excessively to the lingual, an anterior cantilever in the porcelain contours is needed for esthetics. If a cemented restoration is used, the implant is placed at more of an angle (45–65 degrees) to the occlusal plane relatively parallel to the adjacent teeth.[34] The mesiodistal position of the implant must be centered within the central axis of the proposed tooth or teeth in the stent to allow normal esthetic contours (line angles and emergence profile), appropriate gingival contours and control of screw access (Fig. 94.4). For single-tooth applications, adequate interproximal bone is needed. For instance, 8 mm of space is needed to provide for a 4 mm implant having 2 mm bone on each side all the way between the alveolar crest to the root apices (Fig. 94.5). Since 1 mm of peri-implant bone is constantly undergoing modeling/remodeling, at least 1 mm of facial and lingual cortical bone is needed on each side of the implant (Fig. 94.6).[38,39] For proper development of the emergence profile, the implant should be positioned apical to the adjacent teeth. First, consider the position of the soft-tissue thickness and interdental alveolar bone morphology adjacent to the teeth on either side of the proposed site. For a central incisor with a normal gingival attachment, this may mean the head of the

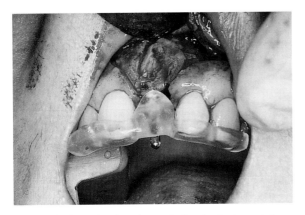

Fig. 94.3 Surgical stent in place demonstrating implant angulation marker through lingual access hole.

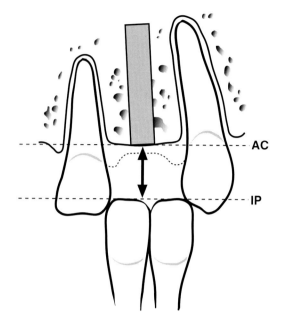

Fig. 94.5 Vertical site selection. A minimum of 7–8 mm of mesiodistal space is needed between teeth (from the height of contour to the apices). Greater than 5 mm of bony vertical height is needed in the mandible and 10–12 mm in the maxillae. A minimum of 7 mm of space (arrow) is needed between the alveolar crest (AC) and the incisal place (IP).

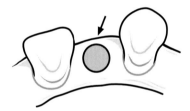

Fig. 94.6 Horizontal site selection. A minimum of 1 mm facial and lingual bone is needed on each side of the implant (arrow). Implants should be greater than 2 mm from adjacent teeth and vital structures along with 3 mm of bone between adjacent implants.

implant is placed 3–4 mm apical to the proximal CEJ (in order to create a transition from the cylindrical implant to the triangular crown) while teeth with round cross-sectional areas (like lateral incisors) can have the implant located 1–2 mm apical to the adjacent CEJs.[3,6,10,34]

The restorative dentist should provisionally select the kind of abutment to be used during the treatment planning stage since the abutment selection will be affected by the amount of vertical space between the crestal bone and the opposing occlusion (Fig. 94.5). For instance, each implant system has minimal heights that can be accommodated by the abutment selected. In the case of the Nobel Biocare system (Westmont, IL), the degree of countersinking of the implant head is dictated by the selected abutment. With the conventional abutment, the minimum ridge (not soft tissue) to occlusal distance is 7 mm. This is slightly less with

the EsthiCone (6.7 mm) or the MirusCone (4.5 mm) while the milled facing for 'UCLA' style direct implant-to-crown abutment has a minimum vertical distance of 3 mm.[3,6,40] Obviously, the determination of ideal implant position and height is based on mounted diagnostic casts, standardized radiographs and clinical examination. Excessive countersinking can result in a restoration that is extremely subgingival, leading to a subgingival environment that is difficult to restoratively manage (impression procedures, cementation, etc.), difficult for the patient to maintain and results in an excessive vertical cantilever. For instance, an excessive vertical cantilever results when the vertical distance from the first screw thread (a common point of stabilized bone remodeling) to an occlusal contact is equal or greater than the length of the implant in bone.[41] This excessive crown length to bone-supported implant leads to rotational bending movements that can cause premature fatigue of the implant components.

Immediate implant placement has been advocated to preserve the residual ridge. A crucial assumption in this approach is that the tooth's position is also the optimal position for the implant. This may not be the case, especially when the tooth was in malocclusion, periodontally involved and/or an effort to decrease the buccal–lingual width of the implant's clinical crown is needed to direct occlusal loading down the long axis of the fixture. Unlike natural teeth, occlusal forces with implants need to be directed down the long axis of the implant rather than the long axis of the crown per se. An alternative to immediate extraction is removal of the tooth followed by the creation of a facial flap and primary closure. Two or three months later, the site is re-entered and an implant placed in the optimal location with the apical two thirds engaged in bone for primary stability.[41,42]

In the partially edentulous and single-tooth situations, the provisional restoration is a key approach to establishing an esthetic and functional result. Following the unloaded healing period, an anatomically contoured provisional restoration should be provided to evaluate esthetics, guide soft-tissue healing, evaluate patient response to treatment and allow a progressive loading of the implant interface (Fig. 94.7).[44-47]

Care in the surgical access to the implant site is important to maintaining the interproximal papillae (see Fig. 94.2). In turn, the placement of an 'anatomic-shaped healing abutment' or custom provisional restoration can be used to guide the healing of the gingival tissues by acting as a template for the approximate emergence architecture of the planned restoration.[47-48] The provisional restoration is critical to the establishment of an esthetic and functional result. In order to maximize the soft-tissue architecture, the provisional

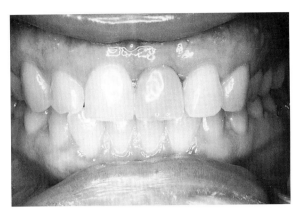

Fig. 94.7 Acrylic resin provisional in place for 8 weeks prior to final impression, allowing the maturation of the gingival architecture.

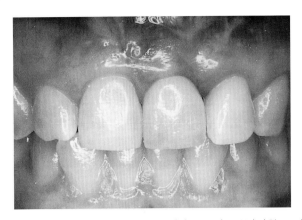

Fig. 94.8 Final all-porcelain crown on tooth (Cera-Adapt Nobel Biocare) demonstrating preservation of interproximal papillae and gingival facial architecture (courtesy of Dr Supanee Buranadham).

restoration can be placed either at the implant uncovering or within a few weeks of stage II. Some restorative dentists request the implant position be transferred to a working model by using an index obtained at implant placement for the laboratory fabrication of a provisional delivered immediately at stage II.[44] In any event, meticulous oral hygiene coupled with the daily use of chlorohexidine rinse (applied to the healing site with a cotton tip applicator or toothbrush) is critical during the first 2 weeks following stage II. Since maturation and stabilization of the gingival contours takes at least 6–8 weeks following the uncovering of the implant, soft-tissue impression procedures should be delayed, especially in critical esthetic areas.[44] Maintaining optimal subgingival health is assisted by using a normal root form for the tooth or teeth to be replaced. Use of appropriate interproximal contacts and gingival embrasure form allows the maturing papillae to adapt to the highly polished acrylic resin of the provisional restoration(s).[47] Thus, the anatomically contoured provisional not only guides soft-tissue healing but also allows for evaluation of esthetics and progressive loading of the implant interface.[4,45,46]

The use of dental implant restorations has revolutionized the relationship between the surgeon and the restorative dentist. Both must be aware of the properties of the implant system chosen and the impact each partner has on the final outcome, the satisfied patient (Fig. 94.8). The role of the restorative dentist is to prescribe the optimal tooth position and prosthesis design based on a complete evaluation of the patient. The surgeon's role is to interpret the prescription and to utilize his/her osseous and soft-tissue restorative skills to establish the objectives of the treatment plan. This is facilitated by ongoing communication of expectations, assumptions and goals by both the restorative dentist and the surgeon.

REFERENCES

1. Adell R, Lekholm U, Rockler B, Branemark P-I 1981 A 15-year study of osseointegrated implants in the treatment of the edentulous jaw. International Journal of Oral Surgery 6:387–416
2. Eckert SE, Laney WR 1989 Patient evaluation and prosthodontic treatment planning for osseointegrated implants. Dental Clinics of North America 33:599–611
3. Haganman CR, Aquilino SA 1996 Restorative implications for optimal implant placement. Oral and Maxillofacial Surgery Clinics of North America 8(3):387–399
4. Stanford CM, Keller JC 1991 The concept of osseointegration and bone matrix expression. Critical Reviews in Oral Biology and Medicine 2(1):83–101
5. Brunski JB 1991 Influence of biomechanical factors at the bone–biomaterial interface. In: Davies JE (ed) The bone-biomaterial interface. University of Toronto Press, Toronto
6. Engelman MJ 1996 Clinical decision making and treatment planning in osseointegration. Quintessence Publishing, Chicago
7. Naert IE 1997 Patient evaluation and treatment planning. Journal of Dentistry 25 (suppl. 1):S5–S11
8. Mericke-Stern R, Zarb G A 1993 Overdentures: an alternative implant methodology for edentulous patients. International Journal of Prosthodontics 6:203–208
9. Naert I, Quiyynen M, Hooghe M, van Steenberghe D 1994 A comparative prospective study of splinted and unsplinted Brånemark implants in mandibular overdenture therapy: a preliminary report. Journal of Prosthetic Dentistry 71:486–492
10. Parel S, Sullivan DY 1989 Considerations for optimal esthetics. In: Parel S, Sullivan D Y Esthetics and osseointegration. Taylor Publishing Co, Dallas
11. Parel S 1996 Prosthesis design and treatment planning for the partially edentulous implant patient. Journal of Oral Implant 22(1):31–33
12. Lewis S, Sharma A, Nishimura R 1992 Treatment of edentulous maxillae with osseointegrated implants. Journal of Prosthetic Dentistry 68(3):503–508
13. Carr AB, Laney WR 1987 Maximum occlusal force levels in patients with osseointegrated oral implant prosthesis and patients with complete dentures. International Journal of Oral and Maxillofacial Implants 2(2):101–108
14. Feine JS, de Grandmont P, Boudrias P et al 1994 Within-subject comparisons of implant-supported mandibular prosthesis: choice of prosthesis. Journal of Dental Research 73(5):1105–1111

15. De Grandmont P, Feine JS, Tache R et al 1994 Within-subject comparisons of implant-supported mandibular prosthesis: psychometric evaluation. Journal of Dental Research 73(5):1096–1104

16. Duckmanton NA, Austin BW, Lechner SK, Klineberg IL 1994 Imaging for predictable maxillay implants. International Journal of Prosthodentics 7:77–80

17. Lechner S, Klineberg I, Duckmanton N 1992 Prosthodontic procedures for implant reconstruction. 1. Diagnostic procedures. Australian Dental Journal 37(5):353–359

18. Lekholm U, Zarb GA 1985 Patient selection and preparation. In: Branemark P-I, Albrektsson T, Zarb GA (eds) Tissue integrated prosthesis. Osseointegration in clinical dentistry. Quintessence, Chicago

19. Jaffin RA, Berman CL 1991 The excessive loss of Branemark fixtures in type IV bone: a 5 year analysis. Journal of Periodontology 62:2–4

20. English CE 1992 The critical A-P spread. Implant Society 3:14–15

21. Skalak R 1983 Biomechanical considerations in osseointegrated prostheses. Journal of Prosthetic Dentistry 49:843–848

22. McAlarney ME, Stavropoulos DN 1996 Determination of cantilever length-anterior–posterior spread ratio assuming failure criteria to be the compromise of the prosthesis retaining screw-prosthesis joint. International Journal of Oral Maxillofacial Implants 11(3):331–339

23. Wadu SG, Penhall B, Townsend GC 1997 Morphological variability of the human inferior alveolar nerve. Clinical Anatomy 10(2):82–87

24. Hansen CA, DeBoer J, Woolsey GD 1992 Esthetic and biomechanical considerations in reconstructions using dental implants. Dental Clinices of North America 36(3):713–741

25. Langer B, Langer L, Herrmann I, Jorneus L 1993 The wide fixture: a solution for special bone situations and a rescue for the compromised implant Part I. International Journal of Oral and Maxillofacial Implants 8:400–408

26. Lazzara RJ 1994 Criteria for implant selection: surgical and prosthetic considerations. Practical Periodontics and Aesthetic Dentistry 6(9):55–62

27. Mecall RA, Rosenfeld AL 1991 The influence of residual ridge resorption patterns on implant fixture placement and tooth position. Part I. International Journal of Periodontics and Restorative Dentistry 11:8–23

28. Weinberg LA 1993 The biomechanics of force distribution in implant-supported prosthesis. International Journal of Oral and Maxillofacial Implants 8(1):19–31

29. Rangert B, Sullivan R 1995 Learning from history: the transition from full arch to posterior partial restorations. Nobelpharma News 9(2):6–7

30. English CE 1993 Biomechanical concerns with fixed partial dentures involving implants. Implant Dentistry 2(4):221–242

31. Parel SM 1993 Intrusion of natural tooth implant bridge abutments: its cause and effect on treatment planning of the partially edentulous patient. Australian Prosthodontics Journal 7:33–38

32. Gunne J, Astrand P, Ahlen K, Borg K, Olsson M 1992 Implants in partially edentulous patients: a longitudinal study of bridges supported by both implants and natural teeth. Clinical Oral Implant Research 3:49–56

33. English CE 1993 Root intrusion in tooth-implant combination cases. Implant Dentistry 2(2):79–85

34. Jansen CE, Weisgold A 1995 Presurgical treatment planning for the anterior single-tooth implant restoration. Compendium 16(8):746–762

35. Olsson M, Lindhe J 1991 Periodontal characteristics in individuals with varying forms of the upper central incisors. Journal of Clinical Periodontics 18:78–82

36. Bahat O, Daftary F 1995 Surgical reconstruction – a prerequisite for long-term implant success: a philosophic approach. Practical Periodontics and Aesthetic Dentistry 7(9):21–31

37. Bahat O, Fontanesi RV, Preston J 1993 Reconstruction of the hard and soft tissues for optimal placement of osseointegrated implants. International Journal of Periodontics and Restorative Dentistry 13:255–275

38. Garetto LP, Chen J, Parr JA, Roberts WE 1995 Remodeling dynamics of bone supporting rigidly fixed titanium implants: a histomorphometric comparison in four species including humans. Implant Dentistry 4:235–243

39. Brunski JB, Hoshaw SJ 1994 Bone modeling and remodeling in relation to maintenance of attachment at bone-dental implant interfaces. In: Davidovitch Z(ed) The biological mechanisms of tooth eruption, resorption and replacement by implants. Harvard University Press, Boston

40. Lewis S, Beumer J, Perri GR, Hornburg WP 1988 Single tooth implant supported restorations. International Journal of Oral and Maxillofac Implants 3(1):25–30

41. Katona TR, Goodacre CJ, Brown DT, Roberts WE 1993 Force-moment systems on single maxillary anterior implants: effects of incisal guidance, fixture orientation and loss of bone support. International Journal of Oral and Maxillofacial Implants 8(5):512–522

42. Garber DA 1996 The esthetic dental implant: letting restoration be the guide. Journal of Oral Implants 22(1):45–50

43. Tarnow D, Fletcher P 1993 The 2–3 month post-extraction placement of root form implants: a useful compromise. Implant Clinical Reviews for Dentistry 2:1–8

44. Touati B 1995 Improving aesthetics of implant-supported restorations. Practical Periodontics and Aesthetic Dentistry 7(9):81–92

45. Stanford C 1994 Biocompatibility, tissue responses and the concept of the interface. In: Worthington P, Lang BR, LaVelle WE (eds) Osseointegration in dentistry: an introduction. Quintessence, Chicago

46. Johansson C, Albrektsson T 1987 Integration of screw implants in the rabbit: a 1-year follow-up of removal torque of titanium implants. International Journal of Oral and Maxillofacial Implants 2:69–75

47. Neale D, Chee WW 1994 Use of provisionals to determine the contour of definitive implant restorations. Journal of Prosthetic Dentistry 71:364–368

48. Bichacho N 1997 Prosthetically guided soft tissue topography surrounding single implant restorations: cervical contouring concept. International Dental Symposium 4:30–35

Avoiding and managing complications in minor oral surgery

STEPHEN F. WORRALL

95

In all things success depends upon previous preparation, and without such preparation there is sure to be failure. (Confucius 550–c 478BC)

INTRODUCTION

The majority of complications involve the operative site and may occur perioperatively or postoperatively. The prevention and management of these categories of complications is the subject of this chapter. While most complications are fortunately minor, occasionally major life-threatening systemic complications such as a respiratory or cardiac arrest will occur. These medical emergencies are often totally unexpected and likely to become more common as the general age of the population increases and more patients with severe underlying medical conditions require oral surgical procedures. It is beyond the scope of this chapter to cover in detail the necessary precautions needed for and the management of patients with complicating medical and dental histories and the reader is referred to the many excellent texts available that cover this subject in depth.[1,2]

In many ways the term 'minor oral surgery' is unfortunate and misleading as it implies that the procedure to be performed is simple and that postoperative sequelae are negligible. It may also give the false impression that less skill and care are required than for the performance of 'major oral surgery'. This is a dangerous misconception. There can be few experienced oral and maxillofacial surgeons who have not been humbled by a lowly third molar tooth. Moreover, complications following such surgery are poorly tolerated by patients whose expectation is that minor surgery should not produce major morbidity.

Following the axiom that prevention is better than cure, the best way to manage complications is not to produce them in the first place. For while a few complications following minor oral surgery are truly unavoidable, most can and should be prevented.

PREOPERATIVE ASSESSMENT AND TREATMENT PLANNING

It is a *sine qua non* of all medical and surgical practice that the clinician must be in possession of the requisite expertise and skill to perform the scheduled procedure. The wise surgeon is aware of any personal limitations in this area and will not elect to perform any operation beyond his or her capabilities. To a certain extent and with some qualifications, this principle may also be applied to managing complications. If a surgeon lacks the ability to remove a fractured and retained root or close an oroantral fistula then one must seriously question the wisdom of embarking on the extraction of the tooth in the first place. Furthermore, all but the simplest of procedures will require the help of a skilled and knowledgeable assistant. This is particularly important for junior surgeons in training who are all too often left to 'finish the list' with only the theater scrub nurse to act as first assistant.

Medical history taking and resuscitation training

The majority of patients who are at increased risk of developing surgical and medical complications should be identified preoperatively following the taking of a comprehensive medical and dental history which should be updated at each subsequent visit. Specific questions should be asked concerning previous cardiac and respiratory diseases, pregnancy, diabetes, excessive bleeding following minor injuries, current and past drug therapy including anticoagulants and steroids, previous local and general anesthetic experience and drug allergies. A history of difficult extractions, postextraction hemorrhage and radiotherapy to the operative area should be taken seriously.

Obviously, the management of the more serious complications of minor oral surgery will be beyond the capability of the relatively inexperienced surgeon, especially if they occur outwith the hospital environment where there is ready access to all the necessary equipment, drugs and support services. In this situation the operating surgeon has a duty of care to the patient to recognize that a complication has arisen and to consult with or refer the patient to a more experienced colleague (usually the local consultant oral and maxillofacial surgeon) for advice and treatment. Depending on the severity of the problem, referral via the telephone rather than the traditional letter may be more appropriate. To err is human but failure to recognize the error and take immediate and appropriate action to remedy it is negligent.

It is essential that all those directly involved in treating patients are fully conversant with the theory and practice of basic life support and resuscitation. This applies to the surgeon who only ever treats patients under local anesthetic as well as those who routinely employ sedation or general anesthesia in their practice. Once learned, basic life support skills must be regularly practiced by the entire surgical team until everyone is fully conversant with their individual roles. Emergency medical and resuscitation equipment must be regularly checked, maintained and serviced.

Simple and seemingly obvious measures such as keeping a list of emergency service contact numbers by the telephone, which should ideally be in the patient treatment area, can save valuable and potentially life-saving minutes should a patient suffer a cardiac arrest.

Surgical equipment

Most minor oral surgical procedures do not require large numbers of instruments. Nonetheless, before embarking on the procedure the surgeon must be satisfied that all the equipment necessary to complete the procedure safely and deal with any complications commensurate with their experience is available, clean and sterile. Perhaps one of the most often neglected items of surgical kit is the operating light. A light that is just adequate to visualize a lower third molar may be totally inadequate when one's attention turns to removing the opposing partially erupted upper third molar, especially if bone needs to be removed in order to facilitate tooth delivery. Lack of adequate lighting can make an otherwise straightforward procedure difficult and a difficult procedure almost impossible. Similar consideration should be given to the suction apparatus to be used. In the United States clinicians are required to have some form of suction apparatus available at all times and also to have a back-up

battery supply in case of mains power failure. While a low-volume salivary aspirator may easily deal with the minimal bleeding consequent on raising a mucoperiosteal flap it will be unable to cope with the sometimes alarming hemorrhage that can arise from a severed nutrient vessel or inferior alveolar artery. The threat to the patient's airway and the likely consequences are obvious.

Radiographs

If damage to vital structures is to be avoided the surgeon must have a very clear understanding of the anatomy of the operative area, including the presence of any local variations that may complicate an otherwise normal procedure (Fig. 95.1). Only then can a surgical treatment plan be produced. This process must take place prior to each and every operative procedure to be performed. Minor oral surgical procedures involving the hard tissues require that information derived from clinical examination of the patient is supplemented by preoperative imaging. For the most part, this means plain radiographs of the area. It is axiomatic that radiographs must show the area to be operated on and they must also be of good quality to enable the differentiation of adjacent structures from each other. A radiograph showing a third molar that is blurred, overexposed and streaked is worse than useless and basing an operation on such a radiograph is foolhardy. For apicectomies an intra-oral radiograph is acceptable providing it also shows the apices of the adjacent teeth on either side of the index tooth. If an apicectomy is to be performed and a cyst enucleated, the entire cyst outline should be visible on the planning radiograph. Radiographs of lower third molars must show:[3,4]

- the entire third molar and hence the type of impaction;
- the entire configuration of the second and first molars if present;

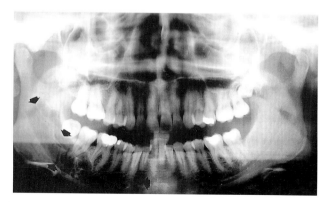

Fig. 95.1 Extensive intrabony arteriovenous malformation in right mandibular body and ramus (courtesy of P J Leopard FDSRCS, FRCS).

- the immediate investing bone and the entire pericoronal space;
- the relationship of the third molar tooth/roots to the neurovascular canal;
- the presence and extent of any associated pathologic changes.

In the majority of situations these requirements will preclude the sole use of the intraoral periapical radiograph for preoperative planning of lower third molar extractions. The use of survey radiographs such as the lateral oblique view and rotational tomography allows these requirements to be met.[3]

The orthopantomogram (OPT) is probably the commonest type of rotational tomogram in use in the United Kingdom and provides an excellent view of all the teeth and related structures on one film. A preoperative OPT or equivalent radiograph is a mandatory investigation prior to extracting any lower third molar, regardless of its eruption status and type of impaction. If there is any doubt over the relationship of the tooth to the neurovascular canal on the preoperative OPT, a high-quality intraoral radiograph of the area should also be obtained. Although perhaps not essential, it is a wise precaution to obtain a radiograph prior to extracting any tooth if unpleasant surprises are to be minimized. Again, the OPT is ideal for this purpose. All radiographs should be indelibly marked with the patient's name or case note number and thoroughly checked to ensure that they are correctly orientated with respect to right and left.

Local anesthesia

Where a local anesthetic is to be given, as with all drugs it is vital to ensure that the solution is unused and not past its expiry date. An aspirating syringe or technique should be used in all cases to avoid intravascular injections. For local anesthetic infiltrations into the periodontal ligament, it is important to use a specially designed syringe that not only delivers small increments of solution but also fully encloses the glass cartridge. Using a normal dental syringe for ligamentous injections will frequently result in fracture or explosion of the local anesthetic cartridge due to the high pressures generated. The dangers to patient and surgeon alike from flying glass are obvious and avoidable.

Occasionally, patients are labeled as being 'resistant' to local anesthetics. This usually centers around failure to achieve surgical analgesia with an inferior alveolar nerve block. Once local infection has been excluded as a cause of failure to achieve surgical analgesia, the commonest cause is faulty technique. If the surgeon is sure that his or her technique is correct, it is likely that there is a local anatomic variation in the region of the lingula. This may be due to an abnormally high or low foramen or the lingula itself may be larger than normal, presenting a physical barrier to the hypodermic needle. Close inspection of the OPT in the region of the lingula will usually show the problem. Thereafter, slight variation in technique, usually injecting a centimeter or so higher, resolves the problem.

If after repositioning the syringe and repeating the injection, surgical analgesia is still not achieved, in order to avoid unwanted toxicity and possible cardiac complications it is important that the surgeon does not continue to inject more and more anesthetic in the blind hope of success. The maximum safe dose of lignocaine containing a vasoconstrictor is 7.0 mg/kg (0.35 ml/kg of a 2% solution) and the total dose of adrenaline should not exceed 200 μg (16 ml of a 1:80 000 solution).[2]

OBTAINING PATIENT CONSENT

Prior to performing any operative procedure the surgeon must obtain the patient's consent for treatment. Failure to obtain consent will leave the surgeon open to a claim for negligence and possible criminal prosecution for battery. Consent must be given voluntarily and the patient must be capable of understanding the proposed treatment, have been appropriately informed beforehand and given the opportunity to ask any questions regarding their treatment.[5] In some circumstances this may require an interpreter to be present and for multilingual information and consent sheets to be available.

It is vital to understand that obtaining consent does not mean simply requesting the patient's verbal permission to submit themselves to treatment. In order for a patient to adequately consent to an operation or treatment, he or she must be fully informed and in possession of and understand the likely consequences and any complications of that treatment. Moreover, it is extremely important that the patient is made fully aware of the advantages and disadvantages of any alternative management strategies to the planned treatment. In many cases this may include no treatment at all. The type of anesthetic to be used and any possible side effects and complications such as drug reactions and phlebitis must also be fully discussed with the patient when obtaining consent.

If a patient suffers a complication of a procedure which he was not warned about preoperatively, without suggesting negligence, the surgeon may be sued for breach of his duty of care to the patient.[5]

Much debate has taken place concerning which complications patients should be explicitly warned about. It has been suggested that patients should be specifically warned about any complication that occurs with a minimum frequency of between 1% and 10%.[6] However, it is currently accepted that patients should receive specific warnings about any temporary condition that occurs in 5% or more of cases and any permanent condition that occurs in 0.5% of cases.[7] This means that all patients should be warned about the risks of postoperative pain, bleeding, bruising, swelling and limitation of function. Patients undergoing lower third molar removal must be warned about the risk of lingual and inferior alveolar nerve anesthesia, paresthesia and dysesthesia. It is thus of some concern that a recent study showed that 4% of UK oral and maxillofacial surgeons did not routinely warn their patients about possible nerve damage following lower third molar surgery.[8]

Similarly, patients undergoing procedures in the territory of the terminal divisions of the facial nerve such as skin biopsies, botulinum toxin injections for masseteric hypertrophy and arthrocentesis/arthroscopy, etc. must be warned about the possibility of permanent facial weakness. It is also important to ensure that patients (especially those caring for young children at home) are aware that they may well need to take leave of absence from work and require help and support for several days postoperatively.

Unfortunately, although giving verbal warnings as outlined above will ensure that the surgeon complies with the 'letter of the law', they may not be sufficient to ensure that he or she complies with the 'spirit of the law'. Almost 50% of patients may fail to recall being verbally warned about at least one complication postoperatively.[5] Patient recall of preoperative warnings and, by implication, the extent to which their consent was fully informed can be increased by the use of written information to supplement the standard verbal warnings.[9,10] Audio and video tapes can also be used during the consultation and while obtaining patient consent. These have the benefit of standardization and ensuring that all the points deemed to be relevant are covered for every patient.

It is important that consent is obtained from the patient not only preoperatively but also in quiet surroundings, before any drugs have been administered and in an area remote from that where the procedure is to be performed.[11] This means that it is unacceptable for a patient to be interviewed and consented by the operating surgeon in the anesthetic room immediately prior to the operation being performed.

The clinician charged with obtaining the patient's consent must have a clear understanding of the procedure to be performed and the possible complications in order to be able to adequately answer patients' questions and concerns. This task is frequently delegated to the most junior member of the team who is often too inexperienced to obtain fully

informed patient consent and has probably never been instructed on the medicolegal requirements of doing so.[12] When completing the proposed treatment section of the consent form, the clinician must always consult the relevant sections in the patient's case notes to be certain that the patient is being consented for the intended treatment. One must never rely on operating theater lists or departmental theater books, etc. for this information. All too often these records will be incorrect due to typographical or transcription errors. If there is any doubt concerning the exact nature of the treatment proposed, the supervising clinician, usually the consultant oral and maxillofacial surgeon, should be consulted.

Everyone involved in obtaining patient consent in the UK should read and understand the National Health Service Executive document *A guide to consent for examination and treatment.*[13]

Children under the age of 16 years (18 in the United States unless the patient is married) may give or withhold their consent for treatment without recourse to their parent or guardian if the clinician believes that they are mentally capable of making an informed decision. Whenever the clinician is not satisfied that a child is able to fully understand the proposed procedures and their complications, consent must be sought from the child's parent or legal guardian except in emergency situations where there is insufficient time to obtain it.[13] In exceptional circumstances and after full discussion with the child's parents in the presence of a witness, if the clinician believes that a parent's refusal to give consent for treatment is likely to prejudice the continuing health of the child, he or she may seek to have the child made a ward of court and request consent from a judge. If time does not permit this process, then the surgeon in charge of the child's care (normally the consultant oral and maxillofacial surgeon) should seek and obtain a written report from a consultant colleague supporting the view that the child's life would be in danger if treatment were to be withheld. Where adult patients lack the mental capacity to give informed consent no one may give consent on their behalf although the law allows treatment to be performed provided it can be demonstrated to be in the best interests of the patient. Such treatments should be discussed with the patient's next of kin where possible but ultimately the decision to proceed with treatment rests with the clinician in charge of the patient's care.

Provided the surgeon follows the above procedures and is demonstrably acting in the patient's best interests, it is unlikely that their actions will be criticized by a court or their professional body.[13] Indeed, in certain circumstances failing to provide necessary treatment may be construed as negligent. If time permits, the surgeon would be wise to consult his or her medical indemnity association to seek expert legal guidance before commencing any treatment for which the patient's written consent has not been obtained.

Having obtained fully informed consent, all warnings and explanations given should be recorded in the case notes and the patient or parent requested to sign a consent form stating that they have been informed of and understand the nature and likely consequences of the procedure. Specimen consent forms which conform to the above standards and guidelines are available for patients being treated within the UK National Health Service.[13] A patient's signature on a consent form in the absence of having obtained fully informed consent is no protection in law against a claim for failing in one's duty of care to the patient.

FINAL CHECKS

Not infrequently, patients will have been on a waiting list for some time prior to their operation. It is vitally important to check that the problem for which they are about to be operated on has not resolved and no longer requires treatment or that the original signs and symptoms have not altered such as to present a different diagnosis and treatment plan to the original ones. In this situation, and if operative treatment is still indicated, the entire process of obtaining informed consent should be repeated.

Written consent should be contemporary with the treatment to be undertaken and where it has been obtained some time in the past, it should be repeated. In the United States some hospitals have their own rules on the appropriate timing of consent prior to treatment although it is left up to the discretion of the individual surgeon when working from his or her own office.

Immediately prior to making the initial incision or the application of forceps and elevators to a tooth, the operating surgeon must recheck the patient's notes and consent form to ensure that the correct procedure is about to be performed at the correct site and on the correct patient! This is particularly important where the operating surgeon is not the person who obtained the patient's consent. Where multiple teeth are to be extracted and in every case of extractions for orthodontic purposes, it is wise for the surgeon to clearly note the teeth to be extracted on a chart or wall board that is legible from the chair/table side to act as a final check before proceeding to extract each and every tooth.

It is imperative that there is adequate surgical access to and exposure of the operative site. Incisions must enable the operator to fully and safely visualize the entire operative area with minimal need for tissue retraction and be sited with due regard to surrounding vital structures and esthetics. All other things being equal, an incision 2 cm long will heal as well and as quickly as one 1 cm long. It thus makes little sense to operate through a 'keyhole' as this will increase the risk of damage to surrounding tissues as a result of traction and tearing.

It should be remembered, particularly by junior surgeons in training, that the operating surgeon is ultimately responsible morally and legally for his or her own actions. This is especially relevant in the hospital setting where, not infrequently, the surgeon performing the operation is not the one who obtained the patient's consent.[8]

On completion of the operation all extracted teeth, roots, instruments, needles and swabs must be accounted for to ensure nothing has been left in the surgical wound. Where a throat pack has been placed preoperatively in order to protect the airway it is the surgeon's responsibility to ensure that this has been removed, to directly inform the anesthetist that he or she has done so and to ensure that it has been recorded in the patient's operation notes. Failure to follow this protocol will one day result in a patient suffering a respiratory arrest shortly after extubation with potentially fatal consequences.

Before discussing individual complications in more detail, it is worth stating that even in the best and most experienced of hands accidents will happen and operations will go wrong. In these situations, having expedited all necessary measures and treatment commensurate with the surgeon's skill and experience, it is vital that every detail is recorded in chronological order and dated in the patient's case notes. Once recorded, alterations to the original entries must not be made. The patient must be fully informed of what has happened, why it happened and the steps that have and will be taken to remedy the situation. In all things, 'honesty is the best policy' and many medicolegal claims can be averted by adopting this strategy.

PERIOPERATIVE COMPLICATIONS

EXTRACTION OF THE WRONG TOOTH

Extraction of the wrong tooth is an avoidable error which can easily be prevented by ensuring that proper identification of the patient and tooth to be extracted is made.[14] Teeth commonly extracted in error are upper canines instead of upper first premolars, lower permanent premolars simultaneously with lower deciduous molars and upper second molars instead of upper third molars. The latter is particularly liable to occur if the upper third molar is partially erupted and difficult to visualize. Being aware of the possibility of these errors and 'counting out' the tooth to be extracted will go some way to minimizing their occurrence. A common source of confusion is the correct identification of one of two molar teeth when the other molar is missing or absent. Although a naming convention exists for just this situation, long-hand notation such as 'the first standing lower right molar' instead of the lower right 7 or 47 may help avoid confusion where the third molar is erupted and the first molar is absent. A similar situation occurs when only one of two unerupted and adjacent teeth is to be extracted. Again, this is commonly requested as part of an orthodontic treatment plan and as such should be avoided at all costs (Figs 95.2, 95.3).

If the wrong tooth is extracted the surgeon should proceed with removing the correct tooth unless the extractions are for orthodontic purposes when it may be better to seek the advice of the patient's orthodontist first. The tooth extracted in error, particularly if it is otherwise healthy, should be immediately replaced in its socket. If mobile, it should be held in place with a custom-made vacuum-formed splint for approximately 4 weeks.[14] It is likely that it will subsequently need to be root filled and if there is any doubt about its prognosis, the advice of a consultant restorative dentist should be sought.

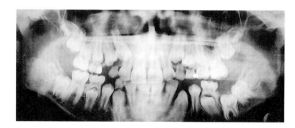

Fig. 95.2 Preoperative OPT. Extraction of the buried lower left first permanent molar had been requested by the patient's orthodontist to facilitate eruption of the unerupted lower left second permanent molar.

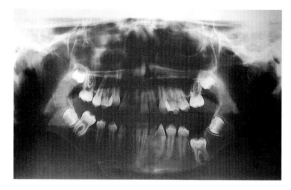

Fig. 95.3 One-year postoperative OPT of the same patient as in Fig. 95.1. The lower left first permanent molar is still present and unerupted. The lower left second permanent molar has been extracted in error, accounting for its 'failure to erupt'.

FRACTURED AND DAMAGED TEETH AND RESTORATIONS

Teeth adjacent to the index tooth may be fractured, loosened in their sockets, subluxed or even extracted by the injudicious application and use of elevators. This is particularly likely to occur if the adjacent tooth rather than the interradicular bone is used as a fulcrum for the elevator and the elevator is being used as a lever against the adjacent tooth. Fracture of the distal root of the upper second molar during elevation of an impacted upper third molar may occur following excessive use of force consequent on inadequate bone removal.

Damage to adjacent tooth roots can occur during bone removal performed for apicectomies and surgical extractions. Close inspection of the preoperative radiographs and noting the long axis of the tooth to be operated on is vital if only the bone overlying the index tooth is to be removed. Special care should be paid to apicectomies on previously post-crowned teeth. Not uncommonly, the long axis of the crown will be divergent from the long axis of the root. If this is not appreciated preoperatively, extensive bone removal in an area distant to the index root apex may be performed and the wrong root apicected. Root apices may be very close together, particularly in the mandibular and maxillary incisor regions. Close attention must be paid to crown/root orientation when apicecting these teeth if collateral damage is to be avoided. Frequently, a sinus will perforate the buccal plate acting as a guide to the site of the root apex beneath it.

Opposing teeth and restorations may be damaged if excessive force is applied to a tooth via forceps or elevators and the tooth suddenly 'gives', resulting in the instrument forcibly contacting teeth in the opposing jaw. Not uncommonly, the distal box of a restoration or an overhanging ledge on an inlay or crown in a lower second molar will be dislodged if the adjacent lower third molar is elevated against it. If possible the restoration should be attended to by the patient's dental surgeon before the third molar is removed. If a restoration is dislodged it is vital that all debris is thoroughly removed from the extraction socket and the tooth dressed with a temporary restoration until such time as it can be made permanent.

Fracture of a tooth or root during exodontia is the commonest complication encountered in minor oral surgery.[3,14] Poor extraction technique, in particular using the wrong extraction forceps, applying the forceps too close to the amelo-cemental junction and too far from the root apex and injudicious use of elevators are undoubtedly the major causes of tooth/root fractures during exodontia. This complication is thus inversely proportional to the experience of the operator. Indeed, complications of all types following the surgical removal of impacted third molars have been reported to be significantly higher when performed by less experienced surgeons.[15] There is thus a strong case to be made for suggesting that ambulatory oral surgery operating lists should be performed by the most senior clinician available if unnecessary complications and unplanned hospital admissions are to be avoided.

Simple exodontia involving forceps and elevators depends on the ability of the index tooth to expand the bony tooth socket walls to facilitate its own delivery. If the alveolar bone is too dense to allow sufficient expansion to occur or the tooth roots are too brittle to expand the bone, failure is assured. In some cases the age, sex, racial origin and physique of the patient may alert the surgeon to the possibility of a difficult extraction although in community-dwelling adults, age is not a risk factor for complications following simple extractions.[16] Patients with a history of 'difficult extractions' often have non-vital and brittle teeth surrounded by dense unyielding bone. These 'glass in concrete' teeth are also better tackled via an elective transalveolar approach. Even then the surgeon may have to use the burr to cut out every last fragment of tooth root due to repeated fractures when elevators are applied.

If preoperative radiographs have not been taken the surgeon will be unaware of the teeth that have grossly curved, divergent, dilacerated, hypercementosed or fused roots. Attempting simple forceps extraction of such teeth will inevitably result in failure to complete the procedure or severe collateral damage. Where these dental conditions are diagnosed on a preoperative radiograph, the surgeon will be forewarned of the problem and can take appropriate measures to circumvent complications. For the most part this will involve electing to remove the tooth via a transalveolar approach following judicious removal of overlying buccal bone (Fig. 95.4).

As a general rule all fractured roots should be removed as soon as they are produced. However, it is important to realize that in some circumstances root removal may do more harm than good, particularly if they are close to structures such as the neurovascular canal, maxillary sinus and lingual plate of the mandible. Small apices, especially if associated with a previously vital and uninfected root, can be safely retained.[17] The advice of the Arabian physician Avicenna (AD 980–1037), 'The cure of a disease must never be worse than the disease itself', is particularly relevant here. If it is elected to leave a root in situ the patient should be informed and the reasons for the decision documented in their case notes.

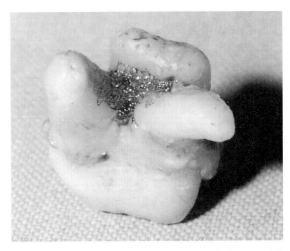

Fig. 95.4 Fully erupted upper third molar with a markedly curved distal root delivered via an elective transalveolar approach.

TOOTH DISPLACEMENT

Instead of the tooth being delivered safely from its socket into the mouth, it may be displaced into any one of a number of potentially hazardous areas including:

- the maxillary sinus
- tissue spaces
- inferior dental canal
- aerodigestive tract.

The maxillary sinus

The apices of the upper premolars and molars are normally close to the floor of the maxillary sinus. Uncontrolled upward pressure from extraction forceps or elevators may force a tooth into the sinus. This is particularly prone to occur with conical single-rooted premolars and the palatal roots of molars, especially when a Coupland elevator is forcibly inserted up the periodontal ligament. If a tooth is displaced into the sinus it is imperative that it is removed as soon as possible. If the tooth cannot be readily visualized then radiographs of the area in two planes at 90 degrees to each other should be taken to locate it (Fig. 95.5, 95.6). The transalveolar route should then be used and the tooth/root delivered into the mouth via inferiorly directed pressure from a suitable elevator. If there is to be any appreciable delay in removal, broad-spectrum antibiotics should be prescribed to minimize the risk of infection and subsequent breakdown of the mucosal repair.

Tissue spaces

It is usually the third molars that fall victim to displacement into adjacent tissue spaces. Unerupted upper third

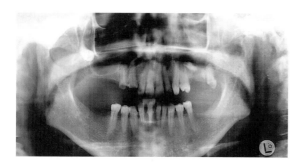

Fig. 95.5 OPT radiograph demonstrating displacement of the upper left second premolar into the left maxillary sinus.

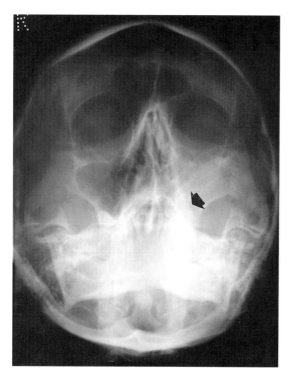

Fig. 95.6 Occipitomental radiograph of the same patient as in Fig. 95.5 confirming the upper left second premolar to be lying within the cavity of the left maxillary sinus.

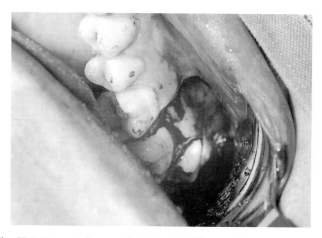

Fig. 95.7 Unerupted upper left third molar following elevation of a buccal mucoperiosteal flap and bone removal. The potential for posterior displacement is obvious.

arguably the most useful instrument in this situation as not only does it physically prevent the upper third molar being displaced posteriorly but it also forms a light-reflective guide channel for the elevator, thus improving visibility and protecting the soft tissues of the lip and commissure which are frequently injured during this maneuver (Fig. 96.8).

Lower teeth are less prone to displacement than uppers but they can be so affected. Lingually placed lower third molars and their roots may occasionally be pushed through a thin or absent lingual plate into the floor of the mouth or below the mylohyoid, from where they can migrate into the neck. Similarly, lingually placed lower premolars, particularly when unerupted, may be displaced into the lingual tissues. The latter situation is prone to occur if these teeth are 'tapped out lingually' using a mallet and elevator. On occasions, direct upwards digital pressure below the mandible will bring the displaced tooth or root into sight and

molars in particular are at risk from this complication but no tooth is immune. The majority of upper third molars have a natural path of withdrawal that takes them posteriorly and inferiorly. When the tooth is erupted this will usually ensure safe delivery into the mouth. However, when the tooth is unerupted and a buccal mucoperiosteal flap has been elevated the tooth may slip behind the maxillary tuberosity and into the pterygomaxillary space from where it may migrate into the deep structures of the neck (Fig. 96.7). To prevent this potentially disastrous situation occurring, it is imperative that an instrument is always placed behind the upper third molar which is kept under direct vision at all times during its extraction. The Laster retractor, inserted around the back of the tuberosity, is

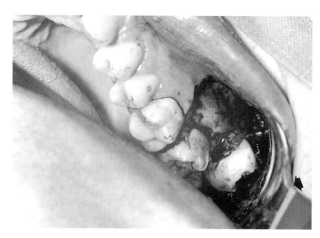

Fig. 95.8 The Laster flap retractor (arrow) provides excellent visibility, prevents posterior displacement of the upper third molar and protects the soft tissues during delivery of the tooth.

facilitate its removal. As with displaced upper teeth, it is vital that the position of the lost tooth or root is located via radiographs before attempting extirpation unless it can be easily and directly visualized immediately postdisplacement, for fear of exacerbating the situation. Radiographs in two planes at 90 degrees should be taken and a lower occlusal and OPT are the radiographs of choice. If the situation cannot be rectified immediately the patient should be placed on antibiotics and referred to a consultant oral and maxillofacial surgeon for urgent assessment and treatment. It may be possible to remove the tooth or root via a standard transalveolar approach but more often the floor of mouth or even extraoral route will be required, depending on its position.

Inferior dental canal

If lower molar roots are fractured during elevation and the decision is taken to proceed with their removal, it is important that they are lifted out of the socket rather than displaced further into its depths by the incorrect use and application of elevators. Overzealous use of the Cryer elevator in particular can gouge out the roof of the inferior dental (ID) canal into which the root can be subsequently pushed. As in all situations, adequate exposure and illumination so as to afford good surgical access are a prerequisite. A fine round burr should be used to remove a channel of bone adjacent to the retained root sufficient to allow its elevation upwards out of the socket. If a root fragment is displaced and not readily visualized, radiographs in two planes should be taken. Again, a lower occlusal and OPT are the radiographs of choice. Once localized, judicious removal of the roof of the ID canal is undertaken until the retained fragment is found. Thereafter a blunt instrument such as a curved Warwick James elevator can be insinuated beneath the fragment which is carefully lifted off the neurovascular bundle.

Aerodigestive tract

It is all too easy for an extracted tooth or dislodged fragment to be swallowed or, worse still, inhaled. Teeth with single conical roots are sometimes ejected from their sockets unexpectedly during exodontia and patients will occasionally move violently just as a tooth is being delivered (especially if they are nervous and/or the depth of analgesia is inadequate). In these circumstances the tooth may disappear over the dorsum of the tongue into the pharynx upon which the patient's gag reflex is activated, compounding the problem. This complication is more likely to occur if surgery is performed with the patient supine and without adequate airway protection. Wherever possible, extractions and surgical procedures performed under local anesthesia with or without sedation in the dental chair should be executed with the patient placed at about 60 degrees to the horizontal. Any tooth or restoration fragments should be immediately removed by the surgeon or the assistant. Where patients are to be treated under general anesthesia, if the airway is not protected via an endotracheal tube or laryngeal mask, etc., the patient should be placed at about 60 degrees and a well-fitting pharyngeal pack placed to protect the airway. In most circumstances this will consist of an opened-out surgical swab or a sponge laid across the back of the tongue to occlude the oropharynx. Even when an endotracheal tube has been placed the airway is still at risk and the pharynx should be occluded with a throat pack. Many anesthetists use ribbon gauze for this purpose which, although adequate for the task, can abrade the delicate mucosal lining of the pharynx both on insertion and removal, adding to the postoperative discomfort. In contrast, two tampons inserted one either side of the endotracheal tube insure complete pharyngeal occlusion without traumatizing the mucosa. As mentioned previously, it is the surgeon's responsibility to ensure that any throat pack is removed on completion of treatment.

If a tooth is dislodged into the unprotected pharynx, with any luck the patient will swallow it and it will pass naturally in several days' time. However, it may well be inhaled and, due to the manner in which the trachea branches at the carina, not infrequently becomes lodged in the right main bronchus. This situation will usually be greeted by violent fits of coughing but may be silent. If such a situation occurs or the tooth cannot be immediately accounted for, an urgent chest and abdominal X-ray should be ordered (two radiographs at 90 degrees). If the patient is being treated outside a hospital environment they should be immediately referred via telephone to the local accident and emergency or oral and maxillofacial unit. If the tooth is seen to be lying in the lung the patient is urgently referred to either a cardiothoracic surgeon or respiratory physician for bronchoscopy. If the tooth is seen within the stomach the patient is reassured that all should be well and is recalled for repeat abdominal X-ray in a week's time. If the tooth has failed to pass a general surgical opinion should be obtained as soon as possible.

FRACTURES AND DISLOCATIONS

Extraction sockets and access cavities

Minor and inconsequential fractures of the tooth socket and inter-radicular bone occur frequently during exodontia.

Provided that any bone chips are removed from the wound, little harm is done. It is important to ensure that the socket edges are smoothed and no sharp spicules remain. Uneven and sharp alveolar ridges are a major source of postoperative discomfort and severely compromise the patient's ability to wear a denture comfortably. One maneuver to be particularly deprecated is the placement of the beaks of extraction forceps outside a tooth socket and then crushing the enclosed bone in order to deliver a fractured and retained root fragment. This causes excessive damage to the bone and often mutilates the overlying mucosa. If large pieces of devitalized alveolar bone or bone dust from rotary instruments are left behind, postoperative pain and infection are almost assured. Following transalveolar surgery of any type, it is vital that the operative area is thoroughly irrigated with copious amounts of 0.9% saline. One should pay particular attention to the depths of buccal mucoperiosteal flaps and the lingual aspect of lower third molar sockets if a lingual flap has been elevated.

Alveolus

The same factors that predispose to fractured teeth also predispose to alveolar fractures, namely poor extraction technique, malformed teeth and dense alveolar bone. Upper canines and upper molars, especially in well-built young males, are particularly prone to result in alveolar fracture. On rare occasions, large sections of buccal or palatal bone may be avulsed with the offending tooth. Again, many cases can be avoided by thorough preoperative clinical and X-ray examination and the avoidance of forceps extractions in high-risk teeth and patients.

Fractures of the maxillary tuberosity are a special subgroup of alveolar fractures. Tuberosity fracture is prone to occur if elevators are used to extract fully erupted upper third molars or excessive force is used during the forceps extraction of lone standing upper molars. In the latter case, loss of neighboring teeth frequently results in marked alveolar bone loss with encroachment of the maxillary sinus floor towards the alveolar crest. If preoperative radiographs suggest tuberosity fracture is likely then an elective transalveolar approach should be used.

Where an alveolar fracture occurs, immediate management will depend on its extent. Small avulsed fragments effectively confined to the extracted tooth socket require no special treatment although the postoperative alveolar form will not be ideal and may compromise future prosthetic rehabilitation. Larger fragments still attached to mucoperiosteum should ideally be replaced and the segment immobilized via archbars or a vacuum-formed splint for approximately 4 weeks, following which the offending tooth is extracted via an elective transalveolar approach. If a substantial alveolar segment is avulsed and detached from the overlying mucoperiosteum it is likely that it will not survive if replaced. Maxillary tuberosity fractures not uncommonly fall into this category. The avulsed bone should be carefully released from any remaining soft tissues using a periosteal elevator. A large oroantral communication is virtually inevitable in this situation. However, following the loss of the bone there is usually sufficient soft tissue to allow for a tension-free closure. Sutures should be left in for at least 10 days and the patient prescribed a broad-spectrum antibiotic together with 0.5% ephedrine nasal drops and enjoined not to blow their nose for 2 weeks for fear of causing the soft-tissue closure to break down. All surgeons who practice exodontia must be able to manage this complication in the manner described on site immediately the problem occurs.

Fractured mandible

This is probably the most feared of all complications following minor oral surgery and, like the majority of them, is largely preventable (Fig. 95.9).

Close inspection of preoperative radiographs will demonstrate the impediments to tooth delivery and facilitate the formation of a treatment plan designed to overcome the problems. Judicious bone removal and tooth division followed by controlled elevation will be successful in virtually all cases. Very rarely, the tooth to be removed may be situated in an area where the bone is extremely thin as a result of pathologic loss or age changes. Even in this situation fracture is not inevitable although it may be prudent to apply direct fixation to the jaw either internally or externally to support the area in the early postoperative period. Patients should be advised to consume a soft diet for several weeks and to return immediately if they become aware of any abnormalities in the jaw. These patients should be treated in a hospital environment with access to the necessary

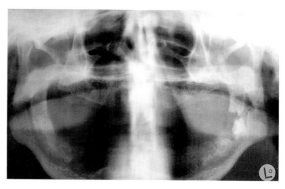

Fig. 95.9 Iatrogenic fracture of the left mandibular angle resulting from the application of excessive and uncontrolled force during the elevation of an ankylosed lower left third molar.

equipment should a fracture occur. If a mandible is fractured unexpectedly and the patient is already under general anesthesia the surgeon should proceed directly to fixing the fracture and fully explain the situation to the patient postoperatively. If the fracture occurs under local anesthesia and outside a hospital environment, the patient should be immediately referred via telephone to the local oral and maxillofacial surgery unit for urgent assessment and treatment.

Temporomandibular joint dislocation

It can be extremely uncomfortable for patients having a lower molar extracted not because of pain at the surgical site but because of traction on the temporomandibular joints (TMJ) consequent on the surgeon pushing down on the tooth with the extraction forceps. It is important that the surgeon fully supports the mandible during extractions in order to relieve stresses on the TMJ. Some patients find even light pressure uncomfortable and in this situation placing a rubber bite prop between the contralateral posterior teeth and asking them to gently bite on it will usually allow the extraction to proceed to completion. Where extractions are performed under general anesthesia it is all too easy to forget the TMJ. On completion of treatment, immediately prior to removing the throat pack, the surgeon should manipulate the mandible into centric occlusion to ensure that it is not dislocated. If it is, then the dislocation should be reduced before the anesthetic is reversed and the patient woken up.

SOFT TISSUE DAMAGE

Mechanical trauma

The rich blood supply to the head and neck region usually ensures that all but the most abused and damaged tissues will eventually heal. However, it cannot be stated too frequently that the key to minimizing surgical complications is meticulous preoperative planning and surgical technique. In particular, gentle handling and respect for the orofacial soft tissues is mandatory. This is particularly important when making elective incisions around the face. Wherever possible, incisions should be placed in the lines of election which are at right angles to the direction of the resultant action of the underlying muscles of facial expression.[18] Gentle handling of the soft tissues, specifically avoiding crushing and tearing the wound margins and approximating the skin edges without tension, is vital to success ('tight enough today – too tight tomorrow'). Patients with a previous history of hypertrophic or keloid scar formation should be treated by

surgeons with considerable expertise in facial soft-tissue surgery.

One of the most disturbing sights to see on a postoperative ward round is the patient who has excoriated and swollen lips and commissures due to careless tissue retraction. This complication, which is more likely to occur under general than local anesthesia, displays an unacceptably casual attitude on the part of the surgeon for the care of his or her patient. Copious amounts of Vaseline or moisturizing cream should be applied to the lips to lubricate them preoperatively and repeated throughout the procedure. Highly polished instruments should be used and the commissures protected with a gauze swab and cheek retractor (Fig. 95.10). The commonest scenario leading to damage to the lips and commissures is when they are trapped between a Howarth periosteal elevator used as a flap retractor and the neck of the elevator being used to extract an upper third molar, especially if the extraction is difficult because of poor visibility and surgical access. It is all too easy to get carried away with the extraction and neglect the soft tissues. The Laster flap retractor provides unparalleled protection in this situation and is highly recommended.

Lacerations to the soft tissues can be caused by careless handling of scalpels, elevators, forceps, scissors and sutures. In fact, any surgical instrument may cause collateral damage if the surgeon loses concentration. Eye protection must always be used when treating patients supine. It is appropriate at this point to condemn the practice of the single-handed operator who, in order to facilitate access to the

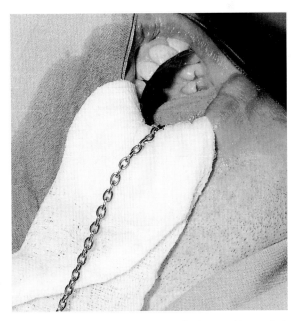

Fig. 95.10 The lips and commissures are easily damaged by surgical instruments including mouth prop chains. Adequate protection can be afforded by the use of moist gauze swabs as demonstrated in this photograph.

mouth, inserts one end of a cheek retractor in the patient's commissure and the other end through the waist tie on the surgical gown. This is an extremely dangerous technique which can easily lead to severe damage to the patient's soft tissues if the operator should slip backwards – a not uncommon occurrence!

Thermal trauma

While all instruments should be autoclave sterilized wherever possible, it is vital to ensure that they are cool before coming into contact with the patient. Surgical handpieces that are not serviced regularly and properly maintained are prone to bearing failure. This will cause the handpiece to overheat in normal use, especially if old burrs are used in an attempt to save money and excess pressure is applied to the blunt burr because it cuts inefficiently. The hot handpiece then comes into contact with the patient's soft tissues, resulting in a deep burn. This is an indefensible disaster and the cosmetic results can be truly appalling. If a surgical handpiece is running hot it should be immediately discarded and sent for repair or condemned. A note to this effect should be recorded in the operating theater equipment log and the surgeon should refuse to use it. If a replacement instrument cannot be provided and there is no other safe way of completing the operation then the procedure should be abandoned and the patient informed of the reason why. If a surgeon injures a patient with an instrument that is known to be defective then he or she will only have themselves to blame when they are sued for negligence.

Poor vigilance while using an electrical cautery or laser is another indefensible cause of damage to surrounding soft tissues. When these instruments are in use, non-conducting and non-reflective retractors should be used and, in the case of lasers, all surrounding areas should be protected by wet swabs. Extreme care should be used when using monopolar cautery to coagulate a blood vessel via a non-insulated pair of tissue forceps in case they should come into contact with the surrounding soft tissues.

Nerves

The terminal branches of the trigeminal and facial nerves are the ones most at risk from accidental damage during minor oral surgical procedures. The inferior dental nerve is at risk of damage during removal of lower third molars, apicectomy of lower premolar and molar teeth, the placement of intraoral implants and soft-tissue surgery around the mental foramen, especially in the elderly where the mental nerve may lie at or close to the alveolar crest. The lingual nerve is at risk during the surgical removal of lower third molars, the placement of intraoral implants and incisions in the floor of the mouth for the removal of submandibular

duct calculi and biopsies, etc. Both nerves may be damaged by inadvertent direct nerve puncture while administering an inferior alveolar nerve block. Less frequently documented is damage to the infraorbital, buccal and incisive nerves. Mention has already been made about the risks to the facial nerve from facial skin incisions, etc.

The incidence of transient inferior alveolar nerve damage following lower third molar removal varies between 1.3%[19] and 7.8%.[20] Between 0.5% and 1% of all lower third molar extractions result in permanent damage to the inferior alveolar nerve.[21] Following lower third molar extraction, the incidence of permanent lingual nerve sensory disturbance necessitating nerve repair lies between 0.3% and 0.8%.[22] The health, social and financial impact to the patient of these and other postoperative sequelae are frequently underestimated by clinicians.[23] It is mandatory that patients are fully warned about these possible complications preoperatively. A few patients when so warned will withhold their consent to undergo surgery.

Potential damage to the inferior dental nerve during third molar extraction can be anticipated in most circumstances by thorough examination of a high-quality preoperative radiograph of the area. Narrowing, loss of definition or acute change in direction of the neurovascular canal in the immediate vicinity of the lower third molar roots is highly suspicious of root notching or actual perforation by the neurovascular bundle (Fig. 95.11). In this situation, unless the tooth is symptomatic or there is an exceptionally good reason for its removal, it should be left in situ. If removal is indicated then a transalveolar approach with wide access to the surgical field and root sectioning should be employed. With careful handling the root can be divided so as to free the entrapped neurovascular bundle (Fig. 95.12).

Forcible elevation of a deeply impacted lower third molar, particularly one with a long mesial root, is clumsy and can crush the contents of the neurovascular canal. This is symptomatic of hasty and ill-planned surgery. It is far better

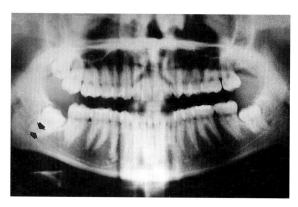

Fig. 95.11 OPT radiograph showing narrowing of the inferior alveolar canal outline in the immediate vicinity of the apices of the lower right third molar.

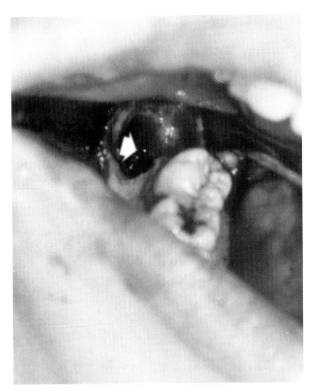

Fig. 95.12 Operative photograph of the lower right third molar socket detailed in Fig. 96.11. The inferior alveolar neurovascular bundle is visible at the base of the tooth socket having been found to be piercing the root apices.

avoid severing the buccal nerve as it crosses the anterior surface of the mandibular ramus in this area.[24] Likewise, avoidance of a buccal-relieving incision by the use of an envelope flap will minimize accidental damage to the buccal nerve in the sulcus while affording excellent surgical access (Figs 96.13, 96.14).

The course of the lingual nerve may be very variable and

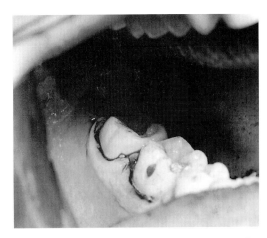

Fig. 95.13 Mucosal incision prior to elevation of an envelope flap. All incisions are placed well away from the lingual and buccal nerves.

and safer to section deeply mesioangular impacted teeth both horizontally and vertically and remove the crown and individual roots separately.

Transient labial paresthesia following lower premolar/molar apicectomies is common as a result of mental nerve traction but permanent damage can and should be avoided. Broadly based, three-sided mucoperiosteal flaps carefully elevated from the bone afford excellent surgical access. Semilunar incisions should never be employed in this area. The mental foramen and the emerging mental nerve must always be identified and protected with a highly polished blunt flap retractor. Bone over the apices of the tooth to be apicected is removed carefully and under constant direct vision. In the case of lower molars it is safest to section the root near its midpoint rather than the apical third as this will take the burr away from the neurovascular canal and also make subsequent amalgam placement easier.

The lingual nerve not uncommonly lies superficially at the alveolar crest in the retromolar triangle. Careless mucosal incisions in this region can easily sever the nerve before any flaps are raised or bone is removed. The distal incision must always be angled laterally to take it away from the lingual aspect of the ramus. Standard teaching is that the incision should be taken up the external oblique ridge. It is important that this incision is kept as short as possible in order to

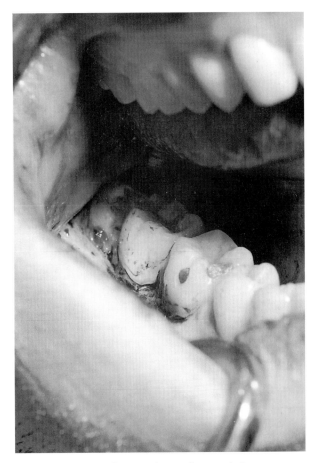

Fig. 95.14 The envelope flap provides excellent surgical access to impacted lower third molars (same case as Fig. 96.13).

in 17.6% of cases it may lie at or above the level of the alveolar crest.[25] Incisions in the floor of the mouth must always be placed with due regard to the direction and level of the lingual nerve. In particular, dochotomy of the submandibular duct to release a calculus must be done with extreme care as occasionally fibrosis around the stricture will have pulled the underlying lingual nerve upwards, placing it at risk from an incision over the duct. Similarly, sutures placed around the duct to prevent distal migration of the calculus can easily damage the lingual nerve if they are placed too deeply in the floor of the mouth.

Debate over how to protect the lingual nerve from damage during lower third molar removal has raged for many years. There is good evidence to show that rather than affording protection to the nerve and reducing lingual nerve damage, the placement of the traditional Howarth periosteal elevator actually increases the frequency of nerve trauma (Fig. 95.15). Robinson et al[22] have demonstrated a highly significant reduction in the incidence of temporary lingual paresthesia when lower third molars were removed without placing a Howarth down the lingual side of the mandible compared to when a Howarth was used. This technique was not associated with an increased incidence of permanent lingual nerve problems. There will undoubtedly be occasions where lingual flap retraction followed by the careful and correct placement of an instrument to protect the lingual nerve is necessary in order to accurately and safely visualize a particular lower third molar. However, avoidance of the routine use of traditional lingual nerve protection via a Howarth is to be recommended wherever possible.

Intraoral implants, particularly mandibular endosseous implants, are emerging as yet another cause of litigation resulting from iatrogenic nerve damage.[26] Poor preoperative planning and imaging together with the careless siting of

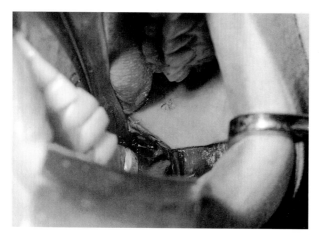

Fig. 95.15 Placement of the traditional Howarth periosteal elevator between the lingual plate and periosteum increases the frequency of transient lingual nerve damage and should be avoided wherever possible.

endosseous implants may damage the inferior alveolar nerve either within the mandibular canal or after its exit from the mental foramen. The prevalence of altered inferior alveolar nerve sensation following the placement of mandibular endosseous implants has been reported to be as high as 36%, of which 23% of cases were transient and 13% of cases were persistent at 6 months or more postimplant placement.[26] Although uncommon, transient lingual nerve paresthesia has also been reported where mandibular endosseous implants have perforated the lingual cortical plate.[27]

Inferior alveolar nerve repositioning to facilitate the placement of endosseous implants posterior to the mental foramen is associated with a very high incidence of temporary inferior alveolar nerve damage. In one series inferior alveolar neurosensory dysfunction was present in 70% of patients at 1 week before falling to 20% at 6 months and 0% at 1 year postoperatively.[28] However, the technique enables the placement of more and longer implants, resulting in increased prosthesis strength and stability, and has a lower permanent dysesthesia rate than when a non-transposed nerve has been accidentally damaged by drilling or implant placement.[29] If such a technique is to be used it is vital that the patient is fully informed about the possibility of temporary and permanent inferior alveolar nerve paresthesia.

The raising of full palatal flaps to gain access to impacted canines or supernumerary teeth can damage the incisive nerves as they exit the nasopalatine foramen. If at all possible, the nasopalatine neurovascular bundle should be preserved intact as division of the nerves produces unpleasant premaxillary mucosal paresthesia which may result in accidental thermal trauma to the premaxillary mucosa from hot food and beverages.

The infraorbital nerve is not commonly involved in procedures typically classified as minor oral surgery. However, it may be damaged by careless retraction of buccal flaps during upper incisor or canine apicectomies. It is also at risk from direct damage from infraorbital nerve local anesthetic blocks. Gentle tissue handling and thorough appreciation of the local anatomy should prevent this complication arising.

Blood vessels

Bleeding from severed vessels is inevitable and if excessive, should be controlled by ligation or electrocautery. If troublesome bleeding occurs from an intrabony vessel this can usually be arrested by crushing the surrounding bone walls with the tips of a curved hemostat or with small amounts of sterile bone wax. Bleeding from the pterygoid plexus can be worrying but will usually respond to direct pressure applied via a gauze swab. Occasionally, profuse bleeding will be encountered from a severed inferior alveolar artery. This may occur because of inadequate preoperative planning, injudicious use of an elevator in the depths of the socket or cutting too close to the neurovascular canal while removing bone or sectioning a tooth. It is vital that adequate suction is always available should this event occur. The socket is packed under pressure with ribbon gauze which invariably will control the situation. This should be left undisturbed for 15 min and then slowly removed. If all bleeding has ceased the socket should be left open for a further 15 min before primary closure is undertaken in case a rebleed occurs shortly after pack removal. If bleeding recurs the socket should be packed with ribbon gauze soaked with BIPP (bismuth subnitrate paraform paste BPC) and left in situ for 24 h.

Very occasionally, a tooth socket may be involved with an arteriovenous malformation. Clinical clues to this possibility include associated cutaneous hemangiomata, marked perioperative bleeding from around the tooth or a patient with the Sturge–Weber syndrome. The surgeon should be very wary if an otherwise healthy tooth becomes mobile, especially if it is a permanent tooth in a child as it may be being pushed out of the socket by an arteriovenous malformation. As always, thorough examination of preoperative radiographs should alert the surgeon to the presence of any local abnormalities (see Fig. 95.1). Any suspicious cases should be referred immediately to a consultant oral and maxillofacial surgeon who can arrange for CT scans and angiograms to be performed if appropriate. If torrential bleeding occurs when a tooth is extracted the tooth should be replaced in the socket and the patient should be instructed to bite firmly together as this will provide the closest fitting socket plug available. Otherwise gauze packing should be used. If the patient is not already in hospital an ambulance should be summoned and immediate transfer to the nearest specialist oral and maxillofacial surgery unit arranged.

It is beyond the scope of this chapter to fully discuss the management of patients taking oral anticoagulants. Suffice it to say that if a patient's INR (international normalized ratio) is greater than 2.0 minor oral surgery may result in persistent bleeding. Irrigating the operative site with 10 ml of a 4.8% solution of tranexamic acid followed by an 8-hourly 2-min mouthrinse for 7 days with 10 ml of the solution has been shown to be highly effective in reducing postoperative bleeding in patients with INRs between 2.1 and 4.0 without having to modify their oral anticoagulation dosage.[30] However, such patients should be referred to a consultant oral and maxillofacial surgeon for treatment as in some cases they will need to be admitted to hospital and heparinized prior to stopping their warfarin before surgery can be safely undertaken. If the INR is less than 2.0 simple extractions with full local hemostatic control should not be problematical. Inferior alveolar nerve blocks should not be used in patients who are anticoagulated.

BROKEN INSTRUMENTS

Modern instruments are manufactured to high standards and are unlikely to fail if they are used correctly and properly maintained. Suture needles, hypodermic needles and surgical burrs are the items that most frequently fail in use.

Suture needles are probably the commonest items to be broken during minor oral surgery. Careless handling and faulty technique probably account for the overwhelming majority of breakages. In order to minimize bending stresses on the suture needle, the surgeon should always select a needle of the appropriate gauge. Attempting to force thin needles through thick and tough tissues will inevitably result in needle fracture. The suture needle should be grasped in the middle of its concavity by the tips of the needle holders and rotated, not pushed, through the tissues. Choice of needle holder is largely a matter of personal preference but serrated instruments such as artery forceps must never be used as needle holders. If the suture needle becomes bent it should be discarded; the surgeon must never attempt to straighten it because if the needle doesn't fracture immediately it is liable to do so when next inserted into the tissues. Suture needles are particularly prone to being damaged when placing interdental sutures as they often engage bone or tooth rather than passing cleanly in between the teeth.

A new disposable hypodermic needle should be used for each patient and should never be intentionally bent or grasped with forceps prior to use. Breakage is uncommon but when it does occur is usually due to either a sudden violent movement by the patient, faulty technique or a structural fault in the needle itself during either an inferior alveolar or posterior superior alveolar nerve block.[4]

All burrs should be clean, sharp and straight. Applying excessive force to a blunt, worn burr generates excessive heat in the substance being drilled, damages the handpiece bearings, hastening their failure, and increases the likelihood of burr fracture. As soon as the surgeon detects that the burr has lost its edge it should be discarded and replaced with a new one.

As a general rule all fragments of broken instruments should be removed immediately before they have time to migrate deeper into the tissues. Whenever administering a local anesthetic injection there should always be a pair of artery forceps readily available in case the needle should break. If the broken end projects into the mouth it is easily grasped with the forceps and removed. Likewise, broken suture needles and burrs are best retrieved with fine artery forceps immediately on fracture. If the fragment cannot be found radiographs in two planes at 90 degrees should be taken of the operative area to locate it. At this point a decision will need to be made as to whether to remove the fragment or leave it in situ, depending on its size and site. Small fragments lying subperiosteally can be safely left as they are unlikely to migrate and cause problems.[4] If the decision is taken to remove the fragment the operative approach will depend on where it is located and a thorough knowledge of the local anatomy is essential if further complications are to be avoided. It should be remembered that small fine foreign bodies can be extremely difficult to locate and that blind exploration of tissue spaces is wont to displace them deeper. The use of image intensification can be very helpful in this situation.

POSTOPERATIVE COMPLICATIONS

PAIN AND SWELLING

Apprehension over the severity and extent of postoperative pain and swelling is extremely common in patients about to undergo minor oral surgery, particularly third molar removal. Instituting active measures to maximize any reduction in postoperative pain and swelling is an integral part of high-quality patient care.

The efficacy of systemic analgesics is greatly enhanced if patients are given regional local anesthetic blocks or infiltrations perioperatively.[31] Inferior dental nerve blocks or local infiltrations, especially of long-acting bupivacaine (Marcain), administered perioperatively for patients undergoing lower third molar removal under general anesthesia improve pain control in the early postoperative period. However, it is vital to warn patients about the possibility of accidental injury from biting or thermal burns from hot food and beverages whenever local anesthetics are administered.

Some degree of postoperative swelling following minor oral surgery is inevitable although its extent is highly variable and unpredictable. This variation is due to patients having widely different inflammatory responses to similar surgical insults independent of operator variability. Postoperative pain and patients' ability to tolerate it is directly correlated with the degree of postoperative swelling present.[32] Llewelyn et al,[33] using magnetic resonance imaging (MRI), have shown that following the removal of third molar teeth patients sustain a mean swelling of almost 1 cm on the first postoperative day.

Postoperative edema can be lessened by careful tissue handling and its extent is dependent on the skill of the surgeon.[34] In particular, retractors and elevators must be used with care. Rotating surgical drills must never be allowed to 'snag' the surrounding soft tissues or abrade the buccal and labial mucosa and the drill tip must be constantly cooled to insure that the bone is never allowed to overheat. Standard air turbine dental handpieces generate very high vent pressures. They must never be used for bone removal or tooth section as the forward-facing air jet can lead to massive emphysema of the surrounding soft tissues with the risk of subsequent pain, swelling, infection and tissue necrosis (Fig. 95.16).

Extraction sockets and pathological cavities must be irrigated with copious amounts of 0.9% saline to remove all bone fragments and debris. Failure to accurately place a retrograde root filling in the root apex and failure to remove excess amalgam from the surgical cavity not only produces an embarrassing 'shotgun' postoperative radiograph but also predisposes to surgical failure from chronic pain and infection. To prevent this error the surgical cavity should be occluded with a strip of ribbon gauze so that only the root apex access cavity is visible. Small volumes of amalgam should then be carefully introduced and condensed immediately. This procedure can be greatly facilitated by using specially designed amalgam carriers and magnifying loupes. On completion the gauze is removed and the cavity thoroughly irrigated and all traces of stray amalgam removed.

Pharmacological treatments can be used as an adjunct to meticulous surgery to reduce postoperative edema. The combination of systemic steroids and non-steroidal anti-inflammatory drugs has been shown to produce marked reduction in postoperative pain and swelling following third molar removal.[35] The administration of 40 mg methylprednisolone intravenously immediately prior to surgery has been

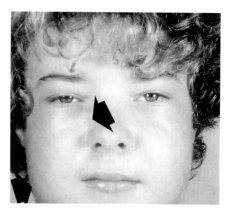

Fig. 95.16 Extensive subcutaneous surgical emphysema following the use of a dental air turbine to remove bone around an impacted lower right third molar tooth (courtesy of A M Corrigan FDSRCS, FRCS).

shown to significantly reduce early postoperative edema and pain and improve patient satisfaction following the removal of impacted lower third molars.[36] No increased morbidity from infection or delayed healing was noted.

Although the hypothalamic–pituitary–adrenal (HPA) axis is acutely depressed following a single intravenous dose of 8 mg of dexamethasone, the HPA response has normalised by 7 days postoperatively.[37] It is the author's practice to administer 8 mg dexamethasone (equivalent to 42.7 mg methylprednisolone (British National Formulary)) intravenously immediately prior to surgery and 400–600 mg ibuprofen 8-hourly postoperatively for all procedures requiring bone removal unless contraindicated for medical reasons.

INFECTION

If infected and abscessed teeth and roots can be extracted easily using forceps or elevators, and providing a local anesthetic injection is not instilled directly into an area of inflammation or acute infection, their loss will hasten the resolution of symptoms by removing the source of infection. Regional local anesthetic blocks can be useful in these circumstances although even then surgical analgesia may not be achievable.

As a general rule the transalveolar approach for the removal of teeth and roots is contraindicated in the presence of acute infection lest the infection be spread to deeper structures. This is particularly so when lower third molars are associated with acute pericoronitis. Injudicious removal can result in a parapharyngeal space infection and upper airway obstruction. Wherever possible, extraction should be deferred until the tooth has been infection free for 2–3 weeks.

In the normal course of events and in the absence of pre-existing infection, postoperative pain and swelling will be on the wane after 48 h or so. However, should the operative site become infected pain, swelling and trismus fail to resolve and usually increase around this time. The infection rate following minor oral surgical procedures is low and in a series of 6713 third molar extractions, was only 3.5%.[38]

Dry socket

Dry socket, also variously termed alveolar osteitis, fibrinolytic alveolitis and alveolitis sicca dolorosa, is a well-recognized complication of exodontia.[4] It is characterized by increasingly severe pain which usually starts on the second or third postoperative day in and around the extraction site, lasting for between 10 and 40 days. The normal postextraction blood clot is lost from the tooth socket, the bony walls of which are denuded and exquisitely sensitive to gentle probing. Halitosis is invariably present. There is great variation in reported incidence rates (1–65%) between series usually due to inconsistency in diagnostic criteria, variation in antimicrobial prophylaxis and study sample heterogeneity. The true incidence rate probably lies somewhere between 3% and 20% of all extractions.

The etiology is multifactorial but essentially it results from lysis of the normal postextraction blood clot. Increased concentrations of both direct and indirect plasminogen activators result in an increased local concentration of plasmin and subsequently an enhanced degradation of fibrin to soluble fragments with clot disintegration and loss. Direct plasminogen activators are released from damaged alveolar bone cells. Bacterial pyrogens and estrogens, particularly those found in oral contraceptives, are potent indirect plasminogen activators. It is thus hypothesized that a dry socket results from a complex interaction between surgical trauma, local bacterial infection and various systemic factors.[39]

Dry socket is a painful, debilitating condition that results in considerable suffering, inconvenience and loss of productivity to the patient. It is also a costly and time-consuming condition for the attending clinician as 45% of patients will require at least four additional postoperative visits.[40]

Several factors have been found to be associated with an increased risk of developing a dry socket.[38,39,40,41,42]

- Extraction of mandibular rather than maxillary teeth
- Extraction of third molars, especially impacted lower third molars
- Singleton extractions
- 'Traumatic' and unduly difficult extractions
- Female sex, especially if concurrently using oral contraception
- Patient aged between 20 and 40 years
- Poor oral hygiene and plaque control
- Active or recent history of acute ulcerative gingivitis or pericoronitis
- Smoking, especially if >20 cigarettes/day
- Increased bone density either locally or generally such as Paget's disease
- Previous history of dry socket(s) following extractions
- Inexperienced surgeon

Clinical application of the above data will minimize the incidence of dry socket. If appropriate, wherever possible oral hygiene measures to reduce plaque levels to a minimum should be instituted and all patients should be given a 0.12% chlorhexidine mouth rinse immediately preoperatively.

Lower third molar extractions should be avoided in the presence of active pericoronitis or acute ulcerative gingivitis. For difficult full or partial bony lower third molar impactions where bone needs to be removed, for immunocompromised patients and those with a history of previous pericoronitis or acute ulcerative gingivitis, appropriate antibiotic prophylaxis should be prescribed. Patients who smoke should be enjoined to cease the habit preoperatively and for at least 2 weeks postoperatively while the extraction sockets heal. Wherever possible, for female patients using oral contraception, extractions should be performed during days 23 through 28 of the tablet cycle.

All extractions should be completed with the minimum amount of trauma, the maximum amount of care and as rapidly as possible commensurate with their degree of difficulty and the experience of the operator. On completion of the procedure, the operative site should be irrigated with copious amounts of sterile saline followed by 15 ml of 0.12% chlorhexidine. Patients should be advised to avoid vigorous mouth rinsing in the immediate postoperative period but to use gentle tooth brushing and 0.12% chlorhexidine mouth rinses for the following 7 days. All patients should be advised to return to the surgery/hospital immediately if they develop increasing pain or a bad taste.

In cases of established dry socket patients should be managed along the following lines. The affected socket(s) should be gently irrigated with warmed 0.12% chlorhexidine and all debris dislodged and aspirated. In extremely painful cases local anesthesia may be required before socket irrigation can be performed. Wherever possible, regional nerve blocks should be employed. The socket should be lightly packed with a dressing that contains an obtundent for pain relief and a non-irritant antiseptic to inhibit bacterial and fungal growth. The dressing should prevent reaccumulation of food debris and protect the exposed bone from irritation. Ideally, the dressing should slowly dissolve without the need for its removal and should not excite a host inflammatory or foreign body response. Numerous commercial agents are available which fulfil these requirements to a greater or lesser extent. Alternatively, sterile $1/4$ inch ribbon gauze impregnated with BIPP can be used although it requires subsequent manual removal by the attending clinician. Providing there are no signs of systemic infection antibiotics are not routinely required. Suitable and effective systemic analgesics should be prescribed and the patient's progress should be reviewed the following day and frequently thereafter until full healing has occurred. Hospitalization is rarely required.

For patients about to undergo surgical removal of full or partial bony impacted third molars, the use of systemic antibiotics confers a significant reduction in postoperative infection rates.[38] If prophylactic antibiotics are to be beneficial they need to be given preoperatively and no more than 2 h prior to the commencement of surgery.[43] There is no point in prescribing postoperative oral antibiotics for clean contaminated procedures (the majority of minor oral surgery) if preoperative systemic antibiotics have been given as they will confer no added benefit. If preoperative systemic antibiotics have not been given, prescribing postoperative oral antibiotics confers no benefit at all. The author's policy is not to use antibiotics for clean contaminated soft-tissue surgery, simple extractions or soft-tissue third molar impactions. For procedures involving bone removal such as third molars and apicectomies and providing there are no medical or pharmacological contraindications, a single intravenous dose of 1.2 g co-amoxiclav is given immediately prior to surgery commencing. Chlorhexidine 0.12% mouthwashes 6-hourly are prescribed for 1 week postoperatively but oral antibiotics are not given.

Osteoradionecrosis

Patients with head and neck cancer who are treated by radiotherapy either as sole modality or as part of a multimodality treatment plan are at risk of developing osteoradionecrosis in bone in the treated area. Osteoradionecrosis results from radiation-induced tissue hypoxia, hypocellularity and hypovascularity.[44,45] Osteoblasts and osteoclasts within the radiotherapized bone may be lethally damaged by the ionizing radiation although they are still able to perform their resting vegetative functions.[44] Because of the extremely slow bone cell turnover rate, this causes few problems until the cells are stimulated to divide. The most common stimulus to divide is provided by tooth extraction which then usually results in massive bone destruction and secondary bacterial infection.

Osteoradionecrosis is an extremely painful, debilitating and indolent disease that makes patients' lives an utter misery. This complication must be avoided at all costs. The most effective way of preventing osteoradionecrosis is to ensure that all patients who are to receive medical irradiation to the head and neck have a thorough oral examination including OPT screening. For head and neck cancer patients this should occur in the context of a multidisciplinary head and neck oncology clinic. Any teeth in the proposed treatment area of doubtful prognosis by virtue of decay or periodontal disease should be scheduled for extraction. If the patient is to undergo surgical resection prior to radiotherapy the ideal time to extract the teeth is during the presurgical examination under anesthetic (EUA). Otherwise the teeth should be extracted under local anesthetic 1–2 weeks prior to commencing radiotherapy.

No matter how careful and thorough the work-up, there will always be circumstances where a patient will require extractions postradiotherapy. Such extractions should be performed by the oral and maxillofacial surgeon attending the oncology clinic and not delegated to the patient's general dental practitioner. Broad-spectrum antibiotics are administered intravenously immediately preoperatively along with 0.12% chlorhexidine mouthwashes and the gingival margins of the teeth to be extracted swabbed with iodine solution. Extractions are performed in the most atraumatic way possible which may involve the elective use of a transalveolar approach and bone removal, depending on the finding on the preoperative radiograph. Postoperative antibiotics and chlorhexidine mouthwashes are commenced and continued until the sockets are healed.

There is extensive evidence that established osteoradionecrosis is best managed by hyperbaric oxygen therapy and subsequent surgical debridement.[46] In patients at high risk of developing osteoradionecrosis it may also be prudent to use a pre-extraction hyperbaric oxygen therapy regime provided that this would not adversely delay starting primary treatment for the patient's head and neck cancer.

Learning without thought is labor lost; thought without learning is perilous. (Confucius 550–c 478 BC)

REFERENCES

1. Scully C, Cawson RA 1993 Medical problems in dentistry, 3rd edn. Wright, Oxford
2. Rowe AHR, Alexander AG 1988 A companion to dental studies, volume 2. Blackwell Scientific, Oxford
3. Tetsch P, Wagner W 1985 Operative extraction of wisdom teeth. Wolf Medical, Munich
4. Killey HC, Seward GR, Kay LW 1975 An outline of oral surgery, part 1. Wright, Bristol
5. Layton SA 1992 Informed consent in oral and maxillofacial surgery: a study of its efficacy. British Journal of Oral and Maxillofacial Surgery 30:319–322
6. Lawton (The Right Hon Lord Justice Lawton) 1983 Legal aspects of iatrogenic disorders: discussion paper. Journal of the Royal Society of Medicine 76:289–291
7. Guralnick WC, Laskin DM 1980 NIH consensus development conference for removal of third molars. Journal of Oral Surgery 38:235–236
8. Williams M 1996 Post-operative nerve damage and the removal of the mandibular third molar: a matter of common consent. British Journal of Oral and Maxillofacial Surgery 34:386–388
9. Humphris GM, O'Neill P, Field EA 1993 Knowledge of wisdom tooth removal: influence of an information leaflet and validation questionnaire. British Journal of Oral and Maxillofacial Surgery 31:355–359
10. O'Neill P, Humphris GM, Field EA 1996 The use of an information leaflet for patients undergoing wisdom tooth removal. British Journal of Oral and Maxillofacial Surgery 34:331–334
11. Poswillo D 1989 Obtaining consent to oral and maxillofacial surgery. Annals of the Academy of Medicine of Singapore 18:616–621
12. Richardson N, Jones P, Thomas M 1996 Should house officers obtain consent for operation and anaesthesia? Health Trends 28:56–59
13. Department of Health NHS Executive 1990 A guide to consent for examination or treatment. Department of Health, London
14. Gillbe GV, Moore JR 1985 Complications of extractions. In: Moore JR (ed) Surgery of the mouth and jaws. Blackwell Scientific, Oxford
15. Sisk AL, Hammer WB, Shelton DW, Joy ED Jr 1986 Complications following removal of impacted third molars: the role of the experience of the surgeon. Journal of Oral and Maxillofacial Surgery 44:855–859
16. Vogler JC, Karuza J, Miller WA 1994 Oral-surgeon-reported incidence of complications related to simple extraction in adults. Special Care in Dentistry 14:92–95
17. Weinberg S 1975 Oral surgery complications in general practice. Journal of the Canadian Dental Association 41:288–299
18. McGreggor IA 1989 Fundamental techniques of plastic surgery, 8th edn. Churchill Livingstone, Edinburgh
19. Schultze-Mosgau S, Reich RH 1993 Assessment of inferior alveolar and lingual nerve disturbances after dentoalveolar surgery, and recovery of sensitivity. International Journal of Oral and Maxillofacial Surgery 22:214–217
20. Rood JP 1992 Permanent damage to inferior alveolar nerves during the removal of impacted mandibular third molars. Comparison of two methods of bone removal. British Dental Journal 172:108–110
21. Blackburn CW, Bramley PA 1989 Lingual nerve damage associated with removal of lower third molars. British Dental Journal 167:103–107
22. Robinson PP, Smith KG 1996 Lingual nerve damage during lower third molar removal: a comparison of two surgical methods. British Dental Journal 180:456–461
23. Bramley P 1981 Sense about wisdoms? Journal of the Royal Society of Medicine 74:867–868
24. Hendy CW, Robinson PP 1994 The sensory distribution of the buccal nerve. British Journal of Oral and Maxillofacial Surgery 32:384–386
25. Kiesselbach JE, Chamberlain JG 1984 Clinical and anatomic observations on the relationship of the lingual nerve to the mandibular third molar region. Journal of Oral and Maxillofacial Surgery 42:565–567
26. Ellies LG, Hawker PB 1993 The prevalence of altered sensation associated with implant surgery. International Journal of Oral and Maxillofacial Implants 8:674–679
27. Berberi A, Le Breton G, Mani J, Woimant H, Nasseh I 1993 Lingual paraesthesia following surgical placement of implants: report of a case. International Journal of Oral and Maxillofacial Implants 8:580–582
28. Rosenquist B 1992 Fixture placement posterior to the mental foramen with transpositioning of the inferior alveolar nerve. International Journal of Oral and Maxillofacial Implants 7:45–50
29. Krogh PHJ 1994 Does the risk of complication make transpositioning of the inferior alveolar nerve in conjunction with implant placement a last resort surgical procedure? International Journal of Oral and Maxillofacial Implants 9:249–250
30. Ramstrom G, Sindet-Pederson S, Hall G, Blomback M, Alander U 1993 Prevention of post-surgical bleeding in oral surgery using tranexamic acid without dose modification of oral anticoagulants. Journal of Oral and Maxillofacial Surgery 51:1211–1216
31. Meyer RA, Chinn MA 1968 Prolonged postoperative analgesia with regional nerve blocks. Journal of Oral Surgery 26:182–184
32. MacGregor AJ, Hart P 1969 Effect of bacteria and other factors on pain and swelling after removal of ectopic mandibular third molars. Journal of Oral Surgery 27:174–179
33. Llewelyn J, Ryan M, Santosh C 1996 The use of magnetic resonance imaging to assess swelling after the removal of third molar teeth. British Journal of Oral and Maxillofacial Surgery 34:419–423

34. Osbon DB 1973 Postoperative complications following dentoalveolar surgery. Dental Clinics of North America 17:483–504

35. Schultze-Mosgau S, Schmelzeisen R, Frolich JC, Schmele H 1995 Use of ibuprofen and methylprednisolone for the prevention of pain and swelling after removal of impacted third molars. Journal of Oral and Maxillofacial Surgery 53:2–7

36. Holland CS 1987 The influence of methylprednisolone on post-operative swelling following oral surgery. British Journal of Oral and Maxillofacial Surgery 25:293–299

37. Williamson LW, Lorson EL, Osbon DB 1980 Hypothalamic-pituitary-adrenal suppression after short term dexamethasone therapy for oral surgical procedures. Journal of Oral Surgery 38:20–27

38. Piecuch JF, Arzadon J, Lieblich SE 1995 Prophylactic antibiotics for third molar surgery. Journal of Oral and Maxillofacial Surgery 53:53–60

39. Birn H 1973 Etiology and pathogenesis of fibrinolytic alveolitis ('dry socket'). International Journal of Oral Surgery 2:211–263

40. Larsen PE 1991 The effect of chlorhexidine rinse on the incidence of alveolar osteitis following the surgical removal of impacted mandibular third molars. Journal of Oral and Maxillofacial Surgery 49:932–937

41. Catellani JE, Harvey S, Erickson SH, Cherkin D 1980 Effect of oral contraceptive cycle on dry socket (localized alveolar osteitis). Journal of the American Dental Association 101:777–780

42. Meechan JG, Macgregor ID, Rogers SN et al 1988 The effect of smoking on immediate post-extraction socket filling with blood and on the incidence of painful socket. British Journal of Oral and Maxillofacial Surgery 26:402–409

43. Classesn DC, Evans RS, Pestotnik SL et al 1992 The timing of prophylactic administration of antibiotics and the risk of surgical wound infection. New England Journal of Medicine 326:281–286

44. Marx RE 1983 Osteoradionecrosis: a new concept of its pathophysiology. Journal of Oral and Maxillofacial Surgery 41:283–288

45. Wood GA, Liggins SJ 1996 Does hyperbaric oxygen have a role in the management of osteoradionecrosis? British Journal of Oral and Maxillofacial Surgery 34:424–427

46. Marx RE 1983 A new concept in the treatment of osteoradionecrosis. Journal of Oral and Maxillofacial Surgery 41:351–357

Index